Retinal
Pharmacotherapy

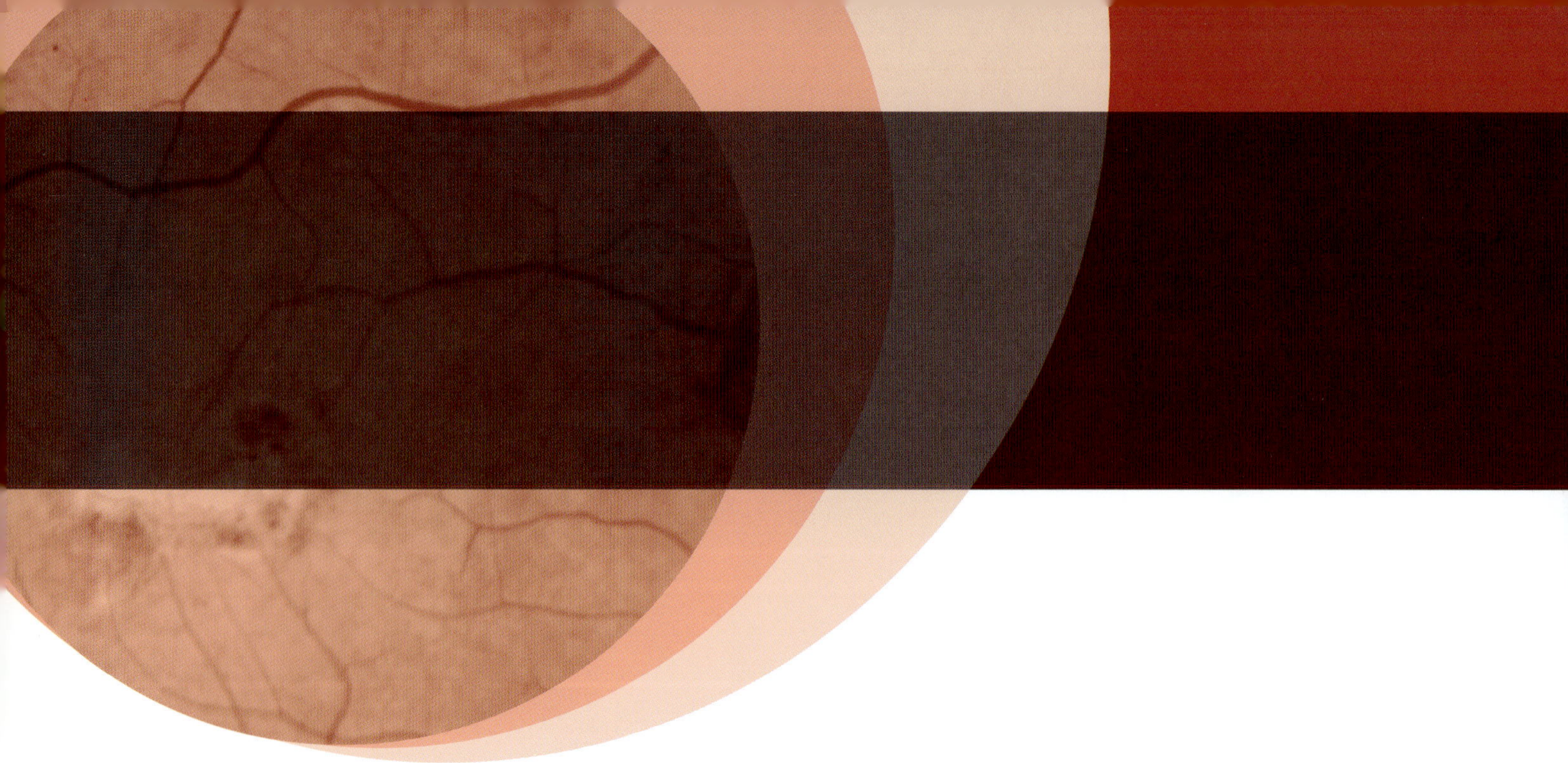

Commissioning Editor: Russell Gabbedy
Development Editor: Alexandra Mortimer
Editorial Assistant: Poppy Garraway
Project Manager: Beula Christopher
Design: Charles Gray
Illustration Manager: Gillian Richards
Illustrator: Cactus
Marketing Managers (UK/USA): Richard Jones / Helena Mutak

Retinal Pharmacotherapy

Quan Dong Nguyen MD, MSc
Associate Professor of Ophthalmology
Diseases of the Retina and Vitreous, and Uveitis
Wilmer Eye Institute
Johns Hopkins University School of Medicine
Baltimore, MD, USA

Eduardo Büchele Rodrigues MD
Department of Ophthalmology
Vision Institute
Federal University of São Paulo
São Paulo, Brazil

Michel Eid Farah MD
Professor of Ophthalmology and Vice-chairman
Retina and Vitreous Department
Vision Institute
Federal University of São Paulo
São Paulo, Brazil

William F. Mieler MD
Professor and Vice-Chairman
Department of Ophthalmology & Visual Sciences
University of Illinois at Chicago
Chicago, IL, USA

SAUNDERS
ELSEVIER

SAUNDERS
ELSEVIER

SAUNDERS is an imprint of Elsevier Inc.

First published 2010

British Library Cataloguing in Publication Data
Retinal pharmacotherapy.
1. Retina–Diseases–Chemotherapy.
I. Rodrigues, Eduardo.
617.7′35061-dc22

ISBN-13: 9781437706031

Library of Congress Cataloging in Publication Data
A catalog record for this book is available from the Library of Congress

Notices

Knowledge and best practice in this field are constantly changing. As new research and experience broaden our understanding, changes in research methods, professional practices, or medical treatment may become necessary. Practitioners and researchers must always rely on their own experience and knowledge in evaluating and using any information, methods, compounds, or experiments described herein. In using such information or methods they should be mindful of their own safety and the safety of others, including parties for whom they have a professional responsibility.

With respect to any drug or pharmaceutical products identified, readers are advised to check the most current information provided (i) on procedures featured or (ii) by the manufacturer of each product to be administered, to verify the recommended dose or formula, the method and duration of administration, and contraindications. It is the responsibility of practitioners, relying on their own experience and knowledge of their patients, to make diagnoses, to determine dosages and the best treatment for each individual patient, and to take all appropriate safety precautions.

To the fullest extent of the law, neither the Publisher nor the authors, contributors, or editors, assume any liability for any injury and/or damage to persons or property as a matter of products liability, negligence or otherwise, or from any use or operation of any methods, products, instructions, or ideas contained in the material herein.

The Publisher

Printed in China
Last digit is the print number: 9 8 7 6 5 4 3 2 1

CONTENTS

FOREWORD

During the past 25 years, our understanding of the molecular mechanisms of ocular diseases has greatly increased. As particular molecules have been implicated in disease processes, treatments that specifically target those molecules have been developed. Some recent successes have fueled research aimed at further elucidating molecular pathogenesis of ocular diseases and translational research aimed at converting recent findings into treatments. Those successes have also awakened the pharmaceutical industry to the unmet needs and potential opportunities related to ocular diseases. Thus, it is likely that new pharmacotherapies for retinal and uveal diseases will continue to become available for the foreseeable future.

In *Retinal Pharmacotherapy*, the editors, Quan Dong Nguyen, Eduardo Büchele Rodrigues, Michel Eid Farah, and William F. Mieler, and the authors have compiled a valuable resource that describes numerous pharmacologic agents that are currently available to treat retinal and posterior uveitic diseases. The Book is organized into six sections. Section 1 is devoted to the basic understanding of the molecular pathogenesis of retinal diseases. Section 2 describes animal models of retinal diseases that are useful for preclinical testing of drugs given by various routes of administration. Clinical features of retinal and posterior uveitic diseases that may be amendable to pharmacotherapy are discussed in Section 3. In Section 4, the appropriate uses of several drugs that have been shown to have therapeutic benefits for retinal diseases are reviewed. Section 5 covers topics that combine pharmacotherapy and surgery for treatment of retinal and posterior uveal diseases. Section 6 discusses value-based medicine, pharmacoeconomics, and the impact of regulatory bodies such as the FDA in the development of pharmacotherapy for retinal diseases.

Retinal Pharmacotherapy contains 53 chapters with contributions from over 120 authors from North America, South America, Europe, Asia, and Australia, many of whom are recognized authorities in the field. It will serve as an important resource for retina specialists, uveitis specialists, and comprehensive ophthalmologists.

Peter A. Campochiaro, MD
George and Dolores Eccles Professor of Ophthalmology
Wilmer Eye Institute
Johns Hopkins University
2009

LIST OF CONTRIBUTORS

Anthony P Adamis MD
Adjunct Professor
Department of Ophthalmology and Visual Sciences
University of Illinois College of Medicine
Chicago, IL, USA

Madeleine KM Adams MB ChB BSc (Hons) MRCOphth
Honorary Research Fellow
University of Melbourne
Centre for Eye Research Australia
Royal Victorian Eye and Ear Hospital
East Melbourne, VIC, Australia

Thomas A Albini MD
Assistant Professor of Clinical Ophthalmology
Bascom Palmer Eye Institute
Miami, FL, USA

Jayakrishna Ambati MD
Professor and Vice Chair
Ophthalmology and Visual Sciences
Professor of Physiology
Dr. E. Vernon Smith and Eloise C. Smith Endowed Chair
University of Kentucky
Doris Duke Distinguished Clinical Scientist
Burroughs Wellcome Translational Research Clinical Scientist
Lexington, KY, USA

Luis Amselem MD
Consultant, Institut de la Mácula i de la Retina
Consultant, Department of Ophthalmology and Visual Sciences
Retinal and Vitreous Surgery
Ocular Oncology
2nd Mayo Hospital
Barcelona, Spain

J Fernando Arévalo MD, FACS
Professor of Ophthalmology
Clinica Oftalmologica Centro Caracas and University of Los Andes
The Arévalo-Coutinho Foundation for Research in Ophthalmology
Caracas, Venezuela

Lluis Arias MD
Consultant
Institut de la Mácula i de la Retina
Centro Médico Teknon
Barcelona, Spain

Helen Dede Ayertey MD
Doctor of Medicine
Center of Ophthalmology
University of Cologne
Cologne, Germany

Paul N Baird BSc (Hons) PhD
Associate Professor of Ophthalmology
University of Melbourne
Centre for Eye Research Australia
Royal Victorian Eye and Ear Hospital
East Melbourne, VIC, Australia

Susanne Binder MD
Professor and Chairman
Department of Ophthalmology
The Ludwig Boltzmann Institute for Retinology and Biomicroscopic Laser Surgery
Vienna, Austria

Fabio Bom Aggio MD
Vision Institute, Department of Ophthalmology
Federal University of São Paulo
São Paulo, Brazil

Melissa M Brown MD, MN, MBA
Director, Center for Value-Based Medicine; Adjunct Senior Fellow, Leonard Davis Institute
Center for Value-Based Medicine
Flourtown, PA, USA

Gary C Brown MD, MBA
Attending Surgeon
Retina Service
Wills Eye Institute
Chief Medical Officer
Center for Value-Based Medicine
Wyndmoor, PA, USA

Richard Brunner MD
Professor of Ophthalmology
Center of Ophthalmology
University of Cologne
Cologne, Germany

J Peter Campbell MD, MPH
Resident in Ophthalmology
Wilmer Eye Institute
Johns Hopkins University School of Medicine
Baltimore, MD, USA

Jose A Cardillo MD
Department of Ophthalmology
Federal University of São Paulo
UNIFESP-EPM
São Paulo, Brazil

Chi-Chao Chan MD
Chief, Section of Immunopathology
Laboratory of Immunology
Chief, Histology Core
National Eye Institute
National Institutes of Health
Bethesda, MD, USA

Pik Sha Chan MD
Attending Physician
Retina and Pediatric Ophthalmology Service
Asian Eye Institute
Makati City, Philippines

Aimee V Chappelow MD
Cole Eye Institute
Cleveland Clinic Foundation
Cleveland, OH, USA

Emily Y Chew MD
Deputy Director
Division of Epidemiology and Clinical Applications
National Eye Institute
National Institutes of Health
Bethesda, MD, USA

Victor Chong MD
Consultant Ophthalmic Surgeon
University of Oxford
Oxford Eye Hospital
Oxford, UK

Hanna R Coleman MD
Staff Clinician, New York Presbyterian Hospital, Columbia
Department of Ophthalmology
Columbia University Medical Center
NY, USA

Gabriel J Coscas MD
Emeritus Professor of Clinical Ophthalmology
Department of Ophthalmology
University of Paris XII
Créteil, France

Yongping Crawford MD PhD
ES Cell Culture
Genentech, Inc.
San Francisco, CA, USA

Emmett T Cunningham Jr MD PhD MPH
Director, The Uveitis Service
California Pacific Medical Center
Adjunct Clinical Professor of Ophthalmology
Stanford University School of Medicine
San Francisco, CA, USA

Hajir Dadgostar MD
Cole Eye Institute
Cleveland Clinic Foundation
Cleveland, OH, USA

Taraprasad Das MD FRCS
Director
LV Prasad Eye Institute
Patia
Bhubaneswar, India

Janet L Davis MD MA
Professor of Ophthalmology
Department of Ophthalmology
Bascom Palmer Eye Institute
University of Miami
Miami, FL, USA

Heidrun L Deissler Dipl-Chem
Head of Research Laboratory
Department of Ophthalmology
University Eye Hospital Ulm
Ulm, Germany

Diana V Do MD
Assistant Professor of Ophthalmology
The Wilmer Eye Institute
The Johns Hopkins University School of Medicine
Baltimore, MD, USA

Michel Eid Farah MD
Professor of Ophthalmology and Vice-chairman
Retina and Vitreous Department
Federal University of São Paulo
Vision Institute
São Paulo, Brazil

Napoleone Ferrara MD
Genentech Fellow
Genentech, Inc.
San Francisco, CA, USA

Robert P Finger MD MIH
Department of Ophthalmology
University of Bonn
Bonn, Germany

Harry W Flynn, Jr. MD
The J Donald M Gass Distinguished Chair in Ophthalmology
Professor of Ophthalmology
Bascom Palmer Eye Institute
University of Miami Miller School of Medicine
Naples, FL, USA

Gildo Y Fujii MD PhD
Professor of Ophthalmology
Londrina State University
Fujii Institute of Ophthalmology
Londrina, Brazil

Gerardo García-Aguirre MD
Assistant Staff
Retina Department
Hospital "Dr. Luis Sánchez Bulnes"
Asociación para Evitar la Ceguera en México (APEC)
Mexico City, Mexico

Thomas W Gardner MD MS
Jack and Nancy Turner Professor of Ophthalmology and Cellular and Molecular Physiology
Department of Ophthalmology
Penn State College of Medicine
Hershey, PA, USA

Gerhard Garhöfer MD
Department of Clinical Pharmacology
Medical University of Vienna
Vienna, Austria

Mauro Goldbaum MD
Executive Director
Eyetech, Inc
São Paulo, Brazil

David T Goldenberg MD
Private Practice
Retinal Consultants of Arizona
Phoenix, AZ, USA

Sandeep Grover MD
Assistant Professor
Director, Inherited Retinal Diseases and Electrophysiology
Department of Ophthalmology
University of Florida
Jacksonville, FL, USA

Robyn H Guymer MBBS PhD FRANZCO
Professor of Ophthalmology
University of Melbourne
Centre for Eye Research Australia
Royal Victorian Eye and Ear Hospital
East Melbourne, VIC, Australia

Zohar Habot-Wilner MD
Doctor of Medicine
Department of Ophthalmology
Tel-Aviv Medical Center
Tel-Aviv, Israel

Seenu M Hariprasad MD
Associate Professor of Surgery
Section of Ophthalmology and Visual Science
Chief, Vitreoretinal Service
Director of Clinical Research and Vitreoretinal Fellowship Program
University of Chicago
Chicago, IL, USA

Jeffrey S Heier MD
Vitreoretinal Specialist
Ophthalmic Consultants of Boston
Boston, MA, USA

Rocío Herrero-Vanrell PhD
Professor of Pharmaceutical Technology
Department of Pharmacy and Pharmaceutical Technology
School of Pharmacy
Universidad Complutense
Madrid, Spain

Alexandra A Herzlich MD
National Institute of Health
Bethesda, MD, USA

Frank G Holz MD
Ophthalmologist, University Eye Hospital
Director
Department of Ophthalmology
University of Bonn
Bonn, Germany

John J Huang MD
Assistant Professor
Director of Ocular Immunology and Uveitis
Faculty of Vitreo-Retina
Director of Clinical Trials and Translational Research
Department of Ophthalmology
Yale University
New Haven, CT, USA

Mohamed Ibrahim MD
Research Fellow
Wilmer Eye Institute
Johns Hopkins University School of Medicine
Baltimore, MD, USA

Hisanori Imai MD
Department of Ophthalmology
Kobe University School of Medicine
Kobe, Japan

Peter Charbel Issa MD FEBO
Department of Ophthalmology
University of Bonn
Bonn, Germany

Peter K Kaiser MD
Professor of Ophthalmology
Cleveland Clinic Lerner College of Medicine
Director, Digital OCT Reading Center
Cole Eye Institute
Cleveland, OH, USA

Jennifer J Kang-Mieler PhD
Associate Professor of Biomedical Engineering
Department of Ophthalmology and Visual Sciences
Illinois Institute of Technology
Chicago, IL, USA

Ravi Keshavamurthy MD
Retina Fellow
Department of Ophthalmology
University of Florida
Jacksonville, FL, USA

Bernd Kirchhof MD
Department of Vitreo-Retinal Surgery
Center of Ophthalmology
University of Cologne
Cologne, Germany

Ainat Klein MD
Medical Doctor
Department of Ophthalmology
Tel-Aviv Medical Center, Sackler Faculty of Medicine
Tel-Aviv University
Tel-Aviv, Israel

Mark E Kleinman MD
Resident in Ophthalmology
Department of Ophthalmology and Visual Sciences
University of Kentucky
Lexington, KY, USA

Tim U Krohne MD FEBO
Ophthalmologist
University Eye Hospital
Bonn, Germany

Baruch D Kuppermann MD PhD
Professor of Ophthalmology
University of California Irvine
Irvine, CA, USA

Malaika M Kurz-Levin MD
University Hospital
Department of Ophthalmology
Medical Retina
Zurich, Switzerland

Oh Woong Kwon MD PhD
Director
The Retina Center
Nune Eye Hospital
Seoul, South Korea

Gabriele E Lang MD
Professor of Ophthalmology
Head of the Division of Medical Retina and Laser Surgery
Department of Ophthalmology
University Eye Hospital Ulm
Ulm, Germany

Susan Lightman PhD FRCP FRCOphth
Professor of Clinical Ophthalmology
Department of Clinical Opthalmology
Institute of Ophthalmology
Moorfields Eye Hospital
London, UK

Richard C Lin MD PhD
Clinical Assistant Professor
Stanford University
Palo Alto Veterans Hospital
Palo Alto, CA, USA

Anat Loewenstein MD
Professor of Ophthalmology
Department of Ophthalmology
Tel Aviv Medical Center
Tel Aviv, Israel

Thorsteinn Loftsson MSPharm PhD
Professor
Faculties of Medicine and Pharmacy
University of Iceland
Reykjavik, Iceland

Tao Lu Lowe PhD
Associate Professor of Pharmaceutical Sciences
School of Pharmacy
Thomas Jefferson University
Philadelphia, PA, USA

Maurício Maia MD PhD
Professor of Vitreoretinal Surgery
Department of Ophthalmology
Federal University of São Paulo
São Paulo, Brazil

Juliana Mantovani Bottós MD
Vision Institute, Department of Ophthalmology
Federal University of São Paulo
São Paulo, Brazil

Mariana Martínez-Castellanos MD
Retina Department
Hospital "Dr. Luis Sánchez Bulnes"
Mexico City, Mexico

Trevor J McFarland BS
Senior Research Assistant
Casey Eye Institute
Oregon Health and Science University
Portland, OR, USA

Gustavo B Melo MD
Vision Institute, Department of Ophthalmology
Federal University of São Paulo
São Paulo, Brazil

Carsten H Meyer MD
Ophthalmologist
University Eye Hospital
Bonn, Germany

Stephan Michels MD MBA
Assistant Professor of Medical Retina
Department of Ophthalmology
Triemli Hospital Zurich
Zurich, Switzerland

William F Mieler MD
Professor and Vice-Chairman
Department of Ophthalmology and Visual Sciences
University of Illinois at Chicago
Chicago, IL, USA

Gauri P Misra MD
Department of Pharmaceutical Sciences
School of Pharmacy
Thomas Jefferson University
Philadelphia, PA, USA

Jordi M Monés MD
Director
Institut de la Mácula i de la retina
Centro Médico Teknon
Barcelona, Spain

Raja Narayanan MD
Consultant
Kanuri Santhamma Vitreoretinal Service
LV Prasad Eye Institute
Hyderabad, India

Jackie K Nguyen MD
Vitreoretinal Surgeon
Private Practice
Eyecare Medical Group
Portland, ME, USA

Quan Dong Nguyen MD MSc
Associate Professor of Ophthalmology
Diseases of the Retina and Vitreous, and Uveitis
Wilmer Eye Institute
Johns Hopkins University School of Medicine
Baltimore, MD, USA

Robert B Nussenblatt MD MPH
Chief
Laboratory of Immunology
National Eye Institute
National Institutes of Health
Bethesda, MD, USA

Masahito Ohji MD
Professor and Chairman
Department of Ophthalmology
Shiga University of Medical Science
Otsu, Shiga, Japan

Timothy W Olsen MD
F Phinizy Calhoun Sr Professor and Chairman
Department of Ophthalmology
Emory University
Director, Emory Eye Center
Atlanta, GA, USA

Mrinali Patel MD
Postgraduate Student (PGY-1)
Memorial Sloan Kettering Cancer Center
NY, USA

Fernando M Penha MD PhD
Postdoctoral Associate,
Bascom Palmer Eye Institute, University of Miami,
Miami, FL, USA
Postdoctoral Associate
Department of Ophthalmology
Federal University of São Paulo
São Paulo, Brazil

Hugo Quiroz-Mercado MD
Professor
Rocky Mountain Lions Eye Institute
University of Colorado Hospital
Aurora, CO, USA

Eduardo Büchele Rodrigues MD
Vision Institute, Department of Ophthalmology
Federal University of São Paulo
São Paulo, Brazil

Mi In Roh MD
Opththalmology Research Fellow
Department of Ophthalmology
Harvard Medical School
Massachusetts Eye and Ear Infirmary
Boston, MA, USA

Juliana V Rossi MD
Retina and Vitreous Vision Institute
Department of Ophthalmology
Federal University of São Paulo
São Paulo, Brazil

Theodor Charles Sauer BS
Duke Medical School
Duke University
Durham, NC, USA

Osamu Sawada MD
Assistant Professor
Department of Ophthalmology
Shiga University of Medical Science
Otsu, Shiga, Japan

Andrew P Schachat MD
Professor of Ophthalmology, Lerner College of Medicine
Vice Chairman
Cole Eye Institute
Cleveland Clinic Foundation
Cleveland, OH, USA

Ursula Schmidt-Erfurth MD
Professor and Chair
Department of Ophthalmology and Optometry
Medical University of Vienna
Vienna, Austria

Hendrik P N Scholl MD MA
Consultant Ophthalmologist
Department of Ophthalmology
University of Bonn
Bonn, Germany

Stephen G Schwartz MD MBA
Associate Professor of Clinical Ophthalmology
Medical Director, Bascom Palmer Eye Institute at Naples
Naples, FL, USA

Syed Mahmood Shah MBBS
Research Scientist
Wilmer Eye Institute
Johns Hopkins University School of Medicine
Baltimore, MD, USA

Chirag Pradip Shah MD MPH
Vitreoretinal Surgery Fellow
Wills Eye Institute
Retina Service
Philadelphia, PA, USA

Carol L Shields MD
Professor of Ophthalmology
Ocular Oncology Service
Wills Eye Hospital
Philadelphia, PA, USA

Jerry A Shields MD
Professor of Ophthalmology
Thomas Jefferson University
Director, Oncology Services
Wills Eye Hospital
Philadelphia, PA, USA

Ravi J Singh MD
Department of Ophthalmology
Penn State College of Medicine
Hershey, PA, USA

Sobha Sivaprasad DM MS DNB FRCS
Consultant Ophthalmologist and Senior Lecturer
Laser and Retinal Research Unit
Kings College Hospital
London, UK

Ricardo Luiz Smith MD PhD
Professor of Anatomy
Department of Morphology and Genetics
Federal University of São Paulo
São Paulo, Brazil

Ji Hun Song MD
Assistant Professor
Department of Ophthalmology
Ajou University School of Medicine
Suwon, South Korea

Gisèle Soubrane MD PhD
Professor and Chair of Ophthalmology
Université de Paris Val de Marne
Créteil, France

Boris V Stanzel MD
Resident in Ophthalmology
University Eye Hospital
Bonn, Germany

Einar Stefánsson MD PhD
Professor and Chairman
Department of Ophthalmology
Landspitali University Hospital
Reykjavik, Iceland

Glenn L Stoller MD
Private Practice
Ophthalmic Consultants of Long Island
Lynbrook, NY, USA

J Timothy Stout MD PhD MBA
Vice President, Oregon Health and Science University
Professor of Genetics, Retina and Vitreous Diseases
Casey Eye Institute
Portland, OR, USA

R C Andrew Symons MB BS PhD FRANZCO
Assistant Professor of Ophthalmology
Department of Ophthalmology
University of Kansas
Prairie Village, KS, USA

John T Thompson MD
Assistant Professor
Wilmer Eye Institute
Johns Hopkins University
Baltimore, MD, USA

Michael T Trese MD
Clinical Professor of Biomedical Sciences, Oakland University, Rochester
Chief Pediatric and Adult Vitreoretinal Surgery, Wm. Beaumont Hospital
Royal Oak, MI, USA

Harvey Siy Uy MD DPBO
Director for Research and Chief, Uveitis Service, Asian Eye Institute
Clinical Associate Professor of Ophthalmology
Jose Rizal Ophthalmology Center
University of the Philippines
Philippine General Hospital
Makati City, Philippines

Monika Voigt MD PhD
Department of Ophthalmology of Créteil
University Paris XII
Créteil, France

Shawn Wilker MD
Assistant Professor of Ophthalmology
Case Western Reserve University
School of Medicine
Cleveland, OH, USA

George A Williams MD
Chair, Department of Ophthalmology
Clinical Professor
Beaumont School of Medicine
Oakland University
Beaumont Eye Institute
Royal Oak, MI, USA

Steven Yeh MD
Vitreoretinal Fellow
Casey Eye Institute
Portland, OR, USA

Ellen Yu-Keh MD
Asian Eye Institute
Makati City, Philippines

Donald J Zack MD PhD
Guerrieri Professor of Genetic Engineering and Molecular Ophthalmology
Johns Hopkins Medical School
Baltimore, MD, USA

David G. Zeballos MD
Retina and Vitreous Service
Clinica Oftalmológica Centro Caracas
Caracas, Venezuela

PREFACE

Retinal Pharmacotherapy has been chosen as the title of this new Book in order to elucidate its dual focus – pharmacology of drugs and therapy of vitreoretinal diseases. It is among the very first books in the field to address the very rapid development of pharmacotherapy, thereby filling the need for a comprehensive reference to aid clinician scientists, retina specialists, and comprehensive ophthalmologists in managing patients and conducting studies.

There have been significant developments and advances in the therapy of vitreoretinal diseases in recent years. Although much progress is still needed, ocular diseases such as age-related macular degeneration, diabetic macular edema, and retinal vein occlusions may now be managed by newly discovered or re-discovered drugs such as corticosteroids or specific monoclonal antibodies. *Retinal Pharmacotherapy* aims to present updated data on the currently existing and upcoming drugs that are employed to treat the many vitreoretinal disorders. We have designed a book that would serve as a reference with basic understanding of retinal physiology and provide information on how certain drugs or classes of drugs may work – how small interfering RNAs aid in the control of angiogenesis and why anti-vascular endothelial growth factor may be effective, among others. The Book also provides a basic framework for new concepts and drugs in the treatment of retinal diseases as well as allowing an understanding of the principles of ocular pharmacotherapy in the retina. It will also facilitate better understanding of novel drugs such as monoclonal antibodies and aptamers (pegaptanib, ranibizumab, bevacizumab, and others). In addition, the Book presents detailed information on the techniques and methods of ocular drug delivery such as intravitreal injections and sustained-release delivery devices.

Throughout the 53 chapters, we have looked at pharmacologic therapies from different points of view with the assistance of authors who are authorities on the topics and who are capable of providing the readers with state-of-the-art information. The Book is divided into major sections including Retinal Molecular Biology, Animal Models and Routes for Retinal Drug Delivery, Retinal Diseases Amenable to Pharmacotherapy, Drugs and Mechanisms and Retinal Diseases, Pharmacotherapy and Surgery, and the Last Words. In "Retinal Molecular Biology," various aspects such as biochemistry, molecular biology, and retinal morphology are presented in great depth as the basis for further comprehension of therapeutic pharmacologic agents. "Animal Models and Routes of Retinal Drug Delivery" presents basic information about animal models employed for research on potential therapeutic agents as well as novel concepts in various routes for retinal drug delivery. In "Retinal Diseases Amenable to Pharmacotherapy," the authors describe retinal diseases that may benefit from pharmacologic approaches in clinical practice. The various chapters in "Drugs and Mechanisms and Retinal Diseases" review different drugs currently used in patients with retinal diseases. The section "Pharmacotherapy and Surgery" illustrates the importance of procedures such as radiotherapy in conjunction with pharmacologic agents. *Retinal Pharmacotherapy* concludes with "The Last Words" where processes to obtain FDA approval, evidence-based medicine, and various therapeutic agents that are in the pipeline for selective diseases such as AMD and DME, are discussed in great detail.

In conclusion, we hope that the Book will bring the ophthalmic scientific community to the frontline of research, diving into diseases of the retina, and will challenge scientists in academia and the pharmaceutical industry to develop innovative strategies for the translation of investigative products into viable therapeutics. Certainly, *Retinal Pharmacotherapy* would not have been successfully produced without the many wonderful colleagues throughout the world who devoted their time and efforts in sharing their expertise in the many chapters. In addition, throughout the many months that were required to bring forth the first edition of *Retinal Pharmacotherapy*, our task was greatly assisted by Mr. Russell Gabbedy, Ms. Alexandra Mortimer, and Mr. Sven Pinczewski of the Editorial Staff at Elsevier, who encouraged and guided us, and occasionally pressured us to meet the various deadlines (and we are so glad they did) during the process, from the time we brought to them the concept of the Book to the time *Retinal Pharmacotherapy* was made available for your use; we certainly owe them our deepest gratitude. Finally, we would like to thank you – our readers and most impartial judges. As this is the first edition of the Book, we are certain that there may be many imperfections. Please kindly share them with us so that the second edition will be more to your satisfaction. Given the lightning rate of progress, we expect to work on the revised edition of *Retinal Pharmacotherapy* very soon!

Quan Dong Nguyen, MD, MSc
Eduardo Büchele Rodrigues, MD
Michel Eid Farah, MD
William F. Mieler, MD

DEDICATION AND ACKNOWLEDGMENTS

– To my parents, Dr. and Mrs. Dong So Nguyen, and my three brothers, Dr. Phong Dong Nguyen, Dr. Chau Dong Nguyen, and Chuong Dong Nguyen, Esquire, for their constant support and encouragement. Through their devotion, I have learned compassion and humility – I am profoundly indebted.

– To my teachers, especially Mrs. Laura Bushar, Dr. Lynda Beck, Mrs. Linda Haskins, Dr. Helen Davies, Dr. George L. Spaeth, Dr. Stuart L. Fine, Dr. C. Stephen Foster, Dr. Charles L. Schepens, Dr. Morton F. Goldberg, and Dr. Peter A. Campochiaro, for their mentorship and guidance. They have guided me along every step, pushed me to my maximum ability, and championed me throughout my career. Without their direction and counsel, I would not have been able to achieve my dreams – I am respectfully grateful.

– To my colleagues, fellows, residents, medical students, and patients, for the challenges they persistently present to me. Together, they bestow upon me the confidence to be the best physician for my patients and the most productive clinician scientist for my profession – I pay them homage.

– Finally, to my wife, partner, and colleague, Dr. Diana Do, for her unconditional love and support, and for her willingness to stand by me throughout the successful as well as the most challenging times. – I owe her so much.

Quan Dong Nguyen

– To my family, Joelma, Rafael Eduardo, Sonia and Elvio, for their dedication and support.

– To those colleagues and Professors I have been in contact for the past few years, who enabled me to grow as a person, doctor and researcher

– Great appreciation to the contributing authors, who offered their expertise and knowledge along with their hard work for the book

Eduardo Büchele Rodrigues

– To my three sons, Michael, Andrew, and Daniel, who understand the value and significance of quality education and hard work

– To the numerous residents and vitreoretinal fellows who continue to ask questions and stimulate all of us to obtain better answers to challenging issues

– To my numerous national and international colleagues for their long-standing support and friendship

– Finally, to Jennifer, who is a uniquely wonderful, special, and talented individual. We make a great team

William F Mieler

– To my family, Ana Luisa, Michelle and Julia, for their dedication and support.

– To our students and trainees (past and present), for their commitment to our research development and the clinical as well as surgical treatments afforded to our patients, the main reason for our work and efforts to create better medicine based on our scientific dreams.

– Special thanks to all the contributing authors, who provided their expertise and knowledge along with their extremely valuable and outstanding collaboration. We, as organizers together with the highly qualified editors from Elsevier, were able to make a beautifully illustrated, as well as exceedingly useful textbook.

– We would particularly like to express our appreciation to our colleagues who offered their suggestions in order to make this book valuable for both clinicians and researchers in the pharmacotherapy of retinal and vitreous diseases.

Michel Eid Farah

CHAPTER

1 Evolving knowledge in pharmacologic treatments

Gisèle Soubrane, MD, PhD, Gabriel J. Coscas, MD, and Monika Voigt, MD, PhD

Modern ocular drug therapy is a result of the extraordinary discoveries and challenges achieved through the last decades in different fields of science such as chemistry, biotechnologies, and physics, to mention a few. The understanding of the pathogenesis of ocular diseases underwent significant changes due to discoveries in medicine, genetics, and cell biology. New insights in the pathology of posterior-segment diseases were obtained by the integration of new imaging techniques such as confocal scanning laser angiography and optical coherence tomography. Within the group of the so-called classic therapies, new molecules emerged, such as antibiotics, nonsteroidal anti-inflammatory drugs, and steroids. Thereby, ocular therapy of diseases like uveitis, endophthalmitis, and diabetic maculopathy improved markedly. Moreover, new treatment concepts appeared with molecules whose mode of action is more complex and sophisticated.[1–3]

MEDICAL TREATMENT

VERTEPORFIN

The beginning of the 21st century was marked by the era of the first medical treatment of exudative age-related macular degeneration (AMD). After years of laser photocoagulation as the gold standard in the therapy of this disease, verteporfin became the first medical treatment.[4,5] Verteporfin (Visodyne, Novartis Pharmaceuticals) is a two-stage process requiring administration of both the photosensitizer for injection and nonthermal red light activation. Verteporfin is transported in the plasma mainly by lipoproteins and appears to accumulate preferentially in proliferating endothelial cells of new vessels, such as in the choroidal neovasculature in the case of the eye. Once verteporfin is activated in the presence of oxygen, highly reactive, short-lived singlet oxygen and reactive oxygen radicals are generated. Light activation of verteporfin results in local damage to neovascular endothelium. Damaged endothelium is known to release procoagulant and vasoactive factors through the lipooxygenase (leukotriene) and cyclooxygenase (eicosanoids such as thromboxane) pathways, resulting in platelet aggregation, fibrin clot formation, and vasoconstriction. The following temporary occlusion of choroidal neovascularization (CNV) has been confirmed in humans by fluorescein angiography and demonstrated a clinical efficacy. However, a collateral damage to retinal structures following photoactivation, including the retinal pigmented epithelium (RPE) and the outer nuclear layer of the retina, can be seen. Unfortunately, photodynamic therapy itself induced a local inflammatory reaction and an increased local production of vascular endothelial growth factor (VEGF), thereby limiting its therapeutic effect. Nevertheless, Visudyne still has some indication as the treatment of choroidal neovessels in myopia.[6–8]

ANTI-VEGF TREATMENT

A new era of ocular neovascular therapy has started.[8,9] Several different approaches regarding anti-VEGF, one of the main factors in ocular neovascularization, are nowadays routine in the treatment of AMD. The importance of VEGF as a therapeutic target derives from its effect on vascular leakage and neovascularization. Gene-based drugs entered the clinical everyday life only in the recent past. The nucleotide sequence of DNA, RNA, or their modifications is used to induce gene expression (gene therapy), suppress translation of the target mRNA (small interference RNA (siRNA), antisense oligonucleotides, ribozymes), or to bind to a specific protein target (aptamers).[10] This approach is interesting as genes express their protein products for prolonged periods, thus a more targeted and long-lasting therapy can be obtained. Currently in ophthalmology clinically used gene-based drugs are Vitravene (Isis Pharmaceuticals) and Macugen (Pfizer). Vitravene is an intravitreally administered phosphorothioate oligonucleotide for the treatment of CMV infection in acquired immunodeficiency syndrome (AIDS) patients. Anti-VEGF aptamers are stable small RNA-like molecules that bind exclusively and with high affinity to the 165-kDa isoform of human VEGF. Sodium pegaptanib (Macugen, Pfizer), can only bind and inhibit the larger VEGF 165 isoform. The aptamer is conjugated to polyethylene glycol to increase its half-life and stability in the vitreous. The same drug is currently in phase II trials for the treatment of diabetic macular edema. Two siRNA molecules (bevasiranib and Sirna-027) that modify the activity of VEGF and its receptor (VEGFR-1) have entered into clinical trials. RNAi is a double-stranded piece of interference RNA that is taken up by chorioretinal cells, activating a protein that breaks down the antisense mRNA. Destruction of VEGF mRNA prevents the production of VEGF protein. The whole process is catalytic, so the RNAi may be a very potent and efficient blockade of VEGF. RNAi may have a long biologic half-life, indicating a much longer interval between intravitreal injections.[11]

OTHER MEDICAL TREATMENTS

Other antiangiogenic therapy approaches are based on proteins like antibodies or enzymes. In contrast to pegaptanib, bevacizumab (Avastin, Genentech), a full-length, humanized monoclonal antibody against VEGF and ranibizumab (Lucentis, Genentech), a recombinant, humanized, monoclonal antibody antigen-binding fragment (Fab), bind and neutralize all the biologically active forms of VEGF. Both drugs are proteins that were genetically modified from the same murine monoclonal antibody against VEGF. The two proteins differ in their component, size, and affinity for VEGF. Whereas bevacizumab is a humanized, murine full-length antibody with two binding sites for VEGF and an Fc fragment, ranibizumab is a humanized, murine antigen-binding fragment (Fab) with only a single affinity-matured binding site for VEGF.

VEGF-Trap (R1R2) is a fusion protein that combines ligand-binding elements taken from the extracellular domains of the receptors VEGFR-1 and VEGFR-2 fused to the Fc portion of immunoglobulin G (IgG). This potent high-affinity VEGF blocker effectively suppresses tumor growth and vascularization *in vivo*.

Several publications demonstrated the fundamental role of the c-raf kinase in cell proliferation, resistance to apoptosis, and its influence on the VEGF pathway. Although this therapy is still at an experimental level, it appears to be a promising method of treating neovascular tissue in AMD and diabetic retinopathy.

The formerly mentioned new therapeutic molecules still require a direct intravitreal injection for usual clinical treatment. Thus, unfortunately, the problem of these potential treatments remains in achieving adequate bioavailibility and prolonged therapeutic tissue concentration.[12]

"PLAYERS" IN OCULAR TREATMENT

The eye is an extraordinary organ. Due to its accessibility and transparency, it offers a unique advantage for pharmacologic and surgical treatments and is therefore very attractive from the perspective of drug delivery. However, its unique structure requires many different therapies, especially in regard to its complex anatomical composition. The eye represents a small multicompartmental system with various tissues, boundaries, and fluid flow factors.[13]

Vitreous, retina, RPE, choroid, and barriers in the anterior segment, such as the stromal tissues of the cornea and the sclera, the corneal epithelium, and endothelium, might affect ocular drug pharmacokinetics. In addition the outer and inner blood–retinal barriers which are formed by RPE and retinal vascular endothelium, respectively, and the internal limiting membrane on the vitreoretinal interface represent further barriers in the posterior segment.

As a result of advances in the understanding of the pathophysiological processes in the retina and choroid, a rapidly growing interest and demand in posterior-segment drug delivery systems can be noticed.[14] Unfortunately, effective treatment methods are not currently available for many of these diseases.

Posterior eye diseases present a major challenge, as they cause impaired vision and blindness for millions of patients all around the world. In industrialized countries, AMD is the major cause of blindness. Almost 2 million people are affected by this disease in the USA alone. Other major diseases of the posterior eye segment include retinal degeneration, diabetic retinopathy, and glaucoma, where loss of vision is caused by death of the retinal ganglion cells. The growing number of patients worldwide and the socioeconomic impact necessitate an earlier and more targeted treatment of these diseases.

Despite extensive research in the field of ocular pharmacotherapy and new promising treatments, the quest for a specific tissue- and disease-targeted therapy is still going on.[15,16]

THE DRUG

The drug itself is of major importance in regard to its pharmaceutical and pharmacokinetical characteristics, including its specific molecular and chemical structure, its hydrophilic or lipophilic behavior, and finally its therapeutic mode of action.[14]

Based on the above characteristics a high ocular penetration should ideally be obtained, resulting in therapeutic targeted tissue concentrations. In addition, the drugs should ensure a prolonged time of action and be safe, with minimal systemic and local toxicity. The transporter vehicle or drug delivery system is designed to enhance ocular tissue penetration and establish controlled drug release. Administration methods should preferably be local, thereby reducing systemic side-effects, and ideally be noninvasive.

ROUTE OF ADMINISTRATION

Although the conventional drug administration forms (eye drops or systemic administration) dominate the field of ocular drug delivery, history has shown that many new pharmaceutical concepts were introduced to clinical practice for the first time in ophthalmology. It was in the 1970s that the term "drug delivery system" appeared. Extensive research was performed during the last decades to improve the drug delivery or transporter vehicle part of the ocular pharmacotherapy system.[3,15–17]

Eye drops

Eye drops have been in use since the times of ancient Egypt for the treatment of ocular conditions. Eye drop administration is still the most used ocular drug delivery method. The inconvenience of this administration method is the need for relatively frequent instillation as ocular drug bioavailability is very low (< 5% of the dose is absorbed). Different types of ocular drops, like suspensions or solution, and ointments were developed to facilitate ocular drug molecules. Nevertheless this administration method could not demonstrate its efficacy in the treatment of the posterior pole diseases and it remains a treatment modality for the anterior segment.

Soluble ophthalmic drug inserts

For these reasons, the application of soluble ophthalmic drug inserts with a prolonged drug delivery was developed. The first inserts were introduced in the 1960s. The matrix of an acrylate-based co-polymer dissolved during a couple of hours after its application to the conjunctival sac. In the early 1970s pilocarpine-releasing Ocusert (Alza) and, later, another insert, Lacrisert (Merck) were developed. The former represents a sophisticated system that releases the drug for a week at constant rate through ethylene vinyl acetate membranes.

Ion drug exchange

Another development was the creation of liquid state delivery systems that forms a drug-releasing gel after its instillation as an eye drop. The concept of ion drug exchange from the surface of microspheres to the tear fluid was put into practice by a product that released betaxolol. Drug-immersed hydrophilic contact lenses and topical ocular liposomes were tested for drug delivery in the 1970s and 1980s, but these approaches resulted in limited improvements, especially in regard to posterior pole drug delivery. Finally, these topical ocular delivery methods failed as possible vehicle devices for treatment of the posterior ocular segment.

Intravitreal injections

In parallel with the discovery and better clinical pathophysiological understanding of posterior-segment diseases, the demand for appropriate treatment increased. New drugs for medication of the posterior ocular segment have emerged, but most drugs are currently delivered by repeated intravitreal injections, such as the anti-VEGF treatments currently used in the treatment of exudative AMD. Unfortunately this invasive drug delivery method can induce vitreal hemorrhages, retinal detachment, or even endophthalmitis. The risk is smaller with periocular drug administration, frequently used in the clinical ophthalmological routine as subconjunctival or peribulbar injections, such as corticoid administration (dexamethasone, triamcinolone), in the treatment of uveitis and chronic inflammatory macular edema. This route, via the conjunctiva and sclera, avoids the counterflow of aqueous humor and the lens barrier, as for drug administration with eye drops. Therefore, this route may be a possible future alternative for drug administration (including proteins and gene-based drugs) to the retina and vitreous if appropriate delivery systems are developed. The sclera is permeable to macromolecules, but choroidal blood flow and the RPE are the major barriers in drug penetration. Delivery of macromolecules is important therapeutically, since antiangiogenic antibodies, oligonucleotides, growth factors, and transgene expression products are all large molecules. Several studies have demonstrated the efficacy of different drug delivery methods via the transscleral route, such as noninvasive application iontophoresis or subconjunctivally placed drug release implants.[18]

Systemic administration

Another major route of drug delivery is via systemic administration. Systemically administered drugs reach the chorioretinal tissue through the blood circulation. However, the outer and inner blood–retinal barriers limit the influx of drugs into the retinal tissue and the vitreous cavity. Therefore, a high rate of drug concentration and frequent administration are required to maintain therapeutic concentrations, which may result in serious side-effects on nontargeted tissues and organs. Therefore, effective, safe, and comfortable methods of drug delivery are needed.

Sustained drug delivery system

This demand revived the interest in ocular-controlled release systems. Currently most research efforts are directed towards a sustained drug delivery system to treat chronic disease. The challenge is to provide a system with an improved ocular drug bioavailability and prolonged duration of activity, yet which presents a minimal risk of ocular complications. Furthermore the final aim is to develop effective drug delivery methods for posterior-segment therapies that would also be applicable for the outpatient use.

Based on experience with drug delivery inserts, used for the anterior segment, and new biophysical and biochemical implant models, the idea of drug transporter vehicles was the increasing focus of clinical ophthalmologic research.[16–18]

Intraocular implants

Emerging methods include polymeric-controlled release injections and implants, nanoparticulates, microencapsulated cells, and iontophoresis. The goal of the implant design is to provide prolonged activity with controlled drug release from the polymeric implant material. Different types of implants such as intraocular or periocular implants are under investigation. Intraocular administration of implants always requires minor surgery. In general, they are placed or injected intravitreally in the area of the pars plana. Although this is an invasive technique, the implants have the benefit of bypassing the blood–ocular barrier to deliver constant therapeutic levels of drug directly to the site of action. Furthermore, it reduces the side-effects associated with frequent systemic and intravitreal injections as their drug release is programmed over a certain period of time. Finally, a significantly reduced drug quantity is required with this route of administration during the treatment period. The ocular implants are classified as nonbiodegradable and biodegradable devices. Nonbiodegradable implants can provide more accurate control of drug release and longer release periods than biodegradable polymers, but nonbiodegradable systems require surgical implant removal with associated risks. Vitrasert and Retisert (Bausch & Lomb) are clinically used nonbiodegradable implants. Vitrasert is the first implantable ganciclovir delivery device which was approved by the Food and Drug Administration (FDA) in 1996. Ethylene vinyl acetate and polyvinyl alcohol (PVA) polymers control the release of ganciclovir. It is effective in controlling the progression of cytomegalovirus retinitis associated with AIDS for a period of 8 months. Retisert is the first marketed fluocinolone acetonide implant for the treatment of chronic noninfectious uveitis of the posterior segment. PVA and silicone laminate control the release of corticosteroid over a 3-year period. Both implant types occasionally showed side-effects like endophthalmitis, increased rate of retinal detachments, cataract formation, and ocular hypertension. The biodegradable implants Surodex and Ozurdex (Allergan) are currently undergoing clinical phase III studies. They are nearly identical polylactic co-glycolic acid (PLGA) implants with different doses of dexamethasone (60 µg for Surodex and 700 µg for Ozurdex). Ozurdex is designed for sustained release of dexamethasone over a period of several months after intravitreal placement.

So far scleral implants have only been studied on an animal model. The device released betamethasone in a constant manner for at least 3 months without detectable drug concentration in the aqueous humor. Surprisingly, this route resulted in a more effective delivery to the macular region than the intravitreal implants. The transscleral delivery system is thus a promising alternative for the treatment of retinal and choroidal diseases.[19,20]

Microparticles and nanoparticles

Another control-releasing strategy is to encapsulate the drug in microparticles or nanoparticles.[21] Usually biodegradable and biocompatible polymers are used, such as polylactide and PLGA, which both are FDA-approved. These systems can provide sustained drug delivery for weeks or even months just by the administration of one single intravitreal injection. To date, some microsphere formulations have been analyzed in preclinical studies, but have not yet undergone clinical trials. Subconjunctival or periocular injections of microspheres were administered to provide transscleral drug delivery instead of invasive intravitreal administration, which can cause vitreal clouding. Targeted microspheres with PKC412, an inhibitor of protein kinase C and of receptors for VEGF, were used to treat CNV.[22] The microsphere system was moreover studied to release pegaptanib sodium (anti-VEGF aptamer). This molecule is already a standard treatment for wet AMD. The pegaptanib-loaded microspheres were either administered through the scleral route or by intravitreal injection.[23,24] Both administration methods released the aptamer over several weeks after injection.

Liposomes

Nanoparticulates and liposomes are suitable for intracellular drug delivery and could thus be used to treat retinal disorders. Liposomes are biocompatible, biodegradable, and can be made of natural lipids. On the one hand, hydrophilic as well as lipophilic drugs can be encapsulated to the lipid walls or the aqueous interior of the liposomes. On the other hand, these carriers can be engineered to target certain cell types. Preclinical experiments have demonstrated the presence of nanoparticles and liposomes in RPE cells probably due to the phagocytic capacity of RPE cells. Nanoparticles are retained within the RPE cells even 4 months after a single intravitreal injection.[25] Liposomes can be prepared with different sizes, stability, and pharmacokinetics. Further, the liposomal surfaces can be modified to allow preferential binding, for example, to the endothelium cells of proliferating neovascular vessels. Liposome technology has been used to develop light-induced systems for retinal disease (for example, Visudyne, Novartis Pharmaceuticals).

Light-induced systems can either be light-activated drugs (i.e., photodynamic therapy) or light-activated delivery systems. So far verteporfin (Visudyne, Novartis Pharmaceuticals) is the only ocular liposomal drug currently in clinical use. Recently another light-induced drug delivery system was combined with a viral transport. This light-induced drug delivery system is based on VP22, a structural protein of herpes simplex virus.[26] The purified VP22 protein binds antisense oligonucleotide of human craf kinase. To obtain a light-induced activation of the drug after intravitreal injection, a fluorochrome is covalently linked to either the protein or to the oligonucleotide. The carriers remain in the cytoplasm of various retinal cell types. Due to transscleral illumination the delivery of free oligonucleotides can be obtained.

Encapsulated cell technology (ECT)

A different promising new drug delivery method is based on the principle of ECT. The concept is to entrap immunologically isolated cells with microcapsules or hollow fibers before their administration into the eye. The genetically engineered cells continuously produce a therapeutic protein at the site of implantation. Thus technology enables the controlled, continuous, and long-term delivery of therapeutic proteins directly to the posterior segment of the eye. The implant is inserted through a small scleral incision and placed at the pars plana. The implant is sutured in order to allow its retrieval when desired. ECT product NT501 (Neurotech) with encapsulated genetically modified human RPE cells which secreted ciliary neurotrophic factor to the vitreous were implanted in the eyes of patient with retinitis pigmentosa for a period of 6 months. An improvement of visual acuity was reported and the device was well tolerated.[27] ECT may have a therapeutic potential as a delivery system for chronic ophthalmic diseases lacking effective therapies, and as a drug vehicle for anti-inflammatory factors.[28] Long-term safety and efficacy have yet to be clinically studied.

Iontophoresis

Finally, iontophoresis should be mentioned as a potent drug delivery system which could be suitable for different drug concepts, such as gene therapy, liposome- or nanoparticle-encapsulated proteins, or other drug molecules.[18] Iontophoresis could be defined as an enforced penetration of charged molecules through a tissue border by applying an electrical field. Iontophoresis generally enhances drug delivery by two mechanisms: electrophoresis and electroosmosis. Iontophoresis is a noninvasive, well-tolerated and safe method. Ocular iontophoresis is classified according to the site of application of the low electrical current for a limited period of time into transcorneal, corneoscleral, or transscleral iontophoresis. Transscleral iontophoresis appears to be more suitable for drug transfer to the posterior segment. The properties of the sclera (hydration, leakiness, low electrical resistance) make iontophoretic delivery feasible at low electric currents or voltages for agents such as nonsteroidal anti-inflammatory drugs, corticoids, immunosuppressive agents, and oligonucleotides. *In vivo* studies have demonstrated its therapeutic efficiency for antisense oligonucleotides in the model of endotoxin-induced uveitis.

A few ocular iontophoresis systems have been investigated recently: Ocuphor (Iomed), Eyegate II Delivery System (EyeGate Pharma), and Visulex (Aciont). These new devices are relatively easy to handle and avoid the adverse effects frequently observed in the past. Eyegate II Delivery System is the first that was used in patients. The iontophoretic technique has the huge advantage of being noninvasive in comparison to intraocular injection drug administration. Hence, the duration of drug action is less prolonged than with intravitreally injected controlled release systems. This could be surpassed in the future by combining iontophoresis with encapsulated drug transport vehicles such as nanoparticles or liposomes. Consequently the enforced and increased intraocular drug penetration resulting from iontophoresis could be combined with the effect of a slow, controlled and targeted drug release obtained by the liposome or other similar encapsulated drug vehicles.

Ocular pharmacology and drug delivery technology is currently facing tremendous challenges and opportunities. Nowadays, drug delivery techniques and pharmacological therapies are clinical routine treatments which, only a decade ago, appeared absolutely futuristic. There is no doubt that further new molecules and treatment strategies with new pathophysiological insights will culminate in a new revolutionary pharmacotherapy.

REFERENCES

1. Emerson MV, Lauer AK. Emerging therapies for the treatment of neovascular age-related macular degeneration and diabetic macular edema. BioDrugs 2007;21:245–257.
2. Chakravarthy U, Soubrane G, Bandello F, et al. Evolving European guidance on the medical management of neovascular age related macular degeneration. Br J Ophthalmol 2006;90:1188–1196.
3. Liu X, Brandt CR, Rasmussen CA, et al. Ocular drug delivery: molecules, cells, and genes. Can J Ophthalmol 2007;42:447–454.
4. Guidelines for using verteporfin (Visudyne) in photodynamic therapy to treat choroidal neovascularization due to age-related macular degeneration and other causes. Retina 2002;22:6–18.
5. Blinder KJ, Bradley S, Bressler NM, et al. Effect of lesion size, visual acuity, and lesion composition on visual acuity change with and without verteporfin therapy for choroidal neovascularization secondary to age-related macular degeneration: TAP and VIP report no. 1. Am J Ophthalmol 2003;136:407–418.
6. Soubrane G. Choroidal neovascularization in pathologic myopia: recent developments in diagnosis and treatment. Surv Ophthalmol 2008;53:121–138.
7. Ruiz-Moreno JM, Amat P, Montero JA, et al. Photodynamic therapy to treat choroidal neovascularisation in highly myopic patients: 4 years' outcome. Br J Ophthalmol 2008;92:792–794.
8. Pece A, Vadalà M, Isola V, et al. Photodynamic therapy with verteporfin for juxtafoveal choroidal neovascularization in pathologic myopia: a long-term follow-up study. Am J Ophthalmol 2007;143:449–454.
9. Pieramici DJ, Rabena MD. Anti-VEGF therapy: comparison of current and future agents. Eye 2008;22:1330–1336.
10. Takeda AL, Colquitt J, Clegg AJ, et al. Pegaptanib and ranibizumab for neovascular age-related macular degeneration: a systematic review. Br J Ophthalmol 2007;91:1177–1182.
11. Patil SD, Rhodes DG, Burgess DJ. DNA-based therapeutics and DNA delivery systems: a comprehensive review. AAPS J 2005;7:E61–E77.
12. Urtti A. Challenges and obstacles of ocular pharmacokinetics and drug delivery. Adv Drug Deliv Rev 2006;58:1131–1135.
13. Ranta V-P, Urtti A. Transscleral drug delivery to the posterior eye: prospects of pharmacokinetic modeling. Adv Drug Deliv Rev 2006;58:1164–1181.
14. Geroski DH, Edelhauser HF. Drug delivery for posterior segment eye disease. Invest Ophthalmol Vis Sci 2004;1:961–964.
15. Del Amo EM, Urtti A. Current and future ophthalmic drug delivery systems. A shift to the posterior segment. Drug Discov Today 2008;13:135–143.
16. Yasukawa T, Ogura Y, Tabata Y, et al. Drug delivery systems for vitreoretinal diseases. Prog Retin Eye Res 2004;23:253–281.
17. Bourges JL, Bloquel C, Thomas A, et al. Intraocular implants for extended drug delivery: therapeutic applications. Adv Drug Deliv Rev 2006;58:1182–1202.
18. Myles ME, Neumann DM, Hill JM. Recent progress in ocular drug delivery for posterior segment disease: emphasis on transscleral iontophoresis. Adv Drug Deliv Rev 2005;57:2063–2079.
19. Kato A, Kimura H, Okabe K. Feasibility of drug delivery to the posterior pole of the rabbit eye with an episcleral implant. Invest Ophthalmol Vis Sci 2004;45:238–244.
20. Okabe K, Kimura K, Okabe J, et al. Intraocular tissue distribution of betamethasone after intrascleral administration using a non-biodegradable sustained drug delivery device. Invest Ophthalmol Vis Sci 2003;44:2702–2707.
21. Moshfeghi AA, Peyman GA. Micro- and nanoparticulates. Adv Drug Deliv Rev 2005;57:2047–2052.
22. Saishin Y, Silva RL, Saishin Y, et al. Periocular injection of microspheres containing PKC412 inhibits choroidal neovascularization in a porcine model. Invest Ophthalmol Vis Sci 2003;44:4989–4993.
23. Carrasquillo KG, Ricker JA, Rigas IK, et al. Controlled delivery of the anti-VEGF aptamer EYE001 with poly(lactic-co-glycolic)acid microspheres. Invest Ophthalmol Vis Sci 2003;44:290–299.
24. Cook GP, Burgess L, Wing J, et al. Preparation and characterization of pegaptanib sustained release microsphere formulation for intraocular application. Association for Research in Vision and Ophthalmology 2006;47:5123.
25. Bourges JL, Gautier SE, Delie F, et al. Ocular drug delivery targeting the retina and retinal pigment epithelium using polylactide nanoparticles. Invest Ophthalmol Vis Sci 2003;44:3562–3569.
26. Normand N, Valamanesh F, Savoldelli M, et al. VP22 light controlled delivery of oligonucleotides to ocular cells *in vitro* and *in vivo*. Mol Vis 2005;11:184–191.
27. Sieving PA, Caruso RC, Tao W, et al. Ciliary neurotrophic factor (CNTF) for human retinal degeneration: phase I trial of CNTF delivered by encapsulated cell intraocular implants. Proc Natl Acad Sci USA 2006;103:3896–3901. Epub 2006 Feb 27.
28. Tao W. Application of encapsulated cell technology for retinal degenerative diseases. Expert Opin Biol Ther 2006;6:717–726.

CHAPTER 2

Retinal anatomy and pathology

Alexandra A. Herzlich, MD, Mrinali Patel, MD, Theodor Charles Sauer, BS, and Chi-Chao Chan, MD

INTRODUCTION

The retina is a thin multilayer of mainly neuronal cells derived from ectoderm. Much like the film of a camera, the retina is charged with the critical task of receiving, modulating, and transmitting visual stimuli from the external world to the optic nerve and, ultimately, the visual cortex of the brain. Adequate conveyance of visual signals depends largely upon the highly specialized anatomy of the retina, and a variety of insults to the retina can generate pathological processes which disrupt this delicate structure and lead to retinal diseases. This chapter provides a brief overview of normal retinal anatomy, as well as key pathological changes seen in major diseases of the retina.

KEY CONCEPTS AND FUNDAMENTALS

NORMAL RETINAL ANATOMY

The retina is a thin, delicate, transparent sheet of tissue derived from neuroectoderm. It comprises the sensory neurons that begin the visual pathway. The neural retina (neuroretina) is divided into nine layers: layer of inner and outer segments of the photoreceptors (rods and cones), external limiting membrane, outer nuclear layer, outer plexiform layer, inner nuclear layer, inner plexiform layer, ganglion cell layer, nerve fiber layer, and internal limiting membrane (Figure 2.1). Light must traverse these many layers before initiating signal transduction in the rods and cones. Below these photoreceptors reside the retinal pigment epithelium (RPE), a monolayer of cuboidal cells characterized by a high concentration of melanosomes from which the cells derive their pigmented color. The RPE cells help to nourish the overlying neurosensory retina, facilitating the diffusion of nutrients from the choroid and the removal of waste or worn-out photoreceptors segments. Each RPE has numerous apical membrane extensions, servicing up to 45 photoreceptors and reaching up to 50% the height of the outer photoreceptor segment. The extracellular space between the photoreceptors and RPE is filled with a glycosaminoglycan ground substance, termed the interphotoreceptor matrix. The basement membrane of the RPE comprises the cuticular portion (inner layer) of Bruch's membrane.

The rod and cone layer is composed of the outer and inner segments of the rod and cone cells, referred to together as the photoreceptor cells. The outer segment contains stacks of membrane discs, which enclose visual pigment molecules and are constantly renewed. New discs are added to the base of the outer segment at the cilium. At the same time, old discs are displaced outwards, eventually being pinched off at the photoreceptor tip and engulfed by the apical processes of the RPE in a diurnal cycle. Anatomically, the outer segment constricts at the cilium, beginning the inner segment, which is divided into the mitochondria-rich outer ellipsoid and Golgi body and ribosome-rich inner myoid. The external limiting membrane, separating the inner and outer segments from the photoreceptor nuclei, is not a true membrane but a series of dashes formed by the terminal bar attachments of the cell bodies of rods, cones, and Müller cells. The outer nuclear layer contains the nuclei of the photoreceptor cells (both rod and cone cells). The outer plexiform layer is formed by the axons of the photoreceptor cells and their synapses with bipolar cells. In the perifovealar area, the axons of the cones take a tangential or oblique course to meet the excentric-positioned neurons of inner retina and ganglion cells, referred to as the nerve fibre layer of Henle.

Several distinct cell types compose the inner neural retina (Figure 2.1). Bipolar cells (glutamatergic or glycinergic neurons) connect the photoreceptor cells ultimately with the dendrites of the ganglion cells in the outer plexiform layer. Horizontal cells are mainly GABAnergic (gamma-aminobutyric acid) neurons that connect to either rod cells or cone cells and synapse with bipolar cells, where on and off responses are generated, to regulate signal transduction. Amacrine cells receive excitatory glutamatergic input from bipolar cells and primarily inhibitory input from other amacrine cells mediated by $GABA_C$ receptors. Amacrine cells can synapse back on to bipolar cells, other amacrine cells, and ganglion cells. Müller cells act as specialized glial cells to form retinal scaffolding, support the inner segments of the photoreceptors, and create the acellular fibrous internal limiting membrane. The nuclear bodies of all these distinct cell types compose the inner nuclear layer. The axons of the bipolar and amacrine cells connect to the dendrites of the ganglion cells to compose the inner plexiform layer. The ganglion cell layer contains the nuclei of the ganglion cells. Their axons en route to the optic disc form the nerve fiber layer. The internal limiting membrane is a basement membrane structure, formed by the footpads of the Müller cells.

The retina measures about 0.4 mm in thickness at the border of the optic nerve head and tends to become thinner toward the periphery until it reaches approximately 0.14 mm at the ora serrata. The clinical macula is a 1.5-mm circular area in the neural retina, 0.35 mm thick on the outside and sloping down to 0.18 mm at the foveola. In this region cones reach a high density: 4000–5000/mm^2 in the macula and 15000/mm^2 in the fovea. Rods reach their greatest density 20° from the fixation point. Foveal cones can match with up to five ganglion cells, while on average the retinal ganglion cells match with roughly 130 different photoreceptors. Metabolic supply is mainly provided to the neural retina by the central retinal artery, which divides into four arteriole branches at the optic disc. The arterioles are 7–8 smooth-muscle cells thick and run in the nerve fiber layer below the internal limiting membrane. Capillary-free zones extend 150 μm around the retinal arteries and within the 400-μm diameter of the foveola. Photoreceptors receive their metabolic supply from the choroid through osmosis across Bruch's membrane and through the RPE.

With age, changes in the normal retina include a shallower optic disc surrounded by focal subtle choroidal atrophy, lipofuscin in the RPE, and few small drusen between the RPE and Bruch's membrane.[1,2]

RETINAL PATHOLOGY

As illustrated above, the retina is an extremely complex structure. One can imagine that its intricate nature can easily result in many different and unique congenital and developmental abnormalities. Similarly, a variety of insults to the retina – including degenerative processes, drug toxicities, inflammation, vascular abnormalities, infection, and neoplastic changes – can result in a broad spectrum of retinal pathology. The

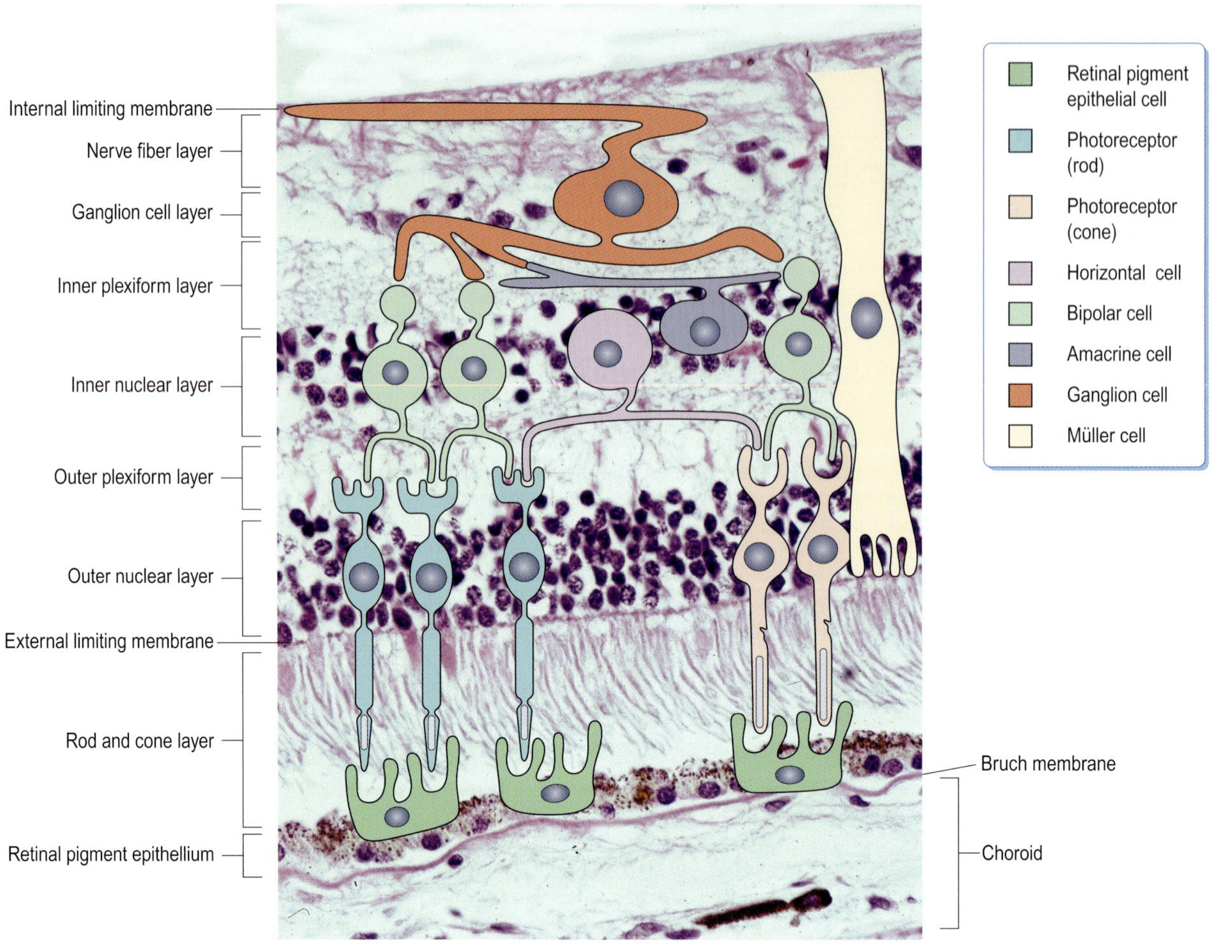

Figure 2.1 Photomicrograph of the retina combined with a diagram of pertinent retinal cells. The 10 layers of the retina (neuroretina and retinal pigment epithelium) are identified along the left and the different cell types in the box on the right. (Hematoxylin and eosin, original magnification, ×200.)

capacity of retinal tissue to respond to such injuries depends largely on the specific cells and tissue involved, as well as the type, duration, and severity of injury or involvement of various diseases.

Congenital abnormalities

Congenital abnormalities can often be severe, as in retinal coloboma, which generally occurs bilaterally and inferonasally. Histological features of the coloboma include absent RPE, atrophic gliotic retina sometimes with rosettes, hyperplastic RPE around the lesion edge, a completely or partially absent choroid, and a scleral alteration that may be thinned or absent, and thus form a staphyloma. A congenital retinal cyst differs in that it is generally located inferotemporally, and lined by gliotic neural retina.

Macular hypoplasia (or aplasia) involves an underdevelopment or absence of the macula, causing irregular distribution of perifoveal capillaries and lack of pigmentation. Retinal dysplasia is characterized by retinal folds and rosettes, which can be focal, multifocal, geographic, or accompanied by retinal detachment.

Oguchi disease, a form of congenital night blindness with onset in childhood, is an autosomal-recessive disorder resulting in an abnormal number of cones in the retina with almost no rods present, especially in the temporal area.[3] In between the photoreceptors and the RPE an amorphous pigment granule substance settles. Restricted light adaptation is also a hallmark of ocular albinism, an X-linked recessive trait. Macromelanosomes develop in the RPE, ciliary body, and iris. Additionally, the foveal pit is nonexistent and there is reduced pigmentation in the retina and iris.[4] Menkes' syndrome is an X-linked disease that affects copper levels in the body. Ocular histology reveals peripheral retinal hypopigmentation and progressive ganglion cell atrophy that is pronounced in the maculae.[5]

A predominant developmental abnormality is retinopathy of prematurity (retrolental fibroplasia), which occurs most frequently in preterm infants weighing less than 1.5 kg. Oxygen levels change following birth, disrupting normal retinal vasculature development and leading to vessel obliteration and subsequent proliferative neovascularization.[6,7] Macular heterotopia and optic disc heterotopia are other developmental abnormalities leading to an abnormal retinal anatomy and visual function.

Dystrophies

Damage confined to the sensory retina is seen in disorders such as rod or cone monochromatism, pericentral cone–rod dystrophy (inverse retinitis pigmentosa), fenestrated sheen macular dystrophy, and X-linked juvenile retinoschisis. In X-linked juvenile retinoschisis there is a bilateral, symmetric, splitting of the nerve fiber layer in macular and peripheral retina (Figure 2.2). Complications include progression to a larger cyst or macular hole, rhegmatogenous retinal detachment, or vitreous hemorrhage. It is mostly missense mutations in the *RS1* gene, that contains six exons encoding a small, 224-amino-acid protein, with an N-terminal secretory leader peptide sequence and a discoidin domain in exons 4–6, that are responsible for the manifestation of X-linked juvenile retinoschisis.[8]

Macular dystrophies usually occur bilaterally. Stargardt's disease, a bilateral, symmetric, slowly progressive dystrophy, proceeds from

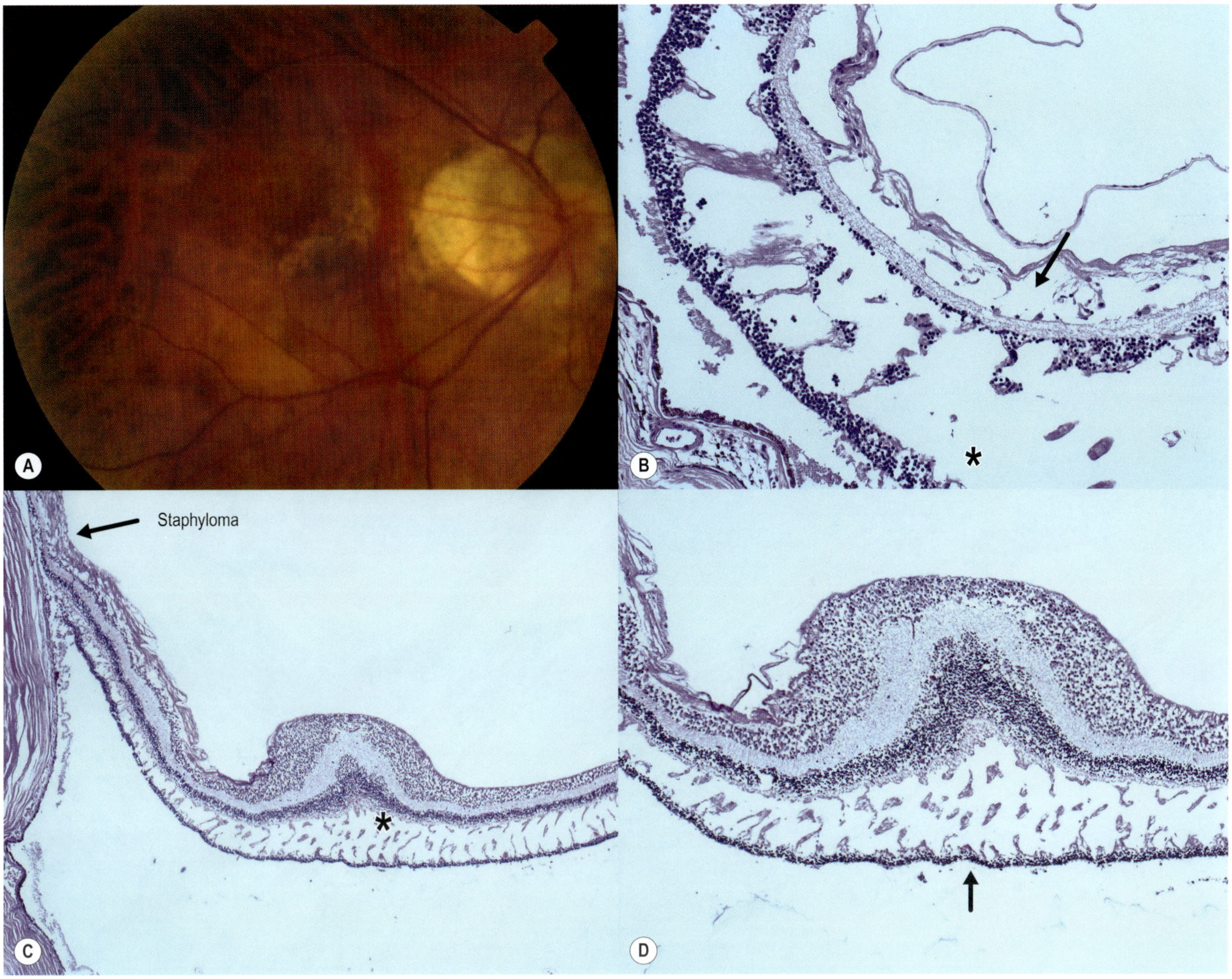

Figure 2.2 Pathological features of retinoschisis. (A) Fundoscopy of a patient with retinoschisis shows retinal splitting, seen as a cartwheel pattern of folds radiating out from the fovea. (B) Photomicrographs of the retina in another patient with retinoschisis shows splitting in the inner plexiform layer (arrow) and the outer plexiform layer (asterisk). (C) Bulging of the thinned sclera forms a staphyloma and retinoschisis (asterisk). (D) Higher magnification illustrating the schisis cavity (arrow) containing amorphous, periodic acid–Schiff (PAS)-positive filamentous material that may be remnants of Müller cells. (PAS, original magnifications, (B) and (D), ×100, (C), ×25.)

the RPE and is characterized by ill-defined yellow-whitish round and linear fishtail or pisiform lesions at the level of the RPE. The main pathology demonstrates loss of RPE and photoreceptors in the macular area. In the RPE there is displacement of nuclei, aggregation of melanin granules, accumulation of mucopolysaccharides, and variation in cell size. In addition, cystoid macular edema and some nodular drusen can be found. When the characteristic lesions are seen throughout the fundus the disorder is known as fundus flavimaculatus. Patients may be genotyped for common mutations in *ABCA4* gene associated with the recessive form of this disease or the gene that codes for *ELOVL4* in the dominant form.[9] Vitelliform dystrophy (Best's disease) will reveal yellowish round lesions that look like the yolk of a fried egg clinically. Pathologically there is RPE and photoreceptor cell atrophy, accumulation of abnormal lipofuscin in residual RPE and deposition of periodic acid–Schiff-positive material in the macula. Best's disease is caused by mutations in *VMD2 (hBEST1)*. Bestrophin, the gene product of *hBEST1*, is a regulatory part of a Ca^{2+} channel or a Ca^{2+}-dependent Cl^- channel.[9] Central areolar pigment epithelial dystrophy is a disturbance of RPE with areas of depigmentation, fine clumping, proliferation with lipid accumulation, and possible complete atrophy of RPE. Atrophy is limited to the central area and not seen in the periphery. Other such disorders of the macula include North Carolina macular dystrophy, familiar drusen, Sorsby's dystrophy, pattern dystrophy of the pigment epithelium of Marmor–Byers, foveomacular vitelliform dystrophy, dominant slowly progressive macular dystrophy of Singerman–Berkow–Patz, butterfly-shaped pigment dystrophy of the fovea, macroreticular dystrophy of the RPE, Sjögren's reticular dystrophy of the RPE, pigment epithelial dystrophy of Noble–Carr–Siegel, and benign concentric annular macular dystrophy.

Diffuse photoreceptor damage is characteristic in either rod–cone or cone–rod dystrophy. In cone–rod dystrophy a loss of photoreceptors occurs mainly in the central macula, along with attenuation of the RPE. Ultrastructure reveals accumulation of abnormal lipofuscin granules in the RPE and enlargement and distortion of the cone photoreceptor pedicles. Retinitis pigmentosa is a classic manifestation of rod–cone dystrophy and presents with photoreceptor atrophy from equator to periphery, RPE migration into the retina, mainly surrounding the retinal vessels, and retinal and optic nerve gliosis. Mutations in the rhodopsin and peripherin/RDS genes account for about 25% of all cases of autosomal-dominant retinitis pigmentosa. The gene for X-linked retinitis pigmentosa, the most severe type of retinitis pigmentosa, has been localized to the Xp21 region.[10]

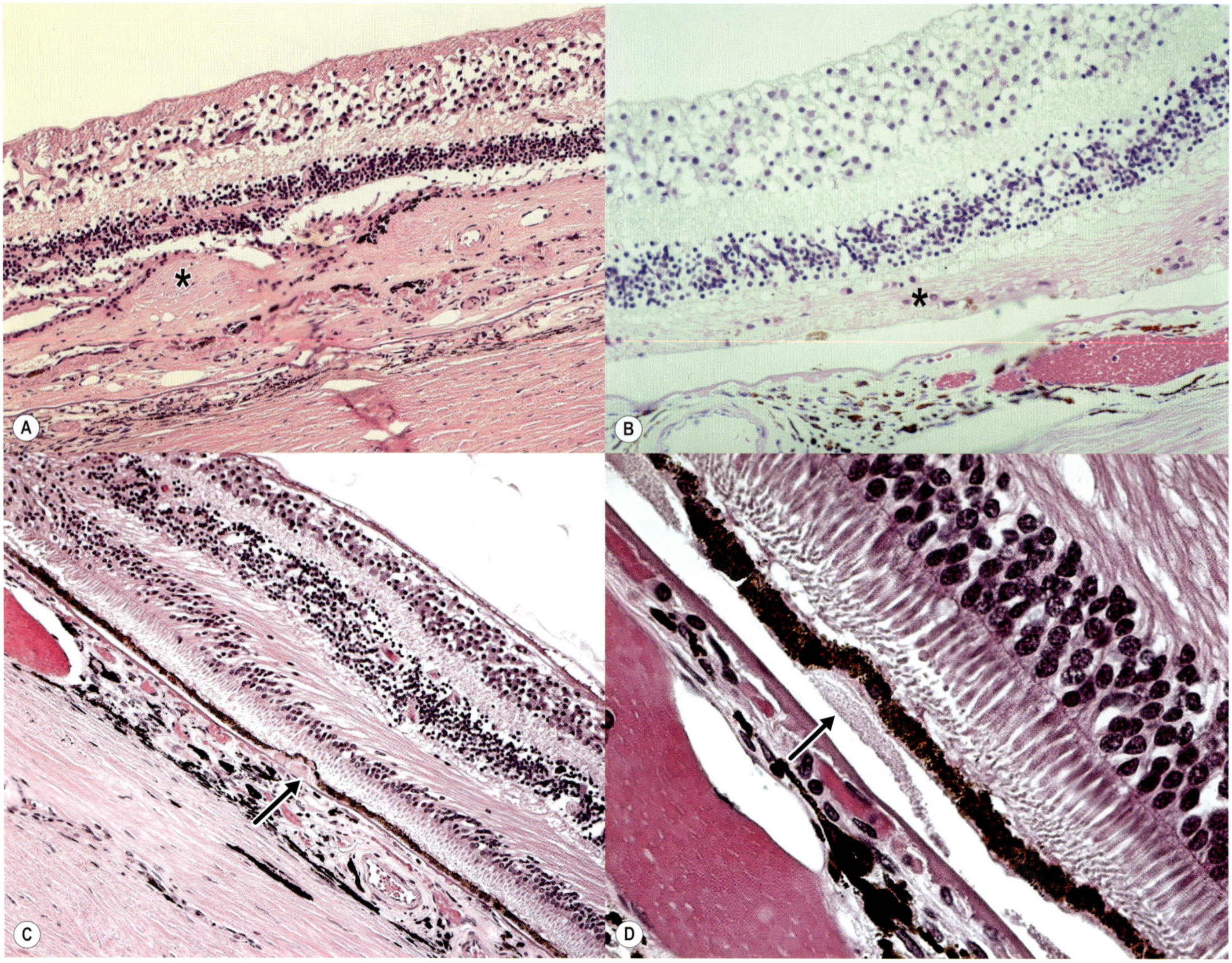

Figure 2.3 Photomicrographs of the retina of four different patients with age-related macular degeneration (AMD) depict the progressive degeneration of the retina. (A) An area (asterisk) of choroidal neovascularization with retinal pigment epithelial (RPE) atrophy, characteristic of wet AMD. (B) An area of geographic atrophy (asterisk), with complete loss of the RPE and outer nuclear layer, seen in dry AMD. (C) A druse (arrow), the hallmark lesion of AMD, a predominantly lipophilic lesion between Bruch's membrane and the RPE. (D) A soft druse at higher power. (Hematoxylin and eosin, original magnifications, (A) and (C), ×50; (B), ×100; (D), ×400.)

Damage confined to the choriocapillaries rather than the retina can be central areolar choroidal dystrophy or choroideremia with pathological features of relative independent degeneration of choriocapillaris, RPE, and retina.[10]

Degenerations

Degenerations can be unilateral and may result from previous disease. Peripheral degeneration refers to degenerative changes that lie parallel to the ora serrata in the peripheral portions of the retina. These changes can be divided into minimal retinal abnormalities or precursors to retinal gliosis. Peripheral retinal degeneration is characterized by cysts and loss of neuronal cells in the retinal inner plexiform layer, among many other particular clinical features. Examples are peripheral cystoid degeneration and cobblestone degeneration, thinning neural retina in areas with chorioretinal adhesion, hypertrophy, and hyperplasia of the RPE at the lesion's margins. Retinoschisis is frequently a bilateral split of at least 1.5 mm at the level of the outer plexiform layer.[11] Lattice degeneration, also a thinning of the retina, is associated with retinal sclerotic vessels and focal neuroretinal atrophy or hypertrophy of the RPE with overlying areas of liquefied vitreous, which can lead to retinal detachments.[12]

Age-related macular degeneration (AMD), a progressive degeneration of the macula seen in elderly patients, can be characterized by multiple drusen, focal RPE alteration, photoreceptor atrophy (dry AMD), RPE serous detachment, choroidal neovascularization leading to exudation or retinal hemorrhages (wet AMD), and fibroglial scars in the late stage (Figure 2.3). Drusen are focal or diffuse hyalin material produced by the RPE. As the drusen progress they can disrupt Bruch's membrane and induce choroidal neovascularization. Several single-nucleotide polymorphisms associated with AMD include *complement factor H (CFH)*, *complement factor B*, *complement factor 2*, *complement factor 3*, *PLEKHA1/ARMS2/HtrA1*, *CX3CR1*, and *vascular endothelial growth factor (VEGF)*.[13]

Severe myopia, exceeding 6 D, can cause stretching of the retina, choroid, and Bruch's membrane with thinning of the sclera in the posterior third due to the elongated globe. The fundus is characterized by abnormal chorioretinal atrophy around the optic disc and Bruch's membrane breaks, which may lead to small hemorrhages that later become pigmented. Clinically this is known as a Fuchs spot. Choroidal

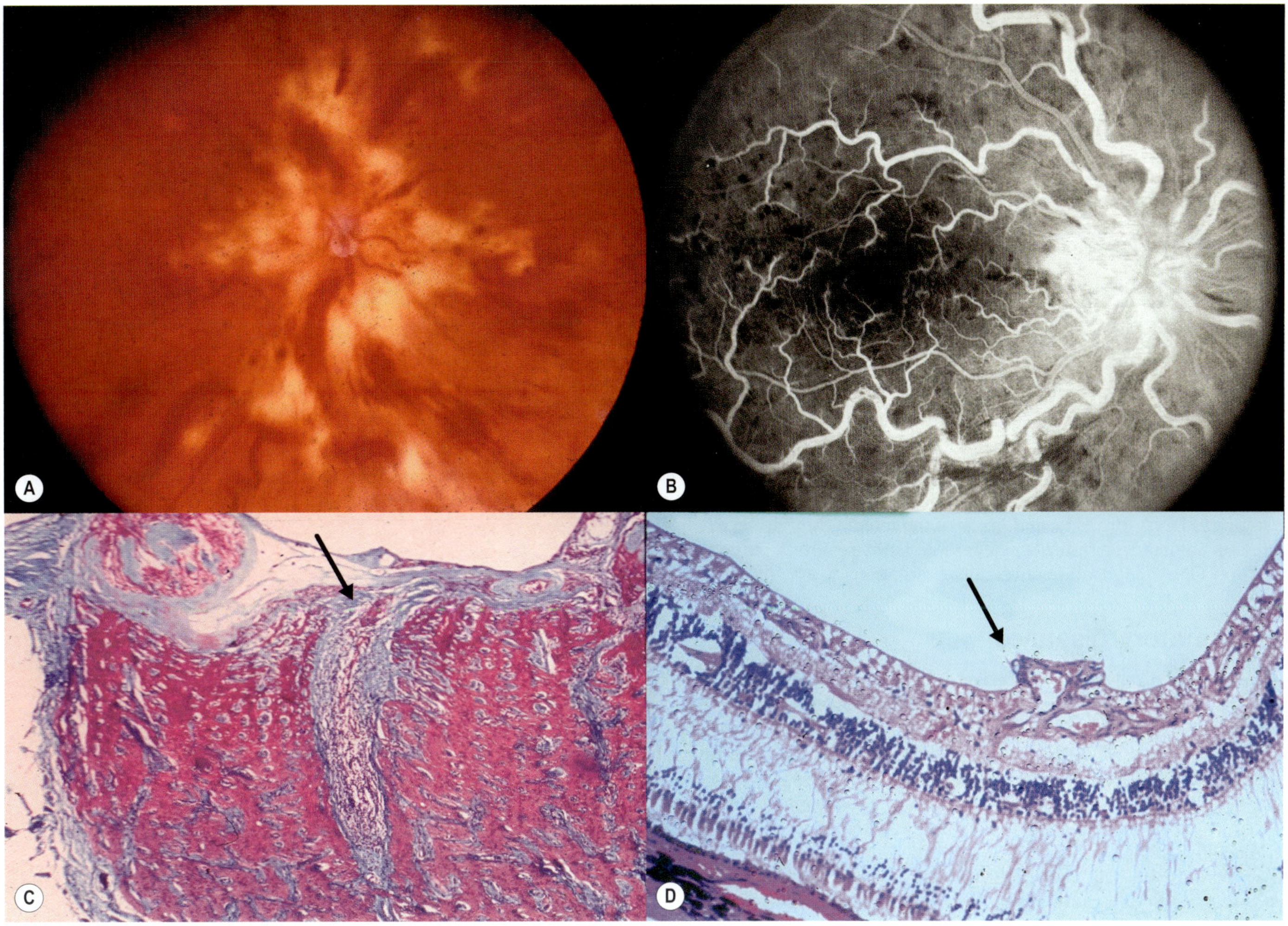

Figure 2.4 Pathological features of central retinal vein occlusion (CRVO). (A) Fundoscopy of a patient with acute CRVO shows hemorrhage and edema surrounding the optic nerve head. (B) Fluorescence angiogram of this patient depicts tortuous retinal arterioles, typical in CRVO. (C) Photomicrograph of the optic nerve head from a patient with CRVO shows the thrombus (arrow) in the central retinal vein at the level of the lamina cribrosa (trichrome Mason, original magnification, ×25). (D) Photomicrograph of retinal neovascularization (arrow) secondary to CRVO. (Hematoxylin and eosin, original magnification, ×100.)

neovascularization may also occur as a complication of the clinical picture.[12]

Vascular diseases

Vascular occlusions lead to serious complications in any organ system: in the eye, early diagnosis and prompt treatment are important. Most retinal vein occlusions are secondary to systemic diseases, most frequently to systemic arterial hypertension. In central retinal vein occlusions, the thrombus often lies at the level of the lamina cribrosa; in branch retinal vein occlusions, the thrombus is frequently at the arteriovenous crossing. Retinal hemorrhages and edema are frequently present (Figure 2.4). Retinal artery occlusions occur less frequently than vein occlusions and are usually secondary to emboli or, less frequently, inflammatory processes. The retinal arteries may appear attenuated or bloodless. The clinically seen gray area is caused by marked edema of the inner layers of the neuroretina. With complete coagulative necrosis of the posterior pole, the choroid-contained blood shows through the central fovea, which has no inner layers, and is clinically visualized as a cherry red spot.[14]

Loss of cell volume control mechanisms resulting in extracellular filtrates can be the cause of macular edema. Some causes of macular edema may be secondary to cataract extraction, such as in Irvine–Gass syndrome, or can be dominantly inherited. Initially reversible, accumulation of fluid is intracellular. Further accumulation of fluid causes the cytoplasm membrane to break and fluid collects extracellularly, causing irreversible damage.[15] Other causes of macular edema include retina vein occlusions, diabetic retinopathy, and uveitis.[16]

Coats' disease, a congenital retinal telangiectasia, also involves vascular abnormalities (Figure 2.5). Telangiectatic retinal vessels with Leber's miliary aneurysms, consisting of fusiform and saccular dilatations of venules and arterioles that surround a diffusely dilated capillary bed, eosinophilic transudate, and rich subneural retinal exudate containing foamy macrophages and cholesterol crystals are seen. It is caused by somatic mutations in the *NDP* gene.[17]

Toxicities

Toxic retinopathy can result due to medications. Chloroquine toxicity can initially occur with macular edema. Later punctate pigment epithelial changes develop, which may progress to bull's-eye maculopathy in the macular region.[18,19] Both phenothiazine and chloroquine toxicity findings may appear similar to those findings associated with retinitis pigmentosa. Tamoxifen toxicity is associated with impairment in color vision, possible retinal vein thrombosis, and fleck-like retinopathy.[19] Gentamicin may also cause ocular toxicity in addition to its usual toxic side-effects.[19] Further details on retina toxicity to drugs applied intraocularly or systemically may be found in Chapters 15 and 16.

Because of the high oxygen consumption of the photoreceptors, high concentration of long-chain polyunsaturated fatty acids in the outer

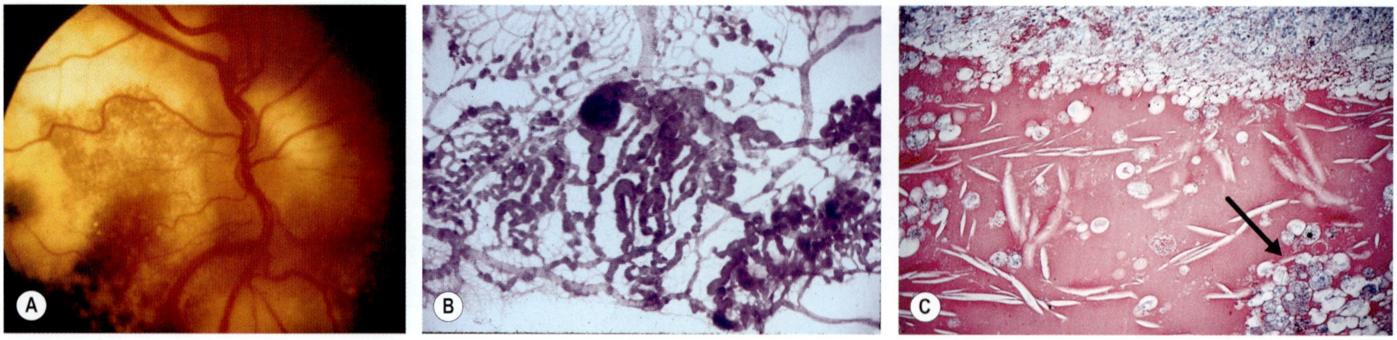

Figure 2.5 Pathological features of Coats' disease. (A) Fundoscopy of a patient with Coats' disease shows mildly dilated retinal vessels, telangiectasias, and exudates. (B) Photomicrograph of Coats' retinal vasculature details the saccular and fusiform dilatations of the abnormal retinal vessels. (Trypsin digestion of the retina, periodic acid–Schiff, original magnification ×50.) (C) Photomicrograph of a Coats' eye shows typical foamy macrophages (arrow) and cholesterol crystals in the retinal exudates. (Hematoxylin and eosin, original magnification, ×200.)

segment, and exposure to visible and ultraviolet light, the retina is highly susceptible to oxidative stress. Free radical formation may result in injury to DNA, proteins, and lipids of the retina. Though the eye has defenses against free radicals, like antioxidants, severe damage to the RPE and DNA may lead to subsequent mutations.[20]

Inflammatory diseases

Inflammatory diseases of the retina and choroid, generally termed "retinitis" or "chorioretinitis," manifest pathologically with inflammatory cells infiltrating the retina and/or choroid. In retinitis there are often dilated blood vessels and increased vascular permeability leading to edema and tissue accumulation of white blood cells, and the inflammation usually occurs near the retinal vessels. Displacement of native retinal tissue by edema leads to swelling and degeneration of neural retinal cells. Retinal hemorrhages and accumulation of microglia and macrophages are also common. If inflammatory vascular occlusion leads to infarction, necrosis results in cystoid bodies due to swelling of nerve fiber axons. The inflammatory healing process can result in the formation of a chorioretinal scar or in hyaline and/or calcareous degenerations. Astrocyte proliferation in the affected areas leads to retinal gliosis. Healing might also involve the development of a fibroglial scar, which during contraction and organization can disrupt the retinal structure, potentially damaging RPE cells and promoting hypertrophy and hyperplasia of nearby RPE.[21,22]

Retinitis comprises both acute and chronic conditions and can remain localized to the retina or can spread to affect the vitreous, optic nerve, and/or uveal tract, particularly the choroid. Retinitis can present as either granulomatous or nongranulomatous. Moreover, retinal inflammations include those caused by both infectious and noninfectious etiologies. Noninfectious etiologies include retinal involvement of inflammatory diseases, such as sarcoidosis, pars planitis, and birdshot retinochoroidopathy. Most of these are autoimmune diseases and entail primarily T-lymphocyte infiltrates. For example, sarcoidosis demonstrates characteristic pathology, including noncaseating granulomas in the retina and choroids (Figure 2.6), infrequently with necrosis, proteinaceous exudates, or hemorrhage into the subretinal space, development of a neovascular membrane from the optic disc to the vitreous cavity, and, occasionally, retinal detachment.[23,24]

Infectious causes include viral, bacterial, fungus and parasitic infection, such as *Candida*, cytomegalovirus (CMV), toxoplasmosis, and onchocerciasis. Pathologically, CMV retinitis manifests with a primary coagulative full-thickness retinal necrosis and scant inflammatory infiltrates. Infected retinal cells were enlarged and contained a large central basophilic intranuclear inclusion, which appears as an "owl eye" due to the presence of a halo separating it from the nuclear membrane, as well as smaller basophilic cytoplasmic inclusions (Figure 2.6). Areas of clinically end-stage CMV retinitis show chorioretinal scarring with total loss of retinal cells.[25] Acute retinal necrosis, most commonly caused by the varicella-zoster virus or the herpes simplex virus, involves acute peripheral necrotizing retinitis, retinal arteritis, and vitritis. On pathology, acute retinal necrosis demonstrates Cowdry type A eosinophilic intranuclear inclusions. Zoster infection is commonly associated with occlusive vasculitis.[26,27]

Neoplasms

Tumors of the retina can arise from any number of cell types, including photoreceptors, RPE, glia, and others. Photoreceptor neoplasms include retinoblastoma and retinocytoma. Retinoblastomas are comprised of undifferentiated cells and possess multifocal growth, including bilateral involvement. They classically form rosettes and pseudorosettes, possess high nuclear-to-cytoplasm ratios, and contain significant areas of necrosis and/or calcification (Figure 2.7).[28] Retinocytomas are rare benign small placoid, noninvasive neoplasms involving cells that have differentiated into photoreceptor elements, numerous fleurettes, lack of mitotic activity, and less necrosis.[29]

RPE tumors include RPE adenoma and RPE adenocarcinoma. Histopathology of RPE adenomas demonstrates an abrupt transition between normal RPE and neoplastic RPE, which consists of polyhedral-appearing epithelial cells with variable pigmentation arranged in papillary, solid, or mixed form. While mitotic figures are rare, nuclear atypia is common. Adenocarcinomas are malignant and appear much like adenomas, but with increased cellular pleomorphism.[30]

Phakomatoses are a group of hereditary disseminated hamartomas, including von Hippel–Lindau (VHL) disease, Wyburn–Mason syndrome, and retinal cavernous hemangioma. One such phakomatosis is VHL disease, an inherited cancer syndrome associated with retinal angiomas, cerebellar hemangioblastomas, renal cysts, pheochromocytomas, pancreatic cysts, epididymal cysts, and retinal hemangioblastomas.[31] These retinal hemangioblastomas appear as a network of endothelium-lined vascular channels among the foamy "stromal" cells, which are the true tumor cells with a mutated or deleted *VHL* gene.[31,32] The complications include leaky capillaries, arteriovenous shunt, hemorrhages, exudates, and retinal detachment.[31]

Retinal detachment

Retinal detachment refers to the separation of the RPE from Bruch's membrane (RPE detachment) or of the photoreceptor layer from the RPE (neurosensory retinal detachment). The two major types of detachment are rhegmatogenous and nonrhegmatogenous retinal detachments; the former arises from a retinal hole or tear, the latter does not usually have a retinal hole or tear and may be either serous or tractional type. Retinal detachments can occur by three major mechanisms: accumulation of fluid beneath the intact retina (nonrhegmatogenous, e.g., hypertension, subneural retinal hemorrhages, choroidal tumors, vascular lesions of the retina), vitreous traction (e.g., secondary to trauma, surgical aphakia, vitreous bands from diabetes mellitus), or accumulation of fluid beneath a broken neural retina (i.e., rhegmatogenous retinal detachment).[33]

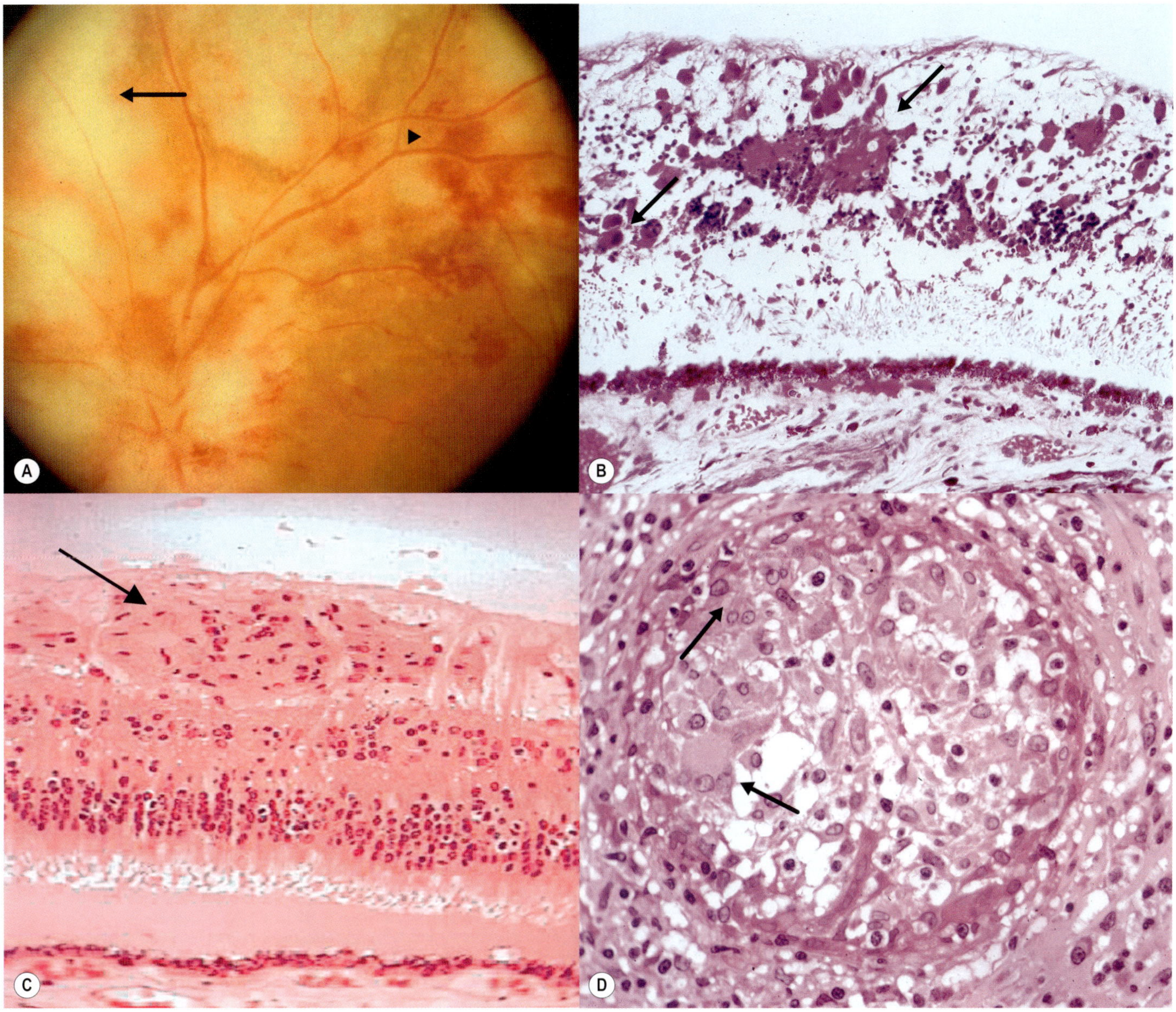

Figure 2.6 Pathological features of infectious and noninfectious retinitis. (A) Fundoscopy of a human eye with cytomegalovirus (CMV) retinitis. Areas of retinal necrosis (arrow) and hemorrhage (arrowhead) near vessels are visible. (B) Photomicrograph of a retina from a patient with CMV retinitis. Widespread retinal necrosis and scant inflammatory infiltrates are visible. Confluent "owl-eye" lesions (arrows) of enlarged CMV-infected cells with a large basophilic inclusion are noted. (Hematoxylin and eosin, original magnification ×100.) (C) Photomicrograph of a retina from a patient with sarcoidosis. Large noncaseating granuloma (arrow) in the inner retina surrounding the retinal vessel is visible. (Hematoxylin and eosin, original magnification ×100.) (D) Photomicrograph of a sarcoidosis granuloma. Magnified view of a retinal granuloma from a patient with sarcoidosis shows numerous multinucleated giant cells (arrows). (Hematoxylin and eosin, original magnification ×200.)

Histologically, detachment of the retina from the RPE leads to neural retinal atrophy (outer > inner retina), due to impaired choroidal blood supply to the outer segments. Early manifestations include loss of photoreceptor outer segments and serous fluid in the subretina. Prolonged detachment leads to photoreceptor cell atrophy, cystic retinal degeneration, retinal thinning, retinal folds, RPE abnormalities, large drusen, choroidal neovascularization, and/or iris neovascularization.[33]

Trauma

Contusions and concussion injuries to the eye by blunt trauma or by a blast can damage neuroretinal and vascular cells. In commotio retinae (Berlin's edema), for example, contrecoup blunt trauma to the globe results in both intra- and extracellular retinal edema. As the edema subsides, RPE degeneration, macular cysts, and photoreceptor degeneration are noted.[34]

Purtscher's traumatic retinopathy can arise from a number of causes, including vascular occlusions, such as from fat emboli after crushing injury or fractures to long bones, compressing injuries to the thorax, raised intracranial pressure, or vasculitis. Purtscher's retinopathy manifests with retina edema, cystoid degeneration, and inner retinal atrophy. Retinal and choroidal vessels may contain occluding material.[35] In the case of fat emboli, adipose globules might also be found in retinal vessels.

Foreign bodies such as metals, vegetable matter, and hair can also cause retinal pathology. These foreign bodies can not only lead to traumatic injury, but, depending on their composition, they can also produce a suppurative reaction resulting in retinal necrosis. Birth injuries and child abuse are other traumatic causes of retinal injury and both manifest largely with retinal hemorrhages.[21,22]

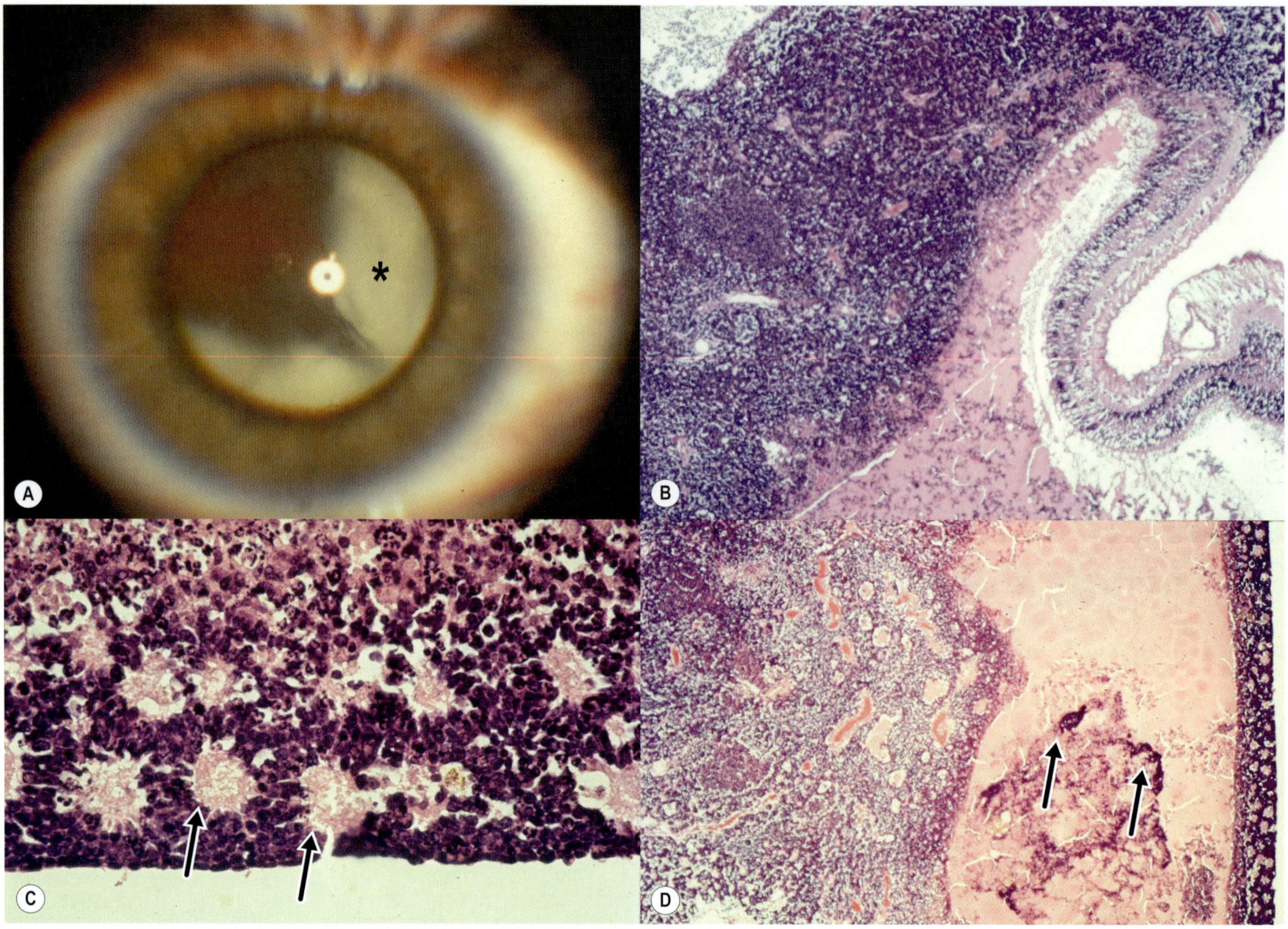

Figure 2.7 Pathological features of retinoblastoma. (A) Photograph of an eye from a patient with retinoblastoma. Pen light examination of a patient with retinoblastoma produces leukokoria, a white reflection (asterisk). (B) Photomicrograph of a retina from a patient with retinoblastoma. Numerous small, basophilic neoplastic cells with high nuclear to cytoplasmic ratios are visible. (Hematoxylin and eosin, original magnification ×50.) (C) Photomicrograph of retinoblastoma tissue. Homer–Wright rosettes (arrows) are noted in a retinoblastoma. (Hematoxylin and eosin, original magnification ×200.) (D) Photomicrograph of a retina from a patient with retinoblastoma. Areas of calcification (arrows) are visible amidst retinoblastoma tissue. (Hematoxylin and eosin, original magnification ×50.)

Involvement of systemic diseases

A multitude of systemic diseases, including blood diseases, genetic metabolic storage diseases, vascular diseases, collagen vascular diseases, and phakomatoses, may present various types of chorioretinal alterations.

Sickle-cell disease manifests with peripheral arteriolar occlusion, peripheral arteriolovenular anastomoses, vascular sclerosis, "sea fan"-shaped neovascular proliferations, fibrous proliferations, vitreous hemorrhage, and/or neural retinal detachment (Figure 2.8).[36] Another blood disease, leukemia, may present with retinopathy, which manifests histologically with leukemic cellular infiltration surrounding by retinal hemorrhages, often accompanied with choroidal infiltration by leukemic cells, even leading to RPE disruption or detachment. Other features include venous congestion and dilation, perivascular infiltration, retinal microaneurysm, capillary loss, and proliferative retinopathy.[37]

Metabolic storage diseases, including mucopolysaccharidoses, mucolipidoses, and sphingolipidoses, can cause hereditary secondary retinal dystrophies. As their name implies, these diseases are marked by the accumulation of storage substance in retinal cells, in particular, ganglion cells, leading eventually to cell injury and death. For example, the autosomal-recessive sphingolipidosis, Tay–Sachs disease, results in the accumulation of ganglioside mainly in retinal ganglion cells, which induce cell death and extracellular deposition of the ganglioside, and finally, develop optic atrophy.[38]

Vascular diseases which lead to retinopathy include hypertension, diabetes, arteriosclerosis, and ocular ischemia due to reduction in blood flow through the ophthalmic or carotid arteries. In the initial vasoconstrictive stage of hypertensive retinopathy, vasospasm and increased arteriolar tone lead to narrowing of retinal arterioles. Consequently, the sclerotic stage of hypertensive retinopathy is associated with intimal thickening, media hyperplasia, and hyaline degeneration, leading to worsened arteriolar narrowing. Subsequently disruption of the blood–retina barrier and necrosis of vascular cells may lead to the development of microaneurysms, hemorrhages, and cystoid degeneration.[39]

Early diabetic retinopathy is initially caused by a loss of pericytes from retinal capillaries, followed by loss of capillary endothelial cells, microaneurysms, and hemorrhages. Ischemia and microinfarction lead to the development of cystoid degeneration. Retinal edema is caused by leakage of plasma from small blood vessels, and retinal exudates are due to resorption of the fluid elements of the leaked plasma secondary to deposition of lipid and lipoprotein components. The ischemic processes might lead eventually to proliferative diabetic retinopathy characterized by retinal neovascularization. If the neovascular membranes extend to the vitreous and hemorrhage into it, visual loss and tractional retinal detachments might ensue. Neovascularization might also occur in the iris (rubeosis irides), impeding aqueous humor outflow and leading to the so-called neovascular glaucoma.[40]

Collagen vascular diseases such as systemic lupus erythematosus (SLE), polyarteritis nodosa, and giant-cell arteritis may also present

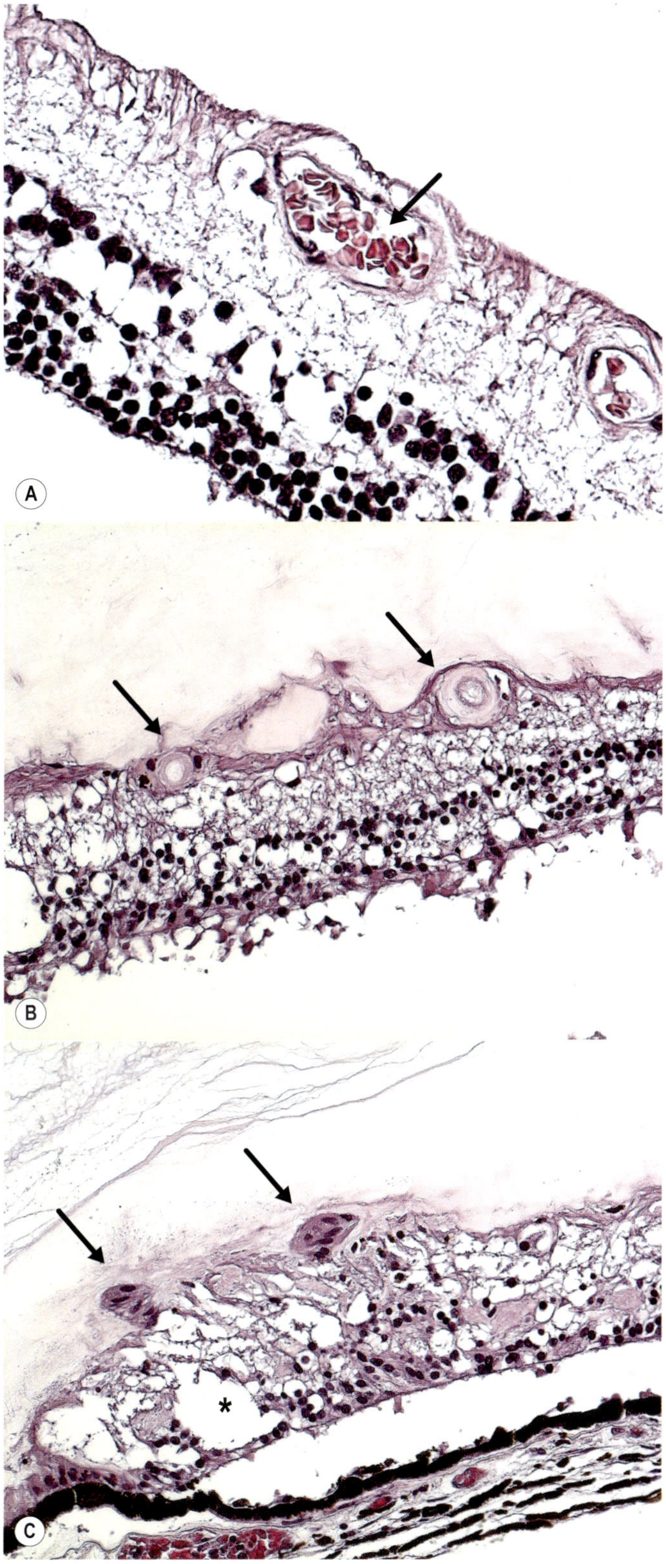

Figure 2.8 Histological representations of sickle-cell disease retinopathy. (A) Photomicrograph of retina from a patient with sickle-cell disease. Sickled red blood cells (arrow) are visible in a retinal vascular lumen. (Hematoxylin and eosin, original magnification ×200.) (B) Photomicrograph of a retina from a patient with sickle-cell disease. Sclerotic blood vessels are visible in the inner retina. (Hematoxylin and eosin, original magnification ×100.)
(C) Photomicrograph of retina from a patient with sickle-cell disease. Retinal "sea fan" neovascularizations (arrows), and retinal cystic degeneration (asterisk) are notable. (Hematoxylin and eosin, original magnification ×200.)

with retinal pathology. The classical histological finding is cystoid bodies. There may also be retinal edema, hard exudates, and/or hemorrhages. Abnormalities in retinal vasculature, including narrowing, dilatation, and microaneurysms, may be noted. Severe occlusive retinopathy or vasculitis due to SLE presents histopathologically with perivascular lymphocytic infiltrates, endothelial swelling, and thrombosis, leading to occlusion of retinal and choroidal vessels. These vascular occlusion processes lead to a proliferative retinopathy with neovascularization, which in turn can lead to vitreous hemorrhage and tractional retinal detachment. Other histopathological features which may be seen include macular exudates and RPE changes.[41]

IMPLICATIONS FOR RETINAL PHARMACOTHERAPY

While the etiologies of retinal diseases vary widely – from developmental anomalies to age-related degenerations and from infectious diseases of the retina to systemic vascular diseases – the ensuing histopathological changes in the retina share some similarities with one another. Neovascularization and inflammation are two key examples of such common denominators. Neovascularization, for instance, is a key histopathological feature with notable clinical consequences in a spectrum of diseases, including retinopathy of prematurity, AMD, retinal detachment, SLE, diabetic retinopathy, and sickle-cell retinopathy, to name a few. These shared features suggest that there are certain major pathological processes – angiogenesis and inflammation, for example – in retinal diseases which may be amenable to therapy. Thus, therapies countering these processes may promise to target multiple, seemingly disparate retinal diseases, providing an added incentive to develop novel therapeutic strategies targeting these key processes.

SUMMARY AND KEY POINTS

The retina comprises the major neurosensory tissue related to the vision process, and includes the photoreceptor cells, which first receive the visual stimuli, the RPE cells, which maintain retinal and especially photoreceptor homeostasis, a variety of neurons such as bipolar cells, amacrine cells, and horizontal cells, which modify the visual stimulus, and ganglion cells, whose axons carry the signal from the retina to the optic nerve and finally to the brain. Retinal pathology, including congenital anomalies, degenerations, dystrophies, toxicities, inflammation, detachments, neoplasms, trauma, and involvement of systemic diseases, result in disruption of this delicate retinal architecture, leading eventually to clinical manifestations. Though the specific array of histopathological changes involved varies from disease to disease, many retinal maladies share certain key pathophysiological changes that may be amenable to pharmacotherapy. However, pharmacotherapy may not be effective once retinal atrophy, the end stage of most retinal diseases, has occurred.

REFERENCES

1. Masland RH. The fundamental plan of the retina. Nat Neurosci 2001;4:877–886.
2. Wassle H, Boycott BB. Functional architecture of the mammalian retina. Physiol Rev 1991;71:447–480.
3. Carr RE. Congenital stationary nightblindness. Trans Am Ophthalmol Soc 1974;72:448–487.
4. Jeffery G. The albino retina: an abnormality that provides insight into normal retinal development. Trends Neurosci 1997;20:165–169.
5. Gasch AT, Caruso RC, Kaler SG, et al. Menkes' syndrome: ophthalmic findings. Ophthalmology 2002;109:1477–1483.
6. Topilow HW, Ackerman AL. Early retinal vessel development and iris vessel dilatation as factors in retinopathy of prematurity. Arch Ophthalmol 1996;114:1160.
7. Wheatley CM, Dickinson JL, Mackey DA, et al. Retinopathy of prematurity: recent advances in our understanding. Br J Ophthalmol 2002;86:696–700.
8. Sikkink SK, Susmito B, Neil RA, et al. X-linked retinoschisis: an update. J Med Genet 2007;44:225–232.

9. Rattner A, Nathans J. Macular degeneration: recent advances and therapeutic opportunities. Nat Rev Neurosci 2006;7:860–872.
10. Phelan J, Bok D. A brief review of retinitis pigmentosa and the identified retinitis pigmentosa genes. Mol Vision 2000;6:116–124.
11. Gehrig A, White K, Lorenz B, et al. Assessment of RS1 in X-linked juvenile retinoschisis and sporadic senile retinoschisis. Clin Genet 1999;55: 461–465.
12. Ballinger R. Peripheral retinal breaks and retinal detachment. Clin Eye Vision Care 1998;10:59–66.
13. Ross RJ, Verma V, Rosenberg KI, et al. Genetic markers and biomarkers for age-related macular degeneration. Expert Rev Ophthalmol 2007;2:443–457.
14. Vallee JN, Massin P, Aymard A, et al. Superselective ophthalmic arterial fibrinolysis with urokinase for recent severe retinal venous occlusion: initial experience. Radiology 2000;216:47–53.
15. Bringmann A, Reichenbach A, Wiedemann P. Pathogenesis of cystoid macular edema. Ophthalmic Res 2004;36:241–249.
16. Lang G. Ophthalmology: A Pocket Textbook Guide. New York: Georg Thieme Verlag; 2000.
17. Black GC, Perveen R, Bonshek R, et al. Coat's disease of the retina (unilateral retinal telangiectasis) caused by somatic mutation in the NDP gene: a role for norrin in retinal angiogenesis. Hum Mol Genet 1999;8:2031–2035.
18. Gola D, Tashjian Jr A, Armstrong E, et al. Principles of Pharmacology: Pathophysiologic Basis of Drug Therapy. Baltimore: Lippincott; 2005.
19. McEvoy GK. American Hospital Formulary Service Drug Reference. Bethesda: American Society of Health-System Pharmacists; 2007.
20. Beatty S, Koh H, Phil M, et al. The role of oxidative stress in the pathogenesis of age-related macular degeneration. Surv Ophthalmol 2000;45:115–134.
21. Yanoff M, Fine B. Ocular Pathology. 5th ed. St. Louis: Mosby; 2002.
22. Spencer W. Ophthalmic Pathology: An Atlas and Textbook. Philadelphia: WB Saunders; 1996.
23. Spalton D, Hitchings R, Hunter P. Atlas of Clinical Ophthalmology. 3rd ed. Spain: Mosby; 2005.
24. Frank KW, Weiss H. Unusual clinical and histopathological findings in ocular sarcoidosis. Br J Ophthalmol 1983;67:8–16.
25. Mansour AM. Ocular pathology in acquired immunodeficiency syndrome. Comp Ther 2002;28:155–159.
26. Culbertson WW, Blumenkranz MS, Haines H. The acute retinal necrosis syndrome: Part 2 – histopathology and etiology. Ophthalmology 1982;89: 1317–1325.
27. Gartry DS, Spalton DJ, Tilzey A, et al. Acute retinal necrosis syndrome. BMJ 1991;75:292–297.
28. Kumar SA. Clinico-pathological observations on retinoblastoma. Indian J Ophthalmol 1975;23:20–22.
29. Margo C, Hidayat A, Kopelman J, et al. Retinocytoma. A benign variant of retinoblastoma. Arch Ophthalmol 1983; 101:1519–1531.
30. Loose IA, Jampol LM, O'Grady R. Pigmented adenoma mimicking a juxtapapillary melanoma. Arch Ophthalmol 1999;117:120–122.
31. Maher ER, Yates JRW, Harries R, et al. Clinical features and natural history of von Hippel–Lindau disease. Q J Med 1990;77:1151–1163.
32. Chan CC, Vortmeyer AO, Chew EY, et al. VHL gene deletion and enhanced VEGF gene expression detected in the stromal cells of retinal angioma. Arch Ophthalmol 1999;117;625–630.
33. Ghazi NG, Green WR. Pathology and pathogenesis of retinal detachment. Eye 2002;16:411–421.
34. Mansour AM, Green WR, Hogge C. Histopathology of commotion retinae. Retina 1992;12:24–28.
35. Agrawal A, McKibbin MA. Purtcher's and Purtscher-like retinopathies: a review. Surv Ophthalmol 2006;51:129–136.
36. Clarkson JG. The ocular manifestations of sickle-cell disease: a prevalence and natural history study. Trans Am Ophthalmol Soc 1992;90:481–504.
37. Reddy SC, Jackson N, Menon BS. Ocular involvement in leukemia: a study of 288 cases. Ophthalmologica 2003;217:441–445.
38. Cogan DG. Ocular correlates of inborn metabolic diseases. J Assoc Med Can 1966;95:1055–1065.
39. Wong TY, Mitchell P. Hypertensive retinopathy. N Engl J Med 2004;351:2310–2317.
40. Frank RN. Diabetic retinopathy. N Engl J Med 2004;350:48–58.
41. Peponis V, Kyttaris VC, Tyradellis C, et al. Ocular manifestations of systemic lupus erythematosus: a clinical review. Lupus 2006;15:3–12.

CHAPTER

3 Retinal biochemistry, physiology, and cell biology

Victor Chong, MD, Ricardo Luiz Smith, MD, PhD, and Sobha Sivaprasad, DM, MS, DNB, FRCS

INTRODUCTION

The vitreous, the vasculature of the retina, macular pigments, phototransduction, retinal pigment epithelium (RPE), the Bruch's membrane (BM), and the extracellular matrix (ECM) all play an important role in the normal function of the retina, as well as in diseases. Understanding the pathophysiology allows us to target treatment. As ocular angiogenesis, immunity, and inflammation are covered elsewhere, those subjects will not be discussed in this chapter.

VITREOUS BIOCHEMISTRY

Vitreous is an important ocular structure in normal physiology and pathologic conditions of the posterior segment.[1] It is a dilute meshwork of collagen fibrils interspersed with extensive arrays of hyaluronan molecules.

Hyaluronan is a major macromolecule of vitreous. It is a long, unbranched polymer of repeating disaccharide linked by glycosidic bonds. Hyaluronan is covalently linked to a protein core: the ensemble is called proteoglycan. Vitreous also contains collagen type II, a hybrid of types V/XI, and type IX collagen in a molar ratio of 75:10:15, respectively. Vitreous collagens are organized into fibrils, with type V/XI residing in the core, type II collagen surrounding the core, and type IX collagen on the surface of the fibril.

The collagen fibrils provide a scaffold-like structure by the hydrophilic hyaluronan. If collagen is removed, the remaining hyaluronan forms a viscous solution; if hyaluronan is removed, the gel shrinks but is not destroyed. The chondroitin sulfate chains of type IX collagen bridge between adjacent collagen fibrils in a ladder-like configuration spacing them apart. Such spacing is necessary for vitreous transparency: keeping vitreous collagen fibrils separated by at least one wavelength of incident light minimizes light scattering, allowing unhindered transmission of light to the retina.

VITREOUS DEGENERATION WITH AGING

During aging, substantial alterations take place in the vitreous body. The gel-to-liquid ratio is reduced with age. In the posterior vitreous, large pockets of liquid vitreous, recognized clinically as "lacunae," are formed. By the age of 80–90 years, more than half the vitreous body is liquid.

Strong adhesion exists between the posterior vitreous cortex and the internal limiting membrane (ILM) of the retina, primarily at the vitreous base and at the posterior pole. Vitreoretinal adhesion appears to be strongest at the disc, fovea, and along retinal blood vessels. With age, there is weakening of vitreoretinal adhesion, most likely due to biochemical alterations in the ECM at the vitreoretinal interface.

These biochemical changes may play a role in the observed weakening of the vitreoretinal interface during aging. Identifying the molecular nature of these changes may provide opportunities for pharmacologic lysis of vitreoretinal adhesion.

PHYSIOLOGICAL AND PATHOLOGICAL CHANGES IN THE VITREORETINAL INTERFACE

Posterior vitreous detachment (PVD) results from weakening of the adhesion between the posterior vitreous cortex and the ILM, in conjunction with liquefaction within the vitreous body. Weakening of the posterior vitreous cortex/ILM adhesion at the posterior pole allows liquid vitreous to enter the retrocortical space via the prepapillary hole. Volume displacement from the central vitreous to the preretinal space causes the observed collapse of the vitreous body.

PVD may exert traction at the vitreoretinal adhesion, leading to hemorrhage, retinal tears, and detachment. Focal attachment in the foveal area can cause vitreomacular traction, with associated diffuse macular edema. Proliferative diabetic retinopathy can be greatly aggravated by anomalous PVD. Effects upon vitreous involve posterior vitreoschisis, where splitting of the posterior vitreous cortex and forward displacement of the vitreous body leave the outer layer of the split posterior vitreous cortex still attached to the retina. This can result in epiretinal membrane, and contribute to macular holes and tractional retinal detachment.

BLOOD–RETINAL BARRIER

As in the central nervous system, the retina is protected against the invasion of circulating macromolecules by cell specialized barriers. Endothelial and epithelial cells display tight junctions forming zonulae occludens which block the transit of such molecules. Disruptions of these barriers are due to alterations in those lining cells affecting the physiologic properties of permeability and transport or the intercellular relationship represented by the tight junctions.

In the eye, there are two systems of barriers: the blood retina–vitreous barrier (BRB) in the posterior segment and the blood–aqueous barrier in the anterior segment. In the ciliary body, nonpigmented cells have zonulae occludens which restrict macromolecule traffic through the fenestrated blood vessels and the iris vessels are continuous with endothelial cells adjoined by tight junctions. Similarly, in the retina, the pigmented retinal epithelium tight junctions block the transit of macromolecules that cross the fenestrated choriocapillaries. Retinal vessels are continuous with endothelial cells displaying tight junctions that perform the barrier function. In the retinal periphery there is a region in the ora serrata margin, where the blood–aqueous barrier joins the BRB.

The maintenance of the retinal milieu microenvironment is essential to preserve visual function. The access of blood-borne molecules in eye tissues and spaces is controlled by cellular transport mechanisms. The BRB is required to maintain retinal homeostasis. Imbalance in the supply and demand of oxygen and nutrients across the BRB leads to pathological angiogenesis. A series of ocular pathologies are accompanied by breakdown of barriers affecting the transport system. Increased vascular permeability underlies the pathology of retinopathy of prematurity, diabetic retinopathy, and age-related macular degeneration. From the pharmacological point of view, the barrier concept has implications on the effectiveness of drug delivery to the retina.[2]

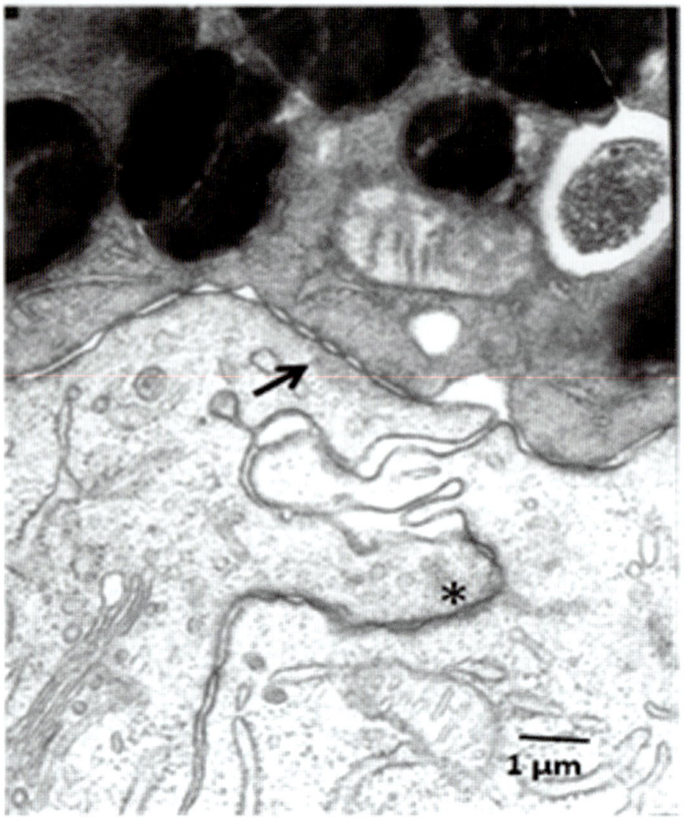

Figure 3.1 Electron micrograph of tight junction between two nonpigmented cells (*) and pigmented and nonpigmented cells at the ora serrata margin (arrow) (chicken eye).

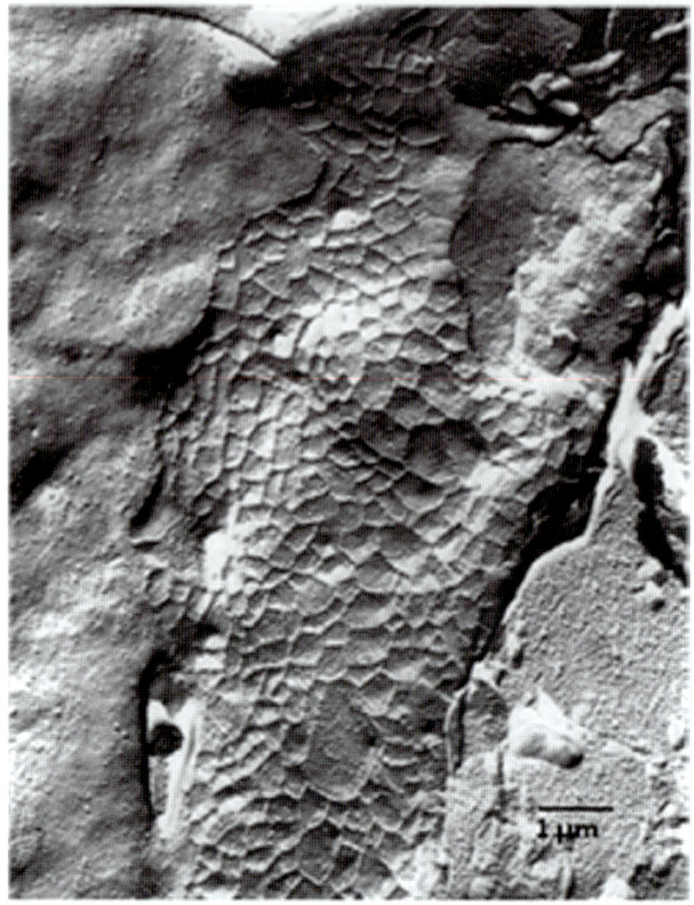

Figure 3.2 Freeze-fracture replica of epithelial tight junction (chicken ciliary body).

TIGHT JUNCTIONS

Tight junctions play an important role in controlling flux across both endothelial and epithelial cells and maintaining the desirable retinal hydration, ionic and solutes balance. They provide both a barrier function restricting the paracellular flux of molecules and a fence function maintaining apical and basolateral membrane composition within a cell. Apparently these junctions may not be necessary to establish cell polarity

The structure of tight junctions is revealed by electron microscopy of ultrathin tissue sections as adjacent cell areas presenting discontinuous fusing points of the outer-membrane leaflets. The intercellular space remains obliterated (Figure 3.1). Freeze-fracture replicas corresponding to the same region reveal the tight junction as a network of anastomosing strands of particles, as seen in the P face (protoplasmic aspect of the intramembrane domain) or complementary grooves in the E face (exoplasmic view) (Figure 3.2).

The molecular components of tight junctions reveal a highly complex assembly of proteins. More than 40 proteins had been found in association with tight junctions, not only functioning as structural components of the paracellular barrier but participating in the regulation of gene expression and cell proliferation. The most studied proteins, particularly related to the BRB, are the ZO-1 (zonula occludens), claudins, occludins, and junction adhesion molecules (JAM). They were extensively demonstrated in epithelia and endothelia, including immunohistochemical location. Claudin and occludin are transmembrane proteins cross-linked with ZO-1, which acts as a scaffold, linking the integral proteins of the tight junction to the actin cytoskeleton, and JAM is suggested to participate as the ultimate sealing molecule of the intercellular space. Other molecules are involved in cell signaling through their association with kinases and Ras or in vesicular trafficking. These tight junction components have been shown to affect several signaling and transcriptional pathways, including self-regulation, changing the expression of structural tight junction proteins which are associated with several disease conditions.[3]

Changes in tight junction proteins have been observed in a wide variety of retinal diseases associated with loss of the BRB. These changes include not only alteration in the content of junctional proteins but also their redistribution and phosphorylation.

BLOOD–RETINA BARRIER DISRUPTION

Many factors contribute to BRB disruption, including inflammatory mediators, neovascularization, vascular endothelial growth factor, and others. Early breakdown of the BRB can be detected in diabetic retinopathy by fluorescein leakage into the vitreous with fluorometric methods.

The passive diffusion permeability of a barrier depends on the physicochemical properties of a substance; its molecular weight and lipophilicity determine bioavailability for a tissue. Tightness of a barrier is evaluated by measuring the transepithelial or transendothelial resistance of cultured cells. *In vitro* model systems represent useful tools for predicting the permeability for certain drugs and molecules.[4]

To reach their targets, therapeutic agents need to cross epithelial and endothelial linings. This is possible by the transcellular and paracellular pathways. The former is employed by lipophilic drugs and by molecules selectively transported by vesicles, channels, pumps, and carriers present in the plasma membrane. Hydrophilic molecules cannot cross biological membranes. Therefore their transport is significantly enhanced if they move through the paracellular pathway. Transit through this route is regulated by tight junctions. To enhance drug delivery across epithelial and endothelial barriers it is necessary to open the paracellular route in a reversible manner. Some patented inventions were designed to alter the tight junctions with peptides homologous to the external loops of integral proteins, antisense oligonucleotides and siRNA for tight junction proteins, toxins and proteins derived from microorganisms that target junction proteins, and with other molecules such as peptides, lipids, heparins, chitosan derivatives, phospholipase inhibitors, and kinase activators.[5]

RETINAL BLOOD FLOW AND VASCULAR CALIBER

Retinal vascular caliber changes may reflect the cumulative structural vascular damage from multiple processes, including aging, long-term hypertension, arteriosclerosis, inflammation, endothelial dysfunction, and other vascular processes. Variations in arteriolar and venular caliber may also be influenced by physiological blood flow parameters such as oxygenation and shear stress.[6]

There are distinct pathophysiological factors influencing retinal arteriolar and venular caliber. The endothelial cells of arterioles and venules are molecularly distinct from the earliest stages of angiogenesis.

MECHANISMS OF RETINAL ARTERIOLAR CALIBER CHANGES

The pathophysiological changes in retinal arterioles in response to blood pressure elevation are well documented. Increased blood pressure initiates vasospasm and an increase in vasomotor tone owing to local autoregulation, leading to elevation in capillary pressure and flow. This is seen as generalized narrowing of the retinal arterioles. With persistent blood pressure elevation, chronic arteriosclerotic changes, such as intimal thickening, media wall hyperplasia, and hyaline degeneration develop. These changes manifest as diffuse arteriolar narrowing and opacification of arteriolar walls seen as "silver wiring," and compression at the venules by arterioles at their junction as "arteriovenous nipping." An exudative stage follows with breakdown of the BRB as a result of autoregulation failure caused by severe elevation in blood pressure. Focal or generalized dilatation of arterioles follows, along with increased permeability, necrosis of smooth muscles and endothelial cells, exudation of blood (hemorrhage) and lipids (hard exudates), and retinal ischemia. Narrowing of the arteriolar caliber is thus part of the initial stages of hypertensive retinopathy. Impairment of autoregulation in the retinal circulation has also been implicated in the pathogenesis of various retinal diseases, including diabetic retinopathy and diabetic macular edema.

The retinal blood vessels have no adrenergic vasomotor nerve supply to initiate changes in vascular tone. Furthermore, retinal blood flow has been postulated to be dependent on myogenic changes in arteriolar tone. Cultured brain endothelial cells can directly interact with smooth-muscle cells and pericytes via gap junctions, and actively regulate arteriolar tone and caliber size by elaborating vasodilators, such as nitric oxide (NO), adenosine, prostanoids, and vasoconstrictors, such as endothelin 1 and angiotensin II, in response to local metabolic needs. Among these factors, NO plays a central role in the maintenance of vascular homeostasis by regulating vascular tone and inhibiting platelet and leukocyte adhesion to endothelial cells. Recent studies have demonstrated that NO synthase may have a vasoregulatory role in the retina.[7]

In diabetes, endothelial dysfunction and inflammation are likely to have a major effect on the retinal microvasculature as well. Both *in vitro* and *in vivo* studies have shown that the synthesis and release of vasoconstrictors by the vascular endothelium are increased in patients with diabetes. This is consistent with the clinical observation that narrower retinal arteriolar caliber predicted the incidence of diabetes, independent of other established factors.

MECHANISMS OF RETINAL VENULAR CALIBER CHANGES

There is less understanding of the pathophysiological mechanisms of retinal venular caliber changes. Epidemiological studies have consistently shown associations of retinal venular caliber with systemic inflammatory markers.

The association of smoking with venular dilation may involve higher carbon monoxide levels and endothelium-dependent relaxation, which may lead to a decrease in oxygen supply to retinal tissue, resulting in retinal venular dilatation. In people with diabetes and hyperglycemia, arteriolar and venular dilation may also reflect hyperperfusion resulting from hyperglycemia and lactic acidosis from retinal hypoxia.

MACULAR PIGMENTS

Three dietary carotenoids, lutein (L), zeaxanthin (Z), and meso-zeaxanthin (meso-Z), accumulate at the macula, where they are collectively referred to as macular pigment. L and Z are not synthesized de novo in humans, and are entirely of dietary origin, whereas meso-Z is primarily formed in the retina from L.[8]

An average western diet contains 1.3–3 mg/day of L and Z combined, with significantly more L than Z (represented by an estimated ratio of 7:1). Approximately 78% of dietary L and Z are sourced from vegetables. L is found in highest concentrations in dark green leafy vegetables, such as spinach, kale, and collard greens. Z is the major carotenoid found in corn, orange peppers, and oranges, with a high mole percentage of both L and Z being found in egg yolk. Possible dietary sources of meso-Z include shrimp, certain marine fish and turtles, none of which is found in a typical western diet.

Macular pigment represents the most conspicuous accumulation of carotenoids in the human body. Z is the predominant carotenoid in the foveal region, whereas L predominates in the parafoveal region. The concentration of meso-Z peaks centrally.

L, Z, and meso-Z are intracellular compounds, separated between the cell cytosol and the cell membrane of the photoreceptor outer-segment membranes, where they are possibly bound to the ubiquitous structural protein tubulin, or to specific xanthophyll-binding proteins. Macular pigment has been shown to reach its maximum concentration within the photoreceptor axon layer (fibers of Henle) of the foveola, whereas outside the foveola, the highest concentrations are found both within the photoreceptor axons and within the inner and outer plexiform layers.

FUNCTIONS OF MACULAR PIGMENTS

Antioxidant

Macular carotenoids are capable of quenching singlet oxygen, free radicals, and triplet-state photosensitizers, thus limiting membrane phospholipid peroxidation. *In vitro* studies of cultured human RPE cells have demonstrated enhanced survival of these cells when they are subjected to oxidative stress in the presence of Z and other antioxidant compounds, as compared with cells subjected to the same conditions in the absence of such antioxidants.

L and Z are more resistant to degradation than other carotenoids when subjected to oxidative stress, an attribute which may facilitate their selective accumulation and slow biological turnover at the macula. Of the macular carotenoids, Z is probably a more potent antioxidant than L.

Optical filter

The absorption spectrum of the macular carotenoids peaks at 460 nm, and thus macular pigment is a filter of blue light and may limit photo-oxidative damage to retinal cells. Both the absorptive characteristics of macular pigment and its location in the anterior portion of individual photoreceptors enable the pigment to attenuate the amount of blue light incident upon the photoreceptor.

It has been estimated that the quantity of visible blue light (460 nm) incident upon the photoreceptors of the macula is substantially reduced as a result of the filtering properties of macular pigment; this reduction is estimated at approximately 40%, but varies from 3 to 100% between individuals.

APOPTOSIS AND RETINAL DEGENERATION

There is convincing evidence that genetic defects in retinitis pigmentosa can lead indirectly to cell death. This is evident, for example, in cone loss in patients with retinitis pigmentosa due to mutations in the *rhodopsin* gene, which is expressed only in rods. It is of interest that in these and other retinal degenerations, photoreceptor cell death occurs by apoptosis. These observations imply that therapeutic modification of the process leading to apoptosis or the apoptotic pathway itself may modify the course of these disorders.

Apoptosis is a common final pathway in retinal degeneration in humans and in animal models (Figure 3.3). Although biochemical aspects are similar in all apoptotic cells (nuclear chromatin condensation, cytoplasmic shrinking, dilated endoplasmic reticulum, membrane blebbing, and internucleosomal DNA fragmentation), different molecular events lead to cell death.

Caspases (cysteine aspartate-specific proteases) are the first proteases identified that coordinate and execute the apoptotic process in many apoptotic systems. These proteins are synthesized as inactive zymogens and are activated by proteolytic cleavage to form a tetramer. Two major pathways, leading to the degradation of key survival proteins, have been described for caspase activation: the extrinsic pathway, initiated by ligand binding to a death receptor and the intrinsic pathway, involving the release of cytochrome c from the mitochondrial intermembrane space into the cytosol.

In retinal degeneration, caspases, calpains, and (LEI)-DNase II have been shown to be activated during photoreceptor cell death in several models.[9] Caspase-1 and -2 were detected in the retinal outer nuclear layer during degeneration in Royal College of Surgeons (RCS) rats, and inhibition of caspase-3 preserved the retina of S334ter rats and tubby mice. In rd mice, calpain mediates apoptosis through caspase-3 activation, and caspase-3 inhibitors preserve the retina.

An unexpected finding was observed during early attempts at retinal transplantation for photoreceptor rescue. Focal injury to the retina appears to protect nearby photoreceptors from degeneration. This was clearly illustrated in the RCS rat in which mechanical injury produced by an injection of saline into the subretinal space or into the vitreous or even insertion of a needle without injection led to protection of photoreceptors near the wound. This protection is not restricted to genetically determined retinal degeneration. Similar photoreceptor rescue by mechanical injury was observed in light-induced retinal damage in the rat. Injury-induced photoreceptor rescue extends beyond the immediate vicinity of the lesion, suggesting that diffusible factors may be involved.

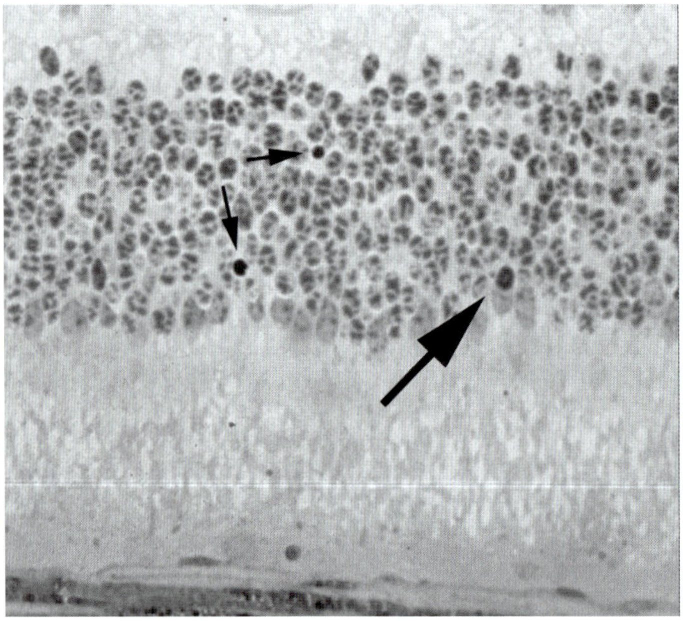

Figure 3.3 Light microscopy of the retina in a canine model of retinal degeneration showing apoptotic cells (arrows).

As mechanical injury to the eye increases the expression of basic fibroblast growth factor and ciliary neurotrophic factor (CNTF) in the rat retina, it is logical to assume that these agents may be responsible, at least in part, for this protection.

CNTF was found to rescue photoreceptors from degeneration when delivered continuously after adeno-associated virus vector transduction; however, it reduces scotopic (rod-dominated) and photopic (cone-dominated) electroretinographic (ERG) amplitudes, which are typically a measure of retinal function. This effect appears to occur in a dose-dependent manner. The continuous delivery of CNTF also results in a reduction of some or all ERG responses in normal mice, rabbits, and rats. Intraocular CNTF injection reduces vision in normal rats. These paradoxical properties of growth factors might limit their therapeutic use.[10]

VISUAL CYCLE

The visual cycle has at least two interlinked components: the retinoid cycle and the electrical amplification cascade.

RETINOID CYCLE

Outer segment of photoreceptors

Visual phototransduction is the photochemical reaction that take place when light (photon) is converted to an electric signal in the retina. Rhodopsin, the visual pigment in the rods, is a membrane protein located in the outer segments of the rods. It contains a chromophore (11-*cis* retinal) that is covalently bound to opsin. On photoactivation, 11-*cis* retinal undergoes photoisomerization to all-*trans* retinal. While still covalently bound to opsin, the compound undergoes a number of conformational intermediates, collectively termed metarhodopsin. It is suggested that metarhodopsin II is important in inactivation of electrical activity.

Retinal pigment epithelium

All-*trans* retinal together with the opsin then diffuses into the interphotoreceptor matrix and enters the RPE, where they are hydrolyzed to all-*trans* retinal and opsin. The all-*trans* retinal is flipped across the membrane by ABCA4 (formerly called ABCR) transporter and then reduces to all-*trans* retinol, which is chaperoned by cellular retinol-binding protein and is esterified by lecithin-retinol acetyl transferase (LRAT). The ester is then chaperoned by RPE65. The all-*trans* retinol is isomerized by retinoid isomerase and retinoid hydrolase to 11 *cis*-retinol.

An alternate cycle exists when some of the all-*trans* retinal remains chaperoned by the opsin and is reduced by all-*trans* retinol dehydrogenase to release all-*trans* retinol. In both cases, all-*trans* retinol moves from the RPE into the outer segment.

Re-entry into the outer segment

Before it enters the rod outer segment again, 11 *cis*-retinol is oxidized to 11-*cis* retinal and diffuses across the interphotoreceptor matrix, chaperoned by interphotoreceptor retinoid-binding protein, where it is conjugated to an opsin to form a new rhodopsin.

Chaperones

The retinal loop indicates that chaperones play an important role at each locus in the cycle, guiding retinoids to their specific site.

PHOTOTRANSDUCTION

Activation

The light activation of rhodopsin generates an amplification cascade that leads to changes in the resting potential of the photoreceptor. There is ongoing outward potassium current through nongated K^+-selective channels. This outward current tends to hyperpolarize the photoreceptor at around –70 mV (the equilibrium potential for K^+). There is also inward sodium current carried by cyclic guanosine monophosphate (cGMP)-gated sodium channels. This so-called "dark current" depolarizes the cell to around –40 mV.

Light activation causes metarhodopsin II to activate transducin, which in turn activates a photoreceptor-specific cGMP phosphodiesterase, resulting in a decrease in intracellular cGMP. It reduces the permeability of plasma membrane cGMP-gated cation channels, leading to hyperpolarization of the photoreceptor cell membrane and decreased neurotransmitter release at synapses with bipolar cells. While in the dark, as cGMP levels are high, cGMP-gated sodium channels remain open, allowing a steady inward current which keeps the cell depolarized at about –40 mV. The depolarization of the cell membrane in the dark allows sodium to exit and calcium to enter and opens voltage-gated calcium channels, releasing glutamate into the synaptic cleft. This excitatory neurotransmitter hyperpolarizes on-center bipolar cells and depolarizes the off-center bipolar cells.

Inactivation

Removing the light stimulus leads to inactivation of the visual cascade. This involves several steps:

- The rhodopsin is phosphorylated by rhodopsin kinase. Arrestin (S-antigen) binds to the phosphorylated proteins, preventing continued activation of transducin.
- GTPase-activating protein (RGS9) interacts with the alpha subunit of transducin, and causes it to hydrolyze its bound guanosine triphosphate (GTP) to guanosine diphosphate (GDP), and thus halts the action of phosphodiesterase, stopping the transformation of cGMP to GMP.
- Guanylate cyclase activating protein (GCAP) is a calcium-binding protein, and as the calcium levels in the cell decrease, GCAP dissociates from its bound calcium ions, and interacts with guanylate cyclase, activating it. Guanylate cyclase then proceeds to transform GTP to cGMP, replenishing the cell's cGMP levels and thus reopening the sodium channels that were closed during phototransduction.
- Metarhodopsin II is deactivated. Recoverin, a calcium-binding protein, is normally bound to rhodopsin kinase. When the calcium levels fall during phototransduction, the calcium dissociates from recoverin, and rhodopsin kinase is released. It phosphorylates metarhodopsin II, which decreases its affinity for transducin.

RETINAL PIGMENT EPITHELIUM AND LIPOFUSCIN

RETINAL PIGMENT EPITHELIUM

An intact RPE is essential for the proper functioning of the visual process. This postmitotic, multifunctional layer is involved in the degradation of photoreceptor outer segments, vitamin A cycle, and support of retinal metabolism and maintenance of the outer BRB. As a consequence of excessive metabolism, high oxygen levels, exposure to light of short wavelength, and free radical formation, the RPE is constantly exposed to insults and cumulative RPE damage.

LIPOFUSCIN

Cells of the RPE phagocytose the membranous discs of the rods and cones. These discs are made of rhodopsin, proteins, and lipids. Rhodopsin consists of 11 *cis*-retinal and opsin. When light-activated, 11-*cis* retinal is converted to all-*trans* retinal and then reduced to all-*trans* retinol to proceed through the visual cycle. However, the excess of all-*trans* retinal reacts with the lipids and proteins of the discs to form lipofuscin.

Formation of lipofuscin

The most widely studied lipofuscin pigments in the RPE are the bisretinoid compound A2E. A2E formation begins in photoreceptor outer segments from nonenzymatic reaction between the membrane lipid, phosphatidylethanolamine, and all-*trans* retinal to form *N*-retinylidene phosphatidylethanolamine (NRPE). After tautomerization, NRPE reacts with a second molecule of all-*trans* retinal to form a pyridinium ring to generate A2PE-H2. This compound autooxidizes and yields A2-PE. The A2-PE is deposited in RPE cells during the normal process of outer-segment phagocytosis and subsequent hydrolysis by phospholipase D generates A2E. A2E is taken up by the lysosomes. When A2E is photoactivated, it fragments and generates a number of photo-oxidation products, including epoxides, furanoid oxides, and cyclic peroxides. Other products of reactions of all-*trans* retinal vary in structure and absorbance spectra. Little is known of these products. The accumulation of lipofuscin increases with age to approximately 70 years. With age, the RPE cells become less efficient in coping with A2E and the associated burden. The lipofuscin fluorescence decreases or reaches a plateau in the eighth decade, probably due to death of lipofuscin-laden RPE cells and the change in ratio of A2E and A2E photo-oxidation products within the cells.

Lipofuscin and RPE atrophy

A healthy RPE is essential for the proper functioning of the rods and cones. Lipofuscin may induce RPE cell death and atrophy in several ways. Blue light (wavelength 435 nm) has been shown to cause damage to RPE cells *in vivo* and *in vitro*. The propensity for RPE cells to be susceptible to blue light-induced damage or death is related to the proportion of A2E accumulation in the cells. This insult is not seen with green light (wavelength 514–532 nm) or in RPE cells devoid of A2E. The light-induced damage may be caused by the direct reaction of the photoactivation molecule with the cellular constituents and through the formation of reactive oxygen species. Antioxidants such as vitamins C and E and Bilberry have been shown to suppress photo-oxidation of A2E in RPE. The RPE cell death pathway involves the activation of caspases and is modulated by the mitochondrial protein Bcl-2. The JNK signaling pathway may have a protective role of photo-oxidation of A2E.

Another hypothesis that explains A2E-induced RPE damage is lysosomal dysfunction. Studies have shown that lipofuscin also causes instability of lysosmal membranes due to membrane blebbing. It also reduces the acidity of the cell organelles, resulting in failure of proteolytic digestion.

Lipofuscin also interferes with the metabolism of phagocytosed lipids of the outer segments within the RPE cells. The A2E-induced alterations in cholesterol homeostasis within the RPE may have several bearings on the aging process as well as in hereditary retinal degeneration and age-related macular degeneration. It is postulated that free cholesterol and the esters extruded from the RPE may contribute to age-related lipid accumulation in the BM and the lipid constituents of drusen and other subretinal deposits. In addition, it may act as a nidus for chronic inflammatory reaction, interfere with the visual cycle, and inhibit other degradative processes and functions of other lipid-dependent receptors and transporters.

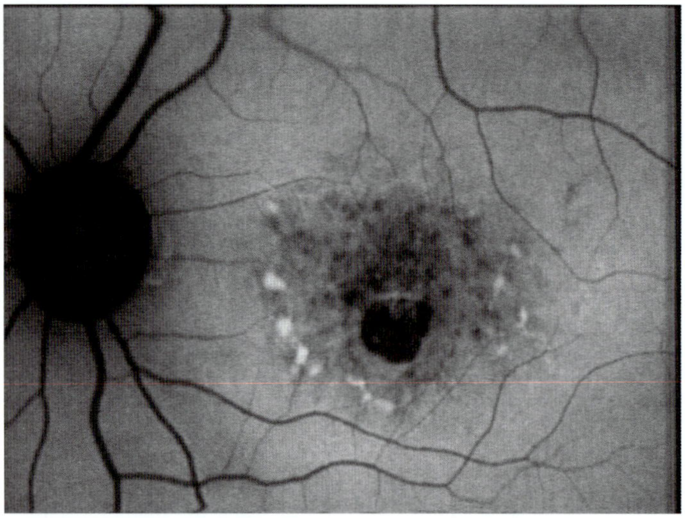

Figure 3.4 Autofluorescence imaging of patient with Stargardt's macular dystrophy showing central atrophy (dark area) with surrounding increased fluorescence spots of lipofuscin accumulation.

Stargardt's disease and lipofuscin

Stargardt's disease, a macular degeneration of juvenile onset, is caused by mutations in both alleles of the ABCA4 (formerly known as ABCR) gene. ABCA4 is a transporter protein called ATP-binding cassette transporter and is expressed in the discs of the outer segments of the rods and cones. In the visual cycle, the all-*trans* retinal formed in the lumen of the disc interacts with phosphatidylamine to form NRPE. The NRPE is flipped across the disc membrane by ABCA4 to be reduced to all-*trans* retinol in the cytosol of the rods. It acts as a flippase for NRPE. So, a loss of ABCA4 function leads to accumulation of NRPE and all-*trans* retinal in the lumen of the discs, with a consequent increase in the formation of lipofuscin (Figure 3.4). Pathologically, Stargardt's disease is associated with accumulation of excessive lipofuscin in the RPE, accounting for the dark choroid on fundus fluorescein angiography. Work with a mouse model of Stargardt's disease, the ABCA4 knockout mouse, has shown that the abundant A2E levels that accompany a loss of ABCA4 activity predispose to RPE atrophy. Short-wavelength visible light adversely affects this disease due to the RPE cell damage caused by the light-assisted generation of photoxidation of A2E.

Age-related macular degeneration and lipofuscin

Lipofuscin in the RPE has been implicated in the pathogenesis of atrophic age-related macular degeneration. In addition to the causes of atrophy mentioned above, photo-oxidation products of A2E may interact with complement at cell surface and activate the alternate pathway of the complement system in the pathogenesis of age-related macular degeneration. The interplay of photo-oxidation of lipofuscin, genetic susceptibility, and environmental factors may play a role in inducing low-grade inflammation in the pathogenesis of age-related macular degeneration. The accumulation of lipofuscin is also shown to activate retinoic acid receptor genes and vascular endothelial growth factor expression that increases the risk of choroidal neovascularization.

MATRIX BIOLOGY

STRUCTURAL COMPOSITION OF THE BRUCH'S MEMBRANE

The BM is a thin (2–4 μm) connective tissue interposed between the metabolically active RPE and its source of nutrition, the choriocapillaris. This pentalaminar structure is classically described as consisting of the basement membrane of the RPE, an inner collagenous zone (ICZ), a fenestrated elastic layer, an outer collagenous zone (OCZ), and the basement membrane of the endothelium of the choriocapillaris.

MACROSCOPIC CHANGES OF THE BRUCH'S MEMBRANE

The fundamental age-related change of BM is increased thickness: thickness is reported to increase by 135% in ten decades. The maximum thickness occurs in the substrata of the OCZ. Disease risk is associated with age-related thickness of the BM. A prolonged choroidal filling phase during fluorescein angiography signals the presence of diffuse BM thickening. In addition, serial measurement of the thickness of BM may be a useful prognostic parameter in longitudinal studies of age-related macular degeneration.

CELL BIOLOGY OF BRUCH'S MEMBRANE

The three anatomical changes that occur in BM with age are the progressive accumulation of debris, lipid deposition, and alteration of the ECM. The deposition of periodic acid–Schiff-positive granular, vesicular, and filamentary deposits in the ICZ of BM has been identified as early as the first decade of life. As age advances, the debris accumulates and contaminates all the collagenous layer of the BM, and is seen on both sides of the elastic lamina, thus forming the bulk of the age-related debris in the collagenous layers, especially in the OCZ. Depending on their proximity to the RPE, deposits may represent incompletely digested waste material emanating from a dysfunctional RPE, an inappropriately directed immune response, or altered remodeling of the membrane.

The proteins identified in the drusen/BM include both locally derived (neural retina, RPE, and choroid) and extracellular nonocular components. The oxidative modifications of some of these components may also be the primary catalyst in drusen formation. The complement system is now known to play a role in the pathogenesis of age-related macular degeneration.

LIPID ACCUMULATION

An age-related exponential accumulation of lipids occurs in the BM. The predominant lipids in the BM consist of phospholipids and fatty acids. About 50% of the phospholipids are phosphatidylcholine, suggesting that the lipids in the BM are more likely of a cellular origin (a potential source being the photoreceptor outer-segment membranes) than from plasma. However, studies using filipin histochemistry and hot-stage polarizing microscopy revealed that lipid content of BM consists of both esterified and unesterified cholesterol, suggesting a vascular origin akin to atherosclerosis.

MATRIX DYSREGULATION

Collagen synthesis increases with age in BM. Newsome et al. found an age-related increase in collagen I in the BM with age.[11] Other collagens noted in the BM include types III, IV, and V. In addition, atypical banding periodicity has been observed in the collagen produced. The ICZ consists more of 640A type collagen while the OCZ contains more 1000A type collagen with age. The meshes formed by the tightly interwoven collagen fibers in the ICZ also become irregular and coarse with age. The long spacing collagen is a material with periodicity ranging between 100 and 140 nm found mainly in the OCZ and which extends as intercapillary pegs to areas where choriocapillaris have undergone age-related atrophy. The increased insoluble collagen may contribute to debris accumulation and serve as a depot for lipoproteins, growth factors, and cytokines.

The amount of noncollagen protein in BM also increases significantly with age, as suggested by an increase in deposition of noncollagen

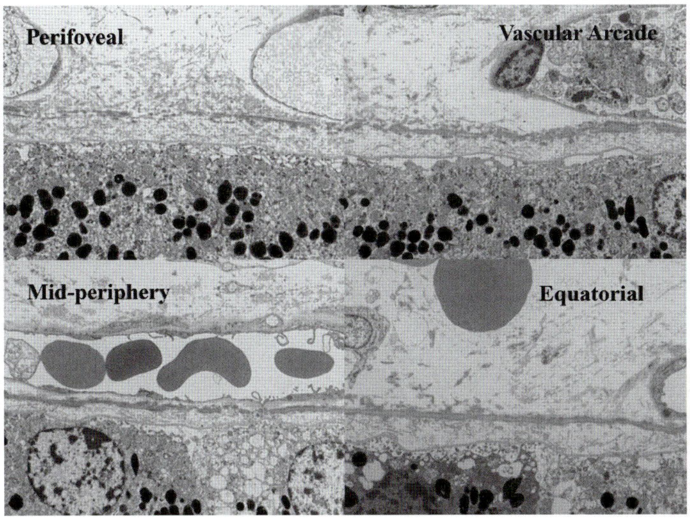

Figure 3.5 Electron microscopy of normal human Bruch's membrane, showing that the elastic layer becomes less porous and thicker from the fovea to the equator.

amino acids in the macular area. The elastic layer becomes basophilic; the elastic fibers increase in number and become more electron-dense. The BM also undergoes calcification and fragmentation, causing the membrane to lose its elasticity and become more brittle. The degree of thinning, calcification, and fragmentation of the elastic layer at the macula corresponds spatially to the distribution of the majority of macular lesions associated with age-related macular degeneration (Figure 3.5), explaining the preponderance of neovascular lesions at the macula.[12] This may explain in part the fact that serum elastin-derived peptides increase with severity of age-related macular degeneration.[13] Elastin fragments are also shown to increase choroidal endothelial cell migration, indicating that both local and systemic abnormalities in elastin physiology may be involved in the pathogenesis of choroidal neovascularization.

An increase in the content and structure of glycosaminoglycans (GAG) in BM has been identified. The increased volume of GAG may be partially responsible for the altered metabolism of the collagens and the resultant increased negative field may also contribute to the decreased filtration across the BM. An increased proportion of heparan sulfate in the basement membranes of the BM and simultaneous decrease in proteoglycan filaments containing chondroitin sulfate and dermatan sulfate associated with the collagen fibrils have been noted.

MATRIX METALLOPROTEINASES

Matrix metalloproteinases (MMPs) are required by BM for ECM remodeling, protein processing, and angiogenesis. The age-related increased collagen content, the release of reactive oxygen radicals by the lipid-laden BM, and the presence of inflammatory cytokines, cellular transformation, and growth hormones may upregulate these enzymes, especially MMP-2 and MMP-9. Plasma MMP-9 levels have been found to be approximately threefold higher than controls, while plasma MMP-2 did not alter significantly between disease and controls.[14] The source of increased MMP-9 in the circulation in age-related macular degeneration subjects remains unclear.

One of the endogenous tissue inhibitors of MMPs (TIMPs) regulates the activation of MMPs and also has other independent actions. Of the four TIMPs characterized to date, TIMP-3 is the only member found exclusively in ECM, explaining the presence of TIMP-3 in the BM. In addition, it binds tightly to sulfated GAGs. Western blotting and quantitative reverse zymography have demonstrated an age-related increase in TIMP-3 in BM and its concentration is shown to correlate with the amount of ECM and the quantity of drusen.[15] In BM, TIMP-3 controls ECM turnover, limits neovascularization, and may play a role in apoptosis. Mutations of TIMP-3 are associated with Sorsby's fundus dystrophy (Figure 3.6), suggesting that mutant TIMP-3 may result in aberrant protein interaction and increased cell adhesiveness, which may cause defective turnover of the BM.[16]

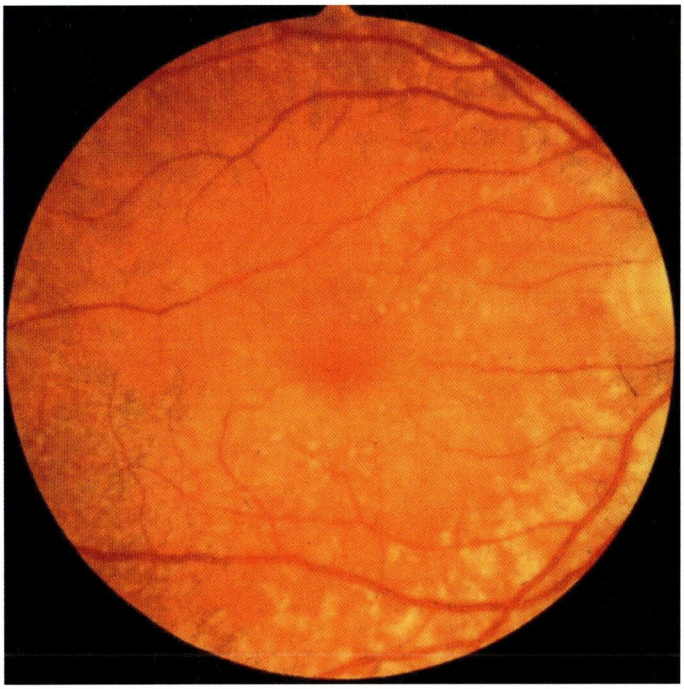

Figure 3.6 Fundus appearance of a patient with Sorsby's fundus dystrophy.

PHARMACOTHERAPY IMPLICATIONS

It is unclear whether the vitreous is a friend or a foe. However, in many circumstances, a controlled separation of the posterior vitreous base and the retina is beneficial. The key here is "controlled" and ideally noninvasive separation. The pathophysiology role in the changes of blood flow in retinal vascular diseases is complex: it remains unclear whether the vascular dilatation commonly seen in these diseases is a beneficial compensation or a cause of further vascular damage. Many drugs can modify the vascular caliber: the therapeutic potential is vast.

The controversy of macular pigments remains unresolved; laboratory evidence does not always translate to clinical benefit. The Age-Related Eye Disease Study (AREDS 2) will give us further insight. Genetic changes of phototransduction are often associated with retinal degeneration, the ability to target and modify the visual cycle or, by reducing apoptosis in reducing cell death, can be potentially useful in treating these diseases by modifying the genetic defect itself.

The abnormal turnover of the ECM, especially in the BM, is clearly implicated in the pathophysiology of age-related macular degeneration. Controlling this aberration will be potentially rewarding.

REFERENCES

1. Sebag J. Molecular biology of pharmacologic vitreolysis. Trans Am Ophthalmol Soc 2005;103:473–494.
2. Cunha-Vaz JG. The blood–retinal barriers system. Basic concepts and clinical evaluation. Exp Eye Res 2004;78:715–721.
3. González-Mariscal L, Betanzos A, Nava P, et al. Tight junction proteins. Prog Biophys Mol Biol 2003;81:1–44.
4. Pournaras CJ, Rungger-Brändle E, Riva CE, et al. Regulation of retinal blood flow in health and disease. Prog Retin Eye Res 2008;27:284–330.
5. Gonzalez-Mariscal L, Hernández S, Vega J. Inventions designed to enhance drug delivery across epithelial and endothelial cells through the paracellular pathway. Recent Pat Drug Deliv Formul 2008;2:145–176.
6. Sun C, Wang JJ, Mackey DA, et al. Retinal vascular caliber: systemic, environmental, and genetic association. Surv Ophthalmol 2009;54:74–95.
7. Berra A, Ganzinelli S, Saravia M, et al. Inducible nitric oxide synthase subserves cholinergic vasodilation in retina. Vis Neurosci. 2005 May-Jun;22(3):371–377.

8. Loane E, Kelliher C, Beatty S, et al. The rationale and evidence base for a protective role of macular pigment in age-related maculopathy. Br J Ophthalmol 2008;92:1163–1168.
9. Perche O, Doly M, Ranchon-Cole I. Caspase-dependent apoptosis in light induced retinal degeneration. Invest Ophthalmol Vis Sci 2007;48: 2753–2759.
10. McGill TJ, Prusky GT, Douglas RM, et al. Intraocular CNTF reduces vision in normal rats in a dose-dependent manner. Invest Ophthalmol Vis Sci 2007;48:5756–5766.
11. Newsome DA, Huh W, Green WR. Bruch's membrane age-related changes vary by region. Curr Eye Res 1987 Oct;6(10):1211–1221.
12. Chong NHV, Keonin J, Luthert PJ, et al. Decreased thickness and integrity of the macular elastic layer of Bruch's membrane corresponds to the distribution of lesions associated with age-related macular degeneration. Am J Pathol 2005;166:241–251.
13. Sivaprasad S, Chong NV, Bailey TA. Serum elastin-derived peptides in age-related macular degeneration. Invest Ophthalmol Vis Sci 2005;46: 3046–3051.
14. Chau KY, Sivaprasad S, Patel N, et al. Plasma levels of matrix metalloproteinase-2 and -9 (mmp-2 and mmp-9) in age-related macular degeneration. Eye 2008;22:855–859.
15. Bailey TA, Alexander RA, Dubovy SR, et al. Measurement of TIMP-3 expression and Bruch's membrane thickness in human macula. Exp Eye Res 2001;73:851–858.
16. Chong NHV, Alexander RA, Gin T, et al. TIMP-3, collagen and elastin immunohistochemistry and histopathology of Sorsby's fundus dystrophy. Invest Ophthalmol Vis Sci 2000;41:898–902.

CHAPTER

4 Ocular angiogenesis: vascular endothelial growth factor and other factors

Anthony P. Adamis, MD

INTRODUCTION

The original visionary proposal by Dr. Judah Folkman[1] that antiangiogenic therapy could offer an approach to the treatment of many cancers ultimately led to a major research effort into the mechanisms which control both physiological and pathological angiogenesis. His work also contemplated the use of antiangiogenic drugs in ophthalmology. A principal focus of this research effort has been the identification of specific molecules involved in the promotion and inhibition of angiogenesis, an effort that has already led to the development of targeted therapies against vascular endothelial growth factor (VEGF). In addition, many other factors have been identified that act as promoters or inhibitors of angiogenesis (Table 4.1). This chapter will focus on those molecules whose roles have been best validated to date, and which possess particular relevance to ocular neovascularization.

PROMOTERS OF ANGIOGENESIS

VASCULAR ENDOTHELIAL GROWTH FACTOR

VEGF in physiologic and pathologic angiogenesis

VEGF (also known as VEGF-A) is a 45-kDa homodimeric glycoprotein belonging to a family that also includes VEGF-B through VEGF-E, platelet-derived growth factor (PDGF), and placental growth factor.[2] Initially isolated as a vascular permeability factor, VEGF was subsequently cloned and found to be a potent proangiogenic factor, acting as a master regulator of angiogenesis (reviewed by Ferrara and Davis-Smyth[3] and Ferrara[2]). VEGF has subsequently been found to act in a wide variety of other physiological contexts,[4] some of which, such as neuroprotection, are completely independent of its role in angiogenesis.

Alternative splicing of the human VEGF gene yields six principal isoforms of 121, 145, 165, 183, 189, and 206 amino acids.[5] The corresponding rodent isoforms are one amino acid shorter.[3] Many studies have focused on characterizing the functions of $VEGF_{121}$, $VEGF_{165}$, and $VEGF_{189}$. $VEGF_{121}$ is freely diffusible, while $VEGF_{189}$ and larger isoforms are found sequestered in the extracellular matrix; $VEGF_{165}$ exists in both diffusible and matrix-bound forms.[2] VEGF acts as a ligand for VEGF receptor 1 (VEGFR1) and VEGFR2; these receptor tyrosine kinases in turn activate downstream signaling cascades.

VEGF acts in many capacities in angiogenesis, including as an endothelial cell mitogen[6] and survival factor,[7] and as a chemoattractant for bone marrow-derived endothelial progenitor cells.[8] In addition, VEGF induces the upregulation of extracellular matrix-degrading enzymes, such as matrix metalloproteinases (MMPs)[9] and plasminogen activator,[10] as well as nitric oxide,[11] a downstream mediator of VEGF signaling.[12] Moreover, VEGF has two additional properties which are of direct relevance for the pathophysiology of ocular neovascular diseases. First, it is the most potent known inducer of vascular permeability,[13] an action related to the edema which often accompanies ocular neovascularization. Secondly, the retinal expression of VEGF, which is produced by a wide variety of retinal cell types,[14–16] is upregulated by hypoxia,[15,17] a response that is believed to be important in maintaining the health of both retinal neurons[18] and the choriocapillaris[17] while also creating a proangiogenic environment.

Reflecting the original focus of Dr. Folkman's proposal on the importance of angiogenesis in cancer growth and metastasis,[1] initial investigations of the role of VEGF in pathological angiogenesis demonstrated that interference with VEGF signaling inhibited tumor growth.[19] Over the course of a decade, a role for VEGF in ocular neovascular disease also was established based on three main lines of evidence: (1) correlations of VEGF elevation with the presence of ocular neovascular disease in the eyes of patients; (2) preclinical studies demonstrating that experimental elevation of VEGF levels in the eye led to neovascularization; and (3) the converse experiment, in which inhibition of VEGF signaling decreased neovascularization.

Correlations between elevations in ocular levels of VEGF and ocular neovascular disease have been reported and include conditions such as iris neovascularization, retinal vein occlusion, diabetic retinopathy (DR), diabetic macular edema (DME), neovascular glaucoma, and retinopathy of prematurity (reviewed by Starita et al.[4]). Elevated expression of VEGF also has been detected in surgically removed maculae[20] and choroidal neovascularization (CNV) membranes of eyes with age-related macular degeneration (AMD).[21]

A variety of approaches have been employed to demonstrate that elevated ocular levels of VEGF are sufficient to induce ocular neovascularization. These have included direct intravitreal injection of VEGF[22] and retinal vein photocoagulation[23] in monkeys; in rodent models, studies have included intravitreal injection of VEGF-expressing vectors,[24] and the use of transgenic mice engineered to overexpress VEGF in the retinal pigment epithelium (RPE).[25]

The experiments demonstrating that VEGF elevations are necessary for the development of ocular neovascularization have also employed various techniques. Agents used to block the actions of VEGF have included VEGFR fusion proteins,[26–28] anti-VEGF antibodies,[29,30] an anti-VEGF monoclonal antibody antigen-binding fragment (Figure 4.1),[31] an aptamer directed against $VEGF_{165}$,[28] and $VEGF_{165}b$, a VEGF variant which binds VEGFR2 but cannot activate it.[32] Agents used to block the ocular production of VEGF or VEGFR1 at the transcriptional or translational level have included small interfering RNAs (siRNAs) specific for VEGF[33] or VEGFR1,[34] and antisense oligonucleotides specific for VEGF.[35] Blocking the actions of VEGF in the eye by various means inhibited neovascularization of the iris,[29] cornea,[30] retina,[26,28,32,34,35] and choroid.[27,31,33,34]

Further detailed investigations into the mechanisms underlying VEGF's importance have revealed that the isoform $VEGF_{165}$ is especially pathogenic. In a murine model of ischemia-associated ocular neovascularization, retinal expression of $VEGF_{165}$ was found to be dramatically elevated compared to other isoforms; moreover, intravitreal injection of a $VEGF_{165}$-specific RNA aptamer was as efficient at inhibiting the pathological neovascularization as injection of a VEGFR-Fc fusion protein that inactivated all VEGF isoforms (Figure 4.2).[28] In addition, $VEGF_{165}$ acts as an especially potent inflammatory cytokine, a property of direct relevance given the importance of inflammation in

Table 4.1 Proangiogenic and antiangiogenic factors

Proangiogenic factors	Antiangiogenic factors
Angiogenin	Angioarrestin
Angiopoietin-1	Angiostatin (plasminogen fragment)
Complement factors C3 and C5	Antiangiogenic antithrombin III
Cryptic collagen IV fragment	Cartilage-derived inhibitor (CDI)
Developmentally regulated endothelial locus 1 (Del-1)	CD59 complement fragment
Fibroblast growth factors: acidic (aFGF) and basic (bFGF)	Endostatin (collagen XVIII fragment)
Follistatin	Fibronectin fragment
Granulocyte colony-stimulating factor (G-CSF)	Growth-related oncogene (Gro-β)
Hepatocyte growth factor (HGF)/scatter factor (SF)	Heparinases
Interleukin-8 (IL-8)	Heparin hexasaccharide fragment
α5 integrins	Human chorionic gonadotropin (hCG)
Leptin	Interferon α/β/γ
Midkine	Interferon-inducible protein (IP-10)
Pigment epithelium-derived growth factor	Interleukin-12
Placental growth factor	Kringle 5 (plasminogen fragment)
Platelet-derived endothelial cell growth factor (PDECGF)	Metalloproteinase inhibitors (TIMPs)
Platelet-derived growth factor-BB (PDGF-BB)	2-Methoxyestradiol
Pleiotrophin (PTN)	Pigment epithelium-derived growth factor
Progranulin	Placental ribonuclease inhibitor
Proliferin	Plasminogen activator inhibitor
Transforming growth factor-α (TGF-α)	Platelet factor-4 (PF4)
Transforming growth factor-β (TGF-β)	Prolactin 16-kDa fragment
Tumor necrosis factor-α (TNF-α)	Proliferin-related protein (PRP)
Vascular endothelial growth factor (VEGF)	Retinoids
	Soluble VEGFR-1
	Tryptophanyl-tRNA synthase fragment
	$VEGF_{xxx}b$
	Tetrahydrocortisol-S
	Thrombospondin-1 (TSP-1)
	Transforming growth factor-β (TGF-β)
	Vasculostatin
	Vasostatin (calreticulin fragment)

Adapted from: Angiogenesis Foundation. Understanding angiogenesis. List of known angiogenic growth factors. Available online at: http://www.angio.org/understanding/content_understanding.html.

pathological neovascularization. Laser injury has been shown to upregulate retinal expression of intercellular cell adhesion molecule-1 (ICAM1), thereby promoting leukocyte adhesion to the vascular endothelium through CD18, the leukocyte ligand for ICAM1.[36] Genetic ablation of either molecule significantly reduced the formation of laser-induced CNV (Figure 4.3).[36] In this context, it is noteworthy that $VEGF_{165}$ was found to be significantly more potent at upregulating ICAM1 expression on endothelial cells than $VEGF_{121}$.[37] In addition, depletion of macrophages has been found to inhibit the development of pathological neovascularization in a rat model of retinopathy of prematurity (Figure 4.4)[28] and in laser-induced CNV.[38] $VEGF_{165}$ was more potent at chemotaxis of monocyte/macrophages than $VEGF_{121}$.[37] Since macrophages produce VEGF,[39] their infiltration serves as an amplification mechanism in further promoting angiogenesis.

Investigational approaches to VEGF inhibition in ocular neovascularization

The extensive research effort into elucidating VEGF's role in ocular neovascularization has provided a sound foundation for the development of anti-VEGF therapies. Three agents, pegaptanib,[40] ranibizumab,[41] and bevacizumab,[42] are already in widespread use, and are discussed in dedicated chapters of this text. A brief account of other approaches currently under evaluation in clinical trials follows.

RNA interference

RNA interference abrogates gene expression through a cellular defense mechanism mediated by double-stranded RNA sequences of at least 21 nucleotides long, resulting in targeted destruction of specific mRNA species.[43] RNA interference has been used to target VEGF mRNA in animal models, leading to suppression of corneal neovascularization[44] as well as CNV induced either by laser[33] or by overexpression of VEGF from a transgene.[45] Sirna-027, an agent targeting the expression of VEGFR1, also has been shown to suppress both retinal and CNV in murine models.[34]

Currently there are two siRNA agents undergoing evaluation in clinical trials for treatment of neovascular AMD. Bevasiranib (Ophi Health), directed against VEGF, has successfully completed a phase II trial and is currently recruiting patients for the phase III COBALT trial in which it will be combined with ranibizumab.[46] In addition, a phase I trial of the anti-VEGFR1 agent AGN211745 (Allergan; previously Sirna-027) has been completed,[47] and enrollment for a phase II trial is ongoing.[48] Recent evidence suggests that antiangiogenic siRNAs work nonspecifically and through a nonclassical siRNA mechanism in suppressing CNV.[49]

Soluble VEGFR fusion protein: VEGF-Trap

Work demonstrating the potential of soluble VEGFR fusion proteins to suppress retinal neovascularization[26] provided a basis for the development of VEGF-Trap, a fusion protein combining components of both VEGFR1 and VEGFR2.[50] VEGF-Trap, which was engineered with a view to optimizing pharmacokinetic properties as well as efficacy, binds to all isoforms of VEGF as well as placental growth factor.[50] Intravitreal injection of VEGF-Trap inhibited laser-induced CNV in mice, as well as preventing VEGF-induced blood–retinal barrier breakdown.[27] It is now being evaluated in a phase III study.[51]

Anecortave acetate

Anecortave acetate is a member of a group of corticosteroids, first isolated in Dr. Folkman's laboratory,[52] that have angiostatic properties but lack conventional anti-inflammatory activity.[53] In a rat retinopathy of prematurity model, anecortave significantly reduced pathologic retinal neovascularization without affecting normal retinal angiogenesis.[54] In other studies with this model, anecortave was found to reduce retinal expression of VEGF,[55] and of insulin growth-factor-1 and its receptor.[56] Anecortave also inhibited VEGFR2 expression in a murine model of retinoblastoma.[57] These findings suggest that the angiostatic effects of anecortave may at least in part be mediated through VEGF signaling pathways.[52]

Anecortave acetate has shown some promise as a treatment for neovascular AMD, administered as a juxtascleral depot either alone[58] or in combination with photodynamic therapy.[59] Although anecortave acetate did not meet its efficacy endpoint in a phase III noninferiority trial comparing it to photodynamic therapy with verteporfin,[58] it remains under study as a prophylactic treatment to slow the progression of neovascular AMD.[60]

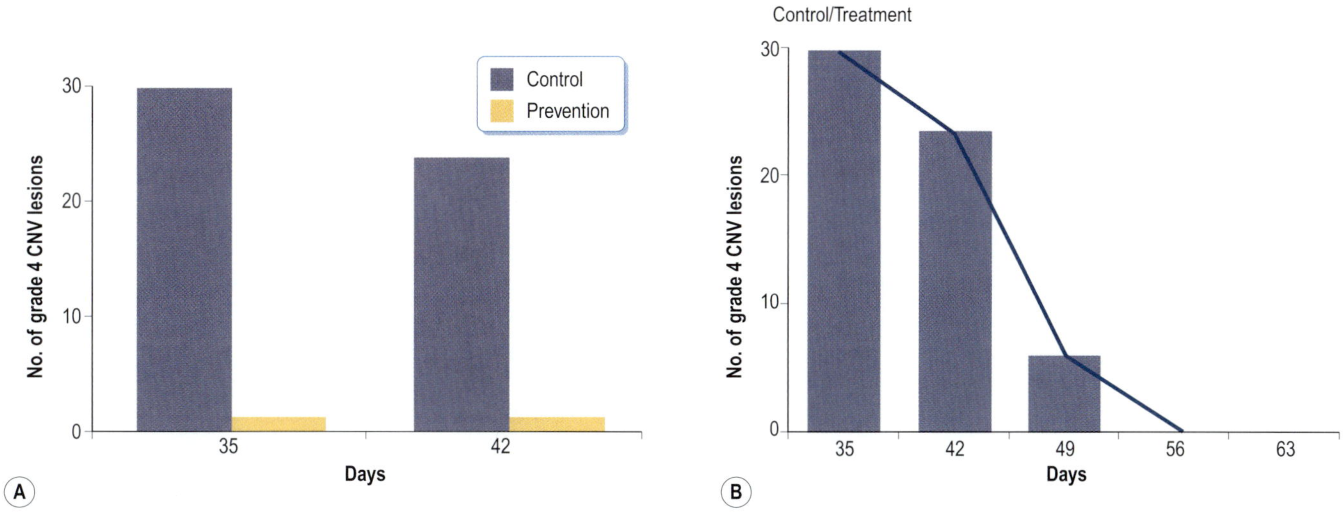

Figure 4.1 Inactivation of all vascular endothelial growth factor (VEGF) isoforms potently inhibits laser-induced choroidal neovascularization (CNV) in the nonhuman primate. (A) Cynomolgus monkeys ($n = 10$) received 500 µg of recombinant humanized monoclonal anti-VEGF antibody (rhuFab VEGF) in one eye and vehicle in the other, every 2 weeks. On day 21, CNV was induced by laser wounding. The bar graph shows the total number of grade 4 CNV lesions in the eyes receiving rhuFab VEGF (gold bar) compared to those in control eyes that received vehicle (blue bar); assessments were made 2 weeks after laser induction (day 35), and 3 weeks after the laser induction (day 42). Adapted from Krzystolik MG, Afshari MA, Adamis AP, et al. Prevention of experimental choroidal neovascularization with intravitreal anti-vascular endothelial growth factor antibody fragment. Arch Ophthalmol 2002;120:338–346.

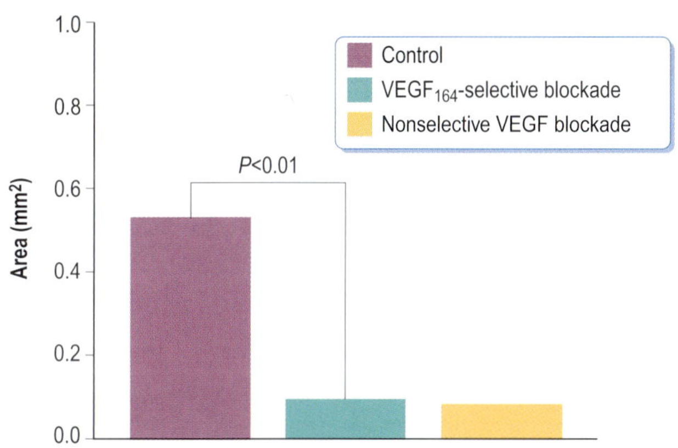

Figure 4.2 Vascular endothelial growth factor ($VEGF_{164/165}$) is especially potent in promoting pathological neovascularization. In a rat model of ischemia-induced retinal neovascularization, intravitreal injection of an aptamer specific for $VEGF_{164/165}$ was as effective in inhibiting pathological neovascularization as a VEGFR1-Fc fusion protein which binds all VEGF isoforms. Adapted from Ishida S, Usui T, Yamashiro K, et al. VEGF164-mediated inflammation is required for pathological, but not physiological, ischemia-induced retinal neovascularization. J Exp Med 2003;198:483–489.

PLATELET-DERIVED GROWTH FACTOR

The PDGF family consists of four related dimeric polypeptides (PDGF-A through PDGF-D)[61] that are structurally related to VEGF.[2] In general they occur as homodimers, although the PDGF-AB heterodimer has also been identified.[61] PDGFs are ligands for two receptor tyrosine kinases, PDGFR-α and PDGFR-β, of which PDGFR-β is principally responsible for signal transduction on cells associated with the vascular system, including endothelial cells, pericytes, and smooth-muscle cells.[62] Similarly, PDGF also has a widespread distribution among these same cell types.[62] In addition to its central role in vascular system development, PDGF signaling is important for processes such as wound healing and central nervous system development.[62]

Studies have revealed a central role for the PDGF-B homodimer in vascular development, as it was found to stimulate the proliferation,[63] and induce capillary tube formation[64] of endothelial cells. PDGF-B is especially critical for the recruitment of mural cells (pericytes and smooth-muscle cells) to the developing vasculature.[65] Genetic ablation of PDGF-B leads to perinatal death from hemorrhages and vascular system abnormalities[66] while ablation of the PDGFR-β gene results in a similar phenotype.[67] Proliferation of mural cells was significantly reduced in mice lacking either PDGF-B or PDGFR-β.[65] Also, administration of an aptamer specific for PDGF-B led first to pericyte loss and then to regression of tumor vessels in a murine tumor model.[68] These findings indicate that PDGF-B produced by endothelial cells is essential for the proliferation, migration, and recruitment of mural cells to the developing capillaries (Figure 4.5).[65]

Studies of ocular neovascularization in mice have provided further evidence in support of this model. Inhibition of PDGF-B signaling, whether by genetic ablation in endothelial cells[69] or PDGFR kinase inhibitors,[70] led to deficient pericyte recruitment in models of retinal[69] and corneal[70] neovascularization.

Studies using three different models of ocular neovascularization, in which PDGF-B and VEGF signaling were blocked by administration of an antibody to PDGFR-β or pegaptanib, respectively, have further delineated the respective roles of these molecules.[71] Physiological retinal angiogenesis was inhibited on postnatal day 3 by blocking PDGF-B, but not by blocking $VEGF_{164}$; however, combined blockade provided greater inhibition. Conversely, VEGF blockade alone inhibited the development of laser-induced CNV, whereas blocking PDGF-B signaling was ineffective on its own; again, greater inhibition occurred if both pathways were blocked. Finally, in a corneal model of neovascularization, PDGF-B blockade between days 10 and 20 postinjury led to detachment of mural cells from corneal neovessels; in contrast, VEGF blockade reduced neovascularization when applied immediately after wounding, but it did not induce regression of vessels after they were established. However, vessel regression was enhanced if both inhibitors were given (Figure 4.6).[71] These experiments suggest that a combination strategy targeting both VEGF and PDGF-B may be more effective, both in treating established neovascularization and in preventing new vessel growth.

FIBROBLAST GROWTH FACTOR 2 (FGF2)

FGF2 (also known as basic FGF) is a heparin-binding growth factor that occurs in several isoforms. FGF2 signals through four receptor tyrosine kinases (FGF receptor 1 through FGF receptor 4) and acts in a variety of developmental processes, including angiogenesis.[72]

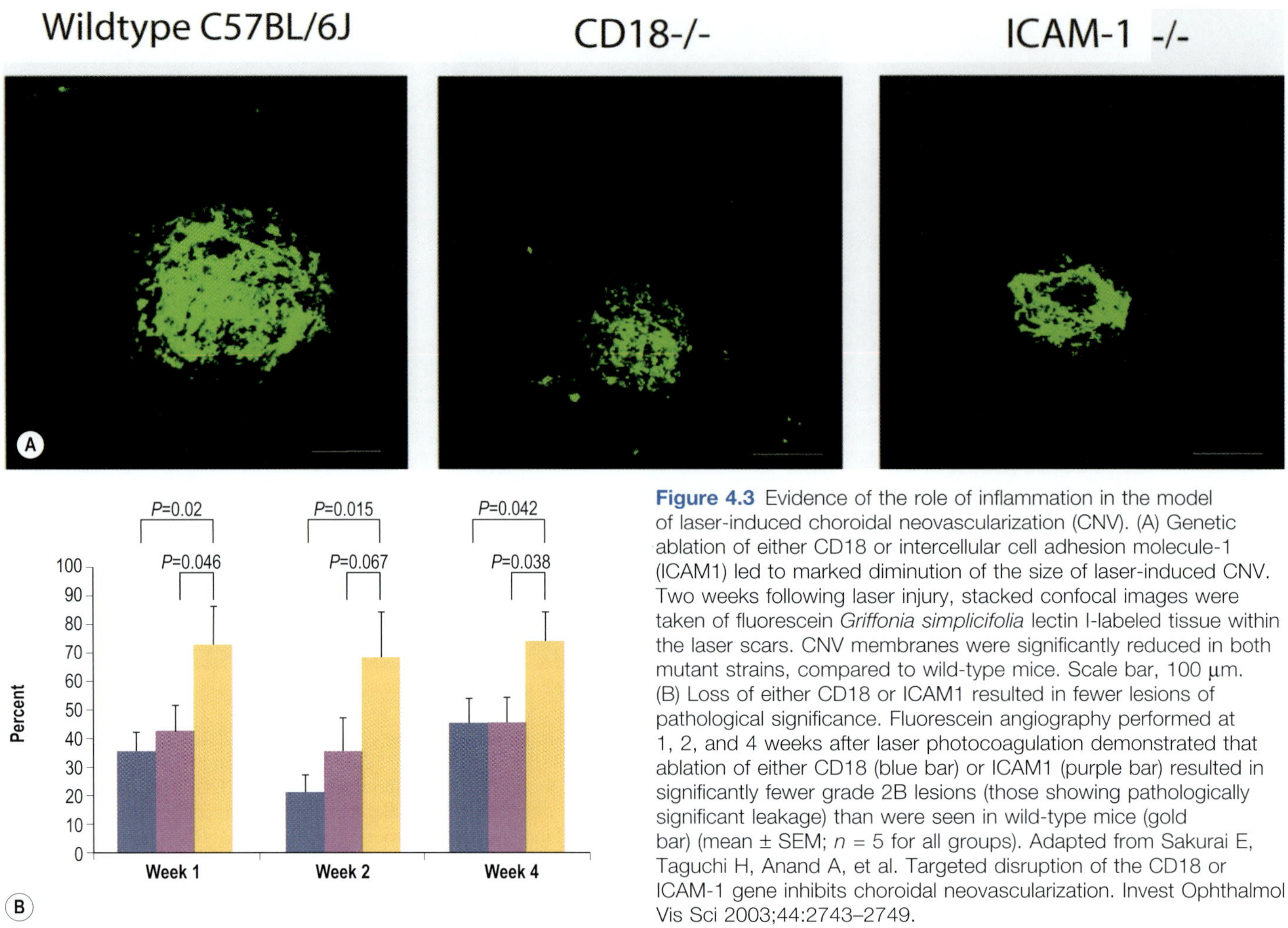

Figure 4.3 Evidence of the role of inflammation in the model of laser-induced choroidal neovascularization (CNV). (A) Genetic ablation of either CD18 or intercellular cell adhesion molecule-1 (ICAM1) led to marked diminution of the size of laser-induced CNV. Two weeks following laser injury, stacked confocal images were taken of fluorescein *Griffonia simplicifolia* lectin I-labeled tissue within the laser scars. CNV membranes were significantly reduced in both mutant strains, compared to wild-type mice. Scale bar, 100 μm. (B) Loss of either CD18 or ICAM1 resulted in fewer lesions of pathological significance. Fluorescein angiography performed at 1, 2, and 4 weeks after laser photocoagulation demonstrated that ablation of either CD18 (blue bar) or ICAM1 (purple bar) resulted in significantly fewer grade 2B lesions (those showing pathologically significant leakage) than were seen in wild-type mice (gold bar) (mean ± SEM; $n = 5$ for all groups). Adapted from Sakurai E, Taguchi H, Anand A, et al. Targeted disruption of the CD18 or ICAM-1 gene inhibits choroidal neovascularization. Invest Ophthalmol Vis Sci 2003;44:2743–2749.

The role of FGF2 in ocular neovascular disease is not well defined. Elevated expression of FGF2 has been detected in CNV membranes from patients with AMD[73] and in epiretinal membranes from patients with proliferative DR.[73] However, exogenous administration of FGF2 produced only subretinal neovascularization that did not penetrate Bruch's membrane in an experimental model of CNV.[74] Other studies found that transgenic mice with elevated retinal FGF2 expression developed CNV following low-intensity laser (sufficient to disrupt photoreceptors but not Bruch's membrane) while wild-type mice did not.[75] Taken together with studies demonstrating that genetic ablation of the FGF2 gene did not inhibit the formation of laser-induced CNV,[76] these findings suggest that FGF2 is in itself not sufficient to provoke CNV in the absence of an additional stimulus and that FGF2 may also not be required to induce CNV.

TUMOR NECROSIS FACTOR-α (TNF-α)

TNF-α is the prototypic member of a superfamily of cytokines that mediate a variety of biological functions, signaling through a correspondingly large family of receptors.[77] Several studies have examined the role of TNF-α as a mediator of angiogenesis, but a unified picture is not yet apparent.

TNF-α has been found to stimulate angiogenesis in the corneas of rats[78] and rabbits.[79] It is not clear if these represent direct or indirect effects since TNF-α has been demonstrated to induce expression of VEGF[80] and VEGFR2[81] potently in cultured endothelial cells. TNF-α also upregulates the synthesis of other factors associated with angiogenesis, including angiopoietin 1 and angiopoietin 2[80] as well as MMP2 and MMP9.[82]

Several studies have assessed the role of TNF-α signaling in angiogenesis. In ischemic-induced neovascularization in the limbs of mice, TNF-α was essential for the mobilization and survival of bone marrow-derived endothelial progenitor cells, induction of VEGF expression and collateral vessel development.[83] In another report, administration of infliximab (a monoclonal antibody to TNF-α)[84] or etanercept (a soluble TNF receptor fusion protein) both inhibited the size of laser-induced CNV in mice.[84] Gene knockout studies, however, have been inconsistent; some studies found a dependence of retinal neovascularization on TNF-α function[85] whereas others did not.[86]

In clinical studies, elevated levels of TNF-α have been found in fibrovascular membranes of patients with proliferative DR[87] and in surgically excised CNV membranes.[88] Intriguingly, intravenous administration of infliximab for treatment of rheumatoid arthritis caused regression of CNV in patients with AMD[89]; moreover, intravenous infliximab also led to reductions in macular edema in patients with DME.[90] It is not clear if these effects of TNF-α are independent of its upregulation of VEGF; if separate pathways are involved, TNF-α inhibition alone or in combination with VEGF inhibition could provide an additional therapeutic option.

EPHS AND EPHRINS

Ephs comprise a large family of receptor tyrosine kinases that are activated upon binding with their cognate membrane-bound ligands, the ephrins.[91,92] EphrinAs are attached to the cell membrane by a glycosylphosphatidyl anchor while the ephrinBs have transmembrane and cytoplasmic signaling domains (Figure 4.7).[93] The Ephs also fall into two

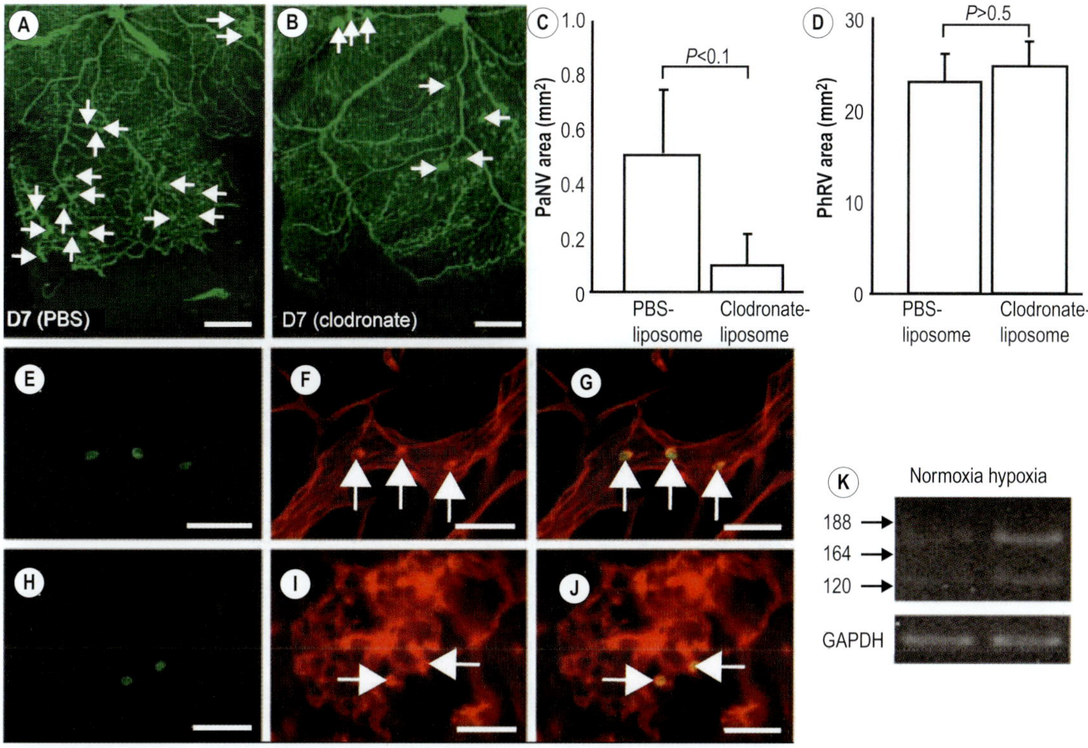

Figure 4.4 Monocytes contribute to pathological retinal neovascularization. In a retinopathy of prematurity model, postnatal day zero (P0) rats were maintained for 10 days in 80% oxygen, interrupted daily by 30 minutes in room air, followed by a progressive return to 80% oxygen. This treatment led to an avascular retina. On P10, corresponding to study day 0 (D0), retinal revascularization was induced by maintaining the rats in room air for an additional 7 days (D7). (A–C) At D7, pathological neovascularization (PaNV; arrows in A and B) was significantly inhibited by treatment with clodronate liposomes compared to control liposomes (n = 8 for both treatments; means ± standard deviation). (D) Physiological neovascular area (PhRV) was not significantly affected by treatment with clodronate liposomes ($P > 0.05$). (E–J) Influx of monocytes was observed just before and during pathological neovascularization. (H–J) Monocytes were labeled with a fluorescein conjugated antibody to CD13 (E and H), while rhodamine-conjugated *Concanavalin* A was used to label the retinal vasculature and adherent leukocytes (F and I). As shown by superposition of these figures (panels G and J), the concanavalin A and CD13 staining co-localized, indicating that the adherent leukocytes were monocytes. (K) In cultured peripheral blood monocytes obtained from retinopathologic rats at D7, exposure to hypoxia (1% oxygen) led to marked increase in expression of vascular endothelial growth factor mRNA compared to exposure to normoxia (21% oxygen). PBS, phosphate-buffered saline. Scale bars: (A and B) 0.5 mm and (E–J) 50 μm. Reproduced from Ishida S, Usui T, Yamashiro K, et al. VEGF164-mediated inflammation is required for pathological, but not physiological, ischemia-induced retinal neovascularization. J Exp Med 2003;198:483–489.

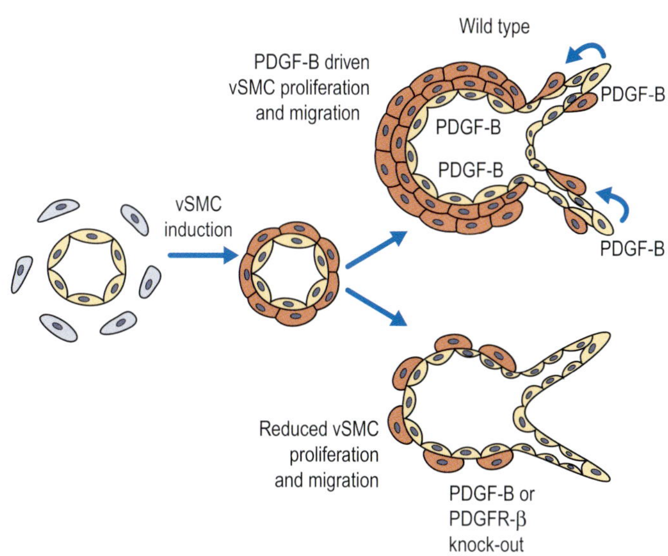

Figure 4.5 Platelet-derived growth factor (PDGF)-B regulates the development of blood vessel walls. During blood vessel development, the nascent endothelial tube (yellow) is surrounded by undifferentiated mesenchymal cells (gray) which are induced to differentiate into vascular smooth-muscle cells (vSMC), and to form a surrounding sheath (red). During further development of the vascular network, with concomitant growth and sprouting of blood vessels, PDGF-B derived from the endothelium further promotes vSMC proliferation and migration. These proliferative and migratory responses are reduced in mice in which PDGF-B or PDGFR-β have been genetically ablated, leading to defective coating of capillaries by pericytes, as well as to vSMC hypoplasia in larger vessels. Reproduced from Hellstrom M, Kalen M, Lindahl P, et al. Role of PDGF-B and PDGFR-beta in recruitment of vascular smooth muscle cells and pericytes during embryonic blood vessel formation in the mouse. Development 1999;126:3047–3055.

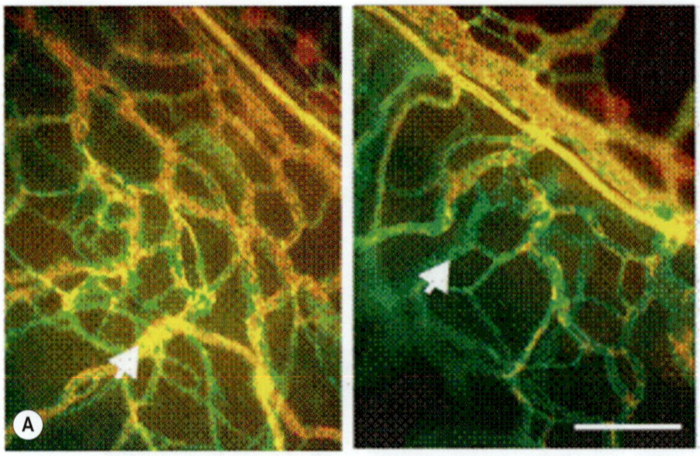

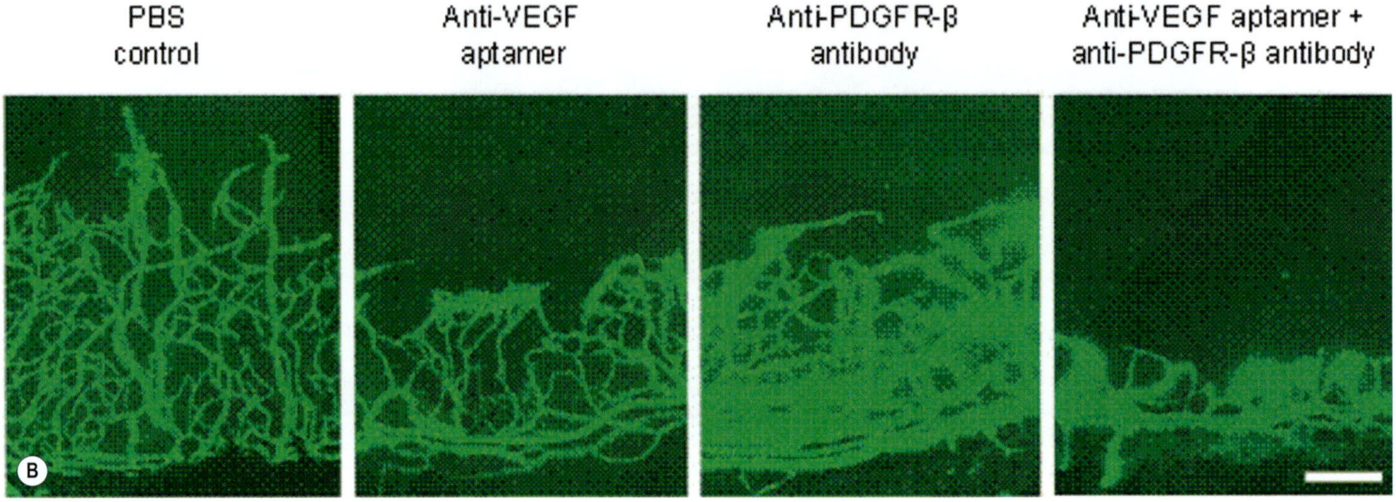

Figure 4.6 The role of platelet-derived growth factor (PDGF)-B on blood vessel growth and mural cell coverage in a corneal neovascularization model. (A) Endothelial cells were labeled by staining with lectin (green) and mural cells were stained with an antibody against smooth-muscle actin (red). Starting at 10 days following corneal injury, mice received daily intraperitoneal injections of an anti-PDGFR-β antibody or phosphate-buffered saline (PBS), and were sacrificed at 20 days postinjury. Treatment with the anti-PDGF-β antibody led to reduced mural cell coverage compared to controls (arrow). Scale bar = 20 μm. (B) Following induction of corneal injury, mice received daily intraperitoneal injections of one of the following: PBS, a polyethylene-glycolated anti-vascular endothelial growth factor (VEGF) aptamer, an anti-PDGFR-β antibody, or both the anti-VEGF aptamer and the anti-PDGFR-β antibody. Neovasculature (green) was stained by fluorescein isothiocyanate-concanavalin A. Neovascularization was significantly reduced by the anti-VEGF aptamer compared with either PBS or the anti-PEGFR-β antibody ($P < 0.01$); inhibition of both VEGF and PDGF-B signaling led to a further significant reduction ($P < 0.05$), compared to inhibition of VEGF signaling alone. Scale bar = 100 μm. Adapted from Jo N, Mailhos C, Ju M, et al. Inhibition of platelet-derived growth factor B signaling enhances the efficacy of anti-vascular endothelial growth factor therapy in multiple models of ocular neovascularization. Am J Pathol 2006;168:2036–2053.

broad groups, EphA and EphB, with the EphAs binding primarily, although not exclusively, to members of ephrinA subclass, while EphBs similarly tend to bind preferentially to ephrinB ligands.

Owing to the association of ephrins to cell membranes, ephrin-Eph signaling requires cell–cell contact. A notable feature of their interaction is that signaling can proceed not only in the forward direction, through activation of Eph kinases, but also in the reverse direction. Their interactions are critical for a wide variety of processes, including proper patterning in the development of the nervous[94] and cardiovascular[91] systems, immune cell trafficking,[95] angiogenesis,[92] and insulin secretion by pancreatic β cells.[96]

There are relatively few studies of ephrinA/EphA signaling in angiogenesis or ocular neovascularization. EphA-deficient endothelial cells were unable to migrate and form capillary tubes,[97] and the administration of soluble EphA2 receptors, which would be expected to block EphA2 signaling, was found to inhibit neovascularization in rodent corneal[98] and retinal[99] models.

There is more support for the importance of ephrinB/ephB interactions in angiogenesis, especially with respect to ephrinB2 and EphB4; ablation of either gene led to defective vascular development.[100,101] Their respective expression patterns are believed to underlie the establishment of arterial or venous identity, with ephrinB2 reported to

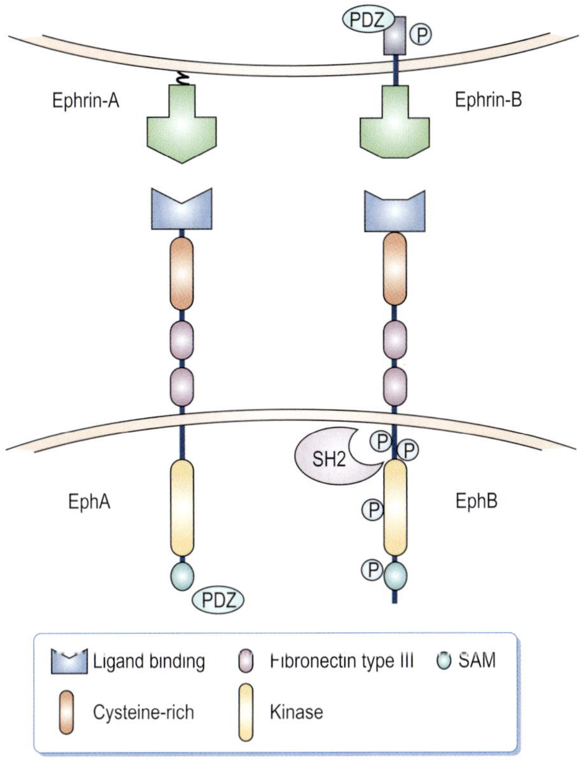

Figure 4.7 Ephrins and their Eph receptors. While both ephrins and Eph receptors are membrane-tethered proteins, ephrinBs traverse the membrane and possess a cytoplasmic signaling domain while ephrinAs do not. Ephrin-Eph binding results in receptor clustering, followed by autophosphorylation of multiple tyrosine residues and docking of downstream effectors through *src*-homology domains. The presence of a sterile alpha motif (SAM) and a PDZ domain (shown here for the carboxy-terminus of EphA, but also present in EphB), promotes ligand-induced receptor clustering. Reproduced from Dodelet VC, Pasquale EB. Eph receptors and ephrin ligands: embryogenesis to tumorigenesis. Oncogene 2000;19:5614–5619.

be expressed primarily on arteries[100] and EphB4 predominantly on veins.[100,101] EphrinB2 also has been found to be involved in recruitment of mural cells to microvessels.[102]

EphrinB2, EphB2, and EphB3 were all expressed in fibroproliferative membranes of patients with retinopathy of prematurity and proliferative DR.[103] However, experimental models have yet to resolve completely the role of EphB/ephrinB signaling in ocular neovascular disease. Angiogenesis was promoted in corneal models by ephrinB2[104] as well as by fusion proteins EphB1-Fc,[105] and ephrinB2-Fc[106]; in contrast, soluble monomeric EphB4[107,108] or ephrinB2 inhibited the development of pathological neovascularization.[108] Further investigation is required to delineate the molecular mechanisms involved in these effects.

NOTCH

Notch is a 300-kDa transmembrane protein, represented in mammals by four members, Notch1 through Notch4. Notch is activated by transmembrane ligands during cell to cell contact; in mammals, these ligands are Jagged1, Jagged2, and the Delta-like family (Dll1 through Dll4, with Dll4 being the most intensively investigated). Ligand binding leads to the proteolytic cleavage of Notch, releasing an intracellular domain that is translocated to the nucleus, inducing transcription of Notch-activated genes.[109,110] Notch signaling plays a key role in pattern formation in a wide variety of tissues, and is essential for such disparate processes as somitogenesis, neurogenesis, and development of the kidney and the cardiovascular system.[109]

Studies on Notch signaling in angiogenesis have identified Dll4 as the principal Notch ligand mediating vascular development.[110] In a study of the developing retinal vasculature, Dll4 was expressed in tip cells at the end of vascular sprouts, as well as in stalk cells, capillaries, arterial endothelium, and mural cells of mature arteries.[111] In addition, inhibition of Dll4/Notch signaling caused dramatic increases in tip cell formation, endothelial cell proliferation, and filopodial extension.[112] Furthermore, heterozygous ablation of the murine *dll4* gene also led to hyperbranching of the retinal vasculature (Figure 4.8)[112] while in a tumor model, blockade of Dll4 led to increased, but poorly organized, tumor vascularity and decreased tumor growth.[113]

Taken together, these findings suggest that Dll4 acts as a negative regulator of VEGF signaling to control aberrant angiogenic sprouting and branching. It remains to be seen whether interference with Notch signaling will provide another means of controlling angiogenesis, independent of VEGF, or whether it leads to excessive sprouting without a reduction in neovascular mass.

ANGIOPOIETINS

The angiopoietins 1 through 4 (Ang1–Ang4) are secreted ligands for Tie2, a receptor tyrosine kinase that is found primarily on endothelial cells and plays an essential role in the development and remodeling of the vasculature. Ang1 and Ang2 are the most intensively investigated members of the group, with Ang1 activating Tie2 and Ang2 usually functioning as a Tie2 antagonist.[114] Genetic ablation of Tie2 was found be embryonically lethal due to vascular defects[115]; similar defects occurred with Ang1 ablation[116] or overexpression of Ang2.[117] Both Ang1 and Ang2 have been studied extensively as potential therapeutic targets for affecting angiogenesis.

Angiopoietin 1

In angiogenesis, Ang1 acts as a chemoattractant for endothelial cells[118] while also promoting endothelial cell sprouting and facilitating tissue invasion by nascent blood vessels through activation of MMPs.[119] In transgenic mice, blood vessels induced by overexpression of VEGF were leaky, while the vessels induced by overexpression of Ang1 were nonleaky; coexpression of both molecules had an additive effect on angiogenesis but the resulting vessels were nonleaky, suggesting that Ang1 may reduce the vascular permeability resulting from chronic inflammation and elevated levels of VEGF.[120] Ang1 also has been found to suppress VEGF-mediated induction of inflammatory markers such as ICAM-1,[121] vascular cell adhesion molecule-1,[121] and tissue factor.[122] These actions are consistent with the overall action of Ang1 as a stabilizer of the quiescent vasculature.[123]

In studies with rodent models, the overexpression of Ang1 was found to inhibit laser-induced CNV and ischemia-induced retinal neovascularization, while also reducing VEGF-mediated retinal vascular permeability,[124] but it had no effect on established neovascularization.[125] Together these studies suggest that intravitreal injection of Ang1 could prove a useful approach in preventing ocular neovascularization and inflammation.

Angiopoietin 2

The principal sites of Ang2 synthesis are endothelial cells,[126] and arterial smooth-muscle cells.[126] Ang2 expression is especially marked at sites of vascular remodeling,[114] and it is upregulated by hypoxia and VEGF.[127,128] Ang2 acts primarily to destabilize the vascular endothelium; it is stored in Weibel–Palade bodies of endothelial cells (Figure 4.9),[95] and is released in response to exogenous stimuli such as proinflammatory cytokines.[129]

Clinically, Ang2 has been found in association with VEGF in highly vascular areas of CNV membranes in patients with a variety of ocular conditions,[130] as well as in the vitreous of eyes of patients with DR.[131] There is evidence that Ang2 and VEGF may act cooperatively in inducing ocular neovascularization. In rodent models, Ang2 enhanced corneal neovascularization in combination with VEGF, while

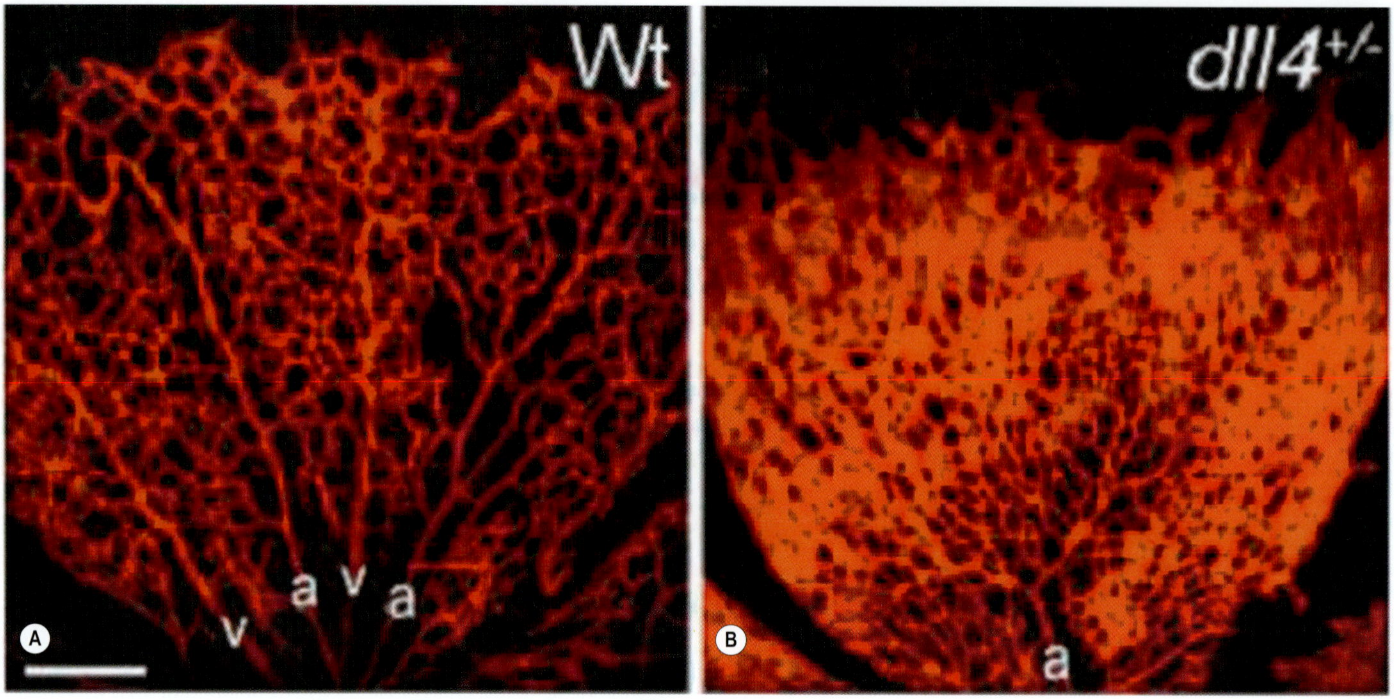

Figure 4.8 Inhibition of Delta4 signaling leads to increased vessel mass. Compared to wild-type (Wt) mice (A), retinal vessels stained at postnatal day 5 in mice for which *dll4* was heterozygously ablated (B) show hyperbranching within the vascular plexus (a, artery; v, vein). Retinal vessels were stained with isolectin B_4. Scale bar, 250 μm. Adapted from Suchting S, Freitas C, le Noble F, et al. The Notch ligand Delta-like 4 negatively regulates endothelial tip cell formation and vessel branching. Proc Natl Acad Sci USA 2007;104:3225–3230.

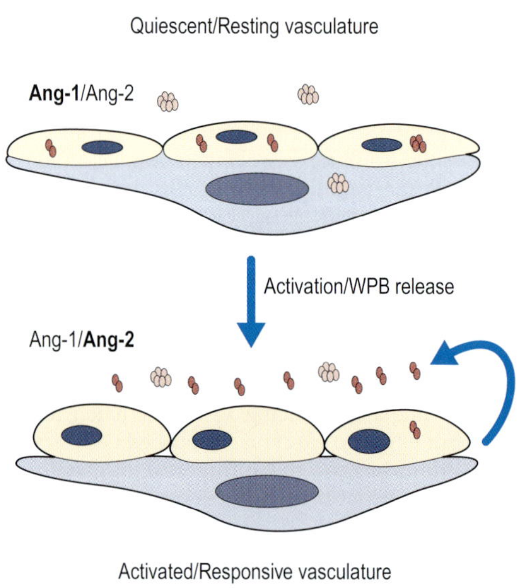

Figure 4.9 Regulation of vascular responsiveness by angiopoietins Ang1 and Ang2. Ang1 (multimeric, white) is secreted constitutively at a low level by mural (periendothelial) cells, and acts on the resting endothelium to sustain a low-level activation of Tie2, thereby helping to maintain the luminal cell surface in an antithrombotic and antiadhesive state (upper panel). Ang2 (dimeric, grey) is stored in Weibel–Palade bodies (WPB) in the endothelium, and during endothelial cell activation is released from them, along with other stored factors, leading to the Ang1/Ang2 ratio being altered more in favor of Ang2 (lower panel). As a result, the endothelial cell layer becomes destabilized and more responsive to proinflammatory stimuli. Reproduced from Pfaff D, Fiedler U, Augustin HG. Emerging roles of the angiopoietin-Tie and the ephrin-Eph systems as regulators of cell trafficking. J Leukoc Biol 2006;80:719–726.

insufficient on its own,[132] and inhibition of Ang2 prevented VEGF-induced corneal neovascularization.[133] Studies also have shown that Ang2 and VEGF can act synergistically to enhance the permeability of retinal endothelium.[134] Depending on the concomitant levels of molecules such as VEGF or Ang1, Ang2 can increase or decrease angiogenesis.[135] In transgenic mice, induction of Ang2 expression in the presence of elevated VEGF levels led to increased neovascularization, whereas induction of Ang2 when VEGF was not elevated led to its regression.[136] These interactions have led to the suggestion that the administration of Ang2, in combination with a VEGF antagonist, might provide a therapeutic approach in treating ocular neovascularization.[137]

ERYTHROPOIETIN

Erythropoietin is a 30-kDa glycoprotein, upregulated by hypoxia, and known primarily for its actions as an inducer of erythropoiesis.[138] Other functions of erythropoietin are being defined, however, including neuroprotection,[139] and promotion of angiogenesis. Erythropoietin has been shown to contribute to angiogenesis in response to ischemia through upregulation of VEGF/VEGFR and in promoting recruitment of endothelial progenitor cells.[140]

Clinical evidence supporting a role for erythropoietin in ocular neovascularization comes from studies demonstrating elevations of erythropoietin in the eyes of patients with DME,[141] and DR, especially in cases of active proliferative disease,[142] and an increased risk of retinopathy of prematurity in infants treated with erythropoietin.[143] Moreover, in a murine model of retinopathy of prematurity, neovascularization was significantly inhibited by a soluble form of the erythropoietin receptor.[142] While these preliminary findings are suggestive, additional evidence is required to establish erythropoietin as a molecular target for antiangiogenesis therapy.

MATRIX METALLOPROTEINASES

MMPs, a large group of enzymes that promote angiogenesis through their degradative action on the extracellular matrix, have been extensively investigated given their importance in tumor vascularization and metastasis.[144] Several studies also have examined their role in promoting ocular neovascularization. In cultured RPE cells, MMP expression was upregulated by angiogenic factors, including VEGF,[82] FGF2,[82] and TNF-α.[82] MMPs were also found to cleave matrix-bound forms of VEGF, releasing soluble fragments and altering its bioavailability.[145] Another MMP action related to angiogenesis involved exposing a cryptic epitope of collagen IV that is needed for full expression of laser-induced CNV in mice.[146]

INTEGRINS

Integrins comprise a family of heterodimeric cell surface receptors that mediate cellular responses to extracellular matrix ligands such as fibronectin and vitronectin. They have been studied intensively for their importance in cancer, where they affect tumor angiogenesis, growth, and metastasis.[147] At least two dozen combinations between different α and β subunits have been identified.

Several studies have defined a role for α_v integrins (particularly $\alpha_v\beta_1$, $\alpha_v\beta_3$, and $\alpha_v\beta_5$) and $\alpha_5\beta_1$ in the pathogenesis of ocular neovascular disease. Expression of $\alpha_v\beta_3$ was identified in active neovascular lesions of eyes with AMD and proliferative DR, while $\alpha_v\beta_5$ was found only in eyes with proliferative DR; neither integrin was expressed on mature quiescent blood vessels.[148] Inhibition of ocular neovascularization by blocking $\alpha_v\beta_3$ integrin responses has been demonstrated in experimental models using peptide antagonists,[149] and a monoclonal antibody conjugated to mitomycin C.[150] Agents that target both $\alpha_v\beta_3$ and $\alpha_v\beta_5$ have also shown utility in preventing experimental ocular neovascularization; these include a peptide antagonist,[148] a peptide conjugated to a proapoptotic sequence,[151] and the small-molecule antagonists, SB-267268,[152] EMD478761,[153] and JNJ-26076713.[154]

Interactions between the $\alpha_5\beta_1$ integrin and its ligand fibronectin have been found to contribute to an angiogenic pathway that is distinct from that of VEGF[155]; moreover, blocking $\alpha_5\beta_1$-mediated responses has been shown to reduce ocular neovascularization in a variety of murine models. JSM5562, a small-molecule antagonist, decreased corneal neovascularization,[156] while the related molecule JSM6427 reduced the formation of laser-induced CNV[157] and ischemia-induced retinal neovascularization.[158] JSM6427 also blocked migration and tube formation in cultured endothelial cells, suggesting a key role for $\alpha_5\beta_1$/fibronectin interactions in these processes.[158] Taken together, these investigations suggest that inhibiting integrin-mediated responses is a promising approach in the treatment of ocular neovascular disease.

COMPONENTS OF THE COMPLEMENT CASCADE

Several lines of evidence have identified a role for the complement cascade in ocular neovascular disease. Genetic studies have identified an association between specific haplotypes of factor H, a regulatory component in complement function, and an elevated risk of developing neovascular AMD.[159] Complement factors C3a and C5a have been detected in the drusen found in the eyes of patients with AMD; furthermore, subretinal deposits of C3a and C5a were generated early in the course of laser-induced CNV in mice.[160]

Studies have demonstrated that genetic ablation of C3[161] or the receptors for C3a and C5a[160] inhibited laser-induced CNV in mice. These findings also correlated with reductions in the levels of VEGF[160,161] and in leukocyte recruitment,[160] supporting the hypothesis that complement-mediated inflammation plays an active role in CNV.

INHIBITORS OF ANGIOGENESIS

Much research has focused on the factors that promote angiogenesis in ocular neovascular disease, yet several naturally occurring endogenous inhibitors also have been identified. These include pigment epithelium-derived factor (PEDF), soluble VEGFR1, the complement regulatory protein CD59, $VEGF_{xxx}b$ isoforms, and the tryptophanyl-tRNA fragment.

PIGMENT EPITHELIUM-DERIVED FACTOR

PEDF is a 50-kDa glycoprotein, highly expressed by the RPE,[162] that exhibits many properties expected of an endogenous inhibitor of angiogenesis. Specifically, PEDF inhibited endothelial cell migration[163] and induced endothelial cell apoptosis *in vitro*[164] and inhibited aberrant blood vessel growth in a murine model of ischemia-induced retinopathy.[164] Moreover, PEDF has been shown to downregulate VEGF expression in endothelial cells,[165] to inhibit VEGF-induced endothelial cell permeability,[166] and to inhibit VEGF-induced signaling through VEGFR1.[167]

Clinical studies have yielded inconsistent findings, in that vitreous PEDF levels have been reported to be lower[168] or, alternately, higher[169] in patients with proliferative DR. While retinal neovascularization in preclinical models was shown to be inhibited by PEDF administered by injection[163] or by expression from a transgene,[170] another study determined that the effects of PEDF on laser-induced CNV were dose-dependent, with inhibition occurring at low doses and promotion seen at higher doses.[171]

PEDF has undergone evaluation in a phase I trial in which a single intravitreal injection of an adenoviral vector expressing human PEDF was administered to patients with AMD; results were favorable, with most subjects experiencing either an improvement or no change in vision at 6 months postinjection.[172] However, until the inconsistencies found in animal models with regard to dose-related promotion of CNV are resolved,[171] particular caution is required in the clinical use of PEDF.

SOLUBLE VEGF RECEPTOR 1

Soluble VEGFR1 is an alternately spliced, secreted isoform that lacks the exons coding for the transmembrane and signaling domains.[173] Since soluble VEGFR1 binds to VEGF and blocks its interaction with VEGF receptors, it acts as a naturally occurring inhibitor of neovascularization and has been found to be essential for preserving corneal avascularity.[174] As previously mentioned, an engineered molecule containing the VEGF-binding domains, both VEGFR1 and VEGFR2 (VEGF-Trap), is being examined clinically as a therapeutic agent.

$VEGF_{XXX}b$ ISOFORMS

$VEGF_{xxx}b$ denotes a family of VEGF isoforms, parallel to those normally considered for their impacts on angiogenesis, but which have an altered carboxy-terminus due to alternative splicing; the resulting variants can bind VEGFR-2, but since they cannot mediate downstream signaling they serve as endogenous competitive inhibitors of VEGF.[175] $VEGF_{xxx}b$ isoforms constituted 64% of the total VEGF in the vitreous of nondiabetic patients and only 12% of the total VEGF in the vitreous of diabetic patients.[176] In studies with murine models of corneal[175] and retinal[32] neovascularization, administration of $VEGF_{xxx}b$ inhibited blood vessel growth. Together, these findings suggest that $VEGF_{xxx}b$ isoforms may be a component of normal homeostasis and that their downregulation may contribute to the pathogenesis of ocular neovascular disease. The efficacy of anti-VEGF agents may thus depend on the local VEGF isoform expression pattern.

COMPLEMENTARY REGULATORY PROTEIN C59

As mentioned previously, the extent of laser-induced CNV in a mouse model was dependent on several components of the complement cascade. Further support for this mechanism has come from a recent study showing that ablation of CD59, a complement regulatory protein, promoted the development of CNV in mice, while intravitreal or intraperitoneal administration of a soluble CD59-Fc fusion protein was inhibitory.[177] These findings suggest that C59 serves as an endogenous inhibitor of ocular neovascularization, by downregulating the complement cascade, and it has been proposed that a soluble form of C59 could serve as a therapeutic agent.

TRYPTOPHANYL-tRNA SYNTHASE FRAGMENT

Tryptophanyl-tRNA synthase fragment (T2-TrpRS) is a 43-kDa natural cleavage product of tryptophanyl-tRNA synthase[178] that was shown to inhibit both physiological retinal angiogenesis and VEGF-induced angiogenesis in murine models.[178] In a retinopathy of prematurity model, T2-TrpRS dramatically inhibited preretinal pathological tuft formation while enhancing physiological revascularization of the obliterated retinal vasculature.[179] These actions may result from its binding to vascular endothelial cadherin, a component of the intercellular junctions between endothelial cells.[180] Recently, the combination of T2-TrpRS and an anti-VEGF aptamer strongly inhibited pathological neovascularization in a retinopathy of prematurity model.[181] This promising combination approach merits further exploration in the treatment of ocular neovascular disease.

OTHER INHIBITORS

As indicated in Table 4.1, there are numerous endogenous factors which have antiangiogenic activity. While the present chapter has focused on certain factors for which evidence supports a role in ocular neovascularization, a comprehensive discussion of endogenous inhibitors is beyond the scope of this chapter. For a comprehensive discussion of these factors, the reader is referred to the review by Zhang and Ma.[182]

SUMMARY

Systematic study of the mechanisms underlying pathological ocular neovascularization in preclinical models as well as in humans has yielded a wealth of knowledge about the numerous proangiogenic and antiangiogenic factors that modulate these processes. A major focus of research has been the role of the angiogenic promoters, the most potent of which (identified to date) is VEGF. VEGF's properties as the principal inducer of vascular permeability and its upregulation in a hypoxic environment also greatly influence the pathology associated with ocular neovascularization. PDGF-B, a molecule structurally related to VEGF, is especially crucial for the recruitment of pericytes and smooth-muscle cells to the developing vasculature and plays a key role in neovascularization of the retina and cornea. The contributions of TNF-α and erythropoietin in angiogenesis have not been as well elucidated.

Investigations involving several other ligand receptor systems have also provided evidence of their contributions to vascular development. These include the Eph kinases and their ephrin ligands, which appear to be critical for establishing arterial and venous identity, and the angiopoietins, Ang1 and Ang2. Overall, Ang1 acts to stabilize the vasculature, and inhibits VEGF-induced increases in vascular permeability, while Ang2 is primarily a destabilizing agent, which, depending on the experimental conditions, can interact with VEGF either to promote neovascularization or to induce its regression. Another signaling pathway, the Dll4-Notch system, also acts to regulate vascular patterning by inhibiting VEGF-induced angiogenic sprouting and branching.

Finally, three other important classes of angiogenic promoters have been identified: the MMPs, integrins, and components of the complement cascade. The MMPs affect VEGF signaling by releasing it from sequestered deposits in the extracellular matrix and also by exposing a cryptic collagen epitope that has been found to promote ocular neovascularization. The integrins, which are well established as mediators of interactions between the extracellular matrix and intercellular components, have recently been shown to be involved in ocular neovascularization as well. With respect to the complement cascade, genetic studies have demonstrated an increased risk of AMD for certain haplotypes of factor H, while preclinical studies have demonstrated roles for factors C3a and C5a in the development of ocular neovascularization.

Several naturally occurring factors have been identified as potential inhibitors of ocular neovascularization. PEDF acts in many assays to inhibit angiogenesis, but it may also promote angiogenesis in some contexts. Endogenous inhibitors of VEGF signaling have also been found; these include soluble VEGFR1 and a group of alternately spliced isoforms, denoted $VEGF_{xxx}b$. Finally, T2-TrpRS, a naturally occurring fragment of the enzyme tryptophanyl-tRNA synthase as well as the complement regulatory protein C59, have been found to inhibit ocular neovascularization in experimental models.

Research investigating the roles of these molecules in regulating angiogenesis has already yielded clinical benefits. Two agents targeting VEGF, pegaptanib and ranibizumab, have received clinical approval for AMD while alternative strategies for inactivating VEGF signaling, including RNA interference and a VEGF receptor fusion protein, are under active study. Infliximab, an antibody against TNF-α, has also shown promise in small-scale clinical studies, while preclinical studies suggest that PDGF-B, components of the complement cascade, and the α_5 integrins are potential molecular targets. Moreover, the endogenous inhibitors may also prove clinically useful. Thus a variety of agents, whether administered alone or as adjunctive therapy with agents targeting VEGF, offer the promise of expanding the range of treatments for ocular neovascular diseases.

Key points

- Systematic study of the mechanisms controlling angiogenesis has led to the identification of a number of proangiogenic and antiangiogenic factors active in ocular neovascularization.
- VEGF has been established as a master regulator of angiogenesis and a potent promoter of vascular permeability, making it an attractive target in treating ocular neovascularization. Two anti-VEGF agents have been approved, with others in clinical trials.
- PDGF-B plays a crucial role in the recruitment of mural cells to developing blood vessels; combination approaches targeting PDGF-B and VEGF are especially effective against ocular neovascularization in preclinical models.
- TNF-α has been shown to promote pathological angiogenesis in preclinical studies while small case series involving TNF-α inhibition have demonstrated therapeutic effects in ocular neovascular disease.
- In keeping with its inflammatory nature, components C3a and C5a of the complement cascade may contribute to the development of ocular neovascularization.
- Integrins are involved in an angiogenic pathway distinct from that of VEGF; small-molecule inhibitors of $\alpha_5\beta_1$ have been shown to reduce ocular neovascularization in preclinical models.
- MMPs promote angiogenesis by degrading the extracellular matrix to facilitate invasion by nascent blood vessels, by releasing matrix-bound growth factors, and by exposing cryptic proangiogenic epitopes.
- Several ligand receptor systems, including the angiopoietins-Tie2, ephrins-Eph kinases, and Delta4-Notch, are all essential for angiogenesis, but further work is required before this knowledge can be exploited in developing new therapies.
- Various endogenous inhibitors of angiogenesis have been identified which may prove useful as therapeutic agents. These include PEDF, complement regulatory protein C59, soluble VEGFR1, a fragment of tryptophanyl-tRNA synthase, and alternatively spliced VEGF isoforms.

REFERENCES

1. Folkman J. Tumor angiogenesis: therapeutic implications. N Engl J Med 1971;285:1182–1186.
2. Ferrara N. Vascular endothelial growth factor: basic science and clinical progress. Endocr Rev 2004;25:581–611.
3. Ferrara N, Davis-Smyth T. The biology of vascular endothelial growth factor. Endocr Rev 1997;18:4–25.
4. Starita C, Patel M, Katz B, et al. Vascular endothelial growth factor and the potential therapeutic use of pegaptanib (Macugen) in diabetic retinopathy. Dev Ophthalmol 2007;39:122–148.
5. Robinson CJ, Stringer SE. The splice variants of vascular endothelial growth factor (VEGF) and their receptors. J Cell Sci 2001;114:853–865.
6. Leung DW, Cachianes G, Kuang WJ, et al. Vascular endothelial growth factor is a secreted angiogenic mitogen. Science 1989;246:1306–1309.
7. Alon T, Hemo I, Itin A, et al. Vascular endothelial growth factor acts as a survival factor for newly formed retinal vessels and has implications for retinopathy of prematurity. Nat Med 1995;1:1024–1028.
8. Csaky KG, Baffi JZ, Byrnes GA, et al. Recruitment of marrow-derived endothelial cells to experimental choroidal neovascularization by local expression of vascular endothelial growth factor. Exp Eye Res 2004;78:1107–1116.
9. Lamoreaux WJ, Fitzgerald ME, Reiner A, et al. Vascular endothelial growth factor increases release of gelatinase A and decreases release of tissue inhibitor of metalloproteinases by microvascular endothelial cells *in vitro*. Microvasc Res 1998;55:29–42.
10. Pepper MS, Ferrara N, Orci L, et al. Vascular endothelial growth factor (VEGF) induces plasminogen activators and plasminogen activator inhibitor-1 in microvascular endothelial cells. Biochem Biophys Res Commun 1991;181:902–906.
11. Uhlmann S, Friedrichs U, Eichler W, et al. Direct measurement of VEGF-induced nitric oxide production by choroidal endothelial cells. Microvasc Res 2001;62:179–189.
12. Papapetropoulos A, Garcia-Cardena G, Madri JA, et al. Nitric oxide production contributes to the angiogenic properties of vascular endothelial growth factor in human endothelial cells. J Clin Invest 1997;100: 3131–3139.
13. Senger DR, Connolly DT, Van de Water L, et al. Purification and NH_2-terminal amino acid sequence of guinea pig tumor-secreted vascular permeability factor. Cancer Res 1990;50:1774–1778.
14. Adamis AP, Shima DT, Yeo KT, et al. Synthesis and secretion of vascular permeability factor/vascular endothelial growth factor by human retinal pigment epithelial cells. Biochem Biophys Res Commun 1993;193: 631–638.
15. Aiello LP, Northrup JM, Keyt BA, et al. Hypoxic regulation of vascular endothelial growth factor in retinal cells. Arch Ophthalmol 1995;113:1538–1544.
16. Famiglietti EV, Stopa EG, McGookin ED, et al. Immunocytochemical localization of vascular endothelial growth factor in neurons and glial cells of human retina. Brain Res 2003;969:195–204.
17. Blaauwgeers HG, Holtkamp GM, Rutten H, et al. Polarized vascular endothelial growth factor secretion by human retinal pigment epithelium and localization of vascular endothelial growth factor receptors on the inner choriocapillaris. Evidence for a trophic paracrine relation. Am J Pathol 1999;155:421–428.
18. Nishijima K, Ng YS, Zhong L, et al. Vascular endothelial growth factor-A is a survival factor for retinal neurons and a critical neuroprotectant during the adaptive response to ischemic injury. Am J Pathol 2007;171:53–67.
19. Kim KJ, Li B, Winer J, et al. Inhibition of vascular endothelial growth factor-induced angiogenesis suppresses tumour growth *in vivo*. Nature 1993;362:841–844.
20. Kliffen M, Sharma HS, Mooy CM, et al. Increased expression of angiogenic growth factors in age-related maculopathy. Br J Ophthalmol 1997;81:154–162.
21. Lopez PF, Sippy BD, Lambert HM, et al. Transdifferentiated retinal pigment epithelial cells are immunoreactive for vascular endothelial growth factor in surgically excised age-related macular degeneration-related choroidal neovascular membranes. Invest Ophthalmol Vis Sci 1996;37: 855–868.
22. Tolentino MJ, Miller JW, Gragoudas ES, et al. Vascular endothelial growth factor is sufficient to produce iris neovascularization and neovascular glaucoma in a nonhuman primate. Arch Ophthalmol 1996;114:964–970.
23. Miller JW, Adamis AP, Shima DT, et al. Vascular endothelial growth factor/vascular permeability factor is temporally and spatially correlated with ocular angiogenesis in a primate model. Am J Pathol 1994;145: 574–584.
24. Spilsbury K, Garrett KL, Shen WY, et al. Overexpression of vascular endothelial growth factor (VEGF) in the retinal pigment epithelium leads to the development of choroidal neovascularization. Am J Pathol 2000;157:135–144.
25. Schwesinger C, Yee C, Rohan RM, et al. Intrachoroidal neovascularization in transgenic mice overexpressing vascular endothelial growth factor in the retinal pigment epithelium. Am J Pathol 2001;158:1161–1172.
26. Aiello LP, Pierce EA, Foley ED, et al. Suppression of retinal neovascularization *in vivo* by inhibition of vascular endothelial growth factor (VEGF) using soluble VEGF-receptor chimeric proteins. Proc Natl Acad Sci USA 1995;92:10457–10461.
27. Saishin Y, Takahashi K, Lima e Silva R, et al. VEGF-TRAP(R1R2) suppresses choroidal neovascularization and VEGF-induced breakdown of the blood–retinal barrier. J Cell Physiol 2003;195:241–248.
28. Ishida S, Usui T, Yamashiro K, et al. VEGF164-mediated inflammation is required for pathological, but not physiological, ischemia-induced retinal neovascularization. J Exp Med 2003;198:483–489.
29. Adamis AP, Shima DT, Tolentino MJ, et al. Inhibition of vascular endothelial growth factor prevents retinal ischemia-associated iris neovascularization in a nonhuman primate. Arch Ophthalmol 1996;114:66–71.
30. Amano S, Rohan R, Kuroki M, et al. Requirement for vascular endothelial growth factor in wound- and inflammation-related corneal neovascularization. Invest Ophthalmol Vis Sci 1998;39:18–22.
31. Krzystolik MG, Afshari MA, Adamis AP, et al. Prevention of experimental choroidal neovascularization with intravitreal anti-vascular endothelial growth factor antibody fragment. Arch Ophthalmol 2002;120:338–346.
32. Konopatskaya O, Churchill AJ, Harper SJ, et al. VEGF165b, an endogenous C-terminal splice variant of VEGF, inhibits retinal neovascularization in mice. Mol Vis 2006;12:626–632.
33. Reich SJ, Fosnot J, Kuroki A, et al. Small interfering RNA (siRNA) targeting VEGF effectively inhibits ocular neovascularization in a mouse model. Mol Vis 2003;9:210–216.
34. Shen J, Samul R, Silva RL, et al. Suppression of ocular neovascularization with siRNA targeting VEGF receptor 1. Gene Ther 2006;13:225–234.
35. Robinson GS, Pierce EA, Rook SL, et al. Oligodeoxynucleotides inhibit retinal neovascularization in a murine model of proliferative retinopathy. Proc Natl Acad Sci USA 1996;93:4851–4856.
36. Sakurai E, Taguchi H, Anand A, et al. Targeted disruption of the CD18 or ICAM-1 gene inhibits choroidal neovascularization. Invest Ophthalmol Vis Sci 2003;44:2743–2749.
37. Usui T, Ishida S, Yamashiro K, et al. VEGF164(165) as the pathological isoform: differential leukocyte and endothelial responses through VEGFR1 and VEGFR2. Invest Ophthalmol Vis Sci 2004;45:368–374.
38. Sakurai E, Anand A, Ambati BK, et al. Macrophage depletion inhibits experimental choroidal neovascularization. Invest Ophthalmol Vis Sci 2003;44:3578–3585.
39. Harmey JH, Dimitriadis E, Kay E, et al. Regulation of macrophage production of vascular endothelial growth factor (VEGF) by hypoxia and transforming growth factor beta-1. Ann Surg Oncol 1998;5:271–278.
40. Ng EW, Shima DT, Calias P, et al. Pegaptanib, a targeted anti-VEGF aptamer for ocular vascular disease. Nat Rev Drug Discov 2006;5: 123–132.
41. Ferrara N, Damico L, Shams N, et al. Development of ranibizumab, an anti-vascular endothelial growth factor antigen binding fragment, as therapy for neovascular age-related macular degeneration. Retina 2006;26:859–870.
42. Lynch SS, Cheng CM. Bevacizumab for neovascular ocular diseases. Ann Pharmacother 2007;41:614–625.
43. Tolentino M. Interference RNA technology in the treatment of CNV. Ophthalmol Clin North Am 2006;19:393–399, vi–vii.
44. Murata M, Takanami T, Shimizu S, et al. Inhibition of ocular angiogenesis by diced small interfering RNAs (siRNAs) specific to vascular endothelial growth factor (VEGF). Curr Eye Res 2006;31:171–180.
45. Cashman SM, Bowman L, Christofferson J, et al. Inhibition of choroidal neovascularization by adenovirus-mediated delivery of short hairpin RNAs targeting VEGF as a potential therapy for AMD. Invest Ophthalmol Vis Sci 2006;47:3496–3504.
46. Bevasiranib Clinical Trial. Safety and efficacy study evaluating the combination of bevasiranib and lucentis therapy in wet AMD. Available online at: ⟨http://clinicaltrialsgov/ct/show/NCT00499590?order=1⟩ 2007; Opko Health, Inc.
47. Sirna Therapeutics. A phase I, open-label, dose escalation trial of a single intravitreal injection of siRNA-027 in patients with subfoveal choroidal neovascularization (CNV) secondary to age-related macular degeneration (AMD). Available online at: ⟨http://clinicaltrialsgov/ct2/show/NCT00363714?term=nct00363714&rank=1;NCT00363714⟩.
48. AGN211745. A study using intravitreal injections of a small interfering RNA in patients with age-related macular degeneration. Available online at: ⟨http://clinicaltrialsgov/ct2/show/NCT00395057?term=NCT00395057&rank=1⟩ Allergan.
49. Kleinman ME, Yamada K, Takeda A, et al. Sequence- and target-independent angiogenesis suppression by siRNA via TLR3. Nature 2008;452:591–597.
50. Holash J, Davis S, Papadopoulos N, et al. VEGF-Trap: a VEGF blocker with potent antitumor effects. Proc Natl Acad Sci U S A 2002;99: 11393–11398.
51. VEGF Trap-Eye. A randomized, double masked, active controlled phase III study of the efficacy, safety, and tolerability of repeated doses of intravitreal VEGF trap in subjects with neovascular age-related macular degeneration. Available online at: ⟨http://clinicaltrialsgov/ct2/show/NCT00509795?term=NCT00509795&rank=1⟩ Regeneron Pharmaceuticals.
52. Crum R, Szabo S, Folkman J. A new class of steroids inhibits angiogenesis in the presence of heparin or a heparin fragment. Science 1985;230: 1375–1378.
53. Clark AF. Mechanism of action of the angiostatic cortisene anecortave acetate. Surv Ophthalmol 2007;52(Suppl. 1):S26–S34.

54. Penn JS, Rajaratnam VS, Collier RJ, et al. The effect of an angiostatic steroid on neovascularization in a rat model of retinopathy of prematurity. Invest Ophthalmol Vis Sci 2001;42:283–290.
55. Yang RL, McCollum G, Bingaman D, et al. The effect of anecortave acetate on VEGF message and protein levels in hypoxic Muller cells and in rat OIR. Invest Ophthalmol Vis Sci 2005;46:e-abstract 4177.
56. Liu C, Gu X, Wang W-H, et al. Local delivery of anecortave acetate inhibits the expression of retinal IGF-1/IGF-1 receptor in the rat OIR model. Invest Ophthalmol Vis Sci 2005;46:e-abstract 4135.
57. Cebulla C, Jockovich M-E, Murray T. Anecortave acetate modulates MMP-2, MMP-9 and Vegf receptor expression in the LHβTAG mouse model of retinoblastoma. Invest Ophthalmol Vis Sci 2005;46:e-abstract 1106.
58. Slakter JS, Bochow TW, D'Amico DJ, et al. Anecortave acetate (15 milligrams) versus photodynamic therapy for treatment of subfoveal neovascularization in age-related macular degeneration. Ophthalmology 2006;113:3–13.
59. Regillo CD, D'Amico DJ, Mieler WF, et al. Clinical safety profile of posterior juxtascleral depot administration of anecortave acetate 15 mg suspension as primary therapy or adjunctive therapy with photodynamic therapy for treatment of wet age-related macular degeneration. Surv Ophthalmol 2007;52(Suppl. 1):S70–S78.
60. Russell SR, Hudson HL, Jerdan JA. Anecortave acetate for the treatment of exudative age-related macular degeneration – a review of clinical outcomes. Surv Ophthalmol 2007;52(Suppl. 1):S79–S90.
61. Fredriksson L, Li H, Eriksson U. The PDGF family: four gene products form five dimeric isoforms. Cytokine Growth Factor Rev 2004;15: 197–204.
62. Heldin CH, Westermark B. Mechanism of action and *in vivo* role of platelet-derived growth factor. Physiol Rev 1999;79:1283–1316.
63. Beitz JG, Kim IS, Calabresi P, et al. Human microvascular endothelial cells express receptors for platelet-derived growth factor. Proc Natl Acad Sci USA 1991;88:2021–2025.
64. Battegay EJ, Rupp J, Iruela-Arispe L, et al. PDGF-BB modulates endothelial proliferation and angiogenesis *in vitro* via PDGF beta-receptors. J Cell Biol 1994;125:917–928.
65. Hellstrom M, Kalen M, Lindahl P, et al. Role of PDGF-B and PDGFR-beta in recruitment of vascular smooth muscle cells and pericytes during embryonic blood vessel formation in the mouse. Development 1999;126: 3047–3055.
66. Leveen P, Pekny M, Gebre-Medhin S, et al. Mice deficient for PDGF B show renal, cardiovascular, and hematological abnormalities. Genes Dev 1994;8:1875–1887.
67. Betsholtz C. Role of platelet-derived growth factors in mouse development. Int J Dev Biol 1995;39:817–825.
68. Sennino B, Falcon BL, McCauley D, et al. Sequential loss of tumor vessel pericytes and endothelial cells after inhibition of platelet-derived growth factor B by selective aptamer AX102. Cancer Res 2007;67: 7358–7367.
69. Enge M, Bjarnegard M, Gerhardt H, et al. Endothelium-specific platelet-derived growth factor-B ablation mimics diabetic retinopathy. Embo J 2002;21:4307–4316.
70. Dell S, Peters S, Muther P, et al. The role of PDGF receptor inhibitors and PI3-kinase signaling in the pathogenesis of corneal neovascularization. Invest Ophthalmol Vis Sci 2006;47:1928–1937.
71. Jo N, Mailhos C, Ju M, et al. Inhibition of platelet-derived growth factor B signaling enhances the efficacy of anti-vascular endothelial growth factor therapy in multiple models of ocular neovascularization. Am J Pathol 2006;168:2036–2053.
72. Okada-Ban M, Thiery JP, Jouanneau J. Fibroblast growth factor-2. Int J Biochem Cell Biol 2000;32:263–267.
73. Frank RN, Amin RH, Eliott D, et al. Basic fibroblast growth factor and vascular endothelial growth factor are present in epiretinal and choroidal neovascular membranes. Am J Ophthalmol 1996;122:393–403.
74. Soubrane G, Cohen SY, Delayre T, et al. Basic fibroblast growth factor experimentally induced choroidal angiogenesis in the minipig. Curr Eye Res 1994;13:183–195.
75. Yamada H, Yamada E, Kwak N, et al. Cell injury unmasks a latent proangiogenic phenotype in mice with increased expression of FGF2 in the retina. J Cell Physiol 2000;185:135–142.
76. Tobe T, Ortega S, Luna JD, et al. Targeted disruption of the FGF2 gene does not prevent choroidal neovascularization in a murine model. Am J Pathol 1998;153:1641–1646.
77. Hehlgans T, Pfeffer K. The intriguing biology of the tumour necrosis factor/tumour necrosis factor receptor superfamily: players, rules and the games. Immunology 2005;115:1–20.
78. Leibovich SJ, Polverini PJ, Shepard HM, et al. Macrophage-induced angiogenesis is mediated by tumour necrosis factor-alpha. Nature 1987;329:630–632.
79. Frater-Schroder M, Risau W, Hallmann R, et al. Tumor necrosis factor type alpha, a potent inhibitor of endothelial cell growth *in vitro*, is angiogenic *in vivo*. Proc Natl Acad Sci USA 1987;84:5277–5281.
80. Hangai M, He S, Hoffmann S, et al. Sequential induction of angiogenic growth factors by TNF-alpha in choroidal endothelial cells. J Neuroimmunol 2006;171:45–56.
81. Giraudo E, Primo L, Audero E, et al. Tumor necrosis factor-alpha regulates expression of vascular endothelial growth factor receptor-2 and of its co-receptor neuropilin-1 in human vascular endothelial cells. J Biol Chem 1998;273:22128–22135.
82. Hoffmann S, He S, Ehren M, et al. MMP-2 and MMP-9 secretion by RPE is stimulated by angiogenic molecules found in choroidal neovascular membranes. Retina 2006;26:454–461.
83. Goukassian DA, Qin G, Dolan C, et al. Tumor necrosis factor-alpha receptor p75 is required in ischemia-induced neovascularization. Circulation 2007;115:752–762.
84. Shi X, Semkova I, Muther PS, et al. Inhibition of TNF-alpha reduces laser-induced choroidal neovascularization. Exp Eye Res 2006;83: 1325–1334.
85. Gardiner TA, Gibson DS, de Gooyer TE, et al. Inhibition of tumor necrosis factor-alpha improves physiological angiogenesis and reduces pathological neovascularization in ischemic retinopathy. Am J Pathol 2005;166:637–644.
86. Vinores SA, Xiao WH, Shen J, et al. TNF-alpha is critical for ischemia-induced leukostasis, but not retinal neovascularization nor VEGF-induced leakage. J Neuroimmunol 2007;182:73–79.
87. Limb GA, Chignell AH, Green W, et al. Distribution of TNF alpha and its reactive vascular adhesion molecules in fibrovascular membranes of proliferative diabetic retinopathy. Br J Ophthalmol 1996;80:168–173.
88. Oh H, Takagi H, Takagi C, et al. The potential angiogenic role of macrophages in the formation of choroidal neovascular membranes. Invest Ophthalmol Vis Sci 1999;40:1891–1898.
89. Markomichelakis NN, Theodossiadis PG, Sfikakis PP. Regression of neovascular age-related macular degeneration following infliximab therapy. Am J Ophthalmol 2005;139:537–540.
90. Sfikakis PP, Markomichelakis N, Theodossiadis GP, et al. Regression of sight-threatening macular edema in type 2 diabetes following treatment with the anti-tumor necrosis factor monoclonal antibody infliximab. Diabetes Care 2005;28:445–447.
91. Zhang J, Hughes S. Role of the ephrin and Eph receptor tyrosine kinase families in angiogenesis and development of the cardiovascular system. J Pathol 2006;208:453–461.
92. Kuijper S, Turner CJ, Adams RH. Regulation of angiogenesis by Eph–ephrin interactions. Trends Cardiovasc Med 2007;17:145–151.
93. Dodelet VC, Pasquale EB. Eph receptors and ephrin ligands: embryogenesis to tumorigenesis. Oncogene 2000;19:5614–5619.
94. Pasquale EB. Eph receptor signalling casts a wide net on cell behaviour. Nat Rev Mol Cell Biol 2005;6:462–475.
95. Pfaff D, Fiedler U, Augustin HG. Emerging roles of the angiopoietin-Tie and the ephrin-Eph systems as regulators of cell trafficking. J Leukoc Biol 2006;80:719–726.
96. Konstantinova I, Nikolova G, Ohara-Imaizumi M, et al. EphA-Ephrin-A-mediated beta cell communication regulates insulin secretion from pancreatic islets. Cell 2007;129:359–370.
97. Brantley-Sieders DM, Caughron J, Hicks D, et al. EphA2 receptor tyrosine kinase regulates endothelial cell migration and vascular assembly through phosphoinositide 3-kinase-mediated Rac1 GTPase activation. J Cell Sci 2004;117:2037–2049.
98. Cheng N, Brantley DM, Liu H, et al. Blockade of EphA receptor tyrosine kinase activation inhibits vascular endothelial cell growth factor-induced angiogenesis. Mol Cancer Res 2002;1:2–11.
99. Chen J, Hicks D, Brantley-Sieders D, et al. Inhibition of retinal neovascularization by soluble EphA2 receptor. Exp Eye Res 2006;82:664–673.
100. Wang HU, Chen ZF, Anderson DJ. Molecular distinction and angiogenic interaction between embryonic arteries and veins revealed by ephrin-B2 and its receptor Eph-B4. Cell 1998;93:741–753.
101. Gerety SS, Wang HU, Chen ZF, et al. Symmetrical mutant phenotypes of the receptor EphB4 and its specific transmembrane ligand ephrin-B2 in cardiovascular development. Mol Cell 1999;4:403–414.
102. Foo SS, Turner CJ, Adams S, et al. Ephrin-B2 controls cell motility and adhesion during blood-vessel-wall assembly. Cell 2006;124:161–173.
103. Umeda N, Ozaki H, Hayashi H, et al. Expression of ephrinB2 and its receptors on fibroproliferative membranes in ocular angiogenic diseases. Am J Ophthalmol 2004;138:270–279.
104. Hayashi S, Asahara T, Masuda H, et al. Functional ephrin-B2 expression for promotive interaction between arterial and venous vessels in postnatal neovascularization. Circulation 2005;111:2210–2218.
105. Huynh-Do U, Vindis C, Liu H, et al. Ephrin-B1 transduces signals to activate integrin-mediated migration, attachment and angiogenesis. J Cell Sci 2002;115:3073–3081.
106. Maekawa H, Oike Y, Kanda S, et al. Ephrin-B2 induces migration of endothelial cells through the phosphatidylinositol-3 kinase pathway and promotes angiogenesis in adult vasculature. Arterioscler Thromb Vasc Biol 2003;23:2008–2014.
107. He S, Ding Y, Zhou J, et al. Soluble EphB4 regulates choroidal endothelial cell function and inhibits laser-induced choroidal neovascularization. Invest Ophthalmol Vis Sci 2005;46:4772–4779.
108. Zamora DO, Davies MH, Planck SR, et al. Soluble forms of EphrinB2 and EphB4 reduce retinal neovascularization in a model of proliferative retinopathy. Invest Ophthalmol Vis Sci 2005;46:2175–2182.
109. Lai EC. Notch signaling: control of cell communication and cell fate. Development 2004;131:965–973.
110. Gridley T. Notch signaling in vascular development and physiology. Development 2007;134:2709–2718.

111. Hofmann JJ, Luisa Iruela-Arispe M. Notch expression patterns in the retina: an eye on receptor-ligand distribution during angiogenesis. Gene Expr Patterns 2007;7:461–470.
112. Suchting S, Freitas C, le Noble F, et al. The Notch ligand Delta-like 4 negatively regulates endothelial tip cell formation and vessel branching. Proc Natl Acad Sci USA 2007;104:3225–3230.
113. Noguera-Troise I, Daly C, Papadopoulos NJ, et al. Blockade of Dll4 inhibits tumour growth by promoting non-productive angiogenesis. Nature 2006;444:1032–1037.
114. Eklund L, Olsen BR. Tie receptors and their angiopoietin ligands are context-dependent regulators of vascular remodeling. Exp Cell Res 2006;312:630–641.
115. Sato TN, Tozawa Y, Deutsch U, et al. Distinct roles of the receptor tyrosine kinases Tie-1 and Tie-2 in blood vessel formation. Nature 1995;376:70–74.
116. Suri C, Jones PF, Patan S, et al. Requisite role of angiopoietin-1, a ligand for the TIE2 receptor, during embryonic angiogenesis. Cell 1996;87: 1171–1180.
117. Maisonpierre PC, Suri C, Jones PF, et al. Angiopoietin-2, a natural antagonist for Tie2 that disrupts *in vivo* angiogenesis. Science 1997;277: 55–60.
118. Witzenbichler B, Maisonpierre PC, Jones P, et al. Chemotactic properties of angiopoietin-1 and -2, ligands for the endothelial-specific receptor tyrosine kinase Tie2. J Biol Chem 1998;273:18514–18521.
119. Kim I, Kim HG, Moon SO, et al. Angiopoietin-1 induces endothelial cell sprouting through the activation of focal adhesion kinase and plasmin secretion. Circ Res 2000;86:952–959.
120. Thurston G, Suri C, Smith K, et al. Leakage-resistant blood vessels in mice transgenically overexpressing angiopoietin-1. Science 1999;286: 2511–2514.
121. Kim I, Moon SO, Park SK, et al. Angiopoietin-1 reduces VEGF-stimulated leukocyte adhesion to endothelial cells by reducing ICAM-1, VCAM-1, and E-selectin expression. Circ Res 2001;89:477–479.
122. Kim I, Oh JL, Ryu YS, et al. Angiopoietin-1 negatively regulates expression and activity of tissue factor in endothelial cells. FASEB J 2002;16: 136–138.
123. Fiedler U, Augustin HG. Angiopoietins: a link between angiogenesis and inflammation. Trends Immunol 2006;27:552–558.
124. Nambu H, Nambu R, Oshima Y, et al. Angiopoietin 1 inhibits ocular neovascularization and breakdown of the blood–retinal barrier. Gene Ther 2004;11:865–873.
125. Nambu H, Umeda N, Kachi S, et al. Angiopoietin 1 prevents retinal detachment in an aggressive model of proliferative retinopathy, but has no effect on established neovascularization. J Cell Physiol 2005;204:227–235.
126. Gale NW, Thurston G, Hackett SF, et al. Angiopoietin-2 is required for postnatal angiogenesis and lymphatic patterning, and only the latter role is rescued by angiopoietin-1. Dev Cell 2002;3:411–423.
127. Mandriota SJ, Pepper MS. Regulation of angiopoietin-2 mRNA levels in bovine microvascular endothelial cells by cytokines and hypoxia. Circ Res 1998;83:852–859.
128. Oh H, Takagi H, Suzuma K, et al. Hypoxia and vascular endothelial growth factor selectively up-regulate angiopoietin-2 in bovine microvascular endothelial cells. J Biol Chem 1999;274:15732–15739.
129. Fiedler U, Reiss Y, Scharpfenecker M, et al. Angiopoietin-2 sensitizes endothelial cells to TNF-alpha and has a crucial role in the induction of inflammation. Nat Med 2006;12:235–239.
130. Otani A, Takagi H, Oh H, et al. Expressions of angiopoietins and Tie2 in human choroidal neovascular membranes. Invest Ophthalmol Vis Sci 1999;40:1912–1920.
131. Watanabe D, Suzuma K, Suzuma I, et al. Vitreous levels of angiopoietin 2 and vascular endothelial growth factor in patients with proliferative diabetic retinopathy. Am J Ophthalmol 2005;139:476–481.
132. Asahara T, Chen D, Takahashi T, et al. Tie2 receptor ligands, angiopoietin-1 and angiopoietin-2, modulate VEGF-induced postnatal neovascularization. Circ Res 1998;83:233–240.
133. Oliner J, Min H, Leal J, et al. Suppression of angiogenesis and tumor growth by selective inhibition of angiopoietin-2. Cancer Cell 2004;6: 507–516.
134. Peters S, Cree IA, Alexander R, et al. Angiopoietin modulation of vascular endothelial growth factor: effects on retinal endothelial cell permeability. Cytokine 2007;40:144–150.
135. Holash J, Maisonpierre PC, Compton D, et al. Vessel cooption, regression, and growth in tumors mediated by angiopoietins and VEGF. Science 1999;284:1994–1998.
136. Oshima Y, Oshima S, Nambu H, et al. Different effects of angiopoietin-2 in different vascular beds: new vessels are most sensitive. FASEB J 2005;19:963–965.
137. Campochiaro PA. Ocular versus extraocular neovascularization: mirror images or vague resemblances. Invest Ophthalmol Vis Sci 2006;47: 462–474.
138. Fisher JW. Erythropoietin: physiology and pharmacology update. Exp Biol Med (Maywood) 2003;228:1–14.
139. Tsai JC, Song BJ, Wu L, et al. Erythropoietin: a candidate neuroprotective agent in the treatment of glaucoma. J Glaucoma 2007;16:567–571.
140. Nakano M, Satoh K, Fukumoto Y, et al. Important role of erythropoietin receptor to promote VEGF expression and angiogenesis in peripheral ischemia in mice. Circ Res 2007;100:662–669.
141. Hernandez C, Fonollosa A, Garcia-Ramirez M, et al. Erythropoietin is expressed in the human retina and it is highly elevated in the vitreous fluid of patients with diabetic macular edema. Diabetes Care 2006;29:2028–2033.
142. Watanabe D, Suzuma K, Matsui S, et al. Erythropoietin as a retinal angiogenic factor in proliferative diabetic retinopathy. N Engl J Med 2005;353:782–792.
143. Brown MS, Baron AE, France EK, et al. Association between higher cumulative doses of recombinant erythropoietin and risk for retinopathy of prematurity. J AAPOS 2006;10:143–149.
144. Deryugina EI, Quigley JP. Matrix metalloproteinases and tumor metastasis. Cancer Metastasis Rev 2006;25:9–34.
145. Lee S, Jilani SM, Nikolova GV, et al. Processing of VEGF-A by matrix metalloproteinases regulates bioavailability and vascular patterning in tumors. J Cell Biol 2005;169:681–691.
146. Jo N, Ju M, Nishijima K, et al. Inhibitory effect of an antibody to cryptic collagen type IV epitopes on choroidal neovascularization. Mol Vis 2006;12:1243–1249.
147. Avraamides CJ, Garmy-Susini B, Varner JA. Integrins in angiogenesis and lymphangiogenesis. Nat Rev Cancer 2008;8:604–617.
148. Friedlander M, Theesfeld CL, Sugita M, et al. Involvement of integrins alpha v beta 3 and alpha v beta 5 in ocular neovascular diseases. Proc Natl Acad Sci USA 1996;93:9764–9769.
149. Luna J, Tobe T, Mousa SA, et al. Antagonists of integrin alpha v beta 3 inhibit retinal neovascularization in a murine model. Lab Invest 1996;75:563–573.
150. Kamizuru H, Kimura H, Yasukawa T, et al. Monoclonal antibody-mediated drug targeting to choroidal neovascularization in the rat. Invest Ophthalmol Vis Sci 2001;42:2664–2672.
151. Lahdenranta J, Sidman RL, Pasqualini R, et al. Treatment of hypoxia-induced retinopathy with targeted proapoptotic peptidomimetic in a mouse model of disease. FASEB J 2007;21:3272–3278.
152. Wilkinson-Berka JL, Jones D, Taylor G, et al. SB-267268, a nonpeptidic antagonist of alpha(v)beta3 and alpha(v)beta5 integrins, reduces angiogenesis and VEGF expression in a mouse model of retinopathy of prematurity. Invest Ophthalmol Vis Sci 2006;47:1600–1605.
153. Fu Y, Ponce ML, Thill M, et al. Angiogenesis inhibition and choroidal neovascularization suppression by sustained delivery of an integrin antagonist, EMD478761. Invest Ophthalmol Vis Sci 2007;48:5184–5190.
154. Santulli RJ, Kinney WA, Ghosh S, et al. Studies with an orally bioavailable alpha V integrin antagonist in animal models of ocular vasculopathy: retinal neovascularization in mice and retinal vascular permeability in diabetic rats. J Pharmacol Exp Ther 2008;324:894–901.
155. Kim S, Bell K, Mousa SA, et al. Regulation of angiogenesis *in vivo* by ligation of integrin alpha5beta1 with the central cell-binding domain of fibronectin. Am J Pathol 2000;156:1345–1362.
156. Muether PS, Dell S, Kociok N, et al. The role of integrin alpha(5)beta(1) in the regulation of corneal neovascularization. Exp Eye Res 2007;85: 356–365.
157. Umeda N, Kachi S, Akiyama H, et al. Suppression and regression of choroidal neovascularization by systemic administration of an alpha5beta1 integrin antagonist. Mol Pharmacol 2006;69:1820–1828.
158. Maier AK, Kociok N, Zahn G, et al. Modulation of hypoxia-induced neovascularization by JSM6427, an integrin alpha5beta1 inhibiting molecule. Curr Eye Res 2007;32:801–812.
159. Donoso LA, Kim D, Frost A, et al. The role of inflammation in the pathogenesis of age-related macular degeneration. Surv Ophthalmol 2006;51:137–152.
160. Nozaki M, Raisler BJ, Sakurai E, et al. Drusen complement components C3a and C5a promote choroidal neovascularization. Proc Natl Acad Sci USA 2006;103:2328–2333.
161. Bora PS, Sohn JH, Cruz JM, et al. Role of complement and complement membrane attack complex in laser-induced choroidal neovascularization. J Immunol 2005;174:491–497.
162. Tombran-Tink J, Shivaram SM, Chader GJ, et al. Expression, secretion, and age-related downregulation of pigment epithelium-derived factor, a serpin with neurotrophic activity. J Neurosci 1995;15:4992–5003.
163. Duh EJ, Yang HS, Suzuma I, et al. Pigment epithelium-derived factor suppresses ischemia-induced retinal neovascularization and VEGF-induced migration and growth. Invest Ophthalmol Vis Sci 2002;43:821–829.
164. Stellmach V, Crawford SE, Zhou W, et al. Prevention of ischemia-induced retinopathy by the natural ocular antiangiogenic agent pigment epithelium-derived factor. Proc Natl Acad Sci USA 2001;98:2593–2597.
165. Zhang SX, Wang JJ, Gao G, et al. Pigment epithelium-derived factor downregulates vascular endothelial growth factor (VEGF) expression and inhibits VEGF-VEGF receptor 2 binding in diabetic retinopathy. J Mol Endocrinol 2006;37:1–12.
166. Yamagishi S, Abe R, Jinnouchi Y, et al. Pigment epithelium-derived factor inhibits vascular endothelial growth factor-induced vascular hyperpermeability both *in vitro* and *in vivo*. J Int Med Res 2007;35: 896–899.
167. Cai J, Jiang WG, Grant MB, et al. Pigment epithelium-derived factor inhibits angiogenesis via regulated intracellular proteolysis of vascular endothelial growth factor receptor 1. J Biol Chem 2006;281: 3604–3613.
168. Ogata N, Nishikawa M, Nishimura T, et al. Inverse levels of pigment epithelium-derived factor and vascular endothelial growth factor in the

vitreous of eyes with rhegmatogenous retinal detachment and proliferative vitreoretinopathy. Am J Ophthalmol 2002;133:851–852.
169. Duh EJ, Yang HS, Haller JA, et al. Vitreous levels of pigment epithelium-derived factor and vascular endothelial growth factor: implications for ocular angiogenesis. Am J Ophthalmol 2004;137:668–674.
170. Mori K, Gehlbach P, Ando A, et al. Regression of ocular neovascularization in response to increased expression of pigment epithelium-derived factor. Invest Ophthalmol Vis Sci 2002;43:2428–2434.
171. Apte RS, Barreiro RA, Duh E, et al. Stimulation of neovascularization by the anti-angiogenic factor PEDF. Invest Ophthalmol Vis Sci 2004;45: 4491–4497.
172. Campochiaro PA, Nguyen QD, Shah SM, et al. Adenoviral vector-delivered pigment epithelium-derived factor for neovascular age-related macular degeneration: results of a phase I clinical trial. Hum Gene Ther 2006;17: 167–176.
173. Kendall RL, Thomas KA. Inhibition of vascular endothelial cell growth factor activity by an endogenously encoded soluble receptor. Proc Natl Acad Sci USA 1993;90:10705–10709.
174. Ambati BK, Nozaki M, Singh N, et al. Corneal avascularity is due to soluble VEGF receptor-1. Nature 2006;443:993–997.
175. Woolard J, Wang WY, Bevan HS, et al. VEGF165b, an inhibitory vascular endothelial growth factor splice variant: mechanism of action, *in vivo* effect on angiogenesis and endogenous protein expression. Cancer Res 2004;64:7822–7835.
176. Perrin RM, Konopatskaya O, Qiu Y, et al. Diabetic retinopathy is associated with a switch in splicing from anti- to pro-angiogenic isoforms of vascular endothelial growth factor. Diabetologia 2005;48:2422–2427.
177. Bora NS, Kaliappan S, Jha P, et al. CD59, a complement regulatory protein, controls choroidal neovascularization in a mouse model of wet-type age-related macular degeneration. J Immunol 2007;178: 1783–1790.
178. Otani A, Slike BM, Dorrell MI, et al. A fragment of human TrpRS as a potent antagonist of ocular angiogenesis. Proc Natl Acad Sci USA 2002;99:178–183.
179. Banin E, Dorrell MI, Aguilar E, et al. T2-TrpRS inhibits preretinal neovascularization and enhances physiological vascular regrowth in OIR as assessed by a new method of quantification. Invest Ophthalmol Vis Sci 2006;47:2125–2134.
180. Tzima E, Reader JS, Irani-Tehrani M, et al. VE-cadherin links tRNA synthetase cytokine to anti-angiogenic function. J Biol Chem 2005;280:2405–2408.
181. Dorrell MI, Aguilar E, Scheppke L, et al. Combination angiostatic therapy completely inhibits ocular and tumor angiogenesis. Proc Natl Acad Sci USA 2007;104:967–972.
182. Zhang SX, Ma JX. Ocular neovascularization: Implication of endogenous angiogenic inhibitors and potential therapy. Prog Retin Eye Res 2007;26:1–37.

CHAPTER

5 Ocular immunity and inflammation

Thomas A. Albini, MD and Janet L. Davis, MD, MA

INTRODUCTION

Many posterior-segment diseases involve inflammatory and immune mechanisms. This chapter provides a basic summary of these mechanisms as a framework for understanding pharmacotherapeutics that may be useful in treating retinal disease.

HISTORY

Like the field of immunology, the field of ocular immunology and inflammation has grown rapidly over the past years. This chapter covers broad concepts in immunology important to ocular disease as well as basic concepts in diagnostic and therapeutic strategies used in ocular inflammatory disease.

KEY CONCEPTS AND FUNDAMENTALS IN MOLECULAR BIOLOGY AND BIOCHEMISTRY

INNATE IMMUNITY

Innate immunity and complement provide immediate protection from pathogens. Although most relevant to eye disease in the protection of the ocular surface from exogenous insults such as infection, the genetically determined intensity of innate complement activation is increasingly understood to be involved in the pathogenesis of age-related macular degeneration (AMD) and assumed to be involved in posterior and panuveitis as well.

Intact surface epithelium, low surface temperature, neutral pH, protective tear-borne enzymes and macrophages, and an intact blink response are important first-line defenses of the external eye. Microbial lipopolysaccharides, peptidoglycans, lipoteichoic acids, mannans, bacterial DNA, double-stranded RNA, and glucans elicit an immediate response from the innate (natural) immune system. In addition, the mammalian immune system recognizes hundreds of pathogen-associated molecular motifs through pattern recognition receptors expressed on macrophages, B lymphocytes, and dendritic cells.[1] Activation of these cells stimulates antigen presentation and upregulation of T lymphocyte costimulatory molecules and results in the slower adaptive (acquired) immune response directed against the invading organism. Finally, pattern recognition molecules coat pathogens and increase recognition by complement and phagocytes. Among the best-characterized pattern recognition receptors are mannan-binding lectin, mannose receptor, Toll-like receptor (TLR), and lipopolysaccharide-binding protein. TLRs have been localized to lymphocytes, eosinophils, mast cells, and epithelial cells of the conjunctiva. More recently, innate immunity via TLRs on intraocular cells has been hypothesized to participate in the development of AMD (Chapter 18).

Over 20 proteins and protein fragments make up the complement system, including serum proteins and cell membrane receptors. Complement activation is destructive to tissue and is rapidly amplified through a triggered-enzyme cascade; several mechanisms prevent its uncontrolled activation and may be particularly important in the retina and choroid. For example, factor H is an important down-regulator of complement located on cell membranes. A common single-nucleotide polymorphism in factor H (Tyr402His) has been strongly associated with AMD.[2] The hypothesis is that this polymorphism results in poorer function of factor H, increased complement activity, and more tissue destruction. Immunologic reactions in the retinal pigment epithelium (RPE) and choroid due to routine immune surveillance of blood-borne infectious agents can be assumed to lead to subsequent damage to ocular tissues if not dampened by protective factors.

ADAPTIVE IMMUNITY

Although polymorphisms in immune response genes may modify the course of intraocular inflammation from any cause, autoimmune, noninfectious uveitis mainly involves adaptive (acquired) immunity through antigen recognition by lymphocytes and typically requires days to establish an effective clonal expansion. A primary response results from the initial contact with the antigen. Secondary, tertiary, and subsequent responses increase in magnitude.

The afferent arm of the immune response occurs in specialized immune organs. Lymphatic vessels are found predominantly in the eyelids and drain into the submandibular lymph nodes.[3] Although when vascularized the cornea may form some lymphatic channels,[4] the remainder of the ocular anatomical structures, with the exception of the conjunctiva and eyelid, do not contain lymphatic channels. Lymphatic drainage from intraocular tissues is minimal, which likely serves to reduce acquired immunity to intraocular proteins except during inadvertent exposure, such as globe rupture or surgery. Nevertheless, extracellular fluid may drain through perivenous spaces of the posterior segment, through the lamina cribrosa, and into the spaces of the optic nerve.[5] There is evidence that antigen injected intravitreally reaches the preauricular lymph node.[6]

Specific cell surface markers distinguish the cells of the adaptive immune system (Table 5.1). Glycoproteins designated as major histocompatibility complex (MHC) molecules – known as human leukocyte antigen (HLA) molecules in humans – present antigens to immunocompetent cells, primarily T lymphocytes. Two classes of MHC molecules exist: class I molecules are found on all nucleated cells and present antigen derived from intracellular components, such as tumor or viral antigens, to cytotoxic cluster of differentiation (CD) 8+ T lymphocytes; class II molecules are found predominantly on professional antigen-presenting cells (APCs), such as dendritic cells, macrophages, and B cells. Class II-bearing cells present extracellular antigens that have been endocytosed, such as fungal or bacterial antigens, to helper CD4+ T lymphocytes (Figure 5.1).

Dendritic cells and macrophages are classic APCs since they constitutively express MHC class II molecules and present antigen to CD4+ T lymphocytes. They also express immunoglobulin G (IgG) receptors that engulf extracellular antigens after they are coated with IgG, a reaction known as opsonization. Moreover, APCs stimulate lymphocytes by cytokine production, such as interleukin-1 (IL-1) and tumor necrosis factor-alpha (TNF-α), and by surface expression of costimulatory

Table 5.1 List of selected cluster of differentiation (CD) antigens

CD antigen	Cellular expression	Functions	Other names
CD1	Cortical thymocytes, Langerhans cells, dendritic cells, B cells, intestinal epithelium, smooth muscle, blood vessels	MHC class I-like molecule with special role in presentation of lipid molecules	
CD2	T cells, thymocytes, NK cells	Adhesion molecule binding CD58 (LFA-3)	T11, LFA-2
CD3	Thymocytes, T cells	Associated with the T-cell antigen receptor (TCR). Required for surface expression and activation TCR	T3
CD4	Thymocyte subsets, Th1 and Th2 cells, monocytes and macrophages	Co-receptor of MHC class II molecule	T4, L3T4
CD8	Thymocyte subsets, cytotoxic T cells	Co-receptor of MHC class I molecule	T8, Lyt2,3
CD 11a	Leukocytes	Subunit of integrin LFA-1	LFA-1
CD 11b	Granulocytes and macrophages	Binds CD 54, complement component iC3b, and extracellular matrix protiens	Mac-1
CD 11c	Granulocytes, macrophages, lymphoctyes		Adhesion molecule, binds fibrinogen
CD 16	Neutrophils, NK cells, macrophages	Low-affinity Fc receptor, mediates phagocytosis and antibody-dependent cell-mediated cytotoxicity	FcγRIII
CD 19	B cells and dendritic cells	CD19 is expressed on B cells from earliest recognizable B-lineage cells but is lost on maturation to plasma cells	
CD 20	B cells	B-lymphocyte surface molecule which plays a role in the development and differentiation of B cells into plasma cells	MS4A1
CD 23	Mature B cells, activated macrophages, eosinophils, follicular dendritic cells, platelets	Low-affinity receptor for IgE	FcεRIII
CD 28	T-cell subsets, activated B cells	Activation of naïve T cells, receptor for co-stimulatory signal. Binds CD80 (B7.1) and CD 86 (B7.2)	
CD 40	B cells, macrophages, dendritic cells, basal epithelial cells	Binds CD 154 (CD 40 L); receptor for co-stimulatory signal for B cells, promotes growth, differentiation, and isotype switching of B cells	
CD 45	All hematopoietic cells	Tyrosine phosphatase	Leukocyte common antigen

For a complete list visit the website of the human leukocyte differentiation antigens (HLDA)/human cell differentiation molecules (HCDM) at www.hlda8.org *or protein reviews provided by the NIH at* www.ncbi.nlm.gov/prow/.
MHC, major histocompatibility complex; NK, natural killer; LFA, lymphocyte function-associated antigen; IgE, immunoglobulin E.

molecules (CD28, CD40) required for successful antigen presentation. These cells secrete a host of other immune mediators, including proteases, collagenases, angiotensin-converting enzyme, lysozyme, IL-6, macrophage colony-stimulating factor, and reactive oxygen and nitrogen species. Specialized macrophages exist in many tissues, such as the Kupffer cells of the liver, dendritic histiocytes of lymphoid organs and uveal tissue, Langerhans cells of the skin, lymph nodes, conjunctiva and cornea, and microglia of the retina and central nervous system.

A subset of lymphocytes, B cells, matures in the bone marrow and produces antibodies. They are the primary cells responsible for adaptive humoral immunity. B lymphocytes can recognize extracellular antigens not processed or presented by other immune cells by means of surface antibody receptors and the antibody which the cell itself produces and secretes. Antibodies are divided into five classes by the characteristics of the constant regions of the antibody molecule. IgM is the initial antibody class produced to a specific antigen. Typically during a second exposure to the same antigen, the B cell is activated either by the surrounding cytokine milieu or by bacterial polysaccharides and lipopolysaccharides, known as T-cell-independent antigens, and the cell switches class production to IgG, IgA or IgE class antibodies. Any particular B cell produces one specific variable region, which recognizes one specific antigen. The fact that an almost infinite range of specificities can be encoded by a finite number of genes is explained by the finding that during B-cell development in the bone marrow, gene segments are randomly, irreversibly joined so as to encode the variable region of the antibody for that particular B cell.

Another subset of lymphocytes matures in the thymus and carries the T-cell receptor (CD3), which allows these T lymphocytes to recognize specific peptides presented by APCs within the peptide groove of either MHC class I or II molecules. T cells are responsible for adaptive cellular immunity. Like antibodies, T-cell receptors that recognize over 10^{18} specific peptides in specific MHC molecules are produced by random combinations of the germline V, D, and J segment genes that make up the variable regions of the T-cell receptor. When mature T cells

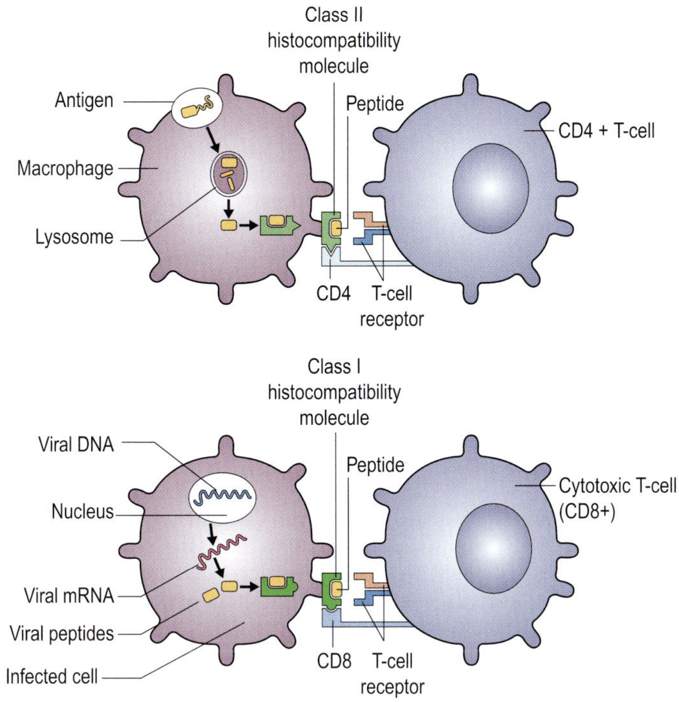

Figure 5.1 Antigen presentation. Top row: A macrophage or other antigen presenting cell (purple) endocytoses extracellular antigens, processes them, and presents peptides derived from these antigens in a binding groove of the major histocompatibility complex (MHC) class II molecule on the cell surface. This complex is recognized by the T-cell receptor (CD3) and CD4 molecules on the helper T-cell surface. Bottom row: infected cells process intracellular antigens such as viral components into viral peptides which are presented in a binding groove of the MHC class I molecule on the cell surface. This complex is recognized by the T-cell receptor (CD3) and CD 8 molecules on the helper T-cell surface.

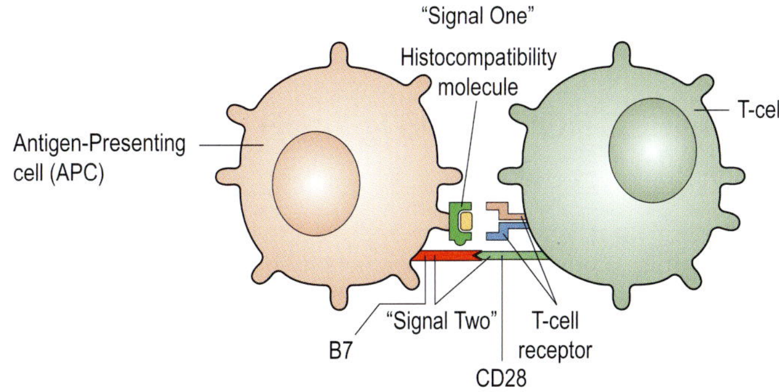

Figure 5.2 Antigen costimulation. In addition to major histocompatibility complex (MHC) class II presentation of antigen to the T-cell receptor (i.e., the first signal), professional antigen presentation also requires a second signal resulting from the engagement of specific coreceptor molecules on the cell surface, B7, and CD28 pictured.

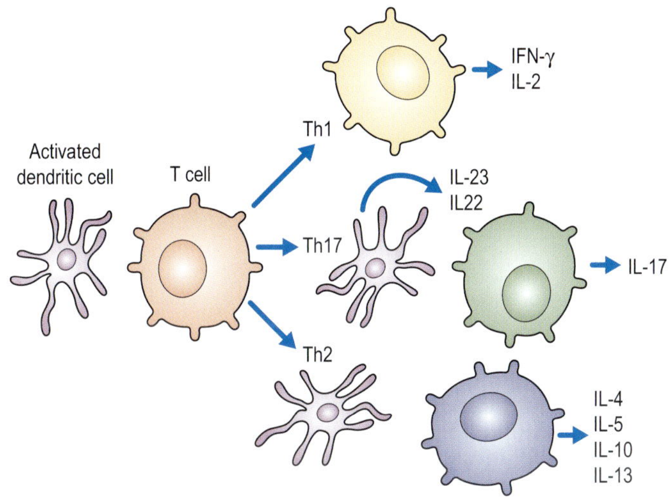

Figure 5.3 T-cell differentiation into Th1, Th2, or Th17 lymphocytes.

are presented with an antigen for which they have a specific T-cell receptor (CD3) by APCs, the T cells undergo clonal expansion, initiating an immune response targeted at the specific antigen. Expression of intraocular proteins in the thymus is necessary for the deletion of autoreactive T-cell clones, resulting in tolerance, and is an important aspect of the immune privilege of the eye.

Subsets of T cells react to antigen in two different ways depending on the co-receptor molecule (either CD4 or CD8) associated with their T-cell receptor (CD3). Cells bearing the CD4 co-receptor promote the immune response through secreted cytokines that activate surrounding lymphocytes and/or macrophages. These cells recognize extracellular antigens that have been processed in intracellular vesicles following ingestion by an APC and presented as peptide in the groove of MHC class II molecules. T cells bearing the CD8 co-receptor are cytocidal, destroying the cells harboring antigen. These cells, called cytotoxic T cells, recognize cytotoxic antigens, such as viral antigens, presented in the groove of MHC class I molecules. In addition to antigen-specific signals mediated through the T-cell receptor and co-receptor molecules, T cells also require antigen-nonspecific costimulation for activation (Figure 5.2). The B7 family of molecules on APCs, which include B7-1 (CD80) and B7-2 (CD86), are recognized by CD28 on T lymphocytes and play important roles in providing costimulatory signals required for development of antigen-specific immune responses.

CD4+ T cells can be divided into four groups: Th1, Th2, Th17 and regulatory T cells (Tregs) (Figure 5.3). Th1 cells are potent clearers of intracellular bacteria such as *Mycobacterium tuberculosis* and *M. leprae* by activating macrophages to fuse bacteria-containing vesicles with lysozymes. They also secrete cytokines that stimulate macrophage migration to the site of infection. Th2 helper cells activate B cells to secrete antibodies, and drive humoral immunity. The term "helper" T cell is often used to describe both Th1 and Th2 cells since Th1 cells "help" activate macrophages and Th2 cells "help" activate B cells. A new subset of CD4+ cells that produce IL-17 have been identified and termed Th17. These cells are stimulated by the combination of IL-6 and transforming growth factor-β (TGF-β). The importance of these cells has yet to be worked out, but they appear to be crucial in the initiation of many autoimmune conditions, including experimental autoimmune uveitis (EAU) – an experimental uveitis following immunization with retinal antigens in animals models.[7] Tregs are regulatory, anti-inflammatory T lymphocytes that are often CD4+ and CD25+ and express the transcription factor forkhead box P3 (FoxP3).[8] They are produced either centrally in the thymus or peripherally.

The differentiation of naïve CD4+ T cells into Th1, Th2, or Th17 cells occurs at the draining lymph node, largely determined by the surrounding cytokines. IL-12 and interferon-gamma (IFN-γ) tend to promote Th1 response, IL-4 and IL-6 promote Th2 differentiation, and IL-6 and TGF-β promote Th17 differentiation. An indication that the Th17 effector may play a role in pathogenesis is the ability to ameliorate inflammation with anti-IL-17 antibodies, and conversely, the enhanced IL-17 response to interphotoreceptor retinoid-binding protein (IRBP), a retinal antigen, observed in the highly EAU-susceptible IFN-γ knockout (KO) mice.[9] IFN-γ KO mice are highly susceptible to EAU but lack a normal Th1 response; this was believed to result from a deviant Th2 response,[10] but may indeed be a manifestation of Th-17 differentiation.

MECHANISMS OF PATHOGENESIS

NONINFECTIOUS POSTERIOR AND PANUVEITIS

The posterior segment of the eye is protected by an efficient blood–retinal barrier produced by tight junctions between RPE cells and retinal vascular endothelial cells. There is no direct lymphoid drainage, although antigens in the posterior segment may reach the anterior chamber and thereby the venous circulation. There are few APCs in the uninflamed posterior segment. Anti-inflammatory molecules abound, including membrane-bound TGF-β, Fas ligand (FasL), B7-CTLA4 interaction, galectin-1, thrombospondin, and complement inhibitors.[11] This aggregate control of immune and inflammatory reactions has been termed immune privilege.

Immune privilege has been mainly studied in the anterior chamber but also exists in the vitreous[12] and subretinal space.[13] Many factors may contribute to the immune privilege of the anterior chamber[14]: absence of blood vessels in the cornea and specialized endothelium of the iris stroma; direct drainage of the anterior-chamber fluid into the venous circulation rather than lymphatic drainage; soluble and cell surface molecules that reduce inflammation; and tolerance-promoting APCs in the iris stroma and trabecular meshwork. Normal murine anterior-chamber fluid has been shown to suppress CD4+ T-cell proliferation, polymorphonuclear leukocyte activation, macrophage activation, and C1q (a subcomponent of complement 1 and complement C (C3). Aqueous TGF-β probably contributes to partial inhibition of the immune response. Corneal endothelial cells have been shown to express CD46, CD55, and CD59, known to inhibit complement activation, as well as FAS ligand, which has been found to promote T-cell apoptosis. Analogous mechanisms likely exist in the posterior segment.

Antigen-specific autoimmune reactions are controlled by tolerance. Central tolerance to self-antigens consists of clonal deletion of the developing T lymphocytes in the thymus that recognize intraocular proteins. Wild-type B10.RIII mice grafted with an IRBP KO thymus had high EAU scores when immunized with a dose of IRBP that induced minimal or no disease in mice with a wild-type thymus.[15] Mice with mutations in a transcription factor known as the "autoimmune regulator" (AIRE) do not express IRBP in the thymus and develop spontaneous uveitis similar to EAU. Double knockouts, which also do not produce IRBP in the retina, do not develop uveitis. Interestingly, humans with mutations in the AIRE transcription factor develop the monogenic recessive disorder autoimmune polyendocrinopathy candidiasis ectodermal dystrophy, but not posterior uveitis. Patients with the syndrome do have corneal disease similar to congenital hereditary endothelial dystrophy (CHED).

Peripheral tolerance is maintained by a number of mechanisms. These include immunologic ignorance, anergy, and T-cell-mediated active suppression. Immunologic ignorance is the inability of small amounts of low-avidity self-antigens to elicit an immune response even if peripheral T cells with the appropriate specificity are present. Anergy is tolerance to self-antigens found in higher concentrations but presented to T cells in the absence of costimulatory signals. The expression of appropriate costimulatory signals is often dependent on the context of antigen presentation. For example, cytokines from nearby neutrophils or natural killer cells that have been activated in an antigen-independent manner, can cause costimulatory molecules to be upregulated on local APCs. Tregs can suppress other lymphocytes via cytokines such as TGF-β or IL-10.[16]

INFECTIOUS RETINITIS AND CHOROIDITIS

The protozoan obligate intracellular parasite *Toxoplasma gondii* commonly infects humans and is a leading cause of posterior uveitis. Infection results in IgM and IgG antibodies but these are insufficient to provide immunity because the organism persists intracellularly. As one would expect, the intracellular parasite elicits a predominantly CD8+ T-cell response. The T cells in turn release cytokines, particularly IFN-γ, that activate macrophages, recruiting them to sites of infection where they function both as effector and APCs. *Toxoplasma* actively invades both phagocytic and nonphagocytic cells, forming a nonfusogenic compartment, called the parasitophosphorus vacule, within the host cell cytosol.[17] By blocking fusion with lysosomes the organism prevents pathogen-derived peptides from being expressed on the host cell's MHC molecules and evading the host immune system. Hence *Toxoplasma* may remain dormant within intracytoplasmic vesicles without exciting an immune response. Intracellular *Toxoplasma* has also been shown to interfere with transcription factors necessary for cytokine expression, including IL-12, IFN-γ, TNF-α, and others.[18] Furthermore, induced apoptotic pathways in macrophages infected with *Toxoplasma* are strongly inhibited, allowing intracellular parasites to survive longer in the host cell.

Herpes simplex virus (HSV), varicella-zoster virus (VZV), and Epstein–Barr virus can cause fulminant acute retinal infections, termed the acute retinal necrosis (ARN) syndrome. Viral infection manifests as fibrinoid necrosis of the retinal vessels with vascular occlusion and focal necrosis of the RPE and retinal layers with overlying vitritis. Areas of necrosis are well defined with sharp borders separating uninvolved retina and viral intranuclear inclusions in retinal cells at the borders. The choroid is inflamed with vascular occlusion. Virus can migrate from the brain to the retina via retrograde axonal transport through the optic nerve from the suprachiasmatic nucleus of the hypothalamus. At this site, it is possible for virus to gain access to the contralateral optic pathway and fellow eye. HSV-specific T cells have been demonstrated and characterized in clinical samples of intraocular fluid derived from patients with ARN.[19] Retinal and choroidal ischemia leads to breakdown of the blood–retina barrier, presumably promoting RPE and fibroblast activation and migration, leading to the development of proliferative vitreoretinopathy. This process, in addition to the development of retinal breaks in areas of retinal necrosis, often leads to retinal detachment. Patients with VZV ARN have inhibited delayed-type hypersensitivity reactions, and intact antibody responses to VZV, a pattern that suggests that the immune privilege of the eye is genetic and involved in pathogenesis.[20]

AGE-RELATED MACULAR DEGENERATION

The inflammatory contribution to AMD has long been suspected. Contributions of cytomegalic infection or macrophage activation were published by Cousins beginning in 2004,[21,22] but real progress was not made until genetic polymorphisms in complement genes were identified as risk factors for AMD.[23] In the protected environment of the subretinal space, natural immunity is ideally tightly regulated to limit complement activation and tissue destruction. Complement factor H polymorphisms may account for 60% of the attributable risk for AMD.[24] Other polymorphisms, and complicated relationships with environmental damage such as smoking and antioxidants, also exist.[25] These discoveries fit well with what was presumed to be a complex genetic predisoposition to AMD, but nonetheless was surprising to many ophthalmologists, who may have presumed that the genes would be related to RPE or matrix. There is undoubtedly a contribution of other aging changes such as progressive choroidal ischemia[26] and systemic inflammatory mediators such as C-reactive protein.[27] The current hypothesis, however, is that inflammation involving the innate immune system is a primary determinant of AMD.

Perhaps even more intriguing is the concept that adaptive immunity may also play a role. Peroxidation products of lipids present in high concentration in Ruysch's complex (RPE–Bruch's–inner choroid) are antigenic. In a mouse model patterned after EAU, immunization with oxidized drusen produces drusen and other changes typical of dry macular degeneration.[28] It is conceivable that a model of wet macular degeneration could be created by immunizing a mouse with the equivalent polymorphisms in the complement system as have been identified in humans to predispose to exudative AMD.

DIABETIC RETINOPATHY

Inflammatory mechanisms are suspected to contribute to the pathogenesis of diabetic retinopathy, in part because of aberrant cytokine levels and adhesion molecules in intraocular specimens.[29,30] Increased adhesion molecules may indicate disruption of the blood–retinal barrier. Increased vascular endothelial growth factor (VEGF) levels in diabetic eyes have been associated with proliferative diabetic retinopathy and macular edema, yet in other vascular beds, low VEGF levels may contribute to pathology.[31] Increased TNF-α is present in both serum and vitreous fluids at higher than normal levels in patients with proliferative diabetic retinopathy. Unlike AMD, strong genetic contributions to diabetic retinopathy have not been identified, and certainly not to genes controlling the inflammatory pathways.[32]

IMPLICATIONS FOR RETINAL PHARMACOTHERAPY

In the previous sections we have discussed innate immunity and complement in macular degeneration, humoral immunity, and T-cell-mediated diseases such as EAU, and infectious uveitis such as ARN with significant destructive immune-mediated components. The treatment of a wide spectrum of ocular diseases therefore involves the pharmacologic modulation of the immune system. This section briefly introduces the immunomodulators used in ocular inflammatory disease. These agents, along with therapeutic monoclonal antibodies, will be discussed further in Section 4.

Corticosteroids bind to specific receptors in the cytosol of immunocompetent cells and then are transported to the nucleus, where they influence DNA transcription and suppress transcription of proinflammatory cytokines, prostaglandins, and other proinflammatory factors. Additionally, corticosteroids at high concentrations reduce calcium and sodium cycling across plasma membranes, which is thought to result in anti-inflammatory effects.[33] Membrane-bound corticosteroid receptors have also been identified and have been shown to exert anti-inflammatory effects. They are only immunosuppressive in high doses.

Antimetabolites reduce DNA synthesis and are immunosuppressive. Methotrexate is a folic acid analog that inhibits folate metabolism via dihydrofolate reductase and suppresses rapidly proliferating cells such as activated lymphocytes. Adenosine release increases T-cell apoptosis due to increased intracellular reactive oxygen species and increased sensitivity to the proapoptic pathways involving CD95, and other mechanisms.[34] Since adenosine release occurs intraocularly without systemic processing, methotrexate is predicted to be effective on intravitreal injection.

Azathioprine, another antimetabolite, inhibits purine synthesis and both DNA and RNA production. Azathioprine undergoes extensive systemic metabolism before incorporation as a thioguanine nucleotide that causes DNA–protein cross-links, single-strand breaks, interstrand cross-links, and sister chromatid exchanges and is unlikely to be useful as an intraocular drug. Thiopurine methyltransferase (TPMT) metabolizes azathioprine; specific polymorphisms in the TPMT gene lead to deficient clearance and increased toxicity. Measurement of TPMT activity can proactively identify patients at higher risk of bone marrow toxicity.[35]

Mycophenolate mofetil (MMF) is a prodrug of mycophenolic acid, an inhibitor of inosine monophosphate dehydrogenase (IMPDH).[36] This is the rate-limiting enzyme in de novo synthesis of guanosine nucleotides. T and B lymphocytes are more dependent on this pathway than other cell types; consequently MMF is more lymphocyte-specific than azathioprine or methotrexate. MMF exerts additional anti-inflammatory effects, such as induced apoptosis of activated T lymphocytes, decreased expression and glycosylation of adhesion molecules involved in lymphocyte recruitment, and inhibited inducible nitric oxide synthetase activity.

Cyclosporine is a fungal protein peptide that binds a cytosolic protein named cyclophilin.[37] The resulting complex then inhibits calcineurin phosphatase, a protein which controls the transcription of IL-2, IL-2 receptor, IL-4, CD40L, and IFN-γ genes. Although cyclosporine has a substantial side-effect profile, it is a T-cell-specific therapy and therefore appropriate for use in a T-cell-mediated process such as noninfectious uveitis.

Tacrolimus is macrolide lactone which also acts by inhibiting calcineurin, but binds to immunophilins. The mechanism of action is similar to cyclosporine, but tacrolimus additionally inhibits cytokine production by activated monocytes and macrophages, thereby increasing its immunosuppressive effect relative to cyclosporine.[38] Sirolimus is also a macrolide lactone[39] that binds to immunophilins, but the resultant complex inhibits the mammalian target of rapamycin (mTOR) protein kinase pathway, rather than calcineurin. Sirolimus acts to block intracellular events associated with CD-28 cross-linking and sustained T-cell activation. Sirolimus blocks cell proliferation even after initial activation in both T cells and B cells. It possesses VEGF-mediated antiangiogenic effects as well and has been shown to inhibit choroidal neovascularization in an animal model, leading to interesting possibilities as both an antiproliferative and immunosuppressive drug for posterior uveitis complicated by neovascularization.[40]

Biologic therapeutic agents mimic the molecular mechanisms of the immune system to regulate disease. Polymorphisms in the TNF-α gene are associated with greater susceptibility to Behçet disease and TNF-α levels are generally increased in Behçet disease.[41] Interferons both activate and control the inflammatory response.[42] Type I interferons consist of at least 13 different IFN-α isotypes and IFN-β, and type II interferons consisting of a single member, IFN-γ. Type I interferons share a common receptor, the IFN-α/IFN-β receptor, whereas type II interferons bind to the IFN-γ receptor. Type I interferons are used therapeutically to exert antiproliferative and proapoptotic affects on lymphocytes, especially in Behçet disease.[43] They initiate transcription of anti-inflammatory mediators such as TGF-β, IL-1 receptor antagonist and soluble TNF receptors as well as many inflammatory cytokines such as TNF-α.

DIAGNOSIS AND ANCILLARY LABORATORY METHODS

Polymerase chain reaction (PCR) has allowed for improved diagnosis of intraocular infections[44] by detection of DNA from vitreous[45] or anterior-chamber fluid. "Universal" panbacterial or panfungal primers can be used first, then narrowed with specific primers.[46,47] Numerous case reports outline the utility of anterior-chamber tap PCR for the identification of cytomegalovirus (CMV),[48,49] HSV, VZV,[50] toxoplasmosis,[51] and tuberculosis[52] from anterior-chamber fluid. Quantifiable PCR technologies such as real-time PCR help avoid false-positives by estimating the initial copies of pathogen DNA.[53] Multiplex PCR technologies allow for the simultaneous assay for multiple primers from one ocular sample.[54] PCR has identified previously unrecognized syndromes, such as CMV anterior uveitis, which may represent a subset of cases of glaucomatocyclitic crisis and Fuchs heterochromic iridocylitis.[55–59] Fomivirsen, a cDNA molecule that interferes with CMV replication, was briefly available as intravitreal injection approved by the Food and Drug Administration for the treatment of CMV retinitis.[47] Identification of other viral targets may lead to other such molecular drugs.[60]

Treatment of AMD already relies heavily on molecular targeting of VEGF. There is a wide range of new therapeutic interventions that can be devised, such as specific complement inhibitors, and other strategies to reduce inflammation.[61] In diabetic retinopathy, links between inflammation and diabetic complications support the use of anti-inflammatory medications such as nonsteroidal anti-inflammatories, corticosteroids, and specific agents directed again TNF-α and VEGF.[62]

SUMMARY AND KEY POINTS

1. Multiple immunologic mechanisms are involved in ocular and vitreoretinal diseases.
2. Experimental studies support the concept of the eye as an immune-privileged site.

3. Anti-inflammatory and immunosuppressive treatments used for ocular inflammatory disease have multiple mechanisms of actions.
4. Molecular diagnostics of ocular fluids is helpful to diagnose intraocular infections with targets amenable to treatment with molecularly specific drugs.

REFERENCES

1. Medzhitov R, Janeway Jr C. Innate immunity. N Engl J Med 2000;343:338–344.
2. Haddad S, Chen CA, Santangelo SL, et al. The genetics of age-related macular degeneration: a review of progress to date. Surv Ophthalmol 2006;51:316–363.
3. Smolin G. The role of tears in the prevention of infections. Int Ophthalmol Clin 1987;27:25–26.
4. Smolin G, Hyndiuk RA. Lymphatic drainage from vascularized rabbit cornea. Am J Ophthalmol 1971;72:147–151.
5. Smolin G, Friedlaender MH. Immunology of ocular tissues. In: Tasman W, editor. Duane's Foundations of Clinical Ophthalmology, vol. 2. New York: Lippincott Williams and Wilkins; 1995 [chapter 26].
6. Hall JM. Specificity of antibody formation after intravitreal immunization with bovine gamma globulin and ovalbumin. I. Primary response. Invest Ophthalmol 1971;10:775–783.
7. Amadi-Obi A, Yu CR, Liu X, et al. TH17 cells contribute to uveitis and scleritis and are expanded by IL-2 and inhibited by IL-27/STAT1. Nat Med 2007;13:711–718.
8. Jiang H, Chess L. Regulation of immune responses by T cells. N Engl J Med 2006;354:1166–1176.
9. Luger D, Silver PB, Tang J, et al. Either a Th17 or a Th1 effector response can drive autoimmunity: conditions of disease induction affect dominant effector category. J Exp Med 2008;205:799–810.
10. Caspi RR. Th1 and Th2 responses in pathogenesis and regulation of experimental autoimmune uveoretinitis. Int Rev Immunol 2002;21: 197–208.
11. Caspi RR. Ocular autoimmunity: the price of privilege? Immunol Rev 2006;213:23–35.
12. Sonoda KH, Sakamoto T, Qiao H, et al. The analysis of systemic tolerance elicited by antigen inoculation into the vitreous cavity: vitreous cavity-associated immune deviation. Immunology 2005;116:390–399.
13. Wenkel H, Streilein JW. Analysis of immune deviation elicited by antigens injected into the subretinal space. Invest Ophthalmol Vis Sci 1998;39: 1823–1834.
14. Streilein JW. Ocular immune privilege: the eye takes a dim but practical view of immunity and inflammation. J Leukoc Biol 2003;74: 179–185.
15. DeVoss J, Hou Y, Johannes K, et al. Spontaneous autoimmunity prevented by thymic expression of a single self-antigen. J Exp Med 2006;203: 2727–2735.
16. O'Garra A, Vieira P. Regulatory T cells and mechanisms of immune system control. Nat Med 2004;10:801–805.
17. Sacks D, Sher A. Evasion of innate immunity by parasitic protozoa. Nat Immunol 2002;3:1041–1047.
18. Sacks D, Sher A. Evasion of innate immunity by parasitic protozoa. Nat Immunol 2002;3:1041–1047.
19. Verjans GM, Feron EJ, Dings ME, et al. T cells specific for the triggering virus infiltrate the eye in patients with herpes simplex virus-mediated acute retinal necrosis. J Infect Dis 1998;178:27–34.
20. Kezuka T, Sakai J, Usui N, et al. Evidence for antigen-specific immune deviation in patients with acute retinal necrosis. Arch Ophthalmol 2001;119:1044–1049.
21. Cousins SW, Espinosa-Heidmann DG, Csaky KG. Monocyte activation in patients with age-related macular degeneration: a biomarker of risk for choroidal neovascularization? Arch Ophthalmol 2004;122:1013–1018.
22. Miller DM, Espinosa-Heidmann DG, Legra J, et al. The association of prior cytomegalovirus infection with neovascular age-related macular degeneration. Am J Ophthalmol 2004;138:323–328.
23. Hageman GS, Anderson DH, Johnson LV, et al. A common haplotype in the complement regulatory gene factor H (HF1/CFH) predisposes individuals to age-related macular degeneration. Proc Natl Acad Sci USA 2005;102:7227–7232.
24. Thakkinstian A, Han P, McEvoy M, et al. Systematic review and meta-analysis of the association between complement factor H Y402H polymorphisms and age-related macular degeneration. Hum Mol Genet 2006;15:2784–2790.
25. Seddon JM, Francis PJ, George S, et al. Association of CFH Y402H and LOC387715 A69S with progression of age-related macular degeneration. JAMA. 2007;297:1793–1800.
26. de Jong PT. Age-related macular degeneration. N Engl J Med 2006;355:1474–1485.
27. Boekhoorn SS, Vingerling JR, Witteman JC, et al. C-reactive protein level and risk of aging macula disorder: the Rotterdam study. Arch Ophthalmol 2007;125:1396–1401.
28. Hollyfield JG, Bonilha VL, Rayborn ME, et al. Oxidative damage-induced inflammation initiates age-related macular degeneration. Nat Med 2008;14:194–198.
29. Adamiec-Mroczek J, Oficjalska-Mlynczak J. Assessment of selected adhesion molecule and proinflammatory cytokine levels in the vitreous body of patients with type 2 diabetes – role of the inflammatory-immune process in the pathogenesis of proliferative diabetic retinopathy. Graefes Arch Clin Exp Ophthalmol 2008;246:1665–1670.
30. Funatsu H, Yamashita H, Noma H, et al. Aqueous humor levels of cytokines are related to vitreous levels and progression of diabetic retinopathy in diabetic patients. Graefes Arch Clin Exp Ophthalmol 2005;243:3–8.
31. Wirostko B, Wong TY, Simó R. Vascular endothelial growth factor and diabetic complications. Prog Retin Eye Res 2008;27:608–621.
32. Patel S, Chen H, Tinkham NH, et al. Genetic susceptibility of diabetic retinopathy. Curr Diabetes Rep 2008;8:257–262.
33. Stahn C, Lowenberg M, Hommes DW, et al. Molecular mechanisms of glucocorticoid action and selective glucocorticoid receptor agonists. Mol Cell Endocrinol 2007;275:71–78.
34. Wessels JA, Huizinga TW, Guchelaar HJ. Recent insights in the pharmacological actions of methotrexate in the treatment of rheumatoid arthritis. Rheumatology 2008;47:249–255.
35. Coulthard S, Hogarth L. The thiopurines: an update. Invest New Drugs 2005;23:523–532.
36. Allison AC, Eugui EM. Mycophenolate mofetil and its mechanisms of action. Immunopharmacology 2000;47:85–118.
37. Matsuda S, Koyasu S. Mechanisms of action of cyclosporine. Immunopharmacology 2000;47:119–125.
38. Miyata S, Ohkubo Y, Mutoh S. A review of the action of tacrolimus (FK506) on experimental models of rheumatoid arthritis. Inflamm Res 2005;54:1–9.
39. Sehgal SN. Sirolimus: its discovery, biological properties, and mechanism of action. Transplant Proc 2003;35(Suppl.):7S–14S.
40. Dejneka NS, Kuroki AM, Fosnot J, et al. Systemic rapamycin inhibits retinal and choroidal neovascularization in mice. Mol Vis 2004;10: 964–972.
41. Ahmad T, Wallace GR, James T, et al. Mapping the HLA association in Behçet's disease: a role for tumor necrosis facto polymorphisms? Arthritis Rheum 2003;48:807–813.
42. Mackensen F, Max R, Becker MD. Interferon therapy for ocular disease. Curr Opin Ophthalmol 2006;17:567–573.
43. Deuter CM, Kötter I, Wallace GR, et al. Behçet's disease: ocular effects and treatment. Prog Retin Eye Res 2008;27:111–136.
44. Van Gelder RN. Cme review: polymerase chain reaction diagnostics for posterior segment disease. Retina 2003;23:445–452.
45. McCann JD, Margolis TP, Wong MG, et al. A sensitive and specific polymerase chain reaction-based assay for the diagnosis of cytomegalovirus retinitis. Am J Ophthalmol 1995;120:219–226.
46. Knox CM, Cevallos V, Margolis TP, et al. Identification of bacterial pathogens in patients with endophthalmitis by 16S ribosomal DNA typing. Am J Ophthalmol 1999;128:511–512.
47. Jaeger EE, Carroll NM, Choudhury S, et al. Rapid detection and identification of *Candida, Aspergillus*, and *Fusarium* species in ocular samples using nested PCR. J Clin Microbiol 2000;38:2902–2908.
48. Chee SP, Bacsal K, Jap A, et al. Clinical features of cytomegalovirus anterior uveitis in immunocompetent patients. Am J Ophthalmol 2008;145: 834–840.
49. van Boxtel LA, van der Lelij A, van der Meer J, et al. Cytomegalovirus as a cause of anterior uveitis in immunocompetent patients. Ophthalmology 2007;114:1358–1362.
50. Tran TH, Rozenberg F, Cassoux N, et al. Polymerase chain reaction analysis of aqueous humour samples in necrotising retinitis. Br J Ophthalmol 2003;87:79–83.
51. Moshfeghi DM, Dodds EM, Couto CA, et al. Diagnostic approaches to severe, atypical toxoplasmosis mimicking acute retinal necrosis. Ophthalmology 2004;111:716–725.
52. Therese KL, Jayanthi U, Madhavan HN. Application of nested polymerase chain reaction (nPCR) using MPB 64 gene primers to detect *Mycobacterium tuberculosis* DNA in clinical specimens from extrapulmonary tuberculosis patients. Indian J Med Res 2005;122:165–170.
53. Dworkin LL, Gibler TM, Van Gelder RN. Real-time quantitative polymerase chain reaction diagnosis of infectious posterior uveitis. Arch Ophthalmol 2002;120:1534–1539.
54. Dabil H, Boley ML, Schmitz TM, et al. Validation of a diagnostic multiplex polymerase chain reaction assay for infectious posterior uveitis. Arch Ophthalmol 2001;119:1315–1322.
55. Chee SP, Bacsal K, Jap A, et al. Clinical features of cytomegalovirus anterior uveitis in immunocompetent patients. Am J Ophthalmol 2008;145: 834–840.
56. de Visser L, Braakenburg A, Rothova A, et al. Rubella virus-associated uveitis: clinical manifestations and visual prognosis. Am J Ophthalmol 2008;146:292–297.
57. Van Gelder RN. Idiopathic no more: clues to the pathogenesis of Fuchs heterochromic iridocyclitis and glaucomatocyclitic crisis. Am J Ophthalmol 2008;145:769–771.

58. van Boxtel LA, van der Lelij A, van der Meer J, et al. Cytomegalovirus as a cause of anterior uveitis in immunocompetent patients. Ophthalmology 2007;114:1358–1362.
59. Vitravene Study Group. Safety of intravitreous fomivirsen for treatment of cytomegalovirus retinitis in patients with AIDS. Am J Ophthalmol 2002; 133:484–498.
60. Andrei G, De Clercq E, Snoeck R. Novel inhibitors of human CMV. Curr Opin Invest Drugs 2008;9:132–145.
61. Fletcher EC, Chong NV. Looking beyond Lucentis on the management of macular degeneration. Eye 2008;22:742–750.
62. Adamis AP, Berman AJ. Immunological mechanisms in the pathogenesis of diabetic retinopathy. Semin Immunopathol 2008;30:65–84.

CHAPTER

6

Complement activation and inhibition in retinal disease

Mark E. Kleinman, MD and Jayakrishna Ambati, MD

INTRODUCTION

Within the past 20 years, a brigade of dedicated researchers from around the world has provided essential insights into the critical niche of immune-mediated inflammation in the pathogenesis of age-related macular degeneration (AMD). Yet, the question has lingered as to whether disease-initiating events are more or less dependent on isolated immune-related responses, unimpeded inflammation, endogenous pathways of age-related cell senescence and oxidative stress, or any of the other numerous molecular derangements that have been identified in the natural history of AMD.[1] There is now an abundant cache of data signifying immune system activation as an impetus in the pathogenesis of this devastating condition.[2] Furthermore, recent rigorous investigations have revealed multiple inciting factors, including several important complement activating components, thus creating a new array of disease-modulating targets for the research and development of molecular therapeutic interventions. While the precise *in vivo* effects of complement activation and inhibition in the progression and treatment of AMD remain to be determined, it is hoped that ongoing clinical trials of the first generation of complement-targeted therapeutics will yield critical data on the contribution of this pathway to the disease process.

HISTORY

The dysregulation of immunologic responses in the pathogenesis of retinal diseases, in particular AMD, have long been under investigation, but it is only recently that specific molecular mechanisms have been elucidated. The phalanx of mammalian immunity is controlled by two intercalated pathways: the innate and adaptive (or acquired) systems. Innate immunity is simply defined as the immediate nonspecific host response upon initial encounter with the pathogen. There is mounting evidence that immune complement, a major humoral component of the innate immune system, plays a major role in AMD pathobiology. Immune complement mediates the opsonization and clearance of pathogens through the classical, alternative, and lectin pathways, all of which feed into a common terminus (Figure 6.1). The alternative and lectin pathways differ from the classical pathway in that no specific antibody–antigen interaction is required for complement-mediated cell lysis.Inappropriate activation of complement occurs in several immunovascular diseases, including glomerulonephritis and rheumatoid arthritis. This immune-mediated inflammation ultimately serves to repair damaged tissue via cellular remodeling, neovascularization, and scar formation. However, when these processes beset the specialized tissues of the eye, they often result in significant vision loss due to hyperplasia of the retinal pigment epithelium (RPE), choroidal neovascularization (CNV), and disciform scarring. Drusen, the hallmark of AMD, actually harbor many of these activated complement factors and other inflammatory mediators that upregulate cytokines critical for CNV.[3] As clinicians and scientists have long suspected, there is now convincing evidence that drusen may not simply precede the pathogenic growth of choroidal blood vessels but actually promote it through specific complement-related mechanisms that are discussed in further detail below.

KEY CONCEPTS IN COMPLEMENT BIOLOGY

Excessive complement activation through the alternative pathway is proposed to contribute significantly to the progression of AMD.[4] There are several critical complement-mediated interactions which drive the feed-forward amplification of the alternative pathway (Figure 6.2). Firstly, factor C3b binds to a diverse array of proteins and polysaccharides present on pathogen membranes.[5] C3b is created upon cleavage of C3 in a reaction carried out by C3 convertase. This enzyme may be formed as a complex of C2a and C4b in the classical or lectin pathways or in the alternative pathway as a complex of the factor D cleaved component of factor B (Bb), properdin (factor P), and hydrolyzed C3.[6] The different forms of C3 convertase channel into a common pathway that supplies the complement cascade with ample C3b, as well as C3a and C5a, both potent anaphylatoxins that mediate leukocyte chemotaxis. It is important to note that the C3a/C5a ligand receptors, C3aR and C5aR, are not only present on circulating proinflammatory leukocytes and mast cells, but also within the retinal nerve fiber and inner plexiform layers.[7] These findings suggest that *in situ* C3a/C5a generation may directly induce cellular alterations of neural retinal elements independent of leukocyte mediation. In the common terminal pathway, a secondary product of C5 cleavage, C5b, assembles with complement factors 6–9 to form the membrane attack complement (MAC) that lyses cells to which it binds. An endogenous soluble complement inhibitor, complement factor H (CFH), is also present and capable of inactivating C3b through factor I binding,[8] thus preventing complement-mediated host cell death in tissues. CFH is expressed in the RPE and choroid[9] and is hypothesized to govern complement-mediated inflammation.

Previously, activation of the classical pathway was not purported to be a major contributory factor in AMD, as little evidence of antibody-mediated complement fixation or localization of specific classical pathway components existed *in vivo*.[10,11] However, there are now several studies reporting genetic association data with classical pathway factors that are mentioned in the next section. Mediators of the lectin pathway, namely the mannose-binding lectin-associated proteases (MASP-1 and -2), are also in early investigations as potential disease modulators of AMD progression and pathologic neovascularization. As modern research strives to unravel the complex interactions of the various complement pathways, the number of potential therapeutic targets for immune-related diseases in the eye and elsewhere will continue to rise. Yet, with only slightly more than a decade worth of advanced biomedical and translational research focused on this problem, there are already a multitude of major molecular discoveries that have propelled the development of specific complement factor-targeted interventions currently in clinical trials.

PATHOGENESIS MECHANISMS AND METABOLISM

Investigations into the molecular mechanisms of AMD pathogenesis have undergone a considerable shift, with numerous laboratories and pharmaceutical ventures now studying the specific mechanisms,

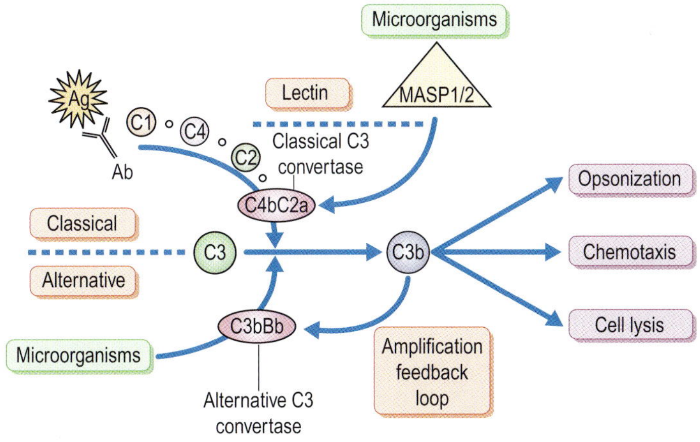

Figure 6.1 Three pathways to complement activation. To date, complement activation is known to occur through the classical, alternative, and lectin pathways. These interrelated molecular cascades share their ability to induce the assembly of C3 convertase, an enzyme that cleaves C3 to its active byproducts, C3a and C3b. C3 activation channels into a terminal pathway via C5 that leads to assembly of the membrane attack complement (MAC). Classical complement activation is initiated by antibody/antigen recognition, C1 binding, and formation of classical C3 convertase, C4bC2a. Conversely, the alternative pathway does not require immunoglobulin and is perpetuated by the binding of C3b to microorganisms and cell surfaces in order to join with cleaved factor B, Bb, and form C3bBb. This complex serves as the alternative form of C3 convertase and regenerates C3b, thereby creating a feedback amplification loop. The lectin pathway is regulated by the proteases mannose-binding lectin-associated proteases (MASP)-1 and -2 which interact via mannose-binding lectin-bound microorganisms to aid in the formation of C3 convertase. All three pathways result in robust host responses to increase opsonization, leukocyte chemotaxis, and cell lysis.

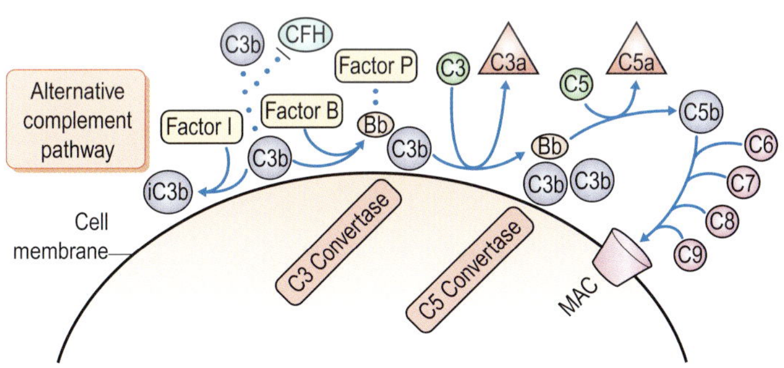

Figure 6.2 The alternative complement pathway. In the alternative pathway of complement activation, C3 convertase is spontaneously produced by hydrolysis of C3 to form C3(H_2O) in a process referred to as "tickover." If complement factor H (CFH) is not sufficient to inhibit cell surface binding, then C3(H_2O) will bind with Bb to form C3 convertase, resulting in activation of the downstream complement cascade. MAC, membrane attack complement.

genome-wide associations, and effects of excessive complement activation. The pioneering studies linking AMD and complement activation found evidence of premature drusen deposition in patients with membranoproliferative glomerulonephritis type II (MPGN-II),[12,13] a disease associated with mutations in the endogenous complement inhibitor, CFH.

CFH quickly advanced to the frontier of AMD biology after a group of independent laboratories simultaneously reported on a panel of single nucleotide polymorphisms (SNPs) within the human CFH gene that dramatically increased AMD risk.[9,14–16] Overall, these studies suggested that CFH accounts for approximately 50% of all cases of AMD. One of the identified mutations, the Y402H variant, was shown to increase AMD risk by nearly threefold in patients of European descent. The Y402H mutation is hypothesized to reduce heparin-binding affinity of CFH on cell membranes, thereby suppressing C3b inhibition and fueling alternative complement pathway activation.[17] Of note, mouse models of CFH deficiency exhibited some visual changes yet only subtle fundoscopic and microscopic features were consistent with human AMD.[18] This weak phenotype may be explained by biological differences between total gene deletion versus expression of the mutant *cfh* gene as well as divergences in human and mouse complement function. Aging of the RPE also decreased expression of CFH, a process postulated to be related to the photo-oxidation of photoreceptor outer segments and the generation of reactive oxygen species, both of which are known to occur in AMD.[19] Subsequent studies confirmed the increased prevalence of AMD in carriers of the CFH variants[20–22] and also identified SNPs in the C2, C3, and factor B genes that were associated with AMD.[23,24] A more recent report demonstrating the genetic association of a SNP of C1 inhibitor (also known as SERPING1) with AMD reinvigorated the hypothesis that classical complement activation is at least partially contributory to AMD progression.[25]

Another widely reported hypothesis is that the formation of inflammatory complement byproducts, most notably C3a and C5a, are responsible for instigating AMD progression. These potent chemoattractant factors were specifically localized to AMD drusen compared to non-AMD peripheral drusen from aged human eyes.[26] In the same study, C3a and C5a upregulated the expression of VEGF-A, a cytokine required for CNV progression. *In vitro*, primary RPE cell isolates treated with C3a or C5a for 8 hours secreted significantly more VEGF-A in both confluent and subconfluent cultures (correlates of healthy and degenerative RPE states, respectively).[26] Whereas an immortalized RPE cell line, D407, exhibited similar responses after C3a/C5a stimulation, primary human choroidal endothelial cells did not. *In vivo*, VEGF-A concentrations in RPE/choroid peaked just 4 hours after intravitreous C3a/C5a administration in a dose-dependent fashion, demonstrating the tissue-localized and rapid response to these anaphylotoxins. The temporal kinetics of this swift inflammatory reaction suggests that the RPE, and perhaps other resident cells, play a major role in VEGF-A production after complement activation (Figure 6.3).

Molecular investigations utilizing the accelerated laser injury-induced mouse model of CNV demonstrated that C3a/C5a levels are selectively increased in the RPE/choroid 12 hours after photocoagulation. With blockade of C3a and C5a, such as in mice that are deficient in C3aR and C5aR, VEGF-A production is suppressed at both 1 and 3 days post-laser. Given that VEGF-A production peaks at 3 days in this animal model, a timepoint which coincides with maximal macrophage infiltration, implementing a strategy to neutralize C3a/C5a signaling may also significantly inhibit leukocyte trafficking. In corroboration with this hypothesis, C3aR/C5aR-deficient mice exhibited decreased neutrophils and macrophages in RPE/choroid tissues after laser injury, resulting in decreased CNV formation. In conclusion, the amplified generation of C3a and C5a fragments during complement activation and the rapid downstream upregulation of VEGF-A may explain the abrupt switch-like progression to neovascular AMD in patients with previously dry fundus exams.

Several other complement-related inflammatory components are present in drusen and RPE/choroid in AMD-affected eyes. C-reactive protein (CRP), an acute-phase protein and commonly employed systemic marker of inflammation that assists in complement-mediated phagocytosis, was elevated in the peripheral blood of patients with AMD,[27] but further data were contradictory[28] perhaps due to patient variability. More recently, CRP has been found to be elevated in the choroid of patients that are homozygous for the CFH risk allele, 402HH.[29] Protein interaction studies of CFH demonstrate that CRP is a binding partner,[30] a function which is significantly reduced with the 402HH gene product.[31,32] Further studies are needed to determine the downstream effects of CRP and CFH interaction, as the current data still do not explain the increase in choroidal CRP in AMD-affected eyes.

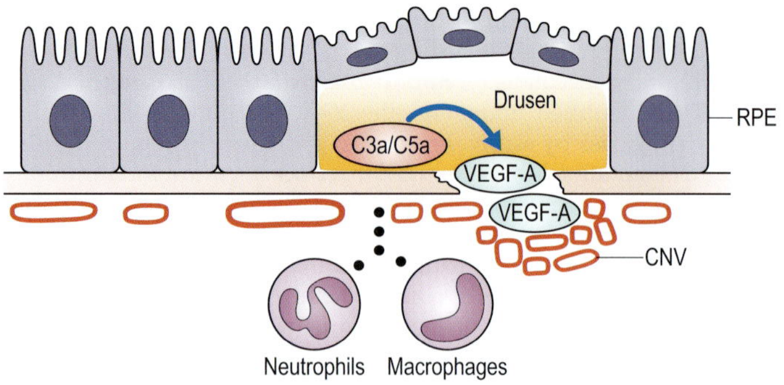

Figure 6.3 Drusen promote choroidal neovascularization (CNV) via C3a/C5a induction of vascular endothelial growth factor (VEGF-A). Complement factors are abundant in drusen and lead to the activation of numerous inflammatory pathways. C3a and C5a upregulate retinal pigment epithelium (RPE) production of VEGF-A which is able to stimulate choroidal endothelial cells to proliferate, migrate, and form leaky vasculature beneath Bruch's membrane, RPE and neural retina. C3a and C5a also function as potent chemoattractants for circulating leukocytes expressing their relative receptors. These include neutrophils and macrophages which accelerate the growth of CNV through cytokine and growth factor release.

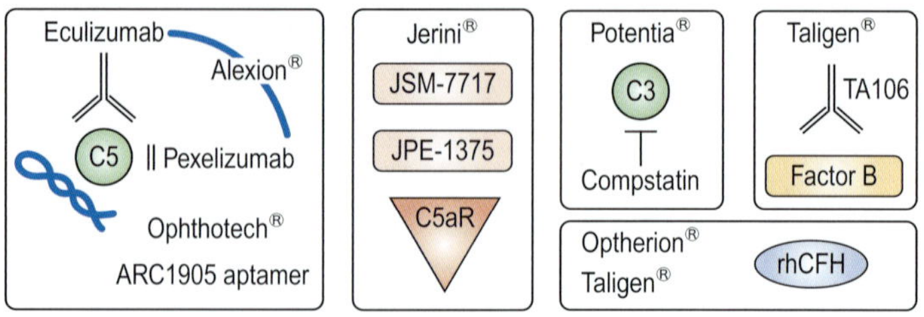

Figure 6.4 Complement factor targets for pharmacologic inhibition in retinal disease. Numerous therapeutic targets for complement pathway inhibition are in preclinical and clinical investigations. Alexion engineered a whole IgG humanized antibody (eculizumab) and single-chain variable fragment (pexelizumab) against C5. Ophthotech developed a pegylated RNA aptamer (ARC1905) that also neutralizes C5. Jerini discovered two peptidomimetics that antagonize C5a receptor and is planning trials to investigate efficacy in the treatment of wet and dry AMD. Potentia revived a previously described small-molecule inhibitor of C3, compstatin, and is currently in phase I trials for the treatment of wet AMD. Optherion is strategically focusing on complement factor H (CFH) repletion using recombinant protein technologies. Taligen is also exploring recombinant human CFH (rhCFH) therapies as well as factor B inhibition using a humanized antibody (TA106).

IMPLICATIONS FOR RETINAL PHARMACOTHERAPY

Even though the field of complement biology within the domain of ophthalmic science is relatively young, a host of new and established pharmaceutical companies are targeting this pathway with novel molecular therapeutics (Figure 6.4). Prior to the genetic association studies of CFH and AMD, the existence of complement activation was identified in rigorous studies demonstrating multiple alternative and terminal complement pathway components in drusen.[33] These provocative data fostered the hypothesis that perhaps a deficiency in endogenous complement inhibition promotes the onset of AMD, leading to several investigations of whether CFH was a major constituent of complement activation during disease progression. In patients with hypofunctional CFH mutations (e.g., Y402H), complement regulation is impaired and *in situ* generation of active complement fragments may result in overdriven assembly of the MAC complexes. Therefore, repletion of CFH utilizing recombinant proteins or genetic engineering is a plausible molecular intervention that is currently being explored by both Optherion and Taligen.

Given that most complement activity channels through C3 and C5, these factors have provided two major targets for therapeutic intervention for AMD. In 2007, the first complement inhibitor approved by the Food and Drug Administration (FDA) came to market, an anti-C5 humanized monoclonal antibody (eculizumab, Solaris) developed by Alexion for the treatment of paroxysmal nocturnal hemoglobinura. The company also developed a short-acting single-chain fragment of this antibody (pexelizumab) that is currently in advanced-phase trials in the treatment of myocardial infarction. While no clinical trials are underway yet evaluating these treatments for AMD, preclinical studies are ongoing and advancement to FDA studies is anticipated within the next few years. Ophthotech is in phase I trials of its anti-C5 aptamer, ARC1905, to study its safety profile and efficacy when used in combination with Lucentis for the treatment of neovascular AMD. Jerini Ophthalmics is targeting the C5a receptor with small-molecule peptidomimetic antagonists and is currently investigating two lead candidates (JPE-1375 and JSM-7717) with promising results in preclinical studies. While several companies have strategized in favor of targeting C5, as there are no known endogenous C5 inhibitors and activation can occur independent of C3, Potentia has rediscovered a small-molecule C3 inhibitor, compstatin (POT-4), and is in phase I trials to treat neovascular AMD. Another company, Taligen, is targeting factor B, an important component in alternative complement pathway amplification, using a humanized monoclonal antibody (TA106), and is currently conducting preclinical studies in animal models of CNV. While there are likely many more startups and lead compounds under investigation at larger pharmaceutical companies, determining the efficacy of complement inhibition in the treatment of neovascular and, perhaps, dry AMD, will be the next major step in improving the molecular and clinical implications of this complex biological pathway within the contexts of this blinding disease.

SUMMARY

Major scientific breakthroughs within the past decade revealed that complement dysregulation may provide a critical component to the inflammatory siege in the pathogenesis of AMD. Many of the specific complement factors responsible for these deleterious effects were identified through genome-wide association and functional studies *in vivo*. CHF, C2, C3, and factor B have all been genetically tied to AMD; however, the association data for CHF remain the most startling with mutations in this endogenous complement inhibitor accounting for approximately 50% of this disease. C3a and C5a, which are generated as byproducts of the common complement pathway and localized to AMD drusen, induce the expression of VEGF-A which is a major cytokine stimulus for CNV. Pharmacologic inhibition of the alternative complement pathway either through introduction of recombinant complement inhibitors or neutralization of specific complement factors is a valuable therapeutic strategy and is being aggressively pursued. In the coming years, further fundamental knowledge will undoubtedly be acquired regarding the role of complement inhibition and the efficacy of the various specific inhibitors as more clinical trials are conducted. Collectively, these data will undoubtedly guide future studies focused on interpreting complement activation and targeted inhibition in retinal diseases with the aim that a molecular therapeutic will be translated into the clinical setting for the benefit of patients suffering from AMD.

REFERENCES

1. Ambati J, Ambati BK, Yoo SH, et al. Age-related macular degeneration: etiology, pathogenesis, and therapeutic strategies. Surv Ophthalmol 2003;48:257–293.
2. Nussenblatt RB, Ferris 3rd F. Age-related macular degeneration and the immune response: implications for therapy. Am J Ophthalmol 2007;144:618–626.

3. Donoso LA, Kim D, Frost A, et al. The role of inflammation in the pathogenesis of age-related macular degeneration. Surv Ophthalmol 2006;51:137–152.
4. Gehrs KM, Anderson DH, Johnson LV, et al. Age-related macular degeneration – emerging pathogenetic and therapeutic concepts. Ann Med 2006;38:450–471.
5. Sahu A, Lambris JD. Structure and biology of complement protein C3, a connecting link between innate and acquired immunity. Immunol Rev 2001;180:35–48.
6. Janeway C. Immunobiology. New York: Garland Science; 2005.
7. Vogt SD, Barnum SR, Curcio CA, et al. Distribution of complement anaphylatoxin receptors and membrane-bound regulators in normal human retina. Exp Eye Res 2006;83:834–840.
8. Jozsi M, Oppermann M, Lambris JD, et al. The C-terminus of complement factor H is essential for host cell protection. Mol Immunol 2007;44: 2697–2706.
9. Hageman GS, Anderson DH, Johnson LV, et al. A common haplotype in the complement regulatory gene factor H (HF1/CFH) predisposes individuals to age-related macular degeneration. Proc Natl Acad Sci USA 2005;102:7227–7232.
10. Johnson LV, Leitner WP, Staples MK, et al. Complement activation and inflammatory processes in drusen formation and age related macular degeneration. Exp Eye Res 2001;73:887–896.
11. Anderson DH, Mullins RF, Hageman GS, et al. A role for local inflammation in the formation of drusen in the aging eye. Am J Ophthalmol 2002;134:411–431.
12. Duvall-Young J, MacDonald MK, McKechnie NM, et al. Fundus changes in (type II) mesangiocapillary glomerulonephritis simulating drusen: a histopathological report. Br J Ophthalmol 1989;73:297–302.
13. Mullins RF, Aptsiauri N, Hageman GS, et al. Structure and composition of drusen associated with glomerulonephritis: implications for the role of complement activation in drusen biogenesis. Eye 2001;15:390–395.
14. Edwards AO, Ritter 3rd R, Abel KJ, et al. Complement factor H polymorphism and age-related macular degeneration. Science 2005;308:421–424.
15. Haines JL, Hauser MA, Schmidt S, et al. Complement factor H variant increases the risk of age-related macular degeneration. Science 2005;308:419–421.
16. Klein RJ, Zeiss C, Chew EY, et al. Complement factor H polymorphism in age-related macular degeneration. Science 2005;308:385–389.
17. Clark SJ, Higman VA, Mulloy B, et al. H384 allotypic variant of factor H associated with age-related macular degeneration has different heparin-binding properties from the non-disease-associated form. J Biol Chem 2006;281:24713–24720.
18. Coffey PJ, Gias C, McDermott CJ, et al. Complement factor H deficiency in aged mice causes retinal abnormalities and visual dysfunction. Proc Natl Acad Sci USA 2007;104:16651–16656.
19. Chen M, Forrester JV, Xu H, et al. Synthesis of complement factor H by retinal pigment epithelial cells is down-regulated by oxidized photoreceptor outer segments. Exp Eye Res 2007;84:635–645.
20. Souied EH, Leveziel N, Richard F, et al. Y402H complement factor H polymorphism associated with exudative age-related macular degeneration in the French population. Mol Vis 2005;11:1135–1140.
21. Francis PJ, Schultz DW, Hamon S, et al. Haplotypes in the complement factor H (CFH) gene: associations with drusen and advanced age-related macular degeneration. PLoS ONE 2007;2:e1197.
22. Kim NR, Kang JH, Kwon OW, et al. Association between complement factor H gene polymorphisms and neovascular age-related macular degeneration in Koreans. Invest Ophthalmol Vis Sci 2008;49:2071–2076.
23. Gold B, Merriam JE, Zernant J, et al. Variation in factor B (BF) and complement component 2 (C2) genes is associated with age-related macular degeneration. Nat Genet 2006;38:458–462.
24. Yates JR, Sepp T, Matharu BK, et al. Complement C3 variant and the risk of age-related macular degeneration. N Engl J Med 2007;357:553–561.
25. Ennis S, Jomary C, Mullins R, et al. Association between the SERPING1 gene and age-related macular degeneration: a two-stage case-control study. Lancet 2008;372:1828–1834.
26. Nozaki M, Raisler BJ, Sakurai E, et al. Drusen complement components C3a and C5a promote choroidal neovascularization. Proc Natl Acad Sci USA 2006;103:2328–2333.
27. Seddon JM, Gensler G, Milton RC, et al. Association between C-reactive protein and age-related macular degeneration. JAMA 2004;291:704–710.
28. McGwin G, Hall TA, Xie A, et al. The relation between C reactive protein and age related macular degeneration in the Cardiovascular Health Study. Br J Ophthalmol 2005;89:1166–1170.
29. Johnson PT, Betts KE, Radeke MJ, et al. Individuals homozygous for the age-related macular degeneration risk-conferring variant of complement factor H have elevated levels of CRP in the choroid. Proc Natl Acad Sci USA 2006;103:17456–17461.
30. Giannakis E, Jokiranta TS, Male DA, et al. A common site within factor H SCR 7 responsible for binding heparin, C-reactive protein and streptococcal M protein. Eur J Immunol 2003;33:962–969.
31. Laine M, Jarva H, Seitsonen S, et al. Y402H polymorphism of complement factor H affects binding affinity to C-reactive protein. J Immunol 2007;178:3831–3836.
32. Ormsby RJ, Ranganathan S, Tong JC, et al. Functional and structural implications of the complement factor H Y402H polymorphism associated with age-related macular degeneration. Invest Ophthalmol Vis Sci 2008;49(5):1763–1770.
33. Mullins RF, Russell SR, Anderson DH, et al. Drusen associated with aging and age-related macular degeneration contain proteins common to extracellular deposits associated with atherosclerosis, elastosis, amyloidosis, and dense deposit disease. Faseb J 2000;14:835–846.

CHAPTER

7

Genetics of retinal disease

Madeleine K.M. Adams, MB, ChB, BSc (Hons), MRCOphth,
Robyn H. Guymer, MBBS, PhD, FRANZCO, and Paul N. Baird, BSc (Hons), PhD

INTRODUCTION

Genetics plays an increasingly important role in our understanding of retinal disease, aiding in diagnosis, furthering our knowledge of pathogenesis, and now proving instrumental in developing specific disease treatments.

Molecular genetics has allowed us to progress beyond merely classifying inherited retinal disease in humans on the basis of their phenotypes, to now being able to define disease at the molecular level. The identification of disease mutations permits the development and testing of functional animal models, with the aim of elucidating disease mechanisms as well as developing new and improved therapeutic agents, including the replacement of the defective gene through gene therapy. Recently two independent clinical trials provided a glimpse of the potential therapeutic power gene therapy may wield in retinal disease. These reported the first successful application of gene therapy to three young adult patients using subretinal injections of recombinant adeno-associated virus vector expressing complementary DNA (cDNA) of the retinal gene RPE65. Partial restoration of vision was achieved in these individuals possessing a rare form of inherited retinal disease, Leber's congenital amaurosis (LCA).[1,2]

Gene discovery in retinal diseases initially centered on those with a mendelian mode of inheritance, and these approaches were very successful in terms of numbers of genes and disease-causative mutations identified. Most recently, major advances in the study of complex retinal diseases such as diabetic retinopathy and age-related macular degeneration (AMD) have also been made, with both of these diseases showing a significant genetic component and a number of disease-associated variants identified. This information together with the ensuing improved knowledge of biological pathways involved in disease pathogenesis has provided a key impetus to the development of new treatment modalities.

This chapter will provide a historical perspective of gene discovery in retinal disease, using illustrative examples to look at the effect genetics has had on our understanding of retinal disease pathogenesis and consequently options for pharmacotherapy. Clearly, space restrictions prevent an indepth analysis, but it is hoped that it will serve to highlight a few aspects of this fascinating and rapidly changing field.

HISTORY OF RETINAL GENE DISCOVERY

Determining the underlying DNA sequence that constitutes a genotype and correlating this with disease phenotype is one of the fundamental aims of genetics. In the last two decades over 190 retinal disease-associated genes and loci have been identified, with hundreds of sequence variants as well as novel variants reported, and the numbers continue to increase (Figure 7.1). There is a startling contrast between the laborious, expensive methods used to unearth the first genes associated with retinitis pigmentosa (RP) in the early 1990s and the current clinic-based gene-specific microarray chips in use today. The latter are typically plated for every reported sequence variant in a number of genes involved in retinal disease. Such retinal gene chips are now in regular use for the study of hereditary retinal disease, based on genes such as RPE65 gene in LCA disease, the ABCA4 gene in Stargardt's disease, and multiple RP genes.[3–5] Using such technology, it is possible to identify known causative mutations within days rather than months and provide readily available clinic-based testing at a diagnostic or research level for a minimal charge. Future advances in this field will invariably include the scaling-up through the use of many more genes on a chip as well as individual whole-genome sequencing once costs are reduced. One can only probe for sequence variants that are already known or characterized for their involvement in retinal disease. Recent reviews of retinal dystrophy screening report, on average, a 50% success in identifying the causative mutation. However, there are still retinal disease pedigrees for which genetic linkage analysis has excluded all currently known loci and for which no known genes are known.[3,4]

The vast majority of hereditary retinal disease genes, including those for RP, LCA, and Stargardt's disease, have been identified through genetic linkage analysis where these genes have been shown to segregate with disease in a mendelian pattern of inheritance in large families or pedigrees. The mapping techniques first developed in the 1980s utilized restriction fragment length polymorphisms (RFLPs) as molecular markers, which were then superseded by distinctive sequences called microsatellite markers. However, prior to completion of the first linkage map, Botstein and Lander realized that most human traits and diseases followed complex modes of inheritance where there was no clearly definable inheritance pattern.[6,7] In addition, as in the case of AMD, linkage analysis may be hampered by the limited availability of multigenerational families due to the late onset of disease. Thus alternative approaches for studying such traits were sought and rapid advances have now been made in the study of complex retinal diseases through the use of single nucleotide polymorphisms (SNPs). These represent biallelic genetic variants randomly spaced across the genome at an average spacing of 1 every 300–400 nucleotides. These markers provide the basis for association studies, which identify the effect a genetic variant has on disease by examining whether there is an increased or decreased frequency of alleles or genotypes in cases when compared to that expected by random distribution, and compared to control individuals who present with no disease trait.[6]

Genome-wide association studies (GWAS) have hugely accelerated the pace of gene discovery in complex traits. GWAS using microarrays or "gene chips" can efficiently probe the genome to detect genomic differences associated with disease or the phenotypic trait of interest. A pioneering GWAS executed by Klein et al.[8] identified a strong association between the Y402H variant in the complement factor H (CFH) gene and AMD, similar results were obtained concurrently by other groups using distinct approaches.[9–12] Although GWAS was instrumental in the discovery of CFH at 1q31, several other genes linked or associated with AMD have also been identified using various genetic techniques. including the LOC387715/HTRA1 genes at 10q26, as well as the CFH-related (CFHR), C2/BF C3, and APOE genes.[13–16] Through the use of better-defined clinical phenotypes and larger cohort size, more powerful genetic studies are now being undertaken to allow genes of moderate effect size to be identified. The GWAS used by Hoh had a mere 100 000 SNPs, which was a figure initially postulated to be sufficient to map the genome effectively. The figure was then revised to 500 000; current gene chips are now in the range of 1 million SNPs.

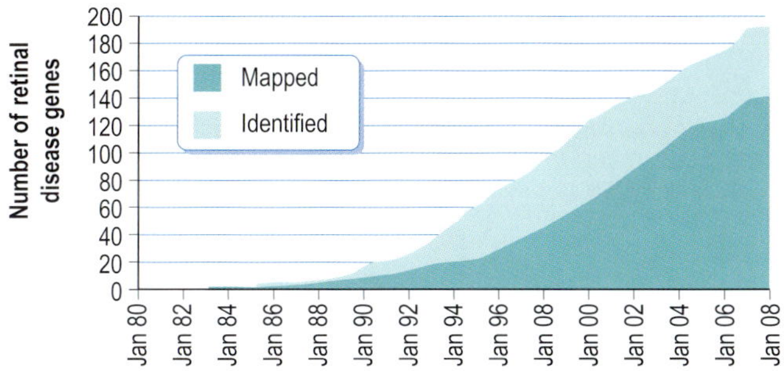

Figure 7.1 Number of mapped and identified retinal disease genes from 1980 to 2008. Reproduced from RetNet, the Retinal Information Network, http://www.sph.uth.tmc.edu/RetNet/, copyright Stephen P Daiger, PhD and The University of Texas Health Science Center, Houston, Texas, with permission.

GWAS of such a scale allow a huge amount of genomic information to be derived without the gold standard of needing complete genome sequencing for all, which, although rapidly approaching, is still just out of reach for most researchers for practical and economic reasons. Resequencing of a gene or locus of interest is now an accessible method to identify specific or novel changes in a gene that have been previously identified in disease.[5,17]

From the first complete sequencing of the human genome in 2001 up until 2004, SNPs were thought to be the major cause of genetic variation among individuals. Most attention had turned from structure to function. However the identification of genome-wide copy number variation (CNVs) has changed this belief. Analogous to chromosomal changes seen in cytogenetics, yet found in phenotypically normal individuals, these submicroscopic structural variants include deletions, duplications, inversions, and translocations which range in scale from a few kilobase pairs (kbp) up to 130 kbp.[18] They are randomly distributed throughout the genome and collectively they are thought to account for a large amount, if not most, of genomic variation. In view of their ubiquity, it is not surprising that the contribution to diseases by CNVs has become increasingly apparent. CNVs (deletions) in CFHR genes 1 and 3 have been shown to reduce the risk of developing AMD,[16] and deletions in PRPF31 have been found to account for at least 5% of autosomal-dominant RP.[3] Data regarding the fine-scale architecture and complexity of CNVs are still being compiled; this information is necessary to create an accurate baseline of genomic variation and to develop specific methods to examine further their disease associations. A step towards this is the first high-resolution map of structural variation, published in recent months.[19] Future GWAS with high densities of SNP markers and the ability to probe simultaneously for CNVs are likely to shed considerably more light on many diseases, including AMD.

Genetic testing improves diagnostic accuracy, provides prognostic information, is used in prenatal screening, and guides therapy, but the ultimate goal is to provide effective genotype-specific treatment, of which defective gene replacement through gene therapy holds the most promise. The precursors to techniques used in human gene therapy emerged in the 1970s and early 1980s. Mammalian genes were subcloned into prokaryotic plasmids and bacteriophages, retroviral vectors were developed and were in common laboratory use by the mid-1980s as a means to transfer genes into mammalian cells. By the late 1980s the stage was set for the first human trials of gene transfer in systemic disease. There have since been encouraging results from animal models and mixed, but promising, results from clinical trials in a range of retinal disease from retinoblastoma to AMD, many of which are still under way. There have also been exciting developments in pharmacotherapy as a direct result of our growing understanding of the pathogenesis of diseases such as AMD. These topics will be examined more closely later in the chapter.

KEY CONCEPTS AND FUNDAMENTS OF GENETIC METHODS IN THE STUDY OF RETINAL DISEASE

A glossary is provided to clarify terms used in genetic studies (Table 7.1).

GENETICS: ILLUMINATING MECHANISMS OF PATHOGENESIS, REVEALING COMPLEXITY

Developing effective, targeted therapy requires an understanding of the mechanisms of disease pathogenesis. Defining diseases on a molecular level has revealed the staggering genetic and pathogenic heterogeneity of retinal dystrophies, and perhaps explains why until now there has been a failure to develop such therapy.

RP: A "COMPLEX" MONOGENIC DISEASE

A spectacular example of such heterogeneity is RP, which is now recognized as not one disease, but a group of neurodegenerative retinal diseases that cause photoreceptor cell death that leads to progressive visual loss and blindness. They are clinically broadly similar despite many different causative genetic mutations and diverse pathogenic pathways; RP has been said to be no more a single disease than "fever of unknown origin." Fifty-three genes have been implicated in the pathogenesis of nonsyndromic RP and the related LCA, and many different mutations have been reported in these genes. There is a great functional diversity in the types of genes that have been implicated in RP; some are eye-specific (e.g., visual transduction cascade, structural proteins, retinoid cycle) or widely expressed (e.g., splicing factors, nucleotide metabolism).[3,4]

Even once a specific gene encoding a particular protein is known, it is not completely straightforward to link genotype and phenotype. An example is the gene encoding peripherin/retinal degeneration slow (RDS) protein. This is a multifunctional protein, important in disc morphogenesis, maintenance of proper disc alignment, and disc shedding. Peripherin/RDS mutations are an important cause of autosomal-dominant (ad) RP, accounting for approximately 9% of cases in northern European populations. To date, 34 different mutations of peripherin/RDS have been implicated in adRP. Transgenic mouse models and *in vitro* experiments have allowed detailed study of the variations in protein products from these different mutations and the resulting phenotypes; it appears that both haploinsufficiency and negative dominance play a role in pathogenesis. All mutations cause photoreceptor and RPE cell death, although the exact mechanisms remain unclear. Some animal studies have shown that distinct mutations affect rods and cones differently. As mentioned above, peripherin/RDS mutations can cause both RP and a range of macular dystrophies, but what is particularly interesting is that an identical mutation can cause completely different phenotypes within the same family[20] (Figure 7.2). These may range widely, from an apparently normal fundus to various macular dystrophies, cone–rod dystrophy as well as adRP, despite an identical causative mutation. Incomplete penetrance has been reported in other families. No satisfactory explanation yet exists for this spectrum in phenotype and variability in penetrance, but it is apparent that there are other factors which exert their influence on the phenotypic outcome: genetic background, environmental influences, and modifier genes have been suggested as plausible candidates.[21]

One such gene suspected of being a modifier gene was ROM1. Three different mutations in the ROM1 gene each cause RP only when co-inherited with a specific missense mutation (Leu185Pro) of peripherin/RDS; this is therefore termed digenic RP. However, mutations in ROM1 have not been found in two families with intrafamilial phenotypic variation,[22] suggesting that other modifier genes are likely to exist.

Table 7.1 **Glossary of genetic terms used**

Term	Description
Adeno-associated virus (AAV) vector	AAV is a small (20-nm) replication-defective, nonenveloped virus of the genus *Dependovirus*, family Parvoviridae. AAV is not currently known to cause disease and consequently the virus causes a very mild immune response. AAV can infect both dividing and nondividing cells. A vector is a gene delivery vehicle, introducing genetic material into a cell
Alleles	One member of a pair or series of different forms of a gene
Association studies	Studies which identify the effect a genetic variant has on disease by examining whether there is an increased or decreased frequency of alleles when compared to that expected by random distribution, and compared to control individuals who present with no disease trait. They can be used on populations rather than families and therefore wield much more power than linkage analysis. Those that use markers across the entire genome are genome-wide association studies (GWAS)
Complex disease	A disease where there is not a single contributory causal gene but many genes presenting in a polygenic pattern with gene effects ranging from small to large; no single gene is enough to invoke disease but each gene provides susceptibility and requires interplay with other factors such as gene–gene or gene–environment interactions to elicit disease. Also referred to as multifactorial disease
Copy number variations (CNVs)	A type of submicroscopic structural variation, randomly distributed throughout the genome, including deletion, duplication, inversion, and translocation, which range in scale from a few kilobase pairs up to 130 kbp. If SNPs are a misprint of a single letter on a page of text, CNVs represent a sentence, paragraph, or page which has been removed or duplicated, sometimes upside down
Digenic disease	Requires mutations on two genes to manifest the phenotype; each mutation alone will not cause disease
Gene therapy	Gene therapy is the insertion of genes into an individual's cells and tissues to treat a disease
Genetic heterogeneity	Describes a disease in which many different genetic mutations produce a phenotype
Genotype	The genetic constitution of a cell, an organism, or an individual, that is the specific allele makeup of the individual, usually with reference to a specific character under consideration
Haplotype	Alleles which cosegregate together in a block through numerous meiotic events in a population; if the block contains a founder mutation or risk variant that is shared by affected individuals through common descent it may be referred to as an ancestral haplotype
Linkage analysis	A relatively coarse measurement of genetic variation, models the distance between a putative disease locus and DNA marker loci. Exists in two forms: classical or parametric, used in mendelian disease, and nonparametric, for diseases with a complex inheritance
Mendelian inheritance	Inheritance of traits in patterns according to Mendel's law. Such traits are often called monogenic. They fall into five categories or modes of inheritance based on where the gene for the trait is located and how many copies of the mutant allele are required to express the phenotype: 1. Autosomal-recessive inheritance (the locus is on an autosomal chromosome and both alleles must be mutant alleles to express the phenotype) 2. Autosomal-dominant inheritance (the locus is on an autosomal chromosome and only one mutant allele is required for expression of the phenotype) 3. X-linked recessive inheritance (the locus is on the X chromosome and both alleles must be mutant alleles to express the phenotype in females) 4. X-linked dominant inheritance (the locus is on the X chromosome and only one mutant allele is required for expression of the phenotype in females) 5. Mitochondrial inheritance
Microarray chips (DNA microarrays)	A collection of DNA probes that are arrayed on a solid support and are used to assay, through hybridization, the presence of complementary DNA that is present in a sample.
Microsatellite	Also known as a short tandem repeat (STR) in DNA. A class of polymorphisms that occurs when a pattern of two or more nucleotides are repeated and the repeated sequences are directly adjacent to each other. The pattern can range in length from 2 to 10 basepairs (bp) (for example (CATG)n in a genomic region) and is typically in the noncoding intron region. Used as molecular markers in linkage analysis prior to the advent of SNPs
Modifier gene	Genetic variants which affect the clinical manifestation of disease; involved in gene–gene interaction, which is sometimes referred to as epistasis
Monogenic trait	A trait which requires one gene to be disrupted to manifest as a phenotype, often used interchangeably with mendelian trait
Penetrance	The percentage of individuals with a specific genotype that possess an associated phenotype
Phenotype	Physical characteristics of an individual
Restriction fragment length polymorphism (RFLP)	RFLP is a difference in homologous DNA sequences that can be detected by the presence of fragments of different lengths after digestion of the DNA samples in question with specific restriction endonucleases. RFLP, as a molecular marker, is specific to a single clone/restriction enzyme combination
RNAi-mediated suppression and codon-modified gene replacement	Gene therapy for dominantly inherited traits. Comprises two elements: gene suppression in conjunction with gene replacement. Suppression is targeted to a site independent of the mutation; therefore, both mutant and wild-type alleles are suppressed. In parallel with suppression, a codon-modified replacement gene refractory to suppression is provided
Sequencing	Process of determining the nucleotide order of a given DNA fragment
Single nucleotide polymorphisms (SNPs)	Nucleotide variations at only a single base, meaning that one base is substituted for another
Subcloning	A technique used in molecular biology to move a particular gene of interest from a parent vector to a destination vector in order to study its functionality

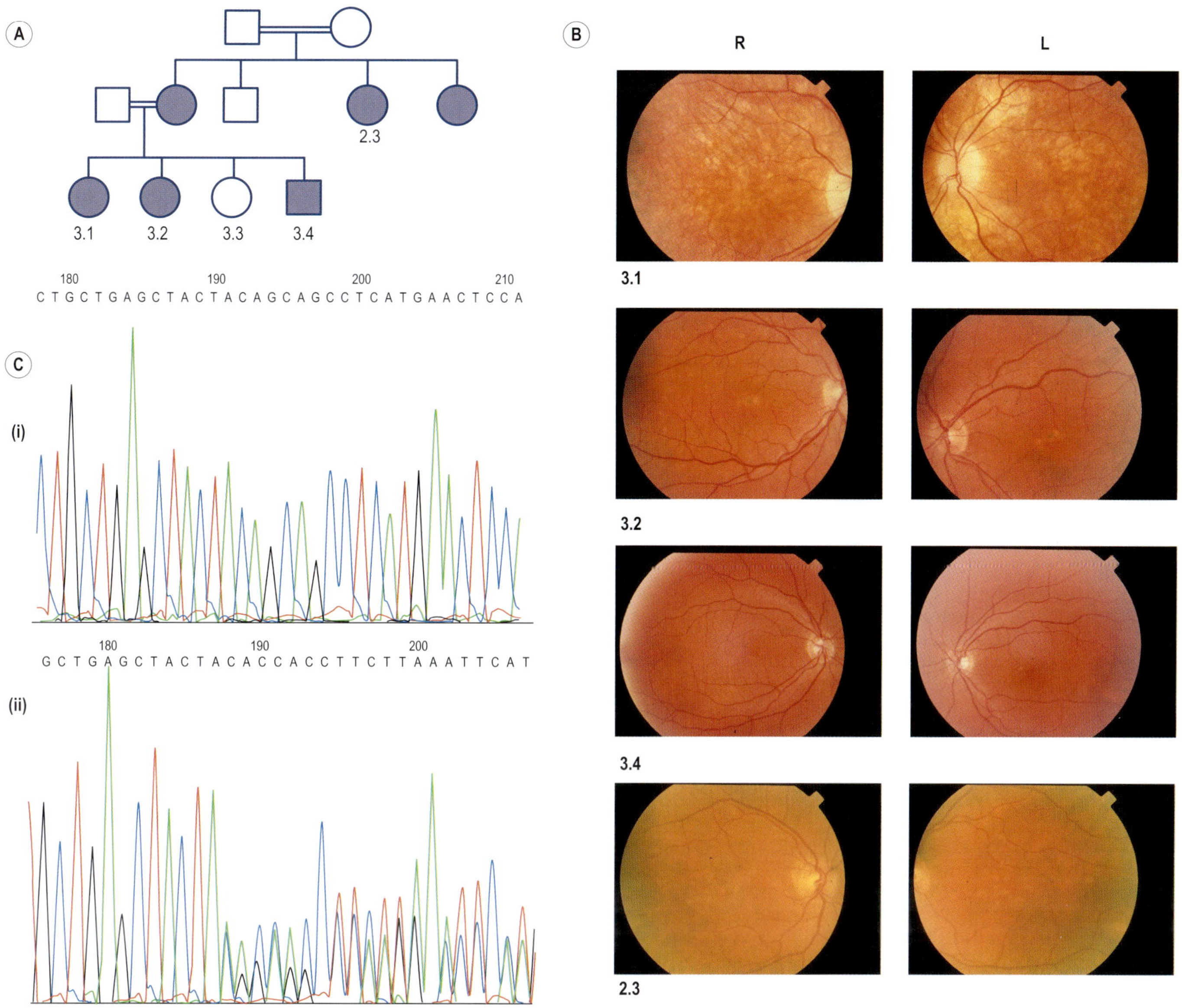

Figure 7.2 Phenotypic variation in individuals in a family with an identical retinal degeneration slow (RDS) mutation. (A) Pedigree of a family in which an RDS mutation is segregating. (B) Fundus photographs: subject 3.1 displays diffuse chorioretinal degenerative changes, in marked contrast to the discrete butterfly dystrophy seen in subjects 3.2, 3.4, and 2.3. (C) DNA sequences of (i) unaffected individual 3.3, and (ii) affected individual 3.4 showing the heterozygous mutation. The mutation is a TAC → TAA (C deletion) causing Tyr → STOP to occur at amino acid position 258 in exon 2 of the RDS gene (this mutation has been previously described by Wells et al.[19]).

Interest in modifier genes has grown with the discovery of a number of families with identical mutations producing distinct phenotypes. In one family with a peripherin/RDS mutation, rod–cone dystrophy was seen in affected male members, whereas female members had a macular disease; this raised the possibility of an X-linked modifier gene. Discordant phenotypes in fraternal (dizygotic) twins with a mutation in the RP GTPase regulator gene (RPGR) have also recently been reported.[23] Modifier genes thus add another layer of complexity to the pathogenic mechanisms of retinal dystrophies. As their effect is small, modifier genes are difficult to identify; GWAS and eventually routine sequencing are likely to further our knowledge in this area. It is possible that modifier genes may prove to be another potential target for gene therapy.

Environmental factors, which have been traditionally considered to exert little or no effect on monogenic disease (and therefore on which little research has been conducted), may also warrant further examination in future studies; some factors, such as light exposure, vitamin A, and dietary fats, are thought to influence macular dystrophies. Our expanding knowledge of the genetics of mendelian diseases and complex traits increasingly blurs the boundaries between them: mendelian traits are not so "cut and dry" in being simply inherited, and complex diseases such as AMD have been found to have a strong genetic component, with genetics unraveling many of its complexities.

SHEDDING LIGHT ON AMD

AMD is a multifactorial disease: in addition to a genetic component, age, diet and other environmental influences such as smoking affect phenotype. Late complications, which can lead to severe visual loss, include choroidal neovascularization (CNV), known as "wet AMD," and geographic atrophy, also known as "dry AMD." The immune system was first implicated in the pathogenesis of AMD in 1999 as a result of some elegant immunocytochemical analyses performed by Hageman et al.[24] on drusen, the hallmark of early AMD. These were found to contain components of the inflammatory process, particularly molecules associated with the alternative pathway of the complement pathway and its regulators, and further analyses strengthened the immune/inflammatory hypothesis by identification of signs of local inflammatory and immune processes, including complement proteins, fibrinogen, vitronectin, and C-reactive protein (CRP). This role of inflammation appeared to be confirmed by three publications published concurrently in 2005 which identified that a polymorphism rs1061170 (representing a tyrosine → histidine change at amino acid 402, i.e., Y402H) in the CFH gene was associated with an increased risk of AMD.[8–10] The CFH gene is located on the regulation of complement activation (RCA) locus on chromosome 1q31. A meta-analysis of multiple association studies revealed heterozygous and homozygous carriers of the risk allele for CFH had a 2.5-fold and a sixfold increase in developing AMD respectively, compared to the nonrisk allele.[25] These studies demonstrate that the inflammatory changes are directly related to the risk of developing disease and not a secondary tissue response.

CFH is an abundant plasma protein comprising 20 repetitive units of 60 amino acids called complement control protein modules or short consensus repeat (SCR) domains. It is produced both in the liver for systemic use and also locally in the RPE. CFH is essential in homeostasis of the alternative complement pathway (AP), which is important in the binding of and destruction of pathogens, tumor cells, and damaged host cells.

Recent work by Ormsby et al.[26] demonstrated that the Y402H polymorphism affected the protein binding of CFH. Their study indicated that the Y402H variant of CFH and CFH related-1 (CFHR1) caused a reduction in binding of CFH and CFHR1 to CRP, but not to RPE cells, as was previously thought. CRP is an acute-phase reactant with both proinflammatory and anti-inflammatory properties; it plays an important part in downregulating the AP by recruiting CFH/CFHR1. A reduction in binding of CFH by CRP would therefore impede the ability of CRP to inhibit AP activation. Individuals with elevated levels of CRP with normal proinflammatory properties but attenuated anti-inflammatory abilities (due to the Y402H polymorphisms) could develop uncontrolled and chronic inflammation. This suggestion correlates with investigations showing an increased risk of AMD in persons carrying both the Y402H variant and a CRP haplotype (a particular signature of SNPs across a gene or part of a gene) which confers a higher serum CRP. The Rotterdam study also revealed an association between elevated serum CRP and the development of early and late AMD.[27]

What are possible triggers of the AP and resultant uncontrolled inflammation? A pathogen would be a likely candidate, as this represents one of the targets of the AP. There is now evidence for a gene–environment interaction between a pathogenic organism, *Chlamydia pneumoniae,* and CFH in the etiology of AMD. Individuals homozygous for the risk allele of CC Y402H with high titers of *C. pneumoniae* were reported as having a 12-fold increased risk of AMD disease progression. Additional analysis using another SNP in the CFH gene previously shown to be associated with AMD progression (SNP rs2274700) revealed a similar effect. Further work will explore the multiple allelic involvement of both CFH variants and other genes in the context of this gene–environment interaction.[28]

Investigation into other genes involved in innate immunity was prompted by the identification of disease-associated variants in the CFH gene. In particular, other genes in either the AP or immune response that have been implicated in AMD include the C2/BF genes for complement factor B on chromosome 6 and, more recently, the C3 gene.[13–16] Not all gene variants are risk, as some have also been shown to confer a protective effect. None of these latter identified genes appear to exhibit such strong association with disease as variants identified in either the CFH or LOC387715/HTRA1 genes.

Far from the RCA locus, the hypothetical LOC387715 and HTRA1 genes on chromosome 10q were first flagged as being associated with AMD in 2005. In 2007 Schaumberg et al.[29] reported that if the CFH risk allele or the A69S risk allele variant in LOC387715 were present, this led to an increased AMD risk of 3.8-fold, whereas having two copies of both risk alleles increased the risk a remarkable 50-fold; the combined effect carried a population-attributable risk of greater than 60%, indicating that at least half of the etiology underlying AMD in the particular population studied was due to variants in these two genes. LOC387715 was until recently referred to as a hypothetical gene as its protein function was not known; Kanda et al. have presented some evidence to suggest that it codes for a 12-kDa protein which localizes to the mitochondrial outer membrane and this locus has been named as ARMS2.[30] However, there is still conjecture as to whether this or the neighboring HTRA1 gene represents the causative gene in this region. Interestingly, a mitochondrial DNA polymorphism A4917G has recently been associated with an increased AMD risk[31] and this raises the question as to whether AMD shares similar pathogenic mechanisms to other age-related neurodegenerative disorders such as Alzheimer's disease and Parkinson's disease, as disruption of mitochondrial function has also been implicated in these two diseases. These findings make it likely that mitochondria will be as intensely studied in AMD as complement over the next few years.

IMPLICATIONS FOR RETINAL PHARMACOTHERAPY

Our increased understanding of the molecular pathogenesis of retinal disorders has facilitated advances in therapeutic strategies, including targeting correction of the primary genetic lesion, delivery of genes to express proteins, or factors to target pathogenic pathways and also gene-independent therapy. A few examples of recent developments are considered below.

GENE THERAPY DIRECTLY TARGETING THE PRIMARY GENETIC LESION

Gene therapy appears to be the most promising approach for retinal dystrophies. The eye is cited as an ideal system for gene therapy for a number of reasons: it is an immune-protective environment, the eye has a small volume to allow concentration of the viral vector, it possesses optically clear media which allow easy visualization, and local administration is readily achievable with minimal systemic exposure. However retinal dystrophies also pose some challenges: extreme mutational heterogeneity (with over 150 different mutations in one RP gene, rhodopsin, alone), and some technical difficulties inherent in treating photoreceptor cells which are targeted in most dystrophies as they have photoreceptor-specific transcripts. Additionally there are potential immune reactions when treating dominantly inherited diseases using gene therapy, therefore most progress has been made in the area of autosomal-recessive (ar) degenerations. Approaches are being developed to circumvent problems with dominance and heterogeneity, such as suppression and replacement using RNAi-mediated suppression in parallel with a codon-modified replacement gene.[32,33]

Recent successes in the treatment of a subtype of LCA2, caused by a mutation in RPE65, have generated hope that rescue of sight by gene therapy may soon be realized. LCA is a genetically heterogeneous group of recessively inherited blinding retinal dystrophies, with onset during childhood. Progression to blindness by the third decade is typical. RPE65 encodes a 65-kDa protein that is a key component of the visual cycle, a biochemical pathway that regenerates the visual pigment after light exposure. A lack of RPE65 results in deficiency of 11-*cis* retinal, rendering rod photoreceptor cells unable to respond to light. Two independent clinical trials in the USA and UK, designed primarily to establish the safety of subretinal delivery of a recombinant adeno-associated virus carrying RPE65 complementary DNA, have reported a modest improvement of vision in some patients following treatment.[1,2] Of a total of six, four had subjective increases in visual function including navigational vision; the three patients in the US trial had improvements in their Snellen visual acuity of 3, 3.5, and 4.5 lines of letters. The patients in the trial were young adults with severe visual loss; the eye with the worse acuity was treated. It seems likely that efficacy will be improved if treatment can be applied in a pediatric population, before amblyopia and retinal degeneration are established. In the naturally occurring animal model of LCA2, the Briard dog (with an rpe65 null mutation), RPE65 gene therapy has been shown to result in long-term rescue (over 5 years) of photoreceptor cells following a single injection.[32] The first successful fetal gene therapy used rpe65 mice; it may be that fetal therapy following prenatal testing is therefore the future for LCA2 treatment.

While there are encouraging results from viral-mediated gene therapy, it is known to have a number of physical limitations, including random integration into the host's genome, immunogenicity of the vector, and limitations in the DNA insert size. These have prompted the development of nonviral methods such as liposomes, compacted DNA nanoparticles, or combinations of both. Nanoparticles have been shown to be nonimmunogenic, noninflammatory, and nontoxic in various tissues, with higher transfection rates than any viral vector. They have had some success in phase I/II clinical trials for cystic fibrosis: ocular-specific nanoparticles for use in retinal dystrophies are being developed.[34]

DELIVERY OF GENES TO TARGET PATHOGENIC PATHWAYS

The multiplicity of mechanisms in the pathogenesis of RP reflecting its genetic heterogeneity prompted a search for therapeutic agents that might be effective in slowing photoreceptor cell death regardless of the causative genetic mutation. One such generic intervention that showed initial promise was through the delivery of the human ciliary neurotrophic factor (CNTF) gene within an encapsulated cell intraocular implant. Although found to be effective in retarding retinal degeneration in a number of transgenic animal models representing different genotypes of RP, it did not prevent photoreceptor cell death in an X-linked canine model. In a recent phase I clinical trial several subjects were reported to show an improvement in visual acuity following treatment, although the trial was not designed or powered to measure the significance of such outcomes. Further trials are required to evaluate whether this could provide either an alternative or an adjunct to primary gene-specific therapy.[35]

Most biological processes represent a balance between endogenous protein agonists and antagonists. When overactivity of a process is found to play a key role in the pathogenesis of a disease, an endogenous antagonist can be used to suppress the process. Gene therapy can therefore be used to transduce DNA into the host cell which stimulates expression of the antagonist. Such an approach circumvents problems with balancing specificity and toxicity of the therapeutic agent, and allows sustained delivery to a targeted organ without systemic effects. This method may be useful in a multifactorial disease such as AMD where no single specific primary genetic lesion may be targeted.

A common model for the wet form of AMD is induction of CNV by disrupting rodent or pig Bruch's membrane with laser. This model has been used to test the delivery of genes to stimulate the endogenous antagonist to vascular endothelial growth factor (VEGF), namely pigment epithelial-derived growth factor (PEDF) using adenovirus as a vector, i.e., AdPEDF. Exogenous anti-VEGF treatments are the current most successful treatment for CNV in our limited armoury, but as they seem to have a relatively transient effect they require frequent administration through intraocular injections and are therefore not without risk. Although AdPEDF also currently requires such injections it carries the advantages of specificity and low toxicity mentioned above and it is hoped it will provide longer-term downregulation of VEGF. Results from animal studies have shown considerable success in suppressing neovascularization. A phase I clinical trial, although not designed to address efficacy, reported promising signs of sustained antiangiogenic activity in treated eyes.[36,37] The risks associated with intraocular injections may be avoided if the development of a new platform for drug delivery is successful. Seagull Technologies is coupling nanotechnology and ultrasound to produce a noninvasive method of retinal drug delivery.[38] Developed primarily for anti-VEGFs, it could also prove to be useful in gene therapy.

GENE-INDEPENDENT THERAPY

The considerable leaps in our understanding of the molecular basis of retinal disease have also allowed new gene-independent therapies to be developed which target specific pathophysiological pathways without stimulating or suppressing genes directly.

Professor Hageman and the company Optherion have worked to create novel therapies for AMD. Optherion's primary therapeutic aim is to replace dysfunctional CFH with normal CFH. This principle has been already proven in another disease, atypical hemolytic–uremic syndrome (HUS). Some types of HUS are caused by factor H deficiency caused by a mutation in the CFH gene. Plasma exchange in these people, which replaces the CFH, is effective in preventing disease episodes and normalizes kidney function. Optherion's products are still in the preclinical stage of development.[39]

Dr. Holer and Dr. Emlen are the co-founders of Taligen, which is another company currently developing AMD treatments that target the AP. Taligen's technologies focus on controlling the amplification of complement activation: a monoclonal antibody which targets factor B (TA106) is designed to inhibit the activation of the alternative pathway of complement, and the targeted inhibitor program (TT30) allows for delivering endogenous inhibitors of the alternative pathway specifically to sites where complement activation is occurring. This targeting technology is designed to provide local regulation of complement activation without triggering systemic complement inhibition, potentially allowing application to a broad range of autoimmune and inflammatory diseases. Taligen has proof-of-concept data using this technology in animal models of CNV, and data demonstrating that targeted delivery of the complement-inhibitory portion of factor H to sites of complement activation with TT30 (CR2~factor H) is equally efficacious in animal models of CNV when given by systemic or by intraocular injection.[40]

The association between *C. pneumoniae* antibody titers, CFH alleles, and AMD risk prompts the question: could prophylactic antibiotics play a role in slowing the development of AMD? Over the last 20 years, the role of *C. pneumoniae* in another complex disease, atherosclerosis, has been evaluated, but it has proven difficult to establish a definite causal role for a common agent in a highly prevalent disease. Many seroepidemiological studies indicate an association between infection and cardiovascular events, yet a recent meta-analysis of 393 papers concluded there is no evidence for the use of antibiotics as a form of secondary prevention for cardiovascular disease.[41,42] Considerable progress towards developing a *C. pneumoniae* vaccine has been made in the past decade, but a vaccine that offers long-lasting immunity in humans is not yet available. For AMD, more research is required to explore the possible role of infection in AMD, including other possible trigger pathogens which may represent therapeutic targets.

Targeting pathways shared by genetically heterogeneous diseases leading to cell death has been proposed as a potential therapy. In RP the final common pathway has been found to be apoptosis of photoreceptors, although it is not yet known whether the same molecular mechanisms are activated during the cell demise in RP caused by different genetic lesions. Inhibiting enzymes involved in apoptosis could potentially provide a generic therapy for RP; further studies in animal models should indicate whether this is viable.[43]

GENOTYPE AS PREDICTOR OF RESPONSE TO TREATMENT

Genotype variation can alter the response to drugs; this information is already in use in several systemic diseases such as human immunodeficiency virus (HIV), Stevens–Johnson, and melanoma. It is probable that genotyping will increasingly be used to guide treatment and predict outcomes in eye disease also. Pharmacogenetic studies in AMD have suggested that CFH genotype may play a role in response to antioxidants and zinc,[44] and also in photodynamic therapy. There are currently studies under way examining possible associations between genotype and failure to respond to current anti-VEGF treatments. It is now technically feasible to identify genetic factors affecting drug response using appropriately designed GWAS performed on responder and nonresponder groups in clinical trials.

SUMMARY: THE FUTURE IS BRIGHT

The advance in our understanding of the molecular basis of retinal disease in the last two decades has been remarkable. From merely classifying disease using phenotypes, we are now aware of over 190 genes important in the pathogenesis of such disease and are moving ever closer to grasping the complexities of how these translate into phenotypes. This progress has been made possible by the collaboration of investigators from diverse disciplines: scientists with expertise in biophysics, molecular biology, and epidemiology as well as geneticists and ophthalmic clinicians who have all worked successfully together to provide answers to many of the questions surrounding inherited retinal disease. With the unprecedented flow of data emerging from GWAS and genome sequencing we will depend increasingly on the input of computer scientists and statisticians. The next 5 years are likely to be as exciting, if not more, so than the last 20, and it is ultimately the patients who should gain most from the long-awaited implementation of our discoveries into effective therapy.

Key points

- Significant advances in our understanding of the genetics of retinal diseases have been made in recent years, aided by microarray chips, GWAS, and the advent of affordable sequencing.
- Inherited retinal diseases of mendelian inheritance have been found to exhibit extreme genetic heterogeneity. Phenotypic variation displayed in pedigrees possessing identical mutations is not yet completely understood; possible mechanisms are modifier genes and environmental factors.
- Diseases of complex inheritance such as AMD are now known to have a strong genetic component. Genetic studies were pivotal in the implication of inflammation and innate immunity, in particular the alternative complement pathway, in the pathogenesis of AMD. This knowledge has inspired the development of therapies for AMD which target these pathways.
- Gene therapy is the most promising approach for the treatment of inherited retinal dystrophies; recent successes in LCA pave the way for further clinical trials.

REFERENCES

1. Bainbridge JWB, Smith AJ, Barker SS, et al. Effect of gene therapy on visual function in Leber's congenital amaurosis. N Engl J Med 2008;358: 2231–2239.
2. Maguire AM, Simonelli F, Pierce EA, et al. Safety and efficacy of gene transfer for Leber's congenital amaurosis. N Engl J Med 2008;358: 2240–2248.
3. Daiger SP, Bowne SJ, Sullivan LS. Perspective on genes and mutations causing retinitis pigmentosa. Arch Ophthalmol 2007;125:151–158.
4. Koenekoop RK, Lopez I, den Hollander AI, et al. Genetic testing for retinal dystrophies and dysfunctions: benefits, dilemmas and solutions. Clin Exp Ophthalmol 2007;35:473–485.
5. Mandal MdNA, Heckenlively JR, Burch T, et al. Sequencing arrays for screening multiple genes associated with early onset human retinal degenerations on a high-throughput platform. Invest Ophthalmol Vis Sci 2005;46:3355–3362.
6. Kruglyak L. The road to genome wide studies. Nat Rev Genet 2008;9:314–318.
7. Lander ES, Botstein D. Mapping complex genetic traits in humans: new methods using a complete RFLP linkage map. Cold Spring Harb Symp Quant Biol 1986;51:49–62.
8. Klein RJ, Zeiss C, Chew EY, et al. Complement factor H polymorphism in age related macular degeneration. Science 2005;308:385–389.
9. Edwards AO, Ritter R III, Abel KJ, et al. Complement factor H polymorphism and age-related macular degeneration. Science 2005;308:421–424.
10. Haines JL, Hauser MA, Schmidt S, et al. Complement factor H variant increases the risk of age-related macular degeneration. Science 2005;308:419–421.
11. Hageman GS, Anderson DH, Johnson LV, et al. A common haplotype in the complement regulatory gene factor H (HF1/CFH) predisposes individuals to age-related macular degeneration. Proc Natl Acad Sci USA 2005;102:7227–7232.
12. Zareparsi S, Branham KE, Li M, et al. Strong association of the Y402H variant in complement factor H at 1q32 with susceptibility to age-related macular degeneration. Am J Hum Genet 2005;77:149–153.
13. Thakkinstian A, Bowe S, McEvoy M, et al. Association between apolipoprotein E polymorphisms and age-related macular degeneration: a HuGE review and meta-analysis. Am J Epidemiol 2006;164:813–822.
14. Yates RWJ, Sepp T, Matharu BK, et al. Complement C3 variant and the risk of age-related macular degeneration. N Engl J Med 2007;357: 553–561.
15. Gold B, Merriam JE, Zernant J, et al. Variation in factor B (BF) and complement component 2 (C2) genes is associated with age-related macular degeneration. Nat Genet 2006;38:458–462.
16. Spencer KL, Hauser MA, Olsen LM, et al. Deletion of CFHR3 and CFHR1 genes in age related macular degeneration. Hum Mol Genet 2008;17: 971–977.
17. Gresham D, Dunham MJ, Botstein D. Comparing whole genomes using DNA microarrays. Nat Rev Genet 2008;9:291–302.
18. Wong KK, deLeeuw RJ, Dosanjh NS, et al. A comprehensive analysis of common copy-number variations in the human genome. Am J Hum Genet 2007;80:91–104.
19. Kidd JM, Cooper GM, Donahue WF, et al. Mapping and sequencing of structural variation from eight human genomes. Nature 2008;453:56–64.
20. Wells J, Wroblewski J, Keen J, et al. Mutations in the human retinal degeneration slow (RDS) gene can cause either retinitis pigmentosa or macular dystrophy. Nat Genet 1993;3:213–218.
21. Boon CJF, den Hollander AI, Hoyng CB, et al. The spectrum of retinal dystrophies caused by mutations in the peripherin/RDS gene. Prog Retin Eye Res 2008;27:213–235.
22. Leroy BP, Kailasanathan A, De Laey JJ, et al. Intrafamilal phenotypic variability in families with RDS mutations: exclusion of ROM1 as a genetic modifier for those with retinitis pigmentosa. Br J Ophthalmol 2007;91: 89–93.
23. Walia S, Fishman GA, Swaroop A, et al. Discordant phenotypes in fraternal twins having an identical mutation in exon ORF15 of the RPGR gene. Arch Ophthalmol 2008;126:379–384.
24. Hageman GS, Mullins RF, Russell SR, et al. Vitronectin is a constituent of ocular drusen and the vitronectin gene is expressed in human retinal pigmented epithelial cells. FASEB J 1999;13:477–484.
25. Thakkinstian A, Han P, McEvoy M, et al. Systematic review and meta-analysis of the association between complement factor HY402H polymorphisms and age related macular degeneration. Hum Mol Genet 2006;15:2784–2790.
26. Ormsby RJ, Rangathan S, Tong C, et al. Functional and structural implications of the complement factor H Y402H polymorphism associated with age related macular degeneration. Invest Ophthalmol Vis Sci 2008;49:1763–1770.
27. Boekhoorn SS, Vingerling JR, Wittmman JCM, et al. C-reactive protein and risk of aging macula disorder. The Rotterdam Study. Arch Ophthalmol 2007;125:1396–1401.
28. Baird PN, Robman LD, Richardson AJ, et al. Gene–environment interaction in progression of AMD: the CFH gene, smoking and exposure to chronic infection. Hum Mol Genet 2008;17:1299–1305.
29. Schaumberg DA, Hankinson SE, Guo Q, et al. A prospective study of 2 major age related macular degeneration susceptibility alleles and interactions with modifiable risk factors. Arch Ophthalmol 2007;125:55–62.
30. Kanda A, Chen W, Othman M, et al. A variant of mitochondrial protein LOC387715/ARMS2, not HTRA1, is strongly associated with age related macular degeneration. Proc Natl Acad Sci 2007;104: 16227–16232.
31. Canter JA, Olson LM, Spencer K, et al. Mitochondrial DNA polymorphisms A4917G is independently associated with age related macular degeneration. PLoS ONE 2008;3:e2091.
32. Rex TS. Rescue of sight by gene therapy – closer than it may appear. Ophthalm Genet 2007;28:127–133.
33. O'Reilly M, Millington-Ward S, Palfi A, et al. A transgenic mouse model for gene therapy of rhodopsin-linked retinitis pigmentosa. Vis Res 2008;48: 386–391.
34. Cai X, Conley S, Naash M. Nanoparticle applications in ocular gene therapy. Vis Res 2008;48:319–324.
35. Sieving PA, Caruso RC, Tao W, et al. Ciliary neurotrophic factor (CNTF) for human retinal degeneration: phase 1 trial of CNTF deleivered by encapsulated cell intraocular implants. Proc Natl Acad Sci 2006;103:3896–3901.
36. Campachiaro PA, Nquyen QD, Shah MS, et al. Adenoviral vector-delivered pigment epithelium derived factor for neovascular age related macular degeneration: results of a phase 1 clinical trial. Hum Gene Ther 2006;17:167–176.
37. Saishin Y, Silva RL, Saishin Y, et al. Periocular gene transfer of pigment epithelium derived factor inhibits choroidal neovascularisation in a human sized eye. Hum Gene Ther 2005;16:473–478.
38. Seagull Technologies. Available online at: <http://www.seagulltechnologies.com.au/>.

39. Optherion. Available online at: <http://www.optherion.com/about-optherion>.
40. Taligen Therapeutics. Available online at: <http://www.taligentherapeutics.com/>.
41. Song Z, Brassard P, Brophy JM. A meta-analysis of antibiotic use for the secondary prevention of cardiovascular diseases. Can J Cardiol 2008;24:391–395.
42. Watson C, Alp NJ. Role of *Chlamydia pneumoniae* in atherosclerosis. Clin Sci (Lond) 2008;114:509–531.
43. Marigo V. Programmed cell death in retinal degeneration. Cell Cycle 2007;6:652–655.
44. Klein ML, Francis PJ, Rosner B, et al. CFH and LOC387715/ARMS2 genotypes and treatment with antioxidants and zinc for age related macular degeneration. Ophthalmology 2008;115:1019–1025.

CHAPTER 8

Vitamins and supplements for age-related macular degeneration

Hanna R. Coleman, MD and Emily Y. Chew, MD

INTRODUCTION

Age-related macular degeneration (AMD) is the leading cause of visual loss in the USA among persons over 65 years of age.[1,2] The incidence is projected to grow at a considerable rate because of the increasing longevity of the US population.[3] The treatment of advanced AMD has progressed significantly over the years, but there is still no effective cure and unfortunately visual impairment continues to be high.[4–7]

HISTORY

A variety of risk factors have been found to be associated with both early- and late-stage AMD,[1,7–15] the most consistent of which are advanced age and smoking. Other risk factors include female gender, light iris color, heredity, cardiovascular health, nutrition status, high body mass index, and lifetime exposure to sunlight. Prevention of modifiable risk factors is a promising approach to reducing the individual's and society's burden of this condition.[16–18]

The possibility that the antioxidant balance can be positively altered by diet or vitamin supplementation has created much interest. Oxidative stress is thought to play a significant role in the pathogenesis of AMD because smoking is known to deplete the body's antioxidative potential.[19] Certain diets and nutritional supplements have already been shown to affect the progression of AMD. Oxidative processes occur in, and are essential to, most biological functions. As such, multiple pathways have evolved to maintain the balance between the necessary free radicals that serve as regulatory molecules and the unchecked highly reactive molecules that can initiate devastating cytotoxic reactions.[20] The retina is extremely susceptible to oxidative stress due to its high oxygen use and its chronic exposure to light. Photoreceptor outer segments in particular are very vulnerable to oxidative damage because of their high content of polyunsaturated fatty acids.[21,22]

The Age-Related Eye Disease Study (AREDS), conducted by the National Eye Institute, was a multicenter randomized, controlled clinical trial of oral supplements. It demonstrated that high doses of antioxidant vitamins, C, E and beta-carotene and zinc can be effective in slowing the progression to advanced AMD by about 25% in participants with intermediate AMD (AREDS category 3: extensive intermediate or large drusen in both eyes) or advanced AMD in one eye (AREDS category 4). The overall risk of moderate vision loss (≥15 letters on the ETDRS chart) was reduced by 19% at 5 years.[23]

In this study, the rate of development of advanced AMD in participants with either no AMD (category 1) or early AMD (AREDS category 2) was exceedingly low, 1.3% in 5 years, and no beneficial effects of the combination treatment were seen. For this reason, the AREDS supplements are only recommended for persons with moderate to severe AMD.

KEY CONCEPTS AND PHARMACOLOGY OF CURRENT DIETARY SUPPLEMENTS

Continuing evidence is accumulating regarding the role of oxidative stress in the pathogenesis of AMD and the mechanisms involved in the process.[24–27] Of particular interest is the occurrence and significance of macular pigment. Macular pigment is composed primarily of lutein and zeaxanthin, both of which are macular xanthophylls and members of the carotenoid family. They are found mostly in green leafy vegetables such as spinach, collard greens, and kale.[28–30] The concentration of macular pigment is greatest at the inner retinal layers of the fovea and the small amounts that are present in the peripheral retina are found in rod outer segments.[17,31] Studies suggest that an inverse relation exists between the risk of AMD and the amounts of lutein and zeaxanthin in the retina.[32–34] A high intake of green leafy vegetables containing lutein and zeaxanthin has also been associated with a reduction in the risk of neovascular AMD.[35–37]

The mechanism of protection of lutein and zeaxanthin is thought to relate to their ability to reflect short-wavelength light. The reduced exposure to these wavelengths may reduce both photochemical and oxidant damage to cellular lipids, proteins, and nuclear material. It has also been postulated that the carotenoids may guard the retina from oxidative stress by modulating light and oxidant exposure via two mechanisms: by absorbing the blue light that may be associated with photochemical damage, and by quenching reactive oxygen species (antioxidative potential).[36,38–42]

At the beginning of the AREDS trial, lutein and zeaxanthin were not commercially available and beta-carotene, although not present in the retina, was used for its antioxidative potential. During the trial, supplementation of beta-carotene was shown to increase the risk of lung cancer and its associated mortality in smokers.[43,44] It also benignly increased the yellowing of the skin. An amendment was made to the AREDS protocol to offer all smokers in the study the chance to stop the medication and consider randomization to placebo or zinc only. The current AREDS formulation with beta-carotene is thus not recommended for smokers. A follow-up clinical trial, AREDS2 (http://www.areds2.org), is currently under way to assess whether lutein and zeaxanthin and/or omega-3 polyunsaturated fatty acids can reduce the risk of developing advanced AMD. AREDS2 will also study the effect of eliminating beta-carotene from the original vitamin formulation on the development and progression of AMD.

Zinc was tested in the original AREDS formulation at high doses of 80 mg and copper was added to offset the common side-effect of copper-deficient anemia. The outcome in the zinc-treated group showed a few letters gained but this was considered to be of questionable clinical significance. The Blue Mountain Eye Study however recently confirmed the AREDS finding of protective influences from zinc against AMD.[45] Zinc treatment was associated with decreased mortality in AREDS (relative risk, 0.73; 95% confidence interval (CI), 0.60–0.89) but the import of this is unknown given the population consisted of motivated volunteers.[46,47] In AREDS, zinc also increased hospitalizations due to genitourinary problems, most commonly prostate enlargement. Other studies have reported that zinc may cause a decrease in high-density lipoprotein ("good") cholesterol or an increase in low-density lipoprotein ("bad") cholesterol, but this was not evident in the AREDS results. Nutritional experts continue to raise concerns about the widespread, common, and chronic use of such a large dose. AREDS2 will study the effects of reducing the dose of zinc from the original AREDS formulation (from 80 to 25 mg) on the development and progression of AMD.

Vitamin E is commonly used at doses of 400 IU. A meta-analysis of 19 studies concerning vitamin E concluded that 400 IU and higher doses were associated with an increased mortality risk.[48] However, a follow-up analysis of studies using 400–440 IU of vitamin E in more than 15 000 participants showed that there was no strong basis for inferring increased mortality among participants exposed to these levels of vitamin E. The pooled risk ratio for these three studies was 0.998 with a risk difference of −1.8 per 10 000 persons in the direction of benefit or reduced mortality. Based on these data, it appears to be safe to take the 400-IU dose of vitamin E found in the AREDS formulation.[49]

EPIDEMIOLOGIC DATA OF ASSOCIATION OF FAT AND ω-3 LCPUFAs WITH AMD

In the Beaver Dam Study, patients with the highest intake of saturated fat and cholesterol were at an 80% increased risk of early AMD. Similar results were found for advanced AMD, but were not statistically significant.[50] Saturated, monounsaturated, polyunsaturated, and trans-unsaturated fats increased the likelihood of progression for the highest fat intake quartile relative compared with the lowest fat intake quartile.

Docosahexanoic acid (DHA) and eicosapentaenoic acid (EPA) are part of the family of omega-3 long-chain polyunsaturated fatty acids (ω-3 LCPUFAs) that are found in high concentrations in the retinal tissue. ω-3 LCPUFAs may influence factors and processes important in the angiogenesis cascade, gene expression, and may be potent regulators of retinal cell survival, inflammation, and energy balance. The main sources of ω-3 LCPUFAs are fish products.

In people reporting the highest levels of ω-3 LCPUFAs and fish intake (two or more servings a week), there is a decreased likelihood of having advanced neovascular AMD relative to people reporting the lowest levels of intake.[51] This was noted especially when intake was in conjunction with lower levels of another fatty acid, linoleic acid. The Blue Mountains Eye Study, a population-based study, showed that eating fish 3 times per week could reduce the incidence of advanced AMD (odds ratio, 0.25; 95% CI, 0.06–1.00).[52] These results and those from other observational analytic investigations[41,53] suggest that modifying diet to include more foods rich in ω-3 LCPUFAs could result in a reduction in the risk of having neovascular AMD.[54–58]

AVAILABLE SUPPLEMENTS FOR MACULAR DEGENERATION

At the time of study development, lutein and zeaxanthin were not commercially available as supplements. Therefore, the supplements evaluated by the AREDS researchers contained:

- 500 mg vitamin C
- 400 mg vitamin E
- 15 mg beta-carotene
- 80 mg zinc as zinc oxide
- 2 mg copper as cupric oxide.

With the availability of the new antioxidants and their benefit reports, several formulations of supplements became available with the original AREDS combination, as well as variations for smokers and with additional antioxidants (Table 8.1).

Table 8.1 Vitamin supplements for age-related macular degeneration

Supplement	Brand name and manufacturer
AREDS formula	Ocuvite PreserVision: Bausch & Lomb
	Icaps AREDS Formula: Alcon
	ProtectRx: ScienceBased Health
	VisiVite Original Formula: VisiVite
	Viteyes Original Formula: Vitamin Health, LLC
AREDS formula for smokers or ex-smokers (without beta-carotene)	Retinavites Smoker's Formula
	MaculaRx Plus (1/10th AREDS beta-carotene dose)
	VisiVite Smoker's Formula (lutein 10 mg)
	Viteyes Smoker's Formula (lutein 10 mg and zeaxanthin 2 mg)
	Preservision Lutein Soft gels (lutein 10 mg)
AREDS lutein and/or zeaxanthin formulas	Ocuvite Lutein (6 mg)
	ICaps Lutein and Zeaxanthin Formula (lutein 4 mg zeaxanthin 4 mg)
	Visivite Premier Ocular formula 2 (lutein 10 mg zeaxanthin 2 mg)

AREDS, Age-Related Eye Disease Study.

IMPLICATIONS OF RETINAL SUPPLEMENT PHARMACOLOGY

Dietary supplements are intended to enhance the diets of some people, but should not aim to replace the important balance of a variety of foods. Physicians and patients need to take diet into consideration when choosing the right supplement. Patients should be counseled to discuss any dietary supplement intake with their primary physician to ensure that there are no interactions with underlying medical conditions as well as with regular prescription and other over-the-counter medicines. If elective surgery is planned, supplement intake should be reviewed in detail several weeks prior.

Dietary supplement products are not reviewed by the government before they are marketed. Manufacturers are responsible for making sure their product is safe before it goes to market, but the Food and Drug Administration (FDA) has the responsibility to take action against any unsafe dietary supplement product. Adverse effects should be reported to the FDA by calling 1-800-FDA-1088, by faxing 1-800-FDA-0178 or online at the FDA website www.fda.gov/medwatch/how.htm. More information on what dietary supplements are and how they are regulated, including the labeling and claims that can be made for supplements, can be found at www.cfsan.fda.gov/~dms/ds-faq.html.[59]

FUTURE DIRECTIONS: AREDS2

Based on all of the available nutritional evidence, the National Eye Institute developed the AREDS2 study, which started enrolling in September 2006 and completed enrollment in September 2008. It is

Table 8.2 The four formulations of the original Age-Related Eye Disease Study (AREDS) formulation that will be tested in the secondary randomization of AREDS2

	1	2	3	4
Vitamin C	500 mg	500 mg	500 mg	500 mg
Vitamin E	400 IU	400 IU	400 IU	400 IU
Beta-carotene	15 mg	0 mg	0 mg	15 mg
Zinc oxide	80 mg	80 mg	25 mg	25 mg
Cupric oxide	2 mg	2 mg	2 mg	2 mg

currently in the follow-up phase. Its primary objective is to determine whether oral supplementation with macular xanthophylls (lutein at 10 mg/day + zeaxanthin at 2 mg/day) and/or ω-3 LCPUFAs (DHA 350 mg and EPA 650 mg for a total of 1 g/day) will decrease the risk of progression to advanced AMD, compared with placebo. AREDS2 will also study the effects of these nutritional supplements on moderate vision loss and on the development of cataracts. The study has enrolled 4203 participants aged 50–85 years, who at the time of enrollment have sufficiently clear lenses for quality fundus photographs and have either bilateral large drusen or large drusen in one eye and advanced AMD (neovascular AMD or central geographic atrophy) in the fellow eye. Of the primary randomization agents, one-quarter of the patients will be assigned placebo, another quarter lutein/zeaxanthin, one-quarter ω-3 LCPUFAs, and the final quarter a combination of the two.

Because the study population in AREDS2 is at least moderately at risk of AMD, all participants will be offered the original AREDS formulation. Because of this opportunity, a second randomization was designed to evaluate the possibility of deleting beta-carotene and decreasing the current dose of zinc. The secondary randomization agents (AREDS-type supplement) formulations are divided into the four inclusion groups listed in Table 8.2. Participants who are smokers are also then included in AREDS2 and they would be randomly assigned to either formulation 2 or formulation 3 in the AREDS supplements in the secondary randomization. It is also recognized that some participants may consider it difficult not to take the original AREDS formulation, the proven formulation for persons with moderate AMD, and they would be allowed to do so. It is also possible that some participants may not be able to tolerate the AREDS formulation and they would also be allowed to withdraw from this secondary randomization.

SUMMARY AND KEY POINTS

The savings gained from preventive therapy for AMD are enormous. It is estimated that about 55 million people in the USA may be at risk of advanced AMD. Of these, 8 million are at high risk, and are thus likely to benefit from the current vitamin formulation of zinc and antioxidant therapy. The economic benefits associated with the prevention of progression to advanced AMD in even a small proportion of cases is significant and will result in major cost savings to individuals and society at large.[60]

- If all 8 million people at a high risk of advanced AMD took the supplement therapy, more than 300 000 of them could be saved from developing loss of vision in the next 5 years.

The evidence that oxidative stress, diet, and nutrition play crucial roles in the pathogenesis of early AMD and its progression to AMD is now compelling. Further studies, like the ongoing AREDS2, are essential in order to find the key micronutrients that may be effective in the prevention of AMD in the future.

- AREDS showed that antioxidant intake reduced the risk of developing advanced AMD by 25% compared with placebo at 5-year follow-up.
- Observational data suggest that higher dietary intakes of lutein, zeaxanthin, and ω-3 LCPUFAs were associated with decreased risk of AMD.

REFERENCES

1. Eye Disease Case Control Study Group. Risk factors for neovascular age-related macular degeneration. Arch Ophthalmol 1992;110:1701–1710.
2. Congdon N, O'Colmain B, Klaver CC, et al. Causes and prevalence of visual impairment among adults in the United States. Arch Ophthalmol 2004;122:477–485.
3. Thylefors B. A global initiative for the elimination of avoidable blindness. Am J Ophthalmol 1998;125:90–93.
4. Macular Photocoagulation Study Group. Argon laser photocoagulation for senile macular degeneration. Arch Ophthalmol 1982;100:912–918.
5. Macular Photocoagulation Study Group. Argon laser photocoagulation for neovascular maculopathy. Three-year results from randomized clinical trials. Arch Ophthalmol 1986;104:694–701.
6. TAP Study Group. Photodynamic therapy of subfoveal choroidal neovascularization in age-related macular degeneration with verteporfin: one-year results of 2 randomized clinical trials – TAP report. Treatment of Age-related macular degeneration with photodynamic Therapy (TAP) study group. Arch Ophthalmol 1999;117:1329–1345.
7. Tomany SC, Klein R, Klein BE. Beaver Dam Eye study. The relationship between iris color, hair color, and skin sun sensitivity and the 10-year incidence of age-related maculopathy: the Beaver Dam Eye Study. Ophthalmology 2003;110:1526–1533.
8. Hyman L, Schachat AP, He Q, et al. Hypertension, cardiovascular disease, and age-related macular degeneration. Age-Related Macular Degeneration Risk Factors study group. Arch Ophthalmol 2000;118:351–358.
9. Klein R, Klein BE, Tomany SC, et al. The association of cardiovascular disease with the long-term incidence of age-related maculopathy: the Beaver Dam Eye Study. Ophthalmology 2003;110:1273–1280.
10. Macular Photocoagulation Study Group. Risk factors for choroidal neovascularization in the second eye of patients with juxta foveal or subfoveal choroidal neovascularization secondary to age related macular degeneration. Arch Ophthalmol 1997;115:741–747.
11. Seddon JM, Cote J, Davis N, et al. Progression of age-related macular degeneration: association with body mass index, waist circumference, and waist–hip ratio. Arch Ophthalmol 2003;121:785–792.
12. Silvestri G, Johnston PB, Hughes AE. Is genetic predisposition an important risk factor in age-related macular degeneration? Eye 1994;8:564–568.
13. Smith W, Mitchell P, Leeder SR. Smoking and age-related maculopathy. Arch Ophthalmol 1996;114:1518–1523.
14. Smith W, Mitchell P, Leeder SR, et al. Plasma fibrinogen levels, other cardiovascular risk factors and age-related maculopathy. The Blue Mountains Eye Study. Arch Ophthalmol 1998;116:583–589.
15. Taylor HR, West S, Munoz B, et al. The long term effects of visible light on the eye. Arch Ophthalmol 1992;110:99–104.
16. Seddon JM. Epidemiology of age-related macular degeneration. In: Ryan SJ, editor. Medical Retina, vol. 2, 3rd edn. St. Louis: Mosby; 2001. pp. 1039–1050.
17. Snellen EL, Verbeek AL, Van Den Hoogen GW, et al. Neovascular age-related macular degeneration and its relationship to antioxidant intake. Acta Ophthalmol Scand 2002;80:368–371.
18. Snow KK, Seddon JM. Do age-related macular degeneration and cardiovascular disease share common antecedents? Ophthalm Epidemiol 1999;6:125–143.
19. Age-Related Eye Disease Study Research Group. Risk factors associated with age-related macular degeneration. A case-control study in the Age-Related Eye Disease Study: Age-Related Eye Disease Study report number 3. Ophthalmology 2000;107:2224–2232.
20. Mayne ST. Antioxidant nutrients and chronic disease: use of biomarkers of exposure and oxidative stress status in epidemiologic research. J Nutr 2003;133:933S–940S.
21. Handleman GJ, Dratz E. The role of antioxidants in the retina and retinal pigment epithelium and the nature of pro-oxidant induced damage. Adv Free Radic Biol Med 1986;2:1–89.
22. Hogg R, Chakravarthy U. Mini-review: AMD and micronutrient antioxidants. Curr Eye Res 2004;29:387–401.
23. Age-Related Eye Disease Study Group. A randomized, placebo-controlled, clinical trial of high-dose supplementation with vitamins C and E, beta carotene, and zinc for age-related macular degeneration and vision loss. AREDS report no. 8. Arch Ophthalmol 2001;119:1417–1436.
24. Beatty S, Koh HH, Henson D, et al. The role of oxidative stress in the pathogenesis of age-related macular degeneration. Surv Ophthalmol 2000;45:115–134.

25. Cai J, Nelson KC, Wu M, et al. Oxidative damage and protection of the RPE. Prog Retinal Eye Res 2000;19:205–221.
26. Roberts JE. Ocular photo toxicity. J Photochem Photobiol 2001;64:136–143.
27. Winkler BS, Boulton ME, Gottsch JD, et al. Oxidative damage and age-related macular degeneration. Mol Vis 1999;5:32.
28. Landrum JT, Bone RA. Lutein, zeaxanthin, and the macular pigment. Arch Biochem Biophys 2001;385:28–40.
29. Snodderly DM, Brown PK, Delori FC, et al. The macular pigment. I. Absorbance spectra, localization and discrimination from other yellow pigments in the primate retinas. Invest Ophthalmol Vis Sci 1984;25:660–673.
30. Snodderly DM, Handelman GL, Adler AJ. Distribution of individual macular pigment carotenoids in the central retina of macaque and squirrel monkeys. Invest Ophthalmol Vis Sci 2000;45:115–134.
31. Bone RA, Landrum JT, Friedes LM, et al. Distribution of lutein and zeaxanthin stereo isomers in the human retina. Exp Eye Res 1997;64:211–218.
32. Beatty S, Murray IJ, Henson DB, et al. Macular pigment and risk for age-related macular degeneration in subjects from a northern European population. Invest Ophthalmol Vis Sci 2001;42:439–446.
33. Bernstein PS, Zhao DY, Wintch SW, et al. Resonance Raman measurement of macular carotenoids in normal subjects and in age-related macular degeneration patients. Ophthalmology 2002;109:1780–1787.
34. Bone RA, Landrum JT, Mayne ST, et al. Macular pigment in donor eyes with and without AMD: a case-control study. Invest Ophthalmol Vis Sci 2001;42:235–240.
35. Moeller SM, Parekh N, Tinker L, et al. Associations between intermediate age-related macular degeneration and lutein and zeaxanthin in the carotenoids in Age-Related Eye Disease Study (CAREDS): ancillary study of the Women's Health Initiative. Arch Ophthalmol 2006;124:1151–1162.
36. Seddon JM, Ajani UA, Sperduto RD, et al. Dietary carotenoids, vitamins A, C, E and advanced age-related macular degeneration. JAMA 1994;272: 1413–1420.
37. Sommerburg OG, Siems WG, Hurst JS, et al. Lutein and zeaxanthin are associated with photoreceptors in the human retina. Curr Eye Res 1999;19:491–495.
38. Eye Disease Case Control Study Group. Antioxidant status and neovascular age-related macular degeneration. Arch Ophthalmol 1993;111:104–109. Erratum appears in: Arch Ophthalmol 1993;111:1228, 1366, 1499.
39. Krinsky NI. Carotenoids as antioxidants. Nutrition 2001;17:815–817.
40. Mares-Perlman JA, Fisher AI, Klein R, et al. Lutein and zeaxanthin in the diet and serum and their relation to age-related maculopathy in the third national health and nutrition examination survey. Am J Epidemiol 2001;153:424–432.
41. Schalch W, Dayhaw-Barker P, Barker FM. The carotenoids of the human retina. In: Taylor A, editor. Nutritional and Environmental Influences of the Eye. Boca Raton: CRC Press, 1999. pp. 215–249.
42. SanGiovanni JP, Chew EY, Clemons TE, et al. The relationship of dietary carotenoid and vitamin A, E, and C intake with age-related macular degeneration in a case-control study. AREDS Report No. 22. Arch Ophthalmol 2007;125:1225–1232.
43. Alpha-Tocopherol, Beta Carotene Cancer Prevention Study Group. The effect of vitamin E and beta carotene on the incidence of lung cancer and other cancers in male smokers. N Engl J Med 1994;330:1029–1035.
44. Omenn GS, Goodman GE, Thornquist MD, et al. Effects of a combination of beta carotene and vitamin A on lung cancer and cardiovascular disease. N Engl J Med 1996;334:1150–1155.
45. Tan JS, Wang JJ, Flood V, et al. Dietary antioxidants and the long-term incidence of age-related macular degeneration: the Blue Mountains Eye Study. Ophthalmology 2008;115(2):334–341.
46. Age-Related Eye Disease Study Group. Associations of mortality with ocular disorders and an intervention of high-dose antioxidants and zinc in the Age-Related Eye Disease Study. AREDS report no. 13. Arch Ophthalmol 2004;122:716–726.
47. Newsome DA, Swartz M, Leone NC, et al. Oral zinc in macular degeneration. Arch Ophthalmol 1988;106:192–198.
48. Miller ER III, Pastor-Barriuso R, Dalal D, et al. Meta-analysis: high-dosage vitamin E supplementation may increase all-cause mortality. Ann Intern Med 2004;142:37–46.
49. Chew EY, Clemons T. Vitamin E and the Age-Related Eye Disease Study supplementation for age-related macular degeneration. Arch Ophthalmol 2005;123:395–396.
50. Mares-Perlman JA, Brady WE, Klein R. Dietary fat and age-related maculopathy. Arch Ophthalmol 1995;113:743–748.
51. Seddon JM, George S, Rosner B. Cigarette smoking, fish consumption, omega-3 fatty acid intake, and associations with age-related macular degeneration: the US Twin Age-Related Macular Degeneration. Arch Ophthalmol 2006;124:995–1001.
52. Chua B, Flood V, Rochtchina E, et al. Dietary fatty acids and the 5-year incidence of age-related maculopathy. Arch Ophthalmol 2006;124:981–986.
53. SanGiovanni JP, Chew EY, Clemons TE, et al. The Age-Related Eye Disease Study Group. The relationship of dietary lipid intake and age-related macular degeneration in a case-control study. AREDS report no. 20. Arch Ophthalmol 2007;125:671–679.
54. Age-Related Eye Disease Study Research Group. The relationship of dietary lipid intake and age-related macular degeneration: a case-control study in the Age-Related Eye Disease Study. AREDS report no. 20. Arch Ophthalmol 2004;122:716–726.
55. Cho E, Hung S, Willett WC, et al. Prospective study of dietary fat and the risk of age-related macular degeneration. Am J Clin Nutr 2001;73:209–218.
56. Herberger RA, Mares-Perlman JA, Klein R, et al. Relationship of dietary fat to age-related maculopathy in the Third National Health and Nutrition Examination Survey. Arch Ophthalmol 2001;119:1833–1838.
57. Seddon JM, Rosner B, Sperduto RD, et al. Dietary fat and risk for advanced age-related macular degeneration. Arch Ophthalmol 2001;119(8): 1191–1199.
58. Smith W, Mitchell P, Leeder SR. Dietary fat and fish intake and age-related maculopathy. Arch Ophthalmol 2000;118(3):401–404.
59. The Eye Digest. Available online at: www.agingeye.net.
60. Lanchoney DM, Maguire MG, Fine SL. A model of the incidence and consequences of choroidal neovascularization secondary to age-related macular degeneration: comparative effects of current treatment and potential prophylaxis on visual outcomes in high risk patients. Arch Ophthalmol 1998;116:1045–1052.

Ocular pharmacokinetic, drug bioavailability, and intraocular drug delivery systems

CHAPTER 9

Rocío Herrero-Vanrell, PhD and Jose A. Cardillo, MD

INTRODUCTION

Successful ophthalmic therapy requires therapeutic concentrations of the active substance on the target site. Depending on the ocular disease the drug must reach a targeted zone where the therapeutic action is completed. For the treatment of ocular surface diseases, such as infection or inflammation, and for anterior-segment diseases, effective concentrations of the drug must be maintained in the cornea and conjunctiva, or in the anterior chamber, respectively. In contrast, to treat chronic ocular diseases as uveitis, macular edema, age-related macular degeneration, retinitis and intraocular malignancy, the active substance must reach the posterior segment of the eye.

Selection of the administration route depends on the location of the target tissue. Topical administration of medication is accepted best by patients. However, these agents present unique and challenging hurdles for drug delivery and only 5% of the administered dose penetrates the eye.[1] For this reason, when higher concentrations of drugs, such as antibiotics, corticoids, antiviral agents, and biopharmaceuticals, are required inside the eye, it is necessary to employ intracameral or intravitreous injections.

A potential barrier to adequate drug delivery after eye drop instillation is diffusion through the cornea.[2,3] Exploiting the permeability of the sclera, periocular routes may also offer a promising alternative to boost drug penetration and tissue targeting.[4–9] Periocular administration includes subconjunctival, sub-Tenon's capsule, peribulbar, posterior juxtascleral, and retrobulbar injections. In these cases, the drug must cross the sclera to reach the intraocular tissues. However, access of drugs to the tissues in the posterior segment of the eye from periocular injections, as well as from doses administered systemically, is repressed by the blood–retina barrier (BRB). Because any disease affecting the posterior segment of the eye may represent visual impairment and blindness, it is necessary to achieve, as fast as possible, effective drug concentrations that are only possible by intravitreous injections.

This chapter comprises an ocular pharmacokinetic overview and describes new topical and intraocular drug delivery systems aimed to obtain successful ocular therapy.

TOPICAL AND PERIOCULAR ADMINISTRATION

Corneal, conjunctival, and scleral routes are used for ocular penetration of active substances administered topically. The topical ophthalmic route is the first therapeutic choice because it is noninvasive and tolerance is generally good. However, drug bioavailability to intraocular tissues is low and only about 5% of the dose is able to reach the anterior segment due to the elimination process of the ocular surface.[1] Furthermore, the conjunctival and scleral routes avoid the counterflow of the aqueous humor and the lens barrier. The sclera is highly permeable to active substances, even several macromolecules. However, transscleral drug penetration to the interior of the eye is limited by choroidal blood flow and the retinal pigment epithelium (RPE) barrier.[2]

The cornea comprises three zones: epithelium, stroma, and endothelium. The thickness in humans is 0.5–0.6 mm in its central portion.[3] A great number of low-molecular-weight substances are able to reach the aqueous humor through the transcorneal route by passive diffusion. The diffusion rate follows Fick's law and is conducted by a concentration gradient, conditioned by the hydrophilic or lipidic nature of the different layers of the cornea and by the nature of the drugs administered (hydrophilic/lipophilic balance).[4] While epithelium and endothelium possess a lipidic nature, the stroma has hydrophilic properties, being highly permeable for hydrophobic or hydrophilic substances respectively. Some substances can pass through the cornea, by the paracellular route. Nevertheless, the tight junctions of corneal epithelial cells limit passage through the intercellular spaces. Absorption promoters can be used to modify the integrity of the tight junctions, improving drug absorption. However, these agents can produce epithelial damage.

Currently the conjunctiva is considered an attractive route for ocular drug absorption.[5] It is a tissue with an endogenous transport machinery to allow penetration of active substances. Furthermore, the conjunctiva surface and pore radius in epithelium are larger than those found in the cornea.

The transscleral route consists of the injection of the drug into a periocular space (subconjunctival, sub-Tenon, peribulbar, posterior juxtascleral, and retrobulbar spaces).[6] Subconjunctival injection has demonstrated poorly sustained vitreous and retinal drug levels in animal studies. Transport barriers in the transscleral route have been categorized as static and dynamic barriers.[7] Static barriers comprise tissues in which the active substance diffuses to reach the retina. In order to get the retina the drug must diffuse through sclera, Bruch's membrane, and RPE. The primary dynamic barriers to transscleral drug delivery are the conjunctival lymphatic/blood vessels and the choroids.

INTRAVITREAL ADMINISTRATION

Intravitreal administration is a direct deposit of the drug in the vitreous by injection. Drugs are mainly eliminated from the vitreous by the anterior route. If the active substance has an adequate permeability in the retinal capillaries and in RPE it can be eliminated from the retina through the BRB to the systemic circulation. Drugs can reach the retina from the choroid, although high systemic doses are needed.

OCULAR PHARMACOKINETICS

Most of the ocular pharmacokinetic studies corresponds to topical administration of active substances and they are based on the determination of the drug concentration in the ocular tissues. The number of compartments depends on the physicochemical properties of the active principle and the tissues. From a clinical point of view, the development of pharmacokinetic models with a small number of parameters is of great interest. If the ocular pharmacokinetic study following a topical administration includes noncompartmental treatments, the most difficult parameter to evaluate is distribution volume because it is necessary to know the whole amount of drug able to reach the aqueous humor. In order to determine the distribution volume, the active substance can be administered in the anterior chamber or by topical infusion.

Incorporation of the drug to systemic circulation after topical administration represents a loss in the biophase. Elimination includes any process that implies a loss of drug from the target tissue, such as distribution to adjacent tissues, drainage of aqueous humor, incorporation in the systemic circulation, and biotransformation. Ocular bioavailability is related to drug access to the target side or biophase, and systemic exposure refers to incorporation of the active substance in the general circulation.

If the drug is in the blood stream through the conjunctival blood capillaries after systemic, topical, or periocular administration, the blood–aqueous barrier limits its access to the anterior chamber. The blood–aqueous barrier is composed of the uveal capillary endothelia and ciliary epithelia. The BRB limits the diffusion of the active substance to the retina. BRB is composed of an outer barrier and an inner barrier. The outer barrier is formed by the RPE the inner barrier by the endothelial cells of retinal vessels. Cells in RPE are connected by tight junctions. Overall flux of active substances across the BRB depends on its concentration gradient, its permeability in the BRB, and the BRB surface area. RPE is a tighter barrier than the sclera for hydrophilic and larger molecules. However, for small lipophilic molecules the RPE and sclera behave similarly.

The most important limitations of ocular pharmacokinetics studies are the sampling and the number of animals. For evaluation of intraocular concentrations each sample comes from one different animal.[8] This means that a large number of animals are necessary to carry out a complete pharmacokinetic study.

TOPICAL FORMULATIONS

In contrast to intestinal mucosa, the ocular surface is not a favorable place for drug penetration. Just after administration of the ophthalmic formulation several processes are triggered. All phenomena are directed to the elimination of the ophthalmic formulation from the ocular surface. Conventional ophthalmic pharmaceutical forms for topical administration include solutions, suspensions, emulsions, aqueous gels, and ointments. Solutions are employed most frequently because they are easily prepared, filtered, and sterilized. Furthermore, the cost of the elaboration process is not as expensive. Slightly viscous liquid formulations are widely employed and solutions with viscosities around 15–18 mPa/s are well accepted by patients. Suspensions are employed for poorly soluble drugs such as corticosteroids. The main disadvantage of ointments are that they produce blurred vision. For this reason they are almost exclusively used at night.

For the past two decades, one of the main objectives in the ocular field has been the optimization of ophthalmic formulations. Efforts have been directed towards the development of systems that are able to improve the bioavailability of the active substance by increasing the contact time of the formulation with the ocular surface or facilitating the transcorneal penetration of the drug. Among the strategies employed to improve ocular bioavailability are formulations of prodrugs, soft contact lenses, inserts and patches, mucoadhesive polymers, *in situ* gelification systems, absorption promoters, vesicular and colloidal systems. Prodrugs are usually obtained by ester linkage of the active substance. In this way the ester penetrates the cornea and hydrolysis occurs in the anterior chamber.

Soft contact lenses are prepared from polymers that act as a reservoir for the drug. Once the device is in contact with the cornea, the active substance is released from the system. Soft lenses are deposited in the conjunctival sac, releasing the drug gradually.

Ophthalmic inserts can be elaborated with biodegradable or nonbiodegradable polymers. Collagen, polyacrylamide, and cellulose derivatives such as hydroxypropylmethylcellulose are the polymers most used for biodegradable inserts. Previously, a nonbiodegradable device (Ocusert) has been developed to release pilocarpine.

Bioadhesive polymers are formulations including anionic or cationic polymers whose end groups are able to interact with the sialic acids of mucins. Then, the ocular contact time of formulation is increased. Among the bioadhesive polymers cellulose derivatives (carboxymethylcellulose), polyacrylic acids (carbopol), and hyaluronic acid are used the most frequently.[9] Due to their good tolerance related to their ocular surface, these polymers are used as components of artificial tears. The *in situ* gel systems are liquid formulations that contain polymers in solution. Once the formulation is instilled the solution changes to gel because of the pH, tears, electrolytes, or increase in temperature. An example is Gelrite, a polysaccharide that is able to form gel systems at low concentration in the presence of cationic molecules of tears.[10]

Absorption promoters are substances that improve the permeability of the epithelium by modifying the cellular membrane or opening the tight junctions of the corneal epithelial cells. Some ionic preservatives, such as benzalconium chloride (BAC) or the sodium salt ethylenediamine tetraacetic acid (EDTA), have been demonstrated to promote the penetration of several substances.[11] However, these substances present adverse effects and can cause damage to ocular surface tissues.

If the active substance is soluble in water it can be included in complex systems such as cyclodextrins (cyclic oligosaccharides). Nanocarriers, such as liposomes, nanoparticles, and dendrimers, are used to enhance ocular drug delivery.[12] They can be administered as eye drops, providing an extended residence time on the ocular surface after their instillation. Liposomes are vesicular systems composed of bilayers of phospholipids organized as cellular membranes. Several substances can be included in the vesicles because they have aqueous and lipid zones. Nanoparticles are polymeric systems of 1–1000 nm size in which the active substance is encapsulated or adsorbed.

The polymers usually employed to prepare nanoparticles for the topical ophthalmic route are poly(acrylic acid) derivatives (polyalquilcyanocrylates), albumin, poly-ε-caprolactone, and chitosan. Dendrimers are macromolecules made up of a series of branches around a small molecule, ending in a large number of cationic or anionic groups. Microemulsions are water and oil disperse systems in which a surfactant and a cosurfactant are employed. The size of the inner phase is less than 1 μm. They have a clear dispersion and are thermodynamically stable.

INTRAOCULAR DRUG DELIVERY SYSTEMS

Pathologies affecting the posterior segment are devastating and the topical treatment is not successful. Therapeutically, success is conditioned for the difficult access to target tissues. When the topical route is employed the cornea, lens, aqueous and BRB yield noneffective drug levels in vitreous, retina, and choroids. Administration of the drug in the vitreous or adjacent structures (transscleral routes) is necessary for prompt effects. While steady-state concentrations are easy to achieve by the oral route, successive intravitreal injections are poorly tolerated, being associated with important side-effects such as vitreous hemorrhage, intraocular pressure increase, optic atrophy, retinal detachment, cataracts, and endophthalmitis. Therefore, the treatment has to be administered promptly and effective concentrations of the active substance maintained as long as possible.

CONVENTIONAL FORMULATIONS

Conventional intravitreal formulations include solutions, vitreous substitutes, and suspensions. However, the main disadvantage of solutions is the impossibility to establish long treatments to maintain drug concentrations in the therapeutic window with a single injection. Moreover intravitreal administration does not eliminate the risk of extraocular infections and infection in the other eye. In the past 20 years substantial effort has been put towards developing new drug delivery systems able to release the drug over a long time, avoiding successive intravitreal injections.

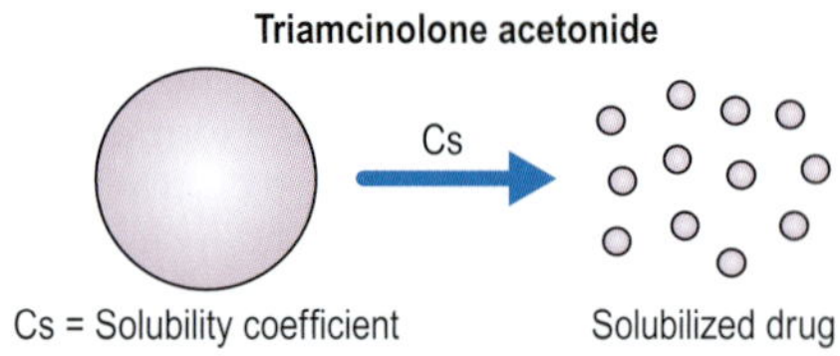

Figure 9.1 Example of a depot system. The poorly soluble drug remains insoluble after intravitreal injection and is slowly solubilized in the aqueous phase (vitreous). The effect is maintained for several months.

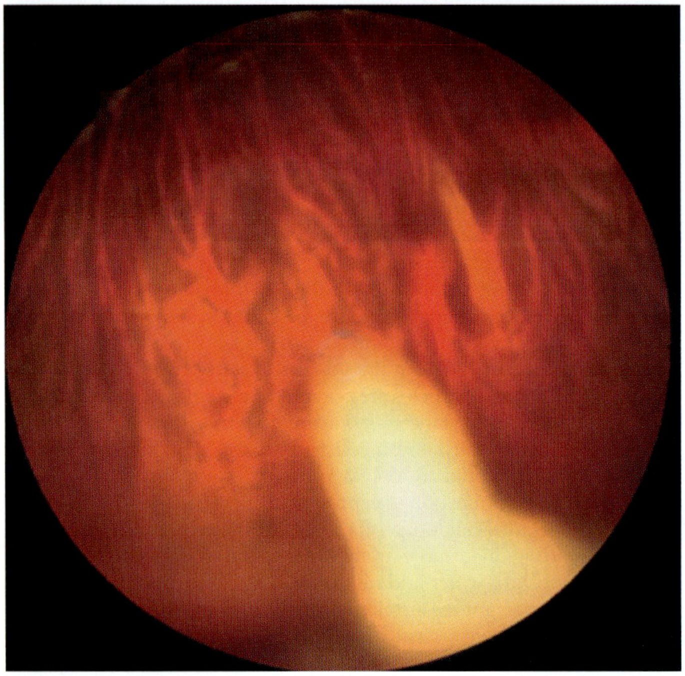

Figure 9.2 Ocular fundus after intravitreal injection of triamcinolone acetonide. (Courtesy of Dr. Jose Manuel Benitez del Castillo.)

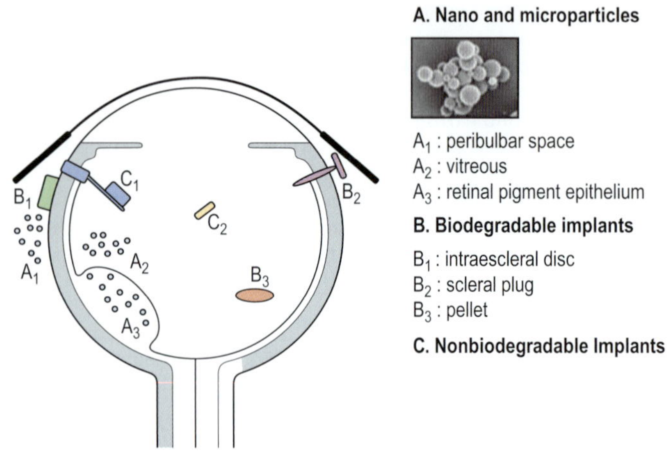

Figure 9.3 Intraocular devices. Adapted from Yasukawa T, Ogura Y, Tabata Y, et al. Drug delivery systems for vitreoretinal diseases. Prog Retin Eye Res 2004;23:253–281.

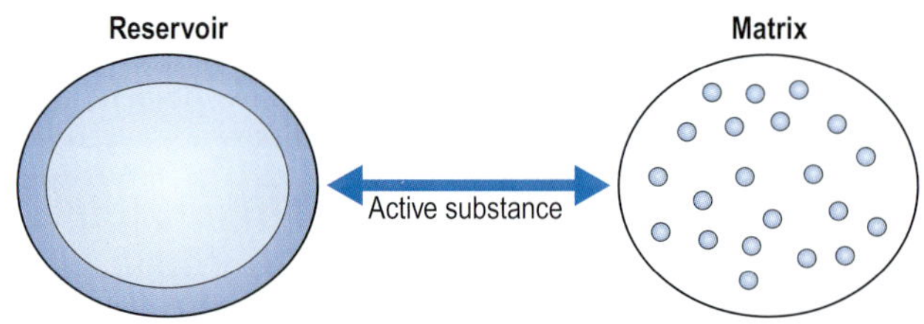

Figure 9.4 Example of reservoir and matrix systems. Reservoir structures include a pellet of the active substance surrounded by a polymeric membrane. Matrix structures are formed by a polymeric network in which the drug is dispersed.

DEPOT FORMULATIONS AND VITREOUS SUBSTITUTES

Currently, depot formulations are employed to treat macular edema and intraocular inflammation. These formulations include poor aqueous solubility drugs such as fluocinolone acetate and triamcinolone acetate that are administered as suspensions. The drug precipitates after injection in the vitreous body (Figure 9.1). Then, the active substance drug is slowly solubilized and the effect lasts for months (Figure 9.2). The main problem in relation to these formulations is the formation of crystalline structures in the proximal areas to the retina. Vitreous substitutes allow the incorporation of lipophilic drugs in vehicles such as silicone oil and aqueous soluble drugs in solutions of hyaluronic acid and cellulosic derivatives.

INTRAOCULAR DRUG DELIVERY SYSTEMS

Intraocular drug delivery systems allow the release of the drug, bypassing the blood–ocular barrier, and are adequate by the intraocular route (Figure 9.3). The main advantage of these preparations is that they can release the drug over a long time with one single administration, having the same effect as multiple injections. Depending on their size, intraocular drug delivery devices must be implanted through a relatively large surgical incision or through a smaller tissue perforation. These pharmaceutical systems are of great interest in the treatment of posterior-segment diseases and they can be prepared from biodegradable or nonbiodegradable polymers. Biodegradable polymers have the advantage of disappearing from the site of action after releasing the drug. The majority of intraocular devices are prepared from nonbiodegradable materials and they are able to release controlled amounts of drugs for months. Nonbiodegradable polymers include silicone, polyvinyl alcohol (PVA) and ethylvinylacetate (EVA). Ocular devices can be classified into reservoir and matrix systems (Figure 9.4). Reservoir structures include a pellet of the active substance surrounded by a polymeric membrane. Matrix structures are a polymeric network in which the drug is dispersed. If the size is larger than 1 mm they are called implants.

NONBIODEGRADABLE IMPLANTS

Examples of nonbiodegradable implants are the Vitrasert and Retisert implants (Bausch & Lomb). Both are reservoir systems. Vitrasert, a reservoir implant loaded with ganciclovir, was approved by the Food and Drug Administration in 1996. The release of the drug is controlled by the EVA and PVA polymers. PVA is a permeable polymer and regulates the release rate of the drug. EVA is non permeable. Once in contact with aqueous fluids the active substance is dissolved and a saturated solution is created in the drug pellet. Then, the drug is released out of the device by diffusion.

As long as the solution in the pellet is saturated with the active substance, the release rate is constant. Vitrasert has been effective in controlling the progression of cytomegalovirus retinitis associated with acquired immunodeficiency syndrome (AIDS) for 8 months. However, this implant has been associated with endophthalmitis and an increased rate of retinal detachment.[13] Retisert ($3 \times 2 \times 5$ mm) is employed for the treatment of chronic noninfectious uveitis of the posterior segment. It is composed of PVA and silicone laminate. The poorly soluble drug (fluocinolone acetonide) is released over a 3-year period.[14,15] The side-effects of this implant are cataract and increased intraocular pressure.

Iluvien (Alimera Sciences and pSivida) is a tube-shaped device (3 mm in length and 0.37 mm in diameter). Its action lasts between 18 and 36 months.[16] Recently a nonbiodegradable intrascleral implant prepared with a copolymer of ethylenvinylacetate and betamethasone has been developed.[16] The device is deposited in the external zone of the sclera and it is connected with the vitreous through a tube of reduced dimensions. The device released the drug for at least 3 months. The reservoir can hold up to 100 mg of the active substance, and can be recharged. In this case it is recommended to introduce an agent to inhibit cellular growth to avoid cellular blockage of the tube. Implants containing genetically modified human RPE cells have been developed (Neurotech). The device NT 501 (6 mm long) is placed in the pars plana through a small incision. The cells included in the device are able to secrete ciliary neurotrophic factor (CNTF). It can be employed for glaucoma, choroidal neovascularization (CNV) and uveitis.[17]

The main disadvantage of nonbiodegradable systems is that they have to be implanted and replaced once the drug is released. Implantation requires a surgical procedure.

INTRAOCULAR BIODEGRADABLE DRUG DELIVERY SYSTEMS

Biodegradable polymers are widely employed in the elaboration of controlled drug delivery systems. These devices release the drug while the polymer is being degraded in the target site. Finally, the device disappears avoiding the need of surgery. These materials have been used to prepare implants, liposomes, and injectable particles (nanoparticles and microparticles). Liposomes are biocompatible and biodegradable vesicles. They can be prepared with natural lipids as phospholipids. Hydrophilic and lipophilic active substances can be encapsulated in the aqueous zone or the lipid walls respectively. The liposomes are taken by phagocytic cells, allowing intracellular drug delivery. The surface of the liposomes can be modified to promote preferential binding (i.e., neovascular vessels).

The administration of liposomes by the intraocular route has been the subject of several studies. Liposomes loaded with a prodrug of ganciclovir inhibited cytomegalovirus retinitis in rabbits.[18] These vesicles have been loaded with oligonucleotides, protecting them from nucleases.[19] Nevertheless, administration of liposomes presents some disadvantages, such as a diminution in visual acuity due to intraocular clouding after intravitreal injection. These side-effects have been described as disappearing after 14–21 days of administration.

Liposomes have been dispersed in thermo-sensible gels of poloxamers to maintain the activity of oligonucleotides and enhance their intracellular penetration.[20] Currently, a liposomal formulation of verteporfin is in clinical use. Visudyne (Novartis Pharmaceuticals) is employed for the treatment of age-related macular degeneration and choroidal neovascularization. Liposomes of verteporfin are administered by intravenous infusion, causing an occlusion of the targeted vessels after its activation through a nonthermal red laser applied to the retina.[21,22] Photrex (Miravant Medical Technologies) contains rostaporfin.[23]

Among the biodegradable polymers employed to prepare intraocular devices poly(lactic) acid and poly (lactic-co-glycolic) acid (PLGA) are the most popular. They are biodegradable and disappear from the injection site after drug delivery. The polymer chain is broken by hydrolysis in the system. The final products, lactic and glycolic acid, are metabolized to carbon dioxide and water mediated by Krebs cycle. These polymers have been employed to obtain implants, scleral plugs, pellets, discs, films, and rods.[13] These implants can be located in different ocular areas such as anterior chamber, peribulbar spaces, scleral surface, or in the vitreous cavity. The size of these devices ranges between 5 mm length and 0.9 mm diameter for scleral plugs; 6 mm length and 0.9 mm diameter for rods; 0.5 mm width and 4 mm diameter for intrascleral discs; and 7 mm length and 0.8 mm diameter for biodegradable implants. Scleral plugs require minimal sclerectomy for implantation.

To date, these devices have not been applied clinically due to potential induction of hypotony and wound-healing delay caused during polymer degradation.[24] Surodex and Ozurdex (Allergan, USA) are used in clinical practice. They are prepared from PLGA and dexamethasone (60 µg for Surodex and 700 µg for Ozurdex). The effects can last for days (surodex) to weeks (Ozurdex) after their implantation. Surodex is indicated for the treatment of postoperative inflammation filtering surgery on eyes with glaucoma. Ozurdex is currently under investigation for the treatment of macular edema related to retinal vein occlusion, diabetic macular edema, and uveitis. A dexamethasone posterior-segment drug delivery system (DDS) with the same composition of Ozurdex has recently been tested releasing 350 or 700 µg of dexamethasone.The implant is inserted into the eye through a small pars plana insertion.[25]

The toxicity and biocompatibility of the PLGA implants have been evaluated after implantation. In all cases low signs or absence of inflammation have been reported. If inflammation is reported it disappears in several weeks. There is no electoretinograph alteration and no evidence of histopathological change in the retina as a consequence of implantation.[26] Injectable particles are classified by size in microparticles (1–1000 µm) and nanoparticles (1–1000 nm). By physical structure, the microparticles are classified as microcapsules and microspheres. Microcapsules have a reservoir structure while in microspheres the drug is dispersed through the polymeric matrix. The release kinetic of the active substance from the polymeric matrix depends on the physicochemical properties of the drug, the characteristics of the polymer, percentage of loaded drug, and the surface area.

The great advantage of the particulate systems is that they can be administered as a conventional intraocular injection. Local administration of micro- and nanoparticles has been carried out by intravitreal[27] and periocular injections.[28] Intraocular administration of microparticles is carried out as a conventional suspension. The needle is chosen depending on the size of the microparticles. Needles most frequently employed are 25–30 G for sizes 1–106 µm and 18 G for particle sizes up to 500 µm.[27] PLGA microparticles have been prepared with different drugs, such as Adriamycin, 5-fluorouracil (5-FU), and retinoic acid for proliferative retinopathy, dexamethasone for uveitis, aciclovir for herpes infection, ganciclovir for cytomegalovirus retinitis, neurotrophic factors for neuroprotection, and inhibitor of protein kinase C (PKC412) for choroidal neovascularization (Figure 9.5).[29,30] PLGA microspheres loaded with triamcinolone have already been injected in humans. Preliminary results have been reported with good tolerance after microparticle injection (Figure 9.6).[31] The vehicle employed to suspend particles was isotonic phosphate-buffered saline.

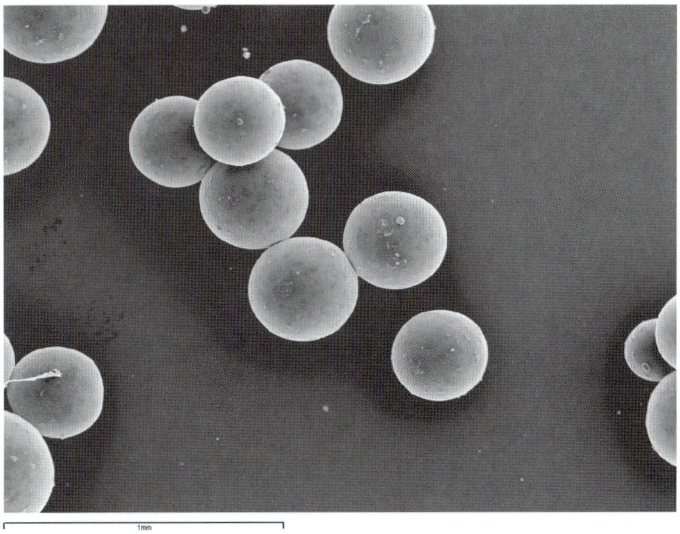

Figure 9.5 Poly(lactic-co-glycolic) acid (PLGA) microspheres loaded with ganciclovir for intravitreal administration. Size 212–300 µm (90 µg ganciclovir/mg microspheres). PLGA inherent viscosity 0.39 dl/g.

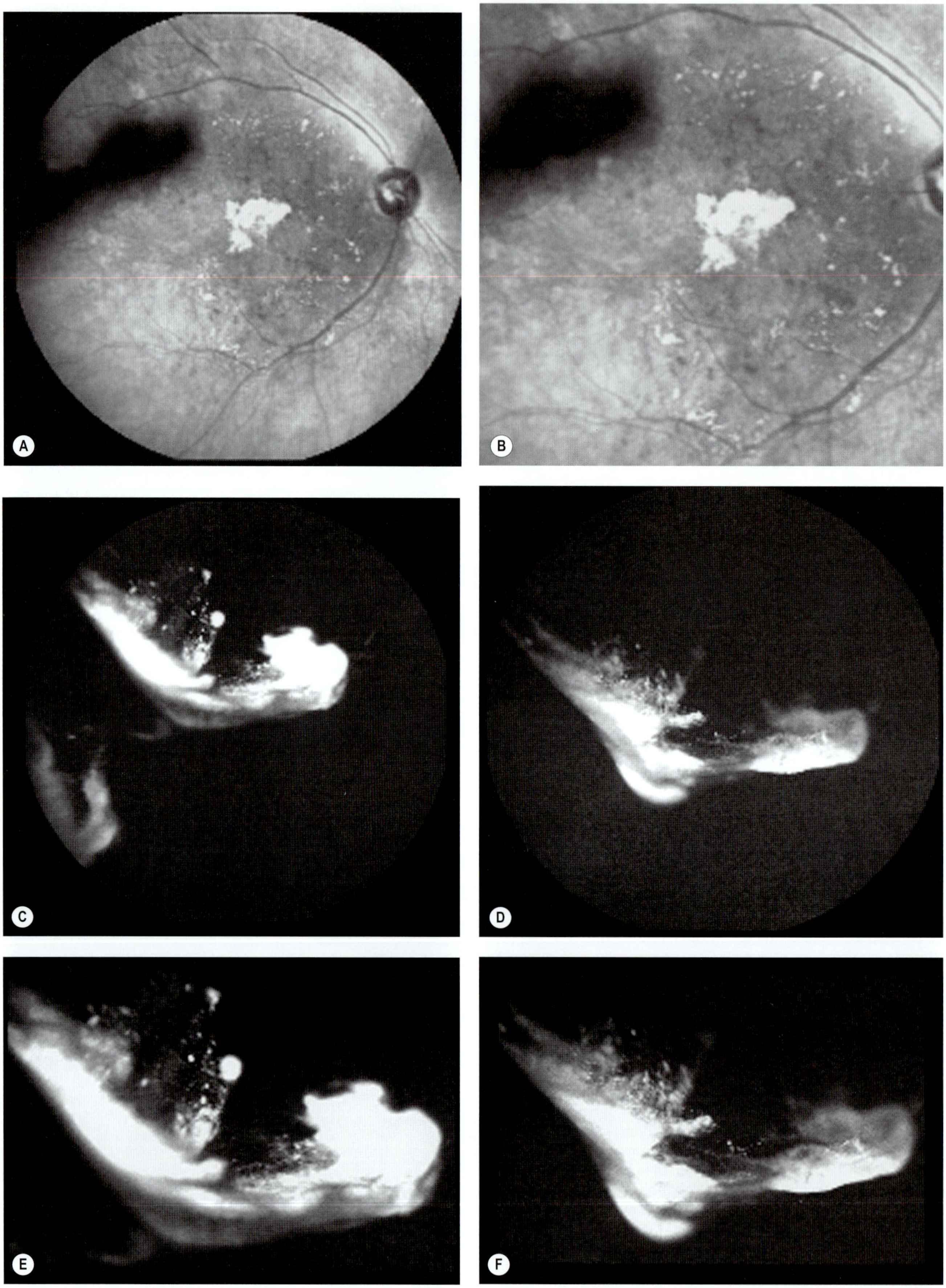

Figure 9.6 (A) Aspect of the microspheres immediately after injection in human eye and (B) 30 days postinjection (note that the visual axis is not obstructed by the system). In detail, the aspect of the microsphere in the vitreous cavity of the same patient (C) 24 hours and (D) 30 days postinjection injection. In high magnification, the spheres (E) 24 hours and (F) 30 days postinjection injection.

Because a significant proportion of microparticles suspended in phosphate-buffered saline tended to adhere to the syringe wall, some researchers have employed viscous solutions of hydroxypropylmethylcellulose (HPMC) and hyaluronic acid (HA). These vehicles are commonly employed as surgical aids in ophthalmology.

Several reactions have been described after administration of PLGA microspheres. Some authors have pointed out the presence of white material that disappeared 20–25 days after injection.[32] However, retinal and choroidal damage were not reported after 35 days of administration. Signs of inflammation have been described associated with intravitreal injection of microparticles. These signs were similar to the ones reported for sutures and disappeared 2–4 weeks after administration.

A secondary concern is regarding the behavior of the spheres and the possibility of causing a visual-impairing vitreous haze following a single intravitreous injection. However, preliminary investigation using triamcinolone microspheres for the treatment of diabetic macular edema in human eyes has showed the opposite. In fact, in contrast to initial fears, the tendency of the microspheres to aggregate and condensate at the site of the injection and leave a free visual axis was clinically observed in all 25 patients.[31] Furthermore, aggregation of microparticles yields in a lower surface area. Then the drug is being released slower from the particles.

Sterility is a critical factor for the intraocular systems. A final sterilization is preferred over aseptic conditions. Nevertheless, devices derived for PLGA are sensitive to most sterilization methods usually employed (heat and ethylene chloride). A few years ago several authors reported the employment of ionizing sterilization methods for PLGA microparticles destined for parenteral and intravitreal injection. Gamma irradiation has a high capacity for penetration and the required dose to achieve sterilization is 25–49 kGy. The dose required to assure sterilization of a pharmaceutical product is 25 kGy. This dose produces a significant reduction of the molecular weight of the polymer affecting the properties of the final product. This problem seems to be solved by using low temperatures during the exposure time of the microparticles to gamma-radiation. This method has presented optimal results with formulations including ganciclovir.[33] Cellular uptake of PLGA micro- and nanoparticles by RPE has been observed.[34] PLA and PLGA microparticles up to 1–2 μm can be phagocytosed by RPE cells.

Nanoparticles have the advantage of cellular entry, which can be used in the delivery of DNA and proteins inside the cells.[35] While particles in the range 200–2000 nm were almost completely retained at the site of administration (subconjunctivally) for at least 2 months, smaller nanoparticles (20 nm) were rapidly cleared from the site of administration.[36] Nanoparticles were retained within RPE cells up to 4 months after intravitreal injection.[37] Albumin has been employed for the elaboration of ganciclovir nanoparticles for intravitreal administration. These particles did not show inflammatory reactions and retinal alterations. The particles were observed in the vitreous cavity and ciliary body for at least 2 weeks after injection. Polymeric nanoparticles are useful for DNA delivery to the eye. Although viral vectors resulted more efficient in gene transfection, nonviral vectors have fewer side-effects.

Other nano systems such as liposomes, self-assembled micelles, dendrimers, and carbon nanostructure nanotubes have been proposed for intraocular drug delivery.[38]

ACKNOWLEDGMENTS

The authors thank Vanessa Andres-Guerrero for technical assistance 920415 and Spanish Ministry of Education (MAT2007-65288) and UCM Research Group 920415 (GR58/08) grants for financial support.

REFERENCES

1. Maurice DM, Mishima S. Ocular pharmacokinetics. In: Sears ML, editor. Handbook of Experimental Pharmacology. Berlin: Springer-Verlag; 1984. p. 19–116.
2. Urtti A. Challenges and obstacles of ocular pharmacokinetics and drug delivery. Adv Drug Deliv Rev 2006;58:1131–1135.
3. Montero JA, Ruiz-Moreno JM, Fernandez-Muñoz M, et al. Effect of topical anesthesics on intraocular pressure and pachymetry. Eur J Ophthalmol 2008;18:748–750.
4. Shirasaki Y. Molecular design for enhancement of ocular penetration. J Pharm Sci 2008;7:2462–2496.
5. Hosoya K, Lee VHL, Kim K. Roles of conjunctiva in ocular drug delivery: a review of conjunctival transport mechanism and their regulation. Eur J Pharm Biopharm 2005;60:227–240.
6. Ranta VP, Urtti A. Transscleral drug delivery to the posterior eye. Prospects of pharmacokinetic modeling. Adv Drug Deliv Rev 2006;58:1164–1118.
7. Robinson MR, Lee SS, Kim H, et al. A rabbit model for assessing the ocular barriers to the transscleral delivery of triamcinolone acetonide. Exp Eye Res 2006:82:479–487.
8. Dib E, Maia M, Longo-Maugeri IM, et al. Subretinal bevacizumab detection after intraviteous injection in rabbits. Invest Ophthalmol Vis Sci 2008;49: 1097–1100.
9. Herrero-Vanrell R, Fernández-Carballido A, Frutos G, et al. Enhancement of the mydriatic response to tropicamide by bioadhesive polymers. J Ocular Pharmacol Ther 2000;16:419–428.
10. Nelson MD, Barlett JD, Karkkainen T, et al. Ocular tolerability of timolol in Gelrite in young glaucoma patients. J Am Optom Assoc 1996;67: 659–663.
11. Chetoni P, Burgalassi S, Monti D, et al. Ocular toxicity of some corneal penetration enhancers evaluated by electrophysiology measurements on isolated rabbit corneas. Toxicol *In Vitro* 2003;17:497–504.
12. Vandervoort J, Ludwig A. Ocular drug delivery: nanomedicine applications. Nanomed 2007;2:11–21.
13. Yasukawa T, Ogura Y, Tabata Y, et al. Drug delivery systems for vitreoretinal diseases. Prog Retin Eye Res 2004;23:253–281.
14. Callanan DG, Jaffe GJ, Martin DF, et al. Treatment of posterior uveitis with a fluocinolone acetonide implant: three-year clinical trial results. Arch Ophthalmol 2008;126:1191–1201.
15. Okabe K, Kimura H, Okabe J, et al. Intraocular tissue distribution of betamethasone after intrascleral administration using a non-biodegradable sustained drug delivery device. Invest Ophthalmol Vis Sci 2003;44: 2702–2707.
16. http://www.alimerasciences.com/medidur_overview.asp.
17. Sieving PA, Caruso RC, Tao W, et al. Ciliary neurotrophic factor (CNTF) for human retinal degeneration: phase I trial of CNTF delivered by encapsulated cell intraocular implants. Proc Natl Acad Sci USA 2006;103:3896–3901.
18. Cheng L, Hostetler KY, Lee J, et al. Characterization of a novel intraocular drug-delivery system using crystalline lipid antiviral prodrugs of ganciclovir and cyclic cidofovir. Invest Ophthalmol Vis Sci 2004;45:4138–4144.
19. Bochot A, Corvreur P, Fattal E. Intravitreal administration of antisense oligonucleotides: potential of liposomal delivery. Prog Retin Eye Res 2000;19:131–147.
20. Fattal E, De Rosa G, Bochot A. Gel and solid matrix systems for the controlled delivery of drug carrier-associated nucleic acids. Int J Pharm 2004;277(11):25–30.
21. Odergren A, Algvere PV, Seregard S, et al. A prospective randomised study on low-dose transpupillary thermotherapy versus photodynamic therapy for neovascular age-related macular degeneration. Br J Ophthalmol 2008;92: 757–761.
22. Antoszyk AN, Tuomi L, Chung CY, et al. Ranibizumab combined with verteporfin photodynamic therapy in neovascular age-related macular degeneration (FOCUS): year 2 results. Am J Ophthalmol 2008;145: 862–874.
23. Chakravarthy U, Soubrane G, Bandello F, et al. Evolving European guidance on the medical management of neovascular age related macular degeneration. Br J Ophthalmol 2006;90:1188–1196.
24. Yasukawa T, Kimura H, Tabata Y, Ogura Y. Biodegradable scleral plugs for vitroretinal drug delivery. Adv Drug Deliv Rev 2001;52:25–36.
25. Gould L, Trope G, Cheng YL, et al. Fifty:fifty poly (DL glycolic acid-lactic acid) copolymer as a drug delivery system for 5-fluorouracilo: a histopathological evaluation. Can J Ophthalmol 1994;29:168–171.
26. Gould L, Trope G, Cheng YL, et al. Fifty:fifty poly (DL glycolic acid-lactic acid) copolymer as a drug delivery system for 5-fluorouracilo: a histopathological evaluation. Can J Ophthalmol 1994;29:168–171.
27. Herrero R, y Refojo M. Biodegradable microspheres for vitreoretinal drug delivery. Adv Drug Deliv Rev 2001;52:5–16.
28. Kompella UB, Bandi N, Ayalasomayajula SP. Subconjunctival nano- and microparticles sustain retinal delivery of budesonide, a corticosteroid capable of inhibiting VEGF expression. Invest Ophthalmol Vis Sci 2003;44:3562–3569.
29. Jiang C, Moore MJ, Zhang X, et al. Intravitreal injection of GDNF-loaded microspheres are neuroprotective in a rat model of glaucoma. Mol Vis 2007;13:1783–1792.
30. Saishin Y, Silva RL, Saishin Y, et al. Periocular injection of microspheres containing PKC412 inhibits thyroidal neovascularization in a porcine model. Invest Ophthalmol Vis Sci 2003;44:4989–4993.
31. Cardillo JA, Souza-Filho AA, Oliveira AG. Intravitreal bioerudivel sustained-release triamcinolone microspheres system (retaac). Preliminary report of its potential usefulnes for the treatment of diabetic macular edema. Arch Soc Esp Oftalmol 2006;81:675–682.

32. Veloso AAA, Zhu Q, Herrero-Vanrell R, et al. Ganciclovir-loaded polymer microspheres in rabbit eyes inoculated with human cytomegalovirus. Invest Ophthalmol Vis Sci 1997;38:665–675.
33. Herrero-Vanrell R, Ramírez L, Fernández-Carballido A y Refojo MF. Biodegradable PLGA microspheres loaded with ganciclovir for intraocular administration. Encapsulation technique, *in vitro* release profiles and sterilization process. Pharm Res 2000;17:1323–1328.
34. Moritera T, Ogura Y, Yoshimura N, et al. Feasability of drug targeting to the retinal pigment epithelium with biodegradable microspheres. Curr Eye Res 1994;13:171–176.
35. Bejjani RA, BenEzra D, Cohen H, et al. Nanoparticles for gene delivery to retinal pigment epithelial cells. Mol Vis 2005;11:124–132.
36. Amrite AC, Kompella UB. Size-dependent disposition of nanoparticles and microparticles following subconjunctival administration. J Pharm Pharmacol 2005;57:1555–1563.
37. Merodio M, Irache HM, Valamenesh F, et al. Ocular disposition and toleranci of ganciclovir/loaded albumin nanoparticles after intravitreal injection in rats. Biomaterials 2002;23:1587–1594.
38. Edelhauser H, Boatright JH, Nickerson JM, et al. Drug delivery to posterior intraocular tissues: third annual ARVO/Pfizer Ophthalmics Research Institute conference. Invest Ophthalmol Vis Sci 2008;49:4712–4720.

CHAPTER

10 Routes for drug delivery to the eye and retina: intravitreal injections and vitrectomy

Carsten H. Meyer, MD, Tim U. Krohne, MD, FEBO, Peter Charbel Issa, MD, FEBO, and Frank G. Holz, MD

INTRODUCTION

THE RATIONALE FOR INTRAVITREAL DRUG DELIVERY

Different approaches have been proposed to deliver drugs into the eye. One of the main challenges is to achieve therapeutic concentrations at the posterior pole. Systemic applications may lead to sufficient concentrations at the retina; however unwanted systemic side-effects are of concern, especially in the long term. Topical applications have the disadvantage that the active agent may not penetrate deep enough into the eye, limiting the therapeutic effect at the posterior pole. Periocular sub-Tenon injections may potentially minimize systemic side-effects, but the drug still has to penetrate the sclera and the blood–retinal barrier (BRB) to reach the intended target in the subretinal space. To overcome these limitations, numerous physicians have suggested intravitreal drug application to achieve locally therapeutic levels with prolonged effective concentrations[1] (Figure 10.1).

HISTORY

Intravitreal drug administrations by single injections or during vitrectomy have become an efficient approach to deliver drugs in therapeutic levels. The advantage of this targeted drug delivery is an immediate and increased therapeutic effect at the intended tissue. Intravitreal injections were initially described by Ohm in 1911[2] to employ an intravitreal air bubble tamponading a retinal tear. Intravitreal application of antibiotics, e.g., sulfanilamide or penicillin, was studied in the early 1940s to treat endophthalmitis. Additional studies, evaluating the appropriate injection technique as well as its feasibility and safety, focused on the treatment of endophthalmitis, submacular hemorrhage, or cytomegalovirus (CMV) retinitis. Triamcinolone acetonide (TA) was the first intravitreally applied drug with widespread application. Most recently, repeated intravitreal injections of antiangiogenic agents like vascular endothelial growth factor (VEGF) inhibitors have become the first-line treatment for exudative age-related macular degeneration (AMD).

The development of additional novel pharmacotherapies has led to an increased use of intravitreal injections. With the recent widespread use of this technique, there has been an increased interest regarding the best approach and application technique.

KEY CONCEPTS AND FUNDAMENTAL POINTS IN RETINAL DRUG DELIVERY

The optimal technique for intravitreal injections is still under evaluation in an attempt to minimize complications and to optimize the "best practice" approach. Extensive clinical experience with intravitreal injection has provided clinicians with an outline of avoidable risks through empirical experience. At present several publications have evaluated the technique of intravitreal injection.[3]

Numerous national boards have defined guidelines on how to perform safe intravitreal injection reliably. The injection should be performed using a standard protocol. While some countries recommend that the injection be applied in an operating room, other countries perform the injection in a conventional examining office under sterile conditions.[4]

STRATEGIES AND IMPLICATIONS FOR RETINAL PHARMACOTHERAPY

PREOPERATIVE PREPARATION

There is now agreement regarding the perioperative management of patients with long-term anticoagulation while undergoing repeated intravitreal injections. A major concern associated with preoperative discontinuation of anticoagulation therapy is the increased risk of thromboembolic or cerebrovascular events.[5]

Previously surgeons discontinued any antiplatelet or anticoagulation therapy perioperatively and determined mild vitreous hemorrhages in less than 0.1%. The low incidence (3/500) convinced them to continue anticoagulation therapy throughout the period of numerous consecutive injections. They performed intravitreal injections with VEGF inhibitors under the currently prescribed anticoagulation therapy.[6,7] During our initial consecutive 3000 injections, no vitreous hemorrhages occurred. Selected eyes received up to 20 consecutive injections. Nineteen percent of our patients were receiving aspirin or warfarin on a regular basis. We found no evidence to suggest that patients undergoing anticoagulation therapy may face persistent vision-threatening vitreal hemorrhages after intravitreal injections.

The Lucentis study trials observed a similar incidence of ocular hemorrhages in patients maintaining warfarin. In the MARINA trial there were a total of 60 warfarin-treated participants, receiving a mean of 22.0 (SD, 3.6) injections.[8] No ocular bleeding was observed during the 1318 consecutive injections. The ANCHOR trial included 25 patients who maintained warfarin. Each patient received a mean of 21.4 (SD, 4.6) injections.[9] The authors concluded that intraocular injections in warfarin-treated patients are unlikely to cause ocular hemorrhages.

Subretinal, vitreal, or subconjunctival hemorrhages (Figure 10.2) after intravitreal injections may relate to the procedure itself, the applied drug, as well as the anticoagulation status of the patient. Small-incision techniques can reduce the risks of hemorrhagic ocular events in the anticoagulated patient. Approximately 10% of all patients with exudative AMD receive warfarin anticoagulation due to concomitant medical conditions. These patients may undergo intravitreal injections without significant risk of hemorrhagic complications while maintaining their anticoagulation therapy.

PROPHYLAXIS OF ENDOPHTHALMITIS: LOCAL DISINFECTION AND TOPICAL ANTIBIOTIC THERAPY

It is mandatory to treat any active external infection, including significant blepharitis, before each intravitreal injection. It has been demonstrated in rabbits that 51 + 4 colony-forming units of *Staphylococcus*

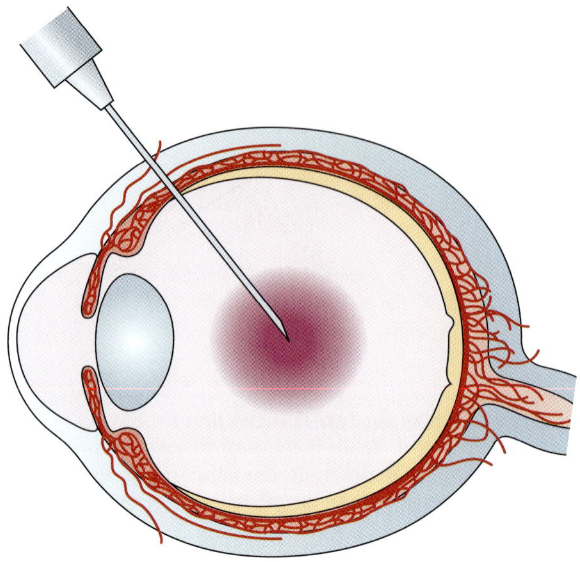

Figure 10.1 Intravitreal injections: via the pars plana route into the mid vitreous.

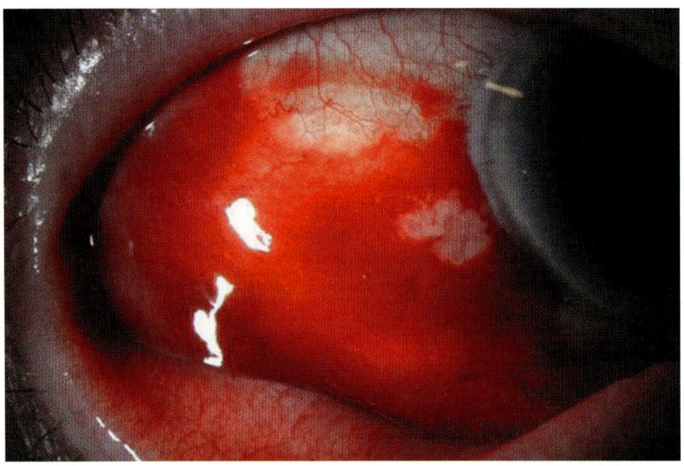

Figure 10.2 Severe hyposphagma after intravitreal injection.

aureus are required to induce endophthalmitis, when injected into the anterior chamber, compared with 19 + 8 colony-forming units when injected into the vitreous. The primary goal of any endophthalmitis prophylaxis is to minimize the present bacterial flora around the surgical entry site. This can be achieved with the topical application of: (1) povidone-iodine; (2) eyelid hygiene; (3) proper isolation of the surgical site; and possibly (4) postoperative antibiotics.[10–14]

The key step to avoid an endophthalmitis is sufficient disinfection of the skin, eyelashes, and conjunctiva. Povidone-iodine reduces significantly the risk of postoperative endophthalmitis in a prospective study of cataract surgery (level II evidence).[15] The lids and lashes are usually disinfected by a povidone-iodine (10%) scrub. A sterile speculum is placed between the lids and three drops of povidone-iodine (5%) are then applied three times several minutes apart over the ocular surface. The various methods of applying povidone-iodine preoperatively have been studied. Two drops of 0.5% povidone-iodine placed on the eye reduced conjunctival bacterial flora significantly by approximately 91% and reduced the prevalence of endophthalmitis significantly after intraocular surgery from 0.24% to 0.06%. Several investigators have also advocated irrigating the conjunctival sac with 1% or 5% povidone-iodine to decrease conjunctival colonization[10]; however it remains unknown whether the application of povidone-iodine drops versus a flush has an impact on preventing endophthalmitis. A surprising finding is the significant increase in bacterial flora with lid scrubs alone compared with a control. There is no consensus among experts whether topical antibiotics should be used preoperatively. Preinjection antibiotic drops may be applied according to the label of the applied drug, although there is no evidence supporting its use before intravitreal injections.

LOCAL TOPICAL ANESTHESIA

Sufficient relief of pain and satisfactory comfort for the patient may be achieved with topical application of lidocaine. The drug may be applied with 2% eye drops, gel, or subconjunctival injection prior to the intravitreal injection. A comparison between topical lidocaine 2% gel and subconjunctival lidocaine 2% injection demonstrated no statistically significant difference in pain scores between the treatment groups ($P = 0.67$, paired test). The effective relief of pain with lidocaine for intravitreal injection is independent of its mode of application (gel versus subconjunctival injection). However, lidocaine gel usually causes less chemosis and hemorrhage compared with subconjunctival anesthesia. Insufficient pain sensation may be released by applying a sterile cotton swab soaked in sterile 4% lidocaine eye drops to the injection area.[16]

SURGICAL TECHNIQUES FOR RETINAL DRUG DELIVERY

THE PROCEDURE AND RECOMMENDED TECHNIQUE

The injection site should be located at the sclera 3.5–4 mm posterior to the limbus. The injection site may differ in repeated injections by approximately one clock-hour, thus avoiding a double penetration through the same site, which may induce a persisting scleral hole with consecutive leaking or vitreous incarceration – vitreous wick.

The angle of the incision through the sclera may be directed on an oblique, tunneled fashion (Figures 10.3 and 10.4), because rectangular radial incisions may remain open, inducing vitreous or drug reflux under the conjunctiva as well as severe chemosis and even hypotony in vitrectomized eyes.[17] We observed persistent unsealed sclerotomies following radial injections using a 30-gauge needle, requiring secondary suturing to seal the penetrating scleral wound.[18]

The depth of the insertion may vary between 5 and 7 mm, so that the tip of the needle is placed in the mid vitreous. The drug should be gently applied into the vitreous cavity, as the jet of a fast injected drug (e.g., recombinant tissue plasmin activation (rTPA), or antibiotics) may damage the perpendicular retinal surface, visible as mild whitening.

The diameter of the needle should be smaller than 25-gauge to reduce the risk of injury to ocular structures or wound leakage. Injections with crystalline TA are frequently applied with 27-gauge needles, while most liquid injections are performed with 30-gauge needles. Experimental studies examined the force required to penetrate the sclera with 27-, 30-, or even 31-gauge needles on a tuberculin syringe and measured almost twice as much force to penetrate the sclera using the 27-gauge needles. Larger needles may not necessarily induce more pain to the patient; however, apparently more trauma, reflux and subconjunctival hemorrhages result. In addition a reduced sharpness of the needle as found in some prefilled syringes induced a deeper inpouching and visible indentation of the eye wall, possibly causing more discomfort to the patient's eye.[19–21]

The injected volume should be limited to 0.15 ml without a routine paracentesis releasing an elevated ocular pressure. Administration of rTPA, anti-VEGF, and SF_6 gas as triple injection for the management of subretinal hemorrhage frequently requires paracentesis to release the elevated eye pressure.

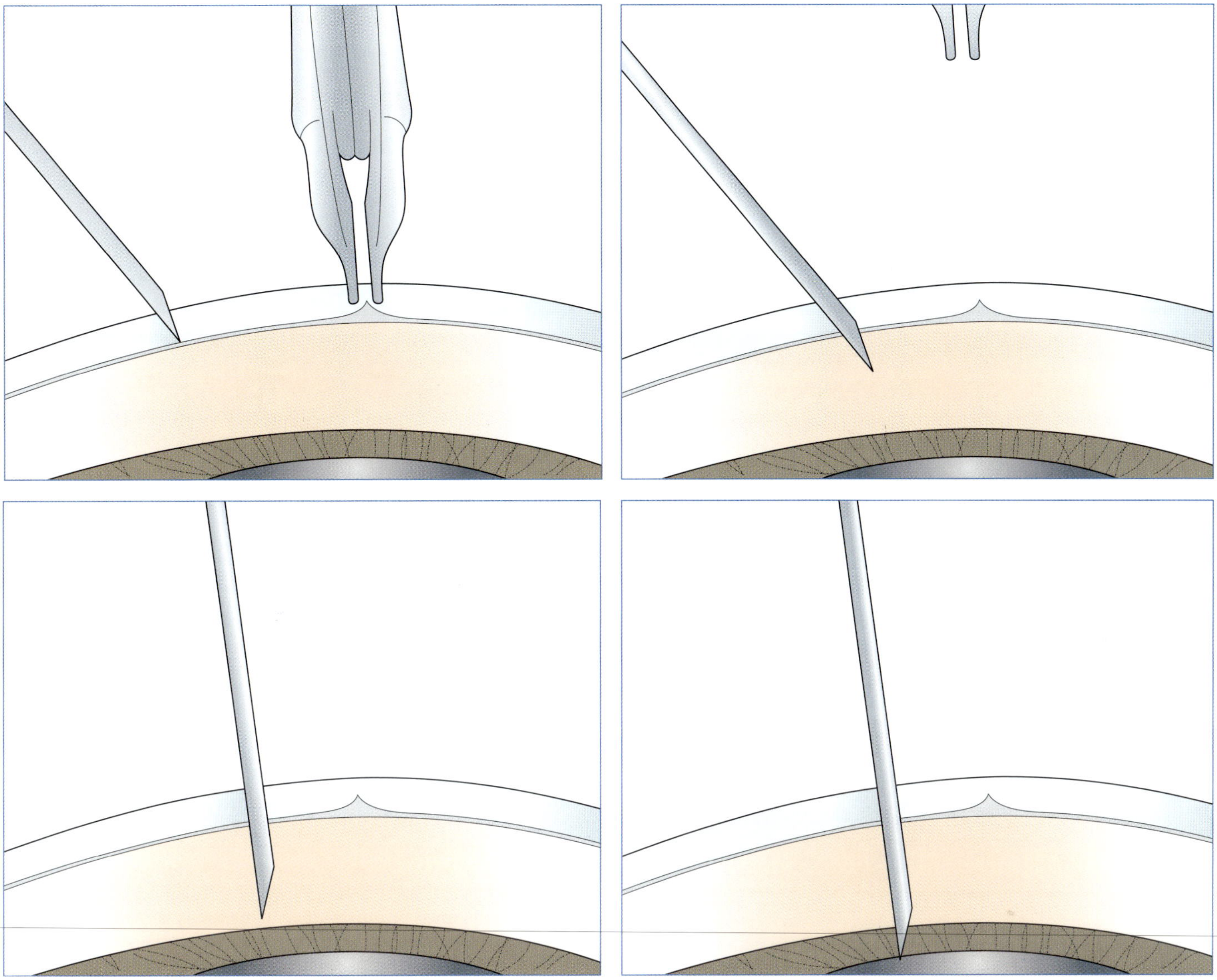

Figure 10.3 Schematic drawing of the injection procedure. The conjunctiva is moved upwards, so that the conjunctival hole and the site of the scleral penetration are not on top of each other. After initial lamellar penetration of the outer sclera, the needle is moved upwards for full-thickness penetration.

COMPLICATIONS WITH THE ROUTE FOR DRUG DELIVERY

PROPHYLAXIS OF ENDOPHTHALMITIS AND POSTOPERATIVE TOPICAL ANTIBIOTICS

The role of topical antibiotics to prevent postoperative endophthalmitis remains controversial. Topical antibiotics may be applied after the injection for a few days, as the break in the conjunctiva and sclera is not completely healed and water-sealed. In addition there may be a synergistic effect between topical antibiotics and povidone-iodine. However, no studies have demonstrated that reducing the conjunctival bacterial count also results in a lower risk for endophthalmitis. Given the paucity of data regarding intraocular infections, there is no evidence supporting the use of antibiotics after intravitreal injections. In fact, there has never been a prospective randomized study showing the benefit of topical antibiotics in preventing endophthalmitis. Such a study would require thousands of patients covering all aspects of the procedure. However, a study of this magnitude is not feasible. There is general agreement that the risk of infectious endophthalmitis following intravitreal injection is small. The exact rate of endophthalmitis after intravitreal injection is unknown due to the paucity of large reported series. The highest reported rate to date is 0.9% for TA and 0.01% for bevacizumab.

OCULAR COMPLICATIONS

A survey on published studies and case series, including more than 15000 intravitreal injections in 4400 eyes, determined a prevalence of endophthalmitis (including pseudo-endophthalmitis) after TA injections of 0.3% per injection and 0.9% per eye. The overall prevalence for retinal detachments was 3.9% per eye or 0.9% per injection. The prevalence of intraocular inflammation (iritis, uveitis, vitritis, and/or anterior-chamber inflammation) was 28.5% per eye and 6.3% (839/13400) per injection. Traumatic cataracts (Figure 10.5), intraocular hemorrhage (i.e., retinal hemorrhage, vitreous hemorrhage, or hyphema) were occasionally reported after intravitreal injection. Temporary hypotony, defined as an intraocular pressure of <4 mmHg, may occur rarely after intravitreal injections and is primarily limited to eyes receiving antiviral therapy. Some cases of retinal artery occlusion have also been reported after intravitreal injections.

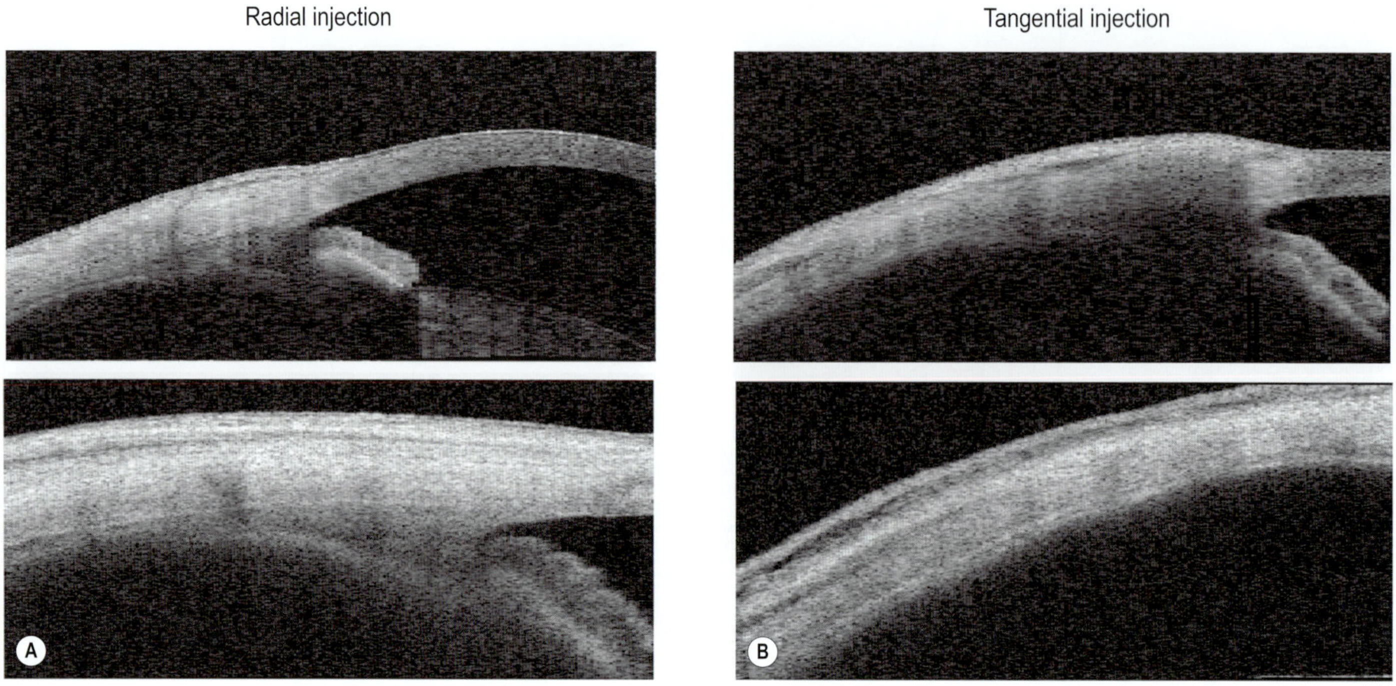

Figure 10.4 Examination of the injection site 15 minutes after injection with the anterior-segment optical coherence tomography (OCT) scan (Visante). The radial injection remains open and visible, whereas the tangential oblique injection is not detected on OCT. (A, two left images) radial injection; (B, two right images) tangential injection.

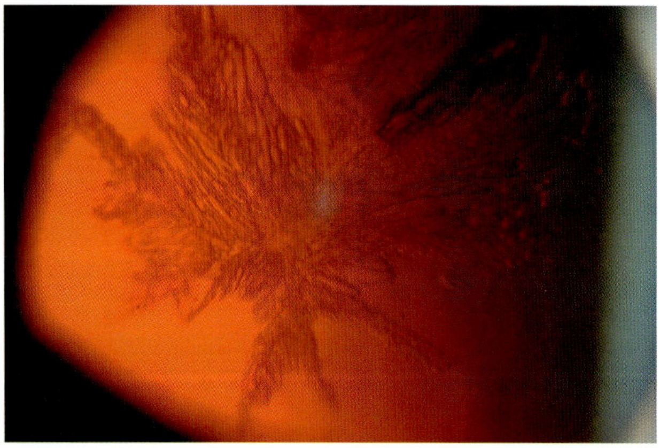

Figure 10.5 Posterior lens touch with a rupture of the posterior capsule.

General guidelines for intravitreal injections were established for the injecting physician. Some aspects are supported by consensus agreement (use of adequate anesthetic, povidone-iodine, and a lid speculum; dilate the pupil; avoid injecting patients with active eyelid or ocular infection; avoid extensive massage of eyelids; avoid prophylactic or postinjection paracentesis) while other parts have less agreement (e.g., most investigators advocate gloves, most prefer povidone-iodine drops over flush, most use no sterile drape). There is no agreement regarding the use of pre- or postinjection topical antibiotics, as well as a specific intraocular pressure level that should not be exceeded before the injection.

PHARMACOKINETICS AND CLEARANCE OF INTRAVITREAL DRUGS

The elimination of intravitreal drugs depends on a number of factors. First, the drug may be eliminated via an anterior route passing into the aqueous humor or a posterior route by active transport across the retina. Zwitterions such as ciprofloxacin and other fluoroquinolones are mainly eliminated by a short elimination half-life through the posterior route. On the other hand, cationic compounds and drugs such as vancomycin and gentamicin show clearing primarily by a passive transport via diffusion in the aqueous humor through the anterior chamber. Second, the mechanism of active transport across the retina is compromised in an inflamed or infected eye. Drugs such as cefazolin that are cleared via the posterior route therefore demonstrated an increased half-life in the vitreous cavity in phakic, nonvitrectomized eyes. Third, the clearance is accelerated in vitrectomized eyes compared to nonvitrectomized eyes, whereas silicone oil-filled eyes show a prolonged elimination of most drugs.

The intravitreal clearance of antibiotics, e.g., 200 µg/0.1 ml moxifloxacin, a fourth-generation fluoroquinolone, was determined to have a half-life of 1.72 hours in rabbit eyes. The mean vitreous concentration was 120.49 + 49.23 µg/ml 1 hour after injection, declining to 20.23 + 5.85 µg/ml at 6 hours and 1.06 + 0.81 µg/ml at 12 hours, respectively.[22] The calculated half-life of 400 mg amikacin injected into the vitreous cavity of rabbit eyes was 25.5 hours in phakic control eyes, 14.3 hours in aphakic eyes, and 7.0 hours in aphakic vitrectomized eyes. Inflammation substantially increased the rate of clearance in aphakic eyes.[23] Vancomycin hydrochloride 1 mg injected into the mid vitreous cavity of rabbit eyes cleared substantially faster from aphakic-vitrectomized eyes (half-life 9.0 hours) compared to aphakic eyes (half-life 8.9 hours) or phakic eyes (half-life 25.1 hours). Inflammation increased the rate of elimination of vancomycin only in the aphakic group.

The intravitreal clearance of antibodies such as rituximab, a monoclonal antibody directed against the CD20 B-cell antigen and approved for the treatment of B-cell lymphoma, takes longer.[24] The pharmacokinetics of 0.1 ml (1 mg) rituximab following intravitreal administration in rabbit eyes demonstrated in a two-compartment model a clearance from the aqueous humor of 1.2 µl/min and a half-life of 4.7 days. The ocular pharmacokinetics of a 1 mg intravitreal injection of C-14-labeled 5-fluorouracil (5-FU) demonstrated a peak level of 664 µg/ml in phakic nonvitrectomized eye which declines to 7.8 µg/ml at 24 hours. For the aphakic vitrectomized eye comparable values are 669 µg/ml at 0.1 hour and 0.21 µg/ml at 24 hours. 5-FU is cleared more than twice as rapidly in aphakic vitrectomized eyes than normal eyes during the first 12 hours following injection.

PHARMACOKINETICS OF INTRAVITREAL CRYSTALLINE TRIAMCINOLONE ACETONIDE

After intravitreal TA injections the drug may persist in the vitreous cavity for months. Its clearance also depends on the status of the vitreous as well as the applied dosage and was initially studied in rabbit eyes, reporting disappearance of 0.5 mg TA after 16.8 days in vitrectomized, compared to 41 days in nonvitrectomized, eyes.

Beer and associates determined the anterior-chamber concentration of TA through an anterior-chamber paracentesis after a single 4-mg TA in humans. They calculated a mean half-life elimination of 3.2 days in vitrectomized eyes compared with 18.6 days in nonvitrectomized eyes.[25] While the concentration after a single 4-mg dose was maintained at a measurable rate for approximately 3 months, a higher 25-mg dose of TA was sustained at detectable levels for up to 9 months in nonvitrectomized eyes and up to 1.5 years in silicone oil-filled vitreous cavity. An intravitreal injection of 20–25 mg of TA can be present in measurable concentrations during the first 6 months at between 3.0 and 436 μg/l and later at 7–12 months between 0.0 and 11.2 μg/l, respectively. A faster clearance of intravitreal TA in the vitrectomized eye must be considered. The clearance of 0.1 ml (0.3 mg) intravitreal TA after 30 days was 0.22 μg/ml in vitrectomized eyes compared to 0.92 ± 1.25 μg/ml in nonvitrectomized eyes. Serum levels of TA obtained 4–92 days after an intravitreal high-dose injection of 20–25 mg did not differ significantly (P = 0.174) after the injection (postoperatively: 0.065 ± 0.21 μg/l).

PHARMACOKINETICS OF VEGF INHIBITORS[26–32]

It is mandatory for a sufficient treatment of vascular AMD to neutralize the elevated VEGF concentration by suitable concentrations of VEGF inhibitors. If the concentration declines, the choroidal neovascularization progresses, and increased leakage may occur. The permeability of the proliferating vessels accelerates, leading to enhanced leakage of subretinal or intraretinal fluid with progression of macular edema and decreased visual acuity. The pharmacokinetics of VEGF inhibitors does not depends neither on age, gender, nor kidney function. An intravitreal injection of 0.5 mg pegaptanib induces a concentration in the vitreous cavity of 350 μg/ml, declining to 1.7 μg/ml within 4 weeks. Studies demonstrated a half-life of pegaptanib by approximately 94 hours in monkeys and 83 hours in rabbits. After monthly injections of 0.5 mg ranibizumab, the highest measured serum concentration was found to be between 0.79 and 2.9 ng/ml and the minimal serum concentration between 0.07 and 0.49 ng/ml. Gaudreault et al. calculated a half-life time of approximately 3 days in rabbit eyes.[27] The concentration of ranibizumab in the vitreous cavity is approximately 90 000 times higher than in the blood serum. There is no indication for any metabolism inside the eye.

Bakri et al injected 1.25 mg bevacizumab in the vitreous cavity in rabbits and determined the intravitreal concentration in the vitreous cavity within 30 days.[28] The concentration peaked with maximal values (400 μg/ml) 3 days after the injection and declined in an exponential function. The concentration declined by a half-life time of 4.32 days and remained >10 mg/ml in the vitreous cavity during the entire 30 days. However, it remains unknown if the animal model is comparable to humans, who have a three-times bigger vitreous cavity (4.5 versus 1.5 ml).

Beer et al.[25] determined the vitreous levels of unbound bevacizumab and unbound VEGF in 2 patients after intravitreal application of bevacizumab. Patient 1 underwent vitrectomy for a retinal detachment 4 weeks after the intravitreal bevacizumab injection. At that time point, the unbound bevacizumab level was 0.16% of the loading dose, a level that was still 3100-fold molar excess of bevacizumab compared to the measured VEGF levels. In patient 2, who underwent vitreous biopsy for endophthalmitis 48 hours after the injection, the unbound bevacizumab level was 53% of the loading dose, which equaled a more than millionfold molar excess compared to measured intravitreal VEGF levels. VEGF concentration was the lower limit of detection in both patients. The calculated half-life of bevacizumab was approximately 3 days. The authors concluded that a single dose of intravitreal bevacizumab is likely to provide a complete intravitreal VEGF blockade for a minimum of 4 weeks.

In 30 nonvitrectomized eyes with cataract and concurrent macular edema we performed cataract surgery 1–53 days after an intravitreal injection of 1.5 mg bevacizumab. During surgery, a sample from the anterior-chamber fluid was obtained and bevacizumab levels quantified by enzyme-linked immunosorbent assay.[29] Concentration of bevacizumab in aqueous humor peaked on the first postinjection day with a mean concentration of 33.3 μg/ml (range 16.6–42.5 μg/ml) and subsequently declined in an exponential fashion. Nonlinear regression analysis determined an elimination half-time of 9.82 days (R^2 = 0.81) .

CLINICAL EXPERIENCE AND RESULTS IN VITRECTOMIZED, AIR-FILLED, OR SILICONE OIL EYES

VITRECTOMIZED EYES

There is only limited experience using VEGF inhibitors in vitrectomized eyes due to the exclusion of those eyes from all phase II/III studies. Intravitreal-applied crystalline TA may have a longer effect compared to dissolved drugs, while the concentration of solute bevacizumab seems to decrease more rapidly, leaving only a minor effect at the retina. Intravitreal injections of solute VEGF inhibitors in vitrectomized eyes are therefore currently not recommended.

Silicone oil tamponade

The clinical management of CMV retinitis and associated retinal detachment often involves the concurrent use of silicone oil and ganciclovir (GCV) implants. Perkins et al. investigated the effect of oil tamponade on intravitreal drug levels achieved with a 5-mg GCV implant in rabbits.[30] Vitreous GCV levels at days 21 and 42 were similar in both the saline- and silicone oil-filled eyes. At day 70, GCV levels were significantly lower in the saline-filled eyes than in silicone-filled eyes. GCV levels may remain for longer in eyes with silicone oil tamponade, supporting the use of combined application.

Silicone oil is also an efficacious delivery system for acetylsalicylic acid in rabbits, extending the duration of the drug in the vitreous cavity.[31]

A combined 5-FU silicone oil intravitreal tamponade was sustained after a conventional three-port lens-sparing pars plana vitrectomy in porcine eyes in a concentration above 1 μg/ml for 5 days. The pharmacokinetics followed a specific release rate constant of 10.7 μg/cm^2.

Gas tamponade

Intravitreal gas bubbles (0.3 ml) in nonvitrectomized eyes may induce a subclinical breakdown of the BRB soon after the gas is absorbed. The effect of intraocular gas tamponade, e.g., perfluoropropane (0.4 ml of 100% C_3F_8), on intravitreal drug levels was studied for sustained-release fluocinolone (FL)/5-FU 10-mg codrug pellet in white rabbits. On postoperative days 4, 7, 21, and 42, there were no statistically significant differences between FL and 5-FU drug levels in eyes containing C_3F_8 as compared with control eyes. Therefore, despite an apparent breakdown of the BRB, intraocular gas tamponade seems to have no significant effect on the intravitreal half-life of these drugs. It is therefore suggested that the concentration of intravitreally applied drugs needs no alteration in the presence of intraocular gas.[32,33]

COMBINATION OF SURGICAL WITH PHARMACOLOGICAL THERAPIES[34–44]

A pars plana vitrectomy combined with pre-, intra-, and postoperative application of drugs has been recommended by numerous authors. The Endophthalmitis Vitrectomy Study demonstrated that early antibiotic drug application may limit the progression of moderate infection, while severe endophthalmitis cases require an early vitrectomy combined with intraoperative application of antibiotics.[3]

PREOPERATIVE DRUG APPLICATIONS

The concept of a planned consecutive intravitreal drug application prior to vitrectomy has been proposed in eyes with severe vitreoretinal adhesions, infections, inflammation, or bleeding, e.g., epiretinal membrane, proliferative vitreoretinopathy, diabetic vitreoretinopathy,[33] retinopathy of prematurity,[35] endophthalmitis, uveitis, or subretinal hemorrhage.

Enzymatic or pharmacologic vitrectomy may induce a cleavage of the posterior hyaloid from the adjacent retinal surface. Dispase, collagenase, hyaluronidase, rtPA[36,38]; RDG peptides,[37] plasmin,[34,35] or microplasmin have been recommended to induce a release of the vitreous from the retina, thus inducing an easier, faster, or less traumatic detachment of the posterior hyaloid. Resolution of a diffuse vitreal hemorrhage may be induced by a liquefaction of the vitreous gel. Highly purified bovine hyaluronidase (Vitrase) has been approved as a complementary approach for the management of vitreous hemorrhage.

Liquefaction of subretinal hemorrhages may be achieved by intravitreal injection of rtPA. Additional SF_6 gas injection can assist the massage of the blood from the subfoveal area towards an inferior location.[38] We proposed a triple injection with rtPA, gas, and anti-VEGF injection in order to occlude the subretinal choroid neovascularization as the primary cause of the bleeding. If the subretinal hemorrhage remains under the fovea or the size of the subretinal hemorrhage is too large, vitrectomy and subretinal lavage of the liquefied blood are recommended. The triple intravitreal injection may increase the intraocular pressure, requiring paracentesis.[39] Koch et al.[45] proposed a minivitrectomy to reduce the volume prior to the drug application. These authors designed a combined 23-gauge vitreous cutter and injection line, Intrector, in order to reduce the vitreous volume, inducing a posterior vitreous detachment and better penetration of the drug through the vitreous cavity and finally consecutive drug application through a single sclerotomy. Initial pilot studies revealed no severe complications using this novel technique. The usefulness of this concept needs additional assessments in further studies.

Eyes with severe nonproliferative diabetic retinopathy or secondary glaucoma (rubeosis iridis) may benefit from intravitreal injected VEGF inhibitors or steroids. Most surgeons apply TA or bevacizumab 3–10 days prior to surgery in order to seal the retinal vessels and reduce the risk of intraoperative bleeding.[40–44,46] However, the fast occlusion of the proliferative vessels can induce traction on the vitreous and retinal surface. Eyes with severe proliferative diabetic retinopathy may therefore develop severe tractional retinal detachments when bevacizumab is applied alone, without subsequent removal of the vitreous gel by vitrectomy.[47] A vitrectomy should be assigned only a few days later, avoiding this devastating complication.

INTRAOPERATIVE DRUG APPLICATIONS

Consecutive drug applications during vitreoretinal surgery have become a frequent maneuver. The selective staining of cellular components in epiretinal membrane or extracellular matrix components on the retinal surface such as the inner limiting membrane (ILM) may be visualized during vitrectomy by a variety of vital dyes (chromovitrectomy). Numerous vital dyes, including indocyanine green, tryphan blue, brilliant blue, patent blue, and triamcinolone, have been proposed to stain the vitreous, epiretinal membranes, or ILM during chromovitrectomy. A better visualization of these semitransparent structures can help to visualize the fine semitransparent structure during surgery, limiting the damage of delicate adjacent structures.[47]

Retinal detachments are frequently treated by removal of the vitreous, drainage of subretinal fluid, and intravitreal gas instillation. Intravitreal gas may assist a permanent reattachment of the retina, sealing the retinal tear during the early postoperative period. The persistence of the gas bubble in the vitreous cavity depends on the type of applied gas. While SF_6 has persisted with different durations in the vitreous cavity, recently, Jackson[48] applied vital dyes into the subretinal space during pars plana vitrectomy in eyes with bullous rhegmatogenous retinal detachments, in order to visualize the retinal break by dye leakage from the subretinal space into the vitreous cavity.

POSTOPERATIVE DRUG APPLICATIONS

Intravitreal drug applications at the end of surgery or early after surgery may support the healing process. A vitrectomy can release the tractional components in diabetic macular edema; however, the edema may persist due to damage of the BRB. Severe uveitis is also frequently associated with a severe breakdown of the BRB. Both indications frequently demonstrate a faster healing process as well as better functional and anatomical improvement after surgery when an intravitreal triamcinolone injection is applied as an adjunct at the end of surgery. The TA crystals may settle on the retinal surface in the inferior quadrant without damaging the retinal surface.[40,41] Unintended application of TA crystals has been observed even in a macular hole early after vitrectomy; however the hole closed without complication and the visual acuity improved to 20/80, demonstrating safety even in this delicate location.

SUMMARY AND KEY POINTS

The rationale for intravitreal drug application is an immediate and increased therapeutic delivery to the targeted tissue. Intravitreal drug application is a safe and effective procedure. Possible side-effects, e.g., elevated intraocular pressure, cataract formation, and endophthalmitis, are limited. The pharmacokinetics depends on the status of the vitreous as well as the structure of the drug. Combined surgical and pharmacological approaches have become an efficient approach to deliver drugs in therapeutic levels to the posterior segment.

REFERENCES

1. Maurice D. Review: practical issues in intravitreal drug delivery. J Ocul Pharmacol Ther 2001;17:393–401.
2. Ohm J. Über die Behandlung der Netzhautablösung durch operative Entleerung der subretinalen Flüssigkeit und Einspritzen vom Luft in den Glaskörper.Graefe Arch Klin Ophthalmol 1911;79:442–450.
3. Aiello LP, Brucker AJ, Chan S, et al. Evolving guidelines for intravitreous injections. Retina 2004;24;S3–S19.
4. Anijeet DR, Hanson RJ, Bhagey J, et al. National survey of the technique of intravitreal triamcinolone injection in the United Kingdom. Eye 2007;21:480–486.
5. Charles S, Rosenfeld PJ, Gayer S. Medical consequences of stopping anticoagulant therapy before intraocular surgery or intravitreal injections. Retina 2007;27:813–815.
6. Meyer CH, Callizo J, Mennel S, et al. Perioperative management of anticoagulated patients undergoing repeated intravitreal injections. Arch Ophthalmol 2007;125:994.
7. Meyer CH, Eter N. Incidence of ocular hemorrhages in anticoagulated patients receiving repeated intravitreal injections. Am J Ophthalmol 2008;145:386–387.
8. Brown DM, Kaiser PK, Michels M, et al. Ranibizumab versus verteporfin for neovascular age-related macular degeneration. N Engl J Med. 2006 Oct 5;355(14):1432–1444.
9. Rosenfeld PJ, Brown DM, Heier JS, et al. Ranibizumab for neovascular age-related macular degeneration. N Engl J Med. 2006 Oct 5;355(14): 1419–1431.
10. Miño de Kaspar H, Chang RT, Singh K, et al. Prospective randomized comparison of 2 different methods of 5% povidone-iodine applications for anterior segment intraocular surgery. Arch Ophthalmol 2005;123:161–165.
11. Meyer CH, Mennel S, Eter N. Incidence of endophthalmitis after intravitreal Avastin injection with and without postoperative topical antibiotic application. Ophthalmologe 2007;104:952–957.

12. Safar A, Dellimore MC. The effect of povidone iodine flush versus drops on conjunctival colonization before intravitreal injections. Int Ophthalmol 2007;27:307–312.
13. Ta CN, Egbert PR, Singh K, et al. Prospective randomized comparison of 3-day versus 1-hour preoperative ofloxacin prophylaxis for cataract surgery. Ophthalmology 2002;109:2036–2041.
14. Ferguson AW, Scott JA, McGavigan J, et al. Comparison of 5% povidone-iodine solution against 1% povidone-iodine solution in preoperative cataract surgery antisepsis: a prospective randomised double blind study. Br J Ophthalmol 2003;87:163–167.
15. Hatch WV, Cernat G, Wong D, et al. Risk factors for acute endophthalmitis after cataract surgery: a population-based study. Ophthalmology. 2009 Mar;116(3):425–430.
16. Kaderli B, Avci R. Comparison of topical and subconjunctival anesthesia in intravitreal injection administrations. Eur J Ophthalmol 2006;16:718–721.
17. Rodrigues EB, Meyer CH, Grumann Jr A, et al. Tunneled scleral incision to prevent vitreal reflux after intravitreal injection. Am J Ophthalmol 2007;143:1035–1037.
18. Rodrigues EB, Meyer CH, Schmidt JC, et al. Unsealed sclerotomy after intravitreal injection with a 30-gauge needle. Retina 2004;24:810–812.
19. Kozak I, Dean A, Clark TM, et al. Prefilled syringe needles versus standard removable needles for intravitreous injection. Retina 2006;26:679–683.
20. Pulido JS, Pulido CM, Bakri SJ, et al. The use of 31-gauge needles and syringes for intraocular injections. Eye 2007;21:829–830.
21. Hochman MN, Friedman MJ. An *in vitro* study of needle force penetration comparing a standard linear insertion to the new bidirectional rotation insertion technique. Quintessence Int 2001;32:789–796.
22. Iyer MN, He F, Wensel TG, et al. Clearance of intravitreal moxifloxacin. Invest Ophthalmol Vis Sci 2006;47:317–319.
23. Mandell BA, Meredith TA, Aguilar E, et al. Effects of inflammation and surgery on amikacin levels in the vitreous cavity. Am J Ophthalmol 1993;115:770–774.
24. Kim H, Csaky KG, Chan CC, et al. The pharmacokinetics of rituximab following an intravitreal injection. Exp Eye Res 2006;82:760–766.
25. Beer PM, Wong SJ, Hammad AM, et al. Vitreous levels of unbound bevacizumab and unbound vascular endothelial growth factor in two patients. Retina 2006;26:871–876.
26. Bakri SJ, Snyder MR, Reid JM, et al. Pharmacokinetics of intravitreal ranibizumab (Lucentis). Ophthalmology 2007;114:2179–2182.
27. Gaudreault J, Fei D, Beyer JC, et al. Pharmacokinetics and retinal distribution of ranibizumab, a humanized antibody fragment directed against VEGF-A, following intravitreal administration in rabbits. Retina 2007;27:1260–1266.
28. Bakri SJ, Snyder MR, Reid JM, et al. Pharmacokinetics of intravitreal bevacizumab (Avastin). Ophthalmology 2007;114:855–859.
29. Krohne TU, Eter N, Holz FG, et al. Intraocular pharmacokinetics of bevacizumab after a single intravitreal injection in humans. Am J Ophthalmol 2008 146:508–512.
30. Perkins SL, Yang CH, Ashton PA, et al. Pharmacokinetics of the ganciclovir implant in the silicone-filled eye. Retina 2001;21:10–14.
31. Kralinger MT, Kieselbach GF, Voigt M, et al. Slow release of acetylsalicylic acid by intravitreal silicone oil. Retina 2001;21:513–520.
32. Perkins SL, Gallemore RP, Yang CH, et al. Pharmacokinetics of the fluocinolone/5-fluorouracil codrug in the gas-filled eye. Retina 2000;20:514–519.
33. Ogura Y, Tsukada T, Negi A, et al. Integrity of the blood–ocular barrier after intravitreal gas injection. Retina 1989;9:199–202.
34. Hirata A, Takano A, Inomata Y, et al. Plasmin-assisted vitrectomy for management of proliferative membrane in proliferative diabetic retinopathy: a pilot study. Retina 2007;27:1074–1078.
35. Tsukahara Y, Honda S, Imai H, et al. Autologous plasmin-assisted vitrectomy for stage 5 retinopathy of prematurity: a preliminary trial. Am J Ophthalmol 2007;144:139–141.
36. Hesse L, Nebeling B, Schroeder B, et al. Induction of posterior vitreous detachment in rabbits by intravitreal injection of tissue plasminogen activator following cryopexy. Exp Eye Res 2000;70:31–39.
37. Oliveira LB, Meyer CH, Kumar J, et al. RGD peptide-assisted vitrectomy to facilitate induction of a posterior vitreous detachment: a new principle in pharmacological vitreolysis. Curr Eye Res 2002;25:333–340.
38. Oshima Y, Ohji M, Tano Y. Pars plana vitrectomy with peripheral retinotomy after injection of preoperative intravitreal tissue plasminogen activator: a modified procedure to drain massive subretinal haemorrhage. Br J Ophthalmol 2007;91:193–198.
39. Meyer CH, Scholl HP, Eter N, et al. Combined treatment of acute subretinal haemorrhages with intravitreal recombined tissue plasminogen activator, expansile gas and bevacizumab: a retrospective pilot study. Acta Ophthalmol 2008;86:490–494.
40. Jonas JB, Söfker A, Degenring R. Intravitreal triamcinolone acetonide as an additional tool in pars plana vitrectomy for proliferative diabetic retinopathy. Eur J Ophthalmol 2003;13:468–473.
41. Cheema RA, Peyman GA, Fang T, et al. Triamcinolone acetonide as an adjuvant in the surgical treatment of retinal detachment with proliferative vitreoretinopathy. Ophthalmic Surg Lasers Imaging 2007;38:365–370.
42. Ishikawa K, Honda S, Tsukahara Y, et al. Preferable use of intravitreal bevacizumab as a pretreatment of vitrectomy for severe proliferative diabetic retinopathy. Eye 2009;23:108–111.
43. Mason 3rd JO, Nixon PA, White MF. Intravitreal injection of bevacizumab (Avastin) as adjunctive treatment of proliferative diabetic retinopathy. Am J Ophthalmol 2006;142:685–688.
44. Rizzo S, Genovesi-Ebert F, Di Bartolo E, et al. Injection of intravitreal bevacizumab (Avastin) as a preoperative adjunct before vitrectomy surgery in the treatment of severe proliferative diabetic retinopathy (PDR). Graefes Arch Clin Exp Ophthalmol 2008;246:837–842.
45. Koch F, Scholtz S, Singh P, et al. Combined intravitreal therapy for age-related macular disease. Klin Monatsbl Augenheilkd. 2008 Dec;225(12):1003–1008.
46. Arevalo JF, Maia M, Flynn Jr HW, et al. Tractional retinal detachment following intravitreal bevacizumab (Avastin) in patients with severe proliferative diabetic retinopathy. Br J Ophthalmol 2008;92:213–216.
47. Rodrigues EB, Meyer CH, Maia M, et al. Vital dyes for chromovitrectomy. Curr Opin Ophthalmol 2007;18:179–187.
48. Jackson TL. Vital staining and retinal detachment surgery. Dev Ophthalmol 2008;42:126–140.

CHAPTER 11

Routes for drug delivery: topical, transscleral, suprachoroidal, and intravitreal gas-phase nanoparticles

Timothy W. Olsen, MD

INTRODUCTION

Targeted drug delivery to the retina is an active area of research, presently under intense investigation. Multiple routes and various methods, devices, and formulations of both pharmaceutical agents and biologics are being investigated. The goal of this research is to provide local drug therapy to the retina, a tissue that is very small, estimated to be 200 µm thick.[1] Gaining access for drug delivery to the retina, given certain anatomical constraints, is challenging. However, if a method for local delivery is achieved for a given condition, therapy to such a small tissue will require extremely small doses relative to the dose that would be required for systemic therapy. Local therapy will minimize systemic drug levels and limit potential systemic toxicity.

Testing local tissue levels with various drug delivery devices and methodologies in humans is not usually possible. The most representative pharmacokinetic human data is obtained by collecting either aqueous or vitreous samples, under strict institutional review board approval, and done in conjunction with a predetermined therapeutic intervention. Computer modeling systems that predict tissue levels in the human eye are also under investigation.[2,3] However, with limited data on tissue barriers, choroidal blood flow, aqueous diffusion kinetics, orbital blood flow, vitreous kinetics and liquefaction, the reliability of determining tissue levels in humans is limited. As more accurate data is acquired, better parameters may be utilized for more sophisticated modeling.

The best possible method to understand the pharmacokinetics of drug delivery to the retina is through carefully designed studies using appropriate animal models. Even using the best possible model, human disease states, such as age-related macular degeneration (AMD) or retinitis pigmentosa (RP) may alter pharmacokinetics in unpredictable ways. Using the most appropriate animal model to study a given therapeutic agent is important. For example, using a rabbit model to study the pharmacokinetics of an intravitreal injection used to treat endophthalmitis is a reasonable approach. On the other hand, using a mouse or rat model to determine topical delivery for a chronic retinal disorder is less optimal. While such a model system may provide an answer to therapeutic efficacy, the pharmacokinetics are much too disparate from the human condition to apply directly to the clinical arena. Simple principles of pharmacokinetics, such as diffusion, variations in diffusional barriers, aqueous kinetics, vitreous liquefaction, and other factors become critical in predicting therapeutic responses to local delivery.

Recent advances in pharmacotherapeutic options for treating disorders of the posterior pole increase the need for effective methods of delivery. Examples of agents that may be useful in treating retinal and optic nerve disorders include anti-vascular endothelial growth factor (anti-VEGF) agents,[4–7] neuroprotectants,[8–10] antioxidants,[11] corticosteroids,[12–14] and other specific biologic agents (e.g., ciliary neurotrophic factor[15–17]).

HISTORY

Topical medications have been available for many years, and represent the mainstay of pharmacotherapy to the eye (Figure 11.1), particularly anterior-segment structures, such as the cornea, conjunctiva, anterior chamber, iris, and ciliary body. However, diffusional barriers limit the ability of topical agents to achieve therapeutic levels to the posterior pole, optic nerve, and retina. The primary barriers for topical drug delivery to the retina include the corneal and conjunctival epithelium,[18] diffusion through the cornea and scleral stroma,[18,19] corneal endothelial barriers,[20] and variations in diffusion from aqueous flow, choroidal blood flow,[21] conjunctival blood flow, and liquefaction of the vitreous. Key variables, such as scleral thickness and surface area, have been documented in humans as well as large-animal models to help in translational studies of pharmacokinetics with direct correlation to the human condition.[19,22,23] Effects from the lens, the internal limiting membrane of the retina, and the blood–retinal barrier also play an important role in pharmacokinetics. Some of the most important work in the investigation of pharmacokinetics of drug delivery was derived from physiologists studying aqueous pathways. For example, pioneering ocular physiologists such as Irving Fatt[24] and Anders Bill,[25] in their studies of uveoscleral outflow facility, originated important principles of transscleral drug delivery (TSDD) that we use today. Essentially TSDD physiology follows pathways identified in uveoscleral outflow studies, in a reverse direction.[26,27]

KEY CONCEPTS

Development and design of drug delivery systems and methodologies need to fit the intended disease. For example, an acute disease process with a short duration is best treated with a pulsed-dose delivery system. Endophthalmitis is an acute disease, requiring a high dose of antibiotic that can be administered with a single intravitreal injection of a therapeutic antibiotic. On the other hand, treating a chronic disease such as glaucoma or atrophic (dry) AMD with a direct intravitreal injection may not be practical, especially given the limited duration of an injection and the need for repeat injections. Exudative (wet) AMD is a subacute phase of a chronic disease and has been treated very effectively with repeated intravitreal injections. However, multiple injections have limitations, including patient tolerability, inconvenience, safety concerns, peak-trough pharmacokinetics, as well as expense. Therefore, treatment of chronic disease or even prolonged subacute disease may be best addressed with a long-acting sustained delivery system or improved drug formulation.

Some concepts that relate to the profile of an ideal delivery system include: (1) sustained and predictable delivery; (2) safety of the device or methodology for the ocular tissues; (3) rechargeable, readily replaceable or regenerative capacity; (4) removable; and (5) compatible with normal visual function. Many systems optimize certain aspects of the ideal system. Matching the delivery system with the underlying disease process is important.

ANIMAL MODELS

Various animal model systems for studying drug delivery to the retina have been studied, each with its own advantages and disadvantages.

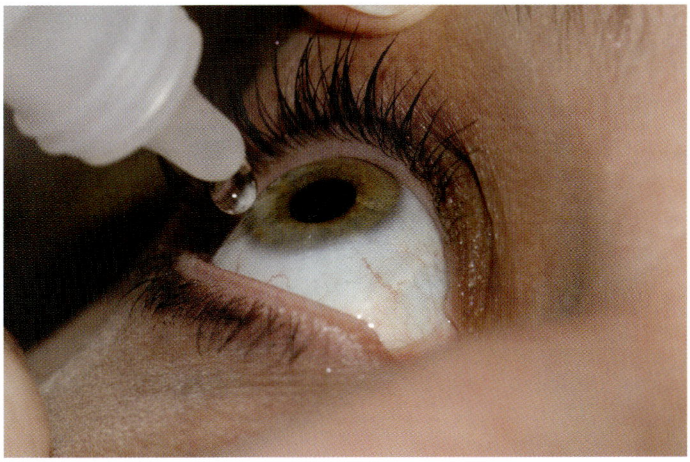

Figure 11.1 Eye drops demonstrated as a primary route for ocular drug delivery. (Courtesy of Robert Myles, CRA.)

Small-animal model systems, such as the mouse or rat, have the unique advantage of a well-defined genotype with defined disease processes. These small animals are also less expensive and easier to maintain. While small animals are ideal for studying a drug's role in the disease, the pharmacokinetics of such small eyes is quite different from those of larger animals. Since the thickness of the sclera, distance for diffusion, and vitreous and lens dimensions are very different from in humans, interpreting the pharmacokinetics from small-animal studies directly to humans is limited.

Larger animals that are commonly employed to study pharmacokinetics in preclinical human studies include the rabbit, primate, pig, cat, or dog. These animal models give a more accurate representation of drug delivery pharmacokinetics that would apply to delivery in the human eye. The rabbit model is commonly employed for such studies. Rabbits are less expensive, easy to handle, and have a relatively large eye. Limitations with the rabbit model include thinner sclera than in humans, a larger lens that alters vitreous diffusional kinetics compared to humans, absence of a macula, and a merangiotic retinal vasculature (essentially an avascular retina).[28]

The pig eye is slightly smaller than a human eye, but has some unique advantages that directly apply to the human eye. For example, pigs have a scleral thickness that is very similar to that in humans.[23] The pig also has a holangiotic retina (vascular pattern very similar to humans), a cone-dense region (area centralis) simulating a macula, a smaller lens than the rabbit, and retinal pigment epithelium with choroid very similar to that in humans.[29] The disadvantage is that pigs are more expensive and more difficult to handle in a lab setting than smaller animals.

Nonhuman primates seem to be the most ideal model system of pharmacokinetics because they have a true macula and anatomy nearly identical to humans; however, there are significant limitations. First, there are the ethical concerns[30] of using large-scale nonhuman primate studies for pharmacokinetics requiring significant animal sacrifice in order to obtain tissue levels. Second, the nonhuman primate sclera is significantly thinner than that in humans.[31] And finally, nonhuman primates are very expensive, require special housing and handling, and are more dangerous to handle.

DRUG DELIVERY MODALITIES

TOPICAL DRUG DELIVERY

The primary barrier to topical drug delivery targeting the retina is the diffusional distance that the drug must overcome in order to achieve therapeutic levels in the retina. The classic example of topical drug delivery for retinal disease is for the treatment of cystoid macular edema (CME). While the center of the macula is the target area of the disease, many times the origin of the pathology is from anterior-segment tissues. Postcataract CME results from inflammation originating during the postoperative period. Inflammatory mediators released from the anterior segment diffuse posteriorly to the fovea, leading to edema and photoreceptor dysfunction.[32] It seems natural that topical therapy, with advantageous pharmacokinetics to treat anterior-segment tissues such as the iris and ciliary body, will lead to resolution of the CME. Therefore, treatment of the CME is achieved primarily by treatment of anterior-segment tissues (indirectly), rather than treating the macula directly. Topical delivery of medications to treat retinal disease could also be effective when the amount of drug required is extremely low. Very potent agents may not require high tissue levels; therefore, the topical route could conceivably be utilized for direct therapy to the macula or optic nerve. Cautious interpretation of data should be considered when examining results of topical therapies for treating macular disease. If pharmacokinetics are done in small-animal models, or in models such as the rabbit with the aforementioned limitations, the data may not be directly applicable to the human eye. Specifically, the thinner sclera and variations in blood flow patterns, globe size, and other parameters of the animal models should be interpreted cautiously to the human condition. Data may be misleading for the translation to posterior-segment tissues of the human eye.

The corneal epithelium, as well as the endothelium, serves as a significant barrier for drug diffusion into the anterior chamber.[33] Some of the epithelial barrier is broken down partially by the preservative benzalkonium chloride, thereby providing increased penetration of various compounds through the epithelium.[34,35] Drugs may be metabolized or even selectively transported[36,37] by cellular mechanisms that affect the overall penetration of drugs via the topical route.[38] The degree of lipophilicity of an agent will also affect the penetration through the corneal epithelium.[39] The crystalline lens, or in some cases, a pseudophakic lens, also serves as a physical barrier for the bulk diffusion of drugs applied topically, for delivery to the retina.

TRANSSCLERAL DRUG DELIVERY

TSDD offers a relatively safe route for posterior-segment drug delivery.[19] This route avoids intraocular manipulation and takes advantage of simple diffusion kinetics through the sclera. Previous work on human scleral permeability[19] suggests that smaller, hydrophilic molecules delivered in thinner equatorial regions of the eye[22] may be the optimal choice for transscleral systems. Adequate quantitative delivery of macromolecules or less hydrophilic compounds may be limited by suboptimal drug diffusion kinetics to target tissue. Such parameters may limit the clinical feasibility of the transscleral route for such molecules.

The kinetics of TSDD have been defined *in vitro*, and proposed to offer a safe route for delivery, namely by avoiding intraocular manipulation and taking advantage of simple diffusion kinetics through the sclera.[19] Data suggest that smaller, more hydrophilic molecules delivered in thinner equatorial regions of the eye[22] may be optimal choices for transscleral systems. Key anatomic scleral parameters have been defined for both the human and the pig model of transscleral delivery.[22,23] An important limitation of TSDD may be adequate quantitative delivery of macromolecules or less hydrophilic compounds due to suboptimal drug diffusion kinetics to the target tissue. These physical restrictions limit the feasibility of the transscleral route for select macromolecules. Drug potency of the specific pharmacologic or biologic agent is an important factor for the relevance of the particular methodology of delivery for a given disease process.

There are some unique advantages of TSDD. First, the sclera is similar to the cornea, without the epithelial or endothelial barriers (assuming one delivers a drug under the conjunctival epithelium). The sclera may serve as a barrier for infectious agents to gain access to the inner coats of the eye as endophthalmitis remains a rare, but potentially dangerous, potential complication of intravitreal injections.[40] In addition, the sclera may also serve as a repository of drug as well as dispersing the drug in various directions by lateral diffusion.[41] Similar to the cornea, the size of the molecule as well as the lipophilicity will also affect overall permeability using the transscleral route.[42,43,44]

SUPRACHOROIDAL DRUG DELIVERY

The suprachoroidal space (SCS) is a potential space (Figure 11.2), limited anteriorly in the region of the scleral spur, and posteriorly by the transscleral connections of the short posterior ciliary vessels to the choroid.[45] There are focal, equatorial connections at the vortex ampulae where venous blood exits the globe. Krohn and Bertelsen have examined the detailed anatomy of the SCS[46,47] and drainage channels from this space.[48] Ophthalmologists and clinicians are well aware of the SCS. The clinical appearance of a choroidal detachment, either serous (fluid-filled) or hemorrhagic (blood-filled), results from a variety of pathologic states, especially following trauma, surgery, and hypotony.

Taking advantage of this space for pharmacologic drug delivery has recently been explored.[49,50] Initial studies used smooth metal cannulae to access the SCS while more recent technologies have been developed to optimize the safety and visualization. Disruption of the retinal pigment epithelium may occur with aggressive intervention in the SCS. Therefore, utilization of small, flexible, illuminated cannulae may offer a safer and more effective methodology to access the SCS for drug delivery in humans[50] (Figure 11.3).

The pharmacokinetics of the SCS are unique. Basically, suprachoroidal drug delivery could be considered an extension of TSDD, with the choroid and retina as the target tissue. Directly accessing the SCS using various methodologies allows for higher therapeutic levels of pharmacologic agents at the level of the outer choroid. Larger molecules, such as antibodies, proteins, and perhaps lipophilic molecules, would not be required to diffuse across the sclera in order to target uveal tissue. The target tissues, namely the choroid and neurosensory retina, receive higher levels than would be expected from an external transscleral system. Drug levels from the depot site in the SCS would decline based on the diffusional pathways as represented from the drug diffusion schematic (Figure 11.4). Drug would also leave the site through choroidal blood flow, aqueous diffusion pathways (uveoscleral diffusional pathways), and into the orbit and surrounding vasculature. Local drug metabolism may also play a role, with drug and drug breakdown products eventually diffusing into the systemic circulation. Theoretically, some drug could also diffuse into the optic nerve and nerve sheath tissues into the central nervous system.[51]

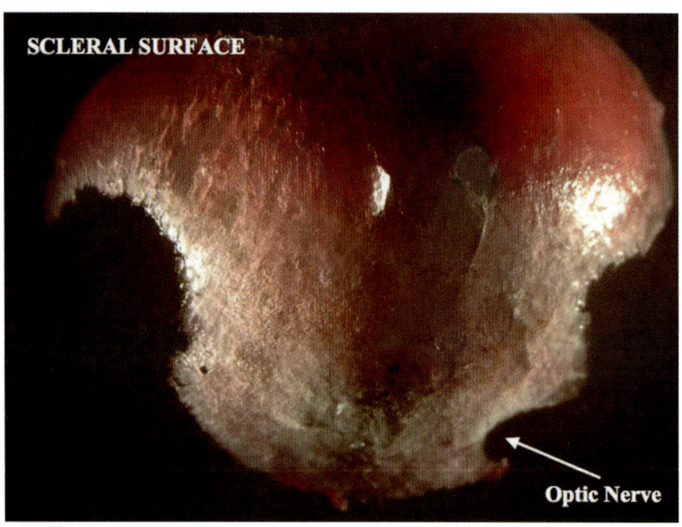

Figure 11.2 A cast of the suprachoroidal space, taken from a pig eye. The cast was formed by injection into the suprachoroidal space (SCS), and digesting away the tissue. Scleral surface designates the outer surface of the SCS. The gap in the cast is the site where the optic nerve exits the globe.

The volume of the SCS, as a potential space for drug delivery, is relatively large, and somewhat expandable (Figure 11.5). Obviously, the space could not expand to the point of interference with visual function, as may occur in pathologic states. Clinicians are well aware of the risk associated with this space, namely the development of acute suprachoroidal hemorrhage, a highly undesirable potential complication of

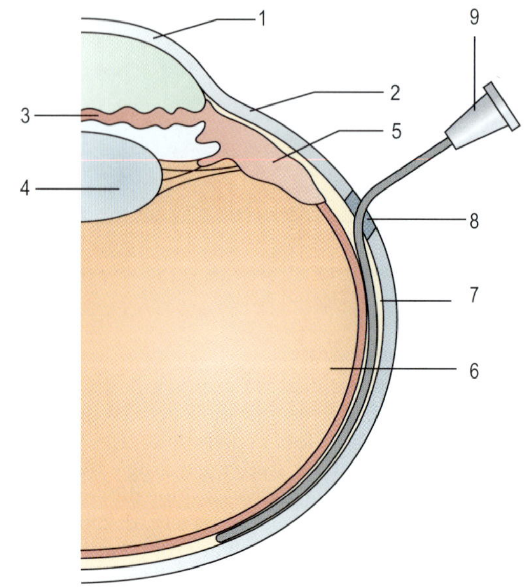

Figure 11.3 Schematic representation of the microcannula (9) entering the suprachoroidal space (7) through a small anterior sclerotomy (8), and extending toward posterior-segment tissues. Other labeled structures include the cornea (1), sclera (2), iris (3), lens (4), ciliary body (5), and retina (6). (Reproduced from Am J Ophthalmol 2006;142:777–787 by permission of Elsevier.)

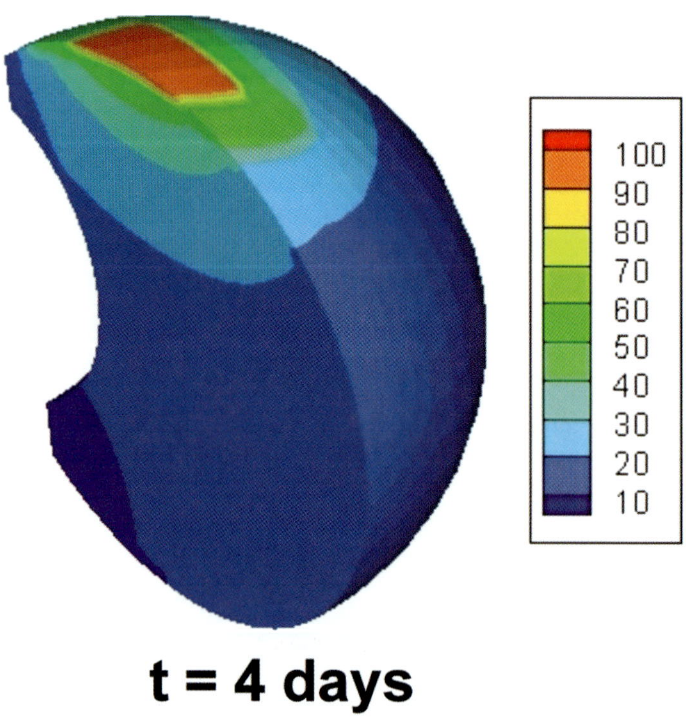

Figure 11.4 An example of a drug diffusion modeling schematic, demonstrating drug distribution from a drug patch at postapplication day 4. (Courtesy of Victor Barocas PhD and Ram Balachandran, University of Minnesota.)

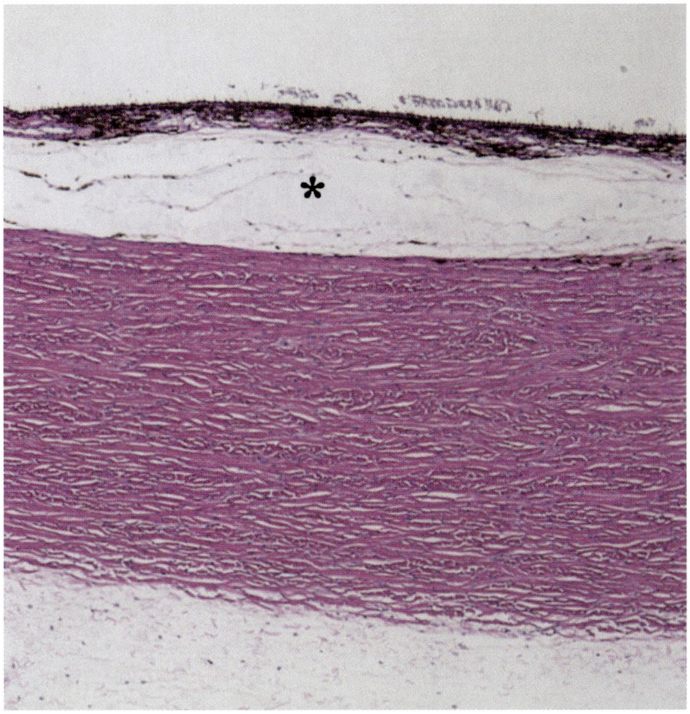

Figure 11.5 Histology of the suprachoroidal space (SCS) in a pig eye. The asterisk (*) indicates the site of separation between the inner sclera and the choroid. *In vivo*, this space is a potential space. In this specimen, the space has been created by injection of Healon into the SCS.

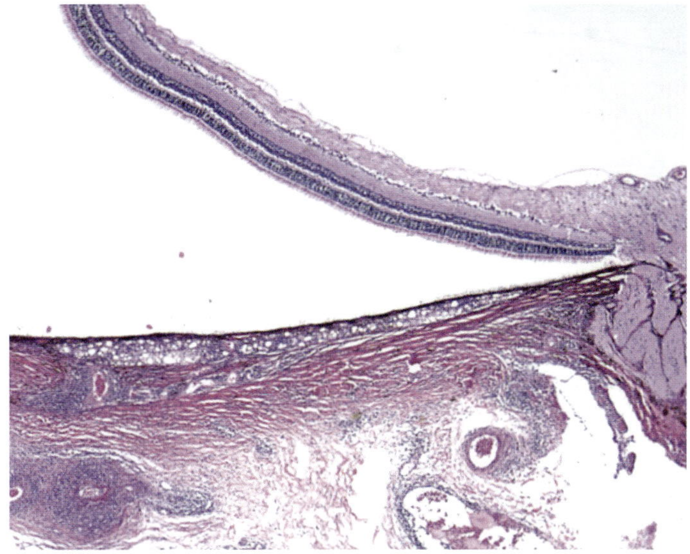

Figure 11.6 Histology demonstrating areas of the posterior pole of an eye in which the cannulae impacted the optic nerve region. Note that there are inflammatory cells and vacuolization of the choroidal tissue, plus inflammation around the vessels outside the globe.

delivery into the SCS. In order to minimize such complications, accessing the space in a delicate and deliberate manner is essential. All efforts to minimize stress and tension in the tissues of the SCS in order to avoid vessel rupture would be important during surgical maneuvers in this space. Indeed, forceful impact of a cannulae into the optic nerve in the pig model has been shown to result in local inflammation (Figure 11.6).[50] In these studies, successful cannulization of the SCS using a novel microcannula technology for delivery of drug to the SCS has been demonstrated to be safe in the pig model with excellent, sustained local tissue levels and low systemic levels (triamcinolone). The technique has been shown to be relatively safe with minimal impact on the choroidal and retinal blood flow as documented with the high-speed confocal scanning laser ophthalmoscopic (cSLO) video angiography, fundus exam, and using wide-field fundus photography, along with short- and long-term histopathologic tissue analysis.

Drug delivery via the SCS using the microcannula technology and methodology may be useful for the treatment of posterior-segment disease, including macular, optic nerve, or even panretinal disease. Proper drug selection and target disease will be critical to determine the clinical role for this route of delivery. Further clinical studies will be necessary to define the role of this technology further in the management of specific posterior-segment disease. Currently, human studies are under way to assess the safety and efficacy in human disease states.

INTRAVITREAL GAS-PHASE NANOPARTICLE DRUG DELIVERY

Intraocular air or gas is commonly deployed in vitreoretinal surgery, due largely to its mechanical properties. Essentially, the intraocular gas bubble serves as a mechanical aid that will tamponade the neurosensory retina, holding the retina in place during reattachment surgery.[52] The surface tension of the gas bubble that surrounds a retinal break may prevent the fluid from disrupting the development of a strong chorioretinal adhesion.[53] By generating nanoparticles and suspending these particles in the gas phase of the intraocular tamponade, a novel methodology for drug delivery is possible.[54] An example of a target disease is proliferative vitreoretinopathy (PVR); however, there are numerous potential applications of this technology. Use of neuroprotectants during retinal detachment surgery, antiproliferative agents to inhibit PVR, antiviral agents or antibiotics for infectious retinitis, or even pneumatic techniques for localized delivery, is also possible.

PVR is the leading cause of retinal redetachment, and requires aggressive surgical means to correct the anatomic abnormalities.[55–60] Some have postulated that mechanical intervention (surgical treatment) will be required until we can control the cellular healing processes with pharmacological intervention.[56] To date, limited therapeutic options are available to modify the healing response that occurs following retinal detachment.

Pharmacologic management of retinal disorders, such as PVR, requires a measured and reliable methodology of drug delivery that will allow for better management of the healing response. Utilizing drug delivery in the gas phase of surgery, through delivery of specific agents, creates a unique opportunity for addressing the healing response at a critical stage. Intravitreal injections of drugs are becoming one of the more common routes of delivery in the clinical setting, especially with the advent of anti-VEGF agents. Delivering an intraocular gas with suspended nanoparticle drug could combine the mechanical aspects of gas tamponade with therapeutic effects of antiproliferative agents for use in pneumatic retinopexy. These approaches require knowledge of the pharmacokinetics and quantifiable delivery amounts. Intravitreal gas-phase nanoparticle technology would also have applications for treating other retinal disorders during vitrectomy, including infectious retinitis, proliferative disorders such as diabetic retinopathy with traction detachments, and immune modulation such as the treatment of uveitis, or even CME by using aerosolized corticosteroids.

Quantification of the aerosol concentration of a given drug, expressed as the mass of drug in a given volume of air as well as the total mass, represents a key parameter for each possible therapeutic agent. Characterization of these parameters allows for more predictable delivery of drug during the gas delivery phase. Other methodologies are available for the fluid phase of delivery and include intravitreal injec-

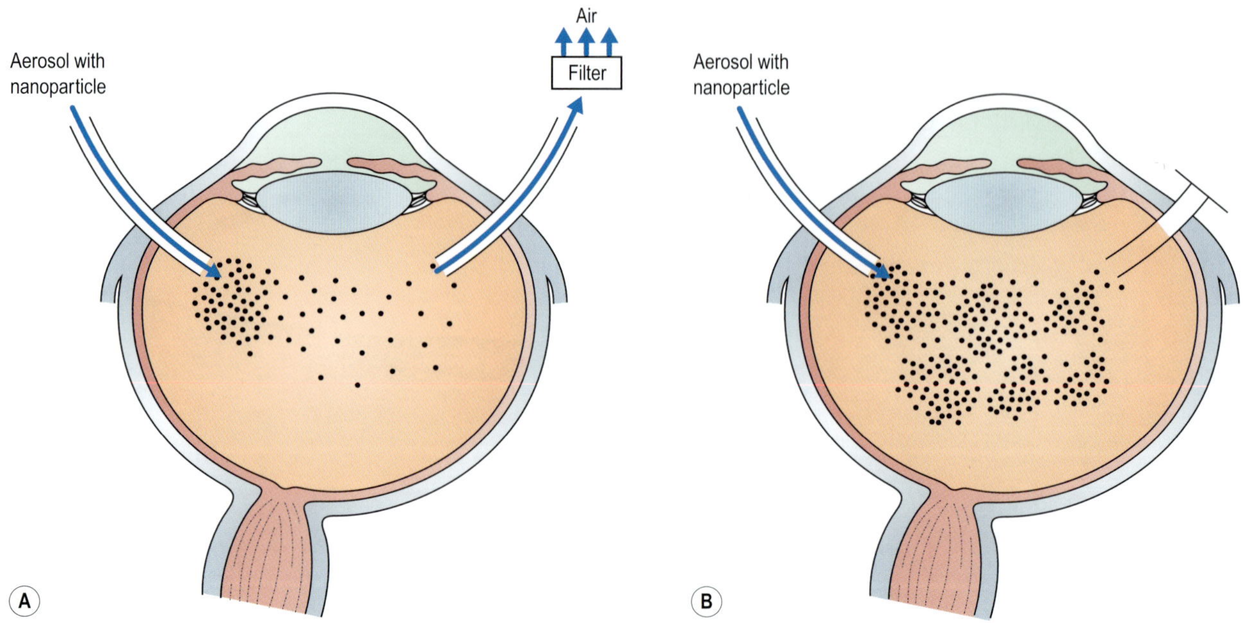

Figure 11.7 Schematic representation of delivering aerosolized nanoparticles in the gas phase of vitrectomy. (A) The flow-through method demonstrates a continuous flow of gas and drug with the exit site filtering out drug before entering room air. (B) The single-fill method shows the globe with aerosolized drug; once full, the sclerotomies are closed. (Reproduced from Zhang G, Feng X, Wabner K, et al. Intraocular nanoparticle drug delivery: a pilot study using an aerosol during pars plana vitrectomy. Invest Ophthalmol Vis Sci 2007;48:5243–5249, with permission; original adapted from National Eye Institute, NEA05.)

tions, implants, biodegradable polymers, or pellets. However, the pharmacokinetics from these methods are unpredictable in gas-filled eyes.

A methodology and pharmacokinetics for the delivery of aerosolized nanoparticles using a tracer dye in the pig model have been characterized.[54] There are two distinct methods of aerosol drug deposition (Figure 11.7). First, the flow-through system utilizes an aerosolized drug passing through the eye continuously with entry through the primary sclerotomy and exit through the secondary sclerotomy. The exit site has a filter to prevent drug from entering room air. This method provides maximal drug deposition because it maintains a higher concentration of intraocular drug to drive diffusion into the retinal tissue. The efficiency of delivery is low, because much of the drug will exit the eye, being filtered at the sclerotomy.

The second method of aerosol delivery is the single-fill method. This involves simply filling the eye or simply injecting the eye with a known concentration of drug, and allowing diffusion of the aerosolized nanoparticle suspension into the retinal tissue. This method results in lower tissue levels because the concentration of the drug within the gas decreases as it diffuses into the retinal tissue. The efficiency of delivery is higher because the drug is essentially trapped in the eye, and will eventually reach a steady state with the tissues.

There are three main mechanisms by which aerosol particles can deposit at the retinal surface: inertial impaction, sedimentation and diffusion.[61] Inertial impaction and sedimentation are more efficient with larger particle size. Diffusion is more efficient with smaller particle size. Both of these principles of transfer lead to a nonuniform deposition pattern. In experimental studies using either the flow-through or single-fill modes of delivery, there does not appear to be a difference in the mass of drug on either the inflow or outflow sides of the retina at any time point.[54] Additionally, evidence suggests that there is greater diffusion into the uveal tissues than into the lens, presumably because the lens is less metabolically active and lacks blood flow. Drug delivery in the gas phase of vitrectomy may increase cataractogenesis, especially dependent upon the pharmacologic agent delivered. Overall, drug would be more selectively deposited into the neurosensory retina and uveal tissues. Logically, increased diffusion of drug removal from the uveal tissue also occurs, as well as diffusion into the sclera and orbital tissues. Time dependence of drug distribution is also important in delivery efficiency. The use of larger molecules or peptides will likely slow the known diffusional pharmacokinetics.

In order to optimize the use of these two methodologies for drug transfer of aerosolized nanoparticles, it becomes clear that each method has unique advantages. The single-fill delivery mode creates a steady state in which the rate of mass deposition in the uvea becomes smaller than the rate of mass transfer from the retina and choroid to the sclera. The use of the single-fill method would be used primarily during pneumatic retinopexy, gas-phase intravitreal injections, or at the conclusion of vitreous surgery. During surgery, the single-fill method would supplement higher tissue drug levels achieved with the flow-through method.

Deposition efficiency is the percentage of drug deposited relative to the total drug available. In the flow-through mode, the amount of drug diffusing into the target tissue increases rapidly because there is a constantly high concentration of drug within the gas phase. Realistic application of this methodology to optimize delivery would utilize the less-efficient flow-through method to get higher tissue levels and then leaving the eye "filled" with aerosolized nanoparticles gas for continued local delivery after the eye is closed. Other technical options include an increase in the particle number concentration that could enhance the delivery capability or a reduced particle size.

Calculating the pharmacokinetics for the delivery of drugs to the retina and choroid in the gas phase may be achieved through modeling systems. For the flow-through method, a model of aerosol particles of uniform concentration, with the assumption that the deposition occurs by diffusion through a boundary layer (stagnant layer), may be assumed. The rate of mass deposition, $\Delta m/\Delta t$, would be given by:

$$\Delta m/\Delta t = DAC/$$

where D is the diffusion coefficient of the aerosol particle, A is the surface area of the chamber, C is the aerosol concentration, and h is the boundary layer thickness.

For single-fill delivery, two models estimate the deposited mass.[54] A pure diffusion model is mathematically represented. The diffusion model has an expression for the mass deposited with time that provides a solution for the diffusion equation with spherical coordinates:

$$M(t) = M_0\left[1 - \frac{6}{\pi^2}\sum_{n=1}^{\infty}\frac{1}{n^2}\exp\left(-\frac{\pi^2 n^2}{R^2}Dt\right)\right]$$

Herein, M_o is the initial mass of aerosol in a hollow sphere of radius (R), $M(t)$ is the mass deposited in time, t (time), and D is the molecular diffusivity.

For deposition by settling, stirred settling seems applicable with an exponential decay in the aerosol concentration. Deposition can be represented as:

$$M(t) = M_0[1 - \exp(-\beta t)]$$

Herein, the deposition rate coefficient, β, is expressed as the terminal velocity of sedimentation divided by the length scale of the enclosure. For the spherical geometry, the following expression for β applies:

$$\beta = \frac{3v}{4R}$$

In this equation, v denotes the settling velocity. The corresponding deposition represents a much faster rate than that observed in animal systems. The stirred settling model lacks an adequate representation of the movement of the gas phase. As particles move downward, they pull the surrounding gas down and a compensatory upward drift of gas fills the void, inhibiting particle deposition. At higher particle concentration, this effect is more significant.

The aerosol delivery of drug nanoparticles represents a novel method to deliver therapeutic agents to the posterior segment during an injection in the clinic or during vitrectomy surgery in the operating room. Drug deposition occurs primarily by diffusion. Careful design of the aerosol generation and delivery parameters (aerosol particle size, delivery mode, and exposure time) and the formulation composition could lead to controlled and sustained release of the therapeutic agents with modification of the wound-healing response. Aerosolized delivery of drugs to the posterior segment is a novel methodology for pharmacologic management of posterior-segment disorders and takes advantage of the gas phase of vitrectomy to treat conditions such as PVR following retinal detachment in high-risk eyes. Additional uses could include antibiotics for endophthalmitis, antiviral for infectious retinitis, antiangiogenic compounds for proliferative disorders, or immunomodulation.

FUTURE DIRECTIONS AND TECHNOLOGIES

Systems will continue to evolve to deliver drugs to the posterior segment. The marketplace will likely drive innovative methods of local drug delivery that will optimize the local tissue effects, minimize systemic risks, and optimize safety. As new agents are developed for targeted disease, such as gene therapy for Leber's congenital amaurosis, more sophisticated delivery systems will be incorporated into our practices.

SUMMARY AND KEY POINTS

Investigation of the pharmacokinetics of drug delivery to the posterior segment of the eye remains a very active area of ophthalmic research. Our clinical interventions as we enter the pharmacologic era of treating posterior-segment disease will continue to change. Significant improvements in visual outcomes and lifestyles for our patients will continue to drive this active area of research. The important points to consider in choosing or developing drug delivery systems include the following: match the delivery modality with the disease process (acute disease, chronic disease, subacute disease); optimize safety; avoid interference with the visual system; allow for replacement or recharging the system; ensure safe and simple removal, and keep the system inexpensive.

ACKNOWLEDGMENT

This study was supported by an unrestricted grant from Research to Prevent Blindness (RPB).

REFERENCES

1. Masland RH. The functional architecture of the retina. Sci Am 1986;255:102–111.
2. Stay MS, Xu J, Randolph TW, et al. Computer simulation of convective and diffusive transport of controlled-release drugs in the vitreous humor. Pharm Res 2003;20:96–102.
3. Xu J, Heys JJ, Barocas VH, et al. Permeability and diffusion in vitreous humor: implications for drug delivery. Pharm Res 2000;17:664–669.
4. Avery RL, Pieramici DJ, Rabena MD, et al. Intravitreal bevacizumab (Avastin) for neovascular age-related macular degeneration. Ophthalmology 2006;113:363–372 e5.
5. Brown DM, Kaiser PK, Michels M, et al. Ranibizumab versus verteporfin for neovascular age-related macular degeneration. N Engl J Med 2006;355:1432–1444.
6. Gragoudas ES, Adamis AP, Cunningham ET Jr, et al. Pegaptanib for neovascular age-related macular degeneration. N Engl J Med 2004;351:2805–2816.
7. Rosenfeld PJ, Brown DM, Heier JS, et al. Ranibizumab for neovascular age-related macular degeneration. N Engl J Med 2006;355:1419–1431.
8. Aktas Z, Gurelik G, Akyurek N, et al. Neuroprotective effect of topically applied brimonidine tartrate 0.2% in endothelin-1-induced optic nerve ischaemia model. Clin Exp Ophthalmol 2007;35:527–534.
9. Chidlow G, Wood JP, Casson RJ. Pharmacological neuroprotection for glaucoma. Drugs 2007;67:725–759.
10. Weinreb RN. Glaucoma neuroprotection: What is it? Why is it needed? Can J Ophthalmol 2007;42:396–398.
11. A randomized, placebo-controlled, clinical trial of high-dose supplementation with vitamins C and E, beta carotene, and zinc for age-related macular degeneration and vision loss: AREDS report no. 8. Arch Ophthalmol 2001;119:1417–1436.
12. Bhisitkul RB, Winn BJ, Lee OT, et al. Neuroprotective effect of intravitreal triamcinolone acetonide against photoreceptor apoptosis in a rabbit model of subretinal hemorrhage. Invest Ophthalmol Vis Sci 2008;49: 4071–4077.
13. Challa JK, Gillies MC, Penfold PL, et al. Exudative macular degeneration and intravitreal triamcinolone: 18 month follow up. Aust N Z J Ophthalmol 1998;26:277–281.
14. Danis RP, Ciulla TA, Pratt LM, et al. Intravitreal triamcinolone acetonide in exudative age-related macular degeneration. Retina 2000;20:244–250.
15. Chong NH, Alexander RA, Waters L, et al. Repeated injections of a ciliary neurotrophic factor analogue leading to long-term photoreceptor survival in hereditary retinal degeneration. Invest Ophthalmol Vis Sci 1999;40: 1298–1305.
16. Sieving PA, Caruso RC, Tao W, et al. Ciliary neurotrophic factor (CNTF) for human retinal degeneration: phase I trial of CNTF delivered by encapsulated cell intraocular implants. Proc Natl Acad Sci USA 2006;103:3896–3901.
17. Tao W, Wen R, Goddard MB, et al. Encapsulated cell-based delivery of CNTF reduces photoreceptor degeneration in animal models of retinitis pigmentosa. Invest Ophthalmol Vis Sci 2002;43:3292–3298.
18. Grass GM, Robinson JR. Mechanisms of corneal drug penetration. I: *In vivo* and *in vitro* kinetics. J Pharm Sci 1988;77:3–14.
19. Olsen TW, Edelhauser HF, Lim JI, et al. Human scleral permeability. Effects of age, cryotherapy, transscleral diode laser, and surgical thinning. Invest Ophthalmol Vis Sci 1995;36:1893–1903.
20. Stiemke MM, McCartney MD, Cantu-Crouch D, et al. Maturation of the corneal endothelial tight junction. Invest Ophthalmol Vis Sci 1991;32: 2757–2765.
21. Robinson MR, Lee SS, Kim H, et al. A rabbit model for assessing the ocular barriers to the transscleral delivery of triamcinolone acetonide. Exp Eye Res 2006;82:479–487.
22. Olsen TW, Aaberg SY, Geroski DH, et al. Human sclera: thickness and surface area. Am J Ophthalmol 1998;125:237–241.
23. Olsen TW, Sanderson S, Feng X, et al. Porcine sclera: thickness and surface area. Invest Ophthalmol Vis Sci 2002;43:2529–2532.
24. Fatt I, Hedbys BO. Flow of water in the sclera. Exp Eye Res 1970;10: 243–249.
25. Bill A. Uveoscleral drainage of aqueous humor: physiology and pharmacology. Prog Clin Biol Res 1989;312:417–427.
26. Kim TW, Lindsey JD, Aihara M, et al. Intraocular distribution of 70-kDa dextran after subconjunctival injection in mice. Invest Ophthalmol Vis Sci 2002;43:1809–1816.
27. Pederson JE, Toris CB. Uveoscleral outflow: diffusion or flow? Invest Ophthalmol Vis Sci 1987;28:1022–1024.

28. Prince JH DC, Eglitis I, Ruskell GL. The Rabbit. Anatomy and Histology of the Eye and Orbit in Domestic Animals. Springfield, IL: Charles C Thomas; 1960. p. 268.
29. Prince JH DC, Eglitis I, Ruskell GL. The Pig. Anatomy and Histology of the Eye and Orbit in Domestic Animals. Springfield, IL: Charles C Thomas; 1960. p. 210–233.
30. Bhogal N, Hudson M, Balls M, et al. The use of non-human primates in biological and medical research: evidence submitted by FRAME to the Academy of Medical Sciences/Medical Research Council/Royal Society/ Wellcome Trust Working Group. Altern Lab Anim 2005;33:519–527.
31. Funata M, Tokoro T. Scleral change in experimentally myopic monkeys. Graefes Arch Clin Exp Ophthalmol 1990;228:174–179.
32. Miyake K, Ibaraki N. Prostaglandins and cystoid macular edema. Surv Ophthalmol 2002;47(Suppl. 1):S203–S218.
33. Yasueda S, Higashiyama M, Yamaguchi M, et al. Corneal critical barrier against the penetration of dexamethasone and lomefloxacin hydrochloride: evaluation by the activation energy for drug partition and diffusion in cornea. Drug Dev Ind Pharm 2007;33:805–811.
34. Green K, Tonjum AM. The effect of benzalkonium chloride on the electropotential of the rabbit cornea. Acta Ophthalmol (Copenh) 1975;53:348–357.
35. Nakashima M, Nakamura T, Teshima M, et al. Breakdown evaluation of corneal epithelial barrier caused by antiallergic eyedrops using an electrophysiologic method. J Ocul Pharmacol Ther 2008;24:43–51.
36. Sakanaka K, Kawazu K, Nishida K, et al. Transport of timolol and tilisolol in rabbit corneal epithelium. Biol Pharm Bull 2006;29:2143–2147.
37. Kawazu K, Midori Y, Shiono H, et al. Characterization of the carrier-mediated transport of levofloxacin, a fluoroquinolone antimicrobial agent, in rabbit cornea. J Pharm Pharmacol 1999;51:797–801.
38. Mannermaa E, Vellonen KS, Urtti A. Drug transport in corneal epithelium and blood-retina barrier: emerging role of transporters in ocular pharmacokinetics. Adv Drug Deliv Rev 2006;58:1136–1163.
39. Ashton P, Clark DS, Lee VH. A mechanistic study on the enhancement of corneal penetration of phenylephrine by flurbiprofen in the rabbit. Curr Eye Res 1992;11:85–90.
40. Karacal H, Kymes SM, Apte RS. Retrospective analysis of etiopathogenesis of all cases of endophthalmitis at a large tertiary referral center. Int Ophthalmol 2007;27:251–259.
41. Kim TW, Lindsey JD, Aihara M, et al. Intraocular distribution of 70-kDa dextran after subconjunctival injection in mice. Invest Ophthalmol Vis Sci 2002;43:1809–1816.
42. Cruysberg LP, Nuijts RM, Geroski DH, et al. *In vitro* human scleral permeability of fluorescein, dexamethasone-fluorescein, methotrexate-fluorescein and rhodamine 6G and the use of a coated coil as a new drug delivery system. J Ocul Pharmacol Ther 2002;18:559–569.
43. Olsen TW, Edelhauser HF, Lim JI, et al. Human scleral permeability. Effects of age, cryotherapy, transscleral diode laser, and surgical thinning. Invest Ophthalmol Vis Sci 1995;36:1893–1903.
44. Ambati J, Canakis CS, Miller JW, et al. Diffusion of high molecular weight compounds through sclera. Invest Ophthalmol Vis Sci 2000;41:1181–1185.
45. Guyer D, Schachat A, Green R. The choroid: structural considerations. In: Ryan S, editor. Retina, 4th edn. China: Mosby, 2006; p. 33–42.
46. Krohn J, Bertelsen T. Corrosion casts of the suprachoroidal space and uveoscleral drainage routes in the human eye. Acta Ophthalmol Scand 1997;75:32-35.
47. Krohn J, Bertelsen T. Corrosion casts of the suprachoroidal space and uveoscleral drainage routes in the pig eye. Acta Ophthalmol Scand 1997;75:28–31.
48. Krohn J, Bertelsen T. Light microscopy of uveoscleral drainage routes after gelatine injections into the suprachoroidal space. Acta Ophthalmol Scand 1998;76:521–527.
49. Einmahl S, Savoldelli M, D'Hermies F, et al. Evaluation of a novel biomaterial in the suprachoroidal space of the rabbit eye. Invest Ophthalmol Vis Sci 2002;43:1533–1539.
50. Olsen TW, Feng X, Wabner K, et al. Cannulation of the suprachoroidal space: a novel drug delivery methodology to the posterior segment. Am J Ophthalmol 2006;142:777–787.
51. Koevary SB. Pharmacokinetics of topical ocular drug delivery: potential uses for the treatment of diseases of the posterior segment and beyond. Curr Drug Metab 2003;4:213–222.
52. Laqua H. Intravitreal gas injection in the management of selected retinal detachment. Klin Monatsbl Augenheilkd 1979;175:32–39.
53. de Juan E Jr, McCuen B, Tiedeman J. Intraocular tamponade and surface tension. Surv Ophthalmol 1985;30:47–51.
54. Zhang G, Feng X, Wabner K, et al. Intraocular nanoparticle drug delivery: a pilot study using an aerosol during pars plana vitrectomy. Invest Ophthalmol Vis Sci 2007;48:5243–5249.
55. Michels RG. Surgery of retinal detachment with proliferative vitreoretinopathy. Retina 1984;4:63–83.
56. Ryan SJ. The pathophysiology of proliferative vitreoretinopathy in its management. Am J Ophthalmol 1985;100:188–193.
57. Lewis H, Aaberg TM, Abrams GW. Causes of failure after initial vitreoretinal surgery for severe proliferative vitreoretinopathy. Am J Ophthalmol 1991;111:8–14.
58. Vitrectomy with silicone oil or perfluoropropane gas in eyes with severe proliferative vitreoretinopathy: results of a randomized clinical trial. Silicone Study Report 2. Arch Ophthalmol 1992;110:780–792.
59. Hakin KN, Lavin MJ, Leaver PK. Primary vitrectomy for rhegmatogenous retinal detachment. Graefes Arch Clin Exp Ophthalmol 1993;231:344–346.
60. McCuen 2nd BW, Azen SP, Stern W, et al. Vitrectomy with silicone oil or perfluoropropane gas in eyes with severe proliferative vitreoretinopathy. Silicone Study Report 3. Retina 1993;13:279–284.
61. Hinds W. Aerosol Technology: Properties, Behavior, and Measurements of Airborne Particles. New York: John Wiley; 1982.

CHAPTER

12 Routes for drug delivery: sustained-release devices

John J. Huang, MD

INTRODUCTION

Vitreoretinal disorders have been gaining attention due to the aging population of the industrialized nations at risk of or suffering from permanent visual loss due to retinal disorders such as age-related macular degeneration (AMD), diabetic retinopathy, and retinal vein occlusion. These disorders are increasing in prevalence together with the increased life expectancy and the incidence of obesity in our population. This is fortunately paralleled by the rapid progress in the biomedical sciences of vitreoretinal disease such as antisense RNA molecules, designer corticosteroids, aptamers, and monoclonal antibodies for the treatment of neovascular AMD and diabetic retinopathy. The current treatments all require repeated intravitreal injections for the delivery of these drugs. The future for the treatment of these chronic posterior-segment conditions will ideally involve drug devices that can safely deliver localized medications at a steady level for a long duration, at 100% bioactivity or efficacy. The device can be replaced or completely biodegraded, and easily applied with other drugs for combination therapies. Currently, several different methods of sustained-release drug devices are available or under testing, including: (1) nonbiodegradable intraocular implants; (2) biodegradable intraocular implants; (3) injectable micro- and nanoparticles; (4) injectable liposomes; and (5) encapsulated cell technology (ECT).[1–5] Each of these methods has advantages and disadvantages based on the need for surgical implantation, duration of drug release, type, and size of the drug molecules (Table 12.1).

HISTORY

The first ophthalmic sustained-release drug was developed in the 1960s in the former Soviet Union. Pilocarpine and mydriatics were embedded in an acrylate co-polymer-based matrix for insertion into the conjunctival fornix. The drug insert provided a delayed release of several hours as the polymer matrix dissolved.[1] Ocusert (Alza), a sustained-release pilocarpine, was introduced in the western world in the 1970s. This insert released the drug for a week at a constant rate of 40 μg/hour through ethylene vinyl acetate membranes.[1] This was followed by Lacrisert (Merck), a sustained-release hydroxypropyl cellulose fornix-based insert for the treatment of dry-eye syndrome. These inserts did not become popular in part due to difficulties with placement of the drug polymer by the elderly population, and extrusion of the inserts. Additional innovations in the drug delivery system included drug-immersed contact lenses and ocular liposomes in the 1970s and 1980s. The early devices in sustained-release technology provided the initial concept for sustained-release ocular drug delivery. Unfortunately, vitreoretinal diseases are not amenable to treatment using the topical delivery system.

KEY CONCEPTS AND FUNDAMENTAL POINTS IN SUSTAINED-RELEASE DRUG DELIVERY

The treatment of retinal disorders has changed significantly during the past decade. Thermal laser photocoagulation therapy for the treatment of diabetic macular edema (DME) and choroidal neovascular complex has been replaced by intravitreal injections of triamcinolone acetonide, dexamethasone, pegaptanib (Macugen), bevacizumab (Avastin), and ranibizumab (Lucentis). The efficacy of these medications has brought new excitement to the field of ophthalmology and hope to patients suffering from retinal disorders. These therapies all have the major disadvantages related to complications of repeated intravitreal injections, such as: endophthalmitis, cataract formation, vitreous hemorrhage, and retinal detachment. Sustained-release technology may offer future patients less frequent dosing for chronic retinal conditions such as AMD, diabetic retinopathy, retinal vein occlusion, and even nonretinal disorders such as glaucoma.

Ocular tissues can be reached by local or systemic drug administration. The surface tissue of the eye limits the penetration of drugs to the targeted tissue. The cornea and conjunctiva epithelium is a barrier to topical medication. The blood–retina barrier limits the delivery of drug from the systemic circulation to the retina. The retinal pigment epithelium (RPE) and the retinal vessel walls form this tight blood–retina barrier. The difference in drug levels between the anterior chamber and the vitreous cavity is several orders of magnitude after topical administration of eye drops. Intravitreal injection can provide a rapid therapeutic dose of medication to the posterior segment. The procedure must be repeated often and is associated with a variety of ocular complications.

The eye is an ideal organ for sustained-release drug delivery devices. Intraocular structures can be easily accessed through an intravitreal drug delivery system or surgical implantation. The blood–retina barrier further helps to localize the intraocular concentration of the drug while minimizing the systemic absorption and side-effects. The eye is also an immunologically privileged site, which limits the amount of inflammation related to the sustained-release device.[1–3]

EXISTING SUSTAINED-RELEASE DRUG DEVICES

Existing intraocular implants are designed to provide consistent release of drug from the polymeric implant for long duration. The intraocular implant must be placed surgically in the pars plana region. The major benefits of intraocular implant are: reduction of systemic side-effects of the medication, decreased risk of repeated intravitreal injections, decreasd total amount of drugs used for treatment, and localized therapeutic drug levels bypassing the blood–retina barrier.[1–5]

The ganciclovir implant (Vitrasert) by Bausch & Lomb was the first intraocular sustained-release drug device approved for the treatment of cytomegalovirus (CMV) retinitis. Before the era of highly active antiretroviral therapy (HAART), CMV retinitis was a common cause of morbidity in acquired immunodeficiency syndrome (AIDS) patients and a harbinger of increased mortality as well. Intravenous and oral administration of ganciclovir and foscarnet is highly effective in the treatment of disease and the prevention of recurrence. Their use was limited by serious side-effects such as myelosuppression and renal toxicity, commonly encountered in AIDS patients. Intraocular administration of ganciclovir minimized these systemic side-effects. The gan-

Table 12.1 **Drug delivery methods**

Method	Advantages	Disadvantages	Clinical examples
Nonbiodegradable implants	Controlled release for long duration	Surgically implanted Require surgical removal Replacement of new implants	Ganciclovir implant Fluocinolone acetonide implant
Biodegradable implants	Do not require removal Designed in various shapes Can be injected	Shorter duration of action Require surgical implantation or injection	Dexamethasone implant
Micro- and nanoparticles	Do not require removal Injection through small-gauge needle	Require injection Clouding of vitreous	
Liposomes	Do not require removal Can be used for large protein and antibody drug molecules	Require injection Clouding of vitreous Unknown long-term effect	
Encapsulated cell technology	May produce protein drug indefinitely	Requires surgical implantation Unknown long-term effect	NT-501

ciclovir implant is composed of a nonbiodegradable polymer that released ganciclovir roughly 1 μg/h over a period of 8 months.[1,6] Uncommon complications related to the surgical implant of the device included retinal detachment, endophthalmitis, and vitreous hemorrhage.[1,2,6,7]

More recently, a fluocinolone acetonide implant (Retisert) by Bausch & Lomb has been approved by the Food and Drug Administration (FDA) for the treatment of chronic uveitis. This is the second nonbiodegradable intraocular polymer implant that requires surgical placement in the pars plana region for the treatment of noninfectious posterior uveitis. Roughly 1 in 5 uveitis patients have posterior-segment inflammation with a risk of vision-threatening complications such as cystoid macular edema, optic nerve edema, retinal vasculitis, retinochoroiditis, and retinal vascular occlusion. Topical corticosteroids are highly effective for the treatment of anterior uveitis, but do not penetrate to a high therapeutic drug level in the vitreous and retina.

Intravenous and oral administration of corticosteroids is equally effective; they are associated with a variety of guaranteed side-effects of systemic corticosteroids. Periocular and intravitreal injection of corticosteroid have been extremely popular among retina specialists for the treatment of DME, neovascular AMD, cystoid macular edema, and retinal vein occlusion. Complications of periocular and intravitreal injection involve orbital fibrosis, ptosis, vitreous hemorrhage, retinal detachment, pseudoendophthalmitis, and endophthalmitis.

The fluocinolone acetonide implant releases a therapeutic level of corticosteroid over a period of 30 months. The FDA-approved implant contains 0.59 mg of fluocinolone acetonide with an initial release of 0.6 μg/day. Over the next 30 days, the drug level gradually decreases to a steady level of 0.3 μg/day.[1,8–10] In a multicenter randomized clinical trial of fluocinolone acetonide implants for the treatment of noninfectious posterior uveitis, the rate of recurrence was decreased from 51.4% before implant to 6.1% after implant.[8] Visual acuity remained stable or improved in 87% of the patients studied. In 21% of patients, there were three or more lines of improvement in visual acuity. More than 50% of patients required pressure-lowering medication and 5.8% required glaucoma surgery during the 34-week follow-up.[8] At 3-year follow-up, implanted eyes demonstrated significantly lowered incidence of cystoid macular edema. Improvement of visual acuity was seen in 28% of eyes versus 15% in the group with standard of care. Adverse results included 92% of phakic patients requiring cataract surgery, increased intraocular pressure in 38% of patients requiring filtering procedure, and 2% requiring removal of the implant for glaucoma management.[1,2,8] (Figure 12.1).

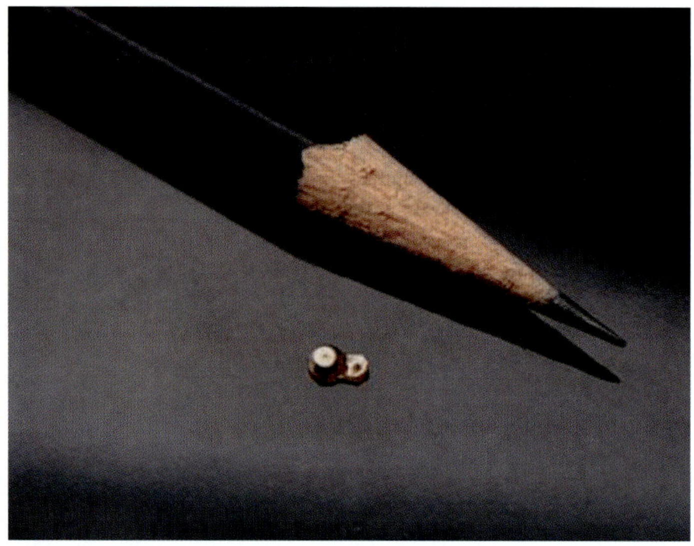

Figure 12.1 Fluocinolone acetonide nonbiodegradable implant (Retisert) from Bausch & Lomb. The device is surgically placed in the pars plana for the treatment of noninfectious uveitis.

BIODEGRADABLE POLYMER IMPLANTS

Currently, the only FDA-approved ganciclovir and fluocinolone acetonide intraocular implants are both nonbiodegradable polymer implants that require surgical implantation and explantation. The advantage of this system is the long duration of activity. Biodegradable implants offer the advantage that the devices do not need to be surgically removed. The drug polymer can be made into different shapes and implanted through small surgical wounds or injected through a small 23-gauge applicator system. A biodegradable dose of 700 μg dexamethasone sustained-release device (Ozurdex®) is currently in clinical trial for the treatment of posterior uveitis, DME, and neovascular AMD. The dexamethasone implant provides an initial burst of highly concentrated dexamethasone, followed by a gradual release over the following 3 months. The clinical effects of the sustained-release dexamethasone for the treatment of macular edema may last up to 6 months. Early pilot studies demonstrated that there was minimal cataract progression and 2% of study patients versus 1% of controls

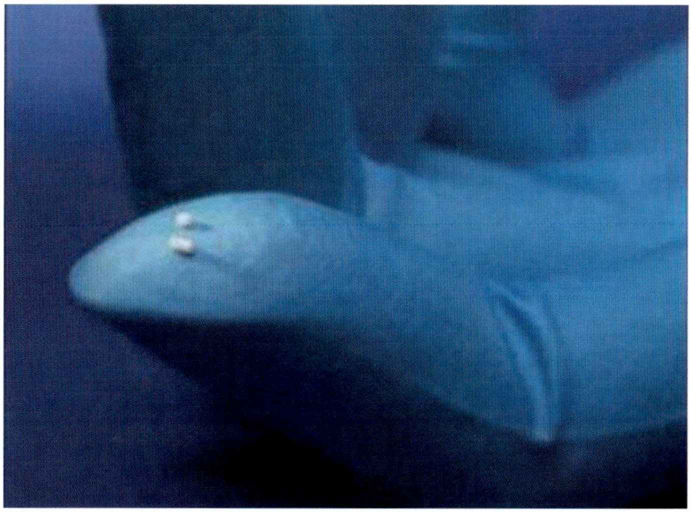

Figure 12.2 Dexamethasone biodegradable implant (Ozurdex®) from Allergan. The implant is injected into the vitreous.

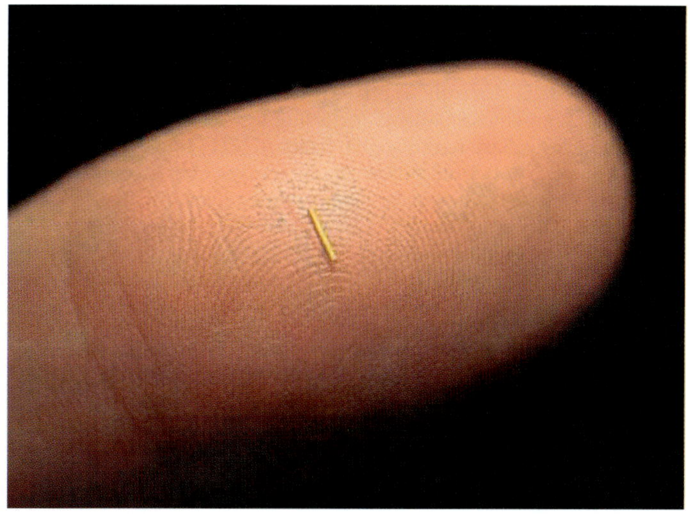

Figure 12.3 Fluocinolone acetonide biodegradable implant (Iluvien) from pSivida. The implant is injected into the vitreous.

developed intraocular pressure elevation of 10 mmHg at 3-months follow-up.[1,2,11] The shorter duration of action and follow-up may explain the significantly lower rates of adverse events. One potential advantage of this system is immediate inflammation control in uveitis patients or treatment of retinal pathology with a gradual steady-state release without the need to explant the device after the drug is completely released. The major disadvantage is the shorter duration of action. Surodex (Oculex Pharmceuticals), a 60-µg dexamethasone implant for the treatment of posttrabeculectomy inflammation, is placed under the scleral flap during surgery. No further development or clinical trial of the implant is currently under way (Figure 12.2).

An injectable sustained-release biodegradable fluocinolone acetonide implant (Iluvien) is currently in phase III clinical trial for the treatment of DME. The implant is a linear tube 3 mm long and 0.37 mm in diameter that can be injected through a 25-gauge needle. The duration of action is between 18 and 36 months.[1] The advantage of this drug delivery system is that it is a minimally invasive procedure for device placement and it is 100% biodegradable. This device shares the same risk of glaucoma and cataract formation consistent with all intraocular corticosteroid implants, in addition to the risk of intravitreal injections (Figure 12.3).

LIPOSOME ENCAPSULATION

Liposome-encased pharmacology is an alternative drug delivery system utilized in other subspecialties of medicine. The liposome is composed of a membrane-like lipid bilayer surrounding an aqueous compartment for the delivery of drugs, including small chemicals, proteins, nucleotides, and plasmid DNA. Liposome vesicles are 25–10 000 nm in diameter.[1,12] There are various methods for the preparation of liposomes, with variations in size, stability, and pharmacokinetics. The chemical compositions of liposome is biocompatible, biodegradable, and can be made of natural lipids. Additional modification of the liposome surface can provide preferential binding to a variety of intraocular structures such as choroidal neovascular membrane, retinal ganglion cells, photoreceptor cells, and the RPE. Liposomes can also be utilized to deliver drug intracellularly through cellular phagocytosis and membrane fusion. The liposome membrane structure is highly stable and can be deformed during injection through a 27- or 30-gauge needle.[1,2,12,13] Liposome encapsulation helps to reduce the intrinsic toxicity of drugs by reducing direct contact of the drug to the intraocular tissue. One limitation of the liposome delivery system is the risk of clouding of the vitreous immediately after injection. The long-term effects of the repeated injection of liposomal vehicle into the vitreous are currently unknown. The current gold standards for the treatment of AMD are ranibizumab and bevacizumab injection every 4–6 weeks. A liposome delivery system can be used to encapsulate large antibody fragments and even small unstable siRNA molecules without degradation and lost of bioactivity.[12–14] In addition, a number of different liposome drugs can be combined together for combination therapy.

MICRO AND NANOPARTICLE COUPLED DRUG DELIVERY

Coupling of the desired drug to microparticles or nanoparticles may be administered through periocular or intraocular injections. Microparticles are 1–1000 µm in size, with nanoparticles ranging from 1 to 1000 nm in size, comprised of biodegradable or biocompatible polymers. The two commonly used polymers are polylactide and polylactic-co-glycolic acid (PLGA); both are approved by the FDA.[1,2,15,16] The duration of the drug and release profile can be adjusted based on the size of the particles: nanoparticles with their larger surface area provide rapid release of the drug whereas microparticles provide a slower release profile. The hydrophobic and hydrophilic properties of the polymer can also be modified to increase or decrease the duration of the drug release profile. The molecular weight of the individual polylactide and PLGA molecule also contributes to the release profile of the coupled drug. In vitrectomized eyes, micro- and nanoparticles will also have a shorter duration of action.

One potential disadvantage of this delivery system is the clouding of the vitreous immediately after injection. Particles larger than 2 µm will sink in the vitreous cavity, similar to triamcinolone acetonide particles in the vitreous cavity after injection.[1,16] The advantage of this drug delivery system is the intrinsic flexibility. Drug particles of varying size can be mixed together to provide any release profile desired. Additional drug particles can be added in a single injection for combination therapies in retinal disorders such as AMD and diabetic retinopathy.

CELLULAR ENCAPSULATION

In ECT, immunologically isolated cells are encased within microcapsules or hollow fibers for intraocular implantation. The implanted microcapsule can provide controlled, continuous delivery of protein drugs to the posterior segment of the eye.[1,17] The device is surgically sutured into the pars plana region and can be retrieved if desired. ECT product NT501 is currently in phase II clinical trial in the treatment of 10 retinitis pigmentosa patients for 6 months. Modified human RPE cells producing ciliary neurotrophic factor (CNTF) into the vitreous of subjects' eyes.[17] ECT could potentially be used to treat glaucoma using neuroprotective agents, macular degeneration using anti-VEGF agents, and uveitis with anti-inflammatory agents. The major concerns with ECT are the long-term safety and efficacy of the device and the need for surgical implantation. The ECT may allow for continuous release of drug molecules definitively without ever needing to be replaced (Table 12.2).

THE FUTURE

We are entering a new era of retina pharmacology where new drugs are rapidly being developed for the treatment of posterior-segment disease. These drugs include small interference RNA (siRNA), aptamers, antibodies, and unique chemical molecules. These new drugs are used to treat a variety of chronic posterior-segment diseases with the requirement for repeated intravitreal injections.[14,18] Sustained-release technology offers the opportunity to provide controlled, continuous long-term release of these new medications, reducing the need for retreatment and the associated procedural risks. Each of these drugs with its unique molecular structure offers a different challenge for the drug delivery device. No single sustained-release drug delivery system will work perfectly with every drug. The ultimate goal is to develop a variety of drug delivery systems to complement and further enhance the efficacy of the available new medications. The ideal sustained-release technology will offer a high level of safety with consistent release over an extended period of time while maintaining 100% drug bioactivity. Minimizing the invasive procedure for the sustained-release drug device is crucial. These systems should be flexible for combining several drugs without the need for multiple procedures.

SUMMARY

Several different technologies exist for sustained-release drug delivery devices, including: (1) nonbiodegradable implants; (2) biodegradable implants; (3) micro- and nanoparticles; (4) liposomes; and (5) ECT. Currently, the only FDA-approved sustained-release devices are the ganciclovir implant for the treatment of CMV retinitis and the fluocinolone acetonide implant for the treatment of noninfectious posterior uveitis. Both implants are nonbiodegradable and require surgical placement. Two biodegradable implants are currently in phase III clinical trial. The dexamethasone and flucinolone acetonide implants can both be shaped and injected using a small-gauge needle or applicator into the vitreous. ECT, currently in phase II clinical trial, utilizes modified RPE cells to produce protein drug molecules in the vitreous. Microparticle, nanoparticle, and liposome technology currently in development may offer the most flexibility for duration of drug release and combination therapy for retinal diseases.

Key points

- Nonbiodegradable implants (fluocinolone and ganciclovir) are the only FDA-approved and available sustained-release devices.
- Biodegradable implants, micro- and nanoparticles, liposomes, and ECT are potential future sustained-release retinal drug delivery systems.
- Future retinal drug delivery modalities will likely utilize a combination of these technologies based on duration of drug release, chemical composition of the drug molecule, size of the drug molecule, and the synergistic activities of multiple drugs.
- Ideal sustained-release technology will offer safety and long duration of action, and maintain continued bioactivity.
- Sustained-release technology may offer treatment for AMD, DME, proliferative diabetic retinopathy, retinal vein occlusion, and uveitis.

Table 12.2 Existing and potential ophthalmic implants

Device name	Active drug	Mode of implantation	Status
Vitrasert	Ganciclovir	Surgical implantation at the pars plana	Clinical application
Retisert	Fluocinolone acetonide	Surgical implantation at the pars plana	Clinical application
Iluvien	Fluocinolone acetonide	Injected in the vitreous	Phase III
Ozurdex	Dexamethasone	Injected in the vitreous	Phase III
Surodex	Dexamethasone	Surgically placed under the scleral flap	Phase III
I-vation	Triamcinolone acetonide	Surgically replaceable screw	Phase II
NT-501	Ciliary neurotrophic factor by modified retinal pigment epithelium cells	Surgical implantation of the microcapsule	Phase II

ACKNOWLEDGMENT

This study was supported by Research to Prevent Blindness, Connecticut Lions Eye Research Foundation, and Allergan Horizon Grant.

REFERENCES

1. Del Amo EM, Urtti A. Current and future ophthalmic drug delivery systems: a shift to the posterior segment. Drug Discov Today 2008;13:135–143.
2. Hsu J. Drug delivery methods for posterior segment disease. Curr Opin Ophthalmol 2007;18:235–239.
3. Urtti A. Challenges and obstacles of ocular pharmacokinectics and drug delivery. Adv Drug Deliv Rev 2006;58:1131–1135.
4. Davis JL, Gilger BC, Robinson MD. Novel approaches to ocular drug delivery. Curr Opin Mol Ther 2004;6:195–205.
5. Bourges JL, Bloquel C, Thomas A, et al. Intraocular implants for extended drug delivery: therapeutic applications. Adv Drug Deliv Rev 2006;58: 1182–1202.
6. Musch DC, Martin DF, Gordon JF, et al. Treatment of cytomegalovirus retinitis with a sustained-release ganciclovir implant. N Engl J Med 1997;335:83–90.
7. Dunn JP, Van Natta M, Foster G, et al. Complications of ganciclovir implant surgery in patients with cytomegalovirus retinitis: the Ganciclovir Cidofovir Cytomegalovirus Retinitis Trial. Retina 2004;24:41–50.
8. Jaffe GJ, Martin D, Callanan D, et al. Flucinolone acetonide implant (Retisert) for noninfectious posterior uveitis: thirty-four-week results of a multicenter randomized clinical study. Ophthalmology 2006;113: 1020–1027.
9. Goldstein DA, Godfrey DG, Hall A, et al. Intraocular pressure in patients with uveitis treated with fluocinolone acetonide implants. Arch Ophthalmol 2007;125:1478–1485.
10. Jaffe GJ, Yang CH, Guo H, et al. Safety and pharmacokinetics of an intraocular fluocinolone acetonide sustained delivery device. Invest Ophthalmol Vis Sci 2000;41:3569–3575.
11. Kuppermann BD, Williams GA, Blumenkranz MS, et al. Efficacy and safety of a novel intravitreous dexamethasone drug-delivery system after applicator or incisional placement in patients with macular edema. Invest Ophthalmol Vis Sci 2006;47:e-abstract 5913.
12. Ebrahim S, Peyman GA, Lee PJ. Applications of liposomes in ophthalmology. Surv Ophthalmol 2005;50:167–182.
13. Bochot A, Fattal E, Boutet V, et al. Intravitreal delivery of oligonucleotides by sterically stabilized liposomes. Invert Ophthalmol Vis Sci 2002;43:253–259.
14. Fattal E, Bochot A. Ocular delivery of nucleic acids: antisense oligonucleotides, aptamers, siRNA. Adv Drug Deliv Rev 2006;58:1203–1223.
15. Moritera T, Ogura Y, Yoshmura N, et al. Biodegradable microspheres containing adriamycin in the treatment of proliferative vitreoretinopathy. Invest Ophthalmol Vis Sci 1992;33:3125–3130.
16. Bourges JL, Gautier SE, Delie F, et al. Ocular drug delivery targeting the retina and retinal pigment epithelium using polylactide nanoparticles. Invest Ophthalmol Vis Sci 2003;44:3562–3569.
17. Sieving PA, Caruso RC, Tao W, et al. Ciliary neurotrophic factor for human retinal degeneration: phase I trial of CNTF delivered by encapsulated cell intraocular implants. Proc Natl Acad Sci 2006;103:3896–3901.
18. Yasukara T, Ogura Y, Tabata Y, et al. Drug delivery system for vitreoretinal diseases. Prog Retin Eye Res 2004;23:253–281.

CHAPTER 13

Microspheres and nanotechnology for drug delivery

Einar Stefánsson, MD, PhD and Thorsteinn Loftsson, MSPharm, PhD

INTRODUCTION

Drug treatment of retinal disease is hampered by difficulties in drug delivery. Regular eye drops are fairly ineffective in delivering drugs to the retina and systemic application may lead to systemic side-effects. Ophthalmologists have resorted to injecting drugs into the vitreous cavity, for example steroids and antibodies against vascular endothelial growth factor. This invasive drug delivery method demands an operating room setting and introduces risks of infection and surgical trauma[1–3] and this is also to some extent true with subconjunctival, sub-Tenons capsule, or suprascleral injections.

In general, drugs can enter the posterior segment of the eye via three distinctive noninvasive routes: (1) through conjunctiva/sclera after topical application; (2) from the cornea and aqueous humor after topical application; and (3) from the systemic circulation after topical, parenteral, oral, or other administration routes that deliver drug to the blood circulation.

In drug development the main emphasis should be on topical and noninvasive methods for drug delivery to the posterior segment of the eye. From the marketing point of view the delivery technology has to be cost-effective, reliable, and applicable to drugs of diverse physicochemical properties. Following is a brief review of microspheres and nanotechnology for drug delivery to the eye followed by an example of topical drug delivery to the posterior segment of the eye.

WHAT IS MICRO AND NANOTECHNOLOGY?

Ophthalmic dosage forms are classified according to their appearance and physical properties into ophthalmic solutions (e.g., the conventional eye drop solutions), gel-forming solutions, powders for solutions, ophthalmic suspensions, ophthalmic ointments, ophthalmic emulsions (e.g., creams), ophthalmic gels, and ocular inserts.[4] This macroscopic classification of ophthalmic dosage forms is not related to their microscopic structure and they can not per se be defined as micro- or nanotechnology. However, examples of micro- and nanotechnological applications for all of these different dosage forms can be found in the scientific literature; some of these forms have been tested in animals and a few in humans (Table 13.1). Micro- and nanotechnological drug formulations are, with some exceptions, classified according to the diameter of their particulates. Microtechnology usually refers to technological devices with dimensions close to 0.1–100 μm (10^2–10^5 nm) and particles between 0.1 and 100 μm are called microparticles. Typical drop size in pharmaceutical emulsions is between 0.1 and 1 μm (10^2–10^3 nm). Simple microemulsions form droplets that are between 5 and 140 nm and, thus, should be more correctly referred to as nanoemulsions. In general, nanotechnology refers to a field of science whose unifying theme is fabrication of devices or matter on a close to molecular scale or dimensions between 1 and 1000 nm. For comparison the diameter of a water molecule is less than 0.3 nm and that of dexamethasone is just over 1 nm. Nanoparticles are particles with at least one dimension less than 100 nm and the size of liposomes is frequently between 10 and 1000 nm.

Microparticles can consist of micronized drug particles for intravitreal injection but more often such particles consist of micronized polymer/drug matrix-like structures, i.e., microspheres, or polymer-coated microparticles, i.e., microcapsules, that are applied topically to the eye surface. Microparticles may be too large for intravitreal injections where nanoparticles with diameter of less than 200 nm have been shown to result in more effective drug delivery to the retina than larger particles.[5] Subconjunctival injection of budesonide microparticles to rats resulted in sustained drug concentration in the retina and vitreous.[6]

Liposomes consist of one or more lipid bilayers and an inner aqueous core. The lipid bilayers are formed by natural or synthetic phospholipids that are similar to those of cellular plasma membranes. Lipophilic drugs are incorporated into the lipid bilayer while hydrophilic drugs are dissolved in the aqueous core. Liposomes are relatively unstable during storage and tend to form aggregates in vitreous causing visual cloudiness for a couple of weeks after intravitreal injection.[7] In spite of these shortcomings, liposomes are regarded as promising vehicles for drug delivery to the posterior segment of the eye. Various drugs, including antiviral drugs and antibiotics, are being encapsulated in liposomes for intravitreal delivery.[8]

Nanoparticles can refer to nanospheres (e.g., drug/polymer matrix) or nanocapsules (e.g., polymer-coated drug particles). Examples of nanoparticles for intravitreal drug delivery include albumin nanoparticles for delivery of ganciclovir and a formivirsen analog,[9] and tamoxifen-loaded nanoparticles.[10] Carbohydrates and oligosaccharides, such as cyclodextrins, form nanoparticles consisting of molecular aggregates. Nanoclusters are nanoparticles formed by molecular aggregation and nanospheres are nanoparticles where the active ingredient is encapsulated by a polymer.

Other micro- and nanotechnological ocular delivery systems have been described, such as microemulsions, that are clear low-viscosity liquid systems for topical drug delivery,[11] and viral vectors used for gene therapy.[12] Then there are micromachines that apply electrical current to deliver drug biological membranes, such as iontophoresis that uses low-voltage continuous electricity to deliver charged drug particles through membranes, and electroporation, that uses high-voltage electrical pulses to induce pores in cell membranes. Most of the work on iontophoresis and electroporation has been carried out on skin and cell membranes.

PERMEATION BARRIERS AND ANATOMICAL CONSIDERATIONS

The eye can be divided into the anterior segment – cornea, aqueous humor, iris, lens, and ciliary body – and posterior segment – vitreous humor, retina, choroid, sclera, and optic nerve. The cornea is a transparent five-layer biomembrane. Outermost is the epithelium, then the Bowman's membrane, stroma (which represents about 90% of the corneal thickness), Descemet's membrane, and finally the endothelium. The main barrier layer towards drug penetration through the cornea is the lipophilic epithelium, which contributes about 90% of the barrier towards hydrophilic drugs and about 10% of the barrier towards lipophilic drugs. The epithelium consists of three to six layers of tightly adherent epithelial cells. The epithelial surface is covered with microvilli.

Drugs penetrate the epithelium either transcellularly (through the cells) or paracellularly (through pores between the cells). The transcellular route predominates for lipophilic drug molecules whereas the paracellular route predominates for hydrophilic molecules and small ions. The pore size has been estimated to be about 1 nm (permeable for drugs with molecular weight (MW) less than about 700 Da) although

Table 13.1

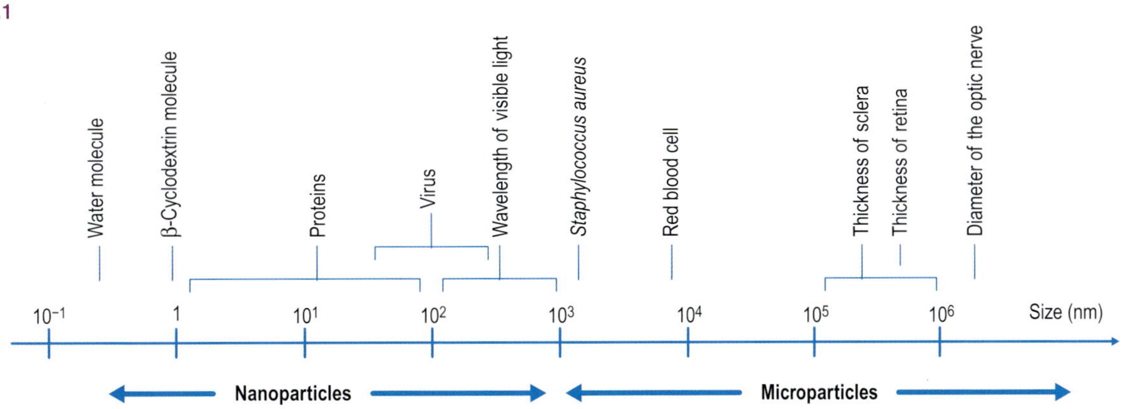

Typical particle diameter	Type of delivery system	Composition
Topical drug delivery:		
~ 2 to 10 nm	Solution	Aqueous dexamethasone/cyclodextrin complex solution[13]
20 to 35 nm	Microemulsion	Timolol in Pluronic F127 microemulsion[14]
$2{\cdot}10^2$ and $5{\cdot}10^3$ nm	Nanosuspension	Corticosteroids as Pluronic F68 stabilized nano- or microparticles[15]
$4{\cdot}10^2$ to $7{\cdot}10^2$ nm	Microsuspension	Maxidex®, Azopt® and Betoptic-S® from Alcon Laboratories[16]
$1{\cdot}10^4$ nm	Microsuspension	Aqueous dexamethasone/cyclodextrin complex suspension[17]
Subconjunctival injection:		
$3.5{\cdot}10^2$ and $3.6{\cdot}10^3$ nm	Nano- and microparticles	Budesonide in a biodegradable DL-polylactide polymer matrix[6]
Intravitreal injection:		
$1.4{\cdot}10^2$ and $3.1{\cdot}10^2$ nm	Nanoparticles	Fluorescence compounds in biodegradable DL-polylactide polymer[18]
$1.5{\cdot}10^2$ and $1.9{\cdot}10^2$ nm	Liposomes	Olegonucleotides in sterically stabilized liposomes[19]

studies have indicated that some pores could be up to 5 nm in diameter.[20,21] However, the porosity (i.e., the pore density on the surface) of the epithelium is rater low, indicating that paracellular permeation is limited by the frequency of a drug molecule hitting a pore. It is believed that most drugs permeate the epithelium via passive diffusion and, although drug transporters have been located in the epithelium, their significance is still unclear.[22] The stroma can, from a drug delivery point of view, be considered to be an aqueous gel where collagen fibrils and glycosaminoglycans form the net structure. It offers little permeation resistance towards hydrophilic drugs but can be the rate-limiting barrier for lipophilic drugs that permeate the epithelium relatively rapidly. The endothelium is a membrane one cell layer thick with large intracellular junctions. It can be regarded as a leaky lipophilic barrier that offers no permeation resistance towards hydrophilic drugs but may offer some resistance towards lipophilic drugs.[23] The Bowman's and Descemet's membranes do not offer any significant resistance towards drug permeation.

The bulbar conjunctiva is a transparent mucous membrane that covers the outer surface of the sclera. It contains numerous microvilli on its surface. Within the bulbar conjunctiva are the goblet cells which secrete mucin, an important component of the tear layer that protects and nourishes the eye surface. The sclera is composed primarily of collagen fibers embedded in mucopolysaccharide matrix, an aqueous structure that resembles the structure of the corneal stroma. The primary route for drug permeation through the sclera is by passive diffusion through an aqueous pathway. The permeability of sclera is similar to that of stroma with no apparent dependence on the drug lipophilicity, i.e., the octanol/water partition coefficient, but a strong dependence on the drug MW, i.e., the hydrodynamic radius of the permeating drug molecule, the permeability coefficient decreasing with increasing MW. Conjunctiva is approximately 15–25 times more permeable and the sclera is approximately 10 times more permeable than the cornea.[24] Both intercellular pore size and pore density in the cornea are much smaller than in the conjunctiva.

The choroid is a vascular layer that lies between the retina and the sclera. It is composed of layers of blood vessels that nourish the back of the eye. The choroidal vasculature can contribute to drug clearance from the eye and, thus, constitute a permeation barrier during drug permeation from the eye surface to the retina and vitreous. The vitreous humor is a clear aqueous gel where the matrix-forming polymer system consists mainly of collagen and hyaluronan with water content of about 99%. Aqueous humor is the fluid that fills the anterior chamber, the space between the iris and the cornea. The aqueous humor has relatively low viscosity and its chemical composition resembles that of blood plasma. Its total volume in human and rabbit eye is between 200 and 300 µl. It is continuously secreted by the ciliary body, flows as a gentle stream (2–5 µl/min) through the pupil, and is drained by the canal of Schlemm.

The eye surface is continuously washed by the tear fluid secreted from the lacrimal glands, the main gland located at the outer portion of the eye orbit. The tear fluid (lacrimal fluid) consists of three layers. The outermost layer is a lipid layer that retards water evaporation from the surface. The central aqueous layer contains mainly water and small amounts of other substances such as proteins. The innermost layer is the mucus, a gel-like fluid containing mainly water (~95%) and mucin.[25] Mucins are large glycoproteins with MW ranging from 0.5 to 20 MDa. Some are membrane-bound but others are not. Mucin forms hydrogen bonds with surrounding water molecules, enhancing water cluster formation and, consequently, decreased water mobility.[26] Following instillation of an eye drop (~35 µl) on to the precorneal area of the eye, the greater part of the drug solution is rapidly drained from the eye surface and the solution volume returns to the normal resident tear volume of about 7 µl. Thereafter, the preocular solution volume remains constant, but drug concentration decreases due to dilution by tear turnover and corneal and noncorneal absorption. Normal tear turnover is about 1.2 µl/min in humans[27] and, thus, after the initial eye drop drainage, the precorneal half-life of topically applied drugs is between 1 and 3 min. As a result, only small percentages of drug dosage in topically applied eye drops are delivered into the intraocular tissues. The major part (50–100%) of the administered dose will be absorbed into the systemic drug circulation, which can cause various side-effects.

THEORETICAL BACKGROUND

Passive drug permeation through multilayer barriers, such as through the tear fluid and through conjunctiva/sclera or cornea, can be described as a series of additive resistances analogous to electric circuits.[28–30] Assuming independent and additive resistances of the individual layers, the total resistance (R_T) of a simple membrane can be defined as:

$$J = P_T \cdot C_V = R_T^{-1} \cdot C_V = (R_D + R_M + R_R)^{-1} \cdot C_V$$
$$= \left(\frac{1}{P_D} + \frac{1}{P_M} + \frac{1}{P_R}\right)^{-1} \cdot C_V \quad (1)$$

where J is the flux of the drug through the membrane, P_T is the overall permeability coefficient, C_V is the drug concentration in the vehicle (i.e., donor phase), R_D, R_M, and R_R and P_D, P_M, and P_R are the resistances and permeability coefficients in the unstirred water layer (UWL) at the donor side (the tear fluid), within the membrane (cornea, conjunctiva, and/or sclera) and in the UWL at the receptor side, respectively.[26,31] If R_R is assumed to be negligible due to relatively rapid removal of drug molecules from the receptor side of the membrane, Equation 2 is obtained:

$$J = \left(\frac{P_D \cdot P_M}{P_D + P_M}\right) \cdot C \quad (2)$$

The relationship between the permeation coefficient (P) and the diffusion coefficient (D) is given by Equation 3:

$$P = \frac{D \cdot K}{h} \quad (3)$$

where h is the thickness (h_D, h_M, or h_R) and K is the partition coefficient between the aqueous phase and the membrane. For P_D and P_R the value of K is unity. Finally D can be estimated from the Stokes–Einstein equation:

$$D \approx \frac{R \cdot T}{6\pi \cdot \eta \cdot r \cdot N} \quad (4)$$

where R is the molar gas constant, T is the absolute temperature, η is the apparent viscosity within the UWL or the lipophilic membrane, r is the radius of the permeating drug molecule, and N is Avogadro's number. Thus, the diffusion constant within the UWL (D_D) will decrease with increasing viscosity of the layer as well as with increasing MW of the drug. For example, small lipophilic drug molecules frequently possess a large permeability coefficient through a lipophilic membrane (i.e., large P_M value) and, thus, may be able to permeate lipophilic membrane (e.g., cornea) much faster that they can be transported through the UWL (e.g., the tear film). Under such conditions, diffusion through the UWL becomes the rate-limiting step in the absorption process. The presence of mucin in the mucus layer not only increases the thickness (h) of this UWL but also its viscosity (η), both of which will increase its resistance (R_D) and consequently decrease permeability (P_D) (Equations 3 and 4). Other surface structures, such as microvilli on the eye surface, can also increase h and η of the UWL. Studies have shown that drug diffusion through mucus is up to 100 times slower than through pure water.[32]

According to Equation 1 there are three major barriers to topical drug delivery into the eye.[31] The first barrier is the rapid decrease of drug concentration (C_V) in the tear fluid due to the lacrimal drainage system. The precorneal half-life of topically applied drugs in simple aqueous eye drop solutions is only between 1 and 3 min. Since passive diffusion is driven by the concentration gradient, i.e., the difference in drug concentration at the outer (C_V) and inner (C_{Aq}) tear layer, this decrease results in a rapid decrease in drug permeability into the eye (Figure 13.1). Increased drug mucoadhesion will increase the precorneal half-life of topically administered drugs. The second barrier is slow permeation of drug molecules through the viscous mucous layer (the UWL) to the membrane surface due to low concentration gradient ($C_V - C_{Aq}$). The amount of dissolved drug in the low-viscosity external layer of the tear film has to be increased (i.e., increase C_V in Figure 13.1). The third barrier to drug delivery is slow drug permeation through the membrane barrier, i.e., cornea or conjunctiva/sclera. The only way to increase drug permeation through the membrane, except by increasing C_{Aq}, is to increase $K_{M/Aq}$ through chemical modifications of the permeating drug molecule (e.g., through formation of prodrugs) or by increasing the diffusion coefficient (D_M) by adding permeation enhancers to the aqueous eye drop solution that temporarily decrease the permeation resistance (i.e., decrease R_M in Equation 1). Somewhat water-soluble microparticles with a diameter of about 20 µm will possess some mucoadhesion and at the same time maintain a constant high drug concentration in the aqueous tear fluid.[31]

CYCLODEXTRINS

Cyclodextrins are oligosaccharides formed by (α-1,4)-linked α-D-glucopyranose units, with a hydrophilic outer surface and a lipophilic central cavity.[33,34] The natural α-, β-, and γ-cyclodextrins consist of

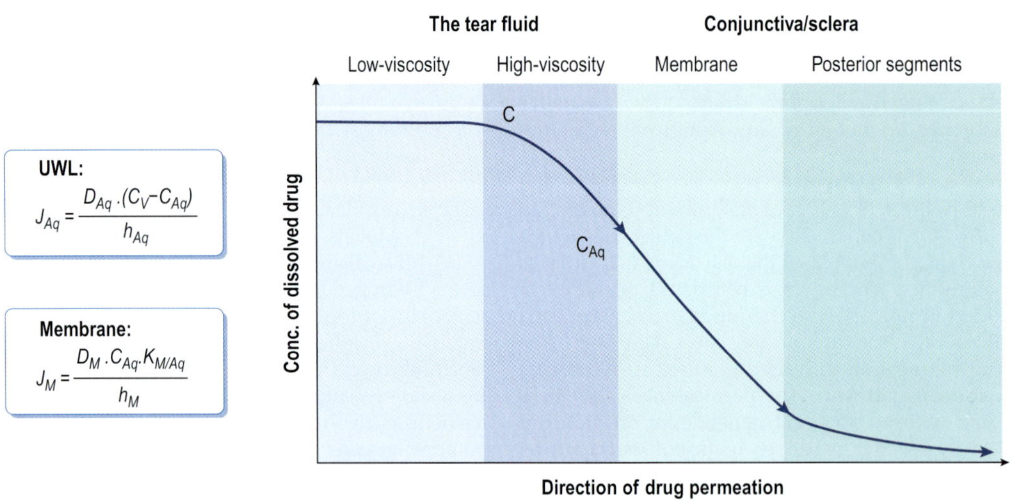

Figure 13.1 UWL, unstirred water layer. Three major barriers to topical drug delivery into the eye. The first is the rapid decrease of drug concentration (CV) in the tear fluid because of the lacrimal drainage system. Passive diffusion driven by the concentration gradient leads to rapid decrease in drug permeability into the eye. The second barrier is slow permeation of drug molecules through the viscous mucous layer (the UWL) to the membrane surface due to low concentration gradient (CV – CAq). The amount of dissolved drug in the low-viscosity external layer of the tear film has to be increased (i.e., increase CV). The third barrier is slow drug permeation through the membrane barrier, i.e., cornea or conjunctiva/sclera.

six, seven, and eight glucopyranose units, respectively. The aqueous solubility of these natural cyclodextrins is somewhat limited and thus several different water-soluble derivatives have been synthesized. Cyclodextrin derivatives which have been applied in ophthalmology include the hydroxypropyl derivatives of β- and γ-cyclodextrin, the randomly methylated β-cyclodextrin, and sulfobutylether β-cyclodextrin.[35] In an aqueous environment, cyclodextrins form inclusion complexes with many lipophilic molecules through a process in which water molecules located inside the central cavity are replaced by either a whole molecule, or more frequently by some lipophilic structure of the molecule. Cyclodextrin complexation of a drug molecule changes the physicochemical properties of the drug, such as its aqueous solubility and chemical stability. Since the cyclodextrin molecule is hydrophilic on the outer surface the complex formation usually increases the water-solubility of lipophilic water-insoluble drugs. Thus, through cyclodextrin complexation it has been possible to formulate lipophilic water-insoluble steroids as aqueous eye drop solutions.[13,35–40] Once included in the cyclodextrin cavity, the drug molecules may be dissociated from the cyclodextrin molecules through complex dilution in the aqueous tear fluid. Since no covalent bonds are formed or broken during the guest–host complex formation, the complexes are in dynamic equilibrium with free drug and cyclodextrin molecules.

Cyclodextrins are able to enhance drug delivery through biological membranes. However, *in vitro* studies have shown that hydrophilic cyclodextrins can only enhance drug delivery through membranes when the permeation resistance of the UWL on the donor side is about equal to or greater than the resistance of membrane barrier, i.e., $R_D \geq R_M$ in Equation 1. This is frequently the case when drugs readily permeate cornea or sclera and the mucinous tear film forms the rate-determining UWL. Conventional penetration enhancers, such as benzalkonium chloride, disrupt the ophthalmic barrier (i.e., reduce R_M), whereas hydrophilic cyclodextrins enhance drug penetration into the eye by carrying the lipophilic water-insoluble drug molecules through the aqueous tear film and thereby increasing drug availability at the membrane surface (i.e., by increasing C and $C - C_{Aq}$; see Figure 13.1). In addition cyclodextrins can form both nano- and microparticles and in some cases large nanoparticles can penetrate human mucus rapidly.[26,31,41]

ANIMAL TESTING OF ROUTES OF DRUG DELIVERY

Dexamethasone is a glucocorticoid that is commonly used as an anti-inflammatory drug in ophthalmology. It is a somewhat lipophilic ($\log P_{(octanol/water)}$ 1.8) and low-MW drug (MW 392.5 Da) that permeates lipophilic biological membranes with relative ease. However, its low aqueous solubility (0.16 mg/ml) hampers its clinical usefulness. Natural cyclodextrins, such as γ-cyclodextrin, are very hydrophilic ($\log P_{(octanol/water)} < -3$) and form water-soluble complexes with dexamethasone. Due to their molecular size and hydrophilicity cyclodextrins do not readily permeate biological membranes and, since the dexamethasone–cyclodextrin complex adopts many of the physicochemical properties of the cyclodextrin molecule, the intact complex does not readily permeate through biological membranes. However, cyclodextrin solubilization of dexamethasone will increase drug availability immediate to the epithelial surface (Figure 13.1).

Dexamethasone was formulated as a dexamethasone–γ-cyclodextrin complex microsuspension.[17] The aqueous solubility of dexamethasone in the formulation is 0.08 mg/ml and the solubility of the complex is about 2.9 mg dexamethasone/ml. The aqueous eye drop formulation contained 1.5% (w/v) dexamethasone in aqueous eye drop suspension that contained 18% (w/v) γ-cyclodextrin. The concentration of dissolved dexamethasone was determined to be 0.1% (w/v) or between 6 and 7% of the total dexamethasone concentration in the eye drops. The mean (± standard deviation) particle size was determined to be 20 ± 10 μm. The reference eye drop formulation was an aqueous 1.5% (w/v) dexamethasone eye drop solution containing randomly methylated β-cyclodextrin as solubilizer.[17,31,42] The eye drops were administered to the left eye but the dexamethasone concentration was determined in both eyes. The concentration difference ($C_{left} - C_{right}$) was used to estimate how much dexamethasone reached various tissues in the left eye via the topical route. Table 13.2 shows that formulating the drug as a suspension, where the solid particles consist of not the pure drug but the drug–cyclodextrin inclusion complexes, increases the drug delivery to the posterior segment of the eye, resulting in greater than threefold increase in the amount of drug reaching the retina. The blood dexamethasone concentration, 2 hours after topical administration, was also much lower when the drug was administered as a cyclodextrin complex suspension, being 45 ± 24 ng/g after administration of the eye drop solution but 10 ± 7 ng/g after administration of the suspension.[17] Interestingly, the amount in sclera was increased by 90% when the drug was administered as suspension whereas it was reduced by 30% in the cornea. Thus, the results indicate that the drug/cyclodextrin delivery system specifically targets sclera and delivery of drugs through sclera to the posterior segment of the eye.

The nature of the solid drug/cyclodextrin particles is also important. Due to their size, the water-soluble drug/cyclodextrin microparticles will not be washed away from the eye surface but adhere to the surface and the surrounding tissue. The particles will dissolve rapidly enough

Table 13.2

Tissue	DEXAMETHASONE CONCENTRATION REACHING THE EYE TISSUE VIA TOPICAL ROUTE (MG/ML)		Increase
	γ-Cyclodextrin	RMβCD	
Anterior segment:			
Cornea	1137	1624	–30%
Aqueous humor	232	567	–59%
Iris-ciliary body	263	505	–48%
Lens	6	14	–57%
Posterior segment:			
Sclera	381	200	90%
Vitreous	25	16	56%
Retina	28	9	210%
Optic nerve	85	46	85%

to maintain the aqueous tear fluid saturated with the drug, i.e., the C_{Aq} in Figure 13.1 will not decrease during drainage of the tear fluid. Particles of lipophilic drugs possessing limited solubility in water will dissolve very slowly in the aqueous tear fluid. Conventional suspensions, even in micronized form, will not possess sufficiently rapid dissolution rates to maintain drug saturation of the aqueous tear fluid. Formulating the drug as more water-soluble drug–cyclodextrin complexes in a microparticle will ensure rapid drug dissolution. This will maintain drug saturation of the aqueous tear fluid (i.e., high C_V and C_{Aq} in Figure 13.1). Consequently this novel formulation technology will not only enhance the flux (J) of drug into the eye but also reduce the amount of drug reaching the systemic circulation via nasal absorption.

FUTURE DIRECTIONS AND TECHNOLOGIES

Cyclodextrin nanoparticle suspension in eye drops offers a new and exciting drug delivery platform for the posterior segment of the eye. It is effective with a variety of drugs, including steroids and sulfonamides, such as carbonic anhydrase inhibitors, and may be used with many small lipophilic molecules. Its potential remains to be studied in clinical trials, where this technology may revolutionize drug treatment for retinal disease.

SUMMARY AND KEY POINTS

Cyclodextrin nanoparticles in eye drops effectively deliver steroids to the retina in rabbits. We have reviewed this aspect of nanotechnology, topical drug delivery to the eye, diffusion barriers, and cyclodextrin chemistry.

We believe that eye drops with cyclodextrin nanoparticles can replace triamcinolone injections in the treatment of macular edema. This technology is firmly based on principles of ocular pharmacology and should be applicable to a variety of drug treatments for the retina and posterior segment of the eye.

REFERENCES

1. Kusaka S, Ikuno Y, Ohguro N, et al. Orbital infection following posterior subtenon triamcinolone injection. Acta Ophthalmol Scand 2007;85:in print.
2. Delyfer MN, Rougier MB, Hubschman JP, et al. Cytomegalovirus retinitis following intravitreal injection of triamcinolone: report of two cases. Acta Ophthalmol Scand 2007;85:in print.
3. Fasolino G, Bamonte G, Patelli F, et al. Retinal pigment epithelial tear after intravitreal injection of triamcinolone acetonide for neovascular pigment epithelial detachment: a mechanical explanation. Acta Ophthalmol Scand 2007;85:575–576.
4. Lang JC, Roehrs RE, Jani R. Ophthalmic preparations. In: Beringer P, Gupta PK, editors. Remington, the Science and Practice of Pharmacy, 21st edn. Philadelphia: Lippincott Williams & Wilkins; 2006. p. 850–870.
5. Sakurai E, Ozeki H, Kunou N, et al. Effect of particle size of polymeric nanospheres on intravitreal kinetics. Ophthalmic Res 2001;33:31–36.
6. Kompella UB, Bandi N, Ayalasomayajula SP. Subconjunctival nano- and microparticles sustain retinal delivery of budesonide, a corticosteroid capable of inhibiting VEGF expression. Invest Ophthalm Vis Sci 2003;44:1192–1201.
7. Booth BA, Denham LV, Bouhanik S, et al. Sustained-release ophthalmic drug delivery systems for treatment of macular disorders. Drugs Aging 2007;24:581–602.
8. Janoria KG, Gunda S, Boddu SHS, et al. Novel Approaches for retinal drug delivery. Expert Opin Drug Deliv 2007;4:371–388.
9. Irache JM, Merodio M, Arnedo A, et al. Albumin nanoparticles for the intravitreal delivery of anticytomegaloviral drugs. Mini-Rev Med Chem 2005;5:293–305.
10. de Kozak Y, Andrieux K, Villarroya H, et al. Intraocular injection of tamoxifen-loaded nanoparticles: a new treatment of experimental autoimmune uveoretinitis. Eur J Immunol 2004;34:3702–3712.
11. Vandamme TF. Microemulsions as ocular drug delivery systems: recent developments and future directions. Prog Retin Eye Res 2002;21:15–34.
12. Campochiaro PA, Nguyen QD, Shah SM, et al. Adenoviral vector-delivered pigment epithelium-derived factor for neovascular age-related macular degeneration: results of a phase I clinical trial. Hum Gene Ther 2006;17:167–176.
13. Kristinsson JK, Friðriksdóttir H, Thórisdóttir S, et al. Dexamethasone-cyclodextrin-polymer co-complexes in aqueous eye drops. Invest Ophthalmol Vis Sci 1996;37:1199–1203.
14. Li C-C, Abrahamson M, Kapoor Y, et al. Timolol transport from microemulsion trapped in HEMA gels. J Coll Interf Sci 2007;315:297–306.
15. Kassem MA, Abdel Rahman AA, et al. Nanosuspension as an ophthalmic delivery system for certain glucocorticoid drugs. Int J Pharm 2007;340: 126–133.
16. Imre L, Resch M, Megyesi M, et al. In-vitro-Untersuchung der Mikrostruktur von handelsüblichen ophthalmologischen Suspensionen mittels HRT-II Rostock Cornea Modul. Ophthalmologe 2007;104:697–704.
17. Loftsson T, Hreinsdóttir D, Stefánsson E. Cyclodextrin microparticles for drug delivery to the posterior segment of the eye: aqueous dexamethasone eye drops. J Pharm Pharmacol 2007;59:629–635.
18. Bourges J-L, Gautier SE, Delie F, et al. Ocular drug delivery targeting the retina and retinal pigment epithelium using polylactide nanoparticles. Invest Ophthalm Vis Sci 2003;44:3562–3569.
19. Bochot A, Fattal E, Boutet V, et al. Intravitreal delivery of oligonucleotides by sterically stabilized liposomes. Invest Ophthalm Vis Sci 2002;43: 253–259.
20. Prausnitz MR, Noonan JS. Permeability of cornea, sclera, and conjunctiva: a literature analysis for drug delivery to the eye. J Pharm Sci 1998;87: 1479–1487.
21. Hämäläinen KM, Kontturi K, Auriola S, et al. Estimation of pore size and pore density of biomembranes from permeability measurements of polyethylene glycols using an effusion-like approach. J Control Rel 1997;49:97–104.
22. Mannermaa E, Vellonen K-S, Urtti A. Drug transport in corneal epithelium and blood–retina barrier: emerging role of transporters in ocular pharmacokinetics. Adv Drug Deliv Rev 2006;58:1136–1163.
23. Ghate D, Edelhauser HF. Ocular drug delivery. Expert Opin Drug Deliv 2006;3:275–287.
24. Hämäläinen KM, Kananen K, Auriola S, et al. Characterization of paracellular and aqueous penetration routes in cornea conjunctiva, and sclera. Invest Ophthalmol Vis Sci 1997;38:627–633.
25. Bansil R, Turner BS. Mucin structure, aggregation, physiological functions and biomedical applications. Curr Opin Colloid Interface Sci 2006;11:164–170.
26. Loftsson T, Vogensen SB, Brewster ME, et al. Effects of cyclodextrins on drug delivery through biological membranes. J Pharm Sci 2007;96: 2532–2546.
27. Sugrue MF. The pharmacology of antiglaucoma drugs. Pharm Ther 1989;43:91–138.
28. Higuchi T. Physical chemical analysis of percutaneous absorption process from creams and ointments. J Soc Cosmetic Chemists 1960;11:85–97.
29. Flynn GL, Carpender OS, Yalkowsky SH. Total mathematical resolution of diffusion layer control of barrier flux. J Pharm Sci 1972;61:312–314.
30. Flynn GL, Yalkowsky SH. Correlation and prediction of mass transport across membranes I: influence of alkyl chain length on flux-determining properties of barrier and diffusant. J Pharm Sci 1972;61:838–852.
31. Loftsson T, Sigurðsson HH, Konráðsdóttir F, et al. Topical drug delivery to the posterior segment of the eye: anatomical and physiological considerations. Pharmazie 2008;63:171–179.
32. Khanvilkar K, Donovan MD, Flanagan DR. Drug transfer through mucus. Adv Drug Deliv Rev. 2001;48:173–193.
33. Loftsson T, Duchêne D. Cyclodextrins and their pharmaceutical applications. Int J Pharm 2007;329:1–11.
34. Brewster ME, Loftsson T. Cyclodextrins as pharmaceutical solubilizers. Adv Drug Deliv Rev 2007;59:645–666.
35. Loftsson T, Stefánsson E. Cyclodextrins in ocular drug delivery. J Drug Deliv Sci Tech 2007;17:3–9.
36. Usayapant A, Karara AH, Narurkar MM. Effect of 2-hydroxypropyl-β-cyclodextrin on the ocular absorption of dexamethasone and dexamethasone acetate. Pharm Res 1991;12:1495–1499.
37. Davies NM, Wang G, Tucker IG. Evaluation of a hydrocortisone/hydroxypropyl-β-cyclodextrin solution for ocular drug delivery. Int J Pharm 1997;156:201–209.
38. Gavrilin MV, Kompantseva EV, Gusova BA, et al. Dexamethasone eye drops based on the products of its interaction with 2-hydroxypropyl-β-cyclodextrin: synthesis and study. Pharm Chem J 1999;33:160–163.
39. Kearse EC, McIntyre OL, Johnson MH, et al. Influence of dehydroepiandrosterone on rabbit intraocular pressure. Ophthalmic Res 2001;33:42–47.
40. Loftsson T, Järvinen T. Cyclodextrins in ophthalmic drug delivery. Adv Drug Deliv Rev 1999;36:59–79.
41. Lai SK, O'Hanlon DE, Harrold S, et al. Rapid transport of large polymeric nanoparticles in fresh undiluted human mucus. Proc Natl Acad Sci USA 2007;104:1482–1487.
42. Sigurdsson HH, Konrádsdóttir F, Loftsson T, et al. Topical and systemic absorption in delivery of dexamethasone to the anterior and posterior segments of the eye. Acta Ophthalmol Scand 2007;85:598–602.

CHAPTER

14 Thermo-sensitive hydrogels

Jennifer J. Kang-Mieler, PhD and William F. Mieler, MD

INTRODUCTION

Since the initial development of hydrogels in 1960, they have been of great interest to biomaterial scientists and tissue engineers. Hydrogels are polymers which have the ability to swell in water or aqueous solvent system, and they hold the solvents in a swollen crosslinked gel system for delivery. Through manipulation of permeation and diffusion characteristics, they can retain hydrophobic and hydrophilic agents, small molecules, and macromolecules. Depending on the specific structure, they can be nondegradable or degradable in application.[1,2] There are numerous advantages that make hydrogels an attractive drug delivery platform.[1,3] The aqueous environment of hydrogels can protect cells and fragile drugs (such as peptides, proteins, oligonucleotides, and DNA). They serve as a good means of transport of nutrients to cells and products from cells. They can also be modified with cell adhesion ligands, and can change physical state (liquid to solid) in response to pH or temperature changes, and, most importantly, they are highly biocompatible.

Among all the hydrogel systems investigated over the years, temperature- and pH-responsive hydrogels have demonstrated great promise in drug delivery due to their novel ability to change physical state. Poly(*N*-isopropylacrylamide) (PNIPAAm) hydrogel is one of the well-known thermo-sensitive materials which has a lower critical solution temperature (LCST) or transition temperature at ~32°C.[4,5] Below the LCST, the hydrogel is swollen and above the LCST, the hydrogel will collapse (shrink). The change in physical state is rapid and reversible, which makes the thermo-sensitive hydrogel an attractive means of drug delivery. Figure 14.1 shows an image of PNIPAAm at room temperature and at body temperature (37°C). At room temperature, the hydrogel exists in a liquid gel-like phase; however, once the temperature is raised beyond its LCST, a solid gel is formed rapidly.

Based on its novel phase transition characteristics, thermo-sensitive hydrogel can be a potential drug delivery platform. The thermo-sensitive hydrogel can encapsulate various agents, including anti-vascular endothelial growth factor (VEGF), antibiotics, and steroids. In the past several years, considerable progress has been made in the treatment of the wet form of age-related macular degeneration and diabetic retinopathy by employing anti-VEGF therapy. While intravitreal anti-VEGF therapy is a very promising treatment, the major drawback is that the treatment must be repeated every 4–6 weeks. Currently, there is no alternative method for delivery of the anti-VEGF agent into the eye; hence, there is a great need and desire to develop a relatively noninvasive delivery method that is more effective and longer-lasting than the current clinical regimen. One possible application of thermo-sensitive hydrogel may be to deliver anti-VEGF agents to the posterior segment. This chapter will address a potential use of the thermo-sensitive hydrogel to deliver to the posterior segment.

CHARACTERISTICS OF THERMO-SENSITIVE HYDROGEL

PNIPAAm is by far the most prominent temperature-responsive hydrogel and can be a powerful drug delivery system.[6–10] However, a potential drawback of PNIPAAm hydrogel is the limited amount of drug released in response to a change in temperature. With a fast response to temperature stimuli, the drug can be released from the hydrogel quickly, and act as an on–off switching release system.[11] In order to address this limitation, several groups have proposed to use poly(ethylene glycol) (PEG) as a pore-forming agent to obtain macroporous PNIPAAm hydrogels.[12–16] PEG is an ideal polymer as it has unique biocompatibility and polymerization characteristics. It is soluble in water and is readily cleared by the body.[17] It can be immobilized either chemically or physically, it is highly resistant to protein adsorption and cell adhesion,[18,19] and it is not readily recognized by the immune system.[20,21] By incorporating PEG in the synthesis, Zhang and colleagues[12] have shown that crosslinked PNIPAAm hydrogels have a homogeneous structure. Zhang and Chu[16] also demonstrated that by introducing PEG diacrylate (PEG-DA) to PNIPAAm, it retained better thermo-sensitive characteristics of PNIPAAm with homogeneous pores. Acrylates are used as end groups because they undergo very rapid photopolymerization.[22] By incorporating PEG-DA with PNIPAAm in the polymerization process, a nondegradable formulation can be achieved.

Crosslinked thermo-sensitive hydrogels potentially offer a better controlled drug delivery system. Investigation was performed to examine whether the crosslinked system retained the thermo-sensitive characteristic of PNIPAAm.[23] Figure 14.2 shows the LCST of PNIPAAm alone and crosslinked thermo-sensitive hydrogels, where LCST was obtained by measuring the average absorbance of the hydrogel as a function of temperature. PNIPAAm alone hydrogel changed its phase (LCST) at ~31°C. Crosslinked hydrogel (PNIPAAm-PEG-DA) changed its phase at ~32°C. By crosslinking with PEG-DA, LCST was shifted by ~1°C due to the increased hydrophilicity[24]; however, the change in temperature is still within an optimal range of injection.

Crosslinked thermo-sensitive hydrogel also retained the swelling/deswelling characteristic of hydrogel. Figure 14.3 shows the equilibrium swelling measurement above and below the LCST. Three different crosslinked thermo-sensitive hydrogels with varying amount of crosslinker (PEG-DA) were used to examine the equilibrium swelling. The hydrogels were weighed before and after swelling to calculate the percentage mass ratio. As the data suggested, the crosslinked thermo-sensitive hydrogels exhibit temperature sensitivity as well as the ability to swell and deswell in response to temperature. This characteristic is important as deswelling (collapsing) of the hydrogel will provide an initial burst release of protein, which will be discussed later in this chapter.

DELIVERY CHARACTERISTICS

In order to release protein in a controlled manner, the pore size of the thermo-sensitive hydrogels becomes an important characteristic to consider. The pore size is one factor that can govern the release rate of the hydrogels and can be modified by the amount of crosslinker PEG-DA added to the system. In order to examine the thermo-sensitive hydrogel's ability to encapsulate and release protein, the effect of crosslink density on the protein release rate was investigated.[23] The protein release rate of thermo-sensitive hydrogel is governed by two factors:

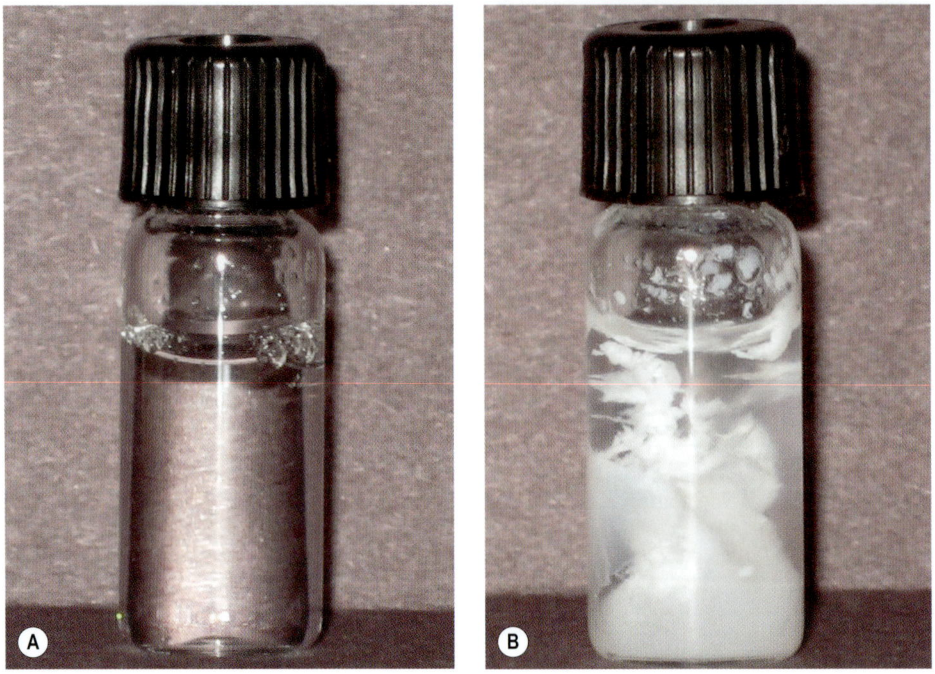

Figure 14.1 Images of crosslinked thermo-sensitive gels. A vial containing the hydrogel (A) at room temperature and (B) at 37°C. For illustration purpose, a high concentration of poly(*N*-isopropylacrylamide) (PNIPAAm) was used to produce the hydrogel. Proposed thermo-sensitive hydrogel is more transparent.

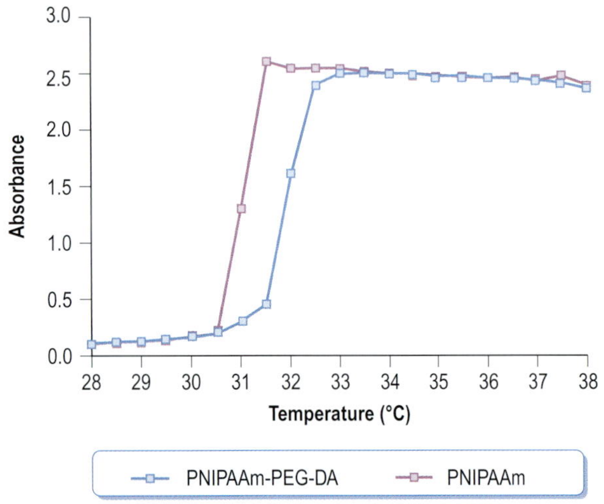

Figure 14.2 Lower critical solution temperature measurement of uncrosslinked hydrogel (pure poly(*N*-isopropylacrylamide) (PNIPAAm) hydrogel) and crosslinked thermo-sensitive hydrogels. PEG-DA, poly(ethylene glycol) diacrylate.

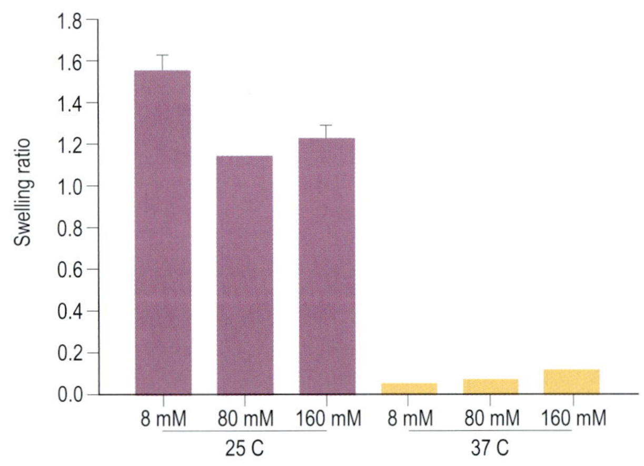

Figure 14.3 Equilibrium swelling ratios for three different crosslinked thermo-sensitive hydrogels at 25°C and 37°C. A ratio of poly(*N*-isopropylacrylamide) and poly(ethylene glycol) diacrylate was varied.

the initial release due to compression of the hydrogel in response to temperature and the pore size of the hydrogel. The initial compression due to change in temperature is difficult to control, though it is partially related to pore size. The pore size or crosslink density is easily controlled by varying the ratio of PNIPAAm and PEG-DA in the polymerization process. A higher PEG-DA concentration in the system yields a higher crosslink density and smaller pore size.

Kang Derwent and Mieler[23] examined two different fluorescently labeled proteins, bovine serum albumin (BSA, 66 kDa) and immunoglobulin G (IgG, 150 kDa) to examine the release rate characteristics of thermo-sensitive hydrogel. The rationale for using BSA and IgG is that their sizes are similar to ranibizumab (Lucentis) and bevacizumab (Avastin), respectively, and this is the key anticipated application of this drug delivery system. The different crosslink densities of thermo-sensitive hydrogel release profiles of BSA and IgG are seen in Figure 14.4. Immediately after temperature change, there was a burst of initial release of proteins, and then the rate of release reached a steady state. Lower crosslink density hydrogels (i.e., hydrogel labeled as 8 mM PEG-DA) released protein faster compared to the higher crosslink density hydrogels. In contrast, the more highly crosslinked hydrogels (i.e., hydrogel labeled as 360 mM PEG-DA) yielded smaller pore size and longer release times.

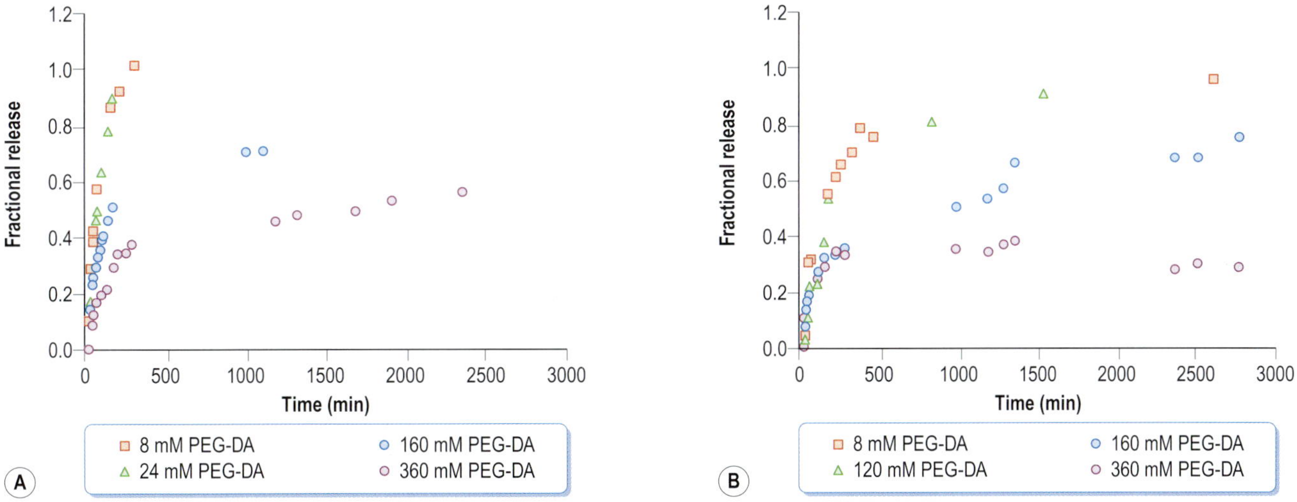

Figure 14.4 Effects of crosslink density on protein release. (A) Bovine serum albumin release profiles and (B) immunoglobulin G release profiles. Different symbols represent different crosslink density, where 8 mM poly(ethylene glycol) diacrylate (PEG-DA) has the lowest density of crosslinker and 360 mM PEG-DA has the highest density of crosslinker.

Figure 14.5 Injection of fluorescein isothiocyanate (FITC)-labeled thermo-responsive hydrogel in a rodent model. (A) Infrared image before the injection. (B) Fluorescein angiography image before the injection. (C) Fluorescein angiography image after the injection. A bright white spot indicates the FITC-labeled thermo-responsive hydrogel.

Even though smaller pore thermo-sensitive hydrogels offer a slower release rate, there is a disadvantage of small pores. If the pore size is small (i.e., there is a high amount of crosslinker in the hydrogel), the hydrogel becomes stiffer in composition. For example, thermo-sensitive hydrogels labeled as "160 mM or 360 mM PEG-DA" in Figure 14.4 were difficult to inject through small-gauge needles (e.g., 27–30-gauge needles) whereas "8 mM PEG-DA" thermo-sensitive hydrogel was able to be injected through small-gauge needles in a rodent model.[23] The inability to inject through small-gauge needles is an important design constraint as the goal is to develop a minimally invasive delivery system to the target sites such as the vitreous cavity or juxtascleral region. Kang Derwent and Mieler[23] have shown that ~8 μM PEG-DA is an optimal ratio of crosslinker in the system, as this offers both thermo-sensitivity as well as the ability to inject through small-gauge needles. These authors' work showed that BSA can be released rapidly during the first 48 hours and then slowly released to about 40% of total encapsulated BSA within 1 week. However, a significant amount of protein was still entrapped within the hydrogel when examined under a fluorescent microscope after 3 weeks. Based on their study, it seems that a significant amount of protein can be further released, if the pore size could be adjusted in a controlled manner. In order to achieve this, a current plan is to add additional copolymer which will slowly degrade, and further extend the delivery time frame. This work is currently in progress.

POTENTIAL DELIVERY SITE

Using the crosslink density proposed by Kang Derwent and Mieler,[23] approximately 3–5 μl of the fluorescein isothiocyanate (FITC)-labeled thermo-sensitive hydrogel was injected via a 30-gauge needle into the vitreous cavity of the adult rat to test if the thermo-sensitive hydrogel could be readily and safely placed there. The scanning laser ophthalmoscope (SLO) images of infrared reflectance and fluorecein angiography were then obtained before and immediately after the injection (Figure 14.5) and weekly for 2 months. Since the hydrogel was labeled with FITC, the hydrogel can be readily seen in the fluorescein angiography image. There was no other fluorescence emitted from any other location of retina, suggesting that the injection was localized. Furthermore, after 2 months, there was no movement of hydrogel location. Future study will include histology as well as evaluation of retinal cellular function via electroretinogram.

TOXICITY TESTING

Pure NIPAAM (unpolymerized form), particularly acrylamide, has been shown to be toxic in the nervous system.[25] However, there are a number of studies that have shown that PNIPAAm (polymerized form) is not toxic.[26,27] This is an important aspect as the application will involve interfacing of hydrogel with living tissue. In work by Kang Derwent and Mieler,[23] the potential toxicity of crosslinked thermo-sensitive hydrogels was examined in a cell culture model. The washes of the hydrogels after polymerization were tested for evidence of possible toxicity. The rationale was that the washes may contain unpolymerized PNIPAAm and other unreacted chemical components of the hydrogel. It is important to determine the number of washes that would be needed in order to prevent any possible toxic effects. Utilizing human umbilical vein endothelial cells (HUVECs), cells were maintained in growth factor supplement medium under standard tissue culture conditions for 3 days to approximately 80% confluence. Cells were then cultured in 0% serum for 24 hours before adding thermo-sensitive hydrogel washes and incubating cells for 48 hours. Growth response to samples was determined by incubating cells in Hank's balanced salt solution with MTS (3-(4,5-dimethylthiazol-2-yl)-5-(3-carboxymethoxyphenyl)-2-(4-sulfophenyl)-2*H*-tetrazolium, inner salt), a tetrazolium salt reduced by only living cells to form an insoluble formazan product. The plate was then incubated for 4 hours before reading at 570 nm in plate reader. Cells were counted and compared to the positive control (Figure 14.6). Compared to the control (20% fetal bovine serum), there was a significant decrease in cell count in response to the first wash of the hydrogel, suggesting that it may contain unpolymerized PNIPAAm or other chemicals which were toxic to the HUVECs. However, after the first wash, there was no significant difference between the second wash and the fifth wash compared to the control. The data suggest that in order to ensure that unpolymerized PNIPAAm is eliminated from the delivery system, multiple washes are needed. Furthermore, after multiple washing of the hydrogels, at least in an *in vitro* system, there is no toxic effect of the thermo-sensitive hydrogels. Further toxicity studies are planned utilizing both *in vitro* retinal cell model and *in vivo* rodent model.

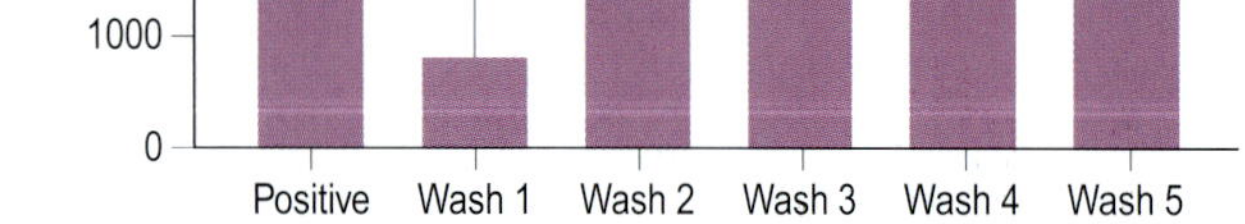

Figure 14.6 Toxicity test of the washes. After overnight polymerization, the hydrogels were washed five times with buffer. Each wash is then added to the cell culture system to test for toxicity. The cell counts from each wash are compared to the positive control. CPM, count per million.

FUTURE DIRECTION

An ideal prolonged drug delivery system would strive to achieve the following criteria: relatively noninvasive delivery method, high encapsulation efficiency of the drug, sustained release, high safety profile, and it should be easy to manufacture, use, and store. A controlled-release system is needed to overcome the complications associated with intravitreal injections. There are numerous advantages of an extended controlled-release system.[28,29] It will significantly decrease the frequency of treatments, and provide sustained and controlled release of drug over an extended period of time. It will also provide protection of the drug from inactivation and degradation, plus provide spatial treatment to localized tissues in the body.

The current investigation by Kang Derwent and colleagues (the current authors) showed that the thermo-sensitive hydrogel can encapsulate protein at a high rate, is nontoxic, and able to release protein for a short period of time. The initial burst of protein delivery governed by convective mass transport can be utilized to act as initial dose delivery. Then, a sustained level of drug will be delivered mainly due to diffusion mechanism. The current system has a limited duration of delivery time; however, when the hydrogels are examined after 3 weeks, a significant amount of protein is still entrapped within the hydrogel complex. The future direction would be to extend the release time and release the remaining protein from the hydrogel network. This could be achieved through the use of degradable crosslinkers. One proposed modification is to extend the central PEG block with oligomers of biocompatible α-hydroxy acids such as oligo(DL-lactic acid) or oligo(glycolic acid) and terminate the molecule with acrylate groups.[30] The degradation kinetics of the crosslinks could be controlled for slow, sustained release of the remaining protein.

SUMMARY AND KEY POINTS

One of the ideal biomaterials to design a localized, sustained-release drug delivery platform that can encapsulate and release anti-VEGF agents may be a thermo-sensitive hydrogel delivery system. Due to its thermo-sensitive characteristic, the hydrogel can be injected in a liquid form to the juxtascleral region or the vitreous cavity via a small-gauge needle. Once exposed to body temperature, the solution rapidly becomes a solid gel that releases the encapsulated protein, for example, anti-VEGF agent. The current investigation showed that the thermo-sensitive hydrogel can encapsulate protein at a high rate, is nontoxic, and is able to release protein for a limited period of time. Further work is required to extend the release time as well as making the system completely biodegradable. This review only discussed a possibility of utilizing thermo-sensitive hydrogel-based drug delivery system for the posterior segment of the eye. However, this hydrogel can be utilized for other ocular drug delivery sites as well as medical drug delivery.

REFERENCES

1. Hoffman AS. Hydrogels for biomedical applications. Adv Drug Deliv Rev 2002;43:3–12.
2. Kim SW, Bae YH, Okano T. Hydrogels: swelling, drug loading and release. Pharm Res 1992;9:283–290.
3. Lee KY, Mooney DJ. Hydrogels for tissue engineering. Chem Rev 2001;101:1869–1880.
4. Heskin M, Guillet JE. Solution properties of poly(N-isopropylacrylamide). J Macromol Sci 1968;2:1441–1455.
5. Dhara D, Chatterji PR. Phase transition in linear and crosslinked poly(N-isopropylacrylamide) in water: effect of various types of additives. J Macromol Sci Rev Macromol Chem Phys 2000;C40:51–68.
6. Shibayama M, Tanaka T. Volume phase transition and related phenomena of polymer gels. Adv Polym Sci 1993;109:1–62.
7. Peppas NA. Hydrogels and drug delivery. Curr Opin Colloid Interface Sci 1997;2:531–537.
8. Gehrke SH. Synthesis, equilibrium swelling, kinetics, permeability and applications of environmentally responsive gels. Adv Polym Sci 1993;110:81–143.

9. Wu XY, Pelton RH, Hamielec AE, et al. The kinetics of poly(N-isopropylacrylamide) microgel latex formation. Colloid Polym Sci 1994;272:467–477.
10. Moselhy J, Wu XY, Nicholov R, et al. *In vitro* studies of the interaction of poly(NIPAm/MAA) nanoparticles with proteins and cells. J Biomater Sci Polym Ed 2000;11:123–147.
11. Bae YH, Okano R, Hsu S, et al. Thermo-sensitive polymers as on-off switches for drug release. Makromol Chem Rapid Commun 1987;8: 481–485.
12. Zhang XZ, Yang YY, Chung TS, et al. Fabrication and characterization of fast response poly(N-isopropylacrylamide) hydrogels. Langmuir 2001;17:6094–6099.
13. Zhuo RX, Li W. Preparation and characterization of macroporous release of proteins. J Polym Sci Part A Polym Chem 2003;41:152–159.
14. Pratt AB, Weber FE, Schmoekel HG, et al. Synthetic extracellular matrixes for *in situ* tissue engineering. Biotechnol Bioeng 2004;86:27–36.
15. Raeber GP, Lutolf MP, Hubbell JA. Molecularly engineered PEG hydrogels: A novel model system for proteolytically mediated cell migration. Biophysl J 2005;89:1374–1388.
16. Zhang XZ, Chu CC. Fabrication and characterization of microgel-impregnated, thermosensitive PNIPAAm hydrogels. Polymer 2005;46:9664–9673.
17. Yamaoka T, Tabata Y, Ikada Y. Accumulation of water-soluble polymers to inflammatory site. Abstr Paper Am Chem Soc 1992;204:114–poly.
18. Allmer K, Hilborn J, Larsson PH, et al. Surface modification of polymers. V. Biomaterial applications. J Polym Sci Polym Chem Ed 1990;28:173–183.
19. Desai NP, Hubbell JA. Biological responses to polyethylene oxide modified polyethylene terephthalate surfaces. J Biomed Mater Res 1991;25:829–843.
20. Fuerteges F, Abuchowski A. The clinical efficacy of poly(ethylene glycol)-modified proteins. J Control Release 1990;11:139–148.
21. Yokoyama M, Okano R, Sakurai Y, et al. Toxicity and antitumor-activity against solid tumors of micelle-forming polymeric anticancer drug and its extremely long circulation in blood. Cancer Res 1991;51:3229–3236.
22. Valdes-Aguilera O, Pathak CP, Shi J, et al. Photopolymerization studies using visible light photoinitiators. Macromolecules 1992;25:541–547.
23. Kang Derwent JJ, Mieler WF. Thermo-responsive hydrogels as a new ocular drug delivery platform to the posterior segment of the eye. Trans Am Ophthalmol Soc 2008;106:206–213.
24. Weir MD, Antonucci JM, Wang FW. Rapid screening of the lower critical solution temperature of injectable hydrogels for tissue engineering applications. Transactions of the 28th Annual Meeting of the Society for Biomaterials 2002: abstract.
25. Hashimoto K, Sakamoto J, Tanji H. Neurotoxicity of acrylamide and related compounds and their effects on male gonads in mice. Arch Toxicol 1981;47:179–189.
26. Takezawa T, Mori Y, Yoshizato K. Cell culture of a thermo-responsive polymer surface. Bio/Technology 1990;8:854–856.
27. Malonne H, Eeckman F, Fontaine D, et al. Preparation of poly(N-isopropylacrylamide) copolymers and preliminary assessment of their acute and subactue toxicity in mice. Eur J Pharm Biopharm 2005;61:188–194.
28. Ghate D, Edelhause HF. Ocular drug delivery. Expert Opin Drug Deliv 2006;3:275–287.
29. Yasukawa T, Ogura Y, Kimura H, et al. Drug delivery from ocular implants. Expert Opin Drug Deliv 2006;3:261–273.
30. Sawhney AS, Pathak CP, Hubbell JA. Bioerodible hydrogels based on photopolymerized poly(ethylene glycol)-co-poly(α-hydroxy acid) diacrylate macromers. Macromolecules 1993;26:581–587.

CHAPTER 15

Retina and ocular toxicity to ocular application of drugs

Eduardo Büchele Rodrigues, MD, Fernando M. Penha, MD, PhD, Gustavo B. Melo, MD, Juliana Mantovani Bottós, MD, and Michel Eid Farah, MD

INTRODUCTION

The periocular and intraocular route of delivery have proved an effective way of providing therapeutic levels of drugs to the retina. Among the local routes for drug delivery, the intravitreal delivery of drugs remains the most important route for pharmacotherapy, as there has been an expanding repertoire of drugs available in the market. However, some disadvantages of intravitreal delivery of drugs and chemicals include the potential for complications from a surgically invasive procedure, short half-lives of many drugs, and risk of retinal toxicity.[1]

The intravitreal delivery of drugs to the retina should be primarily evaluated in terms of toxicity issues. A key step to evaluate preclinical retinal biocompatibility of a new drug for human therapy concerns cell culture and animal studies. Cell culture models with retinal pigment epithelial or neuroretinal cells, i.e., R28 cells, may allow systematic evaluation of drug toxicity in a controlled fashion. Preclinical toxicity studies in animals may be designed to expose a limited number of animals to the highest possible dose of a compound to determine potential toxic effects. In that method, visual electrophysiological techniques and histology examination may identify unwanted adverse effects of therapies of the posterior segment, thereby playing an important role in these early stages of drug development.[2]

Even with the availability of cell culture and electrophysiology tests, there have been problems in evaluating the safety of such drugs and compounds by the lack of a standard agreed-on methodology. Some pharmacologic agents are often off-label use of compounds that have been developed for systemic use, not as primary intraocular agents. With the expanding use of intraocular drugs there has been a long list of conflicting publications in the scientific literature about their safety, including clinical studies in patients, *in vivo* studies in animals, and *in vitro* studies. The multiple methods of evaluation of drugs or compounds to be used in the eye lead to much confusion about their toxicity. For example, in a cell culture system a chemical agent may be found to be safe at certain concentrations, while when *in vivo* evaluation systems have been used, specific signs of damage may arise. These observations may result from the complexity and difficulty of the intraocular milieu to replicate in a cell or tissue culture system. Moreover, some investigators have attributed different results of toxicity evaluation to factors unrelated to the drug or chemical, such as pH, osmolarity, or the preservative of the solution carrying the drug as well as interspecies variability in the preclinical evaluation of drug retinal toxicity.[3,4] In this chapter the retina toxicity issues of local ocular delivery of common drugs used for therapy of retinal diseases will be presented.

HISTORY

In 1911, Ohm first reported the technique of intravitreal injection to administer air for the repair of rhegmatogenous retinal detachment. The fear of harming the retina with intravitreal drug application hampered further developments and clinical use of such methods for several decades. However, later in the 1970s, intravitreal injections again arose as a common approach in the therapy of sight-threatening endophthalmitis. At this stage, the safety, clearance, and efficacy of various antibiotics such as aminoglycosides and cephalosporins were demonstrated using electrophysiology and histopathology on laboratory and clinical studies. In 1987, the first case report described benefit from delivery of ganciclovir sodium to a patient with cytomegalovirus retinitis secondary to acquired immunodeficiency syndrome (AIDS).[5] Later, in 1998, fomivirsen sodium (Vitravene) was licensed by the US Food and Drug Administration (FDA) by intravitreal injection in the treatment of cytomegalovirus retinitis. Further studies were performed in the 1980s and 1990s of intravitreal administration of 5-fluorouracil for patients with proliferative retinopathy, dexamethasone to diabetic retinopathy after vitrectomy, and tissue plasminogen activator for the management of submacular hemorrhage.[6,7] Although the safe dosages of 5-fluorouracil, dexamethasone, and tissue plasminogen activator have been found after numerous reports on animal experiments, only intravitreal injection of tissue plasminogen activator was considered safe and of benefit in those initial clinical studies.

ANIMAL TESTING FOR DRUG DELIVERY SAFETY

Assessing retinal drug toxicity with animal models has become increasingly important in retinal pharmacotherapy. Investigation of animal models using the standard tools of light microscopy and histopathological analysis are critical benchmarks for the study of development and disease. In animals, since behavioral assessment of visual function is not always easily obtained, the electroretinogram may be used to quantify possible functional damage of pharmacologic drugs.[8] When using animal models, one of the great limitations is the interspecies differences in retinal anatomy and physiology. For instance, the quantity and ratio of retinal cells including photoreceptor populations may vary from species to species and should be considered when designing the experiment protocol and for its interpretation. Also, most rodents used in toxicology are essentially nocturnal species, whereas the nonrodent species (e.g., dogs, pigs and monkeys) are usually diurnal.

The rat eye has become increasingly important as an animal model because its anatomy shows great similarities to the human eye.[9] The development and adult structure of the eye are similar in rodents and primates. However, the rodent retina is rod-dominant without a cone-rich macula; the electroretinogram and therapeutic mechanisms of the drugs in rodent model may be for instance different than the human retina.[10] On the other hand, in the mouse eye, their relative small size makes clinical and laboratory examination more challenging than for larger animals. However, useful genetic tools and resources as well as microimaging technologies have emerged to meet those needs in mouse research. In addition, the search for mouse models of ocular diseases has been productive, and experimental studies in mice are proving useful in understanding retinal toxicity mechanisms.[11]

The rabbit eye is a great animal model to study the pharmacokinetics and toxicity of drugs injected intravitreally into the eye. Toxicological studies to evaluate the effect on the retina of subretinal drug injection may also use the rabbits as animal model.[3] However, there are differences in the anatomy of the rabbit eye that have to be considered when extrapolating the results of this study to humans.[2] Compared with humans, the rabbit has a lower mean scleral thickness, higher choroidal flow rates, smaller vitreous cavity, and a poorer vascularized retina. The rabbit eye has lower volume and surface area for drug clearance: the volume of the human eye is 3.9 ml compared with the rabbit's eye of 1.5 ml. Furthermore, albino rabbits are preferred over pigmented animals because ocular pigmentation may protect against the toxic effects of the drug. On an ultrastructural level retinal layers in normal rabbits present reasonable degree of vacuolization which may impair analysis of retina toxicity to drugs. Nevertheless, rabbits are the most commonly applied animal model to study retinal toxicity of drugs for intravitreal injection.[12]

The cat has served as an important research model for neurophysiology and retinal degenerative disease processes. In addition, felines may also be useful for the study of retinal toxic reactions after intravitreal injections of drugs such as human recombinant tissue-type plasminogen activator in the management of subretinal hemorrhage.[13] Anatomically, some diameters of intraocular structures in cats may be similar to those of humans. Their vitreous volume is quite similar to that of human eyes, whereas the transverse and anteroposterior diameters of the globe are around 22.30 mm. The transverse diameter of the cornea averages 16 mm. The volume of the anterior chamber varies from 0.8 to 1.0 ml, and the depth of the anterior chamber is very large, around 4.5 mm. Some recognized characteristics of the cat eye are a considerably larger lens than humans. Also, the vascular supply in the cat eye is different from that of human eyes: there is no central retinal artery and cats have a vascularized inner retina. The single medial and lateral long posterior ciliary arteries pass around the globe within the sclera to form a large vascularized plexus in the pars plana region with the anterior ciliary arteries. The ora ciliaris retina, corresponding to ora serrata in humans, is approximately 6 mm behind the limbus in the cat eye. The large vessels of the plexus can be seen through the sclera, and in attempts to avoid these vessels, the sclerotomies of pars plana vitrectomy should be done as far posterior as possible.[14]

The pig eye may also be a good model for toxicology study because the size and anatomy are similar to those of the human eye.[15] There has been interest in evaluating the suitability of the pig as a model of ocular diseases, since it is phylogenetically close to the human and is much more available, cheaper, and less ethically barren than the monkey. The porcine retina is even more similar to the human retina than that of other large mammals such as the dog or cow. Some examples of similarities in anatomical and histological characteristics of pigs in comparison to humans include nontapetal fundus with a holangiotic vascular pattern and retinal layers of similar thickness. The pig retina has four main arteriovenous branches that arborize to the retinal periphery. Unlike human eyes, these vessels do not typically form a single central artery and vein before reaching the lamina cribrosa, making the pig eye a poor disease model for central retinal vein occlusion. With the conceptions of the lack of a fovea, the porcine retina shares some significant similarities within the photoreceptor mosaic of humans and other primates. Otherwise, the porcine optic nerve structure is similar to that of a human, containing a prominent lamina cribrosa, as well as the retinal blood vessels and vascular supply. Additionally, tools employed for diagnostics in ophthalmology, such as optical coherence tomography, corneal topography imaging, or multifocal electroretinography can easily be applied to the pig eye.

The macula can only be found in primates and birds, and the animal model for macular degeneration and macular toxicity is therefore mostly limited to monkeys. The size and macroscopic eye measurements of primate eyes depend on the species of primate; some species like common marmoset monkeys (*Callithrix jacchus*) exhibit very small ocular dimensions which may impair surgical techniques for investigation in local drug therapy. In the retina ultrastructure some differences among primates' eyes include density and distribution of mitochondria, as well as the complexity of on/off cones. Overall, cynomolgus monkeys (*Macaca fascicularis*) and rhesus macaque (*Macaca mulatta*) have been competently used to analyze the safety and efficacy of intravitreal injection of drugs and chemical compounds for various decades.[2]

MAJOR CLASSES OF DRUGS AND THEIR SAFETY PROFILE AFTER LOCAL OCULAR APPLICATION FOR RETINA THERAPY

CORTICOSTEROIDS

Corticosteroids are powerful drugs widely used in ophthalmology, including in the therapy of retinal diseases. In the past two decades much research has been performed to evaluate the indications of various types of steroids for vitreoretinal diseases. However, beyond efficacy, one of the most important issues for the application of corticosteroids is finding the limitation of their side-effects.

Fluocinolone acetonide is a synthetic corticosteroid with low solubility in aqueous solution. Experiments in rabbits provided the preclinical toxicity profile of fluocinolone to the retina. Clinical examination, electroretinography, or histologic examination determined the safety of both 2 and 15 mg synthetic fluocinolone acetonide in one preclinical study. Neither electroretinographic alterations nor histology alterations were observed in this *in vivo* investigation. However, further clinical experience with implants containing 2 or 6 mg fluocinolone acetonide for therapy of uveitis revealed that a considerable amount of patients do experience complications, which include glaucoma, cataract, and retinal vein occlusion.[16]

A series of contradicting studies have recently been published regarding retinal toxicity after intravitreal triamcinolone acetonide injection. On the one hand, in various experiments intravitreal injection of 4, 16, 20, or 30 mg triamcinolone acetonide promoted normal histological and electroretinographic retinal findings after 7 months. In contrast, in one investigation the authors injected escalating doses from 0.5 to 20 mg of suspended preservative-free triamcinolone acetonide in rabbits, and found at doses 4 mg or higher prominent retinal damage manifested by destruction of photoreceptor outer segments and retinal pigment epithelium/photoreceptor interdigitation.[17] Only a few studies have thus far addressed the subretinal toxicity of triamcinolone acetonide: in one investigation the researchers examined subretinal injection of 3 mg/ml triamcinolone acetonide in primate eyes and described neither ultrastructural nor cellular retinal damage, but Maia et al. in a morphologic study disclosed disturbance to photoreceptor segments after subretinal injection of preservative-free triamcinolone acetonide, although no clinical abnormality on fundoscopy or angiography examination was observed.[18] These opposite findings suggest that other factors may contribute to intravitreal retinal toxicity of triamcinolone acetonide (Figure 15.1).

Much controversy exists in animal studies whether triamcinolone acetonide itself or the vehicle plays the most significant role in retinal damage. Some colleagues demonstrated severe damage to photoreceptor only in a group with triamcinolone acetonide with vehicle compared with preservative-free triamcinolone acetonide. In contrast to these results, other authors revealed a safer profile of the vehicle only; they reported normal retinal structure after intravitreal injection of vehicle only in rabbits.[17,18] It is also unclear which chemical element from the vehicle solution of triamcinolone acetonide may induce retinal injury, although research so far has focused only on the organic colorless preservative benzyl alcohol. Other than benzyl alcohol, the vehicle of commercially available triamcinolone acetonide contains a second preservative named polysorbate at 0.4 mg/ml. Future studies should elucidate the safety of triamcinolone acetonide vehicle and whether benzyl alcohol, polysorbate, sodium carboxymethycellulose, or other factors such as pH or osmolarity pose the higher risk to the retina.

Clinical experience in recent years unraveled the risks of patients injected with intravitreal or periocular triamcinolone acetonide. The two most frequent complications are cataract and glaucoma, which in most patients can be managed by surgery and topical eye drops. Much less common complications are endophthalmitis and pseudoendophthalmitis, encountered in around 0.5% of patients.

Dexamethasone is a synthetic glucocorticoid class of steroid hormones with potent anti-inflammatory and immunosuppressant activities. In a classic work performed by Kwak and D'Amico, the authors

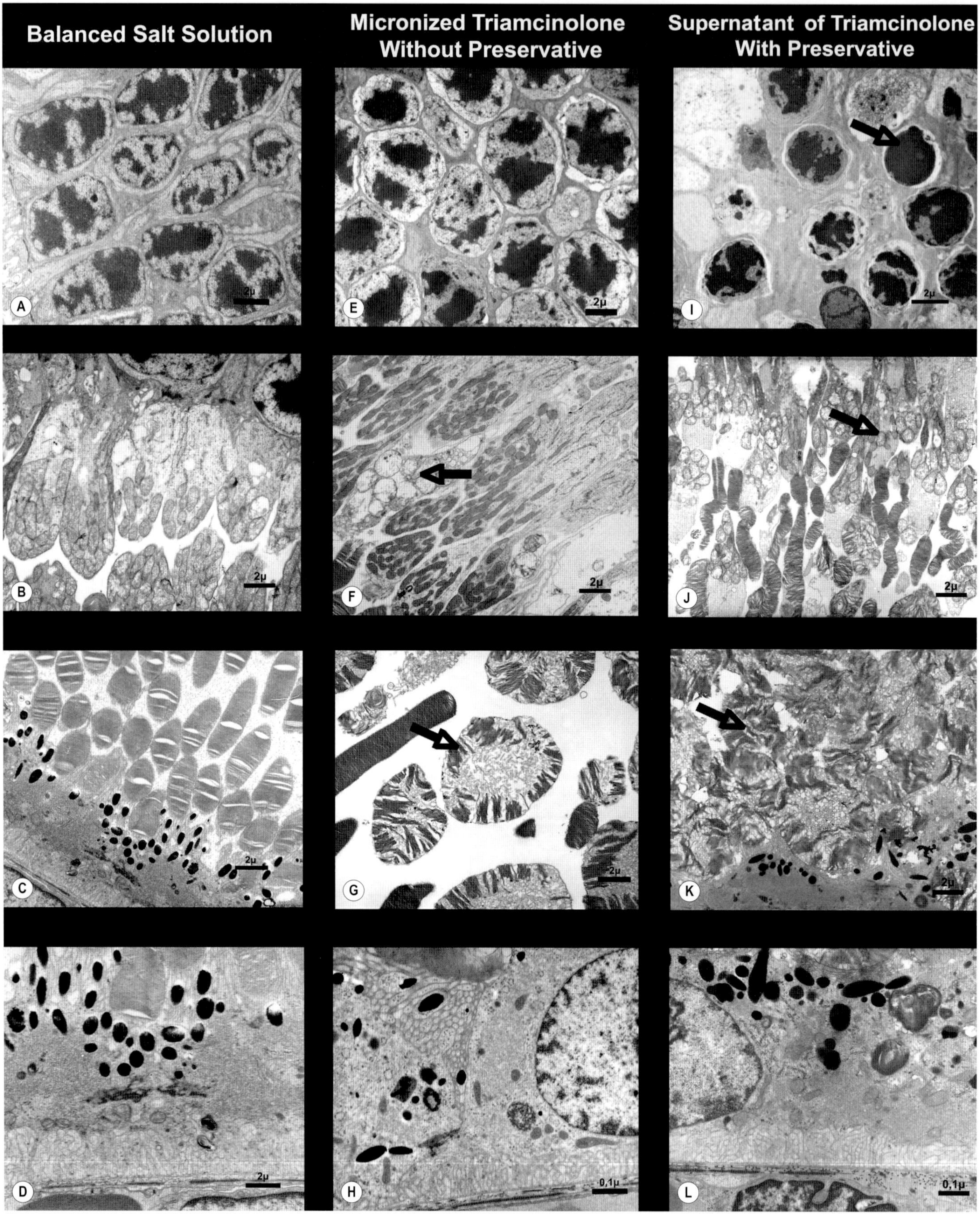

Figure 15.1 After subretinal injection of control, preservative-free triamcinolone, and triamcinolone with preservative, different types of retinal cells manifest various signs of damage. The damage induced by the preservative is more severe in neuroretinal posterior cells than that caused by the drug itself.

evaluated the retina toxicity of dose ranging from 440 to 4000 mg dexamethasone in rabbit eyes. Their study found that, at 440 μg dose, only a transient increase in staining of the Müller cells was observed, which normalized after 2 days.[19] However, recent research in cell culture agreed with these previous works, as they found that a higher dose of 800 μg dexamethasone promoted the reduction of the number of retinal cells. Those experimental works provided the basis for the safety profile of dexamethasone in humans; however future studies should determine whether the dose of 400 or 800 μg is safer in the therapy of edematous, proliferative, and neovascular retinal diseases.

ANTIBIOTICS

The most common application of antibiotics in retina therapy refers to infectious endophthalmitis and uveitis. Postoperative endophthalmitis following cataract surgery is the main indication of intravitreal injection of antibiotics, even though in many cases there may not be knowledge of the microorganisms responsible for the infection. Posterior-segment viral uveitis is usually treated with systemic or intravitreal injections of aciclovir, valaciclovir, and ganciclovir. Every intravitreally injected antibiotic drug might potentially lead to retinal toxicity, which will be addressed in further detail. Table 15.1 summarizes the safe doses of antibiotics when applied locally.

Amikacin used to be one of the most commonly used agents in the treatment of endophthalmitis in the past. Nowadays, it is well known that the aminoglycosides may pose a high risk of toxic effects to the retina. *In vitro* studies with isolated retinas showed that the b-wave of the electroretinography has been reduced in amplitude in the presence of low-dose (1 mg/ml) and completely eliminated by high-dose gentamicin (10 mg/ml). In *in vivo* electroretinographic studies in animals, intraocular administration of gentamicin eliminated the b-wave and reduced the c-wave amplitude. Histopathologic evaluation demonstrated diffuse disruption of the nerve fiber layer and the inner plexiform layers in eyes exposed to the strong aminoglycoside antibiotic. Regarding amikacin, an animal study disclosed retinal toxicity manifested by macrophages in the subretinal space, disorganization of the outer segments and retinal pigment epithelium, and discontinuities in Bruch's membrane after repeated intravitreal injection of 400 μg amikacin. Further experience demonstrated that repetitive injections in nonvitrectomized eyes may result in increasing retina toxicity. Later on, many cases of macular infarction after intravitreal injection of aminoglycosides as amikacin have been reported in humans.[20] This has led ophthalmologists to search for other Gram-negative targeted antibiotics for routine intravitreal injections (Figure 15.2).

Ceftazidime, a third-generation cephalosporin, emerged as a good alternative to aminoglycosides for the treatment of endophthalmitis. An

Table 15.1 Safe doses: concentrations of locally applied antibiotics for intraocular injections

Drug	Topical	Subconjunctival	Intravitreal
Amikacin	10 mg/ml	25 mg	400 μg
Cefazolin	50 mg/ml	100 mg	2250 μg
Ceftazidime	50 mg/ml	100 mg	2000 μg
Ceftriaxone	50 mg/ml	–	–
Clindamycin	50 mg/ml	15–50 mg	1000 μg
Gentamicin	8–15 mg/ml	10–20 mg	100–200 μg
Imipenem	5 mg/ml	–	–
Penicillin G	100 000 U/ml	0.5–1 million units	300 units
Piperacillin	12.5 ng/ml	100 mg	–
Tobramycin	8–15 mg/ml	10–20 mg	–
Vancomycin	20–25 mg/ml	25 mg	1000 μg

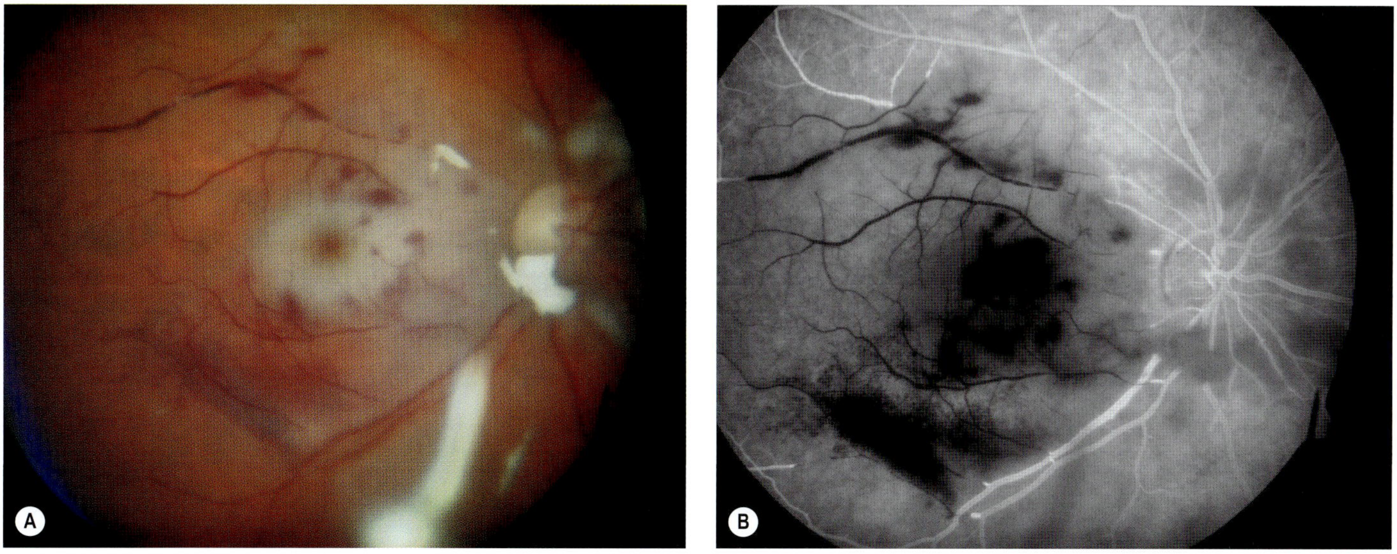

Figure 15.2 (A) Red-free fundus picture showing extensive damage of neurosensorial retina and its vasculature as well as whitening and hemorrhages of the posterior pole after intravitreous injection of gentamicin. (Courtesy of Harry Flynn.) (B) Fluorescein angiography demonstrating signs of vasculitis, vascular occlusion, and capillary nonperfusion after intravitreous injection of gentamicin.

in vivo animal study with monkeys showed no toxicity at the commonly used concentration of 2.25 mg ceftazidine, but others showed that ceftazidime may not be toxic in vitrectomized rabbit eyes.[21] However, it appears that the cephalosporin may cause some degree of toxicity at otherwise nontoxic concentrations in a silicone-filled eye. Based on those preliminary data, surgeons have applied ceftazidime intravitreally in doses up to 2.25 mg for the therapy of endophthalmitis.

Vancomycin remains the antibiotic of choice targeting highly pathogenic Gram-positive microorganisms, usually applied in patients intravitreally in the dose of 1 mg in 0.1 ml. *In vivo* animal studies have shown no toxic effect of this antibiotic when used in an infusion solution that was given intraocularly after or during vitrectomy in rabbit. However, in a silicone-filled eye, nontoxic concentrations of vancomycin may cause toxicity, so vitreous status should be evaluated when vancomycin is the antibiotic of choice as well. In the clinical practice, vancomycin has been associated with postoperative cystoid macular edema when infused as intracameral injection for prophylaxis during cataract surgery.

The ocular toxicity of another class of antibiotics, the quinolones, has been investigated in the recent past. Intravitreal injection of ciprofloxacin has not been associated with toxicity at therapeutic levels of 100–500 μg in rabbits, and significant retina damage has been present only at 2 mg.[22] The fourth-generation quinolones, which include moxifloxacin and gatifloxacin, have had greater attention for clinical use. An *in vitro* study showed that, at concentrations higher than 160 μg/ml, moxifloxacin induced adverse effects on primary retinal pigment epithelium and neuronal retinal cell proliferation and viability. Further studies *in vivo* showed that intravitreal injection of moxifloxacin did not cause retinal toxicity up to 100 μg/ml in mice or 150 μg in rabbits.[23] *In vivo*, intravitreal injection of the other quinolone, gatifloxacin, at doses varying from 50 to 400 μg caused no retinal toxicity assessed clinically and microscopically in rabbits. Clinical experience on retina toxicity studies revealed that the current recommended dose for intracameral injection of ciprofloxacin is less than 25 μg. In humans intravitreal injections of ciprofloxacin 100 μg, ofloxacin 50 μg/ml, trovafloxacin 25 μg or less, moxifloxacin 160 μg/0.1 ml or less, and pefloxacin 200 μg/0.1 ml are considered nontoxic to the retina and intraocular structures.[24]

Fungal infections are difficult-to-treat causes of endophthalmitis. Amphotericin B has traditionally been used for treatment, either systemically or intravitreally, usually injected at doses varying from 1 to 50 μg. In one study with application of escalating doses from 10, 20, 30, and 50 μg, the three higher doses of amphotericin B appeared to be associated with stronger degrees of retina toxicity.[25] Based on the animal experiments, intravitreal amphotericin B in doses of 5 or 10 μg remains an appropriate therapeutic option for patients with severe fungal injection, for instance secondary to *Aspergillus*.

An alternative to amphotericin is the use of intravitreal fluconazole. An *in vitro* study showed no toxicity at a 20 μg/ml exposure to fluconazole. Further animal data revealed no retinal toxicity resulting from vitrectomy with a 2 mg/ml fluconazole infusion in an experimental model of candidal endophthalmitis. For a single intravitreal injection fluconazole at a concentration of 100 μg and above caused harmful retinal changes with disorganization of the photoreceptor outer segments. Clinical experience revealed that intravitreal injection of 10 μg/0.1 ml fluconazole may be the safe dosage for intraocular fungi injection.[25]

For the therapy of cytomegalovirus infections ganciclovir is a commonly used antiviral medication. Ganciclovir dosages of up to 200 μg/0.1 ml appear to be safe for serial intravitreal injections in rabbit eyes following vitrectomy and silicone oil insertion. In unvitrectomized eyes ganciclovir in doses above 300 μg induced severe morphologic retinal damage, although at lower doses of 200 μg ganciclovir promoted only small functional damage characterized by changes on electroretinography b-wave in rabbits. Similar to other types of antibiotics, ganciclovir also induced sporadic cases of macular infarction in patients. A case report of inadvertent intravitreal injection of a high dose of ganciclovir (40 mg/0.1 ml) for cytomegalovirus retinitis in a patient with AIDS led to permanent retinal damage and visual loss.[26] Currently ganciclovir has been injected with consecutive intravitreal injections in doses varying from 400 μg to 4 mg for therapy of intraocular viral infections.

MONOCLONAL ANTIBODIES AND FRAGMENTS

The two anti-vascular endothelial growth factor (VEGF) monoclonal antibodies (mAbs), bevacizumab (Avastin, Genentech), and ranibizumab (Lucentis, Genentech), were shown to promote clinical control of ocular neovascularization in the last few years. Although endovenous administration of anti-VEGF mAbs has demonstrated acceptable toxicity profile, their intraocular injection has decreased the risk of systemic complications. In addition, intravitreal injection of anti-VEGF agents may increase the amount of drug available to intraocular tissues such as the retina.

In vitro cellular assays exposed to various concentrations of bevacizumab (0.08 μg/ml to 1 mg/ml) have shown little toxic effects to neuronal cells like the ganglion cells, neuroretinal cells, as well as retinal pigment epithelial cells. To study the effects of bevacizumab on various types of retinal cells, one investigation exposed cultured adult porcine neurosensory retinas joined to the retinal pigment epithelial/choroid layer to three doses of bevacizumab (0.25, 0.5, and 1.25 mg/ml) for 3 days. Their results showed no toxic effects on ganglion or photoreceptor cells observed at any concentration of bevacizumab. However, they observed significantly enhanced smooth-muscle actin expression in retina blood vessels in the presence of bevacizumab, which may imply a loss of smooth-cell modulation in normal retinal vessels by VEGF.[27] In contrast to those data, others found no toxicity to microvascular retinal cells *in vitro* after their exposure to 0.125, 0.25, 0.50, and 1 mg/ml of bevacizumab for up to 24 hours.

A large body of animal studies has been released about the biocompatibility and safety of bevacizumab and ranibizumab for ophthalmology. Consecutive experimental investigation in rats, rabbits, and primates revealed that intravitreal bevacizumab at various concentrations up to 3 mg/ml demonstrated no functional or morphologic toxicity to the retina.[28] However, a few recent experimental publications demonstrated some signs of retinal damage after intravitreal bevacizumab. In primates, intravitreal bevacizumab application induced choriocapillaris abnormalities manifested by reduced choriocapillaris endothelial cell fenestrations by densely packed thrombocytes and leukocytes within the vascular lumen. Moreover, Manzano et al. reported signs of ocular inflammation after intravitreal injection of high-dose bevacizumab at 5 mg in rabbits' eyes.[28] Also in rabbits, intravitreal 1.25 mg or 3 mg bevacizumab has caused both mitochondrial changes in the inner segments of photoreceptors and intensive apoptotic protein expression of bax and caspase on immunohistochemistry in comparison to control, although on light microscopy and electroretinographic examination no signs of toxicity were detected. The clinical relevance of such apoptotic retinal findings is yet to be clarified. The preclinical safety of ranibizumab has been evaluated in primate eyes, 0.5 mg injection of the monoclonal antibody fragment promoted reduced leakage from choroidal neovascularization whereas no signs of retinal toxicity have been encountered.

Intraocular bevacizumab and ranibizumab injection has promoted few clinically relevant ocular side-effects to date. In contrast to the crystalline steroid drug triamcinolone acetonide, intravitreal bevacizumab has not been shown to induce glaucoma or cataract progression. Further clinical experience with intravitreal bevacizumab revealed few sporadic cases of uveitis, vitreous hemorrhage, retinal pigment epithelium tears, or endophthalmitis.[29]

Clinically Rosenfeld et al. suggested the maximum tolerated dose of ranibizumab is 0.5 mg, as higher doses above 1 mg promoted clinically relevant intraocular inflammation.[30] Additional clinical investigation disclosed that intravitreal ranibizumab has induced few severe complications such as endophthalmitis, uveitis, vitreitis in the fellow eye, while minor reported ocular events were conjunctival bleeding, eye pain, and floaters. In 2008 a head-to-head comparison of ranibizumab versus bevacizumab to treat advanced age-related macular degeneration funded by the National Eye Institute started, and this should clarify

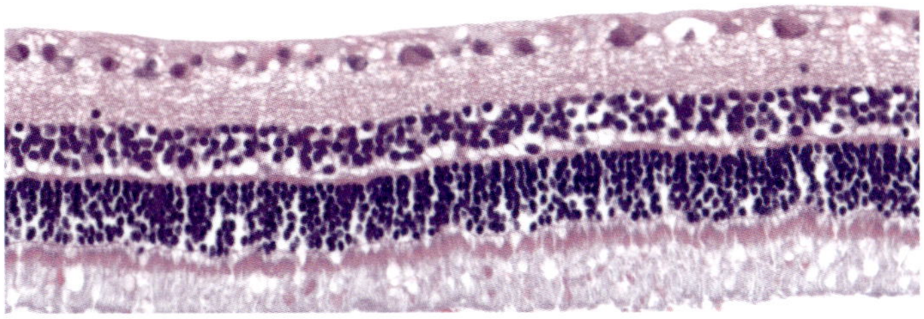

Figure 15.3 A 20× hematoxylin and eosin histopathologic section from rabbit eye injected with 0.5 mg adalimumab showing normal retina histology. (Courtesy of RP Manzano and GA Peyman.)

the safety issue differences between the two monoclonal antibodies (http://www.nei.nih.gov/news/statements/amd_therapy.asp).

Three antitumor necrosis factor agents, infliximab, etanercept, and adalimumab, have been shown to promote clinical control of uveitis and other inflammatory eye diseases. Although infliximab and etanercept have been mainly applied as systemic administration, in the future antitumor necrosis factor monoclonal antibodies may be used intraocularly for the management of severe intraocular inflammatory and angiogenic diseases. Intravitreal injections of infliximab in concentrations lower than or equal to 1.7 mg have been shown to be safe to the retinal tissue in preliminary animal studies, although future detailed research should elucidate the intraocular safety and pharmacokinetics of infliximab and its vehicle.[31]

The pharmacokinetics and safety of intravitreal etanercept delivery in concentration of 100 μg have been investigated in rabbits in one study. Clinical examination, and electroretinography and histology examination revealed no evidence of toxicity and peak retinal concentrations at 4 weeks and still detectable in 8 weeks. Another investigation on the intraocular safety of different doses of etanercept revealed that the antimonoclonal antibodies in doses up to 2.5 mg have promoted no retinal damage.[32] Recent research demonstrated the safety profile of intravitreal injections of various doses of adalimumab in rabbits. Their results showed normal retinal examination in eyes having received saline solution, 0.25 or 0.5 mg adalimumab; however 1 mg adalimumab injection induced inflammatory changes, retinal histopathologic alterations, and significant electroretinographic reduction. In summary, most studies suggest a dose-dependent retina toxicity profile of intravitreal antitumor necrosis factor monoclonal antibodies and further evaluation should unravel the exact safe dosage for each drug (Figure 15.3).

Few additional MAbs such as rituximab, daclizumab, efalizumab, and alemtuzumab showed positive results in animal and early clinical studies, and may represent useful adjuvant therapies for ocular lymphoma or ocular inflammation. Rituximab (Rituxan, Genentech) is the chimeric MAb anti-CD20 antigen approved by the FDA as subcutaneous infusion for patients with recurrent low-grade B-cell lymphoma. A small clinical series revealed rituximab to be an effective treatment for patients with refractory scleritis, orbital inflammation, intraocular and extraocular lymphoma. The intravitreal injection of rituximab in concentrations up to 1 mg induced neither retinal damage in rabbits nor clinical signs of toxicity in a small series of 5 patients.[33] Comprehension of intraocular safety of rituximab may enable intravitreal injection for therapy of uveal/oculocerebral lymphoma and uveitis.

NONSTEROIDAL ANTI-INFLAMMATORY DRUGS

Nonsteroidal anti-inflammatory drugs have cystoid macular edema as their main indication for retina therapy. They may be used either systemically or topically, and topical ketorolac, diclofenac, and nepafenac are used more frequently. The use of both diclofenac and ketorolac intravitreal injections has been assessed in rabbits. Diclofenac formulated in hyaluronan was toxic to the retina at doses equal to or above 540 μg, as evidenced by indirect ophthalmoscopy, and light and electron microscopy.[34] Electroretinography showed no toxic signs of intravitreal injection of 400 μg of this formulation after 25 days. Another study showed no signs of toxicity, either electroretinographically or histologically, of intravitreal injections of up to 300 μg of diclofenac and 3000 μg of ketorolac after 8 weeks.[35] Preservative-free ophthalmic solution of 0.25% or 0.5% (500 μg) ketorolac tromethamine in 0.1 ml was nontoxic to the retina in animals when assessed up to 4 weeks after injection, as shown by microscopic and electroretinographic evaluation. However, intravitreal use of nonsteroidal anti-inflammatory drugs has not been assessed in depth in humans to date. Unlike corticosteroids, the nonsteroidal anti-inflammatory drugs may not be associated with intraocular pressure rise.

ENZYMES AND FIBRINOLYTICS

Pharmacologic vitreolysis refers to the capacity of altering the molecular organization of the vitreous to achieve posterior vitreous detachment induction and liquefaction. Some agents investigated include tissue plasminogen activator, plasmin, microplasmin, and hyaluronidase. In both rabbits and cats injected with tissue plasminogen activator (doses from 50 to 100 μg), in some animals mild to severe vitreous inflammation with or without vitreous strands has been observed. Reduced scotopic A-waves and B-waves on electroretinography, diffuse pigment alterations, severe photoreceptor losses coupled with retinal pigment epithelium necrosis, and proliferation with pigment clumping have been documented. The clinical experience available points out that doses of 25–50 μg of intravitreal tissue plasminogen activator injection may be safe to the retina.

Pharmacologic vitreolysis with this agent may be a useful adjunct to vitreous surgery and could be used to induce posterior vitreous detachment without vitreous surgery. In animals plasmin (1–4 IU) has been found overall safe, except for intraocular inflammation and transient electroretinography reduction. Clinical experience showed that the safety profile of human plasmin is not easy to determine due to the variable amount of enzyme activity obtained from fresh autologous plasma. Intravitreal injection of recombinant microplasmin in doses from 12.5 to 250 μg in the rabbit induces no electroretinography or retinal ultrastructural abnormalities. ThromboGenics (Euronext Brussels), a biotechnology company focused on vascular disease, announced recently the results of the Microplasmin in Vitrectomy (MIVI-I) phase IIa trial, which covered 60 patients. Preliminary results available for all patients through 28 days after vitrectomy revealed that microplasmin was generally well tolerated, even up to the highest dose tested (125 μg).[36]

Hyaluronidase cleaves the glycosidic bonds of hyaluronan as well as other mucopolysaccharides, resulting in dissolution of the hyaluronan and collagen complex and subsequent vitreous liquefaction. Intravitreal injection of hyaluronidase in doses of 20 IU or less does not appear to affect the biomicroscopic morphology or function of ocular structures adversely in preclinical investigation in rabbits. A preservative-free, highly purified ovine hyaluronidase formulation (Vitrase, Ista Pharmaceuticals) has been evaluated in phase III clinical trials. Patients were randomized in a 1:1:1 ratio to intravitreal injection with saline, 55 IU hyaluronidase, and 75 IU hyaluronidase in a 50-ml volume. Overall, intravitreal application of hyaluronidase was well tolerated; dose-dependent iritis was the most common adverse event, occurring in 62% of eyes treated with 55 IU and in 59% of eyes treated with 75 IU. The iritis was often self-limited and did not result in a serious adverse event in any hyaluronidase-treated eye.[36]

MISCELLANEOUS ANTI-INFLAMMATORY AND ANTIANGIOGENIC AGENTS

Some forms of drugs are characterized by a wide variety of actions due to the complex chemical structure and receptor affinity. Two examples of such drugs are thalidomide and methotrexate and thalidomide. Thalidomide is a glutamic acid derivative with proven efficacy in animal models of retinal ischemia, retinal neovascularization, uveitis, and diabetic retinopathy. On the other hand, methotrexate is an antimetabolite and antifolate drug used in the treatment of cancer and autoimmune diseases. Due to its large variety of effects, the agent could be applied in a large variety of ophthalmic diseases; however, so far methotrexate may be indicated mainly in the therapy of primary intraocular lymphoma as routine therapy.

Few consecutive researchers investigated the safety of methotrexate in animals. As early as in 1985, it has been shown that 600 µg methotrexate added to other chemotherapeutic agents such as doxorubicin, 5-fluorouracil, and bleomycin enhanced the risk of retina toxicity. However, in one recent study, the ocular pharmacokinetics and retinal toxicity of intravitreal methotrexate sodium at 400 µg were studied in New Zealand white rabbits.[37] This research group reported that intravitreal methotrexate, combined with fluorouracil and dexamethasone, showed no evidence of retina toxicity determined by electroretinography and histologic examination. Frenkel et al. released their 10-year experience with frequent intravitreal injection of 400 µg/0.1 ml methotrexate. The effective agent rarely induced adverse reactions, the most common being self-limited corneal epitheliopathy, while the vitreoretinal involvement of lymphoma can be controlled effectively.[38] In another retrospective case series, complications that occurred during the period of treatment with intravitreal methotrexate included cataract (73%), corneal epitheliopathy (58%), maculopathy (42%), vitreous hemorrhage (8%), and optic atrophy (4%). However, no patient had irreversible loss of vision that could be definitely attributed to the intravitreal injection of methotrexate. Overall, the intravitreal use of methotrexate in dose up to 400 µg seems to be a safe approach in clinical practice. Although no preclinical investigation has been performed to investigate the retinal biocompatibility of thalidomide for local ocular application, one case report demonstrated corneal endothelium toxicity after oral use of the powerful agent.[39]

SUMMARY AND KEY POINTS

Ocular toxicity caused by the exposure of the retinal tissue to a high concentration of drug for a certain period of time remains an important topic in the approach of intravitreal injection in the therapy of retinal diseases. In the evaluation of drug safety for retinal pharmacotherapy, both exposure concentration and exposure time can be important, but the toxic effect may also be directly related to the transient drug distribution inside the vitreous body. The retina is subject to the risk of drug-induced toxicities owing to its rich blood supply, complex well-organized neuroretinal organization, and lifelong exposure to focused light rays. To enable its physiological functions in the risk of harming, the retina is protected by specific defense mechanisms including the endogenous detoxifying system cytochrome p450 and the blood–retinal barrier. An understanding of these cellular and molecular principles is a key aspect in elucidating the pathological pathways leading to retinotoxicity.

Currently, there are several approved drugs for intravitreal use, such as ranibizumab (Lucentis, Genentech) and pegaptanib (Macugen, Pfizer). However, there are numerous off-label uses of drugs and substances injected in the eye, but the scientific literature remains confusing with regard to intraocular properties and toxicology of off-label drugs such as commercial triamcinolone, antibiotics, antivirals, and tissue plasminogen activator.

Due to the difficulties in evaluating the toxic effect of drugs in the human eye, animal data such as rabbit experiments are used by ophthalmologists as a guideline for designing an administration regime. The toxic level of drug is established by making histologic slides of eye tissues and observing morphologic changes of retinal tissue. In addition, visual electrophysiological recordings, performed at single-cell, tissue, whole-animal, and human patient levels, can provide important information at various stages in the development of new drugs. The evolution of electrophysiological techniques permits them to be used to conduct studies that follow the standards required for good laboratory practice. An expanding number of laboratories are using these procedures and are consequently acquiring the expertise necessary to establish procedures that follow these standards. Regulatory institutions may play a role in the evaluation of preclinical drug safety. Progresses on standardized methods and conditions to evaluate such drugs are an important topic in retinal pharmacotherapy. In the future, such advances in ocular toxicity methods will have a substantial impact on the research of novel drugs in the treatment of vitreoretinal diseases.

ACKNOWLEDGMENTS

The authors acknowledge Dr. Harry Flynn for providing Figures 2A and 2B as well as Dr. Roberta Manzano and Prof. Peyman for providing Figure 3 of this chapter.

REFERENCES

1. Ghate D, Edelhauser HF. Ocular drug delivery. Expert Opin Drug Deliv 2006;3:275–287.
2. Kozak I, Cheng L, Silva GA, et al. Testing of intraocular drugs for clinical use. Invest Ophthalmol Vis Sci 2007;48:4861–4863.
3. Penha FM, Maia M, Eid Farah M, et al. Effects of subretinal injections of indocyanine green, tryptan blue, and glucose in rabbit eyes. Ophthalmology 2007;114:899–908.
4. Rodrigues EB, Meyer CH, Mennel S, et al. Mechanisms of intravitreal toxicity of indocyanine green dye: implications for chromovitrectomy. Retina 2007;27:958–970.
5. Friedman AH, Orellana J, Freeman WR, et al. Cytomegalovirus retinitis: a manifestation of the acquired immune deficiency syndrome (AIDS). Br J Ophthalmol 1983;67:372–380.
6. Blankenship GW. Evaluation of a single intravitreal injection of dexamethasone phosphate in vitrectomy surgery for diabetic retinopathy complications. Graefes Arch Clin Exp Ophthalmol 1991;229:62–65.
7. Vander JF. Tissue plasminogen activator irrigation to facilitate removal of subretinal hemorrhage during vitrectomy. Ophthalmic Surg 1992;23:361–363.
8. Tzekov RT, Serrato A, Marmor MF. ERG findings in patients using hydroxychloroquine. Doc Ophthalmol 2004;108:87–97.
9. van der Zypen E. Experimental morphological study on structure and function of the filtration angle of the rat eye. Ophthalmologica 1977;174:285–298.
10. Rosolen SG, Kolomiets B, Varela O, et al. Retinal electrophysiology for toxicology studies: Applications and limits of ERG in animals and ex vivo recordings. Exp Toxicol Pathol 2008;60:17–32.
11. Hawes NL, Smith RS, Chang B, et al. Mouse fundus photography and angiography: a catalogue of normal and mutant phenotypes. Mol Vis 1999;5:22.
12. Li Q, Wang J, Yang L, et al. A morphologic study of retinal toxicity induced by triamcinolone acetonide vehicles in rabbit eyes. Retina 2008;28:504–510.
13. Hrach CJ, Johnson MW, Hassan AS, et al. Retinal toxicity of commercial intravitreal tissue plasminogen activator solution in cat eyes. Arch Ophthalmol 2000;118:659–663.
14. Bragadóttir R, Narfström K. Lens sparing pars plana vitrectomy and retinal transplantation in cats. Vet Ophthalmol 2003;6:135–139.
15. Beauchemin ML, Babel J. Proceedings: a preliminary study on the ultrastructure of the pig retina. Exp Eye Res 1973;17:400.
16. Holekamp NM, Thomas MA, Pearson A. The safety profile of long-term, high-dose intraocular corticosteroid delivery. Am J Ophthalmol 2005;139:421–428.
17. Yu SY, Damico FM, Viola F, et al. Retinal toxicity of intravitreal triamcinolone acetonide: a morphological study. Retina 2006;26:531–536.
18. Maia M, Penha FM, Farah ME, et al. Subretinal injection of preservative-free triamcinolone acetonide and supernatant vehicle in rabbits: an electron microscopy study. Graefes Arch Clin Exp Ophthalmol 2008;246:379–388.
19. Kwak HW, D'Amico DJ. Evaluation of the retinal toxicity and pharmacokinetics of dexamethasone after intravitreal injection. Arch Ophthalmol 1992;110:259–266.
20. Almeida LN, Canêdo MG, Almeida RN, et al. Macular infarction after intravitreal injection of amikacin: case report. Arq Bras Oftalmol 2005;68:837–840.
21. Campochiaro PA, Green WR. Toxicity of intravitreous ceftazidime in primate retina. Arch Ophthalmol 1992;110:1625–1629.
22. Wiechens B, Grammer JB, Johannsen U, et al. Experimental intravitreal application of ciprofloxacin in rabbits. Ophthalmologica 1999;213:120–128.
23. Aydin E, Kazi AA, Peyman GA, et al. Intravitreal toxicity of moxifloxacin. Retina 2006;26:187–190.
24. Thompson AM. Ocular toxicity of fluoroquinolones. Clin Exp Ophthalmol 2007;35:566–577.
25. Khan FA, Slain D, Khakoo RA. Candida endophthalmitis: focus on current and future antifungal treatment options. Pharmacotherapy 2007;27:1711–1721.
26. Saran BR, Maguire AM. Retinal toxicity of high dose intravitreal ganciclovir. Retina 1994;14:248–252.
27. Kaempf S, Johnen S, Salz AK, et al. Effects of bevacizumab (Avastin) on retinal cells in organotypic culture. Invest Ophthalmol Vis Sci 2008;49:3154–3171.

28. Manzano RP, Peyman GA, Khan P, et al. Testing intravitreal toxicity of bevacizumab (Avastin). Retina 2006;26:257–261.
29. Rodrigues EB, Shiroma H, Meyer CH, et al. Metrorrhagia after intravitreal injection of bevacizumab. Acta Ophthalmol Scand 2007;85:915–916.
30. Rosenfeld PJ, Schwartz SD, Blumenkranz MS, et al. Maximum tolerated dose of a humanized anti-vascular endothelial growth factor antibody fragment for treating neovascular age-related macular degeneration. Ophthalmology 2005;112:1048–1053.
31. Giansanti F, Ramazzotti M, Vannozzi L, et al. A pilot study on ocular safety of intravitreal infliximab in a rabbit model. Invest Ophthalmol Vis Sci 2008;49:1151–1156.
32. Kivilcim M, Peyman GA, Kazi AA, et al. Intravitreal toxicity of high-dose etanercept. J Ocul Pharmacol Ther 2007;23:57–62.
33. Kitzmann AS, Pulido JS, Mohney BG, et al. Intraocular use of rituximab. Eye 2007;21:1524–1527.
34. Shen WY, Constable IJ, Chelva E, et al. Inhibition of diclofenac formulated in hyaluronan on angiogenesis *in vitro* and its intraocular tolerance in the rabbit eye. Graefes Arch Clin Exp Ophthalmol 2000;238:273–282.
35. Kim SJ, Adams NA, Toma HS, et al. Safety of intravitreal ketorolac and diclofenac: an electroretinographic and histopathologic study. Retina 2008;28:595–605.
36. Trese MT. Enzymatic-assisted vitrectomy. Eye 2002;16:365–368.
37. Velez G, Yuan P, Sung C, et al. Pharmacokinetics and toxicity of intravitreal chemotherapy for primary intraocular lymphoma. Arch Ophthalmol 2001;119:1518–1524.
38. Frenkel S, Hendler K, Siegal T, et al. Intravitreal methotrexate for treating vitreoretinal lymphoma: 10 years of experience. Br J Ophthalmol 2008;92:383–388.
39. Srinivasan S, Perez-Gomez I, O'Donnell C, et al. Corneal endothelial abnormalities associated with thalidomide toxicity. Cornea 2005;24:103–105.

CHAPTER

16

Retinal toxicity of systemic and topical medications

Richard C. Lin, MD, PhD and William F. Mieler, MD

INTRODUCTION

Medications are employed with the intent of providing a specific benefit for their usage. In a select number of cases, however, there are unintended consequences in organs or systems, far beyond the initial target. This chapter will review the use of systemic medications (along with select topical agents) which can lead to unwanted retinal consequences.

KEY CONCEPTS AND FUNDAMENTALS

A wide variety of systemic medications are capable of inducing retinal toxicity. Fortunately, in the majority of cases the loss of visual function is minimal or reversible following discontinuation of the inciting drug. Nevertheless, permanent or progressive visual loss may occur in some instances. We present only those medications known to produce a well-described change. The medications can be grouped according to the type of retinal toxicities they produce: disruption of the retina and retinal pigment epithelium (RPE), vascular damage or occlusion, retinopathies characterized by macular edema and/or macular folds, crystalline retinopathies, induction of uveitis and/or hypotony, and functional toxicities without specific, visible retinal changes. The medications are listed in Table 16.1, and the most prominently encountered agents will be discussed throughout the course of this chapter. Also briefly discussed is the retinal toxicity of several topical ocular medications.

PHARMACOLOGY, BIOCHEMISTRY, AND TYPE OF IMPACT ON THE RETINA

DISRUPTION OF THE RETINA AND RETINAL PIGMENT EPITHELIUM

Phenothiazines

Thioridazine

Thioridazine is a piperidine antipsychotic drug that was previously widely used in the treatment of schizophrenia and psychosis. Due to concerns about cardiotoxicity and retinopathy at high doses, this drug is now prescribed less than previously and is mostly used for refractory cases.

Blurred vision, dyschromatopsia (reddish or brownish discoloration of vision), and nyctalopia characterize acute toxicity with thioridazine.[1] In the earliest stages the retinal appearance may be normal or display only mild granular pigment stippling (Figure 16.1). An intermediate stage is characterized by circumscribed nummular areas of RPE loss from the posterior pole to the midperiphery[2] (Figure 16.2). In late stages of thioridazine toxicity, widespread areas of depigmentation alternating with hyperpigmented plaques, vascular attenuation, and optic atrophy are seen[3] (Figure 16.3).

Photography and fluorescein angiography (FA), visual field testing, and electrophysiologic testing are useful ancillary tests in screening and monitoring for possible thioridazine toxicity. FA highlights disruption of the choriocapillaris and zones of pigment rarefaction (Figures 16.2 and 16.3). Visual field testing can reveal mild constriction, paracentral scotomas, or ring scotomas. Electroretinography (ERG) is either normal or shows decreased oscillatory potentials in early stages of toxicity. In the later stages, both the rod and cone functions of the ERG, as well as the electro-oculography (EOG), are markedly abnormal.[4] Multifocal ERG (mfERG) may provide an even better means of detecting early change and monitoring such patients, though such data are currently lacking.

Retinal toxicity from thioridazine is dependent more on the total daily dose than on the cumulative amount of drug received. With higher daily doses, toxicity can occur rapidly, even within the first 2 weeks of therapy.[5] Toxicity is rare at dosages less than 800 mg/day. Nonetheless, a few cases have been reported with lower doses given over several years. As a result, any patient taking thioridazine, regardless of the daily dose, should be monitored for the development of visual symptoms or retinal changes.

At the earliest sign of toxicity, thioridazine should be discontinued. However, the early retinal changes associated with thioridazine often progress despite discontinuation of therapy. It is unclear whether this degeneration represents continued toxicity of the drug or a delayed expansion of chorioretinal scarring secondary to areas of subclinical, preexisting damage. Visual function, in contrast to retinal appearance, usually improves over the first year after drug cessation. In addition, if the drug is stopped early, ERG testing may actually improve over the first year[6]; this undoubtedly would not occur if thioridazine caused persistent toxicity.

The mechanism of thioridazine-mediated retinal toxicity probably involves damage to both the RPE and the retina. Many phenothiazines bind melanin granules of the RPE and uveal tissue, but not all commonly instigate retinal toxicity.[7–9]

Historically, the compound piperidyl-chlorophenothiazine hydrochloride (NP-207) had a similar chemical structure to thioridazine, including the same piperidyl side chain. NP-207 was never marketed however, because of the pronounced pigmentary retinopathy that developed during early clinical trials.[10] This piperidyl side chain is not present in other phenothiazines, which in general exhibit much less evidence of retinal toxicity. Experimental studies demonstrate that phenothiazines alter enzyme kinetics and inhibit oxidative phosphorylation with subsequent abnormalities in rhodopsin synthesis.[11–13] Other studies suggest that thioridazine toxicity may be due to direct effects on the retina rather than the RPE. For instance, histopathologic studies indicate that atrophy and disorganization of photoreceptor outer segments occur primarily, with a secondary loss of the RPE and choriocapillaris.[14]

Given the many antipsychotic medications available today, thioridazine is no longer widely employed. If one encounters a patient on this medication, and there is any degree of retinal pigmentary alternation, a discussion regarding the use of alternative agents should be entertained with the patient's psychologist or psychiatrist.

Table 16.1 Patterns of retinal toxicity

Disruption of the retina and retinal pigment epithelium	
Phenothiazines	Clofazamine
Thioridazine	DDI (2,3 di-deoxyinosine)
Deferoxamine	
Chlorpromazine	Corticosteroid preparations
Chloroquine derivatives	Chemotherapeutic agents
Chloroquine	Cisplatin and BCNU
(Carmustine)	
Hydroxychloroquine	Denileuken diftitox
Quinine sulfate	Potassium iodate
Vascular damage or occlusion	
Quinine sulfate	Ergot alkaloids
Oral contraceptives	Aminoglycosides (intravitreal)
Chemotherapeutic agents	Procainamide
Interferon	
Gemcitadine	
Cisplatin and BCNU (carmustine)	
Cystoid macular edema and retinal edema/folds	
Nicotinic acid	Hydroxychlorothiazide
Sulfa antibiotics	Triamterene
Acetazolamide	Metronidazole
Chemotherapeutic agents	Topiramate
Paclitaxel, docetaxel	
Crystalline retinopathy	
Methoxyflurane	Nitrofurantoin
Canthaxanthine	Talc
Chemotherapeutic agent	
Tamoxifen	
Uveitis	
Cidofovir	Rifabutin
Miscellaneous (subjective ocular effects)	
Digoxin	Sildenafil
Methanol	

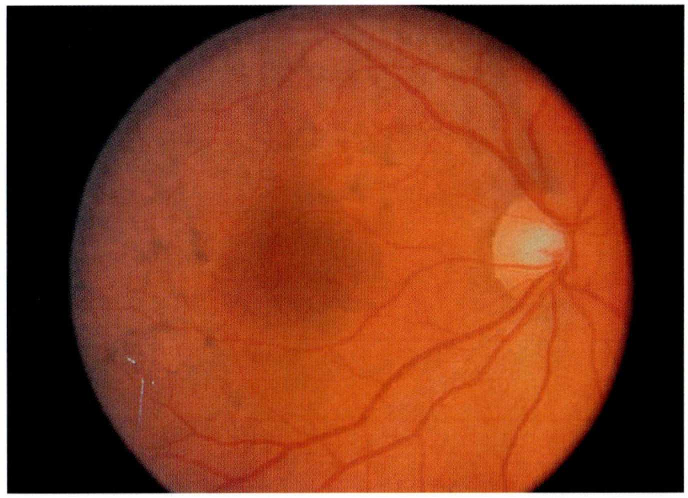

Figure 16.1 Color photograph of right eye. Mild pigment mottling in a patient on thioridazine. Visual acuity is normal.

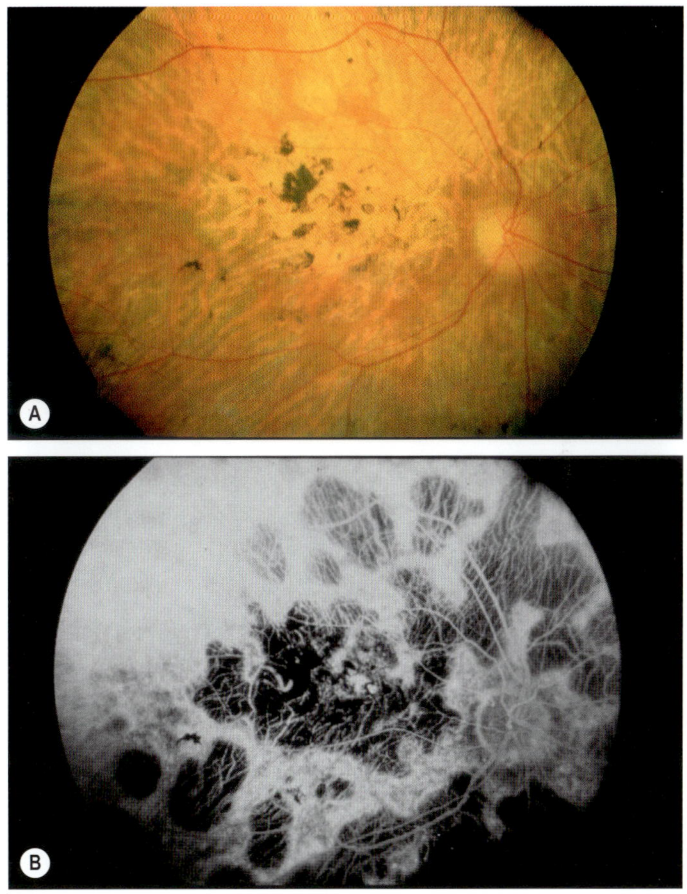

Figure 16.2 (A) Color photograph of right eye, showing nummular areas of pigment loss in a patient on thioridazine. (B) Fluorescein angiography documents nummular loss of retinal pigment epithelium, along with the underlying choriocapillaris.

Chlorpromazine

Chlorpromazine is a phenothiazine antipsychotic medication similar to thioridazine but lacks the piperidyl side chain. The compound binds strongly to melanin and can cause hyperpigmentation in the skin, conjunctiva, cornea, lens, and retina (Figure 16.4).[15–18] Other ocular effects include oculogyric crisis, miosis, and blurred vision caused by paralysis of accommodation. Usual doses range from 40 to 75 mg/day, but dosages up to 800 mg/day are not uncommon.

Retinal toxicity from chlorpromazine is rare. When massive doses are given (e.g., 2400 mg/day for 12 months), pigmentary changes may occur in the retina with attenuation of retinal vessels and optic nerve pallor (Figure 16.5). Similar to thioridazine, the development and extent of toxicity are more closely related to daily dosage than total amount of drug taken. Like thioridazine, chlorpromazine is also not widely used today, and has been largely supplanted by the newer atypical antipsychotic medications.

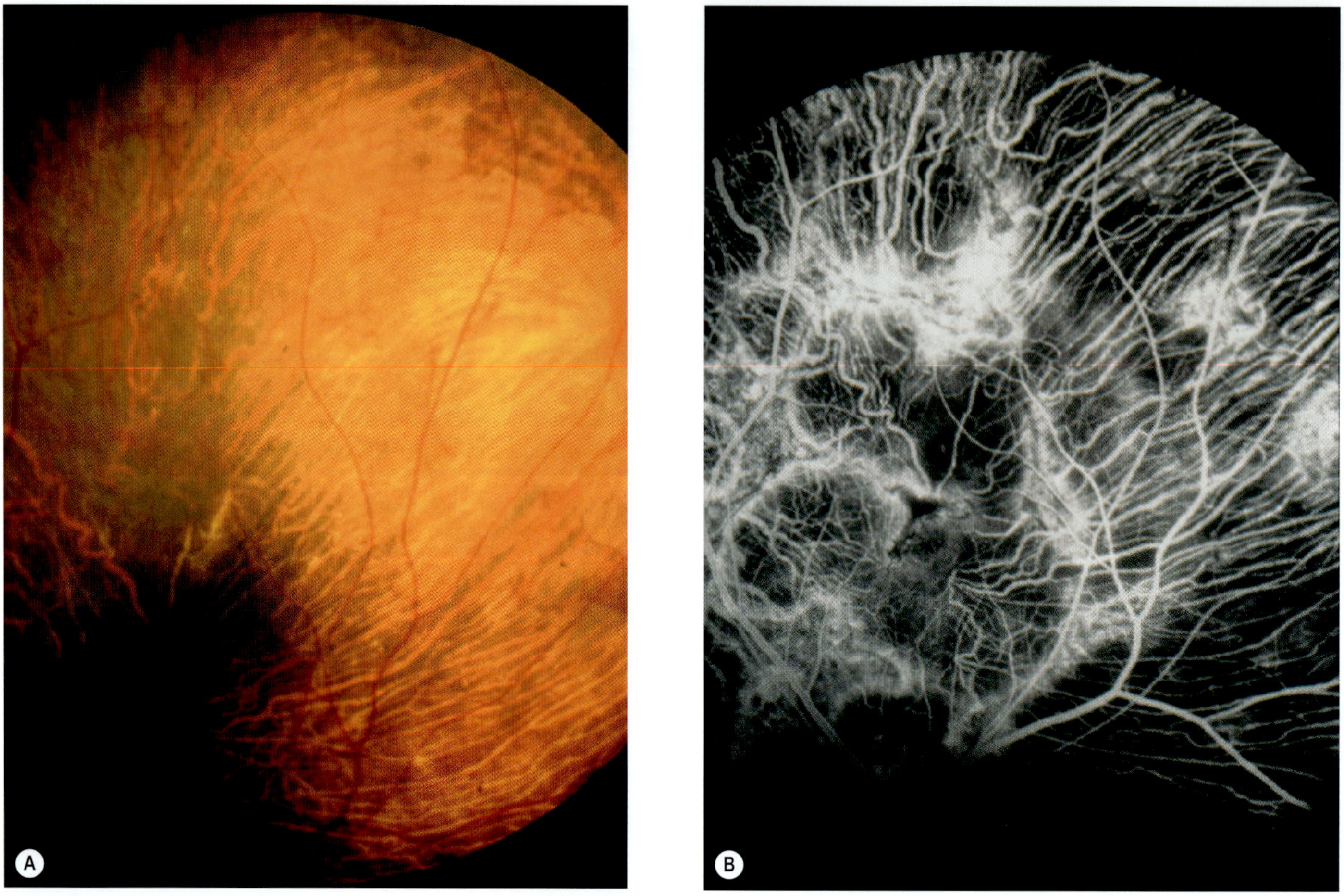

Figure 16.3 (A) Color photograph depicting late-stage thioridazine toxicity, with virtually complete loss of retinal pigment epithelium and underlying choriocapillaris. (B) Fluorescein angiography allows for direct visualization of the large choroidal vessels.

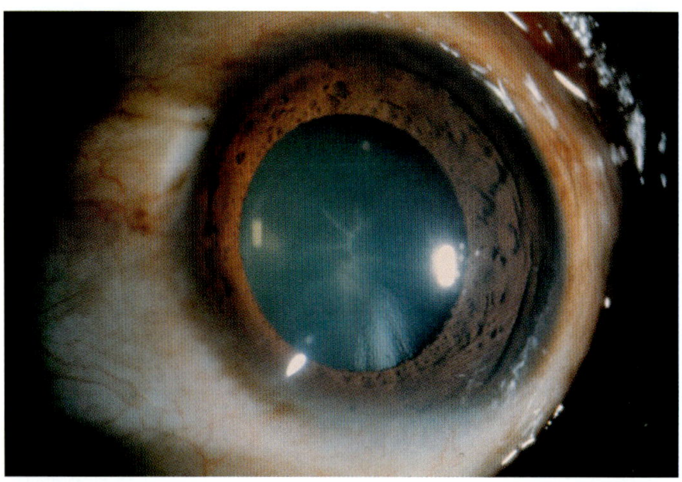

Figure 16.4 Color photograph depicting pigment deposition in the anterior lens capsule in a patient on chlorpromazine. The patient was visually asymptomatic.

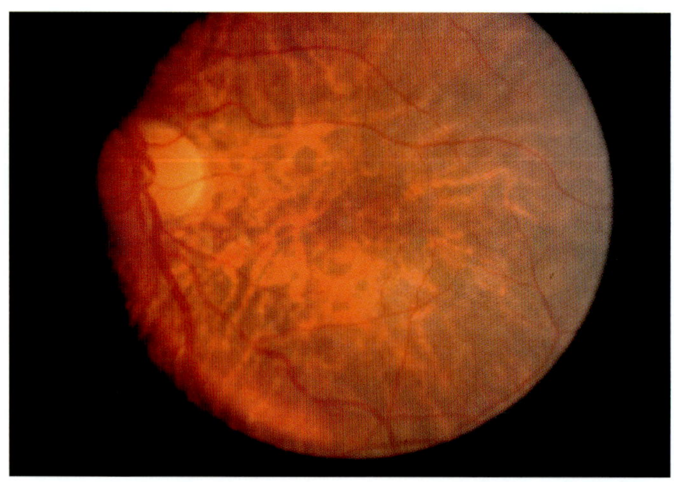

Figure 16.5 Color photograph of left eye of a patient on chlorpromazine. Mild disc pallor is seen along with slight vascular attenuation and diffuse pigment mottling.

Chloroquine derivatives

Chloroquine

Chloroquine was first used as an antimalarial drug in World War II. Currently it is prescribed for treatment of amebiasis, rheumatoid arthritis, systemic lupus erythematosus, and for prophylaxis against malaria. Retinal toxicity with degeneration of the RPE and neurosensory retina as a result of long-term daily use of chloroquine has been well described.

A paracentral scotoma may be the earliest manifestation of retinal toxicity and can precede the development of any ophthalmoscopic or ERG abnormality.[19] Subtle macular pigment stippling with a loss of the foveal light reflex (Figure 16.6) usually appears on fundus examination before the development of a classic bull's-eye maculopathy, in which a ring of depigmentation surrounded by an area of hyperpigmentation is seen centered on the fovea (Figure 16.7). Visual acuity decreases when the RPE abnormalities involve the center of the fovea. The peripheral retina can display pigment mottling, which may, in severe cases, develop into the appearance of primary tapetoretinal degeneration with narrowed retinal vessels, optic disc pallor, and eventual blindness (Figure 16.8).

FA can be helpful in the demonstration of pigment abnormalities in the macula (Figures 16.6 and 16.7), though it is not an essential aid in the diagnosis. There is minimal evidence of damage to the choriocapillaris on FA in the areas of pigment disturbance. The ERG and EOG may be abnormal early, although the EOG is sometimes supernormal initially.[20]

Most cases of chloroquine retinopathy have developed when a higher than currently recommended (3 mg/kg/day using lean body weight) dose was used.[21] A daily dose exceeding 250 mg with a total cumulative dose between 100 and 300 g is customarily needed to produce toxicity.[22] One study showed a 19% incidence of chloroquine retinopathy in patients taking a mean daily dose of 329 mg.[23] On the other hand, with strict adherence to a low dose per day, the incidence of retinal abnormalities is minimal even when cumulative doses reach over 1000 g.[24] The American Academy of Ophthalmology has issued recommendations for screening for chloroquine and/or hydroxychloroquine retinopathy, and these recommendations are discussed below in the section on hydroxychloroquine.

After the cessation of chloroquine treatment, early subtle macular changes can revert to normal. Although far advanced cases may progress despite discontinuation of the drug, most patients remain stable with long-term follow-up.[25,26] Chloroquine, however, is very slowly excreted from the body. It has been detected in the plasma, red blood cells, and urine of patients 5 years after their last known ingestion.[27] This prolonged presence may account for the rare cases of delayed onset of chloroquine retinopathy seen up to 7 years or longer after discontinuation.[28,29]

The precise mechanism of chloroquine-mediated retinal toxicity is unknown. Like the phenothiazines, chloroquine is bound by melanin and concentrated in the RPE and uveal tissues.[30] Possible explanations include inhibition of critical enzymes and interference with the metabolic function of the RPE and photoreceptors.[31,32] Histopathologic sections demonstrate loss of RPE pigmentation with an accumulation of pigment-laden cells in the outer retinal layers with damage and reduction of photoreceptors.[33] Electron microscopic studies reveal more widespread damage to the retina, especially the ganglion cell layer.[34]

Hydroxychloroquine

Given the incidence of toxicity with chloroquine, most rheumatologists prefer hydroxychloroquine for the treatment of rheumatoid arthritis and systemic lupus erythematosus. Although it can produce a retinopathy indistinguishable from chloroquine, its occurrence is rare.[35–38] For instance, in a recent prospective cohort study of 400 patients treated for a mean of 8.7 years, only two developed features of retinal toxicity.[39]

Relatively few cases of hydroxychloroquine toxicity have been well documented, involving decreased visual acuity, paracentral scotoma, and a bull's-eye maculopathy (Figure 16.9). Many of these patients received above the recommended daily dosage of 6.5 mg/kg/day (based on ideal body weight), but the classic retinal findings have been reported at lower doses as well.[40–42] All of the patients with toxicity at lower doses were taking hydroxychloroquine for longer than 5 years.

Several authors have questioned the utility of screening for hydroxychloroquine toxicity given the low yield, high cost, and the difficulty in diagnosing the condition early enough to prevent damage.[43–46] Nevertheless, toxicity does occur, and if retinal and functional changes are detected early, severe visual impairment can be averted.[47,48] Use of static perimetry through the vertical meridian with a red test object may

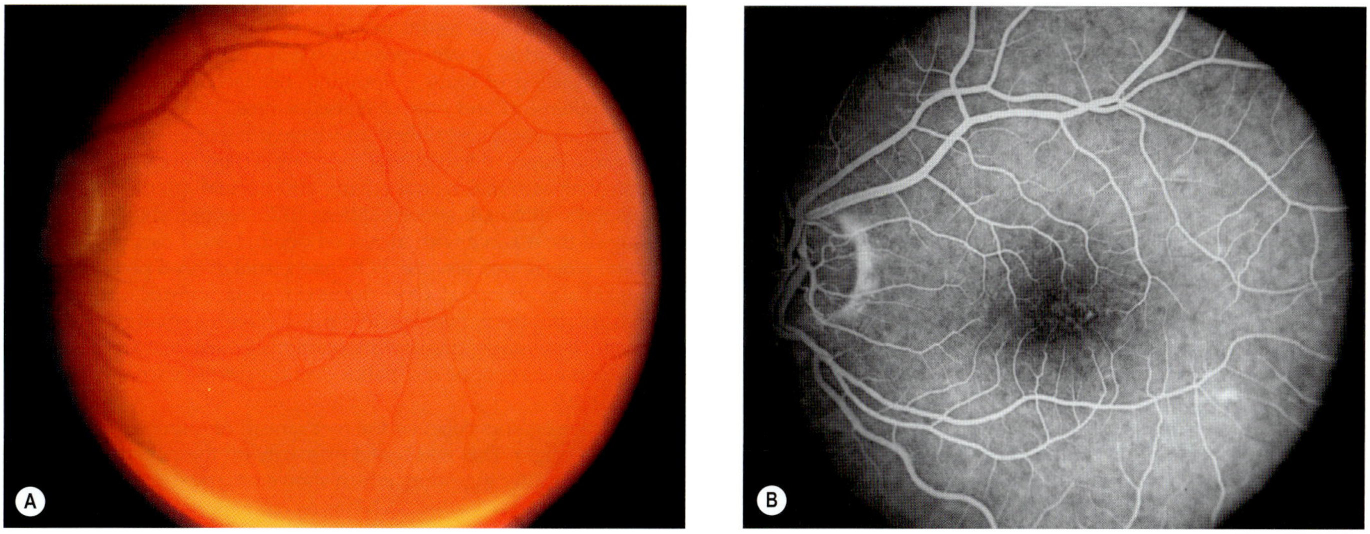

Figure 16.6 (A) Color photograph of left eye showing very early macular pigment mottling in a patient on chloroquine. (B) Fluorescein angiography shows transmission defects in the macular region corresponding to the punctate areas of pigment mottling seen clinically, though there is no bull's-eye lesion.

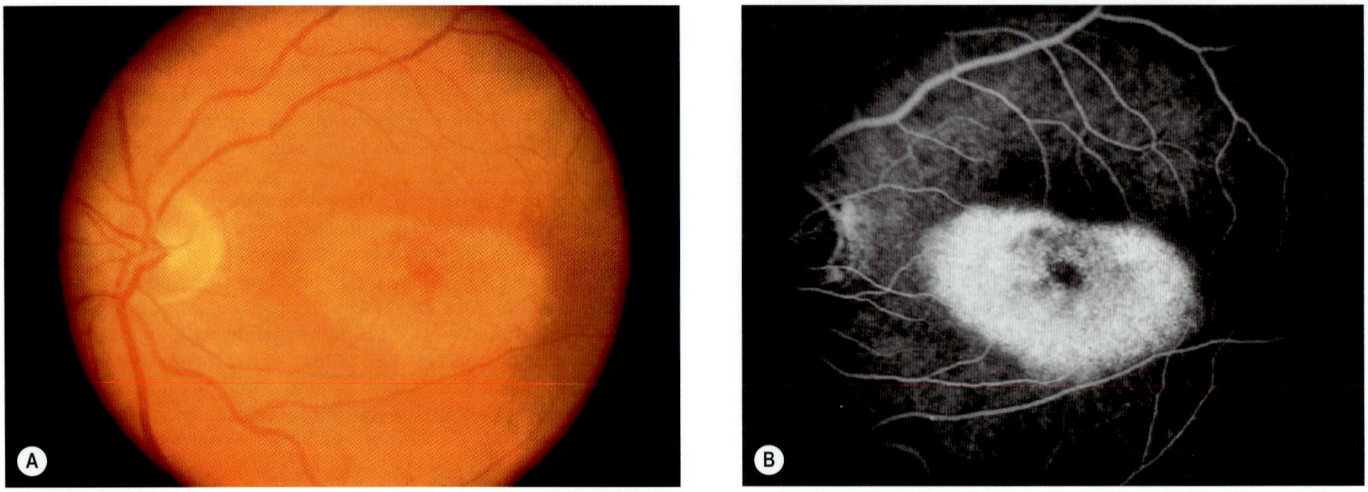

Figure 16.7 (A) Color photograph of left eye revealing a full-blown macular bull's-eye lesion secondary to chloroquine. The patient had bilateral lesions, with loss of central vision. (B) Fluorescein angiography reveals a transmission defect centrally corresponding to the bull's-eye circle of pigment loss.

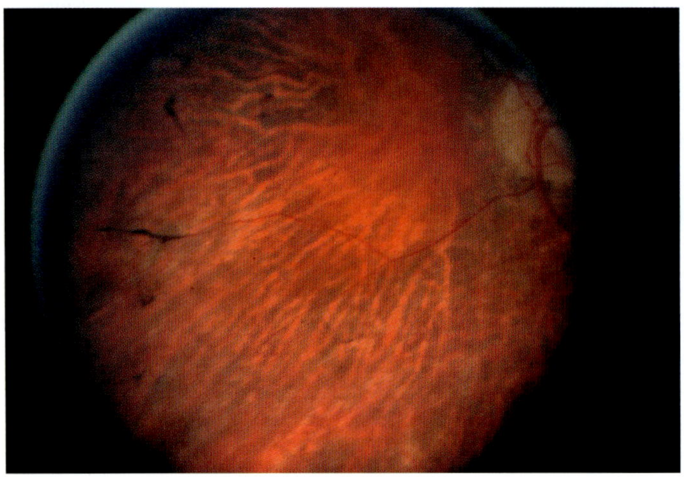

Figure 16.8 Color photograph of left eye documenting end-stage chloroquine retinal toxicity, with disc pallor, vascular attenuation, diffuse pigment mottling, and pigment deposition along the peripheral retinal vessels (similar to retinitis pigmentosa). Visual acuity was 20/200.

be the best method to detect an early paracentral scotoma.[49] These changes usually occur before visible retinal abnormalities and therefore should be performed on follow-up examinations. The Amsler grid is also useful in detecting an early paracentral scotoma and may be substituted for static perimetry.[50] In addition, the grid can be given to patients so that they can monitor their visual function at home. Recent data suggest that mfERG evaluation may detect toxicity at its earliest stages, before changes occur in visual acuity, color vision testing, Amsler grid, or visual field testing.[51]

In 2002, the American Academy of Ophthalmology published guidelines for screening and monitoring for chloroquine or hydroxychloroquine retinopathy. Included is a baseline ocular examination performed at the commencement of therapy.[52] Static perimetry or Amsler grid testing is also recommended at baseline. Retinal photography and FA are optional, and may be helpful for patients with preexisting macular pathology. Color vision testing is also optional. Follow-up screening examinations during the first 5 years of therapy can be performed as part of routine ophthalmic examinations (interval to be determined by age of the patient). If the dosage of hydroxychloroquine utilized is higher than 6.5 mg/kg/day (or >3 mg/kg/day for chloroquine), or if the patient is obese, has renal or liver dysfunction, has concomitant macular disease, or is more than 60 years of age, screening should be performed at least annually. After 5 years of therapy, screening should be performed at least annually in all patients. If ocular toxicity occurs and is recognized at an early stage, efforts should be made to communicate this directly to the prescribing physician so that alternatives can be discussed with the patient. In almost all cases, cessation of the drug should be suggested, as there is no specific treatment once retinopathy develops.

Quinine sulfate

Quinine sulfate was first used for the treatment of malaria in World War II, but it is currently prescribed for the management of nocturnal muscle cramps or "restless leg syndrome." The recommended daily dose is less than 2 g. Signs of systemic toxicity occur with doses greater than 4 g, and the fatal oral dose is generally in excess of 8 g. Ocular toxicity with quinine develops after an overdose, either by accidental ingestion or by attempted abortion or suicide. Very rarely, chronic ingestion at low levels results in ocular toxicity.[53]

With an overdose, a syndrome known as cinchonism is rapidly produced, consisting of nausea, vomiting, headache, tremor, and sometimes hypotension and loss of consciousness. When patients awake they often are completely blind and have dilated, unreactive pupils.[54] In the acute stages of toxicity, retinal examination reveals mild venous dilation with minimal retinal edema and normal arterial caliber. The FA displays minimal abnormalities. ERG testing shows an acute slowing of the a-wave with increased depth, loss of oscillatory potentials, and a decreased b-wave. EOG and visual evoked potential (VEP) testing are also abnormal. Over the next few days visual acuity gradually returns, but the patient is oftentimes left with a small central island of vision. There is a progressive attenuation of the retinal arterioles with the development of optic disc pallor over the next few weeks to months (Figure 16.10).

Early investigators believed the mechanism of quinine toxicity to be vascular in origin. This was based primarily on the retinal appearance several weeks after ingestion, which showed marked arteriolar attenuation and optic disc pallor.[55,56] More recent experimental and clinical studies have demonstrated minimal involvement of the retinal vasculature in the early stages of quinine toxicity.[57] Furthermore, ERG and histopathologic studies document that the site of toxicity is likely the retinal ganglion, bipolar, and photoreceptor cells. It has been suggested

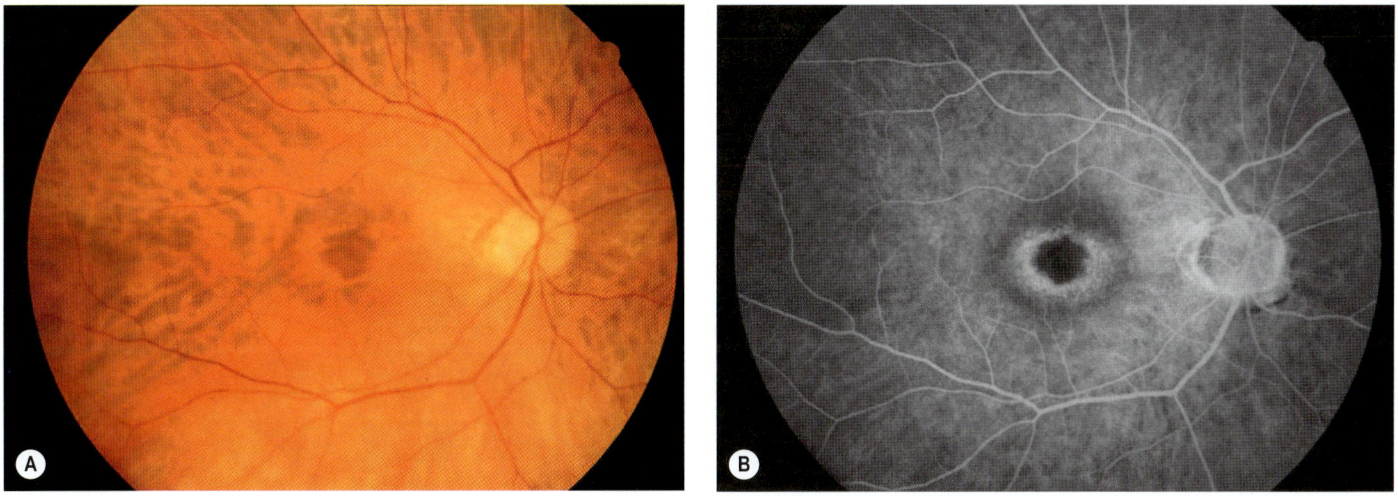

Figure 16.9 (A) Color photograph of right eye of a patient taking hydroxychloroquine for rheumatoid arthritis. She had never been on chloroquine. The patient's dose of medication far exceeded 6.5 mg/kg/day, as she weighed less than 100 lb (45 kg), yet was on a full dose of medication. (B) Fluorescein angiography reveals a classic bull's-eye macular lesion.

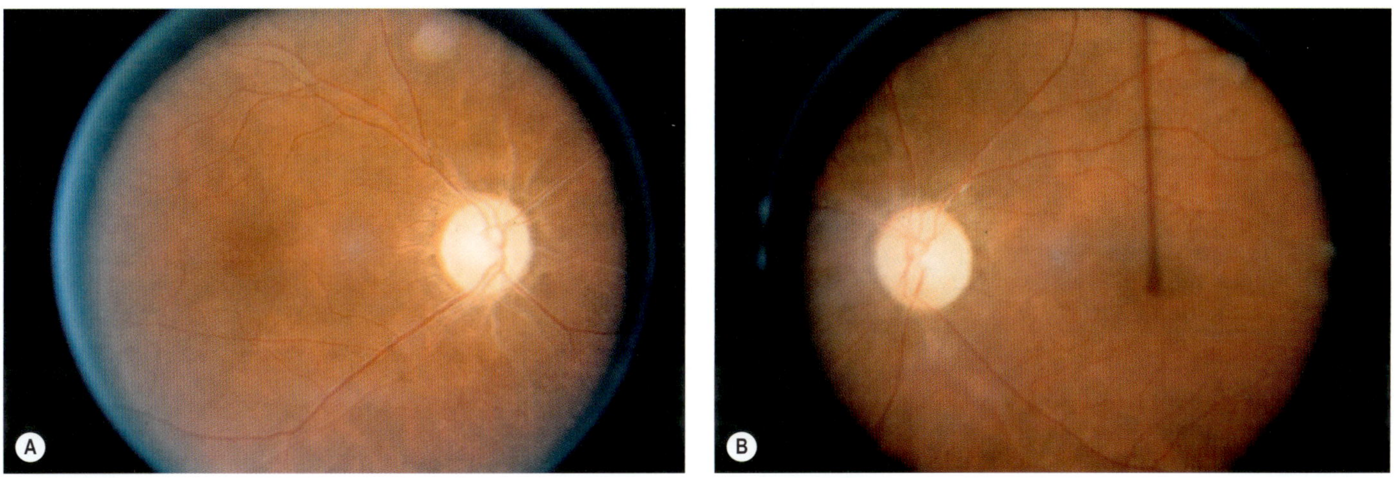

Figure 16.10 (A) Color photograph of right eye, and (B) color photograph of left eye showing the result of quinine toxicity in a patient who attempted suicide. The images reveal prominent disc pallor, vascular attenuation, and mild diffuse retinal pigment mottling.

that quinine may act as an acetylcholine antagonist and disrupt cholinergic transmission in the retina.[58]

Clofazimine

Clofazimine is a red phenazine dye that has been used to treat dapsone-resistant leprosy, psoriasis, pyoderma gangrenosum, discoid lupus, and, more recently, *Mycobacterium avium*–complex (MAC) infections in acquired immunodeficiency syndrome (AIDS) patients. With treatment over several months, clofazimine crystals may accumulate in the cornea. Two cases of bull's-eye maculopathy with pigmentary retinopathy (Figure 16.11) have been reported in AIDS patients with doses of 200–300 mg/day (total dose of 40–48 g).[59,60] Visual acuity was mildly affected, with reduced scotopic, photopic, and flicker ERG amplitudes. Cessation of treatment may result in the clearance of the corneal deposits but does not appear to affect the retinopathy.

2′,3′-dideoxyinosine (DDI)

A mid peripheral pigmentary retinopathy has been noted in three children with AIDS receiving high-dose therapy with the antiviral DDI.[61] The cases were associated with ERG and EOG changes. The retinal toxicity stabilized after discontinuation of the medication.

Deferoxamine

Deferoxamine is a chelating agent used to remove excess iron from the body. Intravenous (IV) and subcutaneous (SQ) administration of deferoxamine has been used to treat patients who require repeated blood transfusions and subsequently develop complications of iron overload. High-dose IV and SQ therapy can produce ocular toxicity, including cataract formation, optic neuropathy, and retinal toxicity, though retinopathy is quite rare. The largest retrospective case series to date includes only 16 patients.[62] In a prospective study of 84 children receiving deferoxamine treatment over a 10-year period, only 1 patient developed toxicity.[63]

Symptoms of deferoxamine toxicity include visual loss, nyctalopia, peripheral and central field loss, photopsias, and metamorphopsia.[64,65] On examination, the retina can be normal initially, or there may be a faint graying of the macula.[66] Pigmentary changes in the macula and periphery develop within a few weeks and are particularly highlighted by FA (Figure 16.12). Macular changes have also been reported to resemble vitelliform maculopathy.[67] The ERG may show delayed rod

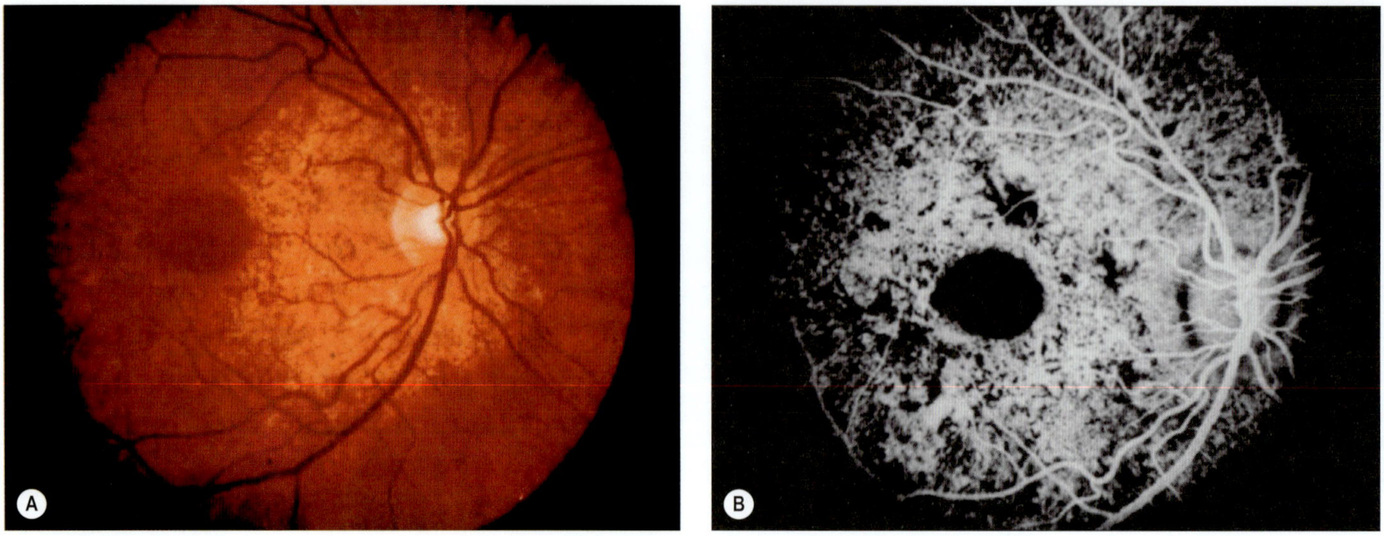

Figure 16.11 (A) Color photograph of right eye of a patient with acquired immunodeficiency syndrome (AIDS), who was treated with clofazimine for atypical *Mycobacterium*. A prominent bull's-eye macular lesion is seen clinically, and (B) readily documented on fluorescein angiography.

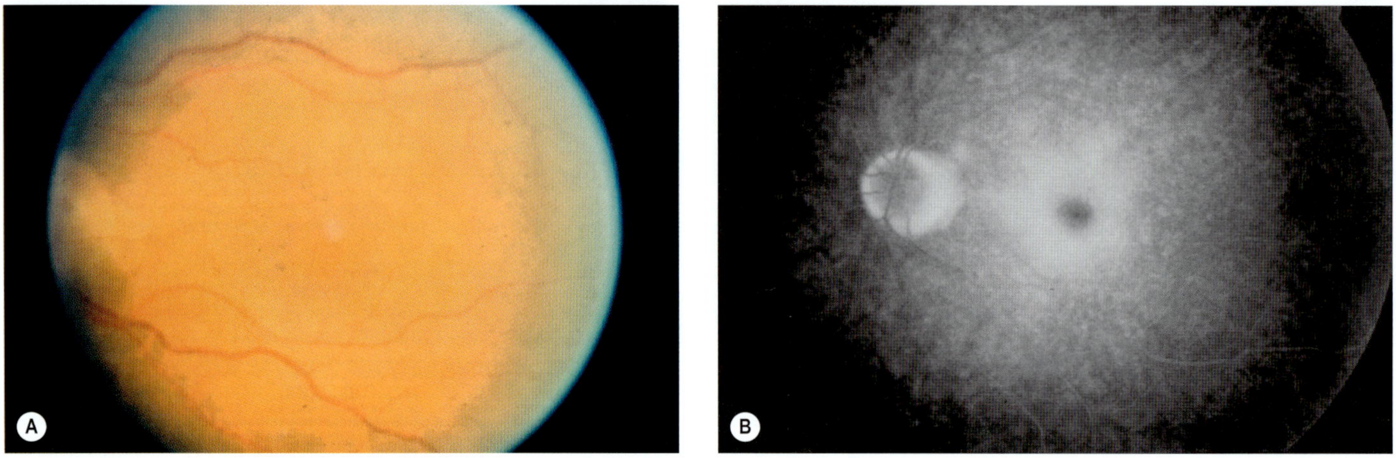

Figure 16.12 (A) Color photograph of left eye showing macular pigment mottling in a patient on deferoxamine, who was being treated for iron overload. (B) Fluorescein angiography shows diffuse central hyperfluorescence corresponding to cystoid macular edema, and also reveals surrounding transmission defects throughout the posterior pole corresponding to the mild pigment mottling seen clinically.

and cone implicit times as well as reduced scotopic and photopic a- and b-wave amplitudes, and the EOG may show a reduced Arden ratio. Return of visual and electrophysiologic function generally occurs following cessation of therapy.

Deferoxamine chelates many metals other than iron, and it is possible that the mechanism of toxicity may involve the removal of copper from the RPE. Histopathologic changes occur primarily in the RPE and include loss of microvilli from the apical surface, patchy depigmentation, vacuolation of the cytoplasm, swelling and calcification of mitochondria, and disorganization of the plasma membrane.[68]

Corticosteroid preparations

The vehicles of several common corticosteroid preparations have been shown to cause retinal necrosis when inadvertently injected into the eye.[69,70] The corticosteroids themselves probably have a minimal toxic effect on the retina, as intravitreal dexamethasone and triamcinolone are very commonly employed today for a variety of conditions.[71] Celestone Soluspan, with its vehicle benzalkonium chloride, and Depo-Medrol, with myristyl gamma-picolinium chloride, caused the most extensive retinal damage in an experimental study comparing several depot corticosteroids.[72] If one of these agents is inadvertently injected, immediate surgical removal should be instituted.

Cisplatin and BCNU (carmustine)

Cisplatin and BCNU are used for the treatment of malignant gliomas and metastatic breast cancer. Three different types of retinal toxicity have been reported with these agents. One type of change consists of a pigmentary retinopathy of the macula with markedly decreased visual acuity and frequently abnormal electrophysiologic testing. This pigmentary change has been reported after administration of combined intraarterial cisplatin and BCNU and with cisplatin alone for malignant glioma.[73,74] These findings probably are the result of platinum toxicity of the retina. Severe bilateral visual loss was reported after IV cisplatin in a patient who received four times the intended dose for treatment of lymphoma.[75] On subsequent histopathologic examination, there was noted to be splitting of the outer plexiform layer.

A second type of retinopathy has been described and consists of cotton-wool spots, intraretinal hemorrhages, macular exudate, and optic neuropathy with disc swelling. This was reported in the setting of high-dose chemotherapy with cisplatin, cyclophosphamide, carmustine, and autologous bone marrow transplantation for metastatic breast cancer.[76]

The third type of change involves a vascular retinopathy or optic neuropathy, which can include arterial occlusion, vasculitis, and papillitis. This has been seen in approximately 65% of patients receiving intraarterial BCNU alone or combined with cisplatin for malignant glioma. These retinal changes are associated with a profound visual loss that begins about 6 weeks after the start of therapy. Other ocular effects may include orbital pain, chemosis, secondary glaucoma, internal ophthalmoplegia, and cavernous sinus syndrome. Injection of medication above the ophthalmic artery can still result in toxicity.[77] The visual loss usually is progressive, and no treatment is known.

Potassium iodate

Overdose of potassium iodate, an iodized salt used for iodine supplementation in areas endemic for goiter, has been shown to cause profound visual loss and extensive retinal pigmentary abnormalities.[78] FA reveals RPE window defects and ERG and VEP testing show marked impairment of retinal function. Visual acuity may improve slowly over several months.

VASCULAR DAMAGE OR OCCLUSION

Quinine sulfate

See section on disruption of the retina and retinal pigment epithelium (above).

Cisplatin and BCNU (carmustine)

See section on disruption of the retina and retinal pigment epithelium (above).

Talc

While talc is not a medicinal agent, talc retinopathy is oftentimes seen in the setting of illicit drug usage. A characteristic retinopathy consisting of small, white, glistening crystals concentrated in the end arterioles of the posterior pole has been described in IV drug abusers (Figure 16.13).[79–81] Drug addicts crush oral medications such as methylphenidate hydrochloride (Ritalin) or methadone HCl and thus create an aqueous suspension by adding water and heating the mixture. The solution is subsequently drawn up into a syringe, with occasional attempts at filtering the mixture with cotton fibers, gauze, or cigarette filters. These oral medications contain talc (hydrous magnesium silicate) as inert filler material; after IV administration, talc particles embolize to the pulmonary vasculature, where the larger particles are trapped. After repeated injections over months to years, collateral vasculature develops, allowing the particles to enter the systemic circulation and embolize to other organs, including the eye. Even before shunt development, particles smaller than 7 μm can traverse the pulmonary capillary bed and enter the retinal circulation.[82] When small particles accumulate in vessel walls, they become visible ophthalmoscopically.[83]

Although talc retinopathy is often asymptomatic, once a large number of talc particles lodge in the small arterioles of the retinal vasculature, a characteristic picture of an ischemic retinopathy begins to develop. Capillary nonperfusion, microaneurysm formation, cotton-wool spots, and venous loops can all be seen.[84] In severe cases optic disc and peripheral neovascularization and vitreous hemorrhage can develop (Figure 16.14).[85,86] An experimental model of talc retinopathy in monkeys has demonstrated with light and electron microscopic techniques that the vascular abnormalities induced are very similar to other ischemic retinopathies seen in humans, such as sickle-cell and hypertensive retinopathy.[87–89]

Once talc retinopathy is diagnosed, an attempt at educating the patient as to the cause of the disorder is indicated. Treatment of neovascularization and vitreous hemorrhage should be undertaken using laser photocoagulation and pars plana vitrectomy (PPV) if necessary in a manner similar to that used for sickle-cell or proliferative diabetic retinopathy. Even if a patient stops IV drug use, the crystals remain visible for many years.

Oral contraceptives

Oral contraceptives have been implicated in some cases of central retinal vein occlusion, retinal and cilioretinal artery obstruction, and retinal edema occurring in young women.[90] The synthetic estrogen and progesterone contained in contraceptive pills are thought to adversely affect coagulation factors and induce a hypercoagulable state leading

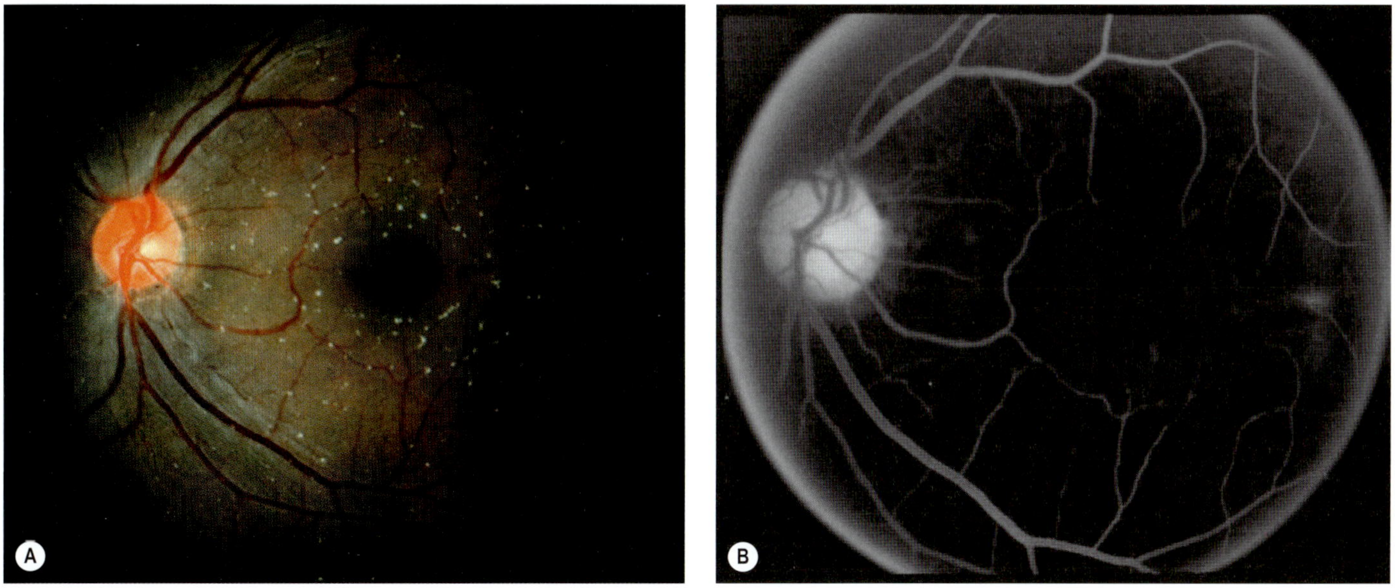

Figure 16.13 (A) Color photograph of left eye revealing numerous intraarterial glistening emboli consistent with talc in an intravenous drug abuser of many years. (B) Fluorescein angiography reveals extensive capillary nonperfusion.

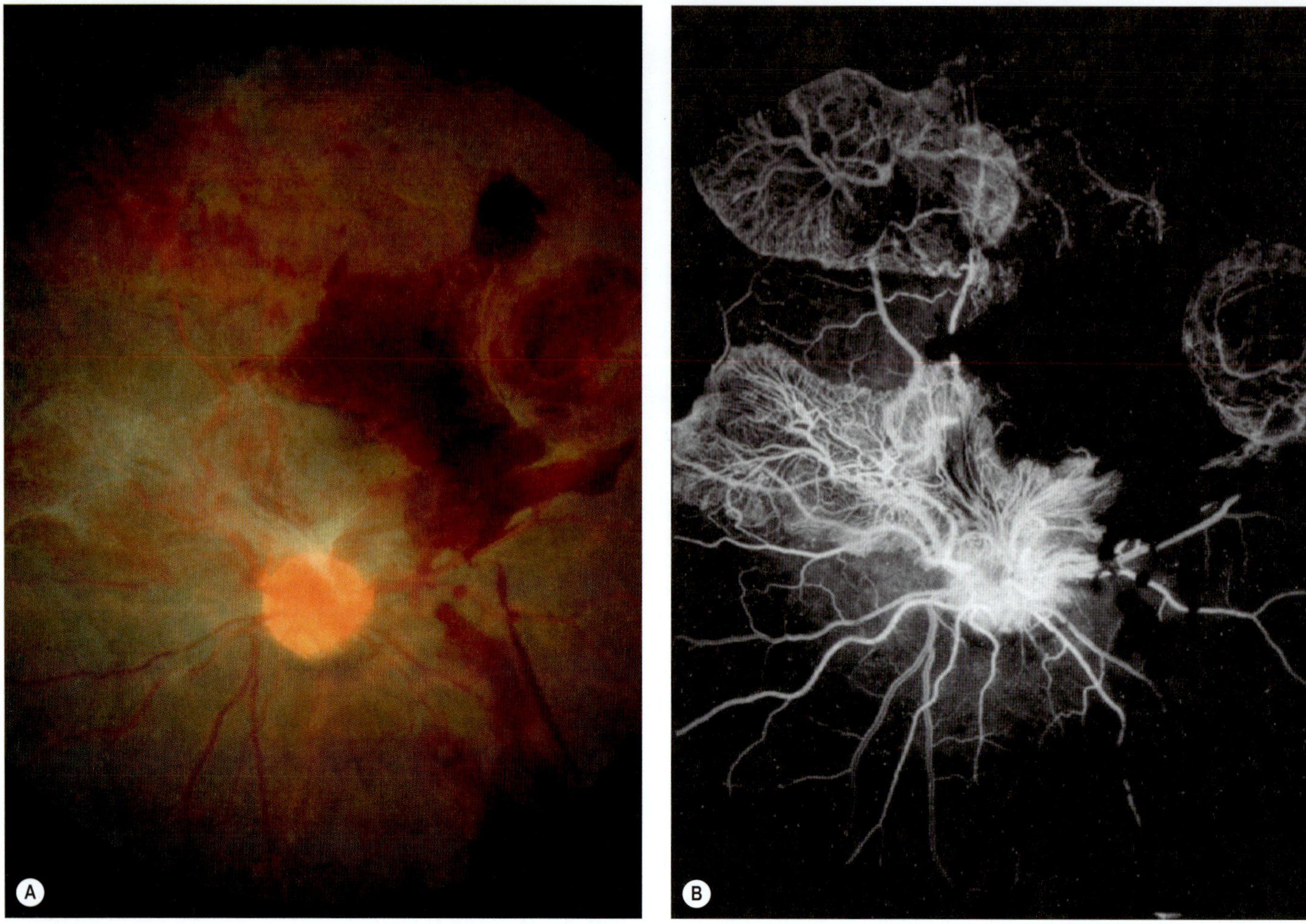

Figure 16.14 (A) Color photograph of left eye showing whorls of retinal neovascularization and preretinal hemorrhage in a patient with a long-standing history of intravenous drug abuse. (B) Fluorescein angiography confirms prominent neovascularization, with extensive mid peripheral nonperfusion of the retina.

to thromboembolic complications. Most of the studies reporting ocular complications are from the 1960s and 1970s, when much higher estrogen concentrations were used. More recent prospective studies have failed to show an increased incidence of ocular complications with this commonly employed medication[91,92] (Figure 16.15).

The use of oral contraceptives has also been associated with a condition called acute macular neuroretinopathy (AMN), in which patients experience a sudden onset of distinct paracentral scotomas.[93,94] Fundus examination reveals brown-red, wedge-shaped, or petaloid parafoveal lesions. FA may show dilated capillaries without leakage. High-resolution optical coherence tomography has demonstrated a thinning in the photoreceptor outer segments.[95] Both vascular and inflammatory factors may contribute to the development of AMN. There is no known treatment, and the scotomas may persist indefinitely despite resolution of the fundus lesions.

Aminoglycoside antibiotics

Retinal toxicity from aminoglycoside antibiotics has been reported after inadvertent intraocular injection of massive doses, intravitreal injection for bacterial endophthalmitis, prophylactic intravitreal injection after PPV, prophylactic subconjunctival injections after routine ocular surgery, and with the use of small amounts in the infusion fluid during cataract extraction.[96–100] Gentamicin is the most toxic antibiotic in the aminoglycoside family, followed by tobramycin and amikacin.[101] Massive doses result in early superficial and intraretinal hemorrhages, retinal edema, cotton-wool patches, arteriolar narrowing, and venous beading (Figure 16.16). FA reveals severe vascular nonperfusion in the acute stages. Visual loss is profound, and late rubeosis iridis, neovascular glaucoma, pigmentary retinopathy, and optic atrophy are common. Intravitreal injection of smaller doses thought to be safe for the eye (100–200 μg) can still cause toxicity with less severe fundus changes. The major preservatives found in injectable gentamicin (methylparaben, propylparaben, sodium bisulfite, and edetate disodium) likely play an additive role in its ocular toxicity.

A number of factors appear to affect the extent of toxicity observed with similar doses of these medications. Peyman et al.[102] found that retinal toxicity could be enhanced with an intravitreal injection directed at the posterior pole with the bevel of the needle pointed toward the retina, and Zachary and Forster[103] demonstrated that an increased rate of injection during intraocular administration could also increase the retinal toxicity observed. One investigator stated that eyes that have undergone previous PPV surgery are at greater risk for gentamicin toxicity, but an experimental model has shown no difference between eyes that had cataract extraction alone compared with those that underwent lensectomy and vitrectomy.[104,105] Finally, increased ocular pigmentation protects the rabbit retina from aminoglycoside toxicity and may explain some of the wide variability seen with intraocular exposure in humans.[106,107]

Although clinical aminoglycoside toxicity appears to affect the retinal vasculature primarily, pathologic studies have revealed that gentamicin in small doses causes the formation of abnormal lamellar lysosomal inclusions in the RPE, and larger doses cause increasing amounts

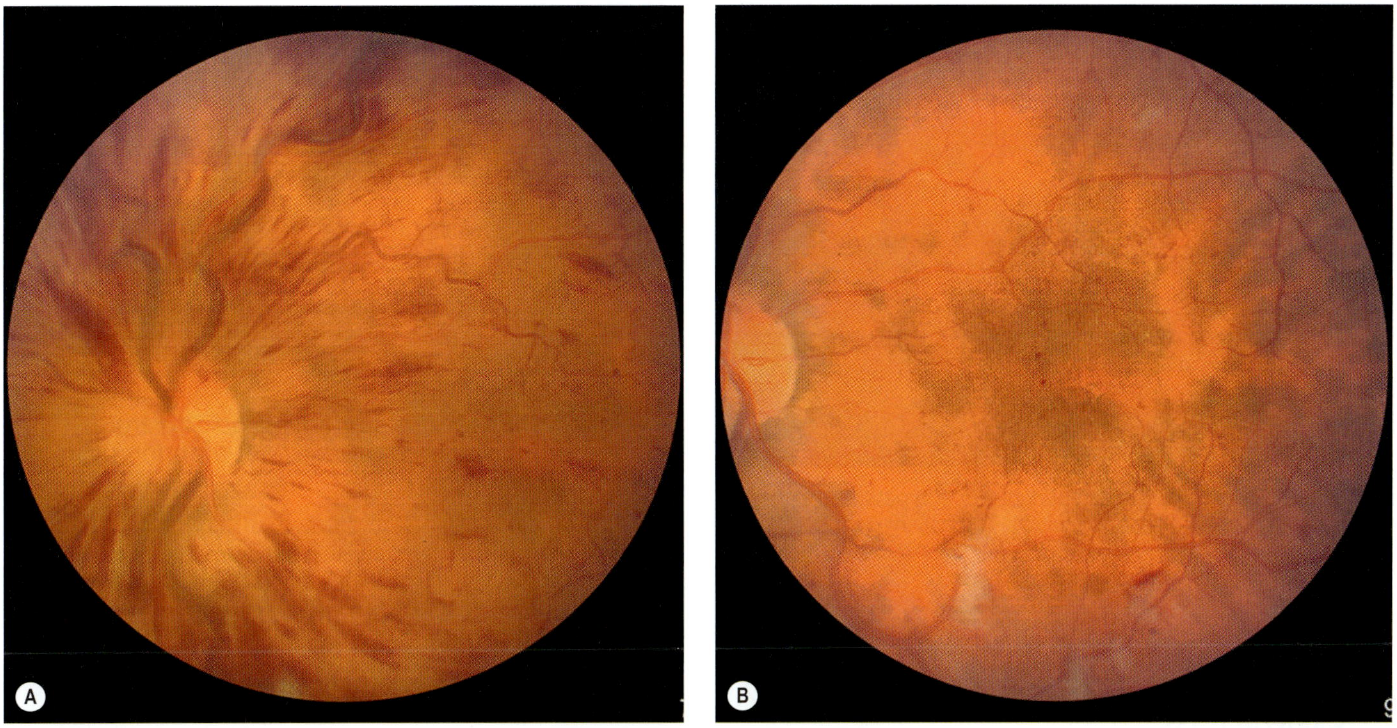

Figure 16.15 (A) Color photograph of left eye of a patient on oral contraceptives who developed a nonischemic central retinal vein occlusion. The patient had hypertension and was 40 years of age. (B) The oral contraceptives were discontinued, and the condition improved without treatment. Vision gradually returned to normal.

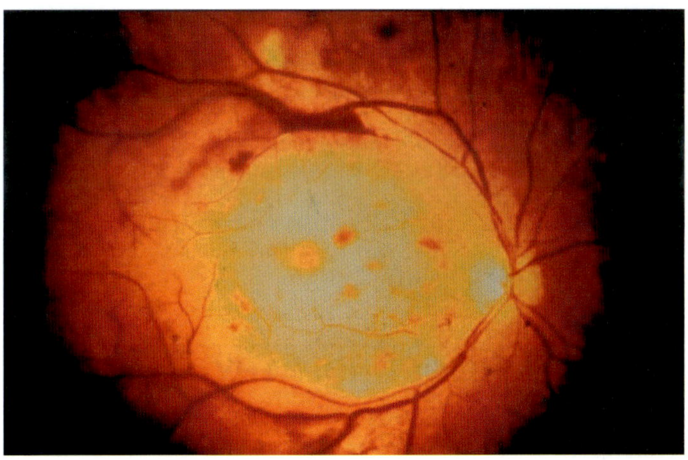

Figure 16.16 Color photograph of right eye of an eye exhibiting gentamicin toxicity. The patient received an intravitreal injection of gentamicin for treatment of endophthalmitis. Note the profound infarction of the posterior retina. The patient did not recover vision beyond hand motions.

of retinal necrosis, first of the outer then inner segments.[108–111] Histopathologically, vessel closure appears to result from granulocytic plugging.

Prevention of aminoglycoside toxicity can be accomplished by abandoning the use of these medications as routine prophylaxis following intraocular surgery, eliminating them from intraocular infusion fluids used in PPV and cataract surgery, and using alternative medications for the treatment of bacterial endophthalmitis. If inadvertent intraocular injection does occur, immediate PPV surgery with posterior-segment lavage should be performed.[112,113] Since there is some evidence that gravity plays a role in the predilection of gentamicin-induced toxicity for the macula, the patient should be placed upright as soon as possible after surgery.[114]

There have been no reported cases of retinal toxicity after systemic administration of aminoglycosides. This is likely due to the poor penetration of aminoglycosides through the blood–retina barrier.[115]

Interferon

Interferon-α is used to treat Kaposi's sarcoma, hemangiomas of infancy, chronic hepatitis C, melanoma, renal cell carcinoma, and in chemotherapy protocols for leukemia, lymphoma, and hemangiomatosis. In the past, it was also briefly employed in the treatment of choroidal neovascular membranes. Interferon therapy has been associated with the development of multiple cotton-wool spots associated with retinal hemorrhages (Figure 16.17).[116–118] Optic disc edema, branch arterial and venous occlusion, central retinal venous obstruction and cystoid macular edema (CME) have been reported with the more severe findings observed in patients receiving high-dose therapy.[119–121] Visual acuity is not usually affected if the retinal findings are limited to cotton-wool spots and intraretinal hemorrhage. Changes are noted within the first 4–8 weeks of therapy and are seen more frequently in diabetic and hypertensive patients.[122] Intravitreal injection of interferon-α-2b is well tolerated in the rabbit eye up to dosages of 1 million units; 2 million units cause a vitreous haze and intraretinal hemorrhages.[123] Interferon toxicity may be caused by an increase in immune complex deposition and activated complement C5a with leukocyte infiltration.

Miscellaneous agents

Ergot alkaloids, when utilized in higher than recommended doses, have been reported to cause retinal vasoconstriction,[124,125] and over-the-counter phenylpropanolamine used in appetite suppressants and decongestants has been implicated in one case of central retinal vein occlusion.[126]

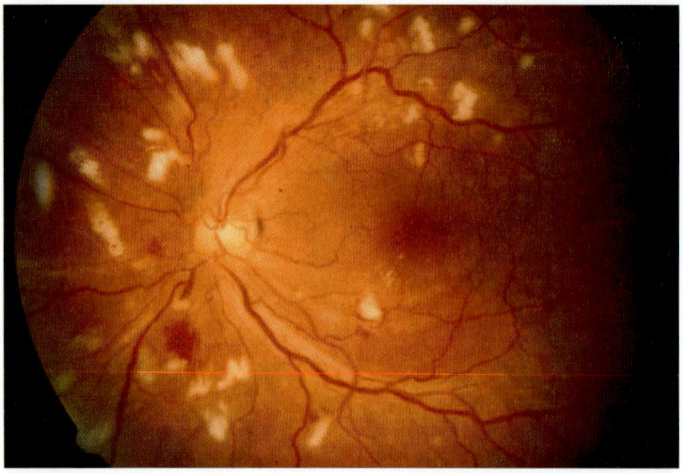

Figure 16.17 Color photograph of right eye of a patient with hepatitis C, receiving interferon therapy. The patient developed multiple cotton-wool spots, though the retinopathy did not progress beyond this stage, and vision remained normal.

CYSTOID MACULAR EDEMA AND RETINAL EDEMA/FOLDS

CYSTOID MACULAR EDEMA

Epinephrine and dipivefrin

The use of epinephrine compounds in glaucoma has decreased with the advent of newer, more efficacious agents. Topical epinephrine can cause macular edema in aphakic eyes, indistinguishable clinically and angiographically from postoperative aphakic CME. In the largest controlled study, 28% of aphakic eyes treated with epinephrine and 13% of untreated aphakic eyes had macular edema, a difference that was statistically significant.[127] Most cases of CME resolve with cessation of epinephrine usage. These medications should be avoided in the treatment of the glaucomatous aphakic and pseudophakic eyes.

Nicotinic acid

High doses of niacin have been used in the past to reduce serum lipid and cholesterol levels; however, better-tolerated 3-hydroxy-3-methylglutaryl-coenzyme A (HMG-CoA) reductase inhibitor agents, have largely curtailed its use. At doses greater than 1.5 g/day, a minority of patients will report blurred central vision, sometimes associated with a paracentral scotoma or metamorphopsia.[128] FA fails to demonstrate vascular leakage despite the typical clinical appearance of CME (Figure 16.18A, B).[129,130] This has led to speculation of a direct toxic effect on Müller cells, resulting in intracellular edema.[131] Optical coherence tomography reveals cystoid spaces in the inner nuclear and outer plexiform layers (Figure 16.18C).[132] With cessation of treatment, the CME resolves, and vision generally returns to normal. Today, an occasional case patient will be seen who is using self-prescribed high doses of niacin, as part of mega-vitamin therapy. Given the rarity of this condition, only patients who are taking high-dose niacin and who have visual symptoms should be evaluated.

Prostaglandin analogues

Latanoprost, bimatoprost, and travoprost are prostaglandin analogues that are used topically to lower intraocular pressure. Although initial human and animal studies did not show an association between latanoprost and CME, recent case reports and studies have documented that approximately 2–5% of susceptible patients with glaucoma may develop CME and anterior uveitis, which resolves after discontinuation of the drug. Subsequently, CME has been shown to develop with the use of all the prostaglandin analogues.[133,134] The preservative used in the drug formulation may also contribute to macular edema.[135] Patients with CME who are taking latanoprost should undergo a trial off the medication before initiating further therapy for the edema. High-risk CME patients, such as those with a history of recent surgery or uveitis, should be managed with other agents.

Retinal edema/folds

Sulfa antibiotics, acetazolamide, ethoxyzolamide, chlorthalidone, hydrochlorothiazide, triamterene, metronidazole

Several medications, most with a structure similar to sulfanilamide (as those listed above), can cause a syndrome of transient acute myopia and anterior-chamber shallowing. This is thought to occur as a result of ciliary body swelling or choroidal effusion, or both, with subsequent forward rotation of the lens-iris diaphragm.[136–138] Retinal folds in the macula are seen in young patients with this syndrome (Figure 16.19A), but FA does not reveal retinal leakage. The folds presumably develop as a result of vitreous traction on the macula that is caused by the forward shift of the lens and iris. The syndrome is generally reversible after discontinuation of the offending medication (Figure 16.19B).

Topiramate

Topiramate is a sulfamate-substituted monosaccharide approved for the treatment of seizures as well as prophylaxis against migraine headaches. This medication was first reported to cause acute myopia and retinal striae in 2001.[139] Subsequently, over 115 cases of myopia, narrow angles, or retinal striae attributable to topiramate have been reported.[140] Signs and symptoms typically occur within 1 month of initiating topiramate therapy, and are usually reversible without any treatment other than discontinuation of the medication. Again, the mechanism is thought to involve ciliochoroidal effusion, forward movement of the lens-iris diaphragm, and vitreous traction on the macula.

CRYSTALLINE RETINOPATHY

TAMOXIFEN

Tamoxifen is an antiestrogen agent used in the treatment of advanced breast carcinoma and as adjuvant therapy after surgical resection of early disease; it has also been tested in clinical trials (at higher dosages) for the treatment of glioblastoma multiforme. Retinal toxicity consisting of decreased visual acuity and color vision, with white intraretinal crystalline deposits, macular edema, and punctate retinal pigmentary changes, can occur.[141] The intraretinal deposits appear to reside in the inner retina and are most numerous in paramacular areas (Figure 16.20), although peripheral crystals can also be seen. Early reports involved patients who had received high doses (60–100 mg/day, total dosage >100 g) of the drug over a period of 1 year.[142] More recent studies have demonstrated that chronic low-dose administration (10–20 mg/day) with as little as 7.7 g total also can cause ocular toxicity.[143–146] Even asymptomatic patients may exhibit intraretinal crystalline formation.[147] Visual function and edema improve after discontinuation of the drug, but the refractile deposits remain.

FA demonstrates late focal hyperfluorescence in the macula consistent with CME. Decreased photopic and scotopic a- and b-wave

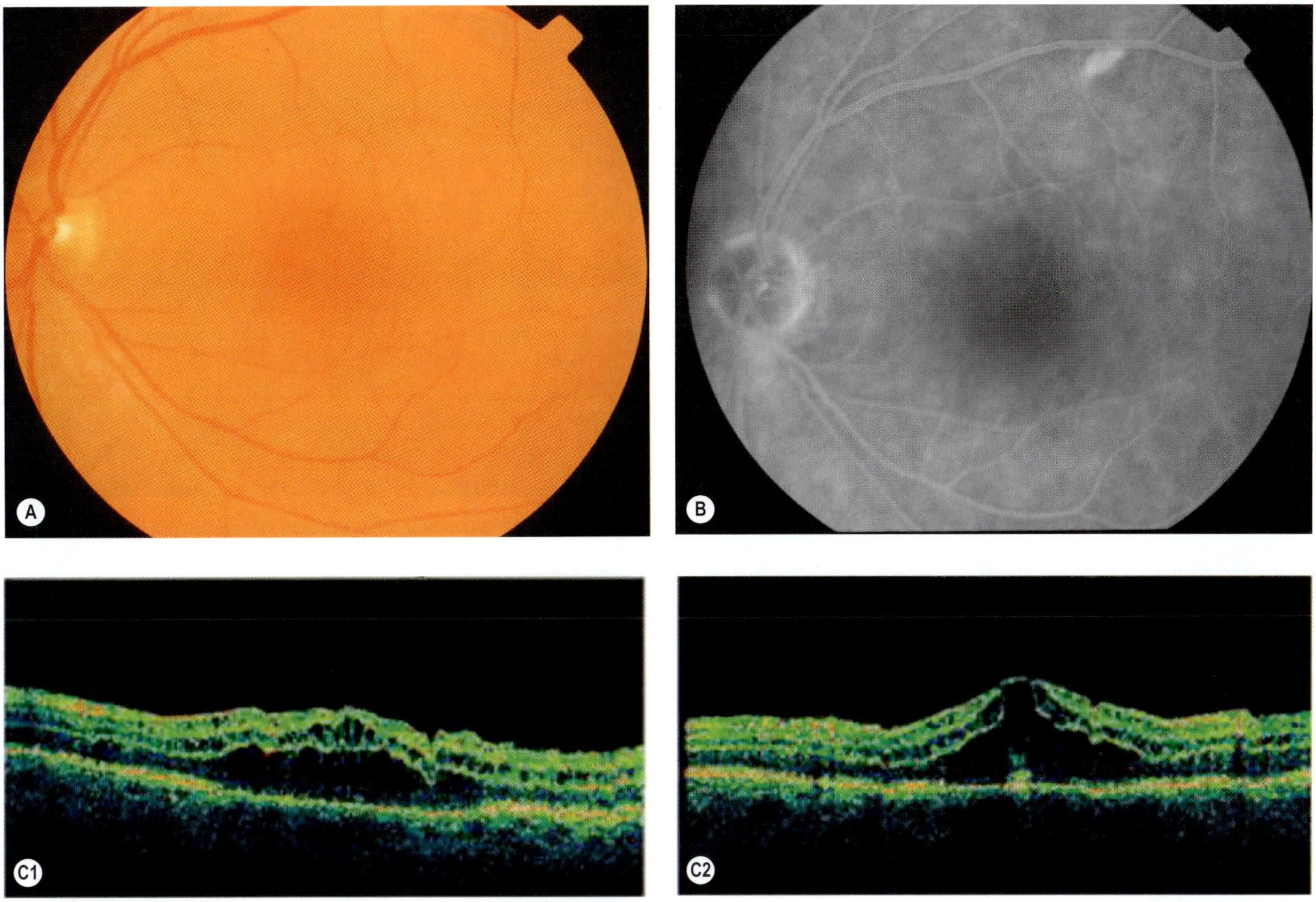

Figure 16.18 (A) Color photograph of left eye of a patient taking a megadose of self-prescribed niacin. There is diminution of the foveal reflex and macular thickening on clinical examination. (B) Fluorescein angiography reveals no evidence of macular leakage, though (C) ocular coherence tomography reveals prominent macular edema. The edema resolved following discontinuation of the niacin, and vision returned to normal.

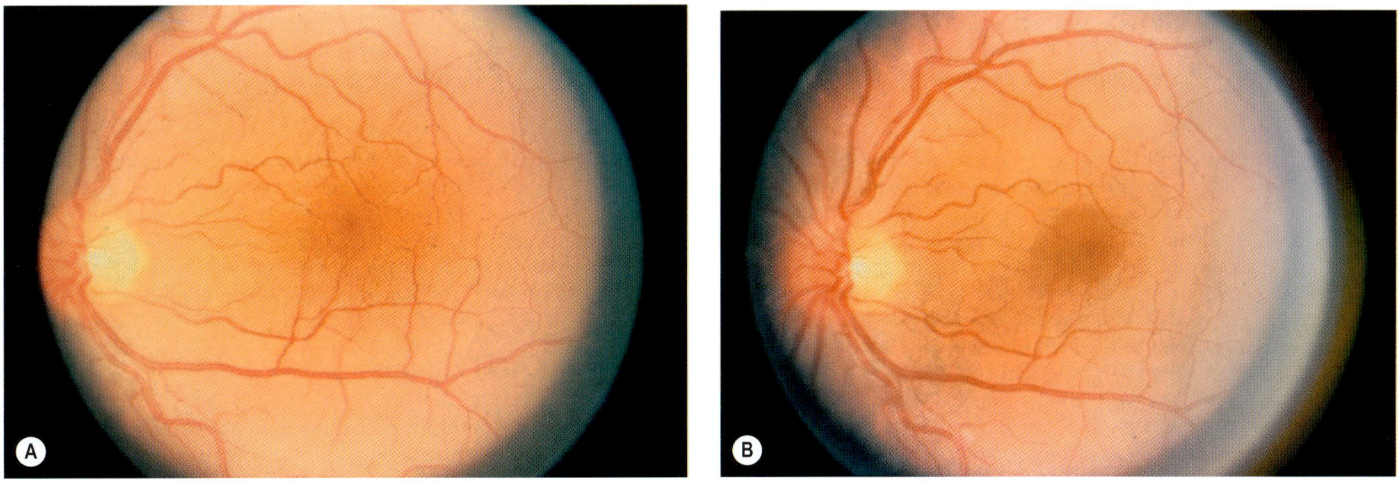

Figure 16.19 (A) Color photograph of left eye showing subtle retinal folds in a patient recently started on chlorthalidone. Vision had dropped to 20/60 left eye with mild metamorphopsia. (B) Once the condition was recognized, the medication was discontinued, and within 2 weeks, the folds had dissipated, and vision returned to normal.

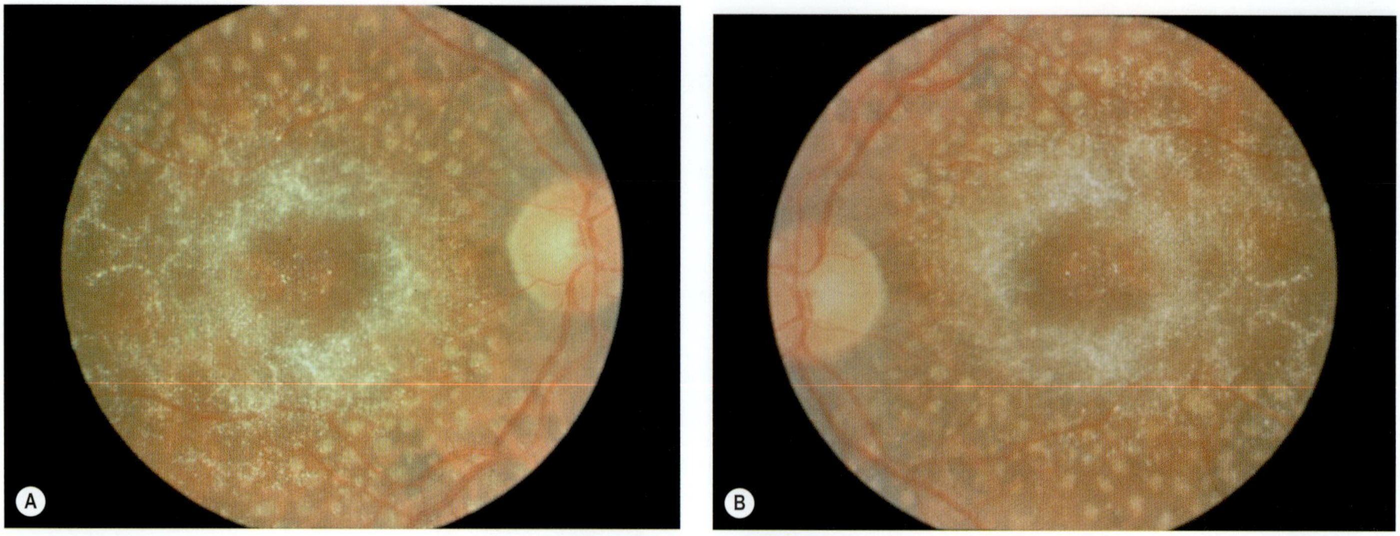

Figure 16.20 (A) Color photograph of right eye, and (B) left eye of a patient on tamoxifen therapy for treatment of metastatic breast carcinoma. Note the prominent ring of perifoveal crystals, though there was no macular edema, and the vision was normal. Since the patient needed the medication as part of her treatment regimen, she was left on it, and did well without loss of vision.

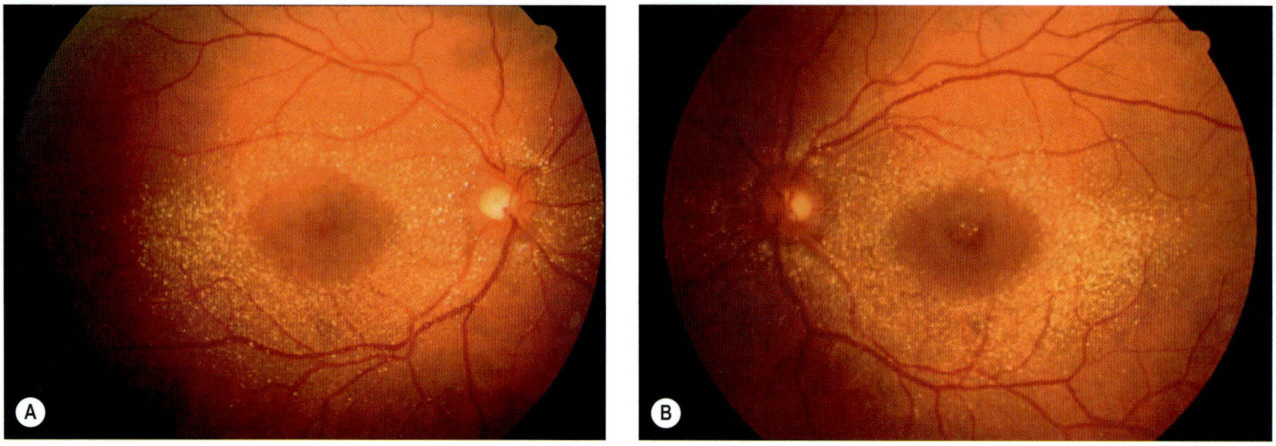

Figure 16.21 (A) Color photograph of right eye, and (B) left eye, of a patient ingesting canthaxanthine for sun-tanning purposes. The patient was visually asymptomatic. Since the agent was not being utilized for medicinal purposes, the canthaxanthine was discontinued. The crystals gradually faded away over a several-year timeframe. (Courtesy of Scott R. Sneed, MD, Traverse City, MI.)

amplitude is noted on ERG testing.[148] Optical coherence tomography reveals hyperreflective inner retinal deposits and a variable amount of macular thickening and cystic spaces.[149]

Decreased vision with bilateral optic disc swelling and retinal hemorrhages has been reported in a patient just 3 weeks after commencement of therapy with tamoxifen. These findings resolved completely after the drug was stopped.[150] It is unclear whether the findings in this patient were related to the more commonly seen toxic effects. With current low-dose therapy (10–20 mg/day), retinal lesions are rare, and routine examination of asymptomatic patients is not indicated; it is estimated that approximately 2–3% of patients on the recommended therapeutic dose of tamoxifen will develop retinal crystals.[151] If a patient taking tamoxifen is noted to have intraretinal crystals, FA should be performed, primarily to rule out juxtafoveal telangiectasis, which can have similar-appearing lesions.[152] Asymptomatic patients with retinal crystals may be monitored. Most patients may be continued on the medication, as it is truly needed in the treatment of their metastatic breast adenocarcinoma. However, if there is confirmed evidence of toxicity causing a visual disturbance, then the medication should be stopped.

The mechanism of tamoxifen toxicity may involve formation of drug–lipid complexes, since the tamoxifen molecule has both hydrophobic and hydrophilic components.[153] In a postmortem examination of an eye with tamoxifen toxicity, light microscopy revealed lesions confined to the nerve fiber and inner plexiform layers, which stained positively for glycosaminoglycans. Small (3–10 μm) intracellular and large (30–35 μm) extracellular lesions were noted on electron microscopy. The lesions appeared to represent products of axonal degeneration.[154]

CANTHAXANTHINE

Canthaxanthine is a naturally occurring carotenoid. It is used as a food-coloring agent, for skin pigmentation in the treatment of vitiligo, and for the treatment of photosensitivity disorders such as erythropoietic protoporphyria, psoriasis, and photosensitive eczema. It also has been used over-the-counter in high doses as an oral tanning agent. Many reports have described a characteristic ring-shaped deposition of yellow-orange crystals in the superficial retina with high doses (usually a total dose greater than 19 g over 2 years) (Figure 16.21).[155–157] The crystals appear more prominently in eyes with preexisting retinal disease and with concurrent use of beta-carotene.[158]

Patients usually are asymptomatic, and FA usually is normal. There have been published reports of both normal and abnormal ERG,

EOG, dark adaptation, and static threshold perimetry.[159–162] Although only clinically evident in the macula, the lipid-soluble crystals are found pathologically in the entire inner retina and ciliary body.[163] The crystals are, as would be expected, larger and more numerous surrounding the fovea. Canthaxanthine crystals are localized to the spongy degeneration of the inner neuropil and are associated with atrophy of the Müller cells. An experimental model of canthaxanthine-induced retinopathy also has demonstrated RPE cell vacuolization and disruption of phagolysosomes.[164]

With discontinuation of treatment, deposits may slowly clear over many years, with corresponding improvement in electrophysiologic parameters.[165,166] This slow reversal correlates with the detection of high plasma levels of canthaxanthine many months after discontinuation of the drug. Rarely, a fundus picture identical to canthaxanthine maculopathy can be seen in patients who have no known history of extradietary canthaxanthine.[167] A high dietary intake concurrent with preexisting retinal disease is thought to partially explain this phenomenon.

METHOXYFLURANE

Methoxyflurane is an inhalational anesthetic, which, if used for extended periods, especially in patients with renal insufficiency, causes irreversible renal failure as a result of deposition of calcium oxalate crystals in the kidney. These crystals are also deposited elsewhere throughout the body. Retinal examination of these patients reveals numerous yellow-white punctate lesions in the posterior pole and periarterially (Figure 16.22).[168,169] The deposits are located histologically in both the RPE and inner retina.[170,171]

TALC

See section on vascular damage or occlusion (above)

NITROFURANTOIN

A single case of crystalline retinopathy following 19 years of nitrofurantoin (Macrodantin) use has been reported.[172]

UVEITIS

RIFABUTIN

Rifabutin is a semisynthetic rifamycin antibiotic that is used for the treatment and prevention of disseminated MAC infection in patients with AIDS. A small percentage of patients treated with higher doses of rifabutin (450 mg/day) for systemic MAC infection, or lower doses (300 mg/day) for prophylaxis against MAC, can develop uveitis. The uveitis usually is bilateral and can be severe enough to cause a hypopyon that simulates infectious endophthalmitis. It can occur from 2 weeks to 14 months after initiation of the drug.[173] Concomitant use of clarithromycin and/or fluconazole, especially when lower doses of rifabutin are used, greatly increases the chance of a uveitic episode. Both systemic fluconazole and clarithromycin elevate rifabutin levels by inhibiting metabolism of the drug via the hepatic microsomal cytochrome P-450.[174] Although most cases have reported mainly an anterior uveitis, posterior vitreitis and retinal vasculitis have been described as well.[175,176]

Rifabutin-associated uveitis can be treated successfully with topical corticosteroids or by decreasing or discontinuing the medication. Long-term use may result in ERG abnormalities.[177] Patients without systemic MAC infection who are taking rifabutin for prophylaxis and also are taking fluconazole or clarithromycin should be warned about the potential for uveitis and counseled as to its signs and symptoms.

CIDOFOVIR

Cidofovir, also known as HPMPC, is a nucleotide analogue that inhibits viral DNA polymerase and is used for the treatment of cytomegalovirus (CMV) retinitis. Cidofovir therapy, with both IV and intravitreous (20 µg) routes of administration, has been associated with an anterior uveitis, hypotony, and visual loss. These complications can be treated and sometimes prevented with the use of topical corticosteroids, cycloplegics, and oral probenecid. Cidofovir has been shown experimentally and clinically to cause a direct toxic effect to the ciliary body, with a resulting iritis and intraocular pressure decrease.[178,179] Although a 10 µg intravitreous dose had fewer side-effects, it is also much less effective against CMV retinitis.[180] Investigations continue to try to determine the optimal dose and route of administration of cidofovir. Fortunately

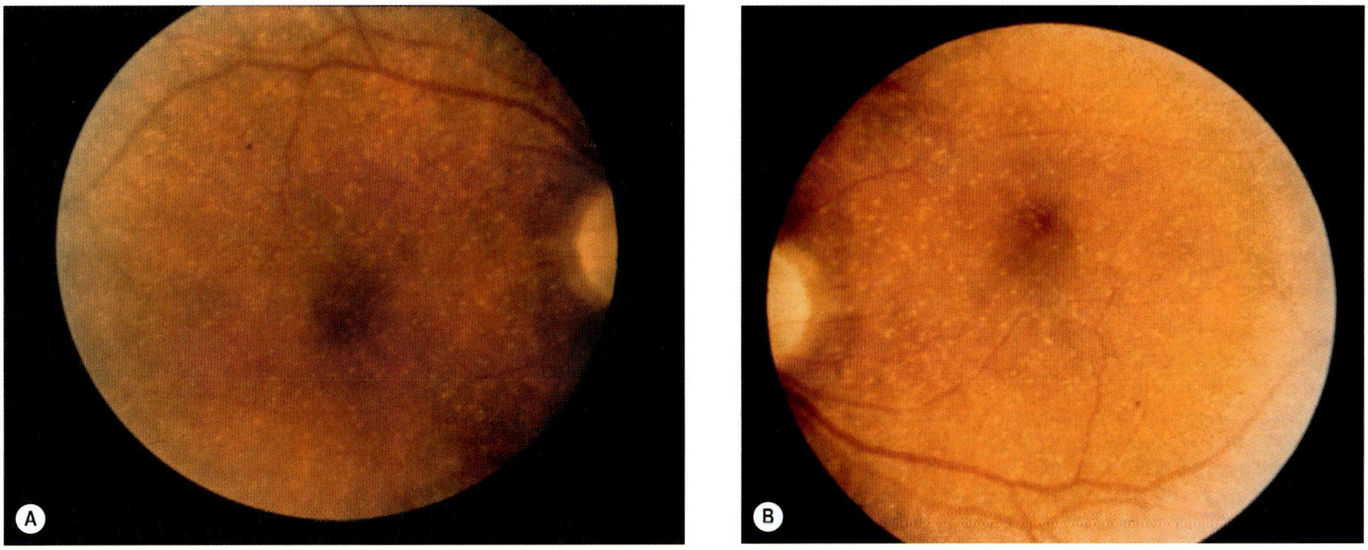

Figure 16.22 (A) Color photograph of right eye and (B) left eye of a patient who developed severe renal failure following prolonged anesthesia which included the use of methoxyflurane. Note the numerous intraretinal crystals dispersed throughout the posterior pole of both eyes. Initially, the crystals appeared to be more intravascular in location.

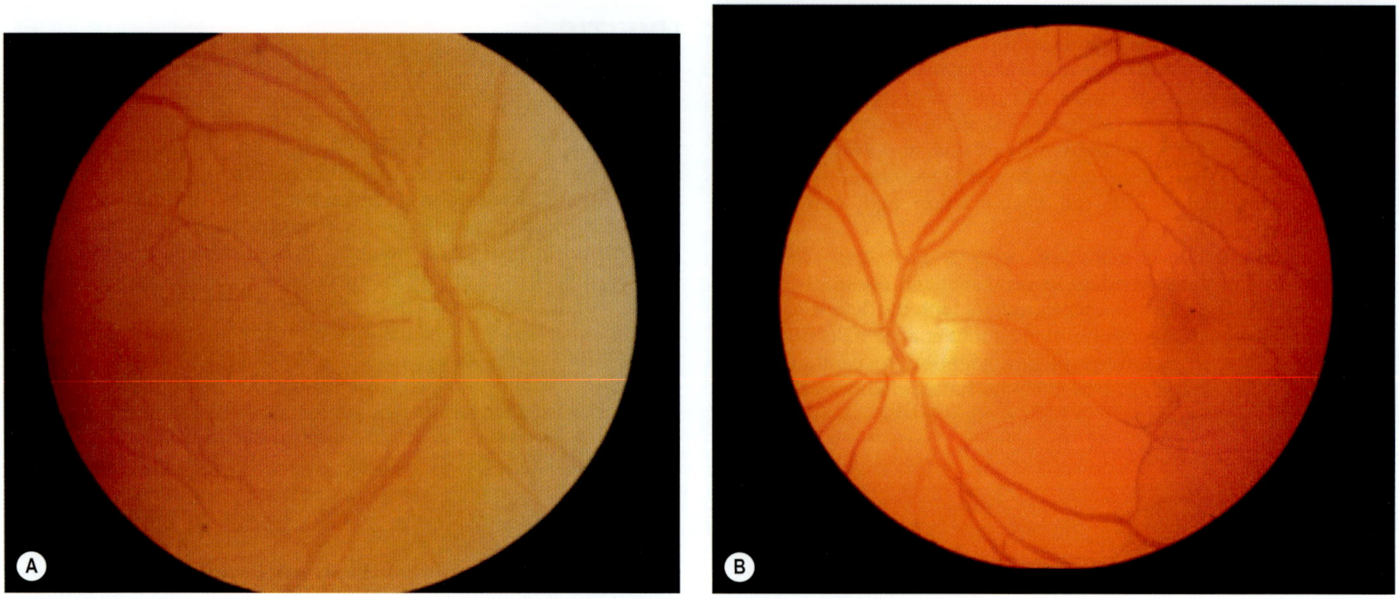

Figure 16.23 (A) Color photograph of right eye, and (B) left eye of a patient with acute methanol toxicity. There is prominent disc congestion and retinal edema, which gradually gave way to optic disc pallor. The patient did not recover useful vision in spite of prompt recognition of the condition.

CMV retinitis is less common since the advent of highly active antiretroviral therapy (HAART). Additionally, CMV retinitis often responds favorably to intravitreal ganciclovir and foscarnet injections, which are not known to cause uveitis.

LATANOPROST

See the section on cystoid macular edema (above).

MISCELLANEOUS (SUBJECTIVE OCULAR EFFECTS)

CARDIAC GLYCOSIDES

Cardiac glycosides such as digoxin are used in the treatment of chronic heart failure and as antiarrhythmic agents. Although these drugs do not cause a characteristic retinal abnormality, ocular symptoms, including blurred vision, scintillating scotomas, and xanthopsia (yellowing of vision), are common.[181,182] These changes probably are caused by direct toxicity to the photoreceptors. The visual symptoms are reversible with discontinuation of the drug.

SILDENAFIL

The widely used erectile dysfunction agent sildenafil is an inhibitor of phosphodiesterase 5 (PDE-5) in the penile corpora cavernosa, but demonstrates cross-activity with the PDE-6 in the photoreceptors as well.[183] A single dose may cause transient and reversible dyschromatopsia,[184,185] though symptoms are generally dose-related. Typically, the fundoscopic examination and FA are normal, but rare reported complications include retinal hemorrhages, retinal vascular occlusion,[186] nonarteritic anterior ischemic optic neuropathy,[187] acceleration of proliferative diabetic retinopathy,[188] and central serous chorioretinopathy.[45,189] Changes commensurate with the above-noted diagnoses may be seen on FA. More reproducible abnormalities, even in asymptomatic subjects, include transient depressions in ERG and mfERG.[190] In most cases, sildenafil appears to cause no apparent long-term retinal damage, although individuals with preexisting retinal disease may be at increased risk.[191,192]

METHANOL

Methanol is occasionally accidently ingested by alcoholics. Visual blurring and field deficits are seen within 12–18 hours. Early retinal findings include optic nerve hyperemia and retinal edema (Figure 16.23), while late findings include optic disc atrophy. Nerve toxicity is mediated by formic acid, a breakdown product of methanol, which directly affects the inner retina and optic nerve.[193] The degree of systemic acidosis correlates well with the extent of visual dysfunction. Early hemodialysis is effective in removing methanol from the body, but if visual recovery is not evident by 6 days, it often remains permanently decreased.

VIGABATRIN

Vigabatrin is used for treatment of epilepsy, and has been associated with optic atrophy and visual field defects.[194,195]

SUMMARY AND KEY POINTS

Although there are thousands of systemic medications, only a small number of these agents produce retinal changes. Retinal toxicity can occur when agents are used at standard therapeutic dosages, or when utilized for nonapproved indications. The mechanism by which toxicity develops is unknown in many cases. With multiple new drugs reaching the market annually, ophthalmologists need to maintain a high index of suspicion that patients' symptoms and clinical findings may be related to one or more of their systemic medications.

REFERENCES

1. Weekley RD, Potts AM, Reboton J, et al. Pigmentary retinopathy in patients receiving high doses of a new phenothiazine. Arch Ophthalmol 1960;64:65–76.

2. Meredith TA, Aaberg TM, Willerson D. Progressive chorioretinopathy after receiving thioridazine. Arch Ophthalmol 1978;96:1172–1176.
3. Miller DF, Bay JW, Lederman RJ, et al. Ocular and orbital toxicity following intracarotid injection of BCNU (carmustine) and cisplatinum for malignant gliomas. Ophthalmology 1985;92:402–406.
4. Miyata M, Imai H, Ishikawa S, et al. Changes in human electroretinography associated with thioridazine administration. Ophthalmologica 1980;181:175–180.
5. Hagopian V, Stratton DB, Busick RD. Five cases of pigmentary retinopathy associated with thioridazine administration. Am J Psychiatry 1966;123:97–100.
6. Marmor MF. Is thioridazine retinopathy progressive? Relationship of pigmentary changes to visual function. Br J Ophthalmol 1990;74: 739–742.
7. Potts AM. Further studies concerning accumulation of polycyclic compounds on uveal melanin. Invest Ophthalmol Vis Sci 1964;3: 399–404.
8. Potts AM. The concentration of phenothiazines in the eye of experimental animals. Invest Ophthalmol Vis Sci 1962;1:522–530.
9. Potts AM. The reaction of uveal pigment *in vitro* with polycyclic compounds. Invest Ophthalmol Vis Sci 1964;3:405–416.
10. Kinross-Wright JT. Clinical trial of a new phenothiazine compound NP-207. Psychiatr Res Rep Am Psychiatr Assoc 1956;4:89–94.
11. Bonting SL, Caravaggio LL, Canady MR. Studies on sodium potassium-activated adenosine triphosphatase. X. Occurrence in retinal rods and relation to rhodopsin. Exp Eye Res 1964;3:47–56.
12. Cerletti A, Meier-Ruge W. Toxicological studies on pheno-thiazine-induced retinopathy. Excerpts Medica Int Congress Ser 1968;145:170–188.
13. Muirhead JF. Drug effects on retinal oxidation: retinal alcohol: NAD oxidoreductase. Invest Ophthalmol Vis Sci 1967;6:635–641.
14. Miller III FS, Bunt-Milam AH, Kalina RE. Clinical-ultrastructural study of thioridazine retinopathy. Ophthalmology 1982;89:1478–1488.
15. DeLong SL, Poley BJ, McFarlane JR. Ocular changes associated with long-term chlorpromazine therapy. Arch Ophthalmol 1965;73: 611–617.
16. Mathalone MBR. Eye and skin changes in psychiatric patients treated with chlorpromazine. Br J Ophthalmol 1967;51:86–93.
17. Siddal JR. The ocular toxic findings with prolonged and high dosage chlorpromazine intake. Arch Ophthalmol 1965;74:460–464.
18. Wolf ME, Richer S, Berk MA, et al. Cutaneous and ocular changes associated with the use of chlorpromazine. Int J Clin Pharmacol Ther Toxicol 1993;31:365–367.
19. Hart WM, Burde RM, Johnston GP, et al. Static perimetry in chloroquine retinopathy: perifoveal patterns of visual field depression. Arch Ophthalmol 1984;102:377–380.
20. Heckenlively JR, Matin D, Levy J. Chloroquine retinopathy. Am J Ophthalmol 1980;89:150.
21. Ochsendorf FR, Runne U. Chloroquine: consideration of maximum daily dose (3.5 mg/kg ideal weight) prevents retinopathy. Dermatology 1996;192:382–383.
22. Tobin DR, Krohel GB, Rynes RL. Hydroxychloroquine: seven-year experience. Arch Ophthalmol 1982;100:81–83.
23. Finbloom DS, Silver K, Newsome DA, et al. Comparison of hydroxychloroquine and chloroquine use and the development of retinal toxicity. J Rheumatol 1985;12:692–694.
24. Mackenzie AH, Scherbel AL. A decade of chloroquine maintenance therapy: rate of administration governs incidence of retinotoxicity. Arthritis Rheum 1968;11:496.
25. Brinkley JR, Dubois EL, Ryan SJ. Long-term course of chloroquine retinopathy after cessation of medication. Am J Ophthalmol 1979;88:1–11.
26. Carr RE, Henkind P, Rothfield N, et al. Ocular toxicity of antimalarial drugs. Am J Ophthalmol 1968;66:738.
27. Rubin M, Bernstein HN, Zvaifler NJ. Studies on the pharmacology of chloroquine. Arch Ophthalmol 1963;70:80–87.
28. Ehrenfeld M, Nesher R, Merin S. Delayed-onset chloroquine retinopathy. Br J Ophthalmol 1986;70:281–283.
29. Sassani JW, Brucker AJ, Cobbs W, et al. Progressive chloroquine retinopathy. Ann Ophthalmol 1983;15:19–22.
30. Bernstein H, Zvaifler N, Rubin M, et al. The ocular deposition of chloroquine. Invest Ophthalmol 1963;2:384–392.
31. Ehrenfeld M, Nesher R, Merin S. Delayed-onset chloroquine retinopathy. Br J Ophthalmol 1986;70:281–283.
32. Ivanina TA, Zueva MY, Lebedeva MM, et al. Ultrastructural alterations in rat and cat retina and pigment epithelium induced by chloroquine. Graefes Arch Clin Exp Ophthalmol 1983;22:32–38.
33. Wetterholm DH, Winter FC. Histopathology of chloroquine retinal toxicity. Arch Ophthalmol 1964;71:82–87.
34. Ramsey MS, Fine BS. Chloroquine toxicity in the human eye: histopathologic observation by electron microscopy. Am J Ophthalmol 1972;73:229–235.
35. Grierson DJ. Hydroxychloroquine and visual screening in a rheumatology outpatient clinic. Ann Rheum Dis 1997;56:188–190.
36. Levy GD, Munz SJ, Paschal J, et al. Incidence of hydroxychloroquine retinopathy in 1207 patients in a large multicenter outpatient practice. Arthritis Rheum 1997;40:1482–1486.
37. Rynes RI. Ophthalmologic considerations in using antimalarials in the United States. Lupus 1996;5:73–74.
38. Coyle JT. Hydroxychloroquine retinopathy. Ophthalmology 2001;108: 243–244.
39. Mavrikakis I, Sfikakis PP, Mavrikakis E, et al. The incidence of irreversible retinal toxicity in patients treated with hydroxychloroquine: a reappraisal. Ophthalmology 2003;110:1321–1326.
40. Falcone PM, Paolini L, Lou PL. Hydroxychloroquine toxicity despite normal dose therapy. Ann Ophthalmol 1993;25:385–388.
41. Mavrikakis M, Papazoglou S, Sfikakis PP, et al. Retinal toxicity in long-term hydroxychloroquine treatment. Ann Rheum Dis 1996;55:187–189.
42. Weiser A, Sandberg MA, Gaadio AR, et al. Hydroxychloroquine retinopathy. Am J Ophthalmol 1991;121:582–584.
43. Easterbrook M, Bernstein H. Ophthalmic monitoring of patients taking antimalarials: preferred practice patterns. J Rheumatol 1997;24: 1390–1392.
44. Morsman CDG, Livesey SJ, Richards IM, et al. Screening for hydroxychloroquine retinal toxicity: is it necessary? Eye 1990;4:572–576.
45. Shipley M, Silman A. Should patients on hydroxychloroquine have their eyes examined regularly? Br J Rheumatol 1997;30:514–515.
46. Silman A, Shipley M. Ophthalmological monitoring for hydroxychloroquine toxicity: a scientific review of available data. Br J Rheumatol 1997;36:599–601.
47. Browning DJ. Hydroxychloroquine and chloroquine retinopathy: screening for drug toxicity. Am J Ophthalmol 2002;133:649–656.
48. Easterbrook M. Hydroxychloroquine retinopathy. Ophthalmology 2001;108:2158–2159.
49. Hart WM, Burde RM, Johnston GP, et al. Static perimetry in chloroquine retinopathy: perifoveal patterns of visual field depression. Arch Ophthalmol 1984;102:377–380.
50. Easterbrook M. The use of Amsler grids in early chloroquine retinopathy. Ophthalmology 1984;91:1368–1372.
51. Maturi RK, Yu M, Weleber RG. Multifocal electroretinographic evaluation of long-term hydroxychloroquine users. Arch Ophthalmol 2004;122:973–981.
52. Marmor MF, Carr RE, Easterbrook M, et al. Recommendations on screening for chloroquine and hydroxychloroquine retinopathy: a report by the American Academy of Ophthalmology. Ophthalmol 2002;109:1377–1382.
53. Horgan SE, Williams RW. Chronic retinal toxicity due to quinine in Indian tonic water. Eye 1995;9:637–663.
54. Brinton GS, Nortona EWD, Zahn JR, et al. Ocular quinine toxicity. Am J Ophthalmol 1980;90:403–410.
55. Bacon P, Spalton DJ, Smith SE. Blindness from quinine toxicity. Br J Ophthalmol 1988;72:219–224.
56. Brinton GS, Nortona EWD, Zahn JR, et al. Ocular quinine toxicity. Am J Ophthalmol 1980;90:403–410.
57. Buchanan TAS, Lyness RW, Collins AD, et al. An experimental study of quinine blindness. Eye 1987;1:522–524.
58. Canning CR, Hague S. Ocular quinine toxicity. Br J Ophthalmol 1988;72:23–26.
59. Craythorn JM, Swartz M, Creel DJ. Clofazimine-induced bull's-eye retinopathy. Retina 1986;6:50–52.
60. Cunningham CA, Friedberg DN, Carr RE. Clofazimine-induced generalized retinal degeneration. Retina 1990;10:131–134.
61. Whitcup SM, Butler KM, Caruso R, et al. Retinal toxicity in human immunodeficiency virus-infected children treated with 2′,3′-dideoxyinosine. Am J Ophthalmol 1992;113:1–7.
62. Haimovici R, D'Amico DJ, Gragoudas ES, et al. The expanded clinical spectrum of deferoxamine retinopathy. Ophthalmology 2002;109: 164–171.
63. Baath JS, Lam WC, Kirby M, et al. Deferoxamine-related ocular toxicity: incidence and outcome in a pediatric population. Retina 2008;28: 894–899.
64. Davies SC, Hungerford JL, Arden GB, et al. Ocular toxicity of high-dose intravenous desferrioxamine. Lancet 1983;2:181–184.
65. Mehta AM, Engstrom RE, Kreiger AE. Deferoxamine-associated retinopathy after subcutaneous injection. Am J Ophthalmol 1994;118:260–262.
66. Gass JDM. Stereoscopic Atlas of Macular Diseases: Diagnosis and Treatment, 4th edn. St. Louis: Mosby, 1997.
67. Gonzales CR, Lin AP, Engstrom RE, et al. Bilateral vitelliform maculopathy and deferoxamine toxicity. Retina 2004;24:464–467.
68. Rahl AHS, Hungerford JL, Ahmed AI. Ocular toxicity of desferrioxamine: light microscopic histochemical and ultrastructural findings. Br J Ophthalmol 1986;70:373–381.
69. Hida T, Chandler D, Arena JE, et al. Experimental and clinical observations of the intraocular toxicity of commercial corticosteroid preparations. Am J Ophthalmol 1986;101:190–195.
70. Pendergast SD, Eliott D, Machemer R. Retinal toxic effects following inadvertent intraocular injection of celestone soluspan. Arch Ophthalmol 1995;113:1230–1231.
71. McCuen II BW, Bessler M, Tano Y, et al. The lack of toxicity of intravitreally administered triamcinolone acetonide. Am J Ophthalmol 1981;91:785–788.

72. Piccolino FC, Pandolfo A, Polizzi A, et al. Retinal toxicity from accidental intraocular injection of depomedrol. Retina 2002;22:117–119.
73. Kupersmith MJ, Seiple WH, Holopigian K, et al. Maculopathy caused by intraarterially administered cisplatin and intravenously administered carmustine. Am J Ophthalmol 1992;113:435–438.
74. Miller DF, Bay JW, Lederman RJ, et al. Ocular and orbital toxicity following intracarotid injection of BCNU (carmustine) and cisplatinum for malignant gliomas. Ophthalmology 1985;92:402–406.
75. Katz BJ, Ward JH, Digre KB, et al. Persistent severe visual and electroretinographic abnormalities after intravenous cisplatin therapy. J Neuroophthalmol 2003;23:132–135.
76. Khawly JA, Rubin P, Petros W, et al. Retinopathy and optic neuropathy in bone marrow transplantation for breast cancer. Ophthalmology 1996;103:87–95.
77. Margo CE, Murtagh FR. Ocular and orbital toxicity after intra-carotid cisplatin therapy. Am J Ophthalmol 1993;116:508–509.
78. Singalavaniga A, Ruangvaravate N, Dulayajinda D. Potassium iodate toxic retinopathy: a report of five cases. Retina 2000;20:378–383.
79. AtLee WE. Talc and cornstarch emboli in eyes of drug users. JAMA 1972;219:49.
80. Murphy SB, Jackson WB, Pare JAP. Talc retinopathy. Can J Ophthalmol 1978;13:152–156.
81. Tse DT, Ober RR. Talc retinopathy. Am J Ophthalmol 1980;90:624–640.
82. Schatz H, Drake M. Self-injected retinal emboli. Ophthalmology 1979;86:468.
83. Zoumalan CI, Marmor MF. Revisiting talc retinopathy. Arch Ophthalmol 2007;125:988.
84. Friberg TR, Gragoudas ES, Regan CDJ. Talc emboli and macular ischemia in intravenous drug abuse. Arch Ophthalmol 1979;97:1089.
85. Brucker AJ. Disk and peripheral retinal neovascularization secondary to talc and cornstarch emboli. Am J Ophthalmol 1979;88:864.
86. Kresca LJ, Goldberg MF, Jampol LM. Talc emboli and retinal neovascularization in a drug abuser. Am J Ophthalmol 1979;87:334.
87. Jampol LM, Setogawa T, Rednam KRV, et al. Talc retinopathy in primates: a model of ischemic retinopathy. I. Clinical studies. Arch Ophthalmol 1981;99:1273–1280.
88. Kaga N, Tso MOM, Jampol LM, et al. Talc retinopathy in primates: a model of ischemic retinopathy. II. A histopathologic study. Arch Ophthalmol 1982;100:1644–1648.
89. Kaga N, Tso MOM, Jampol LM. Talc retinopathy in primates: a model of ischemic retinopathy. III. An electron microscopic study. Arch Ophthalmol 1982;100:1649–1657.
90. Vessey MP, Hannaford P, Mant J, et al. Oral contraception and eye disease: findings in two large cohort studies. Br J Ophthalmol 1998;82:538–542.
91. Garg SK, Chase P, Marshall G, et al. Oral contraceptives and renal and retinal complications in young women with insulin-dependent diabetes mellitus. JAMA 1994;271:1099–1102.
92. Petersson GJ, Fraunfelder FT, Meyer SM. Oral contraceptives. Ophthalmology 1981;88:368–371.
93. Bos PJ, Deutman AF. Acute macular neuroretinopathy. Am J Ophthalmol 1975;80:573–584.
94. Turbeville SD, Cowan LD, Gass JD. Acute macular neuroretinopathy: a review of the literature. Surv Ophthalmol 2003;48:1–11.
95. Monson BK, Greenberg PB, Greenberg E, et al. High-speed, ultra-high-resolution optical coherence tomography of acute macular neuroretinopathy. Br J Ophthalmol 2007;91:119–120.
96. Balian JV. Accidental intraocular tobramycin injection: a case report. Ophthalmic Surg 1983;14:353–354.
97. Campochiaro PA, Conway BP. Aminoglycoside toxicity – a survey of retinal specialists: implications for ocular use. Arch Ophthalmol 1991;109:946–950.
98. Campochiaro PA, Lim JI. Aminoglycoside toxicity in the treatment of endophthalmitis. Arch Ophthalmol 1994;112:48–53.
99. McDonald HR, Schatz H, Allen AW, et al. Retinal toxicity secondary to intraocular gentamicin. Ophthalmology 1986;93:871–877.
100. Rosenbaum JD, Krumholz DM, Metz DM. Gentamicin retinal toxicity after cataract surgery in an eye that underwent vitrectomy. Ophthalmic Surg Laser 1997;28:236–238.
101. D'Amico DJ, Caspers-Velu L, Libert J, et al. Comparative toxicity of intravitreal aminoglycoside antibiotics. Am J Ophthalmol 1985;100: 264–275.
102. Peyman GA, Vastine DW, Crouch ER, et al. Clinical use of intravitreal antibiotics to treat bacterial endophthalmitis. Trans Am Acad Ophthalmol Otolaryngol 1974;78:862–875.
103. Zachary IG, Forster RK. Experimental intravitreal gentamicin. Am J Ophthalmol 1976;82:604–611.
104. Rosenbaum JD, Krumholz DM, Metz DM. Gentamicin retinal toxicity after cataract surgery in an eye that underwent vitrectomy. Ophthalmic Surg Laser 1997;28:236–238.
105. Talamo JH, D'Amico DJ, Hanninen LA, et al. The influence of aphakia and vitrectomy on experimental retinal toxicity of aminoglycoside antibiotics. Am J Ophthalmol 1985;100:840–847.
106. Kane A, Barza M, Baum J. Intravitreal injection of gentamicin in rabbits: effect of inflammation and pigmentation on half-life and ocular distribution. Invest Ophthalmol Vis Sci 1981;20:593–597.
107. Zemel E, Loewenstein A, Lei B, et al. Ocular pigmentation protects the rabbit retina from gentamicin-induced toxicity. Invest Ophthalmol Vis Sci 1995;36:1875–1884.
108. Brown GC, Eagle RC, Shakin EP, et al. Retinal toxicity of intravitreal gentamicin. Arch Ophthalmol 1990;108:1740–1744.
109. Conway BP, Tabatabay CA, Campochiaro PA, et al. Gentamicin toxicity in the primate retina. Arch Ophthalmol 1989;107:107–112.
110. D'Amico DJ, Libert J, Kenyon KR, et al. Retinal toxicity of intravitreal gentamicin: an electron microscopic study. Invest Ophthalmol Vis Sci 1984;25:564–572.
111. Hines J, Vinores SA, Campochiaro PA. Evolution of morphologic changes after intravitreous injection of gentamicin. Curr Eye Res 1993; 12:521–529.
112. Chu TG, Ferreira M, Ober RR. Immediate pars plana vitrectomy in the management of inadvertent intracameral injection of gentamicin: a rabbit experimental model. Retina 1994;14:59–64.
113. Burgansky Z, Rock T, Bartov E. Inadvertent intravitreal gentamicin injection. Eur J Ophthalmol 2002;12:138–140.
114. Lim JI, Anderson CT, Hutchinson A, et al. The role of gravity in gentamicin-induced toxic effects in a rabbit model. Arch Ophthalmol 1994;112:1363–1367.
115. Fiscella RG, Gieser J, Phillpotts B, et al. Intraocular penetration of gentamicin after once-daily aminoglycoside dosing. Retina 1998;18:339–342.
116. Guyer DR, Tiedeman J, Yannuzzi LA, et al. Interferon-associated retinopathy. Arch Ophthalmol 1993;111:350–356.
117. Kawano T, Shegehira M, Uto H, et al. Retinal complications during interferon therapy for chronic hepatitis C. Am J Gastroenterol 1996;91:309–313.
118. Schulman JA, Liang C, Kooragayala LM, et al. Posterior segment complications in patients with hepatitis C treated with interferon and ribavirin. Ophthalmology 2003;110:437–442.
119. Kiratli H, Irkee M. Presumed interferon-associated bilateral macular arterial branch obstruction. Eye 2000;14:920–922.
120. Tokai R, Ikeda T, Miyaura T, et al. Interferon-associated retinopathy and cystoid macular edema. Arch Ophthalmol 2001;119:1077–1079.
121. Hejny C, Sternberg P, Lawson DH, et al. Retinopathy associated with high-dose interferon alfa-2b therapy. Am J Ophthalmol 2001;131: 782–787.
122. Wilson RL, Ross RD, Wilson LM, et al. Interferon-associated retinopathy in a young, insulin-dependent diabetic patient. Retina 2000;20: 413–415.
123. Kertes PJ, Britton WA, Addison DJ, et al. Toxicity of intravitreal interferon alpha-2b in the rabbit. Can J Ophthalmol 1995;30:355–359.
124. Gupta DR, Strobos RJ. Bilateral papillitis associated with Cafergot therapy. Neurology 1972;22:793.
125. Mindel JS, Rubenstein AE, Franklin B. Ocular ergotamine tartrate toxicity during treatment of Vacor-induced orthostatic hypotension. Am J Ophthalmol 1981;92:492–496.
126. Gilmer G, Swartz M, Teske M, et al. Over-the-counter phenylpropanolamine: a possible cause of central retinal vein occlusion. Arch Ophthalmol 1986;104:642.
127. Thomas JV, Gragoudas ES, Blair NP, et al. Correlation of epinephrine use and macular edema in aphakic glaucomatous eyes. Arch Ophthalmol 1978;96:625–628.
128. Fraunfelder FW, Fraunfelder FT, Illingworth DR. Adverse ocular effects associated with niacin therapy. Br J Ophthalmol 1995;79:54–56.
129. Gass JDM. Nicotinic acid maculopathy. Am J Ophthalmol 1973;76:500–510.
130. Millay RH, Klein ML, Illingworth DR. Niacin maculopathy. Ophthalmology 1988;95:930–936.
131. Jampol LM. Niacin maculopathy. Ophthalmology 1988;95:1704–1705.
132. Spirn MJ, Warren FA, Guyer DR, et al. Optical coherence tomography findings in nicotinic acid maculopathy. Am J Ophthalmol 2003;135: 913–914.
133. Holló G. The side effects of the prostaglandin analogues. Expert Opin Drug Safe 2007;6:45–52.
134. Arcieri ES, Santana A, Rocha FN, et al. Blood-aqueous barrier changes after the use of prostaglandin analogues in patients with pseudophakia and aphakia: a 6-month randomized trial. Arch Ophthalmol 2005;123: 186–192.
135. Miyake K, Ibaraki N. Prostaglandins and cystoid macular edema. Surv Ophthalmol 2002;47 (Suppl. 1):S203–S218.
136. Grinbaum A, Ashkenazi I, Avni I, et al. Transient myopia following metronidazole treatment for trichomonas vaginalis. JAMA 1992;267: 511–512.
137. Ryan EH, Jampol LM. Drug-induced acute transient myopia with retinal folds, Retina 1986;6:220–223.
138. Soylev MF, Green RL, Feldon SE. Choroidal effusion as a mechanism for transient myopia induced by hydrochlorothiazide and triamterene. Am J Ophthalmol 1995;120:395–397.
139. Sen HA, O'Halloran HS, Lee WB. Case reports and small case series: topiramate-induced acute myopia and retinal striae. Arch Ophthalmol 2001;119:775–777.

140. Fraunfelder FW, Fraunfelder FT, Keates EU. Topiramate-associated acute, bilateral, secondary angle-closure glaucoma. Ophthalmol 2004;111: 109–111.
141. Alwitry A, Gardner I. Tamoxifen maculopathy. Arch Ophthalmol 2002;120:1402.
142. Kaiser-Kupfer MI, Kupfer C, Rodrigues MM. Tamoxifen retinopathy. Cancer Treat Rep 1978;62:315–320.
143. Chang T, Gonder JR, Ventresca MR. Low-dose tamoxifen retinopathy. Can J Ophthalmol 1992;27:148–149.
144. Griffiths MFP. Tamoxifen retinopathy at low dosage. Am J Ophthalmol 1987;104:185–186.
145. Pavlidis NA, Petris C, Briassoulis E, et al. Clear evidence that long-term, low-dose tamoxifen treatment can induce ocular toxicity. Cancer 1992;69:2961–2964.
146. Noureddin BN, Seoud M, Bashshur Z, et al. Ocular toxicity in low-dose tamoxifen: a prospective study. Eye 1999;13:729–733.
147. Heier JS, Dragoo RA, Enzenauer RW, et al. Screening for ocular toxicity in asymptomatic patients treated with tamoxifen. Am J Ophthalmol 1994;117:772–775.
148. McKeown CA, Swartz M, Blom J, et al. Tamoxifen retinopathy. Br J Ophthalmol 1981;65:177–179.
149. Bourla DH, Sarraf D, Schwartz SD. Peripheral retinopathy and maculopathy in high-dose tamoxifen therapy. Am J Ophthalmol 2007;144:126–128.
150. Ashford AR, Donev I, Tiwari RP, et al. Reversible ocular toxicity related to tamoxifen therapy. Cancer 1988;61:33–35.
151. Nayfield SG, Gorin MB. Tamoxifen-associated eye disease: a review. J Clin Oncol 1996;14:1018–1026.
152. Kalina RE, Wells CG. Screening for ocular toxicity in asymptomatic patients with tamoxifen. Am J Ophthalmol 1995;119:112–113.
153. McKeown CA, Swartz M, Blom J, et al. Tamoxifen retinopathy. Br J Ophthalmol 1981;65:177–179.
154. Kaiser-Kupfer MI, Kupfer C, Rodrigues MM. Tamoxifen retinopathy: a clinicopathologic report. Ophthalmology 1981;88:89–93.
155. Chang TS, Aylward W, Clarkson JG, et al. Asymmetric canthaxanthine retinopathy. Am J Ophthalmol 1995;119:801–802.
156. Lonn LI. Canthaxanthine retinopathy. Arch Ophthalmol 1987;105: 1590–1591.
157. Espaillat A, Aiello LP, Arrigg PG, et al. Canthaxanthine retinopathy. Arch Ophthalmol 1999;117:412–413.
158. Cortin P, Boudreault G, Rousseau AP, et al. La retinopathie a la canthaxanthine. II. Facteurs prédisposants. Can J Ophthalmol 1984;19:215–219.
159. Boudreault G, Cortin P, Corriveau LA, et al. La retinopathie a la canthaxanthine. I. Etude clinique de 51 consommateurs. Can J Ophthalmol 1983;18:325–328.
160. Harnois C, Cortin P, Samson J, et al. Static perimetry in canthaxanthine maculopathy. Arch Ophthalmol 1988;106:58–60.
161. Metge P, Mandirac-Bonnefoy C, Bellaube P. Thesaurismose retinienne a la canthaxanthine. Bull Mem Soc Fr Ophtalmol 1984;95:547–549.
162. Weber U, Goerz G, Hennekes R. Carotenoid retinopathie. I. Morphologische und funktionell Befunde. Klin Monatsbl Augenheilkd 1985;186:351–354.
163. Daicker B, Schiedt K, Adnet JJ, et al. Canthaxanthin retinopathy: an investigation by light and electron microscopy and physiochemical analysis. Graefes Arch Clin Exp Ophthalmol 1987;225:189–197.
164. Scallon LJ, Burke JM, Mieler WF, et al. Canthaxanthine-induced retinal pigment epithelial changes in the cat. Curr Eye Res 1988;7:687–693.
165. Harnois C, Samson J, Malenfant M, et al. Canthaxanthine retinopathy: anatomic and functional reversibility. Arch Ophthalmol 1989;107: 538–540.
166. Leyon H, Ros A, Nyberg S, et al. Reversibility of canthaxanthin deposits within the retina. Acta Ophthalmol 1990;68:607–611.
167. Oosterhuis JA, Remky H, Nijman NM, et al. Canthaxanthine-retinopathie ohne Canthaxanthine-einnahime. Klin Monatsbl Augenheilkd 1989;194:110–116.
168. Bullock JD, Albert DM. Fleck retina: appearance secondary to oxalate crystals from methoxyflurane anesthesia. Arch Ophthalmol 1975;93:26–31.
169. Novak MA, Roth AS, Levine MR. Calcium oxalate retinopathy associated with methoxyflurane abuse. Retina 1988;8:230–236.
170. Albert DM, Bullock JD, Lahav M, et al. Flecked retina secondary to oxalate crystals from methoxyflurane anesthesia: clinical and experimental studies. Trans Am Acad Ophthalmol Otolaryngol 1975;79:817–826.
171. Wells CG, Johnson RJ, Qingli L, et al. Retinal oxalosis: a clinicopathological report. Arch Ophthalmol 1989;107:1638–1643.
172. Ibanez HE, Williams DF, Boniuk I. Crystalline retinopathy associated with long-term nitrofurantoin therapy. Arch Ophthalmol 1994;112:304–305.
173. Tseng AL, Walmsley SL. Rifabutin-associated uveitis. Ann Pharmacother 1995;29:1149–1155.
174. Saran BR, Maguire AM, Nichols C, et al. Hypopyon uveitis in patients with acquired immunodeficiency syndrome: treatment for systemic *Mycobacterium avium* complex infection with rifabutin. Arch Ophthalmol 1994;112:1159–1165.
175. Arevalo JF, Russack V, Freeman WR. New ophthalmic manifestations of presumed rifabutin-related uveitis. Ophthalmic Surg Laser 1997;28: 321–324.
176. Chaknis MJ, Brooks SE, Mitchell KT, Marcus DM. Inflammatory opacities of the vitreous in rifabutin-associated uveitis. Am J Ophthalmol 1996;122: 580–582.
177. Ponjavic V, Granse L, Bengtsson Stigmar E, et al. Retinal dysfunction and anterior segment deposits in a patient treated with rifabutin. Acta Ophthalmol Scand 2002;80:553–556.
178. Banker AS, Arevalo JF, Munguia D, et al. Intraocular pressure and aqueous humor dynamics in patients with AIDS treated with intravitreal cidofovir (HPMPC) for cytomegalovirus retinitis. Am J Ophthalmol 1997;124: 168–180.
179. Taskintuna I, Banker AS, Rao NA, et al. An animal model for cidofovir (HPMPC) toxicity: intraocular pressure and histopathologic effects. Exp Eye Res 1997;64:795–806.
180. Taskintuna I, Rahhal FM, Arevalo F, et al. Low-dose intravitreal cidofovir (HPMPC) therapy of cytomegalovirus retinitis in patients with acquired immune deficiency syndrome. Ophthalmology 1997;104:1049–1057.
181. Blair JR, Mieler WF. Retinal toxicity associated with commonly encountered systemic agents. Int Ophthalmol Clin 1995;35:137–156.
182. Weleber RG, Shults WT. Digoxin retinal toxicity: clinical and electrophysiologic evaluation of a cone dysfunction syndrome. Arch Ophthalmol 1981;99:1568–1572.
183. Ballard SA, Gingell CJ, Tang K, et al. Effects of sildenafil on the relaxation of human corpus cavernosum tissue *in vitro* and on the activities of cyclic nucleotide phosphodiesterase isozymes. J Urol 1998;159:2164–2171.
184. Goldstein I, Lue TF, Padma-Nathan H, et al. Oral sildenafil in the treatment of erectile dysfunction. N Engl J Med 1998;338:1397–1404.
185. Gabrieli CB, Regine F, Vingolo EM, et al. Subjective visual halos after sildenafil (Viagra) administration: Electroretinographic evaluation. Ophthalmology 2001;108:877–881.
186. Tripathi A, O'Donnell NP. Branch retinal artery occlusion: Another complication of sildenafil. Br J Ophthalmol 2000;84:928.
187. Pomeranz HD, Smith KH, Hart Jr WM , et al. Sildenafil-associated nonarteritic anterior ischemic optic neuropathy. Ophthalmology 2002;109:584–587.
188. Burton AJ, Reynolds A, O'Neill D. Sildenafil (Viagra) a cause of proliferative diabetic retinopathy? Eye 2000;14:785–786.
189. Allibhai ZA, Gale JS, Sheidow TS. Central serous chorioretinopathy in a patient taking sildenafil citrate. Ophthalmic Surg Lasers Imaging 2004;35:165–167.
190. Luu JK, Chappelow AV, McCulley TJ, et al. Acute effects of sildenafil on the electroretinogram and multifocal electroretinogram. Am J Ophthalmol 2001;132:388–394.
191. Laties AM, Fraunfelder FT. Ocular safety of Viagra (sildenafil citrate). Trans Am Ophthalmol Soc 1999;97:115–125.
192. Marmor MF. Sildenafil (Viagra) and ophthalmology. Arch Ophthalmol 1999;117:518–519.
193. Treichel JL, Murray TG, Lewandowski MF, et al. Retinal toxicity in methanol poisoning. Retina 2004;24:309–312.
194. Frisen L, Malmgren K. Characterization of vigabatrin-associated optic atrophy. Acta Opthalmol Scand 2003;81:466–473.
195. Malmgren K, Ben-Menachem E, Frisen L. Vigabatrin visual toxicity: evolution and dose dependence. Epilepsia 2001;42:609–615.

17 Non-neovascular age-related macular degeneration

Stephan Michels, MD, MBA, Gerhard Garhöfer, MD, and Malaika M. Kurz-Levin, MD

INTRODUCTION

Age-related macular degeneration (AMD) is one of the diseases affecting the choroid and retinal pigment epithelium (RPE) as well as the retina which has lately experienced many significant transitions. This is true for the pathogenesis, identification of risk factors, early detection of patients at risk, therapeutic options, public awareness, and socioeconomic impact.

The recent discoveries of genetic variants associated with an increased risk for AMD, especially the Y402H polymorphism of complement factor H (CFH) and a modification in the promoter region of HtrA serine peptidase 1 (HTRA1), have led to a completely new understanding of the disease.[1–5] These findings clearly indicate that genetic predisposition is the key factor in the etiology of AMD. Several risk factors have been recognized in the past, but seem less relevant compared to genetic predisposition. Genetic screening for AMD will become most valuable for identifying patients with increased risk for AMD at a young age, possibly allowing early preventive measures. Therapies aiming to modulate the complement cascade, especially the alternative pathway, are currently under intensive investigation with the goal of changing the course of AMD. Paroxysmal nocturnal hematuria (PNH), a rare disease of the complement system, has been shown to be effectively and safely treated by complete inhibition of the complement system using eculizumab, and may serve as a spearhead for AMD.[6] The increase in patients with nonneovascular AMD, especially in industrialized countries, demonstrates that better diagnostic tools and treatments are desperately needed for this form of AMD.

DISEASE PREVALENCE AND INFLUENCE

Several large epidemiologic studies have evaluated the prevalence of nonneovascular or so-called dry AMD. There is some variation in the prevalence of nonneovascular AMD depending on the exact definition of AMD, the age range of the populations evaluated, and genetic as well as environmental variations. Common to all studies is the higher prevalence of early AMD and an increasing prevalence with age. In the early 1990s in the USA the National Health and Nutrition Examination Survey (NHANES) showed a prevalence of 9.2% for all types of AMD in a population 40 years and older. Nonneovascular AMD is considered to make up about 85% of AMD cases. When pooling the prevalence found in large epidemiologic studies inside and outside the USA, the prevalence of AMD in the USA is estimated to be 1.75 million citizens in 2003, increasing to 2.95 million in 2020.[7] So far epidemiologic studies outside the USA have indicated that the occurrence of AMD might be generally lower than in the USA, as shown for example in the Rotterdam Study and the Blue Mountains Eye Study. Recently new epidemiologic studies on AMD have shifted the focus to two new areas of interest. First, certain populations, e.g., Norway and Greenland, seem to have a significantly higher prevalence of AMD than others. In a population aged at least 60 years, born and living in Greenland, the prevalence of any form of AMD was found to be 52.3%.[8] These studies indicate a strong impact of genetic and/or environmental factors and show the socioeconomic relevance of the disease. Lately the association of variants of CFH has been confirmed in many populations.

The second focus is on the prevalence of AMD in Asia. Little was known about AMD in India and China. The reasons for an increasing prevalence of AMD in Japan have not been conclusive. Prevalence of early AMD in a Japanese population is now at the level of the Australian population evaluated in the Beaver Dam Eye Study.[9] Epidemiologic studies in different Chinese populations found a prevalence of AMD above 10% and increasing with age. However, in contrast to Caucasian populations, the frequency of the CFH risk allele seems to be significantly lower in Asian populations.

Overall the impact of AMD is enhanced by increasing life expectancy in most of the large populations throughout the world. Nonneovascular AMD is commonly associated with gradual vision loss. Irreversible severe vision loss can occur, and the risk of progression to neovascular AMD should not be neglected.

RISK FACTORS

Before the discovery of a strong association of CFH and HTRA1 polymorphisms with AMD, several observational studies revealed that AMD shares a number of risk factors with atherosclerosis, among which age and smoking are the most important. However, atherosclerosis itself has not been consistently confirmed to be a risk factor for AMD. Several worldwide epidemiologic studies have found that with age there is an increasing risk for any type of AMD. Cigarette smoking is the most relevant modifiable, dose-dependent risk factor for AMD. A prospective study on cigarette smoking and risk of AMD found a risk ratio of 2.46 for current smokers (at least 20 cigarettes per day) compared to nonsmokers.[10] There is evidence that smoking in addition to variants of CFH and HTRA1 multiplies the risk for AMD.[11] Homozygosis for Y402H in addition to smoking increased the risk for advanced AMD to have an odds ratio (OR) of 10.2.[12] Further modifiable risk factors are a high body mass index (BMI) and fat intake. A BMI of at least 30 has been shown to have an OR of 2.1 for AMD. Again, homozygosis for Y402H polymorphism was found to multiply the OR to 5.9. There is ongoing controversy about dietary fats and their associated risk for AMD. Total fat intake has been consistently associated with an increased risk for AMD or AMD progression. Inconsistency of data with regard to vegetable or animal fats and their associated risk for AMD may be due to different regional fat preferences and regional differences in fat processing. A meta-analysis on the effect of lipid-lowering agents in the development of AMD found no clear evidence for an AMD risk reduction.[13] Interestingly there is a growing body of evidence that higher fish/omega-3 fatty acid consumption may have a protective effect for AMD.

Gender and socioeconomic status have not been shown to be a risk factor for AMD, whereas ethnicity may determine the risk for AMD. Black and Hispanic populations appear to have a lower prevalence for AMD than non-Hispanic white populations. Some Asian populations appear to have a prevalence for AMD comparable to white populations in western industrialized countries. These findings have been an indicator for a strong genetic component of the disease in the past.

Ocular risk factors such as refractive error, iris color, or cataracts have been investigated for a potential associated risk for AMD, but studies have either shown no association or have been contradictory. However, the strongest controversy concerns cataract surgery and progression of AMD.[14] It is mostly based on the question whether the removal of the natural lens, the major barrier to wavelengths of 300–400 nm (near ultraviolet radiation), leads to an increased risk of AMD progression. Several experimental animal studies provide compelling evidence for light toxicity on the retina. However, epidemiologic studies have been contradictory. Most modern intraocular lenses (IOLs) absorb ultraviolet radiation (below 400 nm). The value of yellow IOLs, attenuating blue light in the wavelength range 400–500 nm, in reducing the potential risk of AMD progression following cataract surgery, remains currently unclear.

A genetic component has long been suspected to be the key risk factor for AMD. But only recently genetic polymorphism in the gene encoding for the CFH located on chromosome 1q32 (region of CFH) and polymorphisms on chromosome 10 (LOC387715/PLEKHA1/HTRA1) were detected, validated, and accounted for a large part of the genetic risk for AMD. Variations in both regions are associated with an increased risk for AMD.[1–5] The associated risk for AMD varies between studies due to inclusion of different stages of AMD, different ethnic populations, and slight variations in the gene loci tested. The risk increases in patients with homozygosis and varies for different types of AMD. In particular, one important single nucleotide polymorphism (SNP) has been identified as a replacement of the amino acid tyrosine with histidine at amino acid 402 in exon 9 (Tyr402His). Individuals who carry a single copy of the histidine allele in the Y402H polymorphism have a two- to fourfold increased risk of AMD; individuals who are homozygous for the risk allele have a five- to sevenfold increased risk for developing AMD. Accordingly the incident rate ratios for LOC387715 were found to be 2.5 and 5.5. Subjects homozygous for both risk alleles even have a 50 times increased risk for AMD. Overall the variations at chromosome 10q26 seem to be more strongly associated with neovascular AMD than the variation at chromosome 1q32.

ETIOLOGY/PATHOGENESIS

In the past four principal pathomechanisms have been postulated for nonneovascular AMD: oxidative stress, impairment of choroidal circulation, degeneration of Bruch's membrane, and chronic inflammation.

The oxidative stress hypothesis as a pathomechanism of AMD is based on the breakdown of protective antioxidant systems within the retina. The key mechanism by which tissue damage due to reactive radicals or light-induced singlet oxygen occurs is the formation of lipid peroxides. Photoreceptors degenerate when exposed to continuous oxidative challenge or when antioxidative defense mechanisms are impaired. Currently the strongest evidence for a correlation of oxidative stress and AMD comes from the Age-related Eye Disease Study (AREDS). It investigated the use of high-dose vitamin C and E, beta-carotene, zinc, and copper on AMD and cataract. Patients with intermediate dry AMD or significant vision loss due to AMD in the second eye showed most risk reduction for progression to advanced AMD and for a three-line decrease in visual acuity.[15]

The choroidal circulation theory goes back to Verhoeff and Grossman, who already in 1937 linked sclerotic changes of the choriocapillaris to AMD.[16] Several studies using different techniques showed an association of reduced choroidal blood flow and AMD.[17–20] As mentioned previously, atherosclerosis and AMD have very similar risk factors. However, choroidal vascular changes can also – without atherosclerosis – occur secondary to impairment of the RPE.

Age-related changes in Bruch's membrane are considered to compromise transport of nutrients and metabolic substances to and from the RPE. Degeneration and thickening of Bruch's membrane with formation of drusen initiate or at least contribute to AMD. Drusen are the characteristic changes of early AMD. These deposits exceed those related to the normal aging process. They are located between the inner collagenous layer of Bruch's membrane and the basement membrane of the RPE. Despite the fact that degenerative changes of the RPE are regarded as the primary cause for the formation of drusen,[21,22] there is indication that a variable degree of drusen composition are of choroidal origin. Interestingly, apolipoprotein E (apoE)-deficient mouse and mouse on a high-fat diet show deposits in Bruch's membrane that are similar to AMD. A polymorphism of the apoE gene was found to be a risk factor for AMD.[23]

The role of inflammation in AMD has moved over the last years increasingly into the center of interest. Evidence for a role of inflammation in AMD was found not only in the retina (recruited macrophages, microglia) and in the blood (C-reactive protein (CRP), fibrinogen) but also in drusen, which were shown to contain complement activators, complement fragments, and membrane attack complex. In 2001, Hageman and co-workers outlined their model on the role of inflammation in AMD, proposing activation and recruitment of choroidal dendritic cells by locally injured RPE cells and subsequent drusen formation.[24] Membranoproliferative glomerulonephritis type II, a rare disease showing activation of the alternate complement pathway and drusen undistinguishable from AMD, was the link to CFH.

Early in 2005 four different groups outlined a strong association of a SNP on chromosome 1q32 and AMD. This Y402H variant in the CFH gene seems to affect the physiologic function of CFH. CFH is a regulator of the alternative complement pathway that blocks C3 activation to C3b and also degrades C3b (Figure 17.1). The absence or malfunction of CFH seems to lead to an increased activation of the alternative complement pathway, likely related to the presence of complement proteins in drusen, as described above. It is currently unclear why this specific variant leads to protein deposition in the retina. Further polymorphisms have been found around CFH that are likely to be associated with AMD. Interestingly CRP is also a binding partner of CFH, and the CRP-binding site of CFH is located in the domain containing the Y402H polymorphism. Patients homozygous for Y402H were found to have a 2.5 times higher level of CRP in their RPE and choroid. The role of CRP in the interplay between CFH and AMD is however not well understood.

In addition to the alternative complement pathway, polymorphisms in neighboring genes on chromosome 10 (PLEKHA1, LOC387715, and HTRA1) have shown association with AMD. The three genes appear to be in linkage disequilibrium. In Asian populations, where neovascular AMD occurs more commonly, a polymorphism in the HTRA1 promoter seems to be far more frequent than variants of CFH. HTRA1 itself is a stress-inducible heat shock serine protease. A role of HTRA1 in the inhibition of the angiogenic tumor growth factor-β (TGF-β) has been proposed, but the mechanisms of action remain unclear.

Further polymorphisms of apoE, complement factor B (CFB) and component C2 (part of the classic complement pathway) have shown evidence for an association with AMD, but less strong than polymorphisms of CFH and the promoter of HTRA1.

The recent findings implicate that genetic predisposition is the key factor in the pathogenesis of AMD. Some relations to pathomechanisms and risk factors postulated in the past appear more evident than others.

DIAGNOSIS AND ANCILLARY TESTING/ DIFFERENTIAL DIAGNOSIS

The diagnosis of nonneovascular AMD is commonly made by retinal examination, showing the characteristic drusen, focal hyper- or depigmentations, and/or areas of atrophy of the RPE. Retinal imaging and subsequent planimetric evaluation has been commonly used to evaluate nonneovascular AMD. Fluorescein angiography (FA) characteristically shows staining of drusen, window defects in areas of RPE atrophy, and focal fluorescein blockage in areas of hyperpigmentation. FA is generally used to exclude neovascular AMD. Within recent years two newer imaging modalities have become valuable in cases with nonneovascular AMD. Fundus autofluorescence (FAF) imaging enables topographic mapping of lipofuscin distribution in the RPE.[25] FAF patterns have been associated with different degrees of RPE atrophy progression. It is however unclear if FAF pattern can serve as a predictive

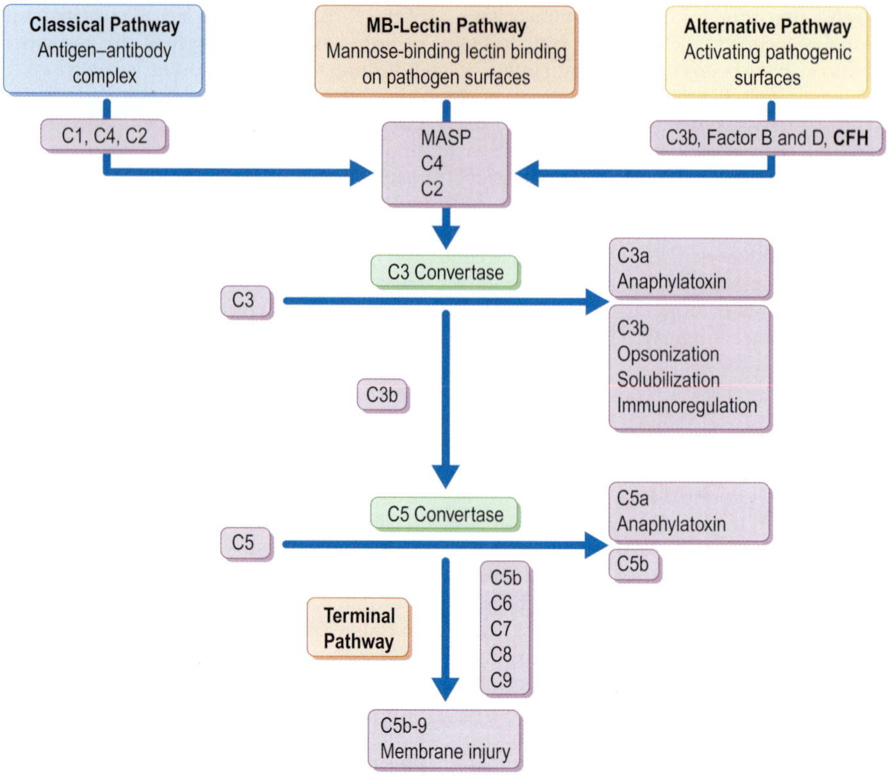

Figure 17.1 Complement cascade.

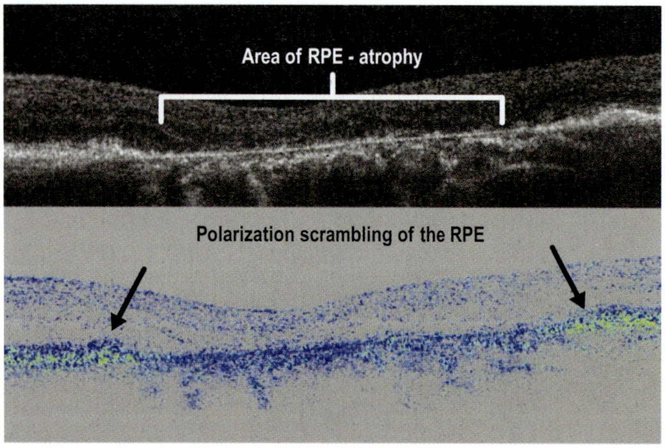

Figure 17.2 Comparison of time domain optical coherence tomography (upper image) and polarization-sensitive optical coherence tomography (lower image) at the exact same location in geographic atrophy.

factor.[26] Optical coherence tomography (OCT), especially the newer spectral domain and ultrahigh-resolution systems, provides further additional information on nonneovascular AMD. The new instruments allow three-dimensional imaging of drusen and show degeneration of photoreceptors overlying RPE atrophy. Further improvements in algorithms will provide detailed evaluation of drusen and RPE changes over time. Polarization-sensitive OCT allows outlining the RPE clearly due to its polarization scrambling properties, as shown in Figure 17.2.[27]

The Amsler grid is a valuable self-testing tool for patients with AMD. It aims for early detection of neovascular AMD, although the main pathological sign when using the Amsler grid, metamorphosia, can also be present in patients with nonneovascular AMD without evidence for any exudative process. More modern technologies such as preferential hyperacuity perimetery have been developed, but detection rates of metamorphopsia have not been convincingly higher than conventional Amsler grid testing. Microperimetry is a valuable tool in outlining retinal sensitivity defects in nonneovascular AMD, but is not very useful in screening patients. In addition anatomic changes associated with new neovascular AMD frequently detectable by OCT commonly precede functional deficits.

Most relevant differential diagnoses are summarized in Table 17.1.

Table 17.1 Differential diagnosis in nonneovascular age-related macular degeneration

Central serous chorioretinopathy (CSC)
Macular dystrophies (Stargardt's disease, pattern dystrophy, vitelliform and pseudovitelliform dystrophies, Malattia leventinese, North Carolina macular dystrophy, Sorsby dystrophy)
Myopic retinal degeneration
Toxic retinopathies (chloroquine retinopathy, clofazimine retinopathy)
Inflammatory maculopathies (multifocal chorioiditis, rubella retinopathy, serpiginous choroidopathy)

SIGNS AND SYMPTOMS

Early-stage AMD is often detected upon routine retinal examination. Those patients are usually not aware of any visual disturbances. The first signs of nonneovascular AMD include the presence of pigmentary abnormalities in the macular area and drusen of variable size and area. Drusen size was defined in AREDS as small (<63 μm), intermediate (≥63 μm, <125 μm), or large (>125 μm, equaling a width of an average large vein at the disc margin). Drusen area was also assessed in AREDS when categorizing the study population into the four predefined categories, as shown in detail in Table 17.2. Pigmentary changes are characterized by increased pigment not considered related to other diseases,

Table 17.2 **Age-related macular degeneration (AMD) categories in the Age-Related Eye Disease Study (AREDS)**

Category	Definition
1	No drusen or drusen < 63 μm with an area <125 μm diameter circle and no pigment abnormalities
2	Small drusen (<63 μm) with an area ≥125 μm diameter circle with possible pigment abnormalities but no geographic atrophy or at least one intermediate-size druse (≥63 μm, <125 μm) or no drusen required if pigment abnormalities present
3a	Intermediate-size druse (≥63 μm, <125 μm) ≥ 360 μm diameter circle if soft indistinct drusen are present, ≥656 μm diameter circle if soft indistinct drusen are absent. Pigment abnormalities can be present but no central geographic atrophy or at least one large druse (≥125 μm) or no drusen required if noncentral geographic atrophy is present
3b	First eye same as 3a; visual acuity <20/32 in second eye not due to AMD
4a	First eye category 1, 2, or 3a; second eye with advanced AMD
4b	First eye category 1, 2, or 3a; visual acuity <20/32 in second eye due to AMD, but no advanced AMD

RPE depigmentation, and noncentral geographic atrophy (GA). For assessing the individual risk of each patient for developing advanced AMD, either nonneovascular or neovascular, it is important to examine the macula carefully at every visit, paying attention to the signs mentioned above. As the classification of AMD according to AREDS is based upon the evaluation of photographs in a central reading center and using a special grid, it is not easily applicable for daily clinical use. A simplified severity scale was therefore developed and tested on the AREDS study population.[28] It does not include drusen area, which in a clinical setting is quite difficult to measure, since a strong association between maximum drusen size and drusen area had been found.[29] Patients without signs of advanced AMD were classified in the simplified severity scale by maximal drusen size and presence or absence of any pigmentary changes in one or both eyes. Bilateral intermediate-size drusen was counted as one risk factor. Small drusen did not count as any risk. The presence of at least one large druse and pigmentary abnormalities in both eyes would sum up to a risk factor of four. The 5-year risk of advanced AMD increases from 0.5% for a patient with 0 risk factors to 3% (one risk factor), 12% (two risk factors), 25% (three risk factors) and 50% (four risk factors). It is not clear to what extent other risk factors such as smoking, genetic predisposition, diet, or supplement use might influence these risks.

The symptoms experienced in nonneovascular AMD vary greatly according to the location and size of changes present. They also depend very much on the involvement of either one or both eyes. Even the presence of large drusen may not cause any visual disturbance as long as the fovea is not directly involved or the other eye is not affected. Confluent centrally located drusen might however cause metamorphosia without the presence of any neovascular changes such as choroidal neovascularization as well as blurred vision. First symptoms in GA are often reading difficulties, increasing when GA involves large areas of the center. In addition, patients will have greater difficulties in dim light as well as marked photophobia. In advanced nonneovascular AMD there can be severe vision loss, including loss of reading ability.

TREATMENT OPTIONS

Currently the treatment options in nonneovascular AMD are limited to trying to prevent disease progression. As mentioned above, oxidative stress in the macular region – no matter what the cause – is considered to be one of the components in the pathogenesis of AMD. The observation that vitamins and minerals with antioxidative properties reduce the risk of AMD progression supports this concept. The potential of antioxidants to scavenger or quench free radicals of different origin may protect photoreceptors and RPE cells. Different antioxidants and minerals have been investigated in nonneovascular AMD.

VITAMIN C

Vitamin C (L-ascorbic acid) is a water-soluble antioxidant and one of the widely used vitamin supplements and is known to act as an antioxidant for several decades. Supplementation of vitamin C reduces light-induced retinal damage[30,31] in animal experiments. The data of human studies are, however, inconclusive. Whereas several reports revealed a correlation between low vitamin C plasma concentration and AMD, others failed to find a protective effect of vitamin C.[32,33]

CAROTENOIDS

Three members of the carotenoid famlily have been proposed to be beneficial for dry AMD. As a first approach, beta-carotene, which is one of the major precursors of vitamin A, has been proven to be an effective antioxidant.[34] The Eye Disease Case-Control Study found that a higher dietary intake of carotenoids was associated with a lower risk for AMD.[33] However, it has been shown that high-dose beta-carotene may increase the risk of cancer, especially in smokers and former smokers.[35] Today, in many preparations targeting dry AMD, beta-carotene has been replaced by lutein and/or zeaxanthin. Lutein and zeaxanthin also belong to the family of carotenoids and are the major components of the macula pigment. Although the exact role of macular pigment remains to be fully elucidated, it has been shown that the macula pigments play a major role in the reduction of light scatter and chromatic aberration in the macula and may protect against the adverse effects of high-energy short-wavelength light. Consequently, it has been hypothesized that dietary supplementation with lutein and/or zeaxanthin might delay the progression of AMD. Preliminary studies using exogenous supplementation of lutein and zeaxanthin have been promising. Lutein and zeaxanthin are part of the protocol evaluated in the recently initiated AREDS 2. Furthermore, all participants will be offered additional treatment with the study formulation used in AREDS 1. Patients, who agree to take this additional supplement will be further randomized to original AREDS 1 medication or modified AREDS 1 medication without beta-carotene or lower levels of zinc.

VITAMIN E

Because vitamin E is mostly given as a combination with other vitamins, the data about vitamin E supplementation alone are sparse. Dietary deficiency of vitamin E has been shown to lead to lipofuscin accumulation in the RPE. Whether this relates to changes seen in AMD has yet to be clarified. The AREDS report indicates that vitamin E, when given in combination with other vitamins and zinc, delays the progression of AMD.[15]

MINERALS

Given that certain minerals such as zinc, copper, iron and others act as cofactors in the human enzymatic antioxidant system, deficiency of these nutritional cofactors negatively affects the antioxidant capacity.

Thus, it has been hypothesized that supplementation of these minerals may be beneficial for patients with AMD. However, direct evidence for a protective role in AMD is sparse and is mainly derived from AREDS, which demonstrates a beneficial role for zinc, especially in combination with other antioxidants.[15]

TREATMENT OUTCOMES AND PROGNOSIS

Epidemiological studies report that people with high vitamin intake are at a reduced risk of developing AMD. However, they do not prove that exogenous supplementation of vitamins and/or minerals is beneficial for patients with dry AMD. To prove the effect of antioxidants on the progression of AMD, large prospective, longitudinal interventional studies are necessary. Until now, evidence for the effectiveness of vitamin and mineral supplementation is mainly based on the AREDS. The study was designed to identify the effect of high-dose vitamin and mineral supplementation on the development of cataract and AMD. This multicenter, prospective, randomized study included 3640 patients aged 55–80 years with AMD from 1992 to 1998.[15] The average follow-up was 6.3 years. The patients were randomized into four groups and received daily oral tablets containing: (1) antioxidants (vitamin C, 500 mg; vitamin E, 400 IU; and beta-carotene, 15 mg); (2) zinc, 80 mg, as zinc oxide and copper, 2 mg, as cupric oxide; (3) antioxidants plus zinc; or (4) placebo. Primary outcomes of the study were progression to advanced AMD and at least moderate visual acuity loss from baseline (15 letters). Comparison with placebo demonstrated a statistically significant odds reduction for the development of advanced AMD with antioxidants plus zinc (regimen 3) (OR, 0.72; 99% confidence interval, 0.52–0.98).[15] Supplementation with antioxidants or zinc alone did not demonstrate a significant odds reduction. It was found however that participants with extensive small drusen, nonextensive intermediate drusen, or pigment abnormalities (category 2) had only a 1.3% 5-year probability to progress to advanced AMD. By excluding category 2 patients, significant odds reduction was also seen for antioxidants or zinc alone. A significant odds reduction for at least moderate vision loss was only seen in patients assigned to antioxidant and zinc (regimen 3) (OR, 0.73; 99% confidence interval, 0.54–0.99).[15] The combination of vitamins and minerals shown in Table 17.3 is currently recommended for nonsmoking patients with nonneovascular AMD of at least AREDS category 2. High-dose supplementation of antioxidants and cofactors is currently not recommended for the general population.

AREDS has several limitations. Given that a combination of antioxidants was used, it is not clear which component is responsible for the beneficial effect. Furthermore, vitamin C, vitamin E, and zinc were included at much higher doses than the recommended daily allowance (www.nal.usda.gov). Thus, it is not entirely clear if a long-term supplementation of such high doses of vitamins could be harmful. In particular, there is evidence that high doses of beta-carotene increase the risk of cancer in smokers and former smokers.[36] To investigate these questions further, the AREDS 2 study started enrolling in the fall of 2006. Its primary objective is to determine whether oral supplementation with lutein/zeaxanthin and/or omega-3 fatty acids in combination with other vitamins may be beneficial for patients with AMD.

Table 17.3 Formulation of high-dose vitamin and mineral supplementation used in the Age-Related Eye Disease Study (AREDS)

Vitamin C	500 mg
Vitamin E	400 IU
Beta-carotene	15 mg
Zinc	80 mg
Copper	2 mg

Table 17.4

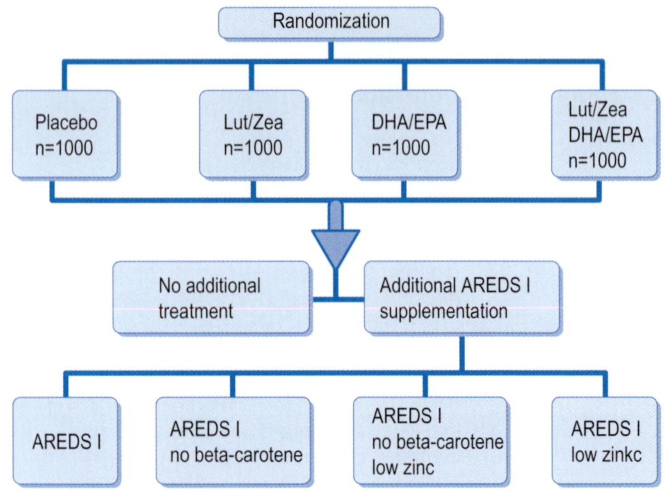

Primary randomization agents AREDS II

	Formulation	Dose
Group 1	placebo	
Group 2	lutein	10 mg
	zeaxanthin	2 mg
Group 3	docosahexaenoic acid	350 mg
	eicosapentaenoic acid	650 mg
Group 4	lutein	10 mg
	zeaxanthin	2 mg
	docosahexaenoic acid	350 mg
	eicosapentaenoic acid	650 mg

SUMMARY AND KEY POINTS

Although significant improvement has been made in understanding the pathogenesis of nonneovascular AMD, many questions remain to be answered. Until now, unfortunately, the available pharmacological approaches, in particular the supplementation of antioxidants and minerals, can only reduce the risk of disease progression but are unable to prevent the disease. Evidence for the effectiveness of high-dose antioxidant vitamin and mineral supplementation in reducing the risk of developing advanced AMD is mainly derived from one single interventional study (AREDS), performed in the USA. The AREDS formulation (Table 17.3) is currently recommended for nonsmoking nonneovascular AMD patients with at least AREDS category 2 findings, based on best evidence available. Whether these results can be applied to other populations with a different nutritional status has yet to be investigated. AREDS 2 has been initiated to evaluate lutein and zeaxanthin as well as omega-3 fatty acids (Table 17.4).

The new insight into the role of polymorphisms in CFH and HTRA1 provides a promising approach to new preventive treatments for nonneovascular AMD, especially when used in combination with genetic risk evaluation. However, this new approach has just entered first clinical trials. Furthermore, infectious and/or inflammatory diseases potentially triggering the disease may play an additional role in the pathogenesis of AMD.

Within the past several years, nonneovascular AMD has truly become a most progressive field for pharmacotherapy. Hopefully, promising treatment and prevention options will soon be introduced into clinical practice.

REFERENCES

1. Klein RJ, Zeiss C, Chew EY, et al. Complement factor H polymorphism in age-related macular degeneration. Science 2005;308:385–389.
2. Edwards AO, Ritter 3rd R, Abel KJ, et al. Complement factor H polymorphism and age-related macular degeneration. Science 2005;308:421–424.
3. Hageman GS, Anderson DH, Johnson LV, et al. A common haplotype in the complement regulatory gene factor H (HF1/CFH) predisposes individuals to age-related macular degeneration. Proc Natl Acad Sci USA 2005;102:7227–7232.
4. Haines JL, Hauser MA, Schmidt S, et al. Complement factor H variant increases the risk of age-related macular degeneration. Science 2005;308:419–421.
5. Zareparsi S, Branham KE, Li M, et al. Strong association of the Y402H variant in complement factor H at 1q32 with susceptibility to age-related macular degeneration. Am J Hum Genet 2005;77:149–153.
6. Rother RP, Rollins SA, Mojcik CF, et al. Discovery and development of the complement inhibitor eculizumab for the treatment of paroxysmal nocturnal hemoglobinuria. Nat Biotechnol 2007;25:1256–1264.
7. Friedman DS, O'Colmain BJ, Muñoz B, et al. Prevalence of age-related macular degeneration in the United States. Arch Ophthalmol 2004;122:564–572.
8. Andersen MV, Rosenberg T, la Cour M, et al. Prevalence of age-related maculopathy and age-related macular degeneration among the inuit in Greenland. The Greenland Inuit Eye Study. Ophthalmology 2008;115:700–707 e1.
9. Kawasaki R, Wang JJ, Ji GJ, et al. Prevalence and risk factors for age-related macular degeneration in an adult Japanese population. The Funagata study. Ophthalmology 2008;115:1376–1381.
10. Christen WG, Glynn RJ, Manson JE, et al. A prospective study of cigarette smoking and risk of age-related macular degeneration in men. JAMA 1996;276:1147–1151.
11. Schaumberg DA, Hankinson SE, Guo Q, et al. A prospective study of 2 major age-related macular degeneration susceptibility alleles and interactions with modifiable risk factors. Arch Ophthalmol 2007;125:55–62.
12. Seddon JM, Hankinson SE, Guo Q, et al. CFH gene variant, Y402H, and smoking, body mass index, environmental associations with advanced age-related macular degeneration. Hum Hered 2006;61:157–165.
13. Chuo JY, Wiens M, Etminan M, et al. Use of lipid-lowering agents for the prevention of age-related macular degeneration: a meta-analysis of observational studies. Ophthalmic Epidemiol 2007;14:367–374.
14. Patel JI. Is cataract surgery a risk factor for progression of macular degeneration? Curr Opin Ophthalmol 2007;18:9–12.
15. A randomized, placebo-controlled, clinical trial of high-dose supplementation with vitamins C and E, beta carotene, and zinc for age-related macular degeneration and vision loss: AREDS report no. 8. Arch Ophthalmol 2001;119:1417–1436.
16. Verhoeff FH, Grossman H. Pathogenesis of disciform degeneration of the macula. Arch Ophthalmol 1937;18:561–585.
17. Ciulla TA, Harris A, Kagemann L, et al. Choroidal perfusion perturbations in nonneovascular age related macular degeneration. Br J Ophthalmol 2002;86:209–213.
18. Mori F, Konno S, Hikichi T, et al. Pulsatile ocular blood flow study: decreases in exudative age related macular degeneration. Br J Ophthalmol 2001;85:531–533.
19. Pauleikhoff D, Spital G, Radermacher M, et al. A fluorescein and indocyanine green angiographic study of choriocapillaris in age-related macular disease. Arch Ophthalmol 1999;117:1353–1358.
20. Uretmen O, Akkin C, Erakgün T, et al. Color Doppler imaging of choroidal circulation in patients with asymmetric age-related macular degeneration. Ophthalmologica 2003;217:137–142.
21. Green WR, McDonnell PJ, Yeo JH. Pathologic features of senile macular degeneration. Ophthalmology 1985;92:615–627.
22. Ishibashi T, Patterson R, Ohnishi Y, et al. Formation of drusen in the human eye. Am J Ophthalmol 1986;101:342–353.
23. Klaver CC, Kliffen M, van Duijn CM, et al. Genetic association of apolipoprotein E with age-related macular degeneration. Am J Hum Genet 1998;63:200–206.
24. Hageman GS, Luthert PJ, Victor Chong NH, et al. An integrated hypothesis that considers drusen as biomarkers of immune-mediated processes at the RPE–Bruch's membrane interface in aging and age-related macular degeneration. Prog Retin Eye Res 2001 Nov;20(6):705–732.
25. Schmitz-Valckenberg S, Holz FG, Bird AC, et al. Fundus autofluorescence imaging: review and perspectives. Retina 2008;28:385–409.
26. Hwang JC, Chan JW, Chang S, et al. Predictive value of fundus autofluorescence for development of geographic atrophy in age-related macular degeneration. Invest Ophthalmol Vis Sci 2006;47:2655–2661.
27. Michels S, Pircher M, Geitzenauer W, et al. Value of polarisation-sensitive optical coherence tomography in diseases affecting the retinal pigment epithelium. Br J Ophthalmol 2008;92:204–209.
28. Age-Related Eye Disease Study Research Group. A simplified severity scale for age-related macular degeneration: AREDS report no. 18. Arch Ophthalmol 2005;123:1570–1574.
29. Davis MD, Gangnon RE, Lee LY, et al. The Age-Related Eye Disease Study severity scale for age-related macular degeneration: AREDS report no. 17. Arch Ophthalmol 2005;123:1484–1498.
30. Organisciak DT, Jiang YL, Wang HM, et al. The protective effect of ascorbic acid in retinal light damage of rats exposed to intermittent light. Invest Ophthalmol Vis Sci 1990;31:1195–1202.
31. Li ZY, Tso MO, Wang HM, et al. Amelioration of photic injury in rat retina by ascorbic acid: a histopathologic study. Invest Ophthalmol Vis Sci 1985;26:1589–1598.
32. SanGiovanni JP, Chew EY, Clemons TE, et al. The relationship of dietary carotenoid and vitamin A, E, and C intake with age-related macular degeneration in a case-control study: AREDS report no. 22. Arch Ophthalmol 2007;125:1225–1232.
33. Seddon JM, Ajani UA, Sperduto RD, et al. Dietary carotenoids, vitamins A, C, and E, and advanced age-related macular degeneration. Eye Disease Case-Control Study Group. JAMA 1994;272:1413–1420.
34. Burton GW, Ingold KU. Beta-carotene: an unusual type of lipid antioxidant. Science 1984;224:569–573.
35. Omenn GS, Goodman GE, Thornquist MD, et al. Risk factors for lung cancer and for intervention effects in CARET, the Beta-Carotene and Retinol Efficacy Trial. J Natl Cancer Inst 1996;88:1550–1559.
36. Omenn GS, Goodman GE, Thornquist MD, et al. Effects of a combination of beta carotene and vitamin A on lung cancer and cardiovascular disease. N Engl J Med 1996;334:1150–1155.

CHAPTER 18

Neovascular age-related macular degeneration

Aimee V. Chappelow, MD and Andrew P. Schachat, MD

DISEASE PREVALENCE AND INFLUENCE

Age-related macular degeneration (AMD) is the leading cause of severe, irreversible vision loss in individuals over the age of 50 years in western societies. Advanced AMD affects an estimated 14 million people worldwide, and as the population ages, the number of individuals with AMD in the USA is expected to increase from 1.75 million in 2000 to 2.95 million in 2020.[1] Choroidal neovascularization (CNV) is the hallmark of "wet" or "exudative" AMD, and is responsible for approximately 90% of cases of severe vision loss due to AMD.

RISK FACTORS

As the nomenclature implies, the prevalence of early and advanced AMD increases with age, from 14.4% in people aged 55–64 years to 36.8% in those older than 75 years.[2] Other systemic risk factors associated with development of AMD include cigarette smoking, Caucasian race, systemic hypertension,[3] elevated serum cholesterol, greater exposure to visible light, and prior history of ischemic stroke.[4] Analysis of demographic data collected from the 4757 Age-Related Eye Disease Study (AREDS) participants confirmed smoking and Caucasian race as risk factors associated with progression from intermediate to advanced AMD.[5] More recently, a role for genetics has been implicated. Homozygosity for a specific polymorphism in the gene for complement factor H has been shown to increase the risk for the development of AMD by a factor of 7.4.[6] Other single nucleotide polymorphisms have been associated not only with an increased risk of progression of AMD, but also with a lower likelihood of response to treatment with antioxidants and zinc (the current standard of care for dry or nonexudative AMD).[7]

A number of studies have assessed the risk for development of CNV in the fellow eye in patients with unilateral neovascular AMD. Risk factors for development of CNV in the fellow eye include the presence of large drusen (>63 μm), five or more soft drusen, focal retinal pigment epithelial (RPE) hyperpigmentation, and definite systemic hypertension.[8] The Macular Photocoagulation Study (MPS) reported a 5-year cumulative incidence rate of neovascular AMD ranging from 7% (if an eye had none of the aforementioned risk factors) to 87% (if all four risk factors were present).[9] The rate of development of CNV in the fellow eye at 1 year ranges from 4 to 12% in various studies.[8] The average age at which neovascular AMD develops is 75 years; given a life expectancy of at least an additional 5–10 years, a significant number of patients will develop bilateral neovascular AMD.

ETIOLOGY/PATHOGENESIS

To date, no single etiology has been identified as causative of neovascular AMD. However, it is thought that the same inflammatory processes that lead to drusen formation also help create a cellular and molecular milieu for CNV.[10] Proposed theories to explain the stimulus for such inflammatory processes include excessive oxidative stress, dietary deficiency, light exposure, and autoimmune mechanisms. Further the drusen itself, composed of cellular remnants of degenerating RPE, serves as a chronic inflammatory stimulus. Many inflammatory mediators, including neutrophils, macrophages, mast cells, and activated microglia, are capable of producing and releasing proangiogenic factors. Through a complex interplay between numerous cellular mediators, stimulation of neovascularization occurs with either a net increase in proangiogenic molecules (transforming growth factor-α (TGF-α), TGF-β, the angiopoietins, and members of the vascular endothelial growth factor (VEGF) family) or a net decrease in antiangiogenic molecules (pigment epithelium-derived factor (PEDF), thrombospondin, and angiostatin). Local hypoxia may also play a role in upregulating VEGF and other growth factors via a separate pathway mediated by hypoxia-inducible factor-1a (HIF-1a).[11]

The VEGF family of proangiogenic factors comprises VEGF-A (often referred to simply as VEGF), VEGF-B, VEGF-C, VEGF-D, and placental growth factor (PlGF)-1 and -2. The biologically active secreted form of VEGF-A is a homodimer that binds VEGF receptor (VEGFR)-1 and VEGFR-2 on vascular endothelial cells, inducing intracellular tyrosine kinase pathways. Multiple biologically active forms of VEGF-A are generated by alternative messenger RNA splicing and proteolytic cleavage. VEGF-A has been detected in elevated levels in both the excised CNV membranes[12] and vitreous of patients with CNV,[13] and is integral to the growth and maintenance of CNV. As such, it has become a popular and effective target for pharmacotherapy in AMD.

Macroscopically, CNV is a neovascular proliferation that grows through breaks in Bruch's membrane and progresses laterally between the RPE and Bruch's membrane. The endothelial cells that make up this neovascular tuft lack normal barrier function, and thus tend to leak fluid, protein, and lipid, which may precipitate within the retina. Further, increased vascular fragility can lead to hemorrhage. Grossniklaus and Gass[14] proposed two different histologic types of subretinal neovascular membranes: type 1 (located beneath the RPE) and type 2 (between the retina and the RPE). Clinical characteristics that distinguished patients with type 2 CNV were younger patient age (<50 years), normal fellow eye, and fundus appearance characterized by a subretinal pigmented halo or pigmented plaque in the area of the lesion and sharply defined borders. Type 1 versus type 2 CNV might have importance during consideration of surgery to remove CNV, but in the pharmacotherapy era the differentiation seems to these authors to be moot.

NATURAL HISTORY

CNV is classified based upon clinical (subfoveal, juxtafoveal, or extrafoveal) and angiographic (classic, occult, predominantly classic, or minimally classic) criteria (Table 18.1). Attempts to define the natural history of each lesion subgroup have been largely achieved by pooling data from fellow eyes in treatment trials rather than through true observational series. Meta-analyses are limited by diversity of reporting formats among individual studies and general paucity of long-term follow-up. With these caveats in mind, the following generalizations can be made.

Table 18.1 Classification of choroidal neovascularization (CNV) in age-related macular degeneration

Basis of classification	CNV subtype	Definition
Angiographic appearance	Classic	Bright focal hyperfluorescence with distinct boundaries discernible in early phases that increases in extent and intensity in late phases
	Occult	1. Fibrovascular pigment epithelial detachment (FVPED): irregular retinal pigment epithelium elevation ± hyperfluorescent stippling early, ± late leakage at lesion borders 2. Late leakage of an undetermined source (LLUS): late leakage without evidence of corresponding classic CNV or FVPED in early or middle frames
Location	Subfoveal	Beneath the center of the FAZ
	Juxtafoveal	Between 1 and 200 μm from the center of the FAZ
	Extrafoveal	≥200 μm from the center of the FAZ
Composition	Predominantly classic	>50% of lesion composed of classic CNV
	Minimally classic	(0% < area of classic CNV < 50%) of total area
	Occult no classic	Lesion comprised solely of occult CNV

FAZ, foveal avascular zone.

Extrafoveal lesions (by definition 200 μm from the foveal avascular zone (FAZ)) tend to progress to subfoveal lesions (between 1 and 199 μm from the FAZ), with the occult variety demonstrating a slower rate of progression of visual loss than the classic variety.[15] Studies have reported 2-year rates of vision loss (3 lines) associated with extrafoveal classic CNV ranging from 56% to 86%.[15] Juxtafoveal CNV progresses to subfoveal CNV in over 90% of patients over the course of 5 years if not treated.[15] Drawing on prospective follow-up data available from the Verteporfin In Photodynamic therapy (VIP) trial, 55% and 69% of eyes with occult with no classic subfoveal lesions lost 3 lines of visual acuity at 12 and 24 months.[16] The Treatment of Age-related macular degeneration with Photodynamic therapy (TAP) trial investigation showed similar rates (54% and 62% loss of 3 lines at 12 and 24 months, respectively) for eyes with subfoveal classic CNV.[17]

In a meta-analysis of 51 studies that pooled data from 4362 patients with any lesion subtype, the proportion of patients with visual acuity worse than 20/200 increased from 19.7% at baseline to 75.7% at 3 years.[18] The same study reported development of neovascular AMD in the fellow eye of 12% and 26.8% of patients by 1 and 3 years, respectively. We are unlikely to gain significant additional natural history data in the current era of highly effective anti-VEGF agents that ethically obviates the use of a noninferiority study design for evaluation of novel potential therapies.

NONPHARMACOLOGIC THERAPIES

Management of sight-threatening subfoveal choroidal neovascular membranes has been approached with variable success through nonpharmacologic methods, including laser photocoagulation and submacular surgery.

Laser photocoagulation causes permanent damage to the retina and RPE, resulting in an absolute scotoma corresponding to the treatment site. It follows that treatment of subfoveal CNV will result in an immediate, irreversible loss of central vision (3 lines, on average). Despite initial losses in visual acuity, the MPS showed that the long-term rate of vision loss due to subfoveal CNV can be slowed with laser treatment of subfoveal CNV such that approximately 30% of treated eyes will be 20/400 or worse at 4-year follow-up, compared to 60% of controls.[19] Laser photocoagulation of extrafoveal and juxtafoveal CNV in AMD has also been shown to result in a modest decrease in the rate of vision loss compared to controls over 3 years (44% versus 63% and 49% versus 58%).[19] It should be noted that only a small proportion of patients meet the eligibility criteria for treatment with photocoagulation according to the MPS since many lesions are poorly demarcated or predominantly hemorrhage. In addition, recurrent CNV occurs in 47–59% of patients, most within 2 years.[20] If the fellow eye has CNV or scar and the patient has high blood pressure and is a smoker, recurrence is almost predictable, reaching about 80% at 5 years.

The Submacular Surgery Trials (SST) investigators randomized 454 study eyes with subfoveal CNV secondary to AMD to observation or surgery. Surgery conferred no benefit over observation with median visual acuity in both groups, declining from 20/100 to 20/400 at 24 months of follow-up.[21] In addition, 39% of eyes in the surgery arm required cataract surgery, compared to 5% of control eyes. Although there may be a small benefit for some subgroups, submacular surgery for neovascular AMD has been largely abandoned.

PHARMACOLOGIC THERAPIES

Beginning with the introduction of photodynamic therapy (PDT) with verteporfin in 1991, advances in the treatment of neovascular AMD over the past two decades have been dominated by novel pharmacotherapies. The era of pharmacologic treatment culminated in the introduction of ranibizumab in 2006, the first therapy approved by the Food and Drug Administration (FDA) for neovascular AMD shown to result in improvement in visual acuity in a percentage of patients. Future therapeutic candidates will be judged in noninferiority trials against the ranibizumab gold standard. Below we review clinical experience and outcomes for important pharmacotherapies currently available for the treatment of neovascular AMD. For additional detail about specific pharmacologic therapies, see Chapter 53.

PDT WITH VERTEPORFIN

PDT involves the intravenous injection of the photosensitive dye verteporfin and its subsequent activation with 689 nm laser light. The efficacy of PDT was investigated in randomized trials with 2 years of follow-up in patients with classic-containing CNV lesions in the TAP Investigation[17] and in patients with occult and minimally classic CNV in the VIP trial.[16] PDT treatment was found to reduce moderate visual loss, especially in patients with predominantly classic lesions. Subgroup analysis suggested a greater treatment benefit in patients with no classic CNV who had either lesions <4 MPS disc areas or visual acuity

<20/50.[16] The treatment strategy that was tested was "treat if there is leaking" on the angiogram. The studies were conducted before optical coherence tomography was available. Over 90% of patients required retreatment at 3 months; however, by year 5 of follow-up, patients were requiring less than one treatment per year. Subjects required about three treatments in the first year and two in the second. In contrast to MPS-style therapy, acute severe vision loss was uncommon, with less than a 4.4% incidence in both the TAP and VIP.

PEGAPTANIB

Pegaptanib is the first FDA-approved therapy for neovascular AMD to target VEGF specifically. A pegylated oligonucleotide aptamer, it was designed to have a high binding specificity for only the $VEGF_{165}$ isoform which is known to stimulate pathologic neovascularization in the eye while not being required for physiologic vascularization. The VEGF Inhibition Study In Ocular Neovascularization (VISION) trials[22,23] consisted of two multicenter controlled replicate trials that randomized a total of 1190 patients regardless of angiographic lesion subtype to receive one of three doses of pegaptanib or sham injection every 6 weeks for 54 weeks. Patients were then re-randomized to continue sham treatments, discontinue sham treatments, or be assigned to two of the three pegaptanib doses every 6 weeks for an additional 54 weeks. All doses were well tolerated and, at 54 weeks, 70% of patients receiving 0.3 mg pegaptanib lost fewer than 15 letters of visual acuity compared to 55% in the sham group ($P < 0.001$).[23] At 102 weeks, patients who continued pegaptanib were half as likely to lose >15 letters of visual acuity than patients who discontinued pegaptanib.[22] Pegaptanib outcomes are similar to PDT outcomes except the drug appears to be helpful for all CNV compositions so a wider range of subjects can be treated.

RANIBIZUMAB

It has been hypothesized that pegaptanib's unique specificity for $VEGF_{165}$ isoform may actually have been its downfall. Its successor, ranibizumab, was developed as a recombinant, humanized monoclonal antibody Fab fragment that binds all active isoforms of VEGF-A with high affinity. Approved by the US FDA in 2006 for the treatment of all angiographic subtypes of subfoveal neovascular AMD, ranibizumab is the first treatment for neovascular AMD that has afforded patients a significant chance for improvement in visual acuity.

The safety and efficacy of ranibizumab in minimally classic and occult subfoveal CNV were evaluated in a 2-year, prospective, randomized, double-masked, sham-controlled trial. The Minimally classic/occult trial of the Anti-VEGF antibody Ranibizumab in the treatment of neovascular Age-related macular degeneration (MARINA) trial[24] randomized 716 patients to receive one of two doses of intravitreal ranibizumab or sham injections every month for 24 months. At 12 months, 95% of patients receiving ranibizumab lost < 15 letters (about 3 lines) of visual acuity compared to 65% of subjects receiving sham injections ($P < 0.001$) (Figure 18.1). At 24 months, this difference was maintained, with 92% and 90% of patients receiving 0.5 mg and 0.3 mg of ranibizumab losing < 15 letters of visual acuity (compared to 52.9% of control subjects). Further, 34% and 25% of patients receiving 0.5 mg or 0.3 mg of ranibizumab gained 15 letters of visual acuity, compared to 5% of control subjects ($P < 0.001$).[24]

The Anti-VEGF antibody for the treatment of predominantly classic choroidal neovascularization in AMD (ANCHOR) trial,[25] another 2-year, randomized, prospective double-masked study, reported similar results for the treatment of predominantly classic CNV with ranibizumab. A total of 423 patients were randomized in a 1:1:1 ratio to receive either monthly intravitreal ranibizumab (0.3 mg or 0.5 mg) or verteporfin PDT on study entry and every 3 months thereafter according to accepted guidelines. At 12 months, 94.3% of patients receiving 0.3 mg of ranibizumab and 96.4% of patients receiving 0.5 mg of ranibizumab lost < 15 letters of visual acuity, compared with 64.3% of controls ($P < 0.001$) (Figure 18.1). Further, 35.7% of the 0.3-mg group

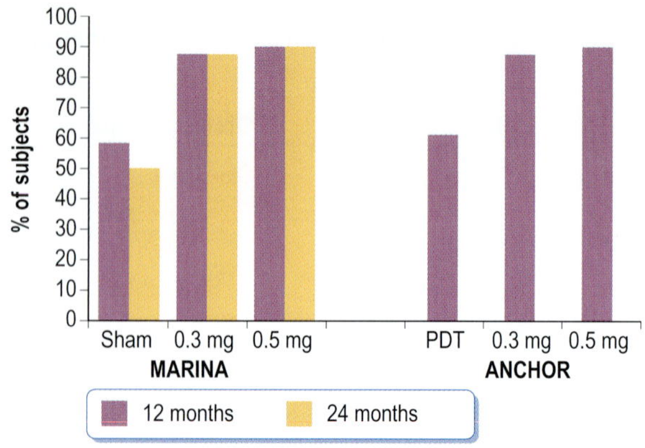

Figure 18.1 Percentage of subjects losing fewer than 15 letters of visual acuity at 12 and 24 months in the Minimally classic/occult trial of the Anti-VEGF antibody Ranibizumab in the treatment of neovascular Age-related macular degeneration (MARINA) trial and at 12 months in the Anti-VEGF antibody for the treatment of predominantly classic choroidal neovascularization in AMD (ANCHOR) trial. 24-month outcomes have not been published for the ANCHOR trial. **P* < 0.001; PDT, photodynamic therapy; 0.3 mg, 0.5 mg, dose of intravitreal ranibizumab.

and 40.3% of the 0.5-mg group gained 15 letters of visual acuity compared to 5.6% of the verteporfin PDT group ($P < 0.001$).[25]

The RhuFab V2 Ocular treatment Combining the Use of Visudyne to evaluate Safety (FOCUS) trial[26] established the superior efficacy of treatment with the combination ranibizumab and verteporfin PDT over treatment with PDT alone. Because the primary goal was the evaluation of treatment safety, patients who were previously treated with PDT were not excluded. All 162 patients received PDT initially then quarterly as needed for 24 months; however patients were also randomized in a roughly 2:1 ratio to receive monthly 0.5-mg ranibizumab injections or sham injections. The study found a distinct benefit of adding bevacizumab, with 90% and 88% of patients receiving bevacizumab losing < 15 letters of VA at month 12 and 24, compared to 68% and 75% for PDT alone ($P < 0.001$, $P < 0.05$) (Figure 18.2). At 24 months, 25% of patients in the bevacizumab + PDT group gained 15 letters, compared to 7% for PDT alone ($P < 0.05$).[26]

Despite the unprecedented consistent efficacy of ranibizumab, the requirement for monthly injections administered for an indefinite period and cost of the drug pose a significant treatment burden.

Several studies have attempted to define alternative dosing strategies for anti-VEGF therapies that decrease dosing frequency without compromising efficacy. The Phase IIIb, multi-center, randomized, double-masked, sham-Injection-controlled study of the Efficacy and safety of Ranibizumab (PIER) study randomized 184 patients with subfoveal CNV of any lesion subtype to receive either sham injections or 0.5 mg ranibizumab monthly for 3 months followed by quarterly dosing for a total of 24 months. For the first 3 months, visual acuity and ocular coherence tomography (OCT) improvements mirrored that observed in the ANCHOR and MARINA trials; however, after 12 months, the mean change in visual acuity from baseline was a loss of 1.6 letters.[27] Thus, scheduled dosing of ranibizumab every 3 months was judged to be inferior to monthly dosing.

Monthly intravitreal ranibizumab for the first 3 months, followed by pro re nata (PRN) OCT-guided therapy, is an alternate dosing strategy for which data appear more promising. The Prospective OCT imaging of patients with Neovascular age-related macular degeneration Treated with intra-Ocular Lucentis (PrONTO) trial[28] treated as such with retreatment decisions based on increase in central retinal thickness (CRT) of at least 100 μm, visual loss associated with edema on OCT, presence of new classic CNV on fluorescein angiography, and presence of new hemorrhage or persistent fluid on OCT. Patients on average received 5.6 injections over the course of the 12-month study period. Further, mean retinal thickness had decreased by 178 μm and visual

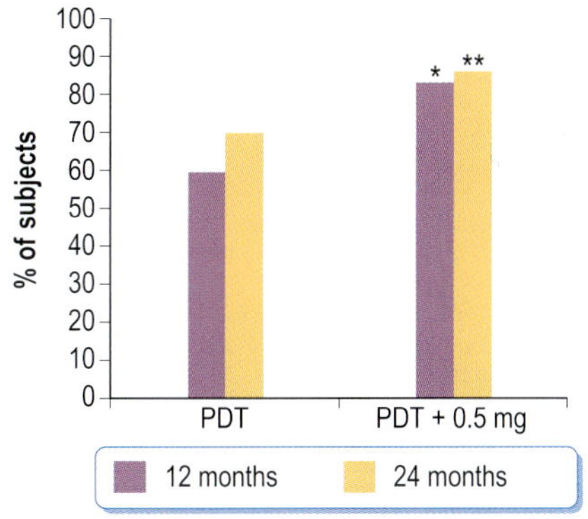

Figure 18.2 Percentage of subjects losing fewer than 15 letters of visual acuity at 12 and 24 months in the RhuFab V2 Ocular treatment Combining the Use of Visudyne to evaluate Safety (FOCUS) trial. $^*P < 0.001$, $^{**}P < 0.05$; PDT, photodynamic therapy; 0.5 mg, dose of intravitreal ranibizumab.

acuity had improved by 9.3 letters, with 35% gaining >15 letters.[28] The ongoing Sustain trial will provide data on the safety and efficacy of ranibizumab administered as three consecutive monthly loading doses followed by retreatment based on visual acuity loss of >5 letters or increase in CRT > 100 μm on OCT. Interim analysis revealed that, of the 531 patients enrolled, the first 69 ranibizumab-naïve patients to complete the 12-month study required a mean (± SD) of 5.3 (±2.2) injections and gained approximately 7 letters of acuity.[29]

BEVACIZUMAB

Around the time that ranibizumab was in phase I/II clinical trials, another nonselective VEGF-A inhibitor, bevacizumab, was approved by the FDA for treatment of metastatic colon cancer. Due to concern about the ability of this large molecule to gain access to CNV by diffusion through retina, it was not initially suggested as therapy for neovascular AMD. However, after animal studies showed leakage of fluorescein-conjugated bevacizumab from laser-induced CNV, Michels et al.[30] initiated a small-scale investigation of off-label intravenous bevacizumab for subfoveal CNV. Twelve-week data showed good tolerability (aside from a 12-mmHg mean increase in systolic blood pressure) and marked improvement in visual acuity, OCT, and angiographic outcomes. Subsequently, several small series of intravitreal administration of bevacizumab[31] echoed the initial favorable reports of safety and efficacy.

Bevacizumab costs physicians approximately $45 per injection while ranibizumab costs approximately $2030. In the USA, the co-pay for Medicare-insured patients is $9 and $406, respectively. In addition to a price ratio of 39:1 with respect to bevacizumab, ranibizumab may also pose the disadvantage of decreased durability per treatment. The intravitreal half-life of bevacizumab and ranibizumab determined in animal studies is 4.32 and 2.88 days.[32] Remission intervals (time until retreatment as indicated by OCT) accordingly were found to be longer for bevacizumab (141 days) compared to ranibizumab (102 days).[33] On the other hand, a longer half-life may have drawbacks with regards to systemic side-effects and toxicity. The reader is referred to Section 4 for additional discussion of the safety of bevacizumab for intravitreal injection.

To date, there have been no randomized double-blinded clinical trials to compare ranibizumab and bevacizumab. However, the Comparison of Age-Related Macular Degeneration Treatments Trial (CATT)[34] which began enrollment in early 2008 will determine which of the following four regimens should be used as the standard of comparison for subsequent clinical trials: bevacizumab or ranibizumab on a fixed dosing schedule of every 4 weeks, or bevacizumab or ranibizumab on a variable (PRN) dosing schedule. A total of 1200 patients with AMD and active subfoveal CNV (without previous treatment) will be enrolled and followed every 4 weeks for 2 years.

COMBINATION THERAPY

While intravitreal anti-VEGF monotherapies offer unprecedented benefit with regard to visual outcome, therapy with monthly intravitreal injection administered for a prolonged period poses significant drawbacks, including additional safety risk, financial burden, and the inconvenience of monthly visits to the ophthalmologist. There is also the theoretical risk of upregulation of VEGF receptors or compensatory upregulation of VEGF production in the setting of long-term use of anti-VEGF therapy. Further, unlike verteporfin PDT, which exerts its effect through a unique angio-occlusive mechanism, anti-VEGF agents fail to destroy existing CNV. Combined therapy with ranibizumab or bevacizumab and PDT offers the potential for a synergistic effect through concomitant elimination of existing CNV and prevention of new CNV. Combination therapy with PDT may also allow for decreased frequency of anti-VEGF therapy.

Augustin et al.[35] reported visual and OCT outcomes for a prospective interventional case series of 104 patients who received one cycle of triple therapy (reduced fluence PDT followed 16 hours later by intravitreal dexamethasone and bevacizumab). Only 5 patients required a second round of triple therapy due to ongoing CNV activity over mean follow-up of 40 weeks (range 22–60 weeks). Further, mean increase in visual acuity was 1.8 lines and mean decrease in retinal thickness was 182 μm.[35] A more recent pilot study of intravitreal triamcinolone acetonide (IVTA) as an adjunct to PDT provides additional support for the role of corticosteroids in the treatment of neovascular AMD. Thirty patients with occult and minimally classic CNV secondary to AMD were randomized to receive either PDT or PDT followed by 12 mg IVTA, with both groups receiving additional PDT as needed quarterly for a year. The difference in visual acuity did not achieve statistical significance at 1 year; however, the mean number of PDT treatments for the IVTA + PDT group (1.13 treatments) was significantly lower than for the PDT alone group (3.6 treatments; $P < 0.001$).[36] However, 40% of patients in the IVTA group required topical glaucoma therapy for intraocular pressure control.

The ongoing Denali trial and its European counterpart, the Mont Blanc trial, are the first large-scale randomized studies to compare ranibizumab monotherapy with ranibizumab combination therapy (with standard or reduced fluence PDT). Approximately 300 patients will be followed for 2 years in order to determine whether combination therapy reduces the frequency of treatments. Primary endpoints will measure the proportion of patients with a treatment-free interval of at least 3 months and best corrected visual acuity at 12 months using the Early Treatment Diabetic Retinopathy Study (ETDRS) protocol.

TREATMENTS UNDER INVESTIGATION

Several new pharmacotherapies aim to halt the angiogenic effects of VEGF by inhibiting the production of either VEGF (bevasiranib) or its receptor (AGN211745). Other potential mechanisms include upregulation of the antiangiogenic factor, PEDF (AdPEDF.11), or blockade of the tyrosine kinase cascade (vatalanib, pazopanib) downstream from the VEGF receptor. VEGF-Trap, which binds existing VEGF like ranibizumab and bevacizumab, is emerging as a potentially important therapy. A recent dose escalation trial (n = 157) reported no ocular adverse events, a 160-μm decrease in CRT, and a 9.3-letter gain at 12 weeks following monthly 0.5-mg intravitreal VEGF-Trap.[37] These and other emerging therapies will be discussed in greater detail in Section 4.

Another newer technique for use in conjunction with ranibizumab involves intraocular application of 24 Gy beta-irradiation directly to CNV via a 20-gauge cannula fitted with a small strand of strontium-90. The low-level radiation preferentially targets the CNV, leaving overlying healthy retina unaffected. Used in combination with ranibizumab, preliminary results have been promising and a prospective randomized trial is under way. Focal radiotherapy combined with ranibizumab both postoperatively and either intraoperatively (n = 22) or preoperatively (n = 12) showed an average 11.4-letter gain in acuity at 9 months for both groups combined. In all, 93% of patients lost less than 15 letters at

9 months, central retinal thickness was reduced from 302 to 218 μm, and no serious adverse events were reported.[38]

SUMMARY AND KEY POINTS

VEGF inhibitors have rapidly become the gold standard for treatment of neovascular AMD characterized by CNV of all lesion subtypes. For the first time, visual outcomes are being reported as gain in letters of vision as opposed to percentage of patients maintaining stable vision or losing less than 3 lines of vision. At the present time, monotherapy with ranibizumab remains the gold standard against which future therapies will be judged. However, there remains room for improvement in the ranibizumab standard, with respect to duration and frequency of treatment, endpoint of therapy, percentage of patients gaining visual acuity, and cost per treatment. Upcoming studies will help better define optimal dosing frequency, follow-up interval, and role for use of other current and emerging therapies in combination with anti-VEGF agents. (For further discussion of emerging therapies, see Chapter 53.)

REFERENCES

1. Friedman DS, O'Colmain BJ, Munoz B, et al. Prevalence of age-related macular degeneration in the United States. Arch Ophthalmol 2004;122:564–572.
2. Klein R, Klein BE, Linton KL. Prevalence of age-related maculopathy. The Beaver Dam Eye Study. Ophthalmology 1992;99:933–943.
3. Hyman L, Schachat AP, He Q, et al. Hypertension, cardiovascular disease, and age-related macular degeneration. Age-Related Macular Degeneration Risk Factors Study Group. Arch Ophthalmol 2000;118:351–358.
4. Tan JS, Mitchell P, Smith W, et al. Cardiovascular risk factors and the long-term incidence of age-related macular degeneration: the Blue Mountains Eye Study. Ophthalmology 2007;114:1143–1150.
5. Clemons TE, Milton RC, Klein R, et al. Risk factors for the incidence of advanced age-related macular degeneration in the Age-Related Eye Disease Study (AREDS). AREDS report no. 19. Ophthalmology 2005;112:533–539.
6. Klein RJ, Zeiss C, Chew EY, et al. Complement factor H polymorphism in age-related macular degeneration. Science 2005;308:385–389.
7. Klein ML, Francis PJ, Rosner B, et al. CFH and LOC387715/ARMS2 genotypes and treatment with antioxidants and zinc for age-related macular degeneration. Ophthalmology 2008;115:1019–1025.
8. Pieramici DJ, Bressler SB. Age-related macular degeneration and risk factors for the development of choroidal neovascularization in the fellow eye. Curr Opin Ophthalmol 1998;9:38–46.
9. Risk factors for choroidal neovascularization in the second eye of patients with juxtafoveal or subfoveal choroidal neovascularization secondary to age-related macular degeneration. Macular Photocoagulation Study Group. Arch Ophthalmol 1997;115:741–747.
10. Nowak JZ. Age-related macular degeneration (AMD): pathogenesis and therapy. Pharmacol Rep 2006;58:353–363.
11. Das A, McGuire PG. Retinal and choroidal angiogenesis: pathophysiology and strategies for inhibition. Prog Retin Eye Res 2003;22:721–748.
12. Kvanta A, Algvere PV, Berglin L, et al. Subfoveal fibrovascular membranes in age-related macular degeneration express vascular endothelial growth factor. Invest Ophthalmol Vis Sci 1996;37:1929–1934.
13. Wells JA, Murthy R, Chibber R, et al. Levels of vascular endothelial growth factor are elevated in the vitreous of patients with subretinal neovascularisation. Br J Ophthalmol 1996;80:363–366.
14. Grossniklaus HE, Gass JD. Clinicopathologic correlations of surgically excised type 1 and type 2 submacular choroidal neovascular membranes. Am J Ophthalmol 1998;126:59–69.
15. Pauleikhoff D. Neovascular age-related macular degeneration: natural history and treatment outcomes. Retina 2005;25:1065–1084.
16. Verteporfin therapy of subfoveal choroidal neovascularization in age-related macular degeneration: two-year results of a randomized clinical trial including lesions with occult with no classic choroidal neovascularization – verteporfin in photodynamic therapy report 2. Am J Ophthalmol 2001;131:541–560.
17. Bressler NM. Photodynamic therapy of subfoveal choroidal neovascularization in age-related macular degeneration with verteporfin: two-year results of 2 randomized clinical trials – TAP report 2. Arch Ophthalmol 2001;119:198–207.
18. Wong T, Chakravarthy U, Klein R, et al. The natural history and prognosis of neovascular age-related macular degeneration: a systematic review of the literature and meta-analysis. Ophthalmology 2008;115:116–126.
19. Argon laser photocoagulation for neovascular maculopathy. Five-year results from randomized clinical trials. Macular Photocoagulation Study Group. Arch Ophthalmol 1991;109:1109–1114.
20. Persistent and recurrent neovascularization after laser photocoagulation for subfoveal choroidal neovascularization of age-related macular degeneration. Macular Photocoagulation Study Group. Arch Ophthalmol 1994;112:489–499.
21. Hawkins BS, Bressler NM, Miskala PH, et al. Surgery for subfoveal choroidal neovascularization in age-related macular degeneration: ophthalmic findings: SST report no. 11. Ophthalmology 2004;111:1967–1980.
22. Chakravarthy U, Adamis AP, Cunningham ET Jr, et al. Year 2 efficacy results of 2 randomized controlled clinical trials of pegaptanib for neovascular age-related macular degeneration. Ophthalmology 2006;113:1508 e1–25.
23. Gragoudas ES, Adamis AP, Cunningham ET Jr, et al. Pegaptanib for neovascular age-related macular degeneration. N Engl J Med 2004;351:2805–2816.
24. Rosenfeld PJ, Brown DM, Heier JS, et al. Ranibizumab for neovascular age-related macular degeneration. N Engl J Med 2006;355:1419–1431.
25. Brown DM, Kaiser PK, Michels M, et al. Ranibizumab versus verteporfin for neovascular age-related macular degeneration. N Engl J Med 2006;355:1432–1444.
26. Antoszyk AN, Tuomi L, Chung CY, et al. Ranibizumab combined with verteporfin photodynamic therapy in neovascular age-related macular degeneration (FOCUS): year 2 results. Am J Ophthalmol 2008;145:862–874.
27. Brown DM, Regillo CD. Anti-VEGF agents in the treatment of neovascular age-related macular degeneration: applying clinical trial results to the treatment of everyday patients. Am J Ophthalmol 2007;144:627–637.
28. Fung AE, Lalwani GA, Rosenfeld PJ, et al. An optical coherence tomography-guided, variable dosing regimen with intravitreal ranibizumab (Lucentis) for neovascular age-related macular degeneration. Am J Ophthalmol 2007;143:566–583.
29. Meyer CH, Eter N, Holz FG, et al. Ranibizumab in patients with subfoveal choroidal neovascularization secondary to age-related macular degeneration. Interim results from the Sustain trial. Invest Ophthalmol Vis Sci 2008;49:e-abstract 273.
30. Michels S, Rosenfeld PJ, Puliafito CA, et al. Systemic bevacizumab (Avastin) therapy for neovascular age-related macular degeneration twelve-week results of an uncontrolled open-label clinical study. Ophthalmology 2005;112:1035–1047.
31. Spaide RF, Laud K, Fine HF, et al. Intravitreal bevacizumab treatment of choroidal neovascularization secondary to age-related macular degeneration. Retina 2006;26:383–390.
32. Bakri SJ, Snyder MR, Reid JM, et al. Pharmacokinetics of intravitreal ranibizumab (Lucentis). Ophthalmology 2007;114:2179–2182.
33. Chang T. Comparison Study of Remission Intervals in Patients Treated with Ranibizumab vs. Bevacizumab for Neovascular AMD. Palm Beach, FL: Macula Society; 2008.
34. Comparison of Age-Related Macular Degeneration Treatments Trial: Lucentis-Avastin Trial (CATT). Available online at: www.clinicaltrials.gov; NCT00593450.
35. Augustin AJ, Puls S, Offermann I. Triple therapy for choroidal neovascularization due to age-related macular degeneration: verteporfin PDT, bevacizumab, and dexamethasone. Retina 2007;27:133–140.
36. Chaudhary V, Mao A, Hooper PL, et al. Triamcinolone acetonide as adjunctive treatment to verteporfin in neovascular age-related macular degeneration: a prospective randomized trial. Ophthalmology 2007;114:2183–2189.
37. Nguyen Q. A Phase II, Randomized, Controlled Dose-Ranging and Interval-Ranging Study of Intravitreal VEGF Trap in Patients with Neovascular Age-related Macular Degeneration. Palm Beach, FL: Macula Society; 2008.
38. Heier J. A Study to Evaluate the Safety and Feasibility of Radiotherapy and Bevacizumab (Avastin®) for the Treatment of Subfoveal Choroidal Neovascularization (CNV) Secondary to Age-Related Macular Degeneration (AMD). Palm Beach, FL: Macula Society; 2008.

CHAPTER

19 Diabetic retinopathy and diabetic macular edema

Gauri P. Misra, MD, Hisanori Imai, MD, Ravi J. Singh, MD, Tao L. Lowe, PhD, and Thomas W. Gardner, MD, MS

INTRODUCTION

This chapter summarizes the pathogenesis, risk factors, diagnosis, signs and symptoms, and treatment options for diabetic retinopathy (DR) and diabetic macular edema (DME). The complex nature of DR has led to a variety of therapies, but treatments for DR and DME are still challenging, particularly in the stages when retinopathy is mild and patients retain good vision.

DIABETIC RETINOPATHY PREVALENCE

DR is one of the major complications of diabetes and is a leading cause of blindness and vision impairment. Approximately 75% of persons suffering from type 1 diabetes develop retinopathy, while approximately 50% of persons with type 2 diabetes may develop retinopathy,[1] and approximately 25% of persons with diabetes may develop macular edema. During the next two decades, over 360 million people worldwide are projected to have diabetes and its complications.[2] Fortunately, the prevalence of severe retinopathy and nephropathy in patients with type 1 diabetes has diminished over the past 35 years due to improved medical care,[3] but the recent epidemic of type 2 diabetes requires a new understanding of the biology of DR and our approach to its prevention and treatment.

RISK FACTORS

The clinical risk factors for DR have long been recognized to include diabetes severity and duration, hypertension, presence of other complications, anemia, hyperlipidemia, insulin resistance/deficiency, and family history of DR (reviewed by Antonetti et al.[4] and Girach and Vignati[5]). While the benefits of decreasing HBA_{1c} or blood pressure levels have been demonstrated in large clinical trials,[6,7] there is presently no integrated index of risk of DR and other complications that include these known variables. Such an integrated index would greatly facilitate the identification of patients who are at increased risk of complications and who merit aggressive systemic and ocular therapy.

In addition to these recognized risk factors there is still much work to be done to determine the potential contribution of genetic factors and the impact of systemic inflammation. For example, a recent study[8] found that a single nucleotide polymorphism in the promoter region of the erythropoietin gene confers a twofold increased risk of proliferative DR and end-stage renal disease versus patients without this mutation. This finding was the result of large-scale genomic screening in three population groups and demonstrates the power of interdisciplinary collaborative studies.

Several studies have demonstrated a relationship between plasma levels of inflammatory markers and DR,[9,10] but it remains unclear if these inflammatory molecules contribute directly to the retinal damage in diabetes or simply reflect the systemic inflammatory state, and if they predict progression of disease or can be employed as markers of treatment response.

ETIOLOGY AND PATHOGENESIS

The etiology and pathogenesis of DR and DME have been the subject of much research and debate for the past three decades. At present the understanding of these processes is undergoing a dramatic shift from a strictly vascular focus to a more comprehensive view of the disease.

The vascular lesions of DR have been emphasized from the first case report of DR in 1855, reviewed by Wolfenbserger and Hamilton,[11] through the development of fluorescein angiography and trypsin digest studies of retinal blood vessels in the early 1960s, and in the classification of DR for the laser treatment trials in the 1970s and 1980s. The microvascular disease approach led to successful development of laser photocoagulation for proliferative retinopathy and DME, but it has not yet produced an approved pharmacologic treatment for DR or DME.

Concurrent with the development of fluorescein angiography and trypsin digest studies, two studies of postmortem human eyes in subjects with DR[12,13] emphasized the degeneration of the retinal neuropil even in regions remote from sites of vascular lesions. Electroretinographic studies subsequently confirmed the impairment of neural retinal function in patients with DR,[14–17] indicating the presence of Müller cell defects, and predicting the risk of progression from severe nonproliferative to high-risk proliferative retinopathy. However, a lack of appreciation of the biology of the transparent retina by clinicians may have limited the clinical application of these findings.

Over the past decade numerous studies of animals and humans have confirmed that all retinal cell types are damaged by diabetes, including loss of inner retinal neurons and their projections,[18,19] dysfunction of Müller cells,[20–22] and astrocytes,[20,23] activation of microglia, resident immune cells of the nervous system,[24,25] and degeneration of the pigment epithelium.[26] Thus, the current biological definition of DR includes all functional and structural changes in the retina due to diabetes. The term "microvascular disease" does not fully describe the retinal features of diabetes and is misleading in its limited scope.

The interrelationships between these retinal cell changes remain to be resolved. Do the vascular changes cause neuronal or glial cell defects, or vice versa, or are all the changes part of a coordinated sequential process? This chicken-and-egg question remains difficult to resolve.

These neuroretinal cell changes have not been well appreciated because they are invisible to clinical examination by ophthalmoscopy, fluorescein angiography, and standard optical coherence tomography. Therefore, new diagnostic methods based on changes in retinal neural cells are now being developed, as discussed below. In eyes with cystoids macular edema the clinical appearance of cysts and corresponding leakage of fluorescein dye suggest that leakage of the perifoveal capillaries likely accounts for macular thickening. However, histologic studies show loss of retinal neurons in addition to foveal cysts; reduction of macular edema may not result in visual improvement if retinal neurons are nonfunctional. Hence, recognizing both the clinical and biological aspects of retinal changes in DME and DR are essential to understanding the mechanisms of vision loss and designing appropriate treatments.

The cell biology of DR and DME is now becoming better understood, but the pathophysiologic processes that lead to the cellular lesions remain highly controversial. Hence, there is currently no well-established unifying hypothesis that accounts for the full range of vascular and neural changes and impairment of visual function. The major concepts are summarized as follows.

First, the basic pathophysiology of diabetes itself deserves emphasis. Diabetes mellitus refers to "honey urine" and reflects the emphasis on glucose accumulation. Clinicians diagnose diabetes based on elevated blood glucose levels because blood glucose concentration correlates closely with clinical symptoms and is measured readily. However, physiologists and biochemists understand both type 1 and type 2 diabetes result from impaired insulin action, which secondarily leads to hyperglycemia, hyperlipidemia, and elevated serum branched-chain amino acids, with catabolic degradation of tissues such as skeletal muscle and adipose.

The role of excess glucose in DR has appropriately received extensive investigation as part of the aldose reductase (polyol) pathway, nonenzymatic glycation and advanced glycation receptor (AGE) activation, protein kinase Cβ activation, oxidative and nitrative stress. Most of these changes have been investigated in rodent models of diabetes, where they seem to have a close connection with vascular changes. However, the promise of aldose reductase inhibitors in diabetic rats was not borne out in diabetic dogs or humans.[27] Likewise, AGE blockers did not demonstrate benefit on diabetes complications in humans and were toxic. The only successful treatment based on a glucose-activated pathway has been the protein kinase Cβ inhibitor, ruboxistaurin,[28,29] but this compound has not received Food and Drug Administration approval as of July, 2009, because a second positive trial has not been completed.

Inflammation is an early and intrinsic feature of systemic insulin resistance and diabetes that involves release of cytokines from adipose tissue that impairs insulin action, and affects patients with both type 1 and type 2 diabetes.[30,31] Interestingly, DR was formerly termed "diabetic retinitis"[32] before the inflammatory component was understood. The clinical picture of DR provides numerous clues to the presence of chronic inflammation, including diffuse vascular dilation, tortuosity, leakage and neovascularization, atrophy of the retinal neural parenchyma, edema of the macula, and eventual fibrosis. Cellular studies reveal activation of microglia[23–25] and leukostasis.[33] Together, these clinical and laboratory-based studies leave little doubt as to the presence of inflammation in DR, even though it is much more insidious than the uveitis associated with other systemic conditions such as sarcoidosis or multiple sclerosis.

The relationship of systemic inflammation to DR is currently unclear. Inflammatory responses are part of the intrinsic immune system reaction to multiple stresses, such as injury or infection, and inflammation is designed to limit the stress. Unrelenting stress and inflammation, however, lead to the clinical features associated with tissue damage that we recognize as "disease." If the intrinsic immune response in diabetes is similar to that in other tissues its activation in diabetes may be designed to maintain cell viability in the presence of metabolic stress. The retina may respond with increased production of growth factors such as vascular endothelial growth factor (VEGF) and erythropoietin, cytokines, complement, and microglial cell activation as a physiologic compensatory response. If the metabolic stress is relieved the inflammation may subside, but prolonged metabolic stress may lead to a maladaptive response in which inflammation would damage tissue because of tissue edema, invasion of circulating immune cells, and fibrosis. Thus, the inflammatory response is probably a two-edged sword with both beneficial and detrimental aspects. At present it is not clear which components of the inflammatory response are critical or which may serve as useful therapeutic targets.

Impaired insulin action is the sine qua non of diabetes and, along with glucagon excess, accounts for numerous tissue changes, including atrophy of skeletal muscle and adipose tissue. Until recently there was very little information on the role of the insulin receptor signaling system in the retina. Biochemical studies show that the receptor is structurally similar to that in the liver, is expressed in all retinal cells, forms heterodimers with the insulin-like growth factor 1 receptor, and has high basal activity relative to other tissues such as the liver.[34,35] In diabetic rodents the basal activity decreases progressively with time, and systemic insulin treatment restores the activity.[36] The impaired activity may predispose the retina to additional metabolic insults from systemic inflammation and hypertension, which also incites inflammation via the retinal rennin–angiotensin system.[37] This dynamically regulated insulin receptor system likely maintains the activity and viability of postmitotic retinal cells but full understanding of this process is currently lacking.

In summary, the etiology of DR is tied closely with the fundamental processes of diabetes itself, but the precise mechanisms that initiate or perpetuate retinal damage and lead to vision impairment remain to be clarified.

DIAGNOSIS AND ANCILLARY TESTING/ DIFFERENTIAL DIAGNOSIS

DR is diagnosed clinically on the basis of visible hemorrhages, microaneurysms, cotton-wool spots, lipid exudates, and neovascularization. Fundus photography and fluorescein angiography have greater sensitivity than ophthalmoscopy because of superior optics, the enhanced contrast of fluorescein angiography, and the ability of the observer to review magnified images without the interference of patients moving or blinking.

The standard clinical features reveal relatively late-stage lesions such as occluded capillaries so new approaches to diagnosing DR and DME are under evaluation – an imperative given the diabetes epidemic. Prevention of vision loss requires better understanding of the fundamental processes that impair vision and improved diagnostic tests to provide parameters to gauge the response to pharmacologic interventions. Retinal dysfunction in diabetes has long been known to begin before the onset of microvascular lesions. Changes in color vision, contrast sensitivity, visual fields, and electroretinography responses have been documented thoroughly[17] over the past three decades. A recent study[38] showed that retinal flavoprotein autofluorescence is increased in patients with diabetes but no retinopathy, and in those with established DR. However, no test of retinal function other than visual acuity has been shown conclusively to predict the onset or progression of retinopathy or vision loss, or to be a useful endpoint for clinical trials. Thus, the understanding of the biology of DR continues to evolve and provides new opportunities to move the timeline of diagnosis and treatment much earlier in the course of diabetes. The process of translating the results of laboratory findings into clinical utility is complex, expensive, slow, and requires new ways of studying DR,[39] but investments in the process should pay substantial dividends in the future.

SIGNS AND SYMPTOMS

DR is unusual among retinal diseases in that the symptoms vary widely and may be out of proportion to the severity of retinal pathology. For example, eyes with mild DME involving the center of the fovea of one eye can have symptomatically decreased vision whereas eyes with severe proliferative retinopathy may have 20/20 acuity and no symptoms until they begin to have vitreous bleeding. This variability and discrepancy between structure and function are the rationale for programs that screen populations at risk to identify and treat asymptomatic patients to reduce the risk of vision loss.[40]

TREATMENT OPTIONS

More than 20 treatment strategies have been proposed for DR and clinical trials of numerous agents are in progress.[41] Nevertheless, the only treatments for which high-quality clinical trial evidence exists are for control of diabetes, control of hypertension, laser photocoagulation, and vitrectomy.[42] That is, at present intraocular steroids and VEGF antagonists, ruboxistaurin, and blood lipid-lowering do not meet this threshold. For example, VEGF neutralizing antibodies have been shown to reduce DME in several case series but the studies generally have short-term follow-up, small cohorts, and few have compared results with standard of care focal or panretinal photocoagulation laser treatment.[43] Indeed, a phase II study of bevacizumab by the Diabetic Retinopathy Clinical Research Network found no benefit, even when combined with focal laser treatment.[44] Likewise, while intravitreal triamcinolone has been used extensively for DME in off-label studies and clinical practice over the past several years, a recent prospective, randomized trial showed it to be less effective than macular photocoagulation over the course of 3 years, even though it was more beneficial after 4 months.[45] Additional treatment trials are under way and are discussed in Section 5.

TREATMENT OUTCOMES AND PROGNOSIS

All treatments for the established vascular lesions of DR reduce the risk of blindness and vision loss but seldom restore normal vision. The continued impact of diabetes, hypertension, and other systemic insults continues to reduce vision. For example, long-term follow-up of patients treated with panretinal photocoagulation in the Diabetic Retinopathy Study retained useful vision that gradually declined over time.[46]

SUMMARY AND KEY POINTS

Retinopathy continues to be a frightening and devastating consequence of diabetes for patients and their families. The prognosis for diabetes and its complications improves with overall enhancements in diabetes management but the ocular complications are still diagnosed and treated late in terms of the biological processes. Fundamentally different approaches to the problem must be taken as the number of persons with diabetes doubles over the next 25 years to prevent a global epidemic of preventable blindness. Surely, laser photocoagulation and vitrectomy will not be able to deal with the burden of disease, particularly in developing nations.

On a more optimistic note, if one considers the major retinal diseases such as age-related macular degeneration, retinitis pigmentosa, and DR, DR is the only one for which large-scale clinical trials have proven the ability to reduce disease incidence and progression.[6,47,48] These studies emphasize the potential to control DR and other complications of disease. Better information is needed on the mechanism of the effects of intensive insulin therapy and how to design and deliver agents to achieve the effect without inducing hypoglycemia or other adverse consequences. Viewing DR as a specific consequence of the metabolic derangement of diabetes provides promise that pharmacotherapy should have a dramatic impact on the risk of vision loss in persons with diabetes.

REFERENCES

1. Kempen JH, O'Colmain BJ, Leske MC, et al. Prevalence of diabetic retinopathy among adults in the United States. Arch Ophthalmol 2004;122:552–563.
2. Wilkinson-Berka J, Miller AG. 2008. Update on the treatment of diabetic retinopathy. Sci World J 2008;6:98–120.
3. Hovind P, Tarnow L, Rossing K, et al. Decreasing incidence of severe diabetic microangiopathy in type 1 diabetes. Diabetes Care 2003;26:1258–1264.
4. Antonetti DA, Barber AJ, Bronson SK, et al. Diabetic retinopathy: seeing beyond glucose-induced microvascular disease. Diabetes 2006;55:2401–2411.
5. Girach A, Vignati L. Diabetic microvascular complications – can the presence of one predict the development of another? J Diabetes Compl 2006;20:228–237.
6. Diabetes Control and Complications Trial Research Group. The effect of intensive treatment of diabetes on the development and progression of long-term complications in insulin-dependent diabetes mellitus. N Engl J Med 1993;329:977–986.
7. Matthews DR, Stratton IM, Aldington SJ, et al. Risks of progression of retinopathy and vision loss related to tight blood pressure control in type 2 diabetes mellitus: UKPDS 69. Arch Ophthalmol 2004;122:1631–1640.
8. Tong Z, Yang Z, Patel S, et al. Promoter polymorphism of the erythropoietin gene in severe diabetic eye and kidney complications. Proc Natl Acad Sci USA 2008;105:6998–7003.
9. Meleth AD, Agron E, Chan CC, et al. Serum inflammatory markers in diabetic retinopathy. Invest Ophthalmol Vis Sci 2005;46:4295–4301.
10. Schram MT, Chaturvedi N, Schalkwijk CG, et al. Markers of inflammation are cross-sectionally associated with microvascular complications and cardiovascular disease in type 1 diabetes – the EURODIAB Prospective Complications Study. Diabetologia 2005;48:370–378.
11. Wolfensberger TJ, Hamilton AM. Diabetic retinopathy – an historical review. Semin Ophthalmol 2001;16:2–7.
12. Bloodworth JMB. Diabetic retinopathy. Diabetes 1962;2:1–22.
13. Wolter JR. Diabetic retinopathy. Am J Ophthalmol 1961;51:1123–1139.
14. Simonsen SE. ERG in juvenile diabetics: a prognostic study. In: Goldberg MF, Fine SL, editors. Symposium on the Treatment of Diabetic Retinopathy. Arlington: US Department of Health, Education and Welfare; 1969. p. 681–689.
15. Bresnick GH. Diabetic retinopathy viewed as a neurosensory disorder. Arch Ophthalmol 1986;104:989–990.
16. Bresnick GH, Palta M. Predicting progression to severe proliferative diabetic retinopathy. Arch Ophthalmol 1987;105:810–814.
17. Ghirlanda G, Di Leo MA, Caputo S, et al. From functional to microvascular abnormalities in early diabetic retinopathy. Diabetes Metab Rev 1997;13:15–35.
18. Barber AJ, Lieth E, Khin SA, et al. Neural apoptosis in the retina during experimental and human diabetes. Early onset and effect of insulin. J Clin Invest 1998;102:783–791.
19. Gastinger MJ, Singh RS, Barber AJ. Loss of cholinergic and dopaminergic amacrine cells in streptozotocin – diabetic rat and Ins2Akita-diabetic mouse retinas. Invest Ophthalmol Vis Sci 2006;47:3143–3150.
20. Barber AJ, Antonetti DA, Gardner TW. Altered expression of retinal occludin and glial fibrillary acidic protein in experimental diabetes. The Penn State Retina Research Group. Invest Ophthalmol Vis Sci 2000;41:3561–3568.
21. Mizutani M, Gerhardinger C, Lorenzi M. Muller cell changes in human diabetic retinopathy. Diabetes 1998;47:445–449.
22. Puro DG. Diabetes-induced dysfunction of retinal Muller cells. Trans Am Ophthalmol Soc 2002;100:339–352.
23. Rungger-Brandle E, Dosso AA, Leuenberger PM. Glial reactivity, an early feature of diabetic retinopathy. Invest Ophthalmol Vis Sci 2000;41:1971–1980.
24. Krady JK, Basu A, Allen CM, et al. Minocycline reduces proinflammatory cytokine expression, microglial activation, and caspase-3 activation in a rodent model of diabetic retinopathy. Diabetes 2005;54:1559–1565.
25. Zeng HY, Green WR, Tso MO. Microglial activation in human diabetic retinopathy. Arch Ophthalmol 2008;126:227–232.
26. Bensaoula T, Ottlecz A. Biochemical and ultrastructural studies in the neural retina and retinal pigment epithelium of STZ-diabetic rats: effect of captopril. J Ocul Pharmacol Ther 2001;17:573–586.
27. Anonymous. A randomized trial of sorbinil, an aldose reductase inhibitor, in diabetic retinopathy. Sorbinil Retinopathy Trial Research Group. Arch Ophthalmol 1990;108:1234–1244.
28. PKC-DRS Study Group. The effect of ruboxistaurin on visual loss in patients with moderately severe to very severe nonproliferative diabetic retinopathy. Initial results of the protein kinase Cbeta inhibitor diabetic retinopathy study (PKC-DRS) multicenter randomized clinical trial. Diabetes 2005;54:2188–2197.
29. Aiello LP, Davis MD, Girach A, et al. Effect of ruboxistaurin on visual loss in patients with diabetic retinopathy. Ophthalmology 2006;113:2221–2230.
30. Greenbaum CJ. Insulin resistance in type 1 diabetes. Diabetes/Metab Res Rev 2002;18:192–200.
31. Wellen KE, Hotamisligil GS. Inflammation, stress, and diabetes. J Clin Invest 2005;115:1111–1119.
32. Dana GW. Type of diabetes mellitus associated with diabetic retinitis. AMA Arch Ophthalmol 1953;50:123–124.
33. Barouch FC, Miyamoto K, Allport JR, et al. Integrin-mediated neutrophil adhesion and retinal leukostasis in diabetes. Invest Ophthalmol Vis Sci 2000;41:1153–1158.
34. Reiter CE, Sandirasegarane L, Wolpert EB, et al. Characterization of insulin signaling in rat retina *in vivo* and ex vivo. Am J Physiol Endocrinol Metab 2003;285:E763–E774.
35. Reiter CEN, Gardner TW. Retinal insulin and insulin signaling: implications for diabetic retinopathy. Prog Retin Eye Res 2003;22:545–562.
36. Reiter CEN, Wu X, Sandirasegarane L, et al. Diabetes reduces basal retinal insulin receptor signaling: reversal with systemic and local insulin. Diabetes 2006;55:1148–1156.
37. Wilkinson-Berka JL. Diabetes and retinal vascular disorders: role of the reninangiotensin system. Expert Rev Mol Med 2004;6:1–18.
38. Field MG, Elner VM, Puro DG, et al. Rapid, noninvasive detection of diabetes-induced retinal metabolic stress. Arch Ophthalmol 2008;126:934–938.

39. Gardner TW, Jackson GR, Quillen DA, et al. Diabetic retinopathy: translating discoveries to treatments. In: Greenbaum C, Harrison LC, editors. Diabetes: Translating Discoveries into Practice. New York: Informa Press; 2009.
40. Stefansson E, Bek T, Porta M, et al. Screening and prevention of diabetic blindness. Acta Ophthalmol Scand 2000;78:374–385.
41. Gardner TW, Antonetti DA. Novel potential mechanisms for diabetic macular edema: leveraging new investigational approaches. Curr Diabetes Rep 2008;8:263–269.
42. Mohamed Q, Gillies MC, Wong TY. Management of diabetic retinopathy: a systematic review. JAMA 2007;298:902–916.
43. Tonello M, Costa RA, Almeida FP, et al. Panretinal photocoagulation versus PRP plus intravitreal bevacizumab for high-risk proliferative diabetic retinopathy (IBeHi study). Acta Ophthalmol 2008;86:385–389.
44. Scott IU, Edwards AR, Beck RW, et al. A phase II randomized clinical trial of intravitreal bevacizumab for diabetic macular edema. Ophthalmology 2007;114:1860–1867.
45. A randomized trial comparing intravitreal triamcinolone acetonide and focal/grid photocoagulation for diabetic macular edema. Ophthalmology 2008;115:1447–1449, e1441–e1410.
46. Blankenship GW. Fifteen-year argon laser and xenon photocoagulation visual results of Bascom Palmer Eye Institute's patients participating in the Diabetic Retinopathy Study. Trans Am Ophthalmol Soc 1990;88:179–185; discussion 185–179.
47. Stratton IM, Kohner EM, Aldington SJ, et al. UKPDS 50: risk factors for incidence and progression of retinopathy in type II diabetes over 6 years from diagnosis. Diabetologia 2001;44:156–163.
48. Sjolie AK, Stephenson J, Aldington S, et al. Retinopathy and vision loss in insulin-dependent diabetes in Europe. The EURODIAB IDDM complications study. Ophthalmology 1997;104:252–260.

CHAPTER

20 Retinal vein occlusion

Osamu Sawada, MD and Masahito Ohji, MD

INTRODUCTION

Retinal vein occlusion (RVO), one of the most frequently occurring retinal vascular disorders in elderly patients, develops predominantly in individuals over age 65 years.[1–3] RVO generally is classified into central RVO (CRVO) and branch RVO (BRVO) according to the site of blockage in the retinal vein. CRVO is divided further into nonischemic and ischemic types according to the perfusion status based on fluorescein angiography. Ischemic CRVO is associated with greater than 10 disc areas in diameter of retinal capillary nonperfusion on fluorescein angiography.[4] Ocular vascular leakage, retinal and iris neovascularization, and intractable elevation of the intraocular pressure may result from progression of ischemic CRVO. Large areas of retinal capillary nonperfusion in BRVO may develop neovascularization followed by vitreous hemorrhage. Macular edema is the major complication of significant visual loss in patients with CRVO and BRVO, and various treatments have been used to improve macular edema and cause regression of intraocular neovascularization. Recent pharmacologic agents primarily have targeted the improvement of macular edema secondary to CRVO and BRVO.[5–15]

DISEASE PREVALENCE

Studies among older population-based samples reported that the prevalences of RVO range from 0.3% (CRVO 6 cases, BRVO 33 cases out of 15 466 persons) in the pooling of two large population-based cardiovascular studies in the Atherosclerosis Risk in Communities Study (12,642 persons aged 51–71 years) and Cardiovascular Health Study (2824 persons aged 73 years and older),[16] 0.7% (BRVO 31 cases, CRVO 7 cases out of 4822 persons aged 43–84 years) in the Beaver Dam Eye Study,[17] to 1.6% (CRVO 18 cases, BRVO 41 cases out of 3654 persons aged 49 years and older) in the Blue Mountains Eye Study.[2]

RISK FACTORS

Systemic risk factors associated with CRVO include systemic vascular diseases (hypertension, diabetes mellitus, and cardiovascular diseases), blood dyscrasias (polycythemia vera, lymphoma, leukemia), paraproteinemias and dysproteinemias (multiple myeloma and cytoglobulinemia), vasculitis (syphilis and sarcoidosis), and autoimmune disease.[18] Medications (oral contraceptives, diuretics, hepatitis B vaccine) also increase the risk of RVO.

Ocular risk factors associated with CRVO include open-angle glaucoma, ischemic optic neuropathy, pseudotumor cerebri, tilted optic nerve heads, and optic nerve head drusen.

The Eye Disease Case-Control Study of 270 patients with BRVO and 1142 controls reported that the systemic risk factors associated with BRVO were hypertension, a history of cardiovascular disease, an increased body mass index at 20 years of age, and higher serum levels of alpha 2-globulin. Ocular risk factors associated with BRVO include open-angle glaucoma and focal arteriolar narrowing and arteriovenous nicking.[19]

PATHOGENESIS

The precise pathogenesis of CRVO remains uncertain. Three occlusive processes have been postulated as pathogenetic: (1) occlusion of the vein by external compression caused by sclerotic adjacent structures (the central retinal artery and fibrous tissue envelope); (2) occlusion by primary wall disease (degenerative or inflammatory in nature); and (3) hemodynamic disturbances resulting from various factors (subendothelial atheromatous lesions in the central retinal artery, arterial spasm, sudden reduction of blood pressure, blood dyscrasias, and further aggravation by arteriosclerosis or unfavorable anatomic relations). These produce stagnated flow in the central retinal vein and result in primary thrombus formation in susceptible eyes.[20]

BRVO always occurs at an arteriovenous crossing, where the retinal artery and vein share a common adventitial sheath. The rigidity of the arteriosclerotic artery caused by underlying arterial disease may compress the vein lumen at the crossing site, resulting in turbulent blood flow and vascular endothelium damage, followed by thrombosis and vein occlusion. Obstruction of the vein elevates venous pressure, which may overload the collateral drainage capacity and lead to macular edema and rupture of the vein wall with intraretinal hemorrhage.[20]

DIAGNOSIS AND ANCILLARY TESTING/ DIFFERENTIAL DIAGNOSIS

CENTRAL RETINAL VEIN OCCLUSION

CRVO is a venous retinal obstructive disease of the central retinal vein, resulting in elevated venous and capillary pressure with stagnated blood flow. The diagnosis is established based on characteristic fundus findings of widespread extensive dot-blot and flame-shaped hemorrhage, engorgement and tortuosity of all branches of the central retinal vein, cotton-wool patches, macular edema, and optic disc edema and hyperemia.

There are two types of CRVO: ischemic and nonischemic. Ischemic CRVO is severe, complete, or total vein obstruction. The fundus has extensive retinal hemorrhaging, venous dilatation and tortuosity, and scattered cotton-wool spots (Figure 20.1). Ischemic CRVO is rarely confused with other entities. Nonischemic CRVO is partial, incomplete, imminent, threatened, incipient, or impending vein obstruction. Nonischemic CRVO can be subtle, because the findings of venous engorgement and tortuosity are mild and cotton-wool patches and optic edema tend to be absent (Figure 20.2). Nonischemic or longstanding CRVO may be similar to the retinopathy of carotid occlusive disease. Although disc edema may be associated with CRVO, it is rare in carotid occlusive disease. Although the veins are engorged in both CRVO and carotid occlusive diseases, they are generally not tortuous in carotid occlusive diseases.

Fluorescein angiography is the most useful ancillary test for the evaluation of ocular neovascularization and macular edema. On fluorescein angiography, eyes with areas of nonperfusion of 10 disc areas or greater should be classified as ischemic (Figure 20.1B). Poor visual acuity (VA) and large areas of retinal capillary nonperfusion are significant factors associated with increased risk of the development of

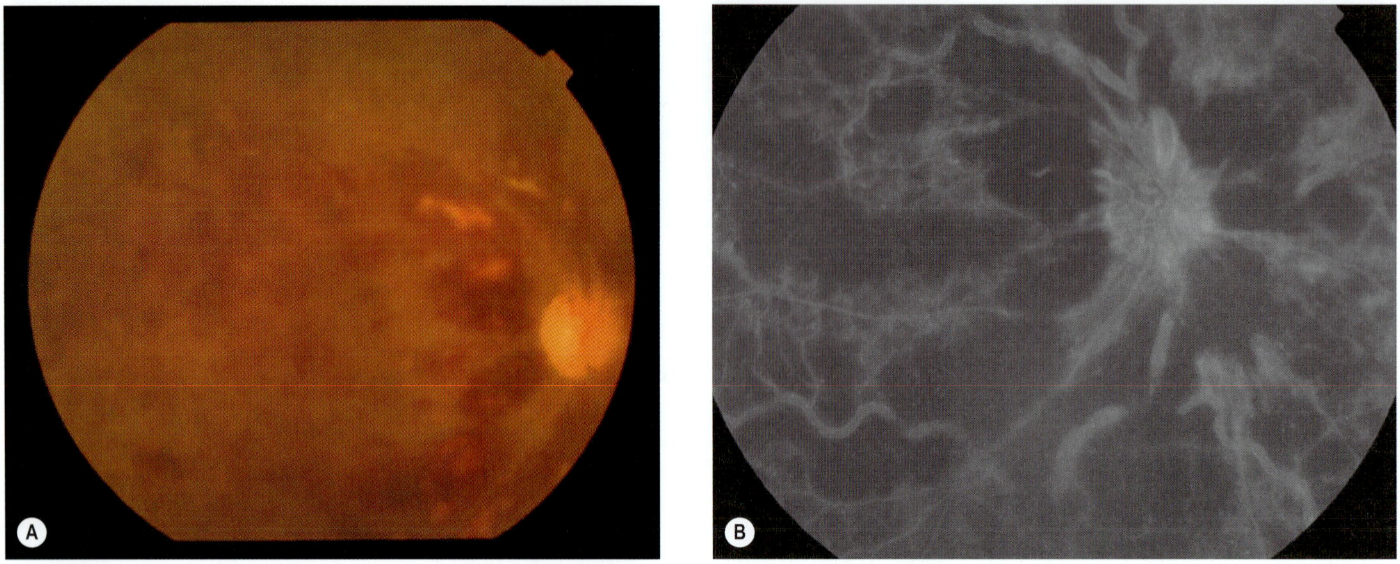

Figure 20.1 (A) Fundus photograph of ischemic central retinal vein occlusion shows an extensive intraretinal hemorrhage with optic disc edema, venous engorgement and tortuosity, and numerous cotton-wool spots. (B) Fluorescein angiogram of the eye shows capillary nonperfusion in all quadrants of the fundus and posterior region.

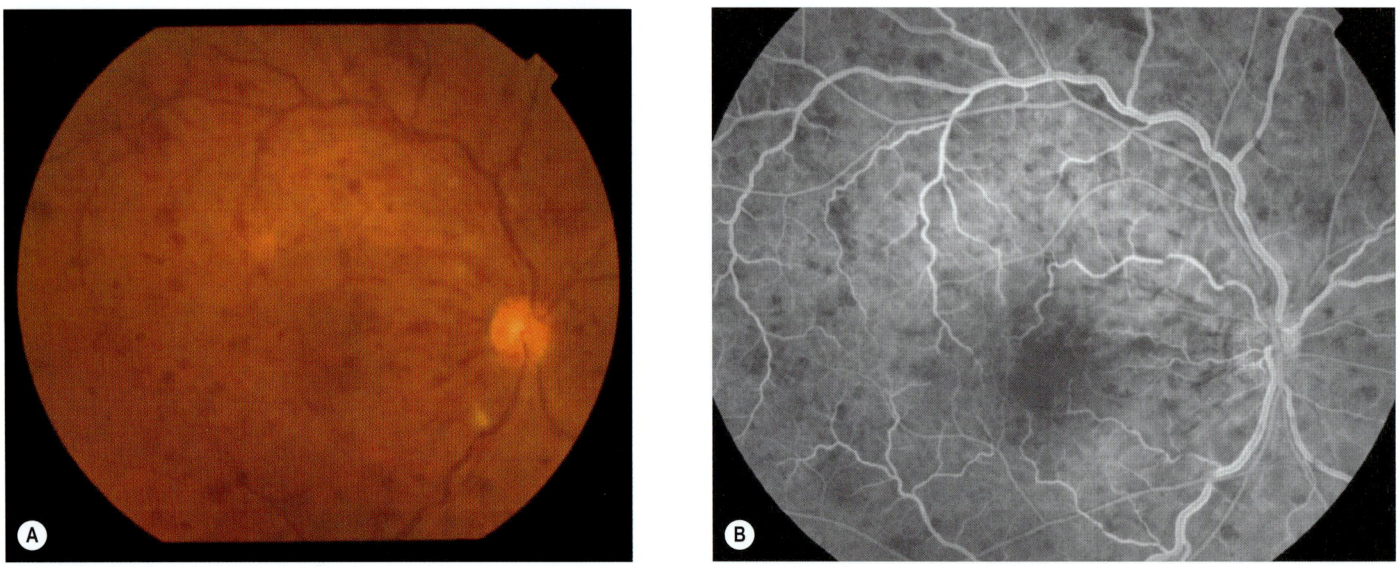

Figure 20.2 (A) Fundus photograph of nonischemic central retinal vein occlusion shows engorgement and tortuosity of all branches of the central retinal vein, intraretinal hemorrhages, and cotton-wool patches. (B) Fluorescein angiogram of the eye shows more clearly the perfused status and engorgement and tortuosity.

iris and anterior-segment neovascularization. Electroretinography is helpful to determine the prognosis.

Optical coherence tomography (OCT) is useful for detecting macular edema and can identify subtle macular edema and offer quantitative data on macular edema that would be helpful for follow-up and research.[21,22]

Because CRVO can be associated with systemic diseases, a general medical evaluation should include an extensive medical history, physical examination with blood pressure measurement, and laboratory evaluation.

BRANCH RETINAL VEIN OCCLUSION

The diagnosis of BRVO is made based on the characteristic findings of flame-shaped and dot-blot hemorrhages on an occluded vein that is dilated and tortuous. The vein occlusion is almost always at an arteriovenous crossing (Figure 20.3).

Fluorescein angiography is a useful ancillary test for evaluating an obstruction site, perfusion status, neovascularization, and macular edema. Indocyanine green angiography may be more useful than fluorescein angiography for detecting sites of obstruction.

It can be difficult to differentiate BRVO from hypertensive retinopathy, diabetic retinopathy, ocular ischemic retinopathy, juxtafoveal retinal telangiectasia, combined branch retinal artery and vein occlusion, and radiation retinopathy. Marked arteriovenous crossing changes and retinal hemorrhages in hypertensive retinopathy may resemble the findings in BRVO. Juxtafoveal retinal telangiectasia may be confused with BRVO with telangiectatic capillaries. Asymmetric diabetic retinopathy may appear similar to BRVO.

Because BRVO is associated with hypertension, a physical examination with blood pressure measurement is recommended.

OCULAR AND SYSTEMIC SIGNS AND SYMPTOMS

Patients with CRVO have unilateral blurred vision, decreased vision, and visual field defects. The VA ranges widely from 20/20 to less than

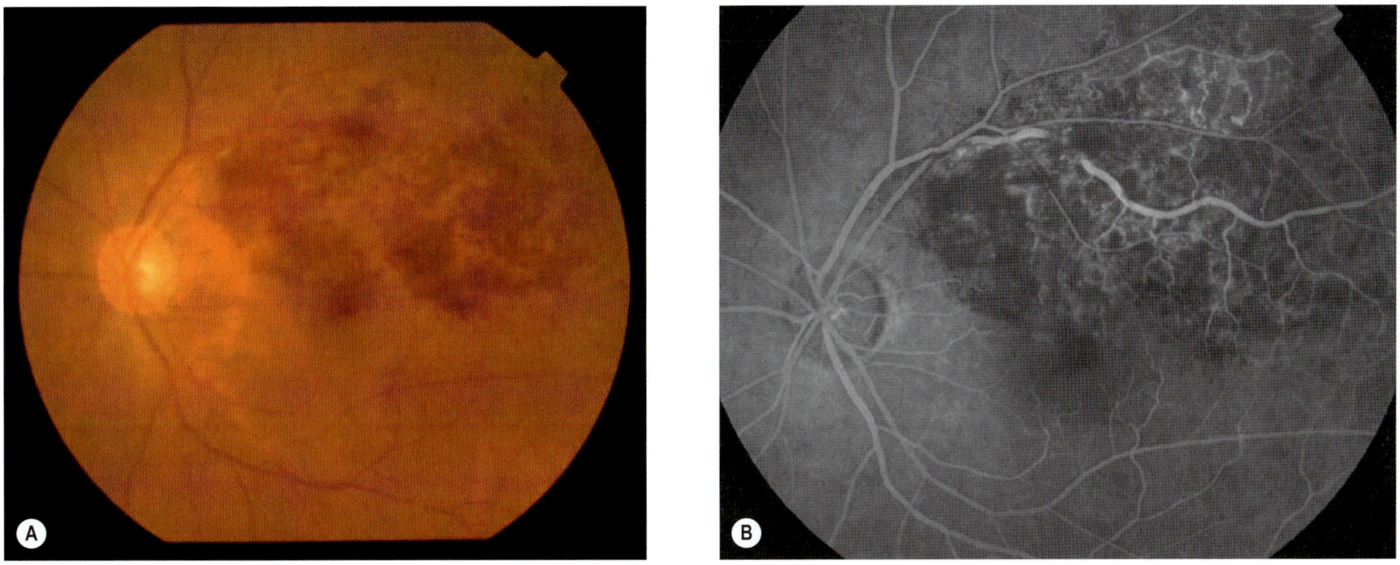

Figure 20.3 (A) Fundus photograph of a superotemporal branch vein occlusion shows the segment pattern of intraretinal hemorrhage. (B) Fluorescein angiogram of the eye in (A) shows dilation of the superotemporal vein and delayed filling-in and areas of capillary nonperfusion superotemporally.

20/200, depending on the disease severity. Patients with ischemic CRVO have severe visual impairment, and the VA usually decreases to 20/200 or less and even to hand motions in some cases. The VA of patients with nonischemic CRVO is better than that in ischemic CRVO and is usually better than 20/200; VA better than 20/40 is not rare. Patients rarely report ocular pain unless rubeotic glaucoma develops.

The symptoms associated with BRVO depend on the amounts and location of damage compromised by the occlusion. Patients with macular involvement report blurred vision and a relative visual field defect. Patients with peripheral occlusions are usually asymptomatic.

Patients with RVO are systemically asymptomatic; however, they may have systemic symptoms due to systemic diseases associated with CRVO, including hypertension and cardiovascular diseases.

TREATMENT OPTIONS

CENTRAL RETINAL VEIN OCCLUSION

Medications for CRVO include tissue plasminogen activator (tPA), corticosteroids, and bevacizumab (Avastin). Other medications of coumadin (warfarin), urokinase, troxerutin, ticlodipine, and pentoxifylline were also reported. Other treatments are hemodilution, laser treatment (including panretinal photocoagulation, grid macular photocoagulation, and chorioretinal venous anastomosis). Radial optic neurotomy (RON) is a surgical option.

BRANCH RETINAL VEIN OCCLUSION

Treatments for BRVO include corticosteroids and bevacizumab (Avastin), laser treatment using grid macular laser photocoagulation, and arteriovenous crossing sheathotomy.

TREATMENT OUTCOMES AND PROGNOSIS

CENTRAL RETINAL VEIN OCCLUSION

It is important to understand the natural course of CRVO. According to the Central Vein Occlusion Study, a randomized multicentered clinical trial of 728 eyes with CRVO, the VA outcomes largely depend on the initial VA. The baseline VA was 20/40 or better (good VA) in 29%, 20/50–20/200 (intermediate VA) in 43%, and 20/250 or worse (poor VA) in 28%, with a median baseline VA of 20/80. Sixty-five percent of patients who had an initially good VA (20/40 or better) maintained good VA at the end of the study. The visual outcomes in eyes with intermediate VA (20/50–20/200) varied: 21% improved to better than 20/50, 41% stayed in the intermediate range, and 38% had worse than 20/200. Patients with poor VA (<20/200) at the first visit had an 80% chance of having VA less than 20/200 at the final visit.[23]

TISSUE PLASMINOGEN ACTIVATOR (tPA)

tPA converts plasminogen to plasmin and destabilizes intravascular thrombi. tPA reduces clot size in occlusive vessels, resulting in dislodgment of the entire thrombus or recanalization of the occluded retinal vein. When used to treat CRVO, tPA has been administered by several routes: systemic, intravitreal, and by endovascular cannulation of retinal vessels. Systemic administration of low-dose (50 mg) tPA resulted in a VA increase of one line or more in 10 (7 CRVO, 3 BRVO) of 14 patients (8 CRVO, 6 BRVO) with RVO.[24] The VA improved 2 lines or more in 10 of 23 patients with CRVO.[25] However, one patient died of an intracranial hemorrhage following tPA administration.[26] Intravitreal administration of tPA is associated with less risk of systemic complications. tPA injected into the vitreous cavity subsequently reaches the retinal vessels. tPA (65–110 μg) was injected intravitreally in 23 patients with CRVO with recent onset of visual symptoms and the VA improved or stabilized in 16 eyes (70%).[27] Another study reported that 4 of 9 patients with CRVO treated with 100 μg of tPA intravitreally had 3 lines or more of VA improvement.[28] However, tPA is associated with retinal toxicity.[29] Endovascular delivery of tPA involved cannulation of retinal vessels and tPA was injected directly into the occluded retinal vein, resulting in release of the suspected thrombus. Pars plana vitrectomy followed by cannulation of a branch vein and, with the help of a stabilization arm, injection of a bolus of 200 μg/ml of tPA toward the optic nerve head improved the VA more than 3 lines in 50% of 28 eyes after a mean follow-up of 12 months. Complications included vitreous hemorrhage in 7 eyes and retinal detachment in 1 eye.[30]

CORTICOSTEROIDS

Corticosteroids improve VA by reducing macular edema. The exact mechanism by which this occurs is unknown, but it is thought to be a combination of anti-inflammatory effects with modulation of cytokine and growth factor production and stabilization of the blood–retinal barrier with reduction of vascular permeability. There is little evidence to support the usefulness of oral corticosteroids for treating macular edema secondary to CRVO.

Intravitreal injection of triamcinolone acetonide (TA), a synthetic corticosteroid, has been used to treat macular edema associated with CRVO and BRVO (Figure 20.4). The intravitreal route of administration allows the drug to reach the target tissue directly, such as the retinal vessels and macular tissue, and does not result in systemic adverse events. A few reports suggested that intravitreal injection had the potential to improve vision loss and retinal thickening in patients with macular edema associated CRVO, but suggested that some patients developed steroid-related complications such as elevated intraocular pressure (IOP) and cataract; injection-related complications such as retinal detachment and endophthalmitis.[5–8] The Standard Care vs Corticosteroid for Retinal Vein Occlusion (SCORE) was multicenter, randomized, clinical trial of 271 participants to compare the efficiency and safety of 1-mg 4-mg doses of preservative-free intravitreal triamcinolone with observation for eyes with macular edema associated with CRVO. The primary outcome in this study, the percentage of participants with a gain in visual acuity letters score of 15 or more from baseline to month 12, was 6.8%, 26.5%, and 25.6% for the observation, 1-mg, and 4 mg respectively. This trial concluded that intravitreal triamcinolone in both a 1-mg and 4-mg dose had better visual outcomes over 12 month than observation and the 1-mg dose had a safety profile superior to 4-mg dose with respect to glaucoma and cataract.[31]"

BEVACIZUMAB

Vascular endothelium growth factor (VEGF) stimulates proliferation of vascular endothelial cells resulting in neovascularization and increases the permeability of the capillaries, causing edema. VEGF concentrations increase in the intraocular fluid of patients with CRVO, with the highest levels seen in patients with iris or anterior neovascularization.[32] Bevacizumab is a full-length humanized monoclonal antibody against all isomers of VEGF and was approved by the Food and Drug Administration for intravenous administration to treat metastatic colorectal cancer.

Intravitreal injection of bevacizumab was used for macular edema due to CRVO (Figure 20.5). Rosenfeld and associates[11] first reported the use of intravitreal bevacizumab to treat macular edema secondary to CRVO. In that study, patients with macular edema due to CRVO were treated with bevacizumab and the VA improved from 20/200 to 20/50. OCT showed resolution of the macular edema within 1 week. The improvements were maintained for 1 month.[11] Another study reported on 46 patients with CRVO who underwent repeated intravitreal injections (1.25 mg) of bevacizumab. The mean VA improved from 20/250 to 20/80 at the 6-month follow-up and the mean central retinal thickness decreased from 535 ± 148 μm at baseline to 323 ±116 μm at the 6-month follow-up visit.[12]

OTHER MEDICATIONS

Ranimizumab

Ranibizumab, a humanized antigen binding portion of a murine anti-VEGF monoclonal antibody with a mature high affinity for all VEGF isoforms, has been approved as an intravitreal treatment for neovascular AMD and is the first such treatment to improve visual acuity (VA) in neovascular AMD.

CRUISE is multicenter, randomized, double-masked, sham injection-controlled Phase III study of 392 participants designed to assess the efficiency and safety profile of ranimizumab for macular edema associated to CRVO. The month 6 result showed that 46.2% (61/132) of patients received 0.3 mg of ranimizumab and 47.7% (62/130) received 0.5 mg of ranimizumab had their vision improved by 15 letters or more compared to 16.9% (22/130) of patients receiving sham injections and mean gain was observed beginning at day seven with an 8.8 and 9.3 letter gain in the 0.3 mg and 0.5 mg study arms of ranimizumab, respectively, compared with 1.1 letters in the sham injection arm.[33]

Coumadin (warfarin)

Coumadin is widely used as an anticoagulant for various systemic diseases such as venous thromboembolism, cardiac arrhythmia, following myocardial infarction, and hematologic abnormalities, among others. However, the efficacy of coumadin for CRVO is not established. It was reported that 13 of 354 patients taking warfarin developed CRVO despite maintaining therapeutic levels of the anticoagulant.[34]

Urokinase

The effect of systemic administration of urokinase is unclear. One study reported the effectiveness of superselective ophthalmic artery fibrinolytic therapy of urokinase for CRVO. Urokinase was infused through a microcatheter into the ostium of the ophthalmic artery via the femoral artery. Six eyes of 26 patients had a significant improvement in VA 24 hours after the fibrinolysis; eyes with combined central retinal artery occlusion and CRVO with recent visual impairment appeared to be the most responsive.[35]

Troxerutin

Troxerutin, a derivative of the naturally occurring bioflavonoid rutin, is thought to inhibit red cell and platelet aggregation, improve erythrocyte deformability, and improve plasma viscosity retinal microcirculation. A double-blind randomized clinical trial compared troxerutin with placebo in 27 patients with CRVO. The limitations of the study included a small number of patients and short follow-up time.[36]

Ticlodipine

Ticlodipine binds to adenosine diphosphate receptors on the platelet surface, resulting in platelet aggregation. A double-blind randomized clinical study that compared the effect of 500 mg/day of ticlodipine with placebo in patients with CRVO found that the treatment group tended to improve compared with placebo, but the results were not significant.[37]

Pentoxifylline

Pentoxifylline can increase red blood cell deformability, reduce blood viscosity, and decrease platelet aggregation and thrombus formation. Pentoxifylline is an oral agent that improves perfusion of occluded vessels and is used to treat systemic vascular diseases. The retinal flow velocity in patients with RVO treated with pentoxifylline improved compared with placebo, but the study had a small number of patients ($n = 8$) and short follow-up (4 weeks), and no visual outcome data were reported.[38]

Hemodilution

In some patients with CRVO, abnormal red cell deformability and increased plasma viscosity and hematocrit and fibrinogen levels were observed. Therefore, reducing hematocrit levels by hemodilution lowers plasma viscosity and may improve retinal microcirculation and perfusion. Several studies have reported significant improvements in VA, arteriovenous passage time, and the clinical appearance by hemodilution.[39,40] However, common adverse effects, including letheargy, fainting spells, and exertional dyspnea, were observed.

Laser treatment

The Central Retinal Vein Occlusion Study Group compared the efficacy of immediate prophylactic panretinal photocoagulation in ischemic CRVO with that of observation only. Iris or angle neovascularization developed in 20% of the early treatment group and 34% in the observed group. Greater resolution of iris or angle neovascularization occurred within 1 month after panretinal photocoagulation in 18 of 32 previously untreated eyes compared with four of 18 eyes that had undergone early prophylactic treatment. Panretinal photocoagulation should be applied promptly after the development of iris or angle neovascularization in eyes with ischemic CRVO.[41] The Central Retinal Vein Occlusion Study Group reported that grid laser photocoagulation for

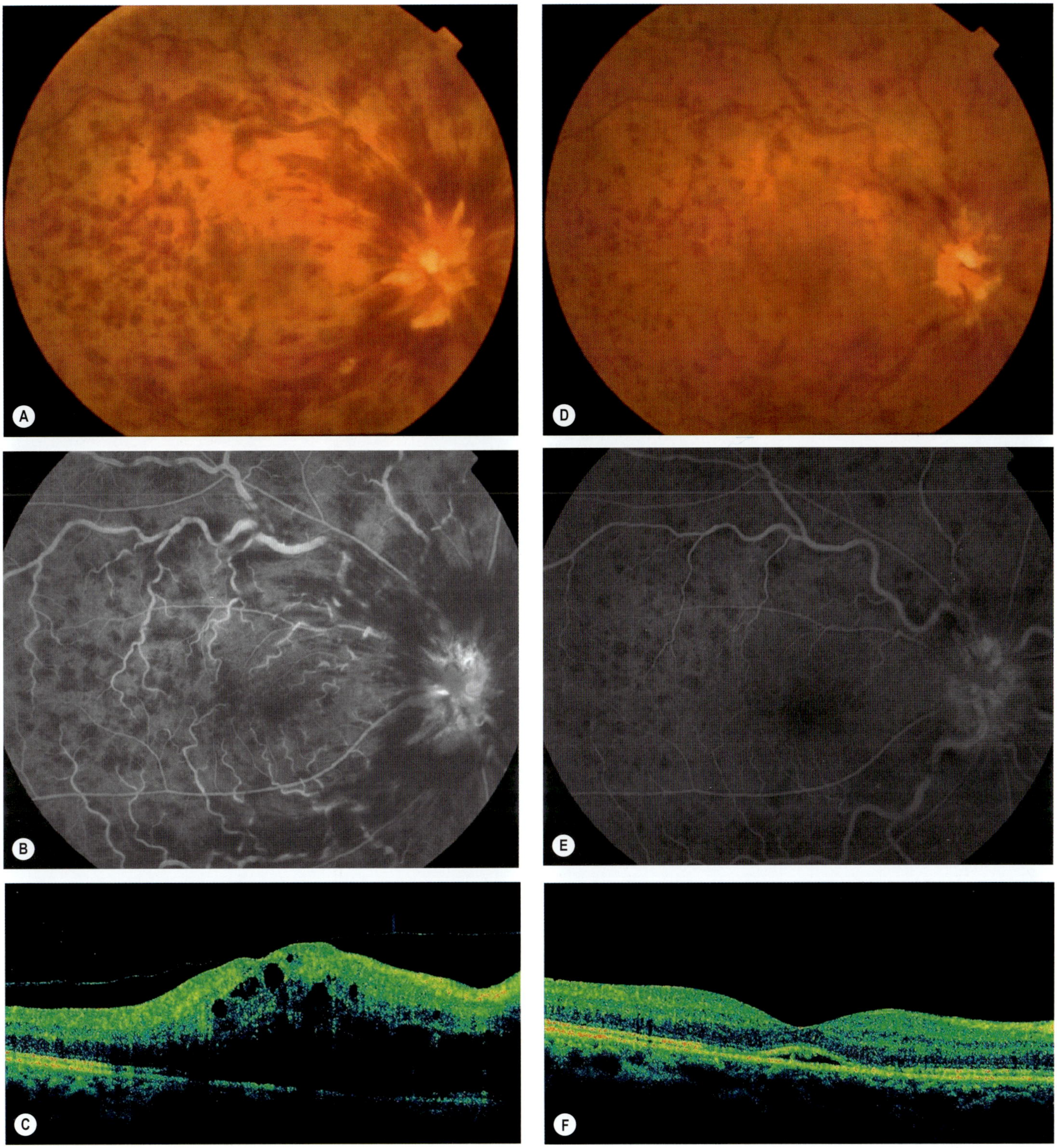

Figure 20.4 (A) Fundus photograph of the eye with macular edema secondary to central retinal vein occlusion shows venous dilatation and tortuosity, optic disc edema, widespread intraretinal hemorrhage, and macular edema at baseline before injection of triamcinolone acetonide (TA). (B) Fluorescein angiogram shows marked distention of the retinal vein, optic nerve head swelling, and intraretinal hemorrhage at baseline before intravitreal injection of TA. (C) Optical coherence tomography (OCT) image shows a large area of macular edema with poor visualization of the retinal pigment epithelium due to shadowing at baseline before intravitreal injection of TA. (D) Fundus photograph 1 month after intravitreal injection of TA (4 mg) shows the resorption of the intraretinal hemorrhage and improved venous dilatation and tortuosity. (E) Fluorescein angiogram 1 month after intravitreal injection of TA (4 mg) shows improved distention of the retinal vein and decreased leakage around the optic nerve head. (F) OCT image a month after intravitreal injection of TA (4 mg) shows a marked improvement in the foveal macular thickness.

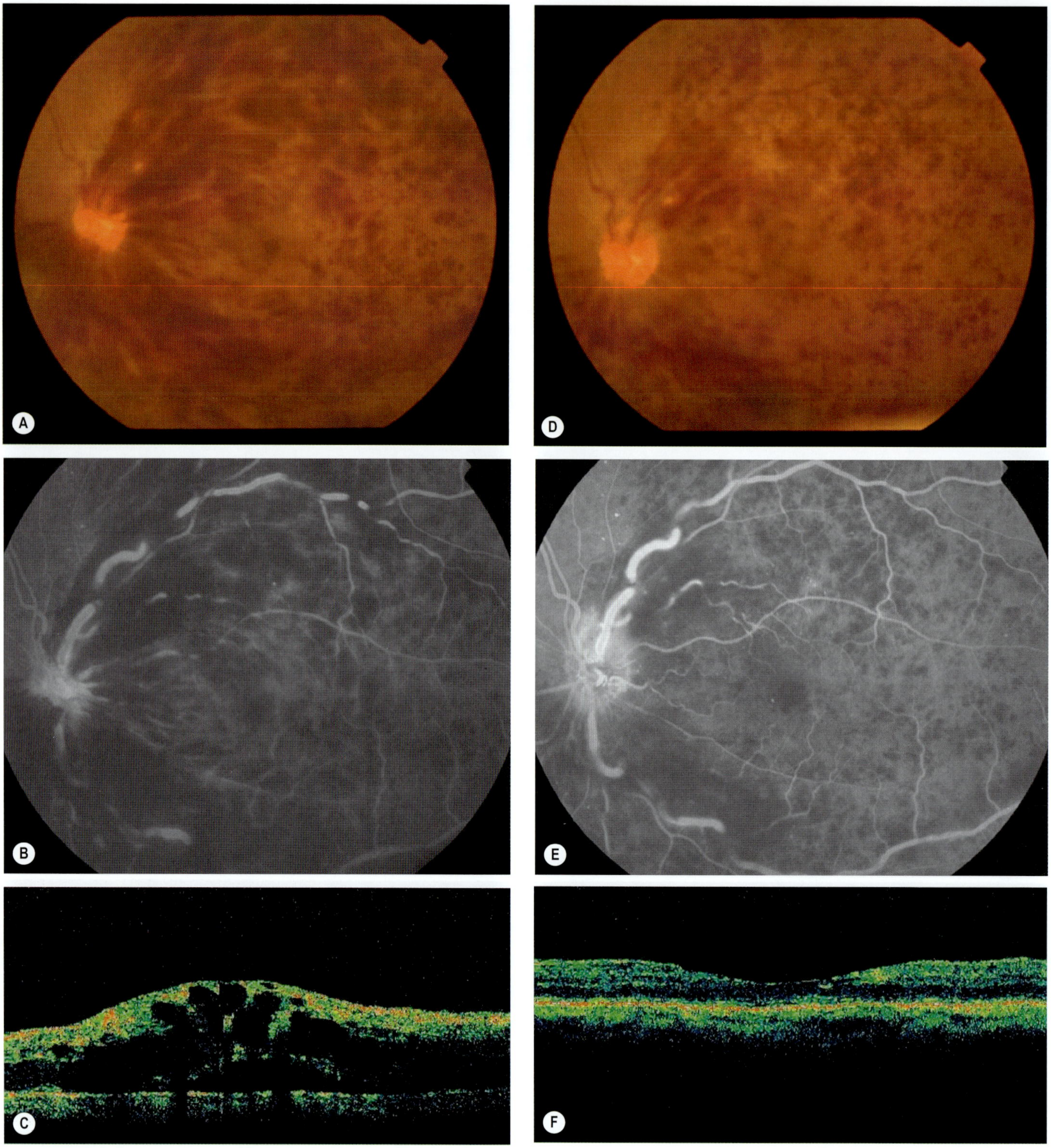

Figure 20.5 (A) Fundus photograph of the eye with macular edema secondary to central retinal vein occlusion shows venous dilatation and tortuosity, optic disc edema, widespread severe intraretinal hemorrhage, and macular edema at baseline before injection of bevacizumab. (B) Fluorescein angiogram shows marked distention of the retinal vein, optic nerve head swelling, and severe intraretinal hemorrhage at baseline before intravitreal injection of bevacizumab. (C) Optical coherence tomography (OCT) image shows a large area of macular edema with poor visualization of the retinal pigment epithelium due to shadowing at baseline before intravitreal injection of bevacizumab. (D) Fundus photograph 1 month after intravitreal injection of bevacizumab (1.25 mg) shows some resorption of the intraretinal hemorrhage and some improvement of the venous dilatation and tortuosity. (E) Fluorescein angiogram 1 month after intravitreal injection of bevacizumab (1.25 mg) shows decrease of the intraretinal hemorrhage and some improvement in the distention of the retinal vein. (F) An OCT image 1 month after intravitreal injection of bevacizumab (1.25 mg) shows a marked decrease and improvement in foveal macular thickness.

macular edema secondary to CRVO caused a significant decrease in macular edema but the VA did not improve in a randomized clinical trial. In that study, eyes with macular edema due to CRVO were randomized to macular grid photocoagulation (77 eyes) or no treatment (78 eyes) and followed every 4 months for 3 years or until the end of the study. This treatment clearly showed reduced macular edema on fundus fluorescein angiography at 1 year (69% of treated versus 0% of untreated eyes). However, there was no difference in VA between the treated (from 20/160 to 20/200) and untreated (from 20/125 to 20/160) eyes.[42]

Chorioretinal venous anastomosis

Chorioretinal venous anastomosis is used to bypass the occluded central retinal vein by creating a chorioretinal anastomosis between a nasal branch retinal vein and the choroidal circulation. Commonly, energy delivered via argon laser is directed at a branch retinal vein to rupture the posterior vein wall and Bruch's membrane. A retrospective consecutive series of 91 patients with nonischemic CRVO was conducted to evaluate the efficacy of and complications associated with laser-induced chorioretinal venous anastomosis and to identify the associated risks. When chorioretinal venous anastomoses were created in 49 eyes, 41 eyes had a 4.3 ± 3.8 line improvement in VA, 8 eyes had no improvement or reduced vision, and 18 eyes had neovascular complications.[43]

In another report of a consecutive series of 8 cases with nonischemic CRVO, successful chorioretinal venous anastomoses were created in 2 eyes, 2 patients had improved VA without a successful treatment, and 6 patients had unchanged or worsened VA. The complications included retinal neovascularization in 3 patients, vitreous hemorrhage in 3 patients, subsequent iris neovascularization in 3 patients, tractional retinal detachment in 2 patients, and neovascular glaucoma in 1 patient.[44] The complications of this technique included immediate internal, subretinal, or vitreous hemorrhage; the long-term complications included vitreous hemorrhage, epiretinal avascular proliferation, fibrovascular proliferation, secondary neovascularization, and tractional retinal detachment. Because some studies reported an increased risk of fibrovascular complications in eyes with ischemic CRVO, laser chorioretinal anastomosis is not recommended for ischemic CRVO.[43,44]

SURGICAL TREATMENT OF CRVO

Radial optic neurotomy (RON)

Opremcak and colleagues hypothesized that CRVO is neurovascular compartment syndrome at the site of the lamina cribrosa. RON, a procedure developed by those investigators, decompresses the scleral outlet via an internal vitreoretinal approach using a radial incision nasal to the optic nerve head.[45] In a report of 117 consecutive cases by Opremcak and colleagues, the Snellen VA improved an average of 2.5 lines in 71% of patients; clinical improvement on fundus examination, fundus photography, and fluorescein angiography was seen in 95%.[46] Postoperatively, chorioretinal anastomosis at the incision site may facilitate more active drainage of retinal edema and hemorrhage compared to laser-induced chorioretinal anastomosis. However, a postoperative visual field defect has been reported, and the potential risk of subintraretinal or vitreous hemorrhage may be problematic.[47]

BRANCH RETINAL VEIN OCCLUSION

Corticosteroids

The effects of intravitreal injection of TA for macular edema secondary to BRVO have been reported (Figure 20.6). Numerous reports suggested that intravitreal injection had the potential to improve vision loss and retinal thickening in patients with macular edema associated BRVO, but suggested that some patients developed steroid-related complications such as elevated intraocular pressure (IOP) and cataract; injection-related complications such as retinal detachment and endophthalmitis.[10,48–59] The Standard Care vs Corticosteroid for Retinal Vein Occlusion (SCORE) was multicenter, randomized, clinical trial of 411 participants to compare the efficiency and safety of 1-mg 4-mg doses of preservative-free intravitreal triamcinolone with grid photocoagulation for eyes with macular edema secondary to BRVO. The primary outcome in this study, the percentage of participants with a gain in visual acuity letters score of 15 or more from baseline to month 12, was 29%, 26%, and 27% for the observation, 1-mg, and 4 mg respectively. This trial concluded that there was no significant difference in terms of visual acuity outcomes among the groups treated with grid photocoagulation, 1-mg of intravitreal triamcinolone, or 4-mg of intravitreal triamcinolone for macular edema secondary to BRVO at 12 months and grid photocoagulation had a safety profile superior to intravitral triamcinolone with respect to the potential for added risks of procedure-related complications.[60]

Bevacizumab

Intravitreal injection of bevacizumab was also used to treat macular edema due to BRVO (Figure 20.7). Twenty-seven consecutive patients with BRVO were treated with intravitreal bevacizumab (1.25 mg/0.05 ml) for macular edema secondary to BRVO. The mean VA improved from 20/200⁻ at baseline to 20/100⁺ at 3 months and, at the last follow-up visit, the mean central 1-mm macular thickness of 478 μm at baseline decreased to 336 at 3 months and 332 μm at the last follow-up visit.[13] There were no significant differences in the number of injections or the anatomic and visual outcomes 6 months after injection of two different doses (1.25 and 2.5 mg) of intravitreal bevacizumab in 45 patients with macular edema secondary to BRVO.[14]

Ranimizumab

Intravitreal injection of ranibizumab was also used to treat macular edema secondary to BRVO.[61] BRAVO is a multicenter, randomized, double-masked, sham injection-controlled Phase III study of 39 participants designed to assess the efficiency and safety profile of ranimizumab for macular edema associated to BRVO. The month 6 result showed that 55.2% (74/132) of patients received 0.3 mg of ranimizumab and 61.1% (80/131) received 0.5 mg of ranimizumab had their vision improved by 15 letters or more compared to 28.8% (38/130) of patients receiving sham injections and mean gain was observed beginning at day seven with an 7.6 and 7.4 letter gain in the 0.3 mg and 0.5 mg study arms of ranimizumab, respectively, compared with 1.9 letters in the sham injection arm.[33]

Laser treatment

The Branch Vein Occlusion Study, a multicenter, randomized, controlled trial supported by the National Eye Institute and the Branch Vein Occlusion Study Group, evaluated if grid macular laser photocoagulation improves VA in eyes with 20/40 or worse vision resulting from macular edema secondary to BRVO. A total of 139 eligible eyes were randomized to either the treated or the untreated control group. The mean VA for patients treated with grid laser was 20/40 to 20/50 compared with 20/70 for the control group (mean follow-up, 3.1 years). Treated patients gained an average of 1.33 lines of VA after 3 years from baseline compared with 0.23 line in the control group. The grid laser group had a significant improvement in VA and gained 2 lines or more of vision over consecutive visits (65% of treated eyes versus 36% of control eyes).[62]

SURGICAL TREATMENT OF BRVO

The obstruction site in BRVO is almost always at an arteriovenous crossing site with the common adventitial sheath of the overlying arteriole and the underlying venule. Removing the compressive factor by sheathotomy may be an effective treatment for BRVO.[63] Osterloh and Charles reported a significant improvement in VA (from 20/200 to 20/25+) over 8 months in the first report of sheathotomy.[64] Mason et al. reported a prospective comparison of 20 eyes treated with vitrectomy and sheathotomy with 20 control eyes (10 observed eyes and 10 laser-treated eyes). In that report, sheathotomy resulted in a significantly better visual outcome (20/250 mean VA at baseline to 20/63 after

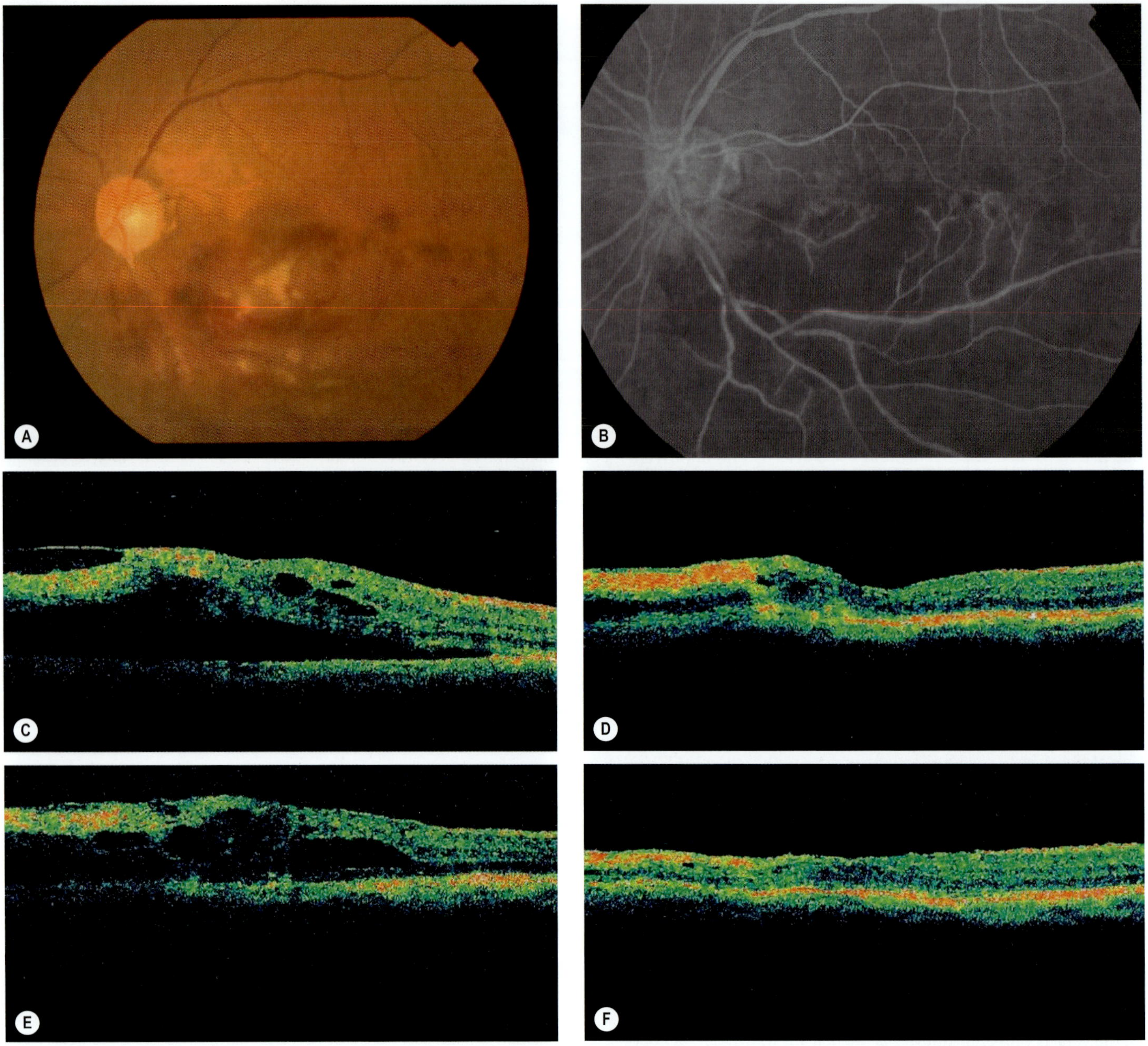

Figure 20.6 (A) Fundus photograph of macular edema secondary to branch retinal vein occlusion before intravitreal injection of triamcinolone acetonide (TA) (4 mg) at baseline shows the intraretinal hemorrhage distributed in an occlusive vein and some cotton-wool patches. (B) Fluorescein angiogram shows dilation of the inferotemporal vein and delayed filling and areas of capillary nonperfusion in the inferotemporal vein. (C) Optical coherence tomography (OCT) image of a patient with macular edema secondary to branch retinal vein occlusion at baseline before intravitreal injection of TA. (D) An OCT image 1 month after intravitreal injection of TA (4 mg). (E) OCT image with recurrence of macular edema 3 months after injection. (F) OCT image 1 month after reinjection of TA (4 mg).

14-months) than a matched control group (20/180 mean VA at baseline to 20/125 after 14 months).[65] However, in a prospective, randomized, comparative, interventional case series of 36 patients who underwent vitrectomy with or without sheathotomy for macular edema due to BRVO with symptoms for 8 weeks or shorter, the median best corrected VA significantly improved from 0.4 at baseline to 0.9 in the vitrectomy group and 1.0 in the sheathotomy group at the final visit. The central foveal thickness also decreased postoperatively in both groups, but the differences between the two groups were not significant. The investigators concluded that vitrectomy with and without sheathotomy improved the long-term visual and anatomic outcomes for patients with macular edema secondary to BRVO and there was no difference between the two groups in the improvement in both VA and central foveal thickness.[66]

SUMMARY AND KEY POINTS

There is limited evidence that oral or systemic anticoagulation or rheologic agents are effective for treating RVO. Intravitreal injection of agents has become a major treatment because it carries less risk than systemic administration and because direct drug delivery to retinal vessels may achieve a better visual outcome. Corticosteroids and anti-VEGF drugs seem to be the major drugs in the medical treatment of RVO, although repeated injections may be needed. The effects of laser photocoagulation and surgery seem to be less than that with medication; however, these could be options in cases refractory to medication.

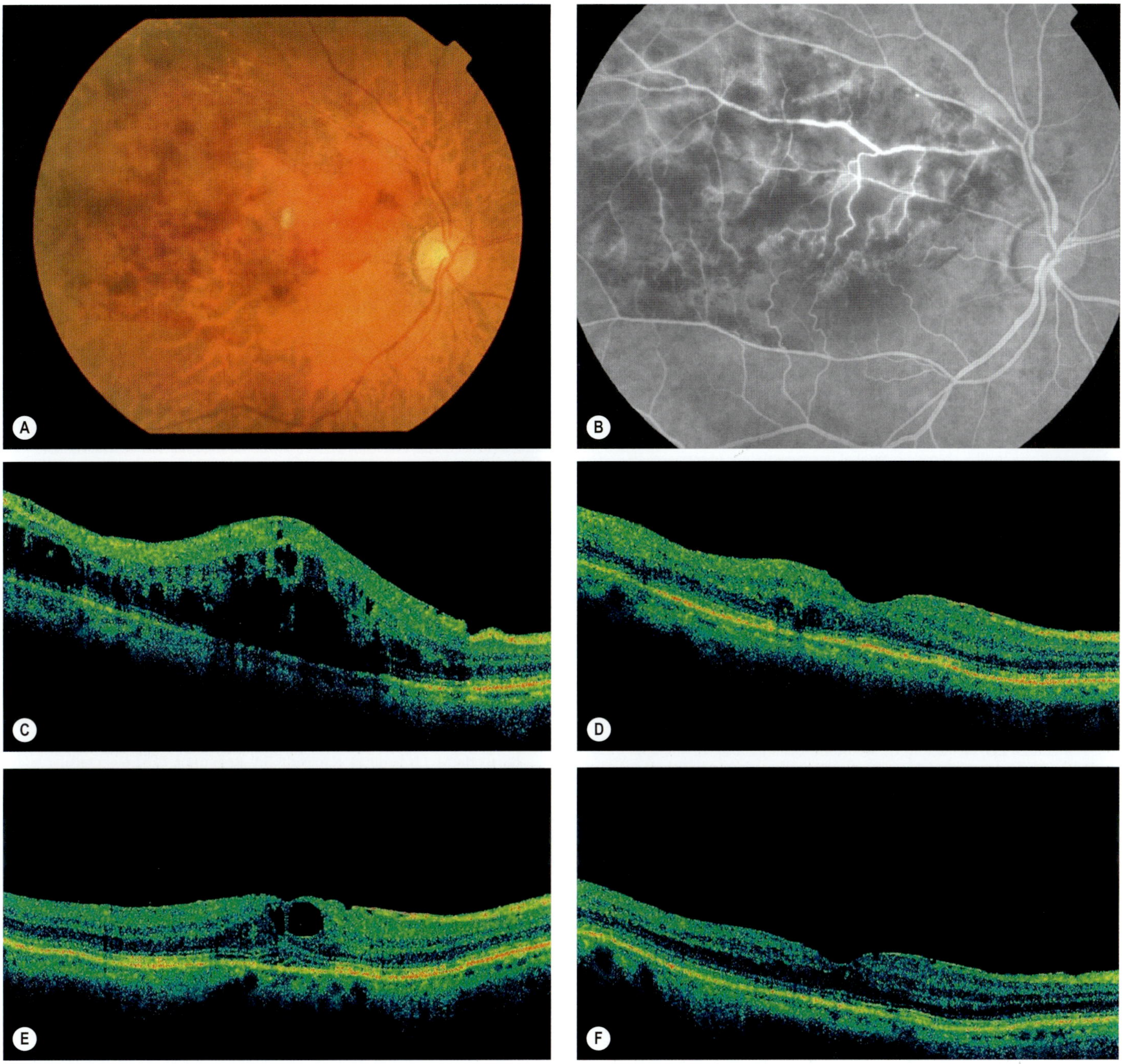

Figure 20.7 (A) Fundus photograph of macular edema secondary to branch retinal vein occlusion before the intravitreal injection of bevacizumab (1.25 mg) at baseline shows the intraretinal hemorrhage distributed in an occlusive vein and some cotton-wool patches. (B) Fluorescein angiogram shows dilation of the superotemporal vein and delayed filling and areas of capillary nonperfusion superotemporally. (C) An optical coherence tomography (OCT) image of a patient with macular edema secondary to branch retinal vein occlusion at baseline before intravitreal injection of bevacizumab. (D) An OCT image 1 month after intravitreal injection of bevacizumab (1.25 mg). (E) An OCT image with recurrence of macular edema 2 months after injection. (F) An OCT image 1 month after reinjection of bevacizumab (1.25 mg).

REFERENCES

1. Hayreh SS, Zimmerman MB, Podhajsky P. Incidence of various types of retinal vein occlusion and their recurrence and demographic characteristics. Am J Ophthalmol 1994;117:429–441.
2. Mitchell P, Smith W, Chang A. Prevalence and associations of retinal vein occlusion in Australia. The Blue Mountains Eye Study. Arch Opthalmol 1996;114:1243–1247.
3. Central Vein Occlusion Study Group. Baseline and early natural history report: the Central Vein Occlusion Study. Arch Ophthalmol 1993;111:1087–1095.
4. Central Vein Occlusive Study Group. Central Vein Occlusion Study of photocoagulation therapy: manual of operations. Online J Curr Clin Trials 1993 Oct;2:92.
5. Greenberg PB, Martidis A, Rogers AH, et al. Intravitreal triamcinolone acetonide for macular oedema due to central vein occlusion. Br J Ophthalmol 2002;86:247–248.
6. Ip MS, Kumar KS. Intravitreous triamcinolone acetonide as treatment for macular edema from central retinal vein occlusion. Arch Ophthalmol 2002;120:1217–1219.
7. Jonas JB, Kreissig I, Degenring RF. Intravitreal triamcinolone acetonide as treatment of macular edema in central vein occlusion. Graefes Arch Clin Exp Ophthalmol 2002;240:782–783.
8. Park CH, Jaffe GJ, Fekrat S. Intravitreal triamcinolone acetonide in eyes with cystoid macular edema associated with central retinal vein occlusion. Am J Ophthalmol 2003;136:419–425.

9. Chen SDM, Lochhead J, Patel CK, et al. Intravitreal triamcinolone acetonide for ischemic macular oedema caused by branch retinal vein occlusion. Br J Ophthalmol 2004;88:154–155.
10. Jonas JB, Akkoyun I, Kamppeter B, et al. Branch retinal vein occlusion treated by intravitreal triamcinolone acetonide. Eye 2005;19:65–71.
11. Rosenfeld PJ, Fung AE, Puliafito CA. Optical coherence tomography findings after an intravitreal injection of bevacizumab (Avastin) for macular edema from central retinal vein occlusion. Ophthalmic Surg Lasers Imaging 2005;36:336–339.
12. Priglinger SG, Wolf AH, Kreutzer TC, et al. Intravitreal bevacizumab injections for treatment of central retinal vein occlusion: six-month results of a prospective trial. Retina 2007;27:1004–1012.
13. Costa RA, Jorge R, Calucci D, et al. Intravitreal bevacizumab (Avastin) for central vein retinal occlusions. IBeVO study. Retina 2007;27:141–149.
14. Rabena MD, Pieramici DJ, Castellarin AA, et al. Intravitreal bevacizumab (Avastin) in the treatment of macular edema secondary to branch retinal vein occlusion. Retina 2007;27:419–425.
15. The Pan-American Collaborative Study Group (PACORES). Comparison of two doses of intravitreal bevacizumab (Avastin) for treatment of macular edema secondary to branch retinal vein occlusion: Results from the Pan-American Collaborative Retina Study Group at 6 months of follow-up. Retina 2008;28:212–219.
16. Wong TY, Larsen EK, Llein R, et al. Cardiovascular risk factors for retinal vein occlusion and arteriolar emboli: the Atherosclerosis Risk in Communities and Cardiovascular Health studies. Ophthalmology 2005;112:540–547.
17. Klein R, Klein BEK, Moss SE, et al. The epidemiology of retinal vein occlusion: the Beaver Dam Eye Study. Trans Am Ophthalmol Soc 2000;98:133–143.
18. Gutman FA. Evaluation of a patient with central retinal vein occlusion. Ophthalmology 1983;90:481–483.
19. The Eye Disease Case-control Study Group. Risk factor for branch retinal vein occlusion. Am J Ophthalmol 1993;116:286–296.
20. Hayreh SS. Retinal vein occlusion. Indian Journal of Ophthalmology 1994:42;109–132.
21. Jaffe GJ, Caprioli J. Optical coherence tomography to detect and manage retinal disease and glaucoma. Am J Ophthalmol 2004;137:156–169.
22. Thomas D, Duguid G. Optical coherence tomography: a review of the principles and contemporary uses in retinal investigation. Eye 2004;18:561–570.
23. The Central Vein Occlusion Study Group. Natural history and clinical management of central retinal vein occlusion. Arch Ophthalmol 1997;115:486–491.
24. Hattenbach LO, Steinkamp G, Scharrer I, et al. Fibrinolytic therapy with low-dose recombinant tissue plasminogen activator in retinal vein occlusion. Ophthalmologica 1988;212:394–398.
25. Hattenbach LO, Wellermann G, Steinkamp GW, et al. Visual outcome after treatment with low-dose recombinant tissue plasminogen activator or hemodilution in ischemic central retinal vein occlusion. Ophthalmologica 1999;213:360–366.
26. Elman MJ. Thrombolytic therapy for central retinal vein occlusion: results of a pilot study. Trans Am Ophthalmol Soc 1996;94:471–504.
27. Lahey JM, Fong DS, Kearney J. Intravitreal tissue plasminogen activator for acute central retinal vein occlusion. Ophthalmic Surg Lasers 1999;30:427–434.
28. Elman MJ, Raden RZ, Carrigan A. Intravitreal injection of tissue plasminogen activator for central retinal vein occlusion. Trans Am Ophth Soc 2001;99:219–223.
29. Yamamoto T, Kamei M, Kunavisarut P, et al. Increased retinal toxicity of intravitreal tissue plasminogen activator in a central retinal vein occlusion model. Graefes Arch Clin Exp Ophthalmol 2008;246:509–514.
30. Weiss JN, Bynoe LA. Injection of tissue plasminogen activator into a branch retinal vein in eyes with central retinal vein occlusion. Ophthalmology 2001;108:2249–2257.
31. The SCRE Research Group. A randomized trial comparing the efficacy and safety of intravitreal triamcinolone with observation to treat vision loss associated with macular edema secondary to central retinal vein occlusion: The Standard Care vs Corticosteroid for Retinal Vein Occlusion (SCORE) Study Report 5. Arch Ophthalmol 2009;127:1101–1114.
32. Aiello LP, Avery RL, Amigg PG, et al. Vascular endothelial growth factor in ocular fluid of patients with diabetic retinopathy and other retinal disorders. N Engl J Med 1994;331:1480–1487.
33. Genentech, Inc., a wholly-owned member of the Roche Group. Two phase III studies of Lucentis in patients with retinal vein occlusion. Retina Congress 2009.
34. Browning DJ Fraser CM. Retinal vein occlusions in patients taking warfarin. Ophthalmology 2004;111:1196–1200.
35. Paques M, Vallee JN, Herbreteau D, et al. Superselective ophthalmic artery fibrinolytic therapy for the treatment of central retinal vein occlusion. Br J Ophthalmol 2000;84:1387–1391.
36. Glacet-Bernard A, Coscas G, Chabanel A, et al. A randomized, double-masked study on the treatment of retinal vein occlusion with troxerutin. Am J Ophthalmol 1994;118:421–429.
37. Houtsmuller AJ, Vermeulen JA, Klompe M, et al. The influence of ticlopidine on the natural course of retinal vein occlusion. Agents Actions 1984;15(suppl):219–229
38. De Sanctis MT, Cesaronr MR, Belcaro G, et al. Treatment of retinal vein thrombosis with pentoxifylline: a controlled, randomized trial. Angiology 2002;53(suppl):S35–S38.
39. Wolf S, Arend O, Bertram B, et al. Hemodilution therapy in central retinal vein occlusion: one year results of a prospective randomized study. Graefes Arch Clin Exp Ophthalmol 1994;232:33–39.
40. Hansen LL, Wiek J, Wiederholt M. A randomized prospective study of treatment of non-ischemic central retinal vein occlusion by isovolaemic haemodilution. Br J Ophthalmol 1989;73:895–899.
41. A randomized clinical trial of early panretinal photocoagulation for ischemic central vein occlusion: the Central Vein Occlusion Study Group N report. Ophthalmology 1995;102:1434–1444.
42. Evaluation of grid pattern photocoagulation for macular edema in central vein occlusion: the Central Vein Occlusion Study M report. Ophthalmology 1995;102:1425–1433.
43. McAllister IL, Douglas JP, Constable IJ, et al. Laser-induced chorioretinal venous anastomosis for nonischemic central retinal vein occlusion: evaluation of the complications and their risk factors. Am J Ophthalmol 1998;126:219–229.
44. Browning DJ, Antoszyk AN. Laser chorioretinal venous anastomosis for nonischemic central retinal vein occlusion. Ophthalmology 1998;105: 670–677.
45. Opremcak EM, Bruce RA, Lomeo MD, et al. Radial optic neurotomy for central retinal vein occlusion: a retrospective pilot study of 11 consecutive cases. Retina 2001;21:408–425.
46. Opremcak EM, Rehmar AJ, Ridenour CD, et al. Radial optic neurotomy for central retinal vein occlusion: 117 consecutive cases. Retina 2006;26: 297–305.
47. Hasselbach HC, Ruefer F, Feltgen N, et al. Treatment of central retinal vein occlusion by radial optic neurotomy in 107 cases. Graefes Arch Clin Exp Ophthalmol 2007;245:1145–1156.
48. Ozkiris A, Evereklioglu C, Erkilic K, et al. The efficacy of intravitreal triamcinolone acetonide on macular edema in branch retinal vein occlusion. Eur J Ophthalmol 2005;15:96–101.
49. Lee H, Shah GK. Intravitreal triamcinolone as primary treatment of cystoid macular edema secondary to branch retinal vein occlusion. Retina 2005;25:551–555.
50. Krepler K, Ergun E, Sacu S, et al. Intravitreal triamcinorone acetonide in patients with macular oedema due to branch retinal vein occlusion: pilot study. Acta Ophthalmol Scand 2005;83:600–604.
51. Hayashi K, Hayashi H. Intravitreal versus retrobulbar injections of triamcinolone for macular edema associated with branch retinal vein occlusion. Am J Ophthalmol 2005;139:972–982.
52. Cekic O, Chang S, Tseng JJ, et al. Intravitreal triamcinolone injection for treatment of macular edema secondary to branch retinal vein occlusion. Retina 2005;25:851–855.
53. Karacorlu M, Ozdemir H, Karacorlu SA. Resolution of serous macular detachment after intravitreal triamcinolone acetonide treatment of patients with branch retinal vein occlusion. Retina 2005;25:856–860.
54. Yepremyan M, Wertz FD, Tivnan T, et al. Early treatment of cystoid macular edema secondary to branch retinal vein occlusion with intravitreal triamcinolone acetonide. Ophthalmic Surg Lasers Imaging 2005; 36:30–36.
55. Chen SDM, Sundaram V, Lochhead J, et al. Intravitreal triamcinolone for the treatment of ischemic macular edema associated with branch retinal vein occlusion. Am J Ophthalmol 2006;141:876–883.
56. Özkiris A, Evereklioglu C, Erkilic K, et al. Intravitreal triamcinolone acetonide for treatment of persistent macular oedema in branch retinal vein occlusion. Eye 2006;20:13–17.
57. Cheng KC, Wu W. Intravitreal triamcinolone acetonide for patients with macular edema due to branch retinal vein occlusion. Kaohsiung J Med Sci 2006;22:321–330.
58. Oh JY, Seo JH, Ahn JK, et al. Early versus late intravitreal triamcinolone acetonide for macular edema associated with branch retinal vein occlusion. Korean J Ophthalmol 2007;21:18–20.
59. Cakir M, Dogan M, Bayraktar Z, et al. Efficacy of intravitreal triamcinolone for the treatment of macular edema secondary to branch retinal vein occlusion in eyes with or without grid laser photocoagulation. Retina 2008;28:465–472.
60. The SCRE Research Group. A randomized trial comparing the efficacy and safety of intravitreal triamcinolone with observation to treat vision loss associated with macular edema secondary to branch retinal vein occlusion: The Standard Care vs Corticosteroid for Retinal Vein Occlusion (SCORE) Study Report 6. Arch Ophthalmol 2009;127:1115–1128.
61. Campochiaro PA, Hafiz G, Shah SM, et al. Ranibizumab for macular edema due to retinal vein occlusions: implication of VEGF as a critical stimulator. Mol Ther 2008;16:791–799.
62. The Branch Vein Occlusion Study Group. Argon laser photocoagulation for macular edema in branch vein occlusion. Am J Ophthalmol 1984;98: 271–282.
63. Kumar B, Yu DY, Morgan WH, et al. The distribution of angioarchitectural changes within the vicinity of arteriovenous crossing in branch retinal vein occlusion. Ophthalmology 1998;105:424–427.
64. Osterloh MD, Charles S. Surgical decompression of branch retinal vein occlusions. Arch Ophthalmol 1988;106:1469–1471.
65. Mason III J, Feist R, White Jr M, et al. Sheathotomy to decompress branch retinal vein occlusion. Ophthalmology 2004;111:540–545.
66. Kumagai K, Furukawa M, Ogino N, et al. Long-term outcomes of vitrectomy with or without arteriovenous sheathotomy in branch retinal vein occlusion. Retina 2007;27:49–54.

CHAPTER 21

Retinal detachment and proliferative vitreoretinopathy

Oh Woong Kwon, MD, PhD, Mi In Roh, MD, and Ji Hun Song, MD

INTRODUCTION

Proliferative vitreoretinopathy (PVR) is a disease entity related to a number of intraocular diseases, including retinal detachment (RD). Several studies have confirmed the hypothesis that PVR occurs as a reparative process induced by retinal breaks and excessive inflammatory reaction. A survey of recently published series suggested that the frequency of PVR remains largely unchanged in primary RD, with the incidence ranging from 5.1 to 11.7%.[1] PVR is the most common cause of failed repair of rhegmatogenous RD and risk factors for PVR are related to several, well-known pre-, intra-, and postoperative clinical situations. Currently, surgery such as pneumatic retinopexy, scleral buckling, and pars plana vitrectomy (PPV) is the mainstream therapeutic modality for RD and PVR. The goal of surgery is to create chorioretinal adhesion around all the retinal breaks and to relive all the tractional force. Single-operation reattachment rates were 73% for pneumatic retinopexy and 82% for scleral buckling after 6 months, and multiple-operation reattachment rates at 2 years were 99% for pneumatic retinopexy and 98% for scleral buckling for RD. Surgical success rates for PVR have improved as techniques and instruments of vitrectomy evolved. The introduction of ancillary techniques such as longer-acting gases and long-term vitreous substitutes like silicone oil elevated the success rate from 35–40% to approximately 60–75% at 6 months. Despite these advances, more than one-fourth of initially successful cases results in redetachment due to recurrent retinal traction. Furthermore, visual results are less satisfactory and only 40–80% of cases with anatomic success achieve ambulatory vision. As a result, PVR remains a difficult problem to manage and continuing efforts have been made to develop other forms of therapy to inhibit the pathologic response causing traction. Recent efforts have been directed toward the chemical inhibition of cellular proliferation and membrane contraction in PVR.

INCIDENCE OF RETINAL DETACHMENT

In normal eyes, RD occurs at a rate of approximately 5 per 100 000 people per year in the USA, and the age-adjusted incidence of idiopathic RD is approximately 12.5 cases per 100 000 per year, or about 28 000 cases per year.[2,3]

ETIOLOGY AND RISK FACTORS FOR RETINAL DETACHMENT

Rhegmatogenous RD develops with: (1) the existence of liquefied vitreous gel; (2) tractional force resulting in retinal breaks; and (3) the presence of a retinal break (Figure 21.1). The most common worldwide etiological factors associated with RD are myopia, cataract removal, and trauma. Approximately 40–50% of all patients with RD have myopia. RD related to myopia tends to occur in patients aged 25–45 years, while nonmyopia RD tends to occur in older individuals. Patients with high myopia (>6 D), which is more common in males than females, have a 5% lifetime risk of RD.

RD occurs at a rate of 5–16 per 1000 cases following cataract surgery, and this comprises approximately 30–40% of all reported RD.[4] The cumulative probability ratio of RD at 20 years after extracapsular cataract extraction or phacoemulsification is reported to be 1.58%, which is four times higher than for patients not undergoing cataract extraction.[5] The risk factors associated with RD in cataract removal are accidental posterior capsule rupture at the time of surgery, young age, increased axial length, a deep anterior chamber, RD in the fellow eye, and male gender.[6,7] While the incidence of RD after clear lens extraction in myopic eyes rises to 8.1%, the incidence of RD decreases to 2.7% with the introduction of small incision coaxial phacoemulsification.[8,9]

Approximately 10–20% of RD is associated with direct ocular trauma. Traumatic detachments are more common in younger people. Although no studies have estimated the incidence of RD in contact sports, certain sports (e.g., boxing and bungee jumping) are associated with an increased risk of RD. There are also a few reports that Nd:YAG laser capsulotomy[10,11] is associated with an increased risk of RD.

As for racial difference in the incidence of RD in pediatrics, while structural abnormalities (56%), previous surgery (51%), trauma (36%), and uveitis (15%) were the main risk factors for RD in USA,[12] high myopia (38%), trauma (31%), structural abnormalities (17%), and previous surgery (5%) were the main risk factors in Asia.[13]

INCIDENCE OF PROLIFERATIVE VITREORETINOPATHY

Published series through the 1990s to early 2000 suggest that the frequency of PVR remains largely unchanged in primary RD, with the incidence ranging from 5.1 to 11.7%.

PATHOGENESIS OF PROLIFERATIVE VITREORETINOPATHY

PVR is the result of growth and contraction of cellular membranes within the hyaloids, retina, and retinal surface.[14] These membranes exert traction and may cause tractional RD that opens otherwise successfully treated retinal breaks, creating new retinal breaks, or promoting proliferation at the posterior vitreous base and anterior cortical vitreous. This in turn causes anteroperipheral traction on the retina with displacement of the peripheral retina toward the pars plana. Membrane contraction on the inner retina causes distortion and folding, resulting in starfolds at the inferior quadrant (Figure 21.2).

RISK FACTORS FOR PROLIFERATIVE VITREORETINOPATHY

Although PVR is the most common cause of failed repair of rhegmatogenous RD, risk factors for PVR are related to several, well-known pre-, intra-, and postoperative clinical situations. A number of factors can increase the risk of PVR, including the preoperative extent of

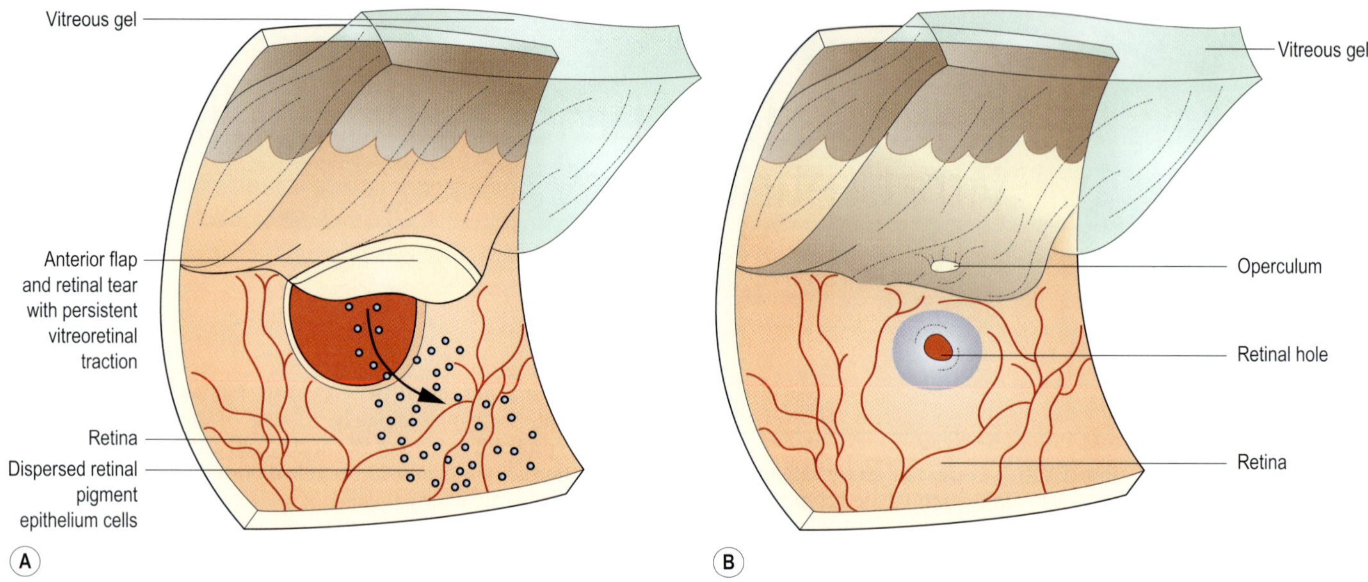

Figure 21.1 Retinal tears due to vitreoretinal traction. Persistent traction frequently causes retinal detachment (A). If the traction results in a break that is not associated with persistent vitreoretinal traction (B), the tear will act as a retinal hole and detachment is unlikely.

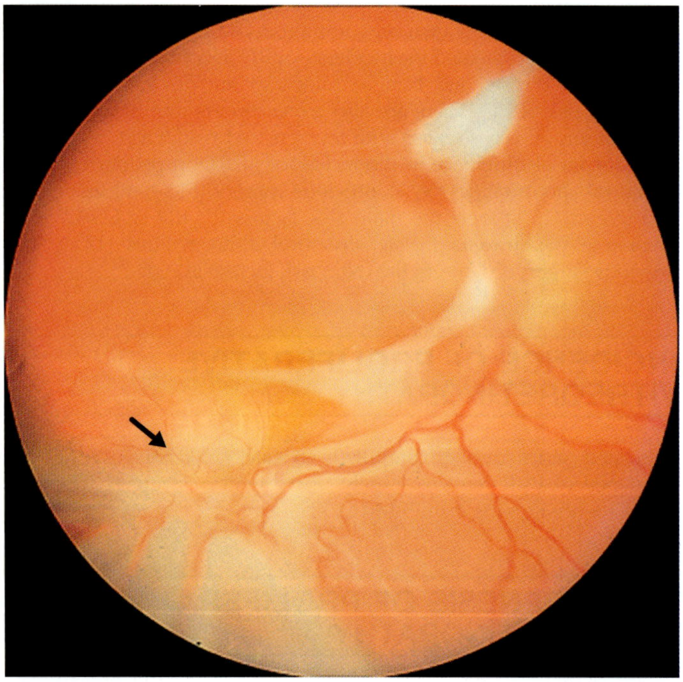

Figure 21.2 Starfold from proliferative vitreoretinopathy. Contraction of a focal retinal surface membrane (arrow) has resulted in the formation of a starfold.

detachment exceeding two quadrants, giant, large, multiple, or undetected retinal breaks,[15] aphakia status, vitreous hemorrhage,[16] preoperative choroidal detachment, previous failed attempts at reattachment, the presence of signs of uveitis, and the preoperative presence of PVR grades A and B.[17] In giant retinal tears, the PVR incidence varies from 16 to 41%, while in penetrating ocular traumas the incidence is 10–45% with a mean of 25%.[1] In eyes with rhegmatogenous RD with grade B PVR, the incidence of severe PVR after surgery was reported to be 25.8% when using cryotherapy and 2.2% when using argon laser photocoagulation.[18] Intraocular hemorrhage during or after surgery, use of air or sulfur hexafluoride (SF_6), excessive cryotherapy, diathermy or photocoagulation,[19] repeated surgical procedures, loss of vitreous during drainage of subretinal fluid, and the use of vitrectomy are also intraoperative risk factors that increase the incidence of PVR.

There are three major wound-healing phases that occur after tissue injury: inflammation, proliferation, and scar modulation.[20] After a retinal break occurs, inflammation proceeds with the breakdown of the blood–retinal barrier. This enables platelets to migrate to the lesion site and release growth factors. Concurrently, extracellular matrix is produced using fibrin and fibronectin.[21] These processes act as chemotactic factors for attracting monocytes. Cells involved in the inflammatory process during wound healing in RD include retinal pigment epithelial (RPE) cells, macrophage-like cells, glial cells, and fibroblast-like cells, and this process triggers the onset of PVR.[22] Of these cell types, RPE cells, which are present in almost all epiretinal membranes, are the key factor in triggering PVR development.[21] RPE cells have a wide range of activities, and can act like fibroblasts and participate in fibrosis,[23] release factors similar to those of glial cells, promote extracellular matrix contraction[24] and synthesize collagen types 1, 2, and 3.[25]

Soluble mediators such as growth factors and cytokines[26] play a role in producing membranes which occur in PVR, and the extracellular matrix components (most importantly, collagen and the elastic fiber family) play a critical role in cellular events, including proliferation, migration, tissue contraction, and tissue remodeling.[25,27] Among the soluble mediators, fibroblast growth factor induces the proliferation of fibroblasts, which synthesize the extracellular matrix, leading to the formation of intravitreal and periretinal membranes. In the final process, membrane contraction occurs, leading to tractional RD.

SIGNS, SYMPTOMS, AND DIAGNOSIS

Rhegmatogenous RD presents as an accumulation of subretinal fluid with one or more retinal breaks. Symptoms such as photopsia and/or increased vitreous floaters with acute posterior vitreous detachment may indicate the development of a retinal break. In symptomatic eyes, retinal tears associated with persistent vitreoretinal traction indicate a high risk for RD which may present with decreased visual acuity and/or restriction of the visual field. The most common presentation of PVR is epiretinal membrane proliferation causing traction, with retinal folds on the retina in an eye with rhegmatogenous RD. Other presentations include multiple retinal breaks, a vitreoretinal traction ring, and contraction of the vitreous base.

It is difficult to diagnose PVR when there is media opacity due to corneal, lenticular, or vitreous opacities. In such cases, ultrasonographic characteristics showing funnel-shaped RD with the opposition of the posterior retina or the presence of an anterior membrane bridging the mouth of the funnel[28] can provide evidence for a diagnosis (Figure 21.3).

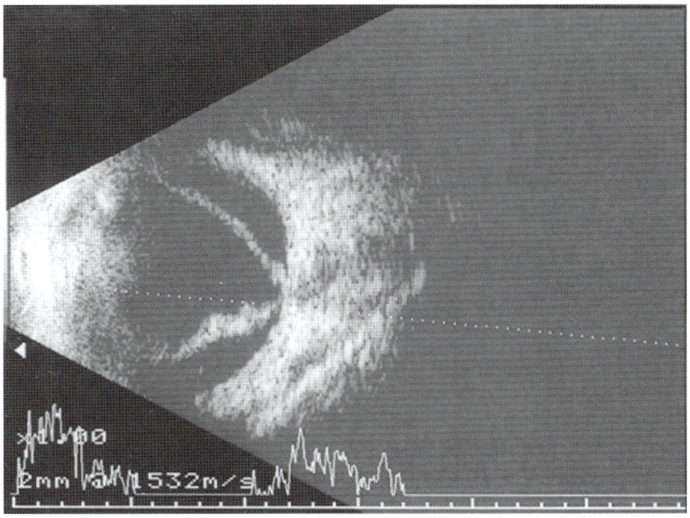

Figure 21.3 Ultrasonograph of an eye with rhegmatogenous reitinal detachment with proliferative vitreoretinopathy.

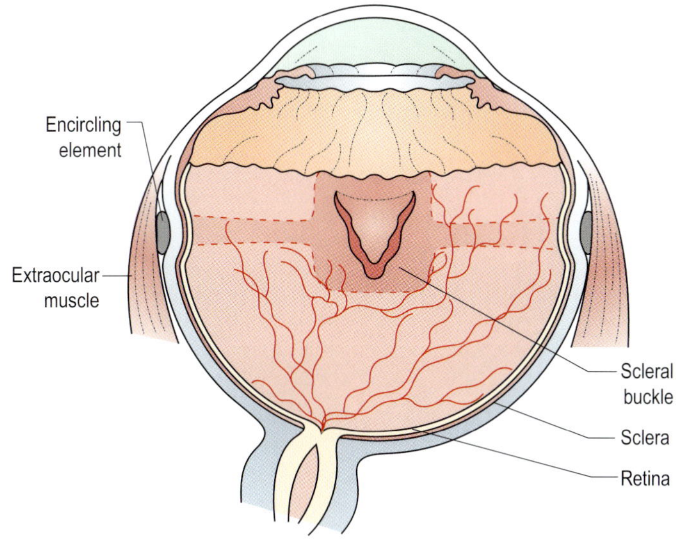

Figure 21.4 Correct position of scleral buckle for flap retinal tear.

Table 21.1 Classification of proliferative vitreoretinopathy (PVR) used in the silicone study

Type no.	Type of contraction	Location of PVR	Summary of clinical signs
1	Focal	Posterior	Starfold
2	Diffuse	Posterior	Confluent irregular retinal folds in posterior retina; remainder of retina drawn posteriorly; optic disc may not be visible
3	Subretinal	Posterior	"Napkin ring" around disc or "clothesline" elevation of retina
4	Circumferential	Anterior	Irregular retinal folds in the anterior retina; series of radial folds more posteriorly; peripheral retina within vitreous base stretched inward
5	Perpendicular	Anterior	Smooth circumferential fold of retina at insertion of posterior hyaloid
6	Anterior	Anterior	Circumferential fold of retina at insertion of posterior hyaloid pulled forward; trough of peripheral retina anteriorly; ciliary processes stretched with possible hypotony; iris retracted

Reprinted with permission from Lean J, Irvine A, Stern W, et al. Classification of proliferative vitreoretinopathy used in the silicone study. The Silicone study group. Ophthalmology 1989;96:765–771.

After diagnosis, PVR should be classified according to the commonly used system presented in Table 21.1. This system distinguishes between anterior and posterior forms of PVR, and identifies proliferation as diffuse, focal, or subretinal. While this system provides information on the anatomical construction of PVR, it does not indicate the biological activity or prognostic factors.[1]

TREATMENT OPTIONS

Currently available surgical options for RD management are pneumatic retinopexy, scleral buckling, and PPV. There remains no consensus regarding the optimal surgical management option, and the choice is generally based on many factors, including the characteristics of the retinal breaks, lens status, various patient factors (e.g., expected compliance with postoperative positioning), and surgeon preference.[29]

The principles of surgical management consist of sealing all retinal breaks by making permanent scars, and relief of vitreoretinal traction. Scleral buckling, including an encircling element and subretinal fluid drainage in some cases, relieves the vitreous traction on the retina and displaces some subretinal fluid from the breaks, resulting in an approximation of a neurosensory retina and RPE (Figure 21.4). Complications of scleral buckling surgery include refractive change, which is typically axial myopia induced by encircling elements, and strabismus, which may be caused by fibrosis and/or altering the action of the rectus muscles. Other complications include infection, extrusion, or intrusion of the buckling element, anterior-segment ischemia, and choroidal detachment. Pneumatic retinopexy is a possible alternative to scleral buckling, and may be used to treat rhegmatogenous RD with retinal breaks in the superior two-thirds of the retina. This procedure involves injecting a gas bubble into the vitreous cavity and positioning the patient's head such that the retinal breaks can be closed by the bubble, while laser photocoagulation or cryotherapy is used for retinopexy. However, the possibility of overlooking an existing retinal break, or creating a new break, could be higher for pneumatic retinopexy compared to scleral buckling.

PPV was previously considered a second-line treatment for primary RD. However, a growing number of surgeons choose primary vitrectomy for rhegmatogenous RD, in part due to the rapid advances in instrumentation. The major advantage of primary vitrectomy is that it allows a direct approach to the release of vitreous traction. Vitrectomy can also remove media opacities, and therefore improve intraoperative visualization and control internal drainage of subretinal fluid. The greatest problem with primary vitrectomy is the possibility of causing new retinal breaks and cataract formation. Furthermore, vitrectomy may be a more expensive procedure because it requires more specialized operating room equipment and instrumentation.[30]

Early surgical failures are mostly the result of failure to seal all retinal breaks, and/or failure to relieve vitreous traction adequately. In contrast, late surgical failures are usually due to PVR, which accounts for

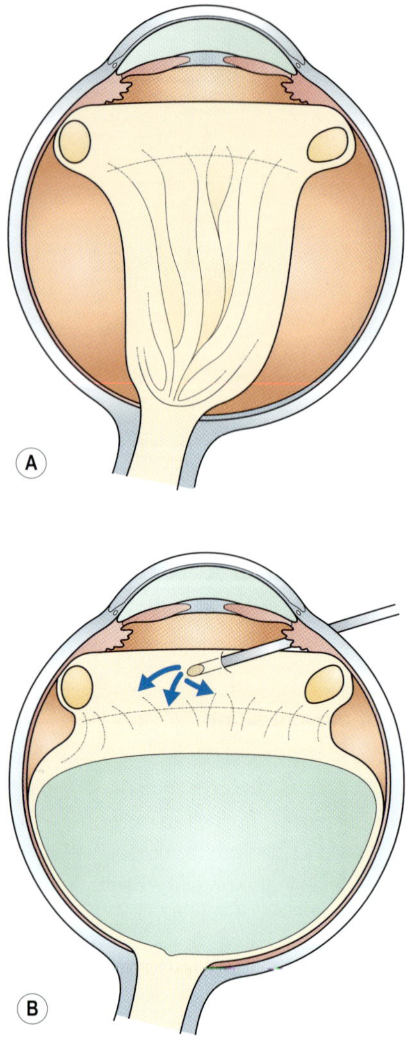

Figure 21.5 Ability of perfluorocarbon liquids to reattach mechanically posterior retina in proliferative vitreoretinopathy. Epiretinal membranes cause folding and shortening of the retina in both anteroposterior and circumferential directions (A). After performing membranectomy on posterior region of the retina, perfluorocarbon liquid may be used to reattach the posterior retina and aid in removal of peripheral epiretinal membrane (B).

the majority of failures following RD surgery. Surgical procedures used to repair RDs associated with PVR include scleral buckling, vitrectomy, membrane peeling, relaxing retinotomies, the use of liquid perfluorocarbons, and internal tamponade with gas or silicone oil (Figure 21.5).[31] In the early stages of PVR, buckling and encircling procedures may close all retinal breaks with release of circumferential traction caused by the vitreous base.[17] A moderately wide, broad silicone band (5–7 mm) extending from the ora serrata to the equator is required to reduce the vitreous traction.[13] In addition, retinopexy with cryotherapy, diathermy, and photocoagulation can be used to treat definite retinal breaks, thus minimizing further RPE cell dispersion, postoperative inflammation, and breakdown of the blood–retinal barrier. While there is no standardized approach to PVR treatment, types 1 and 2 affecting fewer than two quadrants (classification system by the Silicone Oil study) can be successfully treated using buckling procedures.

PPV is indicated in cases with no definite retinal breaks with tractional membranes causing RD, or in cases where the retinal breaks cannot be sealed by scleral buckling alone.[14] However, in complex PVR cases, it is necessary to perform a vitrectomy with membrane peeling and a gas or silicone oil tamponade.[32] Moreover, a relaxing retinotomy and retinectomy may be required to attach the retina to the RPE in such complex cases.[33] Once all traction is relieved, photocoagulation is applied to the edges of the retinotomy site with the addition of long-term tamponades. Most severe cases involving advanced anterior PVR have used a posterior 360° retinotomy combined with an extensive peripheral retinectomy and silicone oil tamponade.[34] However, the results have not been encouraging due to reproliferation causing recurrent macular detachment. Surgical means to reduce the risk of PVR include removal of vitreous collagen, which is the stratum to cell attachment, using wide-angle viewing systems and heavy liquids, and application of dyes which aim at a more thorough and less traumatic removal of vitreous and periretinal membranes.[35] In addition, recent efforts have been directed toward the pharmacological inhibition of cellular proliferation and membrane contraction in PVR.

PROGNOSIS WITH THE VARIOUS TREATMENT OPTIONS

It appears that the surgical success rates for pneumatic retinopexy are either similar to or slightly lower than those for scleral buckling, and the risk of late redetachment is similar for pneumatic retinopexy and scleral buckling.[30] In a 2-year follow-up study, single-operation reattachment rates were 73% for pneumatic retinopexy and 82% for scleral buckling after 6 months, and multiple-operation reattachment rates at 2 years were 99% for pneumatic retinopexy and 98% for scleral buckling.[36]

More recently, a few prospective randomized trials revealed that there was no statistically significant difference in single-operation success rates or visual outcomes when comparing primary vitrectomy with scleral buckling for the treatment of rhegmatogenous RD.[37,38] However, faster foveal reattachment may be an advantage of PPV. In a nonrandomized series of 33 cases of macular-off RD, serial optical coherence tomography examinations showed no primary vitrectomy patients had subfoveal fluid while approximately one-third of scleral buckling patients had subfoveal fluid after the operation.[39]

Surgical success rates for PVR have improved as vitrectomy techniques and instruments have evolved. The introduction of ancillary techniques such as longer-acting gases and long-term vitreous substitutes like silicone oil have elevated the success rate from 35–40% to approximately 60–75% at 6 months.[40,41] Despite these advances, more than 25% of initially successful cases result in redetachment due to recurrent retinal traction. Furthermore, visual results are less satisfactory and only 40–80% of cases with anatomic success achieve ambulatory (5/200 or better) vision.[42] As a result, PVR remains a major problem, and continuing efforts have been made to develop other forms of therapy to inhibit the pathological response causing traction. Recent efforts have been directed towards chemical inhibition of cellular proliferation and membrane contraction for PVR.

ADJUNCTIVE THERAPIES

Although PVR is currently primarily managed surgically, ongoing efforts seek to identify adjuvant therapies that might inhibit PVR development. No matter how thoroughly vitrectomy is performed, it is virtually impossible to prevent some level of cell adhesion and pathological change. Control of the biological processes involved in proliferation and wound-healing would improve the success rate of surgery for primary RD and PVR.

Daunorubicin was the first adjunct agent to be studied in a randomized controlled trial for the management of PVR, and was found to reduce the number of reoperations within 1 year.[43] Recent advances in the sustained release of daunomycin achieved by a single intravitreal application of liposome encapsulation[44] may be very useful for future treatment strategies.

A randomized controlled trial in the UK reported that adjuvant 5-fluorouracil and heparin prevented PVR. In that study, the combination treatment resulted in a significant reduction in the rate of postoperative PVR development.[45] However, subsequent studies failed to show any benefit of this combination treatment, and indeed one of the study results showed worse outcomes in macula-sparing RDs patients.[46,47]

Many drugs, such as colchicine, corticosteroids, retinoids, and heparin, might be useful for inhibiting PVR development at specific stages. More detailed understanding of the pathophysiology underlying PVR may lead to the development of effective prophylactic and/or adjunct therapies. Further work is necessary to identify optimal adjunct therapies for the management of RD and PVR.

SUMMARY AND KEY POINTS

Current methods of surgical management of RD and PVR are pneumatic retinopexy, scleral buckling, and PPV. The principles of surgical management consist of sealing all retinal breaks and relief of vitreoretinal traction. However, although surgical success rates for PVR have improved as vitrectomy techniques and instruments have evolved, more than 25% of initially successful cases result in retinal redetachment due to recurrent tractional proliferation. This of course, results in suboptimal visual results as well.

Recent efforts have therefore been directed toward pharmacologic inhibition of cellular proliferation and membrane contraction with drugs such as daunorubicin, 5-fluorouracil, and heparin. Pharmacologic inhibition of the pathologic response involved in cell adhesion, proliferation, and membrane contraction would most likely improve the surgical success rate for RD. Moreover, better understanding of the processes leading to retina damage after detachment, and knowledge of how to protect or rehabilitate such retinas, may ultimately result in better visual outcomes, even in relatively long-standing macular-off retinal detachments.

REFERENCES

1. Charteris DG, Sethi CS, Lewis GP, et al. Proliferative vitreoretinopathy – developments in adjunctive treatment and retinal pathology. Eye 2002;16:369–374.
2. Ivanisevic M, Bojic L, Eterovic D. Epidemiological study of nontraumatic phakic rhegmatogenous retinal detachment. Ophthalmic Res 2000;32:237–239.
3. Subramanian ML, Topping TM. Controversies in the management of primary retinal detachments. Int Ophthalmol Clin 2004;44:103–114.
4. Ramos M, Kruger EF, Lashkari K. Biostatistical analysis of pseudophakic and aphakic retinal detachments. Semin Ophthalmol 2002;17:206–213.
5. Erie JC, Raecker ME, Baratz KH, et al. Risk of retinal detachment after cataract extraction, 1980–2004: a population-based study. Trans Am Ophthalmol Soc 2006;104:167–175.
6. Bhagwandien AC, Cheng YY, Wolfs RC, et al. Relationship between retinal detachment and biometry in 4262 cataractous eyes. Ophthalmology 2006;113:643–649.
7. Tuft SJ, Minassian D, Sullivan P. Risk factors for retinal detachment after cataract surgery: a case-control study. Ophthalmology 2006;113:650–656.
8. Colin J, Robinet A, Cochener B. Retinal detachment after clear lens extraction for high myopia: seven-year follow-up. Ophthalmology 1999;106:2281–2284; discussion 2285.
9. Alio JL, Ruiz-Moreno JM, Shabayek MH, et al. The risk of retinal detachment in high myopia after small incision coaxial phacoemulsification. Am J Ophthalmol 2007;144:93–98.
10. Jahn CE, Richter J, Jahn AH, et al. Pseudophakic retinal detachment after uneventful phacoemulsification and subsequent neodymium: YAG capsulotomy for capsule opacification. J Cataract Refract Surg 2003;29:925–929.
11. Ranta P, Tommila P, Kivela T. Retinal breaks and detachment after neodymium: YAG laser posterior capsulotomy: five-year incidence in a prospective cohort. J Cataract Refract Surg 2004;30:58–66.
12. Weinberg DV, Lyon AT, Greenwald MJ, et al. Rhegmatogenous retinal detachments in children: risk factors and surgical outcomes. Ophthalmology 2003;110:1708–1713.
13. Wang NK, Tsai CH, Chen YP, et al. Pediatric rhegmatogenous retinal detachment in East Asians. Ophthalmology 2005;112:1890–1895.
14. Ryan SJ. Retina. 4th ed. Philadelphia: Elsevier/Mosby; 2006.
15. Girard P, Mimoun G, Karpouzas I, et al. Clinical risk factors for proliferative vitreoretinopathy after retinal detachment surgery. Retina 1994;14:417–424.
16. Duquesne N, Bonnet M, Adeleine P. Preoperative vitreous hemorrhage associated with rhegmatogenous retinal detachment: a risk factor for postoperative proliferative vitreoretinopathy? Graefes Arch Clin Exp Ophthalmol 1996;234:677–682.
17. Retina Society Terminology Committee Classification. The classification of retinal detachment with proliferative vitreoretinopathy. Ophthalmology 1983;90:121–125.
18. Bonnet M, Guenoun S. Surgical risk factors for severe postoperative proliferative vitreoretinopathy (PVR) in retinal detachment with grade B PVR. Graefes Arch Clin Exp Ophthalmol 1995;233:789–791.
19. Jaccoma EH, Conway BP, Campochiaro PA. Cryotherapy causes extensive breakdown of the blood–retinal barrier. A comparison with argon laser photocoagulation. Arch Ophthalmol 1985;103:1728–1730.
20. Wiedemann P, Weller M. The pathophysiology of proliferative vitreoretinopathy. Acta Ophthalmol Suppl 1988;189:3–15.
21. Casaroli Marano RP, Vilaro S. The role of fibronectin, laminin, vitronectin and their receptors on cellular adhesion in proliferative vitreoretinopathy. Invest Ophthalmol Vis Sci 1994;35:2791–2803.
22. Baudouin C, Hofman P, Brignole F, et al. Immunocytology of cellular components in vitreous and subretinal fluid from patients with proliferative vitreoretinopathy. Ophthalmologica 1991;203:38–46.
23. Lee SC, Kwon OW, Seong GJ, et al. Epitheliomesenchymal transdifferentiation of cultured RPE cells. Ophthalmic Res 2001;33:80–86.
24. Glaser BM, Cardin A, Biscoe B. Proliferative vitreoretinopathy. The mechanism of development of vitreoretinal traction. Ophthalmology 1987;94:327–332.
25. Hiscott P, Sheridan C, Magee RM, et al. Matrix and the retinal pigment epithelium in proliferative retinal disease. Prog Retin Eye Res 1999;18:167–190.
26. Wiedemann P. Growth factors in retinal diseases: proliferative vitreoretinopathy, proliferative diabetic retinopathy, and retinal degeneration. Surv Ophthalmol 1992;36:373–384.
27. Jerdan JA, Pepose JS, Michels RG, et al. Proliferative vitreoretinopathy membranes. An immunohistochemical study. Ophthalmology 1989;96:801–810.
28. Fuller DG, Laqua H, Machemer R. Ultrasonographic diagnosis of massive periretinal proliferation in eyes with opaque media (triangular retinal detachment). Am J Ophthalmol 1977;83:460–464.
29. Schwartz SG, Flynn HW. Primary retinal detachment: scleral buckle or pars plana vitrectomy? Curr Opin Ophthalmol 2006;17:245–250.
30. Saw SM, Gazzard G, Wagle AM, et al. An evidence-based analysis of surgical interventions for uncomplicated rhegmatogenous retinal detachment. Acta Ophthalmol Scand 2006;84:606–612.
31. Pastor JC. Proliferative vitreoretinopathy: an overview. Surv Ophthalmol 1998;43:3–18.
32. Ryan SJ. Traction retinal detachment. XLIX Edward Jackson Memorial Lecture. Am J Ophthalmol 1993;115:1–20.
33. Iverson DA, Ward TG, Blumenkranz MS. Indications and results of relaxing retinotomy. Ophthalmology 1990;97:1298–1304.
34. Federman JL, Eagle Jr RC. Extensive peripheral retinectomy combined with posterior 360 degrees retinotomy for retinal reattachment in advanced proliferative vitreoretinopathy cases. Ophthalmology 1990;97:1305–1320.
35. Kirchhof B. Strategies to influence PVR development. Graefes Arch Clin Exp Ophthalmol 2004;242:699–703.
36. Tornambe PE, Hilton GF, Brinton DA, et al. Pneumatic retinopexy. A two-year follow-up study of the multicenter clinical trial comparing pneumatic retinopexy with scleral buckling. Ophthalmology 1991;98:1115–1123.
37. Ahmadieh H, Moradian S, Faghihi H, et al. Anatomic and visual outcomes of scleral buckling versus primary vitrectomy in pseudophakic and aphakic retinal detachment: six-month follow-up results of a single operation – report no. 1. Ophthalmology 2005;112:1421–1429.
38. Brazitikos PD, Androudi S, Christen WG, et al. Primary pars plana vitrectomy versus scleral buckle surgery for the treatment of pseudophakic retinal detachment: a randomized clinical trial. Retina 2005;25:957–964.
39. Wolfensberger TJ. Foveal reattachment after macula-off retinal detachment occurs faster after vitrectomy than after buckle surgery. Ophthalmology 2004;111:1340–1343.
40. Chang S, Coleman DJ, Lincoff H, et al. Perfluoropropane gas in the management of proliferative vitreoretinopathy. Am J Ophthalmol 1984;98:180–188.
41. Sell CH, McCuen 2nd BW, Landers 3rd MB, et al. Long-term results of successful vitrectomy with silicone oil for advanced proliferative vitreoretinopathy. Am J Ophthalmol 1987;103:24–28.
42. Sun JK, Arroyo JG. Adjunctive therapies for proliferative vitreoretinopathy. Int Ophthalmol Clin 2004;44:1–10.
43. Wiedemann P, Hilgers RD, Bauer P, et al. Adjunctive daunorubicin in the treatment of proliferative vitreoretinopathy: results of a multicenter clinical trial. Daunomycin Study Group. Am J Ophthalmol 1998;126:550–559.
44. Shinohara K, Tanaka M, Sakuma T, et al. Efficacy of daunorubicin encapsulated in liposome for the treatment of proliferative vitreoretinopathy. Ophthalmic Surg Lasers Imaging 2003;34:299–305.
45. Asaria RH, Kon CH, Bunce C, et al. Adjuvant 5-fluorouracil and heparin prevents proliferative vitreoretinopathy: Results from a randomized, double-blind, controlled clinical trial. Ophthalmology 2001;108: 1179–1183.
46. Wickham L, Bunce C, Wong D, et al. Randomized controlled trial of combined 5-fluorouracil and low-molecular-weight heparin in the management of unselected rhegmatogenous retinal detachments undergoing primary vitrectomy. Ophthalmology 2007;114:698–704.
47. Garcia RA, Sanchez JG, Arevalo JF. Combined 5-fluorouracil, low-molecular-weight heparin, and silicone oil in the management of complicated retinal detachment with proliferative vitreoretinopathy grade C. Ophthalmic Surg Lasers Imaging 2007;38:276–282.

CHAPTER 22

Posterior Uveitis

Harvey Siy Uy, MD, DPBO, Ellen Yu-Keh, MD, and Pik Sha Chan, MD

INTRODUCTION

Uveitis comprises a group of diseases characterized by inflammation of the uveal tract, which is composed of the iris, ciliary body, and choroid. These structures comprise the vascular coat of the eye and play many essential roles in the proper functioning of the visual system, such as control of the amount of light entering the eye, aqueous humor formation, accommodation, aqueous outflow, and blood supply to the photoreceptors and outer retina. Uveal inflammation frequently results in visual dysfunction and visual loss. Pharmacotherapy is the mainstay of uveitis treatment and preserves vision by reducing and preventing inflammation, thereby protecting ocular tissues from damage. This chapter discusses the key diagnostic features and pharmacotherapeutic approaches for the management of common posterior uveitis entities.

DISEASE PREVALENCE AND INFLUENCE

Uveitis is a significant cause of ocular morbidity worldwide and affects individuals of all ages and both genders.[1–5] The largest study conducted in North America estimated the incidence of uveitis to be 52.4/100000 person-years and the prevalence to be 115.3/100000 population.[3] Epidemiological data estimate the incidence of chronic, noninfectious posterior uveitis to range from 14 to 17/100000.[5] The economic burden of uveitis and its treatment is likely to be increasingly heavy as young populations mature. A study of Medicare data from elderly patients revealed that, in the 1990s, the cumulative prevalence of uveitis increased from 511/100000 to 1231/100000, with anterior uveitis accounting for most cases. The same study estimated the average incidence of posterior uveitis to be 76.6/100000 and the incidence of panuveitis and endophthalmitis to be 41.7/100000.[6]

Uveitis is believed to be the fourth leading cause of blindness among the working population (ages, 20–60 years). Visual impairment has been reported to involve approximately 35–70% of uveitis patients, unilateral visual loss to involve approximately 14–50%, and bilateral visual loss to involve 4–50% of patients.[2,6] Uveitis is responsible for many ocular complications, such as cystoid macular edema (CME), cataract, glaucoma, and retinal detachment (RD). The frequency of complications increases with disease duration. In the course of the disease, surgery is performed in about half of all patients.[2,7]

RISK FACTORS

The risk factors for developing a particular kind of uveitis are multifactorial and not fully identified but include genetic, racial, geographic, and environmental factors.[8] The association of major histocompatibility haplotypes with particular uveitis entities highlights the importance of genetic factors on development of uveitis. For example, the human leukocyte antigen (HLA)-A29 genotype is associated with birdshot chorioretinopathy (BSRC) while HLA-B51 is associated with Behçet's disease. Racial or ethnic background also determines risk for developing a particular type of uveitis. For example, Asians are predisposed to developing Vogt–Koyanagi–Harada (VKH) disease, while Caucasians are prone to develop BSRC.

The risk factors for visual loss or impairment due to uveitis are varied but the most significant ones include panuveitis, posterior uveitis, bilateral inflammation, duration of disease, delay in presentation to subspecialist, increased patient age, and development of complications (CME, cataract, glaucoma).[6,9] In one large series, juvenile rheumatoid arthritis and sarcoidosis were the systemic conditions most associated with visual loss.[2]

PATHOGENESIS

Inflammation is a protective response of the human body which aims to remove causes of injury such as microbial agents and toxins, as well as byproducts of injury such as damaged and dead cells and tissues. The components of the immune system comprise the main participants in the inflammatory process, including cellular (leukocytes, lymphocytes) and humoral (antibodies, cytokines) elements. Immune system activation produces the classic inflammatory features of warmth, redness, pain, swelling, and malfunction. The underlying processes causing these signs include vasodilation, increased blood flow, extravasation of plasma proteins, emigration of cellular elements from the circulation, secretion of chemical mediators of inflammation (prostaglandins, leukotrienes, nitric oxide, complement factors, histamines, lysozomal enzymes, platelet-activating factors). When inflammation is inappropriately directed or prolonged, damage to the normal body tissues may occur, leading to disease and morbidity.

In most cases of uveitis, permanent visual morbidity does not result from a single episode but from recurrent episodes of inflammation or prolonged disease, which produce cumulative tissue damage. The most common cause of severe visual loss among uveitis patients is CME, which occurs in about half of patients with posterior uveitis.[2,9] Other significant causes of visual loss include cataract, glaucoma, RD, and chorioretinal scarring. Onset of these complications and resulting visual outcomes are correlated with the frequency and duration of inflammatory episodes.[9,10] In order to preserve as much visual function as possible, the goal of pharmacotherapy for posterior uveitis should be total elimination of inflammation through appropriate and adequate management. Fortunately, the range of available pharmacotherapeutic modalities has expanded such that the vast majority of uveitis conditions are amenable to treatment.

SPECIFIC DISEASES: DIAGNOSIS AND PHARMACOTHERAPY

In this section, we discuss the diagnostic features of common, posterior-segment inflammatory conditions and discuss currently available treatments. The principles of treatment and therapeutic agents discussed here are applicable to other, less common uveitis entities such as retinal vasculitis, white-dot syndromes, and intermediate uveitis, The pharmacokinetic features and dosages of each drug are discussed in more detail in another section of this book.

Diagnosis of uveitis can be a confusing and frustrating process even for experienced clinicians. Careful history-taking, comprehensive review of systems, ocular examination, and targeted laboratory workup are essential steps for diagnosis. In order to generate a differential diagnosis, the gathered data are classified according to descriptive categories, such as demographic data, location of uveitis, and clinicopathologic features. When applicable, specific laboratory tests are then obtained to aid in arriving at a final, sometimes, "best guess" diagnosis. A correct diagnosis can be crucial in timely selection and institution of potentially sight-saving pharmacotherapy. The diagnostic features of the common noninfectious posterior uveitis entities are summarized in Table 22.1.

Since their introduction in the 1950s, corticosteroids have remained a mainstay of treatment for all types of noninfectious uveitis and are typically used for initial control of inflammation. However, their long-term systemic use is limited by the development of side-effects such as cushingoid syndrome, hyperglycemia, hypertension, gastrointestinal ulceration, and osteoporosis (Figure 22.1). For posterior-segment involvement, high drug levels of corticosteroids may be achieved by using the periocular, intravitreal, and systemic routes of administration.[11] New intraocular devices have been developed and, when implanted, provide a sustained and controlled dose of steroids inside the eye (Retisert, Bausch & Lomb, Rochester, NY and Ozurdex, Allergan, Irvine, CA). These nonsystemic routes of administration minimize systemic side-effects.

Nonsteroidal anti-inflammatory drugs such as diclofenac sodium, ketorolac, and nepafenac are utilized to reduce mild inflammation, resolve CME, and minimize the incidence of corticosteroid-related side-effects. They can be administered systemically or topically and may be combined with corticosteroids as steroid-sparing agents.[11]

Immunosuppressive agents are used for the treatment of several posterior uveitis entities (Table 22.2). They can be used as steroid-sparing agents or added to corticosteroid therapy when an inadequate response is obtained. The International Uveitis Study Group has recommended that Adamantiades–Behçet disease (ABD), chronic VKH syndrome, and serpiginous choroidopathy (SPC) be considered absolute indications for immunosuppressive therapy due to their unacceptable long-term prognosis.[12,13] In 2000, Jabs and Rosenbaum and a panel of inflammation experts published guidelines for corticosteroids, immunosuppressive and biologic drugs for patients with ocular inflammation.[11] The following sections summarize their recommendations and incorporate newer information regarding pharmacotherapy of common posterior uveitis entities.

ADAMANTIADES–BEHÇET DISEASE

Diagnostic features

ABD is a major cause of posterior uveitis in the Mediterranean and Asian regions. ABD is classically diagnosed in the presence of oral ulcers (Figure 22.2), genital ulcers, and uveitis. The International Study Group for Behçet's Disease diagnostic criteria include recurrent oral ulcers (at least 3 times per year) plus any two of the following: recurrent genital ulcers, ocular inflammation, skin involvement (erythema nodosum, superficial migratory thrombophlebitis), or a positive pathergy (skinprick) test.[13] Other systemic manifestations of ABD include: arthritis, epididymitis, neuropsychiatric symptoms, gastrointestinal, and vascular lesions. ABD may manifest as anterior uveitis with or without hypopyon. Posterior-segment involvement may manifest as vitritis, retinal vasculitis, focal necrotizing retinitis, and posterior uveitis. Left untreated, the visual outcomes are uniformly poor, with approximately 3 of 4 patients developing blindness within 3.5 years of onset.[14]

While there is no universally accepted laboratory test for ABD, there is an association between ABD and HLA-B51.[15] During acute inflammation, fluorescein angiography (FA) demonstrates leakage from inflamed retinal vessels and the optic disc (Figure 22.3). Areas of capillary nonperfusion, neovascularization, telangiectasia, and edema may also be identified. Indocyanine green angiography (ICGA) may demonstrate subclinical choroidal involvement.[16] The differential diagnosis of different posterior-segment clinical findings is outlined in Table 22.3.

Treatment modalities

Corticosteroid treatment alone does not change the long-term visual outcome but only delays the onset of blindness. For this reason, the early use of immunosuppressive drugs has been advocated for posterior uveitis due to ABD.[17] There is excellent, level I evidence to show that azathioprine and cyclosporine-A (CSA) are effective in reducing the frequency and severity of uveitis attacks resulting from ABD.[2,11,18,19] Low-dose CSA has been recommended as first-line immunomodulatory therapy with or without low-dose corticosteroids. Cyclophosphamide

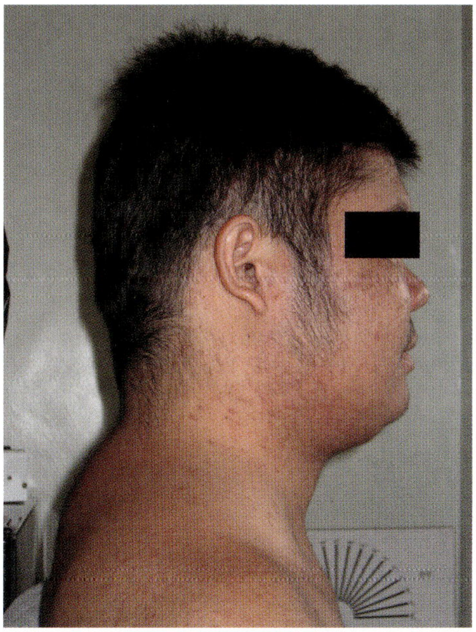

Figure 22.1 Moon facies, buffalo hump, acne, and hirsutism in a patient maintained on oral corticosteroids.

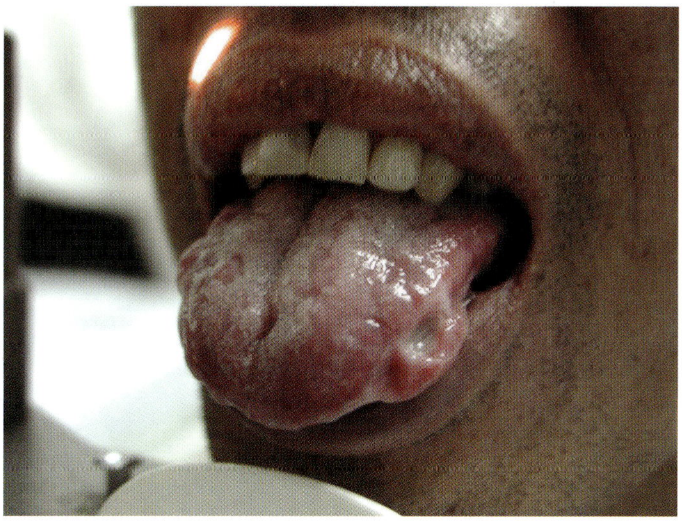

Figure 22.2 Oral ulcers in a patient with Adamantiades–Behçet disease.

Table 22.1 Clinical features of noninfectious posterior uveitis*

Noninfectious uveitis syndromes with systemic manifestations	
Behçet's disease	**Ocular manifestations** *Early* Vitreous cells, retinal vasculitis (affecting arteries and veins), central or branch vein occlusion, retinal hemorrhage or exudates, macular edema, choroidal infarcts, papillitis *Late* Posterior vitreous detachment, vascular sheathing, attenuated retinal vessels, neovascularization, vitreous hemorrhage, epiretinal membranes, RPE alterations, chorioretinal scarring, tractional retinal detachment, retinal or optic atrophy **Systemic manifestations** Oral ulcers, skin lesions (erythema nodosum, pseudofolliculitis, cutaneous hypersensitivity, thrombophlebitis), genital ulcers, arthritis, intestinal ulcers, epididymitis, vascular disease (obliteration, occlusion, aneurysm), neuropsychiatric symptoms
Sympathetic ophthalmia	**Ocular manifestations** *Early* Vitritis, multiple yellow-white peripheral choroidal lesions, serous retinal detachment, papillitis *Late* Retinal and optic atrophy, subretinal neovascularization or fibrosis, choroidal atrophy **Systemic manifestations (uncommon)** Alopecia, poliosis, vitiligo, dysacousis, cerebrospinal fluid pleocytosis
Vogt–Koyanagi–Harada syndrome	**Ocular manifestations** *Early* Vitritis, diffuse choroiditis, focal areas of subretinal fluid, bullous serous retinal detachments, optic disc hyperemia *Late* Sunset glow fundus, nummular chorioretinal depigmented scars, retinal pigment epithelium clumping, subretinal neovascularization **Systemic manifestations** Neurological/auditory findings, meningismus (malaise, fever, headache, nausea, abdominal pain, stiffness of neck and back), tinnitus, cerebrospinal fluid pleocytosis, alopecia, poliosis, vitiligo
Sarcoidosis	**Ocular manifestations** *Early* Vitritis, retinal vasculitis (periphlebitis) ± yellow perivenous exudates, multifocal chorioretinal lesions, choroidal nodules, exudative retinal detachment, cystoid macular edema *Late* Venous sheathing, chorioretinal atrophy, retinal neovascularization, subretinal neovascularization **Systemic manifestations** Hilar adenopathy, pulmonary disease, lymphadenopathy, skin involvement (erythema nodosum, granulomatous sarcoid nodules), splenomegaly, arthritis, parotid disease, central nervous system involvement (cranial nerve palsies, neuropathy, myopathy, aseptic meningitis)
Noninfectious uveitis syndromes without systemic manifestations	
Birdshot retinochoroidopathy	**Ocular manifestations** *Early* Vitritis, distinct cream-colored depigmented "birdshot" lesions, retinal vasculitis (venules), cystoid macular or disc edema *Late* Chronic cystoid macular edema, retinal and subretinal neovascularization, optic atrophy, epiretinal membrane

Table 22.1 Clinical features of noninfectious posterior uveitis*— cont'd

Noninfectious uveitis syndromes without systemic manifestations	
Serpiginous choroidopathy	**Ocular manifestations** *Early* Vitritis, deep peripapillary or macular gray-green or cream-colored chorioretinal lesion with indistinct borders ± neurosensory retinal detachment, inactive scar with active inflammation of distal edge *Late* RPE clumping, prominent choroidal vessels, serpentine-shaped chorioretinal atrophy, choroidal neovascularization, subretinal fibrosis
White-dot syndromes	
Acute posterior multifocal placoid pigment epitheliopathy	**Ocular manifestations** *Early* Vitritis, multiple cream-colored plaques at level of RPE, vasculitis, papillitis *Late* RPE mottling or depigmentation, choroidal neovascularization (rare)
Multifocal choroiditis with panuveitis	**Ocular manifestations** *Early* Significant vitritis, punched-out chorioretinal lesions, cystoid macular edema, disc edema *Late* Chorioretinal scarring, choroidal neovascularization, peripapillary pigmentary changes
Punctate inner choroidopathy	**Ocular manifestations** *Early* No vitreous inflammation, punched-out chorioretinal lesions *Late* Chorioretinal scarring, choroidal neovascularization
Subretinal fibrosis and uveitis	**Ocular manifestations** *Early* Vitritis, multiple whitish-yellow subretinal lesions with indistinct borders, cystoid macular edema, papillitis *Late* Punched-out atrophic scars, pigmented chorioretinal scars, coalescence of lesions with subretinal fibrosis, subretinal neovascular membranes, serous retinal detachment
Multiple evanescent white-dot syndrome	**Ocular manifestations** *Early* Vitreous cells, small discrete white dots at the level of RPE, granular appearance of macula, cystoid macular edema, optic disc edema *Late* RPE changes, choroidal neovascularization (rare)

**Ocular clinical manifestations are divided into two categories. Early manifestations include posterior-segment findings during acute or recurrent inflammation; late manifestations include ocular complications of posterior uveitis.*

RPE, retinal pigment epithelium.

Table 22.2 Pharmacotherapeutic agents for common posterior-segment uveitis entities

Posterior uveitis entity	Pharmacotherapeutic agent
Adamantiades Behçet's disease	Corticosteroids Cyclosporine A Azathioprine Cyclophosphamide Tacrolimus Chlorambucil Infliximab Adalimumab
Birdshot chorioretinopathy	Azathioprine Mycophenolate mofetil Cyclosporine A Intravenous immunoglobulin Infliximab Daclizumab
Multifocal choroiditis and panuveitis	Corticosteroids Methotrexate Cyclosporine A Azathioprine Chlorambucil Sirolimus
Sarcoidosis	Corticosteroids Methotrexate Azathioprine Cyclosporine A Mycophenolate mofetil Infliximab Daclizumab
Serpiginous choroidopathy	Corticosteroids Cyclosporine A Azathioprine Cyclophosphamide Chlorambucil
Vogt–Koyanagi–Harada syndrome	Corticosteroids Methotrexate Cyclosporine A Tacrolimus Azathioprine Intravenous immunoglobulin Mycophenolate mofetil
Sympathetic ophthalmia	Corticosteroids Cyclosporine A Tacrolimus Azathioprine

Table 22.3 Differential diagnosis of posterior uveitis based on clinical findings

Clinical finding	Differential diagnosis
Chorioretinal lesions (multifocal)	**Noninfectious** VKH, sympathetic ophthalmia, BSCR, MCP, sarcoidosis, serpiginous choroiditis, white-dot syndromes (APMPPE, MEWDS, PIC), subretinal fibrosis, and uveitis **Infectious** Tuberculosis, syphilis
Chorioretinal lesions (focal)	**Noninfectious** Serpiginous choroiditis **Infectious** Toxoplasmosis, toxocariasis, tuberculosis, sarcoidosis
Retinal vasculitis Primarily affecting arteries	**Noninfectious** Systemic lupus erythematosus, polyarteritis nodosa, frosted-branch angiitis **Infectious** Syphilis, ARN, PORN
Primarily affecting veins	**Noninfectious** BSCR, Eale's disease, sarcoidosis **Infectious** Toxoplasmosis, tuberculosis
Affects both arteries and veins	**Noninfectious** Behçet's disease
Retinitis	**Noninfectious** Sarcoidosis **Infectious** Toxoplasmosis, toxocariasis, syphilis, tuberculosis, ARN, CMV, retinitis, DUSN
Neurosensory detachment	**Noninfectious** VKH, sympathetic ophthalmia, posterior scleritis, SLE **Infectious** Syphilis, CMV retinitis, SFU, ARN, toxocariasis

VKH, Vogt–Koyanagi–Harada syndrome; BSCR, birdshot retinochoroidopathy; MCP, multifocal choroiditis and panuveitis; APMPPE, acute posterior placoid pigment epitheliopathy; MEWDS, multiple evanescent white-dot syndrome; PIC, punctate inner choroidopathy; ARN, acute retinal necrosis; PORN, progressive outer retinal necrosis syndrome; CMV, cytomegalovirus; DUSN, unilateral subacute retinitis; diffuse SLE, systemic lupus erythematosus; SFU, subretinal fibrosis and uveitis syndrome.

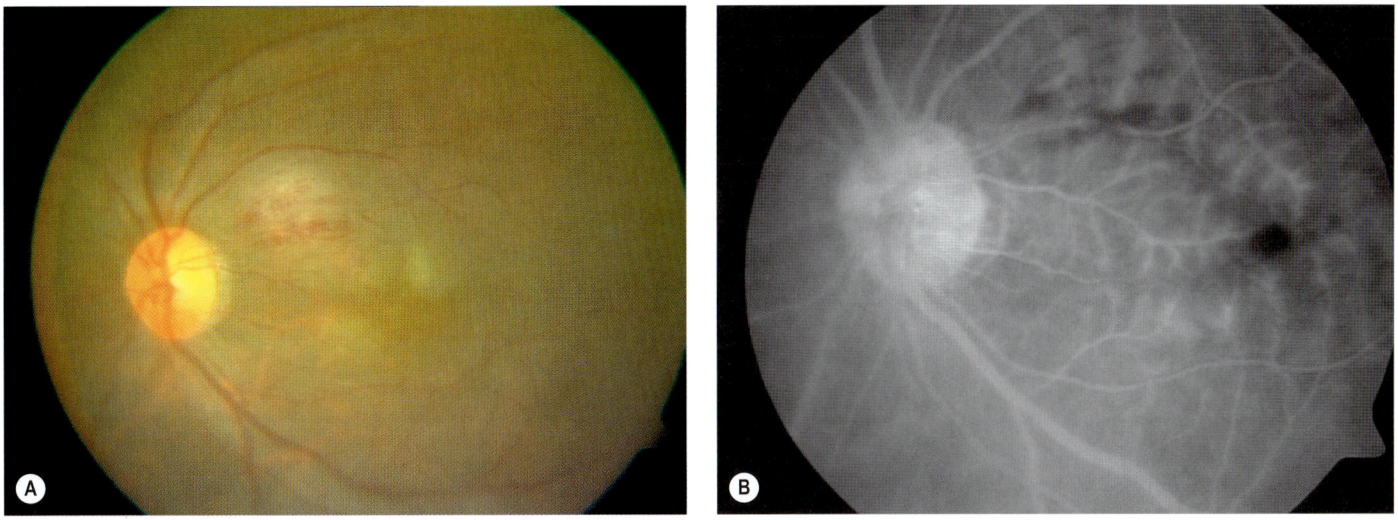

Figure 22.3 (A) Color photograph and (B) fluorescein angiogram showing vasculitis in the macular area in Adamantiades–Behçet disease.

and tacrolimus are alternative agents for patients who are unresponsive to or intolerant of first-line agents. Chlorambucil is an effective option, but is now considered a second-line agent, and should be used with caution because of its potential for toxicity.

Recently, several case series have reported successful control of refractory ABD using anti-tumor necrosis factor (TNF) drugs infliximab and adalimumab.[20,21] Intravitreal triamcinolone acetonide (IVTA) injections have been shown to resolve CME due to ABD.[22] A novel localized treatment modality for ABD and other posterior uveitis disorders is the fluocinolone acetonide implant (Retisert, Bausch & Lomb, Rochester, NY), which has been demonstrated to reduce the frequency of uveitis recurrence, improve visual outcome, and reduce the need for adjunctive therapy in patients with noninfectious posterior uveitis.[23] Potential adverse effects of IVTA and fluocinolone acetonide implant include cataract progression and glaucoma. The choice of which drug to use will depend on individual features such as tolerance and response to treatment.

BIRDSHOT RETINOCHOROIDOPATHY

Diagnostic features

BSCR is characterized by bilateral, multiple, hypopigmented postequatorial retinal pigment epithelial (RPE) and choroidal inflammatory lesions associated with low-grade inflammation. The main clinical diagnostic criteria for BSRC include: (1) bilateral disease; (2) at least three peripapillary "birdshot lesions" inferior or nasal to the optic disc in one eye; (3) low-grade anterior-segment intraocular inflammation (<1+ cells); and (4) low-grade vitreous inflammatory reaction (<2+ vitreous haze). Supportive findings for BSCR include: presence of the HLA-A29 haplotype, retinal vasculitis, and CME. Exclusion criteria for BSRC include keratic precipitates, posterior synechiae, and presence of other inflammatory diseases that can cause multifocal choroidal lesions.[24] BSCR patients may present with disturbances in night and color vision as well as decreased visual acuity.

ICGA usually demonstrates retinal and choroidal spots more numerous than clinically detected or seen on FA and may be more helpful in assessing disease activity and progression.[25] Electroretinogram abnormalities were associated with recurrence of inflammation[26] and improvement with therapy,[27] and may be a useful adjunct in therapeutic decision making. Visual field (VF) abnormalities appear to be associated with retinal damage, and automated VF testing may be an objective measure to monitor activity.[28] The most common VF patterns reported were multiple foci and arcuate defects. Optical coherence tomography (OCT) can be used to evaluate the macula in BSCR to determine causes of central vision loss such as macular thinning,[29] CME, epiretinal membrane, and choroidal neovascularization (CNV). BSCR must be differentiated from the white-dot syndromes and other causes of multifocal choroidal lesions (Table 22.3).

Treatment modalities

Periocular steroids are beneficial in acute exacerbation of inflammation and in the treatment of CME. However, the use of corticosteroid-sparing immunosuppressive agents is recommended for the treatment of BSCR because progressive deterioration of retinal function and poor visual prognosis have been associated with corticosteroid monotherapy. Low-dose azathioprine has been reported to be more effective than corticosteroids but does not lead to a durable remission. A combination of mycophenolate mofetil and CSA has been recommended as first-line therapy for BSCR.[30] Alternative treatment agents for BSCR include intravenous immunoglobulin,[31] and cytokine inhibition with infliximab[32] and daclizumab.[33]

MULTIFOCAL CHOROIDITIS AND PANUVEITIS (MCP)

MCP is a type of idiopathic posterior-segment chorioretinal inflammatory condition which exhibits: (1) bilateral, multiple (up to several hundred) choroidal lesions ranging in size from 50 to 350 μm, arranged singly, in clumps or in linear clusters, situated in the posterior pole and/or the periphery; (2) vitritis; (3) absence of systemic disease; (4) absence of features associated with other ocular diseases (e.g., HLA-A29 and abnormal electrocardiogram suggesting BSRC); (5) peripapillary changes, atrophy, or pigmentation; and (6) anterior uveitis. MCP predominantly affects young, healthy female adults and has no familial or racial predilection. Patients may complain of decreased visual acuity, photophobia, floaters, and photopsia usually affecting both eyes. MCP is a significant cause of visual impairment and visual loss: up to 38% of patients having 20/200 or worse visual acuity were reported in one series. The retinal complications of MCP include CNV, which is the most common cause of vision loss, as well as epiretinal membrane and CME.

FA will demonstrate the yellow or gray active lesions of MCP to be hypofluorescent in the early frames and hyperfluorescent in the late frames. CNV is a complication of MCP which can be confirmed by FA or ICGA. VF testing may show blind-spot enlargement or central scotoma. Electroretinography may demonstrate depressed rod and cone function.

Treatment modalities

Due to its chronic and recurrent course, MCP can result in permanent visual loss even with corticosteroid therapy. The use of immunosuppressive drugs (methotrexate, cyclosporine and/or azathioprine, and chlorambucil), instead of low-dose corticosteroids, was associated with a significant (83%) reduction in the risk of posterior-segment complications and with a significant (92%) reduction in the risk of blindness. Improved visual outcome among patients with MCP is obtained by reducing the risk of sight-threatening posterior-pole complications, especially CNV.[34] Sirolimus, an immunosuppressive agent with antiangiogenic properties, has been demonstrated to reduce fluid and leakage associated with CNV associated with MCP.[35] Subfoveal and juxtafoveal CNV may be treated successfully using photodynamic therapy, with most treated patients experiencing stabilized or improved visual acuity.[36]

SARCOIDOSIS

Diagnostic features

Ocular sarcoidosis involves both anterior and posterior segments and may affect up to 50% of patients with systemic sarcoid. Involvement of the anterior segment occurs in 85% of ocular sarcoid patients and may manifest as conjunctival "millet seed" nodules, granulomatous anterior uveitis, iris nodules, secondary glaucoma, and posterior synechiae. Posterior-segment involvement may manifest as vitritis, intermediate uveitis, posterior or panuveitis. When vitritis is present, cellular infiltration and accumulation may produce the appearance of snowballs or "string of pearls." Periphlebitis with yellowish perivenous exudates (candle wax drippings) is a hallmark of sarcoidosis. Punched-out focal or multifocal choroidal lesions have also been reported. Retinal ischemia may result in neovascularization and should be differentiated from other nonuveitic causes such as retinal vein occlusion, diabetes mellitus, and sickle-cell retinopathy.

FA may demonstrate retinal vascular staining, retinal neovascularization, or CME. ICGA may additionally demonstrate hypofluorescent choroidal lesions, leakage from choroidal blood vessels, or diffuse late zonal hypofluorescence.

Almost all organ systems can be affected by sarcoidosis, with the lung being the most frequently involved extraocular site. Definitive diagnosis is established by histopathologic evidence of classic noncaseating granulomas. Biopsy material can be collected from ocular and orbital structures such as conjunctiva and lacrimal gland, and from nonocular organ systems involved. Blood and imaging studies are less invasive, and are used by clinicians to make a presumptive diagnosis of sarcoidosis. Angiotensin-converting enzyme (ACE) is secreted by macrophages within granulomas and is useful in monitoring disease activity. Levels may be increased in serum, tears,[37] and aqueous humor.[38] In patients with suspected ocular sarcoidosis but with normal or equivocal chest radiograph, serum ACE level combined with whole-body gallium scan increases the diagnostic specificity to 100%.[39] A chest computed tomography is also useful in suspected sarcoidosis with negative radiographs.[40] Other studies used in the evaluation of patients with suspected sarcoidosis include serum lysozyme, serum and urinary calcium levels, and skin testing to demonstrate anergy; other imaging tools include gadolinium-enhanced magnetic resonance imaging[41] and positron emission tomography.[42]

Treatment modalities

Systemic corticosteroids are a mainstay of treatment and are indicated for anterior and posterior uveitis, neovascularization, and orbital disease refractory to topical steroids. Early use of systemic steroids may be sight-saving. Periocular steroids may be helpful, especially in the treatment of CME. Methotrexate, azathioprine, cyclosporine, and mycophenolate mofetil have been shown to be effective in controlling sarcoidosis-associated uveitis, enabling decrease or discontinuation of oral corticosteroid. Refractory ocular sarcoidosis, despite systemic immunosuppressive therapy, has been found to respond to anti-TNF monoclonal antibody (infliximab),[32] and humanized immunoglobulin monoclonal antibody (daclizumab).[43] Retinal neovascularization responds well to panretinal photocoagulation. IVTA may be useful in resolving refractory CME.

SERPIGINOUS CHOROIDOPATHY

Diagnostic features

SPC is a rare, idiopathic, bilateral, chronic, progressive, recurrent inflammation of the RPE, choriocapillaris, and choroid. SPC affects patients of both genders and all races and predominantly presents between ages 30 and 60. The presenting symptoms of SPC include painless blurring of central vision and scotoma formation. A mild vitritis may be observed. In active disease, the fundus exhibits striking focal or multifocal, cream or gray-colored, deep retinal lesions of varying sizes with irregular borders. These lesions involve both RPE and choroidal layers. As the active lesion resolves, the involved areas develop areas of RPE and choroidal atrophy containing hyperpigmented clumps. New lesions usually occur at the borders of the inactive lesions. These lesions usually begin in the peripapillary area and extend outward in a serpentine pattern.

There is no confirmatory laboratory test for SPC, but the peripapillary, serpentine fundus lesions are characteristic. However, macular serpiginous and atypical ampiginous variants can be other presentations. On FA, active lesions exhibit blocked fluorescence in early frames and diffuse leakage and staining in late frames. Although FA can differentiate active from healed lesions, ICGA is useful in monitoring disease progression and response to therapy. ICGA can reveal subclinical lesions not detectable clinically or by FA. ICGA is better at demonstrating persistent choroidal activity even with angiographic disappearance of retinal activity.[44] VF testing may show scotomas, which are usually dense in active lesions and become less dense as the lesions resolve.[45]

Treatment modalities

Systemic or periocular corticosteroids may resolve active disease but do not prevent disease progression[46] nor influence long-term visual outcomes, which depend on prevention of recurrences and resulting macular involvement. Mixed results are reported with CSA monotherapy, but treatment may result in clinical remission and disease cessation in some patients. Azathioprine combined with corticosteroids,[47] or triple-agent therapy with CSA, azathioprine, and prednisone,[48] has been reported to result in rapid remission of active disease. Alkylating agents (cyclophosphamide or chlorambucil), initially combined with oral corticosteroids, were also shown to be effective in controlling inflammation and inducing remission in patients who failed to respond to oral corticosteroids or triple-agent therapy.[49] Long-term therapy with azathioprine, CSA, and cyclophosphamide was noted to prolong remission.[50] Use of interferon alpha-2a has been reported for SPC unresponsive to other immunomodulatory therapy.[51]

VOGT–KOYANAGI–HARADA SYNDROME

Diagnostic features

VKH is a multiorgan disease affecting different organ systems, including ocular, nervous, auditory, and integumentary. VKH has worldwide distribution but is more common among darkly pigmented races such as Asians, blacks, Hispanics, and Native Americans. Females are slightly more affected than males.

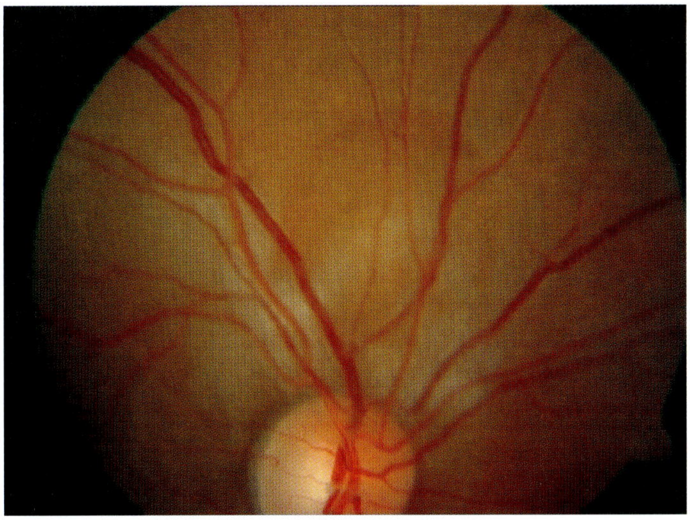

Figure 22.4 Fundus photography demonstrating multiple foci of exudative retinal detachment in a patient with Vogt–Koyanagi–Harada syndrome.

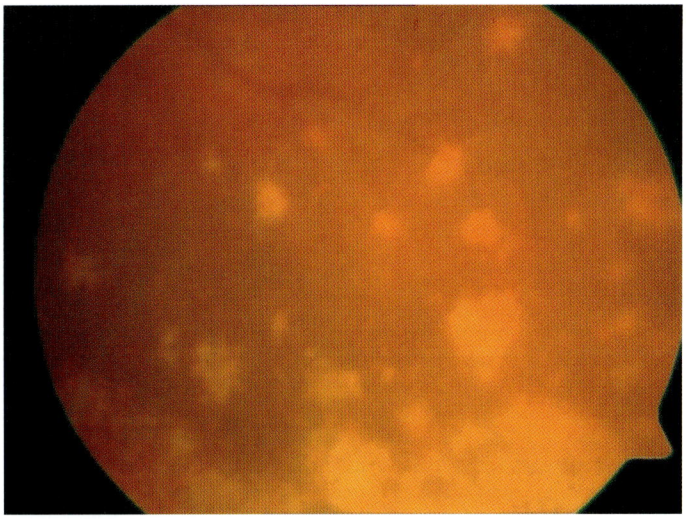

Figure 22.5 Chorioretinal depigmented lesion in the retinal periphery of an 8-year-old boy with Vogt–Koyanagi–Harada syndrome.

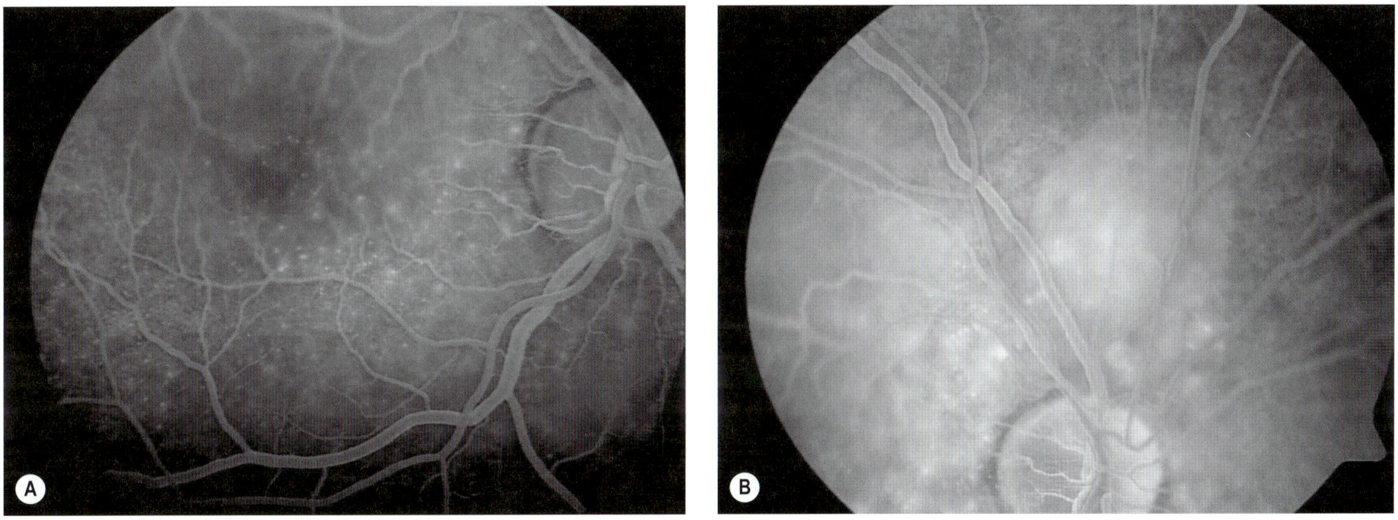

Figure 22.6 Fluorescein angiogram of patient in Figure 22.4 demonstrating (A) multifocal areas of pinpoint "starry night" leakage and (B) pooling of dye within subretinal fluid.

The revised diagnostic criteria developed in 2001 by an international panel[52] categorized VKH as complete (criteria 1–5 present), incomplete (criteria 1–3, and either 4 or 5 present), or probable (isolated eye disease with criteria 1–3 present) based on the following criteria:

1. Lack of penetrating ocular trauma or surgery preceding the uveitis onset
2. Lack of clinical or laboratory evidence of other ocular diseases
3. Bilateral ocular involvement (either 3a or 3b must be met, depending on the stage of disease when the patient is examined):
   a. Early manifestations of disease, including diffuse choroiditis (with or without anterior uveitis, vitreous inflammatory reaction, or optic disc hyperemia), which may manifest as focal areas of subretinal fluid or bullous serous RDs (Figure 22.4)
   b. Late manifestations of disease, including history or signs of prior early disease, ocular depigmentation (sunset glow fundus or Suguira's sign), nummular chorioretinal depigmented lesions (similar to Dalen–Fuchs nodules) (Figure 22.5), or RPE clumping and/or migration, or recurrent or chronic anterior uveitis.
4. Neurological/auditory findings (which may have resolved by the time of evaluation) include meningismus (malaise, fever, headache, nausea, abdominal pain, stiffness of the neck and back, or a combination of these factors), tinnitus, and cerebrospinal fluid pleocytosis
5. Integumentary findings, including alopecia, poliosis, or vitiligo. There is evidence pointing to T-cell-mediated damage to retina melanocytes.

In the acute stage, FA characteristically demonstrates multiple punctate hyperfluorescent dots at the RPE level which gradually enlarge, producing a "starry night" appearance (Figure 22.6A). Pooling of subretinal fluid in multiple areas of localized RD is another prominent feature (Figure 22.6B). Optic nerve hyperfluorescence is frequently visualized as well. B-scan ultrasonography may demonstrate diffuse choroidal thickening, serous RD, vitreous opacities, and posterior scleral thickening. Magnetic resonance imaging may differentiate VKH from posterior scleritis, a major cause of multifocal exudative RD.

The major ICGA findings in active disease include: (1) early choroidal stromal vessel hyperfluorescence and leakage; (2) multiple mid-phase hypofluorescent dark dots; (3) fuzzy vascular pattern of large stromal vessels; and (4) disc hyperfluorescence. With treatment, the hypofluorescent spots decrease in number and disappear as disease activity subsides. The other ICGA findings also diminish with response to treatment. ICGA is useful to detect subclinical choroidal inflammation[53] and guide therapy.[54] OCT may be utilized to quantify objectively the amount of subretinal fluid and resolution with treatment. Sympathetic ophthalmia (SO) can present similar to VKH, thus any history of penetrating ocular trauma or surgery should be thoroughly elicited.

Treatment modalities

Corticosteroids constitute the primary treatment for acute disease. VKH responds well to systemic steroids, although some reports suggest that use of immunomodulatory therapy as first-line therapy is associated with a superior visual outcome compared to using corticosteroid alone.[55]

Treatment of VKH typically requires an average of 6 months or longer, and the addition of a second, steroid-sparing agent allows the corticosteroid dose to be decreased, thereby preventing steroid-related complications. Methotrexate, cyclosporine, tacrolimus, azathioprine, and mycophenolate mofetil are the immunomodulatory agents used to treat VKH in reported series. The use of intravenous immunoglobulin has also been reported.[56] In pediatric VKH cases, methotrexate was used as a steroid-sparing agent in steroid-resistant cases, with good results.[57] Triple therapy with methotrexate, cyclosporine, and corticosteroid was necessary in one pediatric VKH case reported.[58] The aggressive, early use of steroids and maintenance using immunosuppressive agents produces fairly good prognosis, with over half of patients having visual outcomes of 20/30 or better. Poor visual outcomes are associated with increased age of onset, poor response to corticosteroids requiring prolonged treatment, and CNV.

SYMPATHETIC OPHTHALMIA

Diagnostic features

Since its description by William MacKenzie in the mid 19th century, SO has generated much interest and has become one of the most well-known forms of uveitis among lay people. SO is a rare form of bilateral panuveitis usually following nonsurgical trauma to one eye (the exciting eye) with consequent inflammation of the nontraumatized (sympathizing) eye. SO may also occur after ocular surgery and radiotherapy. The onset of SO occurs within 1 year of the inciting event in 90% of cases, but may occur decades later.

SO presents as granulomatous uveitis with anterior-chamber inflammation, mutton-fat keratic precipitates, vitritis, and posterior-segment abnormalities. Yellow lesions (Dalen–Fuchs nodules) are seen in the periphery of the choroid, sometimes becoming confluent. Secondary glaucoma or cataract may develop.

Classic histopathological features of SO include granulomatous uveal tract infiltration and collections of inflammatory cells under the RPE (Dalen–Fuchs nodules). Monocytes, or T-helper and B lymphocytes, may be the major cellular components in the choroidal infiltrates. The clinical presentation may be similar to VKH, thus it is important to determine if there is any history of penetrating trauma or surgery. ICGA has been used as adjunct to FA in evaluating response to therapy with hypofluorescent spots present in active disease resolving with therapy.[59] OCT may be utilized to document decrease in subretinal fluid with treatment.

Treatment modalities

Earlier reports suggested that early enucleation of the inciting eye was beneficial in preventing SO. More recent studies have reported good visual outcomes with aggressive, early, and adequate immunosuppressive therapy. High-dose systemic steroids should be the initial treatment. Relapses are common with SO, hence the need for prolonged duration of treatment with corticosteroids and gradual tapering of steroid dosage only after prolonged, close follow-up. Good results have been reported on the use of tacrolimus,[60] cyclosporine, and/or azathioprine,[61,62] combined with corticosteroids for SO. Chlorambucil has also been used for intractable SO with induction of remission.[63]

SUMMARY AND KEY POINTS

Advances in drug development have greatly expanded the spectrum of inflammatory eye diseases amenable to pharmacotherapy. The great majority of patients with noninfectious, posterior-segment uveitis do respond to corticosteroids or currently available immunosuppressive agents. In many instances, early, aggressive, and appropriate treatment of intraocular inflammation makes a huge difference as to whether the patient retains or loses vision. The challenge to clinicians is to diagnose the disease condition correctly and early and enable their patients to have access to specialized care. The chronic, relapsing, insidious nature of posterior uveitis demands careful attention by caregivers. As the pathophysiological processes of these conditions become clearer, promising new treatments will be developed that provide more effective and safer treatments for uveitis patients.

Key points

- Uveitis is a leading cause of visual impairment worldwide.
- Pharmacotherapy is the primary means of treating posterior uveitis.
- Aggressive anti-inflammatory therapy is crucial for sight preservation in autoimmune posterior uveitis.
- Choice of pharmacotherapeutic agent is based on specific disease entity and patients' clinical profiles.
- Appropriate drug selection and careful monitoring provide safe, effective treatment.
- New immunosuppressive drugs and devices provide alternative modalities for drug resistance or drug intolerance.

REFERENCES

1. Weiner A, BenEzra D. Clinical patterns and associated conditions in chronic uveitis. Am J Ophthalmol 1991;112:151–158
2. Rothova A, Suttorp-van Schulten MS, Frits Treffers W, et al. Causes and frequency of blindness in patients with intraocular inflammatory disease. Br J Ophthalmol 1996;80:332–336.
3. Gritz DC, Wong IG. Incidence and prevalence of uveitis in northern California. The Northern California Epidemiology of Uveitis Study. Ophthalmology 2004;111:491–500.
4. Uy HS, Tam IW. Patterns of uveitis in a Philippine eye clinic. Phil J Ophthalmol 2005;30:37–41.
5. Baarsma GS. The epidemiology and genetics of endogenous uveitis: a review. Curr Eye Res 1992;1(suppl):1–9.
6. Reeves SW, Sloan FA, Lee PP, et al. Uveitis in the elderly: epidemiological data from the National Long-term Care Survey Medicare Cohort. Ophthalmology. 2006 Feb;113:307.
7. Durrani OM, Tehrani NN, Marr JE, et al. Degree, duration, and causes of visual loss in uveitis. Br J Ophthalmol 2004;88:1159–1162.
8. Rosenberg KD, Feuer WJ, Davis JL. Ocular complications of pediatric uveitis. Ophthalmology 2004;111:2299–2306.
9. Chang JH, Wakefield D. Uveitis: a global perspective. Ocul Immunol Inflamm 2002;10:263–279.
10. Dana MR, Merayo-Lloves J, Schaumberg DA, et al. Prognosticators for visual outcome in sarcoid uveitis. Ophthalmology 1996;103:1846–1853.
11. Jabs DA, Rosenbaum JT. Guidelines for the use of immunosuppressive drugs in patients with ocular inflammatory disorders: recommendations of an expert panel. Am J Ophthalmol 2000;130:492–513.
12. Kitaichi N, Miyazaki A, Iwata D, et al. Ocular features of Behçet's disease: an international collaborative study. Br J Ophthalmol 2007;91:1579–1582.
13. International Study Group for Behçet's Disease. Criteria for diagnosis of Behçet's disease. Lancet 1990;335:1078–1080.
14. Mamo JB. The rate of visual loss in Behçet's disease. Arch Ophthalmol 1970;84:451–452.

15. Ohno S, Ohguchi M, Hirose S, et al. Close association of HLA-Bw51 with Behçet's disease. Arch Ophthalmol 1982;100:1455–1458.
16. Matsuo T, Sato Y, Shiraga F, et al. Choroidal abnormalities in Behçet disease observed by simultaneous indocyanine green and fluorescein angiography with scanning laser ophthalmoscopy. Ophthalmol 1999;106: 295–300.
17. Kim EC, Foster CS. Immunomodulatory therapy for the treatment of ocular inflammatory disease: evidence-based medicine recommendations for use. Int Ophthalmol Clin 2006;46:141–164.
18. Yazici J, Pazarli H, Barnes CG, et al. A controlled trial of azathioprine in Behçet's syndrome. N Engl J Med 1990;322:281–285.
19. Masuda K, Nakajima A, Urayama A, et al. Double-masked trial of cyclosporine versus colchicines and long-term open study of cyclosporine in Behçet's disease. Lancet 1989;1:1093–1096.
20. Accorinti M, Pirraglia MP, Paroli MP, et al. Infliximab treatment for ocular and extraocular manifestations of Behçet's disease. Jpn J Ophthalmol 2007;51:191–196.
21. Mushtaq B, Saeed T, Situnayake RD, et al. Adalimumab for sight-threatening uveitis in Behçet's disease. Eye 2007;21:824–825.
22. Atmaca LS, Yalçindag FN, Ozdemir O. Intravitreal triamcinolone acetonide in the management of cystoid macular edema in Behçet's disease. Graefes Arch Clin Exp Ophthalmol 2007;245:451–456.
23. Jaffe GJ, Martin D, Callanan D, et al. Fluocinolone acetonide implant (Retisert) for noninfectious posterior uveitis: thirty-four-week results of a multicenter randomized clinical study. Ophthalmology 2006;113: 1020–1027.
24. Levinson RD, Brezin A, Rothova A, et al. Research criteria for the diagnosis of birdshot chorioretinopathy: results of an international consensus conference. Am J Ophthalmol 2006;141:185–187.
25. Howe LJ, Stanford MR, Graham EM, et al. Choroidal abnormalities in birdshot chorioretinopathy: an indocyanine green angiography study. Eye 1997;11:554–559
26. Zacks DN, Samson CM, Loewenstein J. Electroretinograms as an indicator of disease activity in birdshot retinochoroidopathy. Graefes Arch Clin Exp 2002;240:601–607.
27. Holder GE, Robson AG, Pavesio C, et al. Electrophysiological characterisation and monitoring in the management of birdshot chorioretinopathy. Br J Ophthalmol 2005;89:709–718.
28. Gordon LK, Monnet D, Holland GN, et al. Longitudinal cohort study of patients with birdshot chorioretinopathy. IV. Visual field results at baseline. Am J Ophthalmol 2007;144:829–837.
29. Monnet D, Levinson RD, Holland GN, et al. Longitudinal cohort study of patients with birdshot chorioretinopathy. III. Macular imaging at baseline. Am J Ophthalmol 2007;144:818–828.
30. Kiss S, Ahmed M, Letko E, et al. Long-term follow-up of patients with birdshot retinochoroidopathy treated with corticosteroid-sparing systemic immunomodulatory therapy. Ophthalmol 2005;112:1066–1071.
31. LeHoang P, Cassoux N, George F, et al. Intravenous immunoglobulin for the treatment of bordshot retinochoroidopathy. Ocul Immunol Inflamm 2000;8:49–57.
32. Theodossiadis PG, Markomichelakis NN, Sfikakis PP. Tumor necrosis factor antagonists: preliminary evidence for an emerging approach in the treatment of ocular inflammation. Retina 2007;27:399–413.
33. Sobrin L, Huang JJ, Christen W, et al. Daclizumab for treatment of birdshot chorioretinopathy. Arch Ophthalmol 2008;126:186–191.
34. Michel SS, Ekong A, Baltatzis S, et al. Multifocal choroiditis and panuveitis: immunomodulatory therapy. Ophthalmol 2002;109:378–383.
35. Nussenblatt RB, Coleman H, Jirawuthiworavong G, et al. The treatment of multifocal choroiditis associated choroidal neovascularization with sirolimus (rapamycin). Acta Ophthalmol Scand 2007;85:230–231.
36. Gerth C, Spital G, Lommatzsch A, et al. Photodynamic therapy for choroidal neovascularization in patients with multifocal choroiditis and panuveitis. Eur J Ophthalmol 2006;16:111–118.
37. Sharma OP, Vita JB. Determination of angiotensin-converting enzyme activity in tears. A noninvasive test for evaluation of ocular sarcoidosis. Arch Ophthalmol 1983;101:559–561.
38. Weinreb RN, Sandman R, Ryder MI. Angiotensin-converting enzyme activity in human aqueous humor. Arch Ophthalmol 1985;103:34–36.
39. Power WJ, Neves RA, Rodriguez A. The value of combined serum angiotensin-converting enzyme and gallium scan in diagnosing ocular sarcoidosis. Ophthalmology 1995;102:2007–2011.
40. Statement on sarcoidosis. Joint Statement of the American Thoracic Society (ATS), the European Respiratory Society (ERS) and the World Association of Sarcoidosis and Other Granulomatous Disorders (WASOG) adopted by the ATS Board of Directors and by the ERS Executive Committee. Am J Respir Crit Care Med 1999;160:736–755.
41. Smedema JP, Snoep G, van Kroonenburg MP, et al. Evaluation of the accuracy of gadolinium-enhanced cardiovascular magnetic resonance in the diagnosis of cardiac sarcoidosis. J Am Coll Cardiol 2005;45:1683–1690.
42. Teirstein AS, Machac J, Almeida O, et al. Results of 188 whole-body fluorodeoxyglucose positron emission tomography scans in 137 patients with sarcoidosis. Chest 2007;132:1949–1953.
43. Gallagher M, Quinones K, Cervantes-Castaneda RA, et al. Biological response modifier therapy for refractory childhood uveitis. Br J Ophthalmol 2007;91:1341–1344.
44. Giovannini A, Mariotti C, Ripa E. Indocyanine green angiographic findings in serpiginous choroidopathy. Br J Ophthalmol 1996;80:536–540.
45. Weiss H, Annesley Jr WH, Shields JA. The clinical course of serpiginous choroidopathy. Am J Ophthalmol 1979;87:133–142.
46. Christmas NJ, Oh KT, Oh DM, et al. Long-term follow-up of patients with serpiginous choroiditis. Retina 2002;22:550–556.
47. Vianna RNG, Ozdal PC, Deschenes J, et al. Combination of azathioprine and corticosteroids in the treatment of serpiginous choroiditis. Can J Ophthalmol 2006;41:183–189.
48. Hooper PL, Kaplan HJ. Triple agent immunosuppression in serpiginous choroiditis. Ophthalmology 1991;98:944–951.
49. Akpek EK, Jabs DA, Tessler HH, et al. Successful treatment of serpiginous choroiditis with alkylating agents. Ophthalmol 2002;109:1506–1513.
50. Akpek E, Baltatzis S, Yang J, et al. Long-term immunosuppressive treatment of serpiginous choroiditis. Ocul Immunol Inflamm 2001;9:153–167.
51. Sobaci G, Bayraktar Z, Bayer A. Interferon alpha-2a treatment for serpiginous choroiditis. Ocul Immunol Inflamm 2005;13:59–66.
52. Read RW, Holland GN, Rao NA. Revised diagnostic criteria for Vogt–Koyanagi–Harada disease: report of an international committee on nomenclature. Am J Ophthalmol 2001;131:647–652.
53. Bacsal K, Wen DS, Chee SP. Concomitant choroidal inflammation during anterior segment recurrence in Vogt–Koyanagi–Harada disease. Am J Ophthalmol 2008;145:480–486.
54. Herbort CP, Mantovani A, Bouchenaki N. Indocyanine green angiography in Vogt–Koyanagi–Harada disease: angiographic signs and utility in patient follow-up. Int Ophthalmol 2007;27:173–182.
55. Paredes I, Ahmed M, Foster CS. Immunomodulatory therapy for Vogt–Koyanagi–Harada patients as first-line therapy. Ocul Immunol Inflamm 2006;14:87–90.
56. Gonzalez-Delgado M, Gonzalez C, Blazquez JI, et al. Intravenous immunoglobulin therapy in Vogt–Koyanagi–Harada syndrome. Neurologia 2004;19:401–403.
57. Soheilian M, Aletaha M, Yazdani S, et al. Management of pediatric Vogt–Koyanagi–Harada (VKH)-associated panuveitis. Ocul Immunol Inflamm 2006;14:91–98.
58. Berker N, Ozdamar Y, Soykan E. Vogt–Koyanagi–Harada syndrome in children: report of a case and review of the literature. Ocul Immunol Inflamm 2007;15:351–357.
59. Saatci AO, Pasa E, Soylev MF, et al. Sympathetic ophthalmia and indocyanine green angiography. Arch Ophthalmol 2004;122:1568.
60. Ishioka M, Ohno S, Nakamura S, et al. FK506 treatment of noninfectious uveitis. Am J Ophthalmol 1994;118:723–729.
61. Chan CC, Roberge RG, Whitcup SM. 32 cases of sympathetic ophthalmia. A retrospective study at the National Eye Institute, Bethesda, Md., from 1982 to 1992. Arch Ophthalmol 1995;113:597–600.
62. Hakin KN, Pearson RV, Lightman SL. Sympathetic ophthalmia: visual results with modern immunosuppressive therapy. Eye 1992;6:453–455.
63. Tessler HH, Jennings T. High-dose short-term chlorambucil for intractable sympathetic ophthalmia and Behçet's disease. Br J Ophthalmol 1990;74:353–357.

CHAPTER 23

Choroidal neovascularization secondary to inflammation, infection, and myopia

Jackie K. Nguyen, MD and Jeffrey S. Heier, MD

INTRODUCTION

Choroidal neovascularization (CNV) represents a pathologic growth of new blood vessels extending from the choroid into the subretinal or subretinal pigment epithelium (subRPE) space. A significant cause of vision loss, CNV results from a wide range of disorders that affect the RPE–Bruch's membrane–choriocapillaris complex.[1] CNV due to age-related macular degeneration (AMD) is the leading cause of irreversible severe vision loss among the elderly in the developed world. In patients younger than 50 years of age, CNV may occur as a secondary manifestation of various inherited and acquired conditions, including angioid streaks, high myopia, trauma, and infectious and inflammatory diseases. Idiopathic CNV refers to neovascularization which develops from an unknown etiology.[2]

DISEASE PREVALENCE

The prevalence of myopia in developed countries is reported to be between 11% and 36%, with degenerative myopia affecting up to one-third of the myopic population. The prevalence of degenerative myopia varies significantly among races and ethnic groups, from 0.2% in Egypt to 18% in Japan.[3] In the United States, myopia affects up to 25% of the population, with approximately 2% demonstrating high myopia.[4] A higher prevalence of myopia has been associated with younger birth cohorts, females, a higher educational level, higher socioeconomic classes, and near working habits.[3] CNV is the most common vision-threatening complication of high myopia, affecting 5–10% of eyes with high myopia.[5,6] In one series, high myopia was the most common cause of CNV in young patients, accounting for 62% of CNV cases in patients younger than 50 years of age.[7]

Presumed ocular histoplasmosis syndrome (POHS) is an inflammatory syndrome associated with systemic infection by *Histoplasma capsulatum*, a dimorphic fungus endemic in the soil in the Ohio and Mississippi river valleys of the United States. Epidemiologic studies have found the prevalence of POHS to range from 1.6 to 5.3%.[8] POHS occurs mostly in Caucasians in the second to fifth decade of life, with some studies reporting a higher prevalence in women.[9] POHS is the second leading cause of CNV in young patients, accounting for 12% of CNV cases in this age group.[7]

CNV due to angioid streaks, or linear breaks in Bruch's membrane, has been found to account for 5% of CNV cases in young patients. The remainder of CNV cases in young patients have been attributed to various hereditary, traumatic, or inflammatory disorders (4%) or considered idiopathic (17%) when no definitive etiology could be determined.[7]

RISK FACTORS

MYOPIA

Degenerative myopia, usually occurring in individuals with greater than 6 diopters of myopia or an axial length greater than 26 mm, is characterized by a progressive elongation of the globe associated with typical chorioretinal degenerative changes in the posterior pole.[3] Increasing axial length, posterior staphyloma, and lacquer cracks have been associated with a higher risk for myopic CNV.[6,10,11] One study found patchy chorioretinal atrophy and lacquer cracks to be the most important lesions in high myopia predisposing to the development of CNV. This study also found a higher incidence of CNV development in the fellow eyes of patients with pre-existing CNV (34.8%) than in eyes of patients without pre-existing CNV (6.1%).[6]

PRESUMED OCULAR HISTOPLASMOSIS SYNDROME

POHS is most common in the Ohio and Mississippi river valleys, where 60–80% of the population have been exposed to *H. capsulatum* and react positively to the histoplasmin skin antigen. The association between POHS and *H. capsulatum* is based on epidemiologic studies demonstrating a positive histoplasmin skin test in most patients with POHS. However, studies have identified patients with typical POHS findings who have not been exposed to *H. capsulatum*, indicating that this organism may be only one of several possible pathogens. Human leukocyte antigen (HLA) subtypes DRw2 and B7 have been found to be associated with POHS, suggesting a possible genetic or autoimmune predisposition to the development of POHS following infection with *H. capsulatum* or other causative pathogens.[8,9,12] Secondary CNV occurs in fewer than 5% of POHS patients with atrophic scars in the macular area. The chorioretinal scars may indicate focal infection or inflammation of the choroid, which leads to a disruption of Bruch's membrane and a stimulus for the development of CNV.[2,9,12]

OTHER INFLAMMATORY CAUSES

Active inflammation may lead directly to CNV, such as in cases of posterior uveitis, serpiginous choroidopathy, sarcoidosis, or syphilis. The most common inflammatory cause of CNV, however, is multifocal choroiditis and panuveitis (MCP), a disease of unknown etiology characterized by fundus lesions similar to those seen in POHS. Patients with MCP may develop CNV during episodes of active inflammation or from macular scars in periods without inflammation.[2] MCP occurs predominantly in myopic women between the second and sixth decades of life. The disease is bilateral in the majority of patients, although it frequently presents asymmetrically.[2,13,14]

ANGIOID STREAKS

Angioid streaks represent linear breaks in a thickened, calcified, and abnormally brittle Bruch's membrane. Angioid streaks may occur in isolation or as an ocular manifestation of several systemic diseases, including pseudoxanthoma elasticum (PXE), Paget's disease (osteitis deformans), sickle cell anemia, and Ehlers–Danlos syndrome. PXE, a primary disorder of elastic tissue, is the most common cause of angioid streaks. Greater than 50% of cases of angioid streaks have PXE, and 80–87% of patients with PXE show evidence of angioid streaks. Angioid streaks have been reported in 8–15% of patients with Paget's disease and in 1–2% of patients with sickle hemoglobinopathy. Angioid streaks almost always occur bilaterally. In surveys of patients with angioid streaks, CNV has been reported to occur in 44–57% of patients.[15–17]

IDIOPATHIC CNV

Patients presenting with idiopathic CNV usually have unilateral CNV and have a low risk of developing CNV in the fellow eye. There are no known ocular or systemic associations with idiopathic CNV.[2]

ETIOLOGY AND PATHOGENESIS

The mechanisms involved in the pathogenesis of CNV are not fully understood. Aging and genetically determined changes in the RPE–Bruch's membrane–choriocapillaris complex are important in inducing CNV, and wound-healing responses are instrumental for their progression and resolution.[1] Studies of eyes with CNV obtained surgically or postmortem have led to the concept that the development of CNV represents a wound repair response to a specific stimulus provided by the underlying disease. There are three basic CNV growth patterns: (1) subRPE, between the RPE and Bruch's membrane (type 1); (2) subretinal, between the retina and RPE (type 2); and (3) both subRPE and subretinal (combined). The type 1 pattern of CNV is the most typical pattern seen in AMD and starts with multiple ingrowth sites. The type 2 growth pattern likely occurs with single or few ingrowth sites and may occur in focal disease processes, such as POHS.[18]

Angiogenesis plays a causal role in the development of CNV in AMD. Vascular endothelial growth factor (VEGF) has been implicated as a major angiogenic stimulus responsible for neovascularization in AMD. VEGF stimulates angiogenesis through the promotion of endothelial cell proliferation and survival, vascular permeability, and recruitment of leukocytes.[19] Although the pathogenesis of CNV formation in other diseases may be different from that in AMD, preliminary evidence showing improvements in response to antiangiogenic therapy suggests that VEGF is also important in CNV attributable to causes other than AMD.

The pathogenesis of CNV due to non-AMD causes is often related to inflammation in close proximity to Bruch's membrane or breaks in Bruch's membrane, as in angioid streaks or lacquer cracks in myopia.[2] The pathogenesis of CNV in POHS is not clearly defined, but is believed to be related to focal infection or inflammation of the choroid at the time of systemic infection or autoimmune trigger. Choroidal scars represent a focal disruption of Bruch's membrane which leads to the formation of CNV. The stimulus that promotes the progression of some atrophic scars to neovascularization, while others remain quiescent, remains unknown.[9,12] The growth of new vessels in cases of inflammation suggests that inflammation, or injury resulting from inflammation, may be a driving stimulus for neovascularization.[2]

DIAGNOSIS AND ANCILLARY TESTING

MYOPIA

Myopic CNV is typically seen on biomicroscopy as a small, flat, grayish, subretinal membrane with hyperpigmented borders. The membranes are usually less than 1 disc diameter in size and are located in the subretinal space (type 2). Most myopic CNV is subfoveal or juxtafoveal with minimal subretinal fluid, hemorrhage, or exudate.

Fluorescein angiography (FA) is used to confirm the diagnosis of CNV. Myopic CNV tends to have a classic pattern of leakage on FA, with transit-phase hyperfluorescence followed by minor leakage in late phases (Figure 23.1). Indocyanine green (ICG), which is minimally absorbed by the RPE and blood, may allow better differentiation of CNV when subretinal hemorrhage or surrounding atrophy is present. FA and ICG angiography also help to detect subtle lacquer cracks.[3,20]

Optical coherence tomography (OCT) produces high resolution cross-sectional images of the retina and is useful in evaluating CNV and other macular pathologies. OCT can aid in treatment decisions by localizing CNV and detecting the presence of associated retinal thickening or subretinal fluid. Fluid accumulation within the neurosensory retina is usually moderate with myopic CNV (Figure 23.1).[3,20]

PRESUMED OCULAR HISTOPLASMOSIS SYNDROME

Presumed ocular histoplasmosis is a clinical diagnosis and relies on observation of characteristic fundus lesions in one or both eyes. The diagnosis of POHS is typically based on the presence of: (1) multiple discrete, atrophic choroidal scars in the macula or periphery that appear "punched out" of the inner layers of the choroid (histo spots); (2) peripapillary atrophy; and (3) CNV, or a fibrovascular disciform macular scar from resolution of CNV (Figure 23.2). In POHS, there is an absence of anterior chamber or vitreous inflammation. On fundus examination, the CNV appears as a yellow-green subretinal discoloration, sometimes surrounded by a pigment ring. In advanced cases, a central disciform scar from subretinal fibrosis is seen, and active CNV can be observed at the peripheral edge of the scar.[8,9,12] Patients with POHS generally have type 2 (subretinal) CNV.

Fluorescein angiography is performed to evaluate for CNV in patients with symptomatic visual loss or any signs of exudation. Areas of RPE atrophy, as with histo spots, will stain on FA. POHS commonly exhibits a classic CNV pattern, with early hyperfluorescence and late leakage (Figure 23.2).[21] OCT is performed to evaluate for intraretinal or subretinal fluid.

ANGIOID STREAKS

Angioid streaks are seen on ophthalmoscopy as irregular dark red to brown bands located deep to the retina and radiating from the optic disc. Fluorescein angiography can help to delineate the presence of angioid streaks when the ophthalmoscopic appearance is subtle. On FA, angioid streaks are variably hyperfluorescent depending on the condition of the overlying RPE (Figure 23.3). Transmission defects are seen in areas of thin RPE overlying an intact choriocapillaris. When present, CNV shows the classic increase in size and intensity of fluorescence as the angiogram progresses. Angioid streaks appear more prominent on ICG than on FA and fundus photography.[15,16]

INFLAMMATORY CAUSES

MCP is characterized by fundus lesions similar to those seen in POHS, including chorioretinal atrophic spots, peripapillary scarring, CNV, and linear streaks in the periphery. However, unlike POHS, patients with MCP have recurrent bouts of intraocular inflammation and are more likely to develop new chorioretinal atrophic lesions. MCP commonly presents with anterior and posterior chamber inflammation, and optic disc swelling may be seen.[2,13]

FA findings for MCP vary with the amount of intraocular inflammation. During quiescent periods, patients show scattered transmission defects in areas of chorioretinal atrophy. During active inflammation, retinal vascular leakage and late staining of the optic nerve may be seen. ICG angiography of active MCP shows numerous hypofluorescent spots and broad areas of hypofluorescence, corresponding to blind spots on visual field testing.[2]

There are two distinct subtypes or closely aligned disorders of MCP: punctate inner choroidopathy, characterized by smaller and more numerous lesions, and diffuse subretinal fibrosis, characterized by a prominent deposition of fibrosis associated with a multifocal choroiditis.[2]

DIFFERENTIAL DIAGNOSIS

AMD is the leading cause of CNV and should be considered in the differential diagnosis in virtually all cases. AMD is usually seen in patients older than 50 years of age. It is typically a bilateral process with associated clinical features of drusen, RPE atrophy, and focal pigmentary changes. Neovascular AMD is characterized by intraretinal or

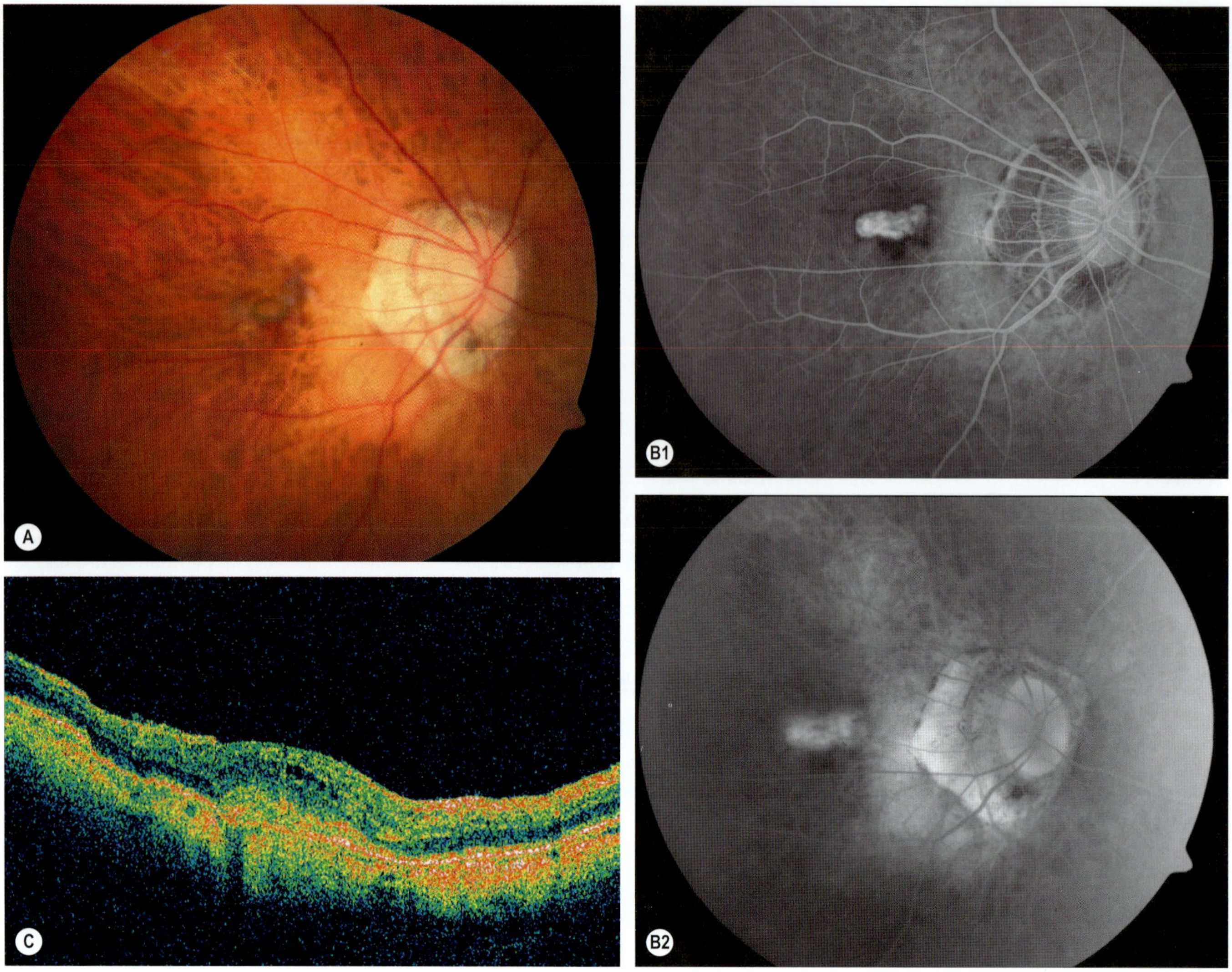

Figure 23.1 Myopic choroidal neovascularization (CNV). (A) Fundus photo showing typical small myopic CNV with surrounding hemorrhage. (B) Fluorescein angiogram showing early hyperfluorescence with late leakage. (C) Optical coherence tomography demonstrating intraretinal fluid.

subretinal fluid accumulation, hemorrhage, lipid exudation, and fibrosis (in the late stages).

CLINICAL SIGNS AND SYMPTOMS

MYOPIA

Typical fundus changes in high myopia include tilted discs, peripapillary atrophy, macular chorioretinal or RPE atrophy, and posterior staphyloma. Lacquer cracks are caused by spontaneous ruptures in Bruch's membrane and are commonly associated with small hemorrhages. The RPE overlying these hemorrhages atrophies, leaving a linear or stellate pattern of RPE loss. Fuchs' spots are submacular slightly raised and pigmented circular lesions which consist of an ingrowth of fibrovascular tissue. CNV is usually seen as a small light-gray round or elliptical macular lesion. Progressive atrophic changes in the macula often cause gradual visual loss by the fifth decade. The development of CNV causes visual loss at a younger age and induces a sudden painless reduction in vision, usually associated with metamorphopsia.[20]

PRESUMED OCULAR HISTOPLASMOSIS SYNDROME

Patients with POHS can be asymptomatic or present with an acute or insidious progressive blurring of central vision and metamorphopsia.[9] Fundus examination reveals multiple "punched-out" atrophic choroidal scars, peripapillary atrophy, and macular CNV or fibrovascular disciform scar, without anterior chamber or vitreous inflammation.[8,9,12]

ANGIOID STREAKS

Patients with angioid streaks are usually asymptomatic unless the macula is involved or CNV is present, leading to decreased vision or symptoms of metamorphopsia. Fundus examination reveals irregular linear dark red or brown bands radiating from the optic disc. A peculiar mottling of the RPE described as "peau d'orange" is commonly seen in the temporal midperiphery in patients with PXE, but has also been observed in patients with angioid streaks who do not have PXE.[15]

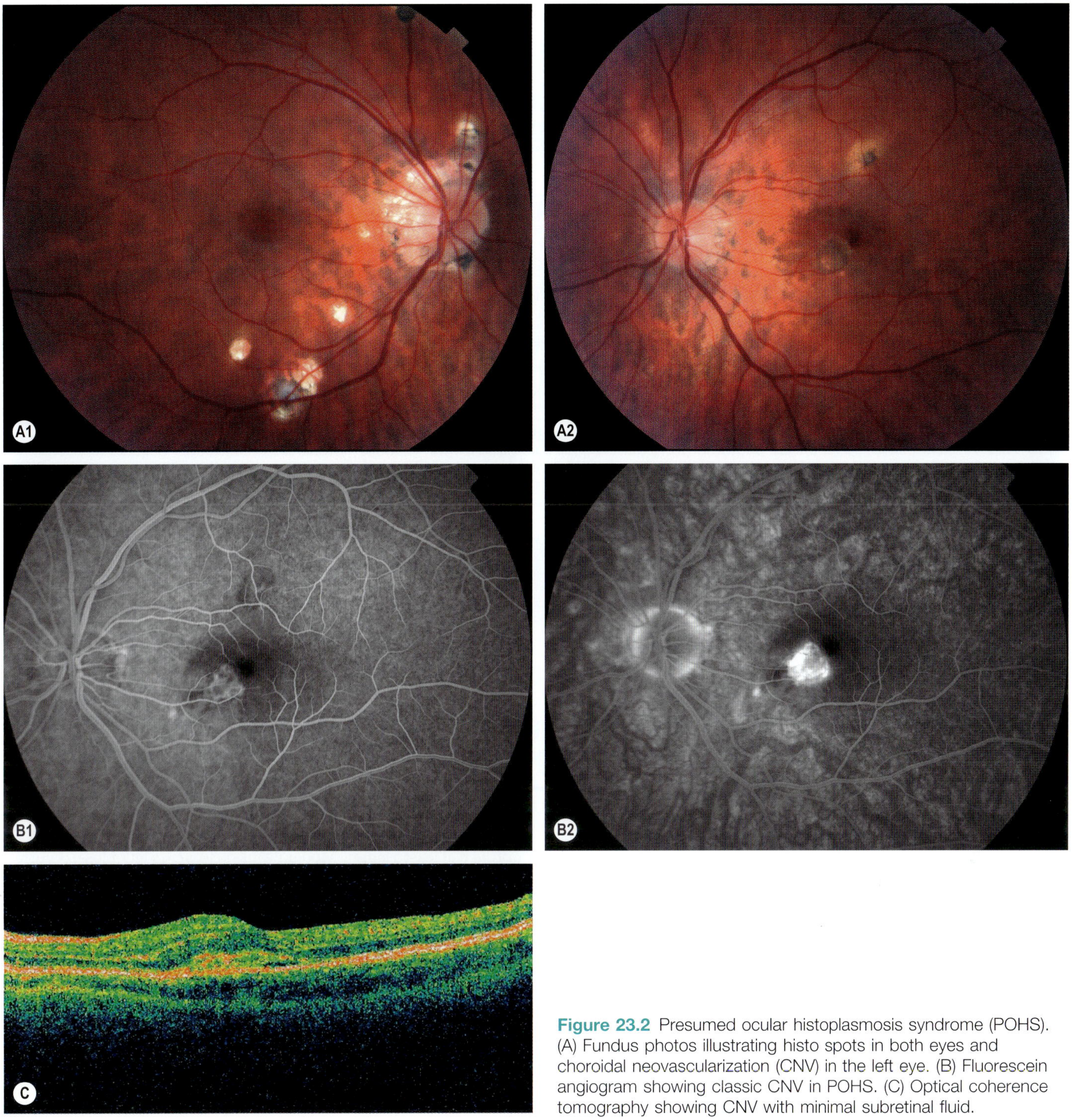

Figure 23.2 Presumed ocular histoplasmosis syndrome (POHS). (A) Fundus photos illustrating histo spots in both eyes and choroidal neovascularization (CNV) in the left eye. (B) Fluorescein angiogram showing classic CNV in POHS. (C) Optical coherence tomography showing CNV with minimal subretinal fluid.

INFLAMMATORY CAUSES

MCP is characterized by chorioretinal atrophic spots, peripapillary scarring, CNV, and linear streaks in the periphery, accompanied by intraocular inflammation. During the active phase, patients may have visual field defects, including enlarged blind spots and isolated scotomas, which resolve with resolution of the acute inflammation. Acute spots are a creamy yellow color, and with time the spots become more atrophic. The spots in MCP are usually smaller and more numerous and variable in size than those seen in POHS.[2]

TREATMENT

Despite its importance as a cause of visual impairment, no effective treatment has been established for CNV secondary to non-AMD-related causes. The design of therapeutic modalities for CNV is limited by the gaps in our understanding of the pathogenesis of CNV. Treatment for non-AMD-related CNV has been based on therapies developed for AMD, a much more common entity with more significant public health implications.[9]

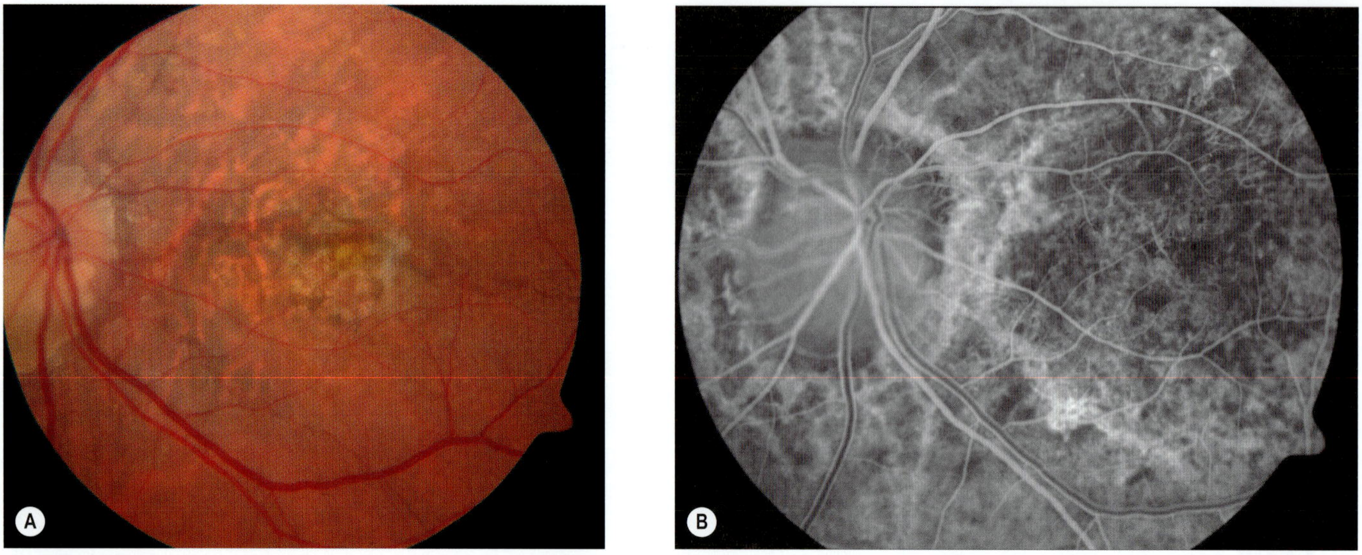

Figure 23.3 Angioid streaks. (A) Fundus photo showing dark red angioid streaks with macular fibrosis from choroidal neovascularization. (B) Fluorescein angiogram demonstrating hyperfluorescence of angioid streaks.

CONVENTIONAL LASER PHOTOCOAGULATION

For many years, thermal laser photocoagulation was the only proven treatment for CNV. Controlled trials showed a benefit from laser photocoagulation in well-demarcated CNV lesions associated with AMD. Laser photocoagulation has therefore been applied to the treatment of CNV due to myopia, POHS, and other non-AMD-related causes with variable results.

Several retrospective studies have demonstrated laser photocoagulation to be of limited benefit in improvement or stabilization of vision in myopic CNV.[22,23] These studies showed that while laser photocoagulation might cause occlusion of the myopic CNV and temporary vision improvement, prominent enlargement of the atrophic photocoagulation scar eventually results in a worse long-term visual prognosis.

In contrast to the results of laser treatment for myopic CNV, the Macular Photocoagulation Study (MPS) demonstrated that argon and krypton laser photocoagulation is effective in treating well-defined extrafoveal and juxtafoveal CNV associated with POHS. Eyes with extrafoveal CNV were randomized to argon laser treatment or to no treatment.[24] Untreated eyes demonstrated 3.6 times the risk of treated eyes of losing 6 lines or more of visual acuity (VA). After 5 years, treated eyes lost a mean of 0.9 lines of VA, compared to a loss of 4.4 lines in observed eyes. Eyes with juxtafoveal CNV secondary to POHS were randomized to krypton laser treatment or no treatment.[25] Approximately 11% of treated eyes lost 6 lines or more of VA compared with 30% of untreated eyes. As laser photocoagulation causes irreversible destruction of the retina and RPE, with resulting scotoma and immediate visual loss, the MPS did not evaluate the efficacy of laser photocoagulation in treating subfoveal CNV from histoplasmosis.

The MPS also demonstrated the benefits of laser photocoagulation in patients with extrafoveal and juxtafoveal idiopathic CNV.[26] Patients with idiopathic CNV were randomly assigned to krypton laser photocoagulation or to observation. After 3 years of follow-up, 10% of treated eyes compared with 37% of untreated eyes lost 6 lines or more of VA.

Retrospective studies of laser photocoagulation of CNV in patients with angioid streaks demonstrated that laser photocoagulation can result in closure of the CNV and either stabilization of VA or slowing of visual loss. A high rate of recurrence was reported, however, with CNV recurring in 77% of eyes.[27,28]

PHOTODYNAMIC THERAPY

Photodynamic therapy (PDT) with verteporfin (Visudyne; Novartis, Basel, Switzerland) consists of an intravenous infusion of verteporfin, a photosensitive drug which is activated by a laser light at 689 nm delivered at an intensity of 600 mW/cm^2 over 83 seconds. PDT causes incomplete occlusion of the treated vessels. The advantage of PDT lies in its ability to target CNV selectively without destroying the overlying retina.[29]

PDT for CNV secondary to pathologic myopia was evaluated in the Verteporfin in Photodynamic therapy (VIP) trial. Patients with subfoveal myopic CNV were randomly assigned to verteporfin or placebo. At 12 months, 72% of verteporfin-treated patients compared with 44% of placebo-treated patients lost fewer than 8 letters, and 32% versus 15% improved at least 5 letters. Moderate vision loss (>15 letter loss) occurred in 14% of PDT-treated eyes compared with 33% of placebo eyes.[30] While the 24-month data showed no statistically significant difference in the percentage of eyes losing at least 8 or 15 letters, the distribution of change in VA was in favor of a benefit for the patients assigned to verteporfin. Improvement by at least 5 letters was observed in 40% of verteporfin cases versus 13% of placebo cases, and improvement by at least 15 letters was seen in 12% of verteporfin cases versus 0 placebo cases. Based on both the 1- and 2-year results, the VIP study group recommended a consideration for verteporfin therapy for subfoveal CNV resulting from pathologic myopia.[31]

The Verteporfin in Ocular Histoplasmosis (VOH) study demonstrated the safety and efficacy of PDT with verteporfin for the treatment of subfoveal CNV in patients with POHS.[32] At 24 months, 22 patients treated with PDT had a median VA improvement of 6 letters. Ten patients (45%) gained 7 or more letters, whereas 4 patients (18%) lost 8 or more letters. There was absence of leakage on FA from classic CNV in 85% of the patients, and no leakage from occult CNV was observed.

PDT with verteporfin for the treatment of CNV secondary to angioid streaks has been evaluated in several retrospective case series, showing that PDT does not significantly prevent the progression of the disease and associated visual loss.[33,34] A small prospective study demonstrated an initial benefit of PDT after 1 year, but there was a progressive decline in vision after 2 years, as well as a failure to prevent subfoveal progression in the majority of cases.[35]

The treatment of CNV associated with idiopathic or inflammatory causes using PDT with verteporfin has been evaluated in several case series. Although the studies have been limited by a small number of patients and a short follow-up, these case series demonstrated that PDT is well tolerated and may be useful in stabilizing or improving vision in young adults with subfoveal or juxtafoveal CNV secondary to idiopathic or inflammatory etiologies.[36,37]

SURGICAL THERAPY

Submacular surgery for myopic CNV has been evaluated in several small case series which showed that surgical removal of myopic CNV can result in improvement or stabilization of vision. However, postoperative recurrence of CNV, RPE atrophy, and marked atrophic scar expansion lead to eventual visual decrease in many eyes following surgical removal of CNV, making this a less attractive option for the treatment of myopic CNV.[38,39]

The Submacular Surgery Trial (group H) was undertaken to evaluate the benefit of surgical therapy for idiopathic or POHS-related CNV.[40] A successful outcome, defined as a final VA better than or no more than 7 letters worse than initial VA, was seen in 46% of eyes in the observation arm and 55% in the surgery arm. In the subgroup of eyes with VA worse than 20/100 at baseline, 76% of eyes in the surgery group versus 50% of eyes in the observation group had a successful outcome. Recurrent CNV developed in 58% of surgical eyes at 24 months. Retinal detachment developed in 4.5% of eyes in the surgery group, and 24% of initially phakic eyes in the surgery arm had cataract surgery during follow-up. Overall, this trial demonstrated no benefit or a smaller benefit to surgery than the trial was designed to detect, although the data indicate that surgery may be advantageous for patients with VA worse than 20/100.

Macular translocation surgery is another surgical therapy for CNV which involves repositioning the neurosensory retina overlying the CNV on to an area of healthier RPE and choriocapillaris. Preliminary experience with limited macular translocation has shown that this treatment modality offers the potential to improve vision in some eyes with subfoveal CNV secondary to myopia, POHS, angioid streaks, idiopathic neovascularization, and multifocal choroiditis. However, a high rate of retinal detachment was seen. Further studies are needed to define the precise role of macular translocation in the management of these conditions.[41]

ANTIANGIOGENIC THERAPY

The development of antiangiogenic therapies represented a major advance in the treatment of CNV. Ranibizumab (Lucentis, Genentech) is a specific affinity-matured, recombinant, humanized, anti-VEGF antigen-binding antibody fragment (Fab) that binds and neutralizes all the biologically active forms of VEGF-A. Ranibizumab was approved by the Food and Drug Administration (FDA) for the treatment of neovascular AMD after several large clinical trials demonstrated the safety and efficacy of intravitreal injections of ranibizumab for neovascular AMD. Ranibizumab therapy was the first treatment for neovascular AMD shown to improve vision for a significant number of patients.[42] Bevacizumab (Avastin, Genentech) is a humanized, murine full-length antibody genetically modified from the same murine monoclonal antibody against VEGF as ranibizumab. Similar to ranibizumab, bevacizumab targets all the biologically active forms of VEGF-A. Bevacizumab is currently approved by the FDA for the treatment of metastatic colorectal cancer. Several case series have demonstrated the safety and efficacy of the off-label use of intravitreal bevacizumab for neovascular AMD.[43,44] Based on encouraging results of ranibizumab and bevacizumab for the treatment of AMD-related CNV, these antiangiogenic therapies have also been used in the treatment of CNV attributable to causes other than AMD.

Several case series have demonstrated promising short-term results using intravitreal bevacizumab for the treatment of CNV in pathologic myopia. Yamamoto et al. reported a retrospective case series of 11 eyes with myopic subfoveal CNV treated with intravitreal bevacizumab.[45] With a mean follow-up of 153 days, VA improved by a mean of 3.5 lines, 8 of 11 eyes achieved 20/50 or better, and mean OCT central foveal thickness decreased by 103 μm. Ruiz-Moreno et al. reported a prospective interventional study of bevacizumab for subfoveal and juxtafoveal myopic CNV in 26 eyes.[46] Patients were treated by three monthly injections with bevacizumab. Mean VA was 20/62 at baseline and 20/38 at month 6. Mean central foveal thickness was 282 μm at baseline and 224 μm at month 6. Leakage from CNV had ceased in all eyes at month 3, with closure of CNV lasting through month 6. No ocular or systemic safety issues were observed in either case series. These case series suggest that intravitreal bevacizumab is a safe and effective treatment for myopic CNV.

A retrospective case series has shown a benefit of intravitreal bevacizumab in patients with CNV associated with presumed ocular histoplasmosis.[47] Twenty-eight eyes underwent intravitreal injection of bevacizumab for the treatment of CNV secondary to POHS. After a follow-up of 22 weeks, mean VA improved from a logMAR VA of 0.65 (Snellen equivalent 20/88) to a final logMAR VA of 0.43 (Snellen equivalent 20/54). Twenty eyes (71%) experienced an increase in VA, 4 eyes (14%) were unchanged, and 4 eyes (14%) experienced a decrease in vision. This series demonstrated that intravitreal bevacizumab may improve or stabilize VA in a majority of patients with neovascular complications of POHS.

The results of intravitreal bevacizumab for the management of CNV in patients with PXE-associated angioid streaks have also been evaluated in an interventional case series of 9 eyes.[48] With a mean follow-up of 6 months, VA improved from a mean of 20/368 at baseline to 20/289 at the final visit. VA either improved or stabilized in all 9 eyes. OCT measurements decreased from a mean of 353 μm at baseline to 201 μm at the last visit. These short-term results support the use of intravitreal bevacizumab for the management of CNV in patients with angioid streaks.

Intravitreal bevacizumab has also been shown to be effective for idiopathic or inflammation-related CNV. Mandal et al. reported a prospective interventional case series of intravitreal bevacizumab in 32 eyes with idiopathic subfoveal CNV.[49] At 12 weeks, mean VA improved from 20/133 to 20/50, and mean central macular thickness decreased from 314 to 236 μm. At the final visit, 59% had a VA improvement of 3 lines or more, 34% remained stable, and 6% lost 3 lines or more. Adan et al. reported on the effects of intravitreal bevacizumab in 9 patients with inflammatory CNV.[50] Bevacizumab injection resulted in CNV closure and a significant decrease in OCT thickness. VA improved in 8 eyes (88.8%) and remained stable in 1 eye (11.2%). No significant ocular or systemic adverse effects were observed in the reported series. These short-term results suggest that intravitreal bevacizumab is safe and effective in idiopathic and inflammatory CNV.

An ongoing multicenter open-label trial has been initiated to evaluate the safety and efficacy of ranibizumab in patients with CNV secondary to causes other than AMD (Heier, unpublished data). Patients are randomized to receive ranibizumab for either 12 monthly injections or three initial injections followed by additional injections administered for persistence or recurrence of CNV. Preliminary results of 20 patients with at least 1-month follow-up show that ranibizumab may be a promising treatment for non-AMD-related CNV. Ten of the 20 patients were randomized to receive 12 monthly injections, and 10 were randomized to receive 3 injections followed by pro re nata (PRN) dosing. In the first group, the mean change in VA compared with baseline was an improvement of 18.3 letters (n = 10) at 1 month and 24.3 letters (n = 3) at 6 months. OCT central retinal thickness decreased by a mean of 113 μm at month 1 (n = 10) and 181 μm at month 6 (n = 3). In the second group, VA improved by a mean of 4.6 letters at 1 month (n = 10) and 16.7 letters at 6 months (n = 3). OCT central retinal thickness improved by 129 μm at month 1 (n = 10) and 215 μm at month 6 (n = 5) (Figure 23.4). Continued follow-up is necessary to confirm the preliminary findings of the safety and efficacy of ranibizumab in non-AMD-related CNV.

SUMMARY AND KEY POINTS

- CNV is a significant cause of vision loss in all age groups.
- In patients younger than 50 years of age, CNV may occur as a secondary manifestation of various inherited and acquired conditions:

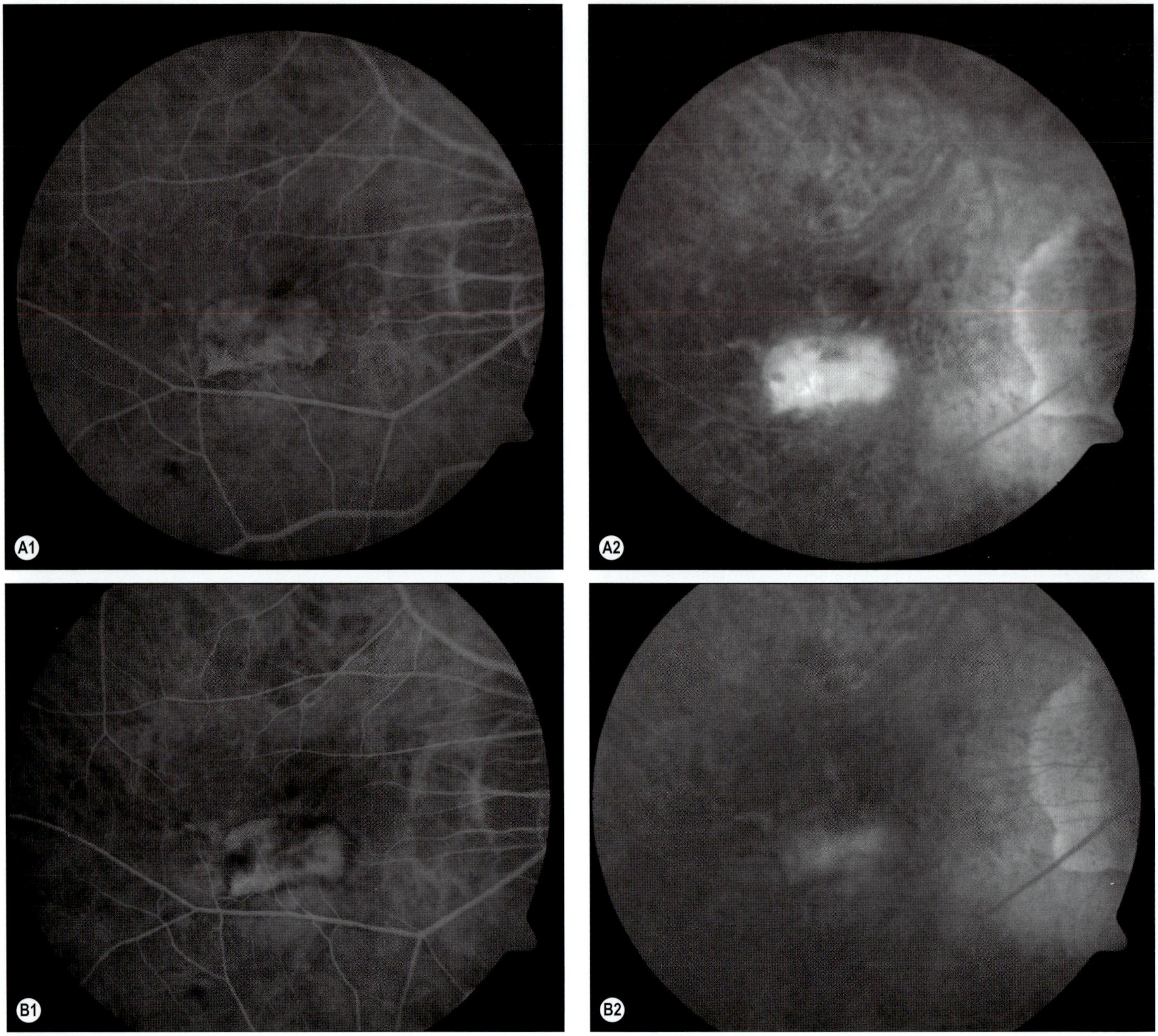

Figure 23.4 (A) Fluorescein angiogram (FA) of myopic choroidal neovascularization. (B) FA showing decreased leakage following ranibizumab treatment.

- High myopia (62%)
- POHS (12%)
- Angioid streaks (5%)
- Various hereditary, traumatic, or inflammatory disorders (4%)
- Idiopathic CNV (17%).

- FA and OCT are useful diagnostic tools in diagnosing and evaluating CNV.
- Treatment options are similar for CNV secondary to AMD:
  - Laser photocoagulation
  - PDT
  - Surgical therapy
  - Antiangiogenic therapy.

REFERENCES

1. Ryan SJ, Hinton DR, Murata T. Choroidal Neovascularization. In: Ryan SJ, editor. Retina, 4th edn. Philadelphia: Elsevier; 2006. p. 991–1009.
2. Spaide RF. Choroidal neovascularization in younger patients. Curr Opin Ophthalmol 1999;10:177–181.
3. Soubrane G, Coscas GJ. Choroidal neovascular membrane in degenerative myopia. In: Ryan SJ, editor. Retina, 4th edn. Philadelphia: Elsevier; 2006. p. 1115–1133.
4. Sperduto RD, Seigel D, Roberts J, et al. Prevalence of myopia in the United States. Arch Ophthalmol 1983;101:405–407.
5. Grossniklaus HE, Green WR. Pathologic findings in pathologic myopia. Retina 1992;12:127–133.
6. Ohno-Matsui K, Yoshida T, Futagami S, et al. Patchy atrophy and lacquer cracks predispose to the development of choroidal neovascularisation in pathological myopia. Br J Ophthalmol 2003;87:570–573.
7. Cohen SY, Laroche A, Leguen Y, et al. Etiology of choroidal neovascularization in young patients. Ophthalmology 1996;103:1241–1244.
8. Hawkins BS, Alexander J, Solomon SD, et al. Ocular histoplasmosis. In: Ryan SJ, editor. Retina, 4th edn. Philadelphia: Elsevier; 2006. p. 1749–1762.
9. Oliver A, Ciulla TA, Comer GM. New and classic insights into presumed ocular histoplasmosis syndrome and its treatment. Curr Opin Ophthalmol 2005;16:160–165.
10. Steidl SM, Pruett RC. Macular complications associated with posterior staphyloma. Am J Ophthalmol 1997;123:181–187.
11. Hotchkiss ML, Fine SL. Pathologic myopia and choroidal neovascularization. Am J Ophthalmol 1981;91:177–183.
12. Prasad AG, Van Gelder RN. Presumed ocular histoplasmosis syndrome. Curr Opin Ophthalmol 2005;16:364–368.

13. Vianna RN, Ozdal PC, Filho JP, et al. Longterm follow-up of patients with multifocal choroiditis and panuveitis. Acta Ophthalmol Scand 2004;82: 748–753.
14. Brown Jr J, Folk JC, Reddy CV, et al. Visual prognosis of multifocal choroiditis, punctate inner choroidopathy, and the diffuse subretinal fibrosis syndrome. Ophthalmology 1996;103:1100–1105.
15. Clarkson JG, Altman RD. Angioid streaks. Surv Ophthalmol 1982;26:235–246.
16. Shields JA, Federman JL, Tomer TL, et al. Angioid streaks. I. Ophthalmoscopic variations and diagnostic problems. Br J Ophthalmol 1975;59:257–266.
17. Deutman AF, Hoyng CB, van Lith-Verhoeven JJC. Macular dystrophies. In: Ryan SJ, editor. Retina, 4th edn. Philadelphia: Elsevier; 2006. p. 1163–1209.
18. Grossniklaus HE, Green WR. Choroidal neovascularization. Am J Ophthalmol 2004;137:496–503.
19. Ng EW, Adamis AP. Targeting angiogenesis, the underlying disorder in neovascular age-related macular degeneration. Can J Ophthalmol 2005;40:352–368.
20. Chan WM, Ohji M, Lai TY, et al. Choroidal neovascularisation in pathological myopia: an update in management. Br J Ophthalmol 2005;89:1522–1528.
21. Ciulla TA, Piper HC, Xiao M, et al. Presumed ocular histoplasmosis syndrome: update on epidemiology, pathogenesis, and photodynamic, antiangiogenic, and surgical therapies. Curr Opin Ophthalmol 2001;12:442–449.
22. Jalkh AE, Weiter JJ, Trempe CL, et al. Choroidal neovascularization in degenerative myopia: role of laser photocoagulation. Ophthalmic Surg 1987;18:721–725.
23. Secretan M, Kuhn D, Soubrane G, et al. Long-term visual outcome of choroidal neovascularization in pathologic myopia: natural history and laser treatment. Eur J Ophthalmol 1997;7:307–316.
24. Argon laser photocoagulation for neovascular maculopathy. Five-year results from randomized clinical trials. Macular Photocoagulation Study Group. Arch Ophthalmol 1991;109:1109–1114.
25. Laser photocoagulation for juxtafoveal choroidal neovascularization. Five-year results from randomized clinical trials. Macular Photocoagulation Study Group. Arch Ophthalmol 1994;112:500–509.
26. Krypton laser photocoagulation for idiopathic neovascular lesions. Results of a randomized clinical trial. Macular Photocoagulation Study Group. Arch Ophthalmol 1990;108:832–837.
27. Lim JI, Bressler NM, Marsh MJ, et al. Laser treatment of choroidal neovascularization in patients with angioid streaks. Am J Ophthalmol 1993;116:414–423.
28. Pece A, Avanza P, Galli L, et al. Laser photocoagulation of choroidal neovascularization in angioid streaks. Retina 1997;17:12–16.
29. Regillo CD. Update on photodynamic therapy. Curr Opin Ophthalmol 2000;11:166–170.
30. Photodynamic therapy of subfoveal choroidal neovascularization in pathologic myopia with verteporfin. 1-year results of a randomized clinical trial – VIP report no. 1. Ophthalmology 2001;108:841–852.
31. Blinder KJ, Blumenkranz MS, Bressler NM, et al. Verteporfin therapy of subfoveal choroidal neovascularization in pathologic myopia: 2-year results of a randomized clinical trial – VIP report no. 3. Ophthalmology 2003;110:667–673.
32. Rosenfeld PJ, Saperstein DA, Bressler NM, et al. Photodynamic therapy with verteporfin in ocular histoplasmosis: uncontrolled, open-label 2-year study. Ophthalmology 2004;111:1725–1733.
33. Heimann H, Gelisken F, Wachtlin J, et al. Photodynamic therapy with verteporfin for choroidal neovascularization associated with angioid streaks. Graefes Arch Clin Exp Ophthalmol 2005;243:1115–1123.
34. Shaikh S, Ruby AJ, Williams GA. Photodynamic therapy using verteporfin for choroidal neovascularization in angioid streaks. Am J Ophthalmol 2003;135:1–6.
35. Browning AC, Amoaku WM, Chung AK, et al. Photodynamic therapy for angioid streaks. Ophthalmology 2007;114:1592.
36. Rogers AH, Duker JS, Nichols N, et al. Photodynamic therapy of idiopathic and inflammatory choroidal neovascularization in young adults. Ophthalmology 2003;110:1315–1320.
37. Wachtlin J, Heimann H, Behme T, et al. Long-term results after photodynamic therapy with verteporfin for choroidal neovascularizations secondary to inflammatory chorioretinal diseases. Graefes Arch Clin Exp Ophthalmol 2003;241:899–906.
38. Uemura A, Thomas MA. Subretinal surgery for choroidal neovascularization in patients with high myopia. Arch Ophthalmol 2000;118:344–350.
39. Ruiz-Moreno JM, de la Vega C. Surgical removal of subfoveal choroidal neovascularisation in highly myopic patients. Br J Ophthalmol 2001;85:1041–1043.
40. Hawkins BS, Bressler NM, Bressler SB, et al. Surgical removal vs observation for subfoveal choroidal neovascularization, either associated with the ocular histoplasmosis syndrome or idiopathic: I. Ophthalmic findings from a randomized clinical trial: Submacular Surgery Trials (SST) Group H Trial: SST report no. 9. Arch Ophthalmol 2004;122:1597–1611.
41. Fujii GY, Humayun MS, Pieramici DJ, et al. Initial experience of inferior limited macular translocation for subfoveal choroidal neovascularization resulting from causes other than age-related macular degeneration. Am J Ophthalmol 2001;131:90–100.
42. Rosenfeld PJ, Rich RM, Lalwani GA. Ranibizumab: phase III clinical trial results. Ophthalmol Clin North Am 2006;19:361–372.
43. Rich RM, Rosenfeld PJ, Puliafito CA, et al. Short-term safety and efficacy of intravitreal bevacizumab (Avastin) for neovascular age-related macular degeneration. Retina 2006;26:495–511.
44. Avery RL, Pieramici DJ, Rabena MD, et al. Intravitreal bevacizumab (Avastin) for neovascular age-related macular degeneration. Ophthalmology 2006;113:363–372 e5.
45. Yamamoto I, Rogers AH, Reichel E, et al. Intravitreal bevacizumab (Avastin) as treatment for subfoveal choroidal neovascularisation secondary to pathological myopia. Br J Ophthalmol 2007;91:157–160.
46. Ruiz-Moreno JM, Gomez-Ulla F, Montero JA, et al. Intravitreous bevacizumab to treat subfoveal choroidal neovascularization in highly myopic eyes: short-term results. Eye 2009 Feb;23(2):334–338.
47. Schadlu R, Blinder KJ, Shah GK, et al. Intravitreal bevacizumab for choroidal neovascularization in ocular histoplasmosis. Am J Ophthalmol 2008 May;145(5):875–878.
48. Bhatnagar P, Freund KB, Spaide RF, et al. Intravitreal bevacizumab for the management of choroidal neovascularization in pseudoxanthoma elasticum. Retina 2007;27:897–902.
49. Mandal S, Garg S, Venkatesh P, et al. Intravitreal bevacizumab for subfoveal idiopathic choroidal neovascularization. Arch Ophthalmol 2007;125:1487–1492.
50. Adan A, Mateo C, Navarro R, et al. Intravitreal bevacizumab (avastin) injection as primary treatment of inflammatory choroidal neovascularization. Retina 2007;27:1180–1186.

CHAPTER 24

Ocular infection: endophthalmitis

Stephen G. Schwartz, MD, MBA, Harry W. Flynn, Jr., MD, and Taraprasad Das, MD, FRCS

INTRODUCTION

Endophthalmitis is characterized by marked inflammation of intraocular fluids and tissues. Severe visual loss may occur, even with prompt and appropriate diagnosis and treatment. Infective endophthalmitis may be categorized by the cause of the infection and the characteristic timing of clinical signs and symptoms.[1] Categorization helps predict the underlying etiology and most likely causative organisms (Table 24.1).

The major category, representing over 70% of cases, is acute-onset, postoperative endophthalmitis, which is defined as endophthalmitis presenting within 6 weeks of intraocular surgery (Figure 24.1).[1] Chronic postoperative endophthalmitis presents more than 6 weeks following intraocular surgery. Filtering bleb-associated endophthalmitis may present months or years following glaucoma filtering surgery.[2] Posttraumatic endophthalmitis occurs following open-globe injuries. Endogenous endophthalmitis occurs from hematogenous spread of systemic infection. Endophthalmitis may be associated with microbial keratitis[3] and following office-based intravitreal injection.[4]

DISEASE INCIDENCE

The incidence of acute-onset postoperative endophthalmitis is in the range of 0.036–0.36% of eyes undergoing intraocular surgery.[5–7] A 2005 survey of 15 920 cataract surgical procedures performed at the Bascom Palmer Eye Institute reported a risk of 0.04% following cataract surgery.[8] An earlier survey reported rates of endophthalmitis of 0.2% following secondary intraocular lens (IOL) implantation, 0.2% after glaucoma surgery, and 0.03% after pars plana vitrectomy (PPV).[9] In the USA, Medicare claims data suggest that the incidence of acute-onset postoperative endophthalmitis may be increasing.[10]

The incidence of endophthalmitis following 20-gauge transscleral PPV was historically lower than that following other types of intraocular surgery. However, the rate of endophthalmitis following small-gauge transconjunctival sutureless vitrectomy may be higher than that following 20-gauge PPV. Three recent retrospective series have reported an incidence of endophthalmitis following 25-gauge transconjunctival sutureless vitrectomy between 0.23% and 1.6%, as compared with an incidence following 20-gauge PPV of 0–0.03%.[11–13]

One series of open-globe injuries has reported an endophthalmitis rate of 6.8%.[14]

The incidence of endophthalmitis following intravitreal injections in prospective clinical trials is in the range of 1% per eye (Table 24.2).[15–18] These reported rates relate to eyes, not to the number of total injections. In these trials, most eyes underwent a series of injections, so the incidence of endophthalmitis per injection is very low. For example, a recent report combining two large randomized clinical trials found an incidence of 0.05% per injection.[19] The published rates of infection following intravitreal triamcinolone acetonide[20] and bevacizumab[21] (Avastin, Genentech, South San Francisco, CA) are generally in the range of 0.1% per injection or less. Recent large, retrospective case series of intravitreal injections of bevacizumab, ranibizumab (Lucentis, Genentech, South San Francisco, CA), and pegaptanib (Macugen, Eyetech, New York, NY) generally report infection rates in the range of 0.05% (Table 24.3).[22]

RISK FACTORS

In acute-onset, postoperative endophthalmitis, preoperative risk factors include immune compromise (e.g., diabetes mellitus or immunosuppressive medications), chronic blepharitis, disease of the lacrimal drainage system, contaminated eye drops, contact lens wear, a contralateral ocular prosthesis, and active infection elsewhere in the body. Intraoperative risk factors include prolonged surgery, secondary IOL implantation, posterior capsular rupture, vitreous loss, iris prolapse, contaminated irrigating solutions or IOLs, and a slightly inferotemporal clear corneal incision. Postoperative risk factors include wound leaks and vitreous incarceration in the wound.

Some authors have suggested that clear cornea wounds are a risk factor for infection,[23] but in a large series from the Bascom Palmer Eye Institute, the surgical technique (clear cornea phacoemulsification versus other methods) did not affect the incidence of endophthalmitis.[8] In general, the clinical course, causative organisms, and visual outcomes from endophthalmitis following clear cornea cataract surgery are similar to those from other methods of cataract surgery.[24]

Using evidence-based medicine criteria, povidone-iodine antisepsis is the only technique to reach category II evidence for prevention of postoperative endophthalmitis.[25]

Risk factors for filtering bleb-associated endophthalmitis include a history of conjunctivitis, contaminated topical glaucoma medications, contact lenses, an inferior filtering bleb, bleb leak, bleb manipulations, and nasolacrimal duct obstruction.[2] Risk factors for posttraumatic endophthalmitis include delayed primary repair (beyond 24 hours), soil-associated injuries, retained intraocular foreign bodies, and breach of lens capsule.[14] Possible, but unproven, risk factors for endophthalmitis following 25-gauge transconjunctival sutureless vitrectomy include unsutured sclerotomy wounds, vitreous wick syndrome, early postoperative hypotony, increasing use of adjuvants (such as intravitreal triamcinolone acetonide), and the reluctance of some surgeons to use subconjunctival antibiotics in these patients. Risk factors for endogenous endophthalmitis include debilitation, immune compromise, and intravenous drug abusers.[26] Microbial keratitis is very infrequently associated with endophthalmitis, unless associated with corneal perforation.

The incidence of endophthalmitis following intravitreal injection can be reduced with a standardized protocol for aseptic injections, including the use of a sterile eyelid speculum and povidone-iodine.[27] For example, in the VISION study, most endophthalmitis cases occurred in the setting of a protocol deviation.[15] Prophylactic topical antibiotics are commonly used, although their efficacy is unproven.[28]

ETIOLOGY/PATHOGENESIS

The etiology of infective endophthalmitis is predicted by the clinical features and past history, and this is summarized in Table 24.1.[29–33] Posttraumatic endophthalmitis is frequently caused by relatively more virulent organisms, such as *Bacillus cereus*.[34]

Endogenous endophthalmitis is more frequently caused by fungi, but bacterial cases may also occur.[26] The most common causative organisms include *Candida albicans* and *Aspergillus* species. In bacterial

Table 24.1 Categories of endophthalmitis, with common causative organisms

Acute-onset postoperative	Coagulase-negative staphylococcus
	Staphylococcus aureus
	Streptococcus species
Delayed-onset (chronic) postoperative	*Propionibacterium acnes*
	Candida parapsilosis
	Coagulase-negative staphylococcus
Filtering bleb-associated	*Streptococcus* species
	Staphylococcus species
	Haemophilus influenzae
Posttraumatic	*Staphylococcus* species
	Bacillus cereus
Endogenous	*Candida albicans*
	Aspergillus species
Following microbial keratitis	Gram-negative organisms
	Staphylococcus aureus
	Fusarium species
Following intravitreal injection	Coagulase-negative staphylococcus

Adapted from Schwartz SG, Flynn HW Jr, Scott IU. Endophthalmitis: classification and current management. Expert Review Ophthalmol 2007;2:385–396.

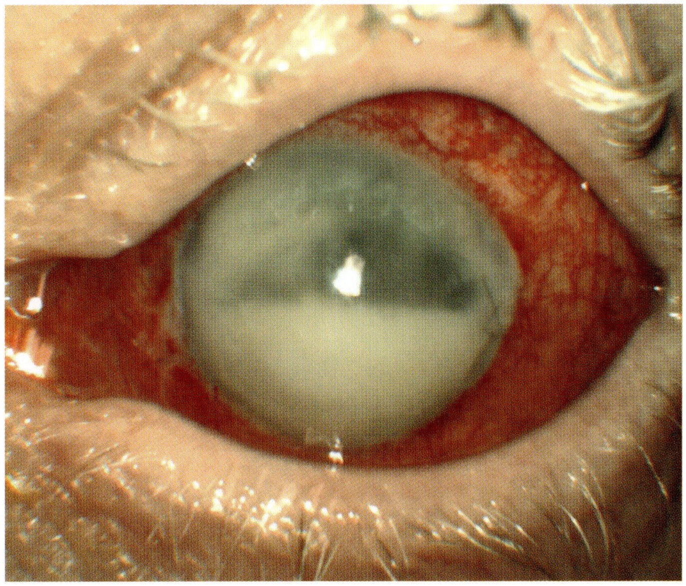

Figure 24.1 Acute-onset endophthalmitis. This patient underwent intraocular lens repositioning and developed coagulase-negative staphylococcus endophthalmitis. Despite vitreous tap and injection, followed by two vitrectomies, the eye lost all visual function.

Table 24.2 Incidence of endophthalmitis following intravitreal injection: selected prospective clinical trials

Study	Medication	Cases	Treated eyes	Incidence
VISION[15]	Pegaptanib sodium (Macugen, OSI/ Eyetech, Melville, NY)	12*	890	1.3%
Ranibizumab phase I/II[16]	Ranibizumab (Lucentis, Genentech, South San Francisco, CA)	1	62	1.6%
ANCHOR[17]	Ranibizumab	2†	277	0.7%
MARINA[18]	Ranibizumab	5‡	477	1.0%

Note: These studies reported incidence per eye (most eyes received a series of injections).

**Two-thirds of cases associated with deviations in injection protocol.*

†In the 0.3-mg group, there were 0/137 cases (0%). In the 0.5-mg group, there were 2/140 cases (1.4%). Pooled data are presented here.

‡In the 0.3 mg group, there were 2/238 cases (0.8%). In the 0.5 mg group, there were 3/239 cases (1.3%). Pooled data are presented here.

Adapted from Schwartz SG, Flynn HW Jr, Scott IU. Endophthalmitis: classification and current management. Expert Rev Ophthalmol 2007;2,385–396.

Table 24.3 Incidence of endophthalmitis following intravitreal injection: selected observational case series

First author	Medication	Cases	Injections	Incidence
Westfall[20]	Triamcinolone acetonide	1	1006	0.099%
Fung[21]	Bevacizumab	1	7113	0.014%
Moshfeghi[52]	Triamcinolone acetonide	8	922	0.87%

Note: these retrospective studies reported incidence rate per injection, not per eye.

Adapted from Schwartz SG, Flynn HW Jr, Scott IU. Endophthalmitis: classification and current management. Expert Rev Ophthalmol 2007;2,385–396.

endogenous endophthalmitis, the most common causative organisms are *B. cereus*, *Staphylococcus aureus*, *Klebsiella*, *Pseudomonas*, and *Streptococcus* species.[35,36]

Traditionally, endophthalmitis associated with microbial keratitis has been caused by Gram-negative organisms, *Staphylococcus aureus*, streptococcal species, and various fungi.[37] Recent outbreaks of *Fusarium* keratitis have been associated with soft contact lenses,[38–40] and recent series of endophthalmitis in eyes with *Fusarium* keratitis have been reported.[3,41]

Infective endophthalmitis following intravitreal injection is typically due to coagulase-negative staphylococci.[22]

DIAGNOSIS AND ANCILLARY TESTING/ DIFFERENTIAL DIAGNOSIS

Infective endophthalmitis is a clinical diagnosis but may be confirmed by evaluation of intraocular fluid specimens. The clinical signs are variable and depend on the infecting organism, the duration of infection, the associated inflammation, and various patient risk factors, such as prior surgery, trauma, and immune status, as previously discussed.

Obtaining intraocular cultures is important in the work-up of endophthalmitis. A vitreous specimen is more likely to yield a positive culture result than a simultaneously acquired aqueous specimen.[42] The vitreous specimen can be obtained by needle biopsy (vitreous tap) or by the use of automated vitrectomy instrumentation. If a needle biopsy approach is selected, a butterfly needle may offer better stability than a tuberculin syringe.[43] A single-port transconjunctival sutureless vitrector has been advocated for the treatment of endophthalmitis in the office setting. This device, the Visitrec vitrectomy unit (Insight Instruments, Stuart, FL), combines the theoretical advantages of standard PPV without the associated delays in treatment or increased expenses.[44,45]

Depending on the volume of the specimen and the clinical setting, alternative culture techniques can be selected.[1] The traditional approach, direct inoculation of the specimen on to culture media, is commonly selected. Culture media may include 5% blood agar, for most common bacterial and fungal pathogens; chocolate agar, for fastidious organisms such as *Neisseria gonorrhoeae* and *Haemophilus influenzae*; Saboraud agar, for fungi; thioglycollate broth; and anaerobic blood agar. Alternatively, the specimen may be injected into blood culture bottles, which are particularly useful in after-hours emergency cases.[46]

The differential diagnosis of marked inflammation following intraocular surgery is listed in Table 24.4. Sterile inflammation may be secondary to retained lens fragments or foreign material introduced during surgery. Retained cortical fragments may cause more severe inflammation than nuclear fragments, and these eyes occasionally present with hypopyon.[47]

Toxic anterior-segment syndrome (TASS) is a sterile inflammatory reaction of moderate to severe intensity, usually within 12–48 hours after intraocular surgery. Typical signs include corneal edema, anterior-chamber cell and flare with fibrin and/or hypopyon, an unreactive pupil, and elevated intraocular pressure (Figure 24.2).[48] TASS may be caused by exposure to various foreign substances, including the IOL, ointments, and disinfecting compounds.[49–51] In some patients, TASS may be difficult to distinguish from infective endophthalmitis. Typically, TASS presents earlier, and the signs are confined to the anterior segment. The corneal edema may be out of proportion to the level of inflammation. TASS may present in a cluster of patients from the same surgical center.

Table 24.4 Differential diagnosis of marked inflammation following cataract surgery

Endophthalmitis
Toxic anterior-segment syndrome (TASS)
Retained lens fragments
Flare-up of pre-existing uveitis
Triamcinolone acetonide particles
Longstanding (dehemoglobinized) vitreous hemorrhage

Adapted from Schwartz SG, Flynn HW Jr, Scott IU. Endophthalmitis: classification and current management. Expert Rev Ophthalmol 2007;2,385–396.

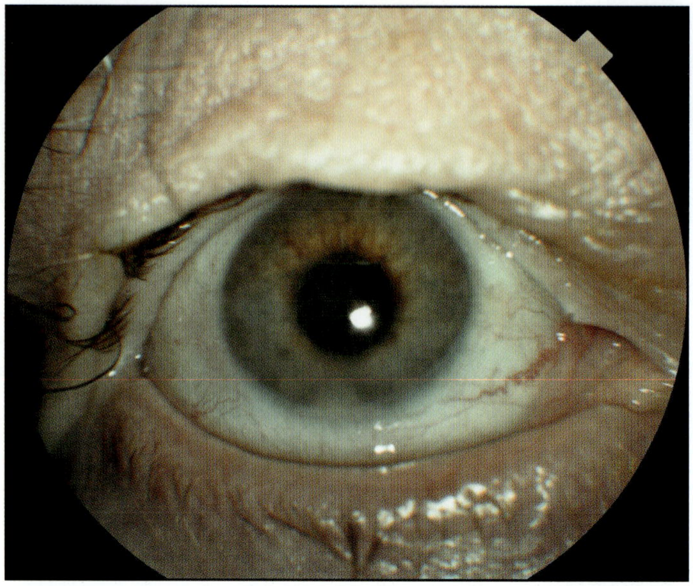

Figure 24.2 Toxic anterior-segment syndrome. Note the small hypopyon and the lack of other inflammatory signs.

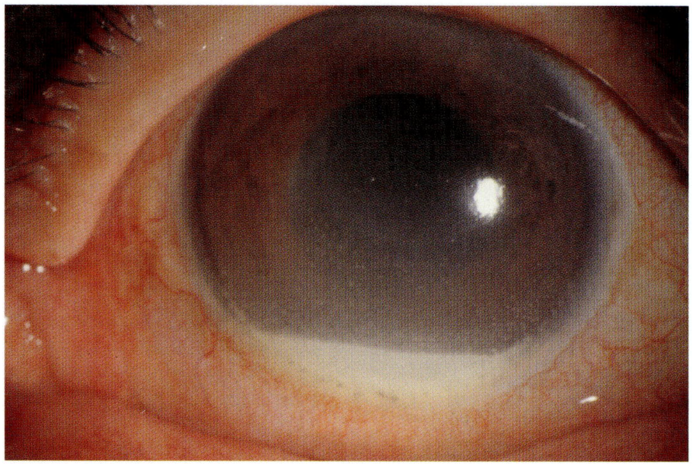

Figure 24.3 Pseudohypopyon following intravitreal injection of triamcinolone acetonide.

Eyes with noninfective foreign material in the anterior chamber may appear similar to eyes with endophthalmitis. For example, particles of triamcinolone may migrate anteriorly, mimicking a hypopyon (Figure 24.3).[52] Intraocular blood, particularly when dehemoglobinized, may be confused with infective material.[53,54]

SIGNS AND SYMPTOMS

OCULAR

In acute-onset postoperative bacterial endophthalmitis, there is typically acute-onset visual loss and redness, associated with marked intraocular inflammation, anterior chamber, fibrin, and hypopyon.[1] Eyelid

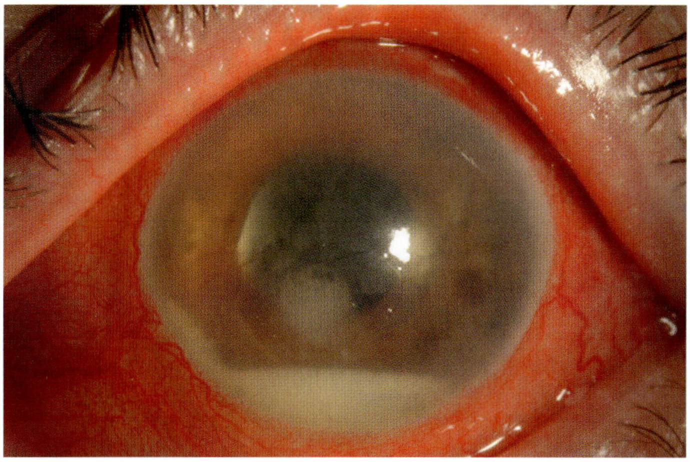

Figure 24.4 Endophthalmitis associated with microbial keratitis.

edema, conjunctival congestion, vitreous inflammation, and retinal periphlebitis may be noted. Chronic postoperative endophthalmitis is typically marked by relatively mild but progressive inflammation and an indolent course. In filtering bleb-associated endophthalmitis, clinical features include purulent bleb involvement, as well as aqueous and vitreous inflammation, including hypopyon.[2]

As compared with bacterial endophthalmitis, fungal endophthalmitis is generally associated with less inflammation, a more indolent course, and less pain. Endogenous endophthalmitis due to *Candida* often manifests as isolated white infiltrates in formed vitreous overlying a localized area of chorioretinitis.

Endophthalmitis following open-globe injuries is often severe and rapidly progressive. In contrast, there is frequently a delay in diagnosis of endophthalmitis associated with microbial keratitis, because of the recognition that many cases of keratitis with hypopyon do not have endophthalmitis. Additionally, the posterior-segment findings (including echography) may be relatively mild or not helpful in establishing the diagnosis. The diagnosis should be suspected when patients with keratitis continue to worsen despite appropriate topical, systemic, and other therapy (including, in some cases, penetrating keratoplasty) (Figure 24.4).

SYSTEMIC

Typically, the systemic findings in infectious endophthalmitis are minimal. An exception is endogenous endophthalmitis, in which there may be systemic signs of infection, such as fever or debilitation.

TREATMENT OPTIONS

In the management of endophthalmitis, safe and effective antimicrobial agents are selected. In most cases, culture results are not available until days after initiation of treatment. Therefore, initial therapy should provide coverage for a broad range of Gram-positive and Gram-negative organisms. Many of the current treatment guidelines originate from the Endophthalmitis Vitrectomy Study (EVS), a randomized, multicenter, clinical trial which treated all patients with intravitreal vancomycin and amikacin; subconjunctival vancomycin, ceftazidime, and dexamethasone; and systemic corticosteroids.[55] The results of the EVS are summarized in Table 24.5.[30,56,57] Several points must be considered when applying these results to clinical practice.

First, the EVS reported a benefit for PPV only in eyes with visual acuity of light perception. However, in selected rapid onset cases with moderate or severe vitreous inflammation, PPV may be considered, even when visual acuity is better than light perception. PPV may be performed using a two-port (end-irrigating light pipe and vitreous cutter) or standard three-port technique. Small-gauge transconjunctival sutureless vitrectomy is becoming more popular for this indication.[58]

Table 24.5 Endophthalmitis Vitrectomy Study (EVS)

1. Enrollment criteria
   - (a) Acute postoperative endophthalmitis (within 6 weeks of surgery)
   - (b) Following cataract surgery or secondary intraocular lens implantation
2. Vitreous tap versus pars plana vitrectomy (PPV)
   - (a) Patients with presenting visual acuity of hand motions (HM) or better
     - (i) No difference in outcomes between vitreous tap and PPV
   - (b) Patients with presenting visual acuity of light perception
     - (i) Better visual outcomes with PPV than with vitreous tap
     - (ii) Statistically significant
   - (c) Diabetic patients with presenting visual acuity of HM or better
     - (i) Slightly better visual outcomes with PPV than with vitreous tap
     - (ii) Not statistically significant
     - (iii) Either PPV or vitreous tap could be considered in this situation
3. Systemic antibiotics
   - (a) Systemic amikacin and ceftazidime offered no additional benefit over the observation group
   - (b) Other systemic antibiotics were not evaluated

Adapted from Schwartz SG, Flynn HW Jr, Scott IU. Endophthalmitis: classification and current management. Expert Rev Ophthalmol 2007;2,385–396.

Second, the EVS only recruited patients with acute-onset endophthalmitis following cataract surgery or secondary IOL implantation. Therefore, these results do not necessarily apply to other forms of endophthalmitis, which are more frequently caused by more virulent organisms. Thus, the benefits of PPV may be more important in these clinical settings.

Third, the antibiotic choices should be tailored to the individual patient. Even though the EVS used intravitreal amikacin, either intravitreal ceftazidime or ceftriaxone may be considered to avoid the risk of aminoglycoside toxicity. Although the EVS used subconjunctival antibiotics, two more recent clinical studies showed no difference in outcomes by using subconjunctival antibiotics in addition to intravitreal antibiotics.[59,60] The EVS reported no benefit from adjunctive systemic amikacin and ceftazidime, but there may be a rationale to use other systemic agents. For example, the fourth-generation fluoroquinolones achieve intraocular drug levels even in the noninflamed eye, although their benefit in endophthalmitis remains unproven.[61] Systemic gatifloxacin (Tequin, Bristol-Myers Squibb, New York, NY) is no longer commercially available because of the associated risks of hypoglycemia and hyperglycemia.[62] Another fourth-generation fluoroquinolone, moxifloxacin (Avelox, Bayer Healthcare, Wuppertal, Germany), is currently available but has the same limitations. Systemic ciprofloxacin may be beneficial for *Pseudomonas* endophthalmitis, because the MIC_{90} of ciprofloxacin is much lower than that of gatifloxacin or moxifloxacin.[63]

Fourth, the EVS treated all patients with systemic corticosteroids. Although systemic corticosteroids may improve final outcomes, caution is advised regarding systemic side-effects, particularly in elderly patients and those with diabetes mellitus.

Fifth, the EVS did not recruit patients with suspected fungal endophthalmitis. Many patients with endogenous fungal endophthalmitis will respond to systemic therapy alone, typically in consultation with an internist or infectious disease specialist. Systemic antifungals may be combined with PPV, which reduces fungal load and perhaps

Table 24.6 Clinically important antifungal agents

Agent	Mechanism of action
Intravitreal	
Amphotericin B	Disrupts fungal cell membranes
Fluconazole*	Inhibits synthesis of fungal cell membranes
Voriconazole	Synthetic inhibitor of synthesis of fungal cell membranes
Intravenous	
Amphotericin B	Disrupts fungal cell membranes
Echinocandins	Disrupt fungal cell wall
Fluconazole	Inhibits synthesis of fungal cell membranes
Voriconazole	Synthetic inhibitor of synthesis of fungal cell membranes
Oral	
Fluconazole	Inhibits synthesis of fungal cell membranes
Itraconazole	Inhibits synthesis of fungal cell membranes
Ketoconazole	Inhibits synthesis of fungal cell membranes
Posaconazole	Inhibits synthesis of fungal cell membranes
Voriconazole	Synthetic inhibitor of synthesis of fungal cell membranes

*Experimental.

increases intraocular penetration of systemic agents. In some patients, intravitreal antifungals are necessary. Traditionally, amphotericin B was used commonly, but some of the newer azole compounds are gaining increased acceptance in many situations. For example, intravitreal voriconazole (VFEND, Pfizer, New York, NY), a synthetic, second-generation triazole, has shown efficacy in some reports.[64] Various antifungal agents are listed in Table 24.6.

TREATMENT OUTCOMES AND PROGNOSIS

In the EVS, the most important predictor of final visual outcome was presenting visual acuity. Patients with presenting visual acuity of light perception or worse had the poorest outcomes.[30] Thus, early treatment of endophthalmitis is associated with improved visual outcomes. Prompt initiation of therapy is more important than any other factor, including PPV versus vitreous tap or the use of adjunctive systemic antibiotics.

Other independent predictors of poorer visual outcomes in the EVS include older age, diabetes mellitus, corneal infiltrate or ring ulcer, abnormal intraocular pressure, iris neovascularization, an absent red reflex, and an open posterior capsule.[65] The presence of a vitreous membrane on echography is associated with a poorer visual prognosis.[66]

SUMMARY AND KEY POINTS

Infective endophthalmitis is uncommon but may cause severe visual loss, even with prompt diagnosis and appropriate treatment. The clinical presentation aids in categorization of the patient, which helps predict the etiology and causative organisms. Endophthalmitis is a clinical diagnosis, but laboratory confirmation is important. A vitreous sample may be obtained either through needle tap or with automated vitrectomy instrumentation, depending on the clinical situation. Prompt institution of safe and effective antimicrobial therapy is important in achieving best visual outcomes.

ACKNOWLEDGMENTS

This study was supported in part by National Institutes of Health center grant P30-EY014801, and by an unrestricted grant to the University of Miami from Research to Prevent Blindness, New York, NY.

Harry W. Flynn, Jr., MD has served as a consultant to Alcon, Eli Lilly, Genentech, Novartis, Optimedica, and Pfizer. Stephen G. Schwartz, MD, MBA has received research funding from Genentech, owns equity in Pfizer, and is co-holder of a patent pending entitled "Molecular targets for modulating intraocular pressure and differentiation of steroid responders versus non-responders."

REFERENCES

1. Doft B. Endophthalmitis Management. Focal Points: Modules for Clinicians. San Francisco: American Academy of Ophthalmology; 1997.
2. Song A, Scott IU, Flynn Jr HW, et al. Delayed-onset bleb-associated endophthalmitis: clinical features and visual acuity outcomes. Ophthalmology 2002;109:985–991.
3. Rosenberg KD, Flynn Jr HW, Alfonso EC, et al. *Fusarium* endophthalmitis following keratitis associated with contact lenses. Ophthalmic Surg Lasers Imaging 2006;37:310–313.
4. Jonas JB, Kreissig I, Spandau UH, et al. Infectious and noninfectious endophthalmitis after intravitreal high-dosage triamcinolone acetonide. Am J Ophthalmol 2006;141:579–580.
5. Lundstrom M, Wejde G, Stenevi U, et al. Endophthalmitis after cataract surgery: A nationwide prospective study evaluating incidence in relation to incision type and location. Ophthalmology 2007;114:866–870.
6. Patwardhan A, Rao GP, Saha K, et al. Incidence and outcomes evaluation of endophthalmitis management after phacoemulsification and 3-piece silicone intraocular lens implantation over 6 years in a single eye unit. J Cataract Refract Surg 2006;32:1018–1021.
7. Kamalarajah S, Silvestri G, Sharma N, et al. Surveillance of endophthalmitis following cataract surgery in the UK. Eye 2004;18: 580–587.
8. Miller JJ, Scott IU, Flynn Jr HW, et al. Acute-onset endophthalmitis after cataract surgery (2000–2004): incidence, clinical settings, and visual acuity outcomes after treatment. Am J Ophthalmol 2005;139:983–987.
9. Eifrig CWG, Flynn Jr HW, Scott IU, et al. Acute-onset postoperative endophthalmitis: review of incidence and visual outcomes. Ophthalmic Surg Lasers 2002;33:373–378.
10. West ES, Behrens A, McDonnell PJ, et al. The incidence of endophthalmitis after cataract surgery among the U.S. Medicare population increased between 1994 and 2001. Ophthalmology 2005;112:1388–1394.
11. Shaikh S, Ho S, Richmond PP, et al. Untoward outcomes in 25-gauge versus 20-gauge vitreoretinal surgery. Retina 2007;27:1048–1053.
12. Kunimoto DY, Kaiser RS. Incidence of endophthalmitis after 20- and 25-gauge vitrectomy. Ophthalmology 2007;114:2133–2137.
13. Scott IU, Flynn Jr HW, Dev S, et al. Endophthalmitis after 25-gauge and 20-gauge pars plana vitrectomy: Incidence and outcomes. Retina 2008;28:138–142.
14. Essex RW, Yi Q, Charles PG, et al. Post-traumatic endophthalmitis. Ophthalmology 2004;111:2015–2022.
15. Gragoudas ES, Adamis AP, Cunningham Jr ET, et al. Pegaptanib for neovascular age-related macular degeneration. N Engl J Med 2004;351: 2805–2816.
16. Heier JS, Antoszyk AN, Pavan PR, et al. Ranibizumab for treatment of neovascular age-related macular degeneration: a phase I/II multicenter, controlled, multidose study. Ophthalmology 2006;133:633–642.
17. Brown DM, Kaiser PK, Michels M, et al. Ranibizumab versus verteporfin for neovascular age-related macular degeneration. N Engl J Med 2006;355(14):1432–1444.
18. Rosenfeld PR, Brown DM, Heier JS, et al. Ranibizumab for neovascular age-related macular degeneration. N Engl J Med 2006;355(14): 1419–1431.
19. Bhavsar AR, Ip MS, Glassman AR, et al. The risk of endophthalmitis following intravitreal triamcinolone injection in the DRCRnet and SCORE clinical trials. Am J Ophthalmol 2007;144:454–456.
20. Westfall AC, Osborn A, Kuhl D, et al. Acute endophthalmitis incidence: intravitreal triamcinolone. Arch Ophthalmol 2005;123:1075–1077.
21. Fung AE, Rosenfeld PJ, Reichel E. The international intravitreal bevacizumab safety survey: using the internet to assess drug safety worldwide. Br J Ophthalmol 2006;90:1344–1349.
22. Schwartz SG, Flynn HW, Scott IU. Endophthalmitis after intravitreal injections. Expert Opin Pharmacother 2009;10:1–8.
23. Wallin T, Parker J, Jin Y, et al. Cohort study of 27 cases of endophthalmitis at a single institution. J Cataract Refract Surg 2005;31:735–741.

24. Lalwani GA, Flynn Jr HW, Scott IU, et al. Acute-onset endophthalmitis after clear corneal cataract surgery (1996–2005): Clinical features, causative organisms, and visual acuity outcomes. Ophthalmology 2008;115:473–476.
25. Ciulla TA, Starr MB, Masket S. Bacterial endophthalmitis prophylaxis for cataract surgery: an evidence-based update. Ophthalmology 2002;109: 13–26.
26. Schiedler V, Scott IU, Flynn Jr HW, et al. Culture-proven endogenous endophthalmitis: clinical features and visual acuity outcomes. Am J Ophthalmol 2004;137(4):725–731.
27. Scott IU, Flynn Jr HW. Reducing the risk of endophthalmitis following intravitreal injections. Retina 2007;27:10–12.
28. Scott IU, Flynn Jr HW. The role of topical antibiotic prophylaxis for intravitreal injections. Arch Ophthalmol 2007;125:974–976.
29. Bannerman TL, Rhoden DL, McAllister M, et al. The source of coagulase-negative staphylococci in the Endophthlamitis Vitrectomy Study: a comparison of eyelid and intraocular isolates using pulsed-field gel electrophoresis. Arch Ophthalmol 1997;115:357–361.
30. Endophthalmitis Vitrectomy Study Group. Results of the Endophthalmitis Vitrectomy Study: a randomized trial of immediate vitrectomy and of intravenous antibiotics for the treatment of postoperative bacterial endophthalmitis. Arch Ophthalmol 1995;113:1479–1496.
31. Clark WL, Kaiser PK, Flynn Jr HW, et al. Treatment strategies and visual acuity outcomes in chronic postoperative *Propionibacterium acnes* endophthalmitis. Ophthalmology 1999;106:1665–1670.
32. Chaudhry NA, Flynn Jr HW, Smiddy WE, et al. *Xanthomonas maltophilia* endophthalmitis after cataract surgery. Arch Ophthalmol 2000;188: 572–575.
33. Scott IU, Lieb DF, Flynn Jr HW, et al. Endophthalmitis caused by *Mycobacterium chelonae*: selection of antibiotics and outcomes of treatment. Arch Ophthamol 2003;121:573–576.
34. Vahey JB, Flynn Jr HW. Results in the management of *Bacillus* endophthalmitis. Ophthalmic Surg 1991;22:681–686.
35. Scott IU, Matharoo N, Flynn Jr HW, et al. Endophthalmitis caused by *Klebsiella* species. Am J Ophthalmol 2004;138:662–663.
36. Miller JJ, Scott IU, Flynn Jr HW, et al. Endophthalmitis caused by *Streptococcus pneumoniae*. Am J Ophthalmol 2004;138:231–236.
37. Scott IU, Flynn Jr HW, Feuer W, et al. Endophthalmitis associated with microbial keratitis. Ophthalmology 1996;103:1864–1870.
38. Alfonso EC, Cantu-Dibildox J, Munir WM, et al. Insurgence of *Fusarium* keratitis associated with contact lens wear. Arch Ophthalmol 2006;124: 941–947.
39. Chang DC, Grant GB, O'Donnell K, et al. Multistate outbreak of *Fusarium* keratitis associated with use of a contact lens solution. JAMA 2006;296(8): 953–963.
40. Iyer SA, Tuli SS, Wagoner RC. Fungal keratitis: emerging trends and treatment outcomes. Eye Contact Lens 2006;32:267–271.
41. Dursun D, Fernandez V, Miller D, et al. Advanced *Fusarium* keratitis progressing to endophthalmitis. Cornea 2003;22:300–303.
42. Donahue SP, Kowalski RP, Jewart BH, et al. Vitreous cultures in suspected endophthalmitis: biopsy or vitrectomy? Ophthalmology 1993;100:452–455.
43. Raju B, Das T, Hyderabad Endophthalmitis Research Group. Simple and stable technique of vitreous tap. Retina 2004;24:803–805.
44. Josephberg RG. Endophthalmitis: the latest in current management. Retina 2006;26(Suppl. 6):S47–S50.
45. Hilton GF, Josephberg RG, Halperin LS, et al. Office-based sutureless transconjunctival pars plana vitrectomy. Retina 2002;22:725–732.
46. Eser I, Kapran Z, Altan T, et al. The use of blood culture bottles in endophthalmitis. Retina 2007;27:971–973.
47. Irvine WD, Flynn Jr HW, Murray TG, et al. Retained lens fragments after phacoemulsification manifesting as marked intraocular inflammation with hypopyon. Am J Ophthalmol 1992;114:610–614.
48. Mamalis N, Edelhauser HF, Dawson DG, et al. Toxic anterior segment syndrome. J Cataract Refract Surg 2006;32(2):324–333.
49. Jehan FS, Mamalis N, Spencer TS, et al. Postoperative sterile endophthalmitis (TASS) associated with the Memory Lens. J Cataract Refract Surg 2000;26:1773–1777.
50. Werner L, Sher JH, Taylor JR, et al. Toxic anterior segment syndrome and possible association with ointment in the anterior chamber following cataract surgery. J Cataract Refract Surg 2006;32:227–235.
51. Duffy RE, Brown SE, Caldwell KL, et al. An epidemic of corneal destruction caused by plasma gas sterilization: the Toxic Endothelial Cell Destruction Syndrome Investigative Team. Arch Ophthalmol 2000;188:1167–1176.
52. Moshfeghi AA, Scott IU, Flynn Jr HW, et al. Pseudohypopyon after intravitreal triamcinolone acetonide injection for cystoid macular edema. Am J Ophthalmol 2004;138:489–492.
53. Nguyen JK, Fung AE, Flynn Jr HW, et al. Hypopyon and pseudoendophthalmitis associated with chronic vitreous hemorrhage. Ophthalmic Surg Lasers Imaging 2006;37:317–319.
54. Schwartz SG, Mieler WF, Holz ER, et al. Intravitreal hemoglobin spherulosis: a rare complication of subretinal hemorrhage. Arch Ophthalmol 2002;120:85–87.
55. Flynn Jr HW, Scott IU. Legacy of the Endophthlamitis Vitrectomy Study (EVS). Arch Ophthalmol 2008;126:559–561.
56. Durand M. Microbiologic factors and visual outcome in the Endophthalmitis Vitrectomy Study. Am J Ophthalmol 1997;124:127–130.
57. Doft DH, Wisniewski SR, Kellsy SF, et al. Diabetes and postoperative endophthalmitis in the Endophthalmitis Vitrectomy Study. Arch Ophthalmol 2001;119:650–656.
58. Tan CS, Wong HK, Yang FP, et al. Outcome of 23-gauge sutureless transconjunctival vitrectomy for endophthalmitis. Eye 2008;22:150–151.
59. Iyer MN, Han DP, Yun HJ, et al. Subconjunctival antibiotics for acute postcataract extraction endophthalmitis: is it necessary? Am J Ophthalmol 2004;137(6):1120–1121.
60. Smiddy WE, Smiddy RJ, Ba'Arath B, et al. Subconjunctival antibiotics in the treatment of endophthalmitis managed without vitrectomy. Retina 2005;25:751–758.
61. Hariprasad SM, Mieler WF, Holz ER. Vitreous and aqueous penetration of orally administered gatifloxacin in humans. Arch Ophthalmol 2004;121:345–350.
62. Park-Wyllie LY, Juurlink DN, Kopp A, et al. Outpatient gatifloxacin therapy and dysglycemia in older adults. N Engl J Med 2006;354:1352–1361.
63. Duggirala A, Joseph J, Sharma S, et al. Activity of newer fluoroquinolones against Gram-positive and Gram-negative bacteria isolated from ocular infections: an *in vitro* comparison. Indian J Ophthalmol 2007;55:15–19.
64. Breit SM, Hariprasad SM, Mieler WF, et al. Management of endogenous fungal endophthalmitis with voriconazole and caspofungin. Am J Ophthalmol 2005;139:135–140.
65. Johnson MW, Doft BH, Kelsey SF, et al. The Endophthalmitis Vitrectomy Study: relationship between clinical presentation and microbiologic spectrum. Ophthalmology 1997;104:261–272.
66. Das T, Kunimoto DY, Sharma S, et al. Relationship between clinical presentation and visual outcome in postoperative and posttraumatic endophthalmitis in south central India. Indian J Ophthalmol 2005;53:5–16.

CHAPTER

25

Retinopathy of prematurity

Gerardo García-Aguirre, MD, Mariana Martínez-Castellanos, MD, and Hugo Quiroz-Mercado, MD

INTRODUCTION

Retinopathy of prematurity (ROP) is a proliferative disorder of the developing retina that continues to be a major cause of blindness in children.

DISEASE PREVALENCE AND INFLUENCE

In the USA, it is among the most prominent causes of blindness in children under 3 years of age.[1] It is estimated that 24% of Latin American children with blindness have ROP.[2]

RISK FACTORS

The main recognized risk factors for developing ROP include birth weight of 1500 g or less (especially of 1250 g or less), gestational age of 32 weeks or less, and prolonged exposure to high concentrations of oxygen after birth.[3]

ETIOLOGY/PATHOGENESIS

NORMAL RETINAL VASCULAR DEVELOPMENT IN HUMANS

Retinal vascular development in humans occurs in two phases, mediated by two different mechanisms.[4,5] The first phase depends on a mechanism known as *vasculogenesis*, and implies *de novo* blood vessel formation from endothelial precursor cells. It occurs at week 14–15 of gestational age and begins with the growth of spindle-shaped cells from the optic nerve. These spindle cells migrate towards the periphery, following the tracts of the future retinal vascular arcades, and form primitive vascular tubes. It is believed that the development of these primitive vascular tubes is independent of vascular endothelial growth factor (VEGF). It has also been suggested that alterations in vasculogenesis lead to zone I ROP, a more aggressive clinical course, and worse prognosis.[6]

The second phase of normal retinal vascular development relies on a process known as *angiogenesis*, which consists of the formation of new blood vessels that originate in previously existing blood vessels. It begins at week 17–18 of gestational age, and features new vessels and capillary networks that form in the perifoveal area and in the leading edge of peripheral retinal vascularization. This second phase is dependent on the production of VEGF by the nonvascularized retina (especially by Müller cells and astrocytes). *In utero*, the nonvascularized retina is in a state of relative hypoxia, which causes a delayed turnover of intracellular hypoxia-inducible factor-1, which in turn increases the transcription of VEGF mRNA, and increased VEGF production. These "physiologically increased" levels of VEGF are the main drive for normal peripheral retinal vascularization, which is commonly almost completed at term.

ABNORMAL RETINAL VASCULARIZATION IN ROP

When a newborn is born preterm, normal peripheral retinal vascularization is usually not yet completed. During increased oxygen exposure (such as when the newborn is under oxygen therapy), the nonvascularized retina becomes hyperoxic, which in turn decreases VEGF production, and normal peripheral retinal vascularization is arrested (stage 1 ROP). When returning to normal oxygen exposure, the nonvascularized retina becomes hypoxic. Hypoxia may then induce increased production of VEGF and degeneration of retinal astrocytes. At this point, a ridge, composed primarily of immature astrocytes, is formed (stage 2 ROP). Astroctye degeneration allows passage of VEGF to the vitreous humor. The abnormally increased levels of VEGF (which are maximally elevated in the border between vascular and avascular retina) promote new vessel formation (stage 3 ROP). These new vessels may bleed, causing vitreous hemorrhage, or may contract, causing partial (stage 4 ROP) or total (stage 5 ROP) retinal detachment. Increased VEGF levels may also induce dilatation or tortuosity in normal retinal vessels ("plus" disease).

ROLE OF GROWTH FACTORS IN ROP

The importance of increased levels of VEGF in the pathogenesis of retinal neovascularization has been corroborated in several animal models which simulate the fluctuating oxygen conditions present in patients with ROP.[7–10]

Increased levels of VEGF in the ocular fluids of human newborns with ROP have been found in two studies. The first study, by Sonmez et al.,[11] measured vitreous levels of VEGF in patients with vascularly active ($n = 12$) and vascularly inactive ($n = 10$) stage 4 ROP that underwent vitrectomy, and compared the levels with vitreous samples ($n = 5$) obtained from controls (vitreous from patients that underwent surgery for congenital cataract), and found a median concentration of 3454 pg/ml (range, 774–8882 pg/ml), 316 pg/ml (range, 105–665 pg/ml), and 59 pg/ml (range, 38–135 pg/ml), respectively ($P < 0.001$).

The second study, performed by our group,[12] measured VEGF levels in the aqueous humor and subretinal fluid of patients with stage 5 ROP that underwent open-sky vitrectomy, and compared them with VEGF levels in the aqueous of controls that underwent surgery for congenital cataract. VEGF levels in the aqueous and subretinal fluid were 85.03 ± 61.42 pg/ml and 1600.63 ± 355.14 pg/ml respectively, while VEGF levels in the aqueous of controls were 15.15 ± 1.89 pg/ml ($P < 0.005$).

Insulin-like growth factor-1 (IGF-1) has also been implicated in the pathogenesis of ROP. IGF-1 is thought to play a permissive role for VEGF-induced normal peripheral retinal vascular development. Lack of IGF-1 in preterm infants has been shown to prevent normal retinal vascular growth in stage 1 ROP, despite the presence of VEGF. As newborns mature, increasing levels of IGF-1 in later stages of ROP allow VEGF-stimulated pathological neovascularization.[13,14]

Prolactin peptides have also been studied in patients with ROP.[15] A 16-kDa fragment of prolactin (16K-PRL), which has antiangiogenic activity, has been found to be elevated in aqueous humor and subretinal fluid of patients with stage 5 ROP who underwent open-sky vitrectomy. It is believed that 16K-PRL is involved in the regression of pathologic neovascularization, and offers a potential target for the treatment of this disease.

DIAGNOSIS AND ANCILLARY TESTING/DIFFERENTIAL DIAGNOSIS

Diagnosis of this disease is clinical. Patients at risk should be examined with their pupils dilated using an indirect ophthalmoscope, a condensing lens, a lid speculum, and a scleral indentator, following a screening protocol.[16] No ancillary tests are usually required, but fundus photographs may be useful for follow-up.

Differential diagnosis of ROP stages 1–3 includes familial exudative vitreoretinopathy, and atypical cases of Coats' disease or Eales' disease. Differential diagnosis of ROP stages 4–5 must be made with causes of leukocoria, including retinoblastoma, persistent fetal vasculature, and Norrie's disease.

SIGNS AND SYMPTOMS

CLASSIFICATION OF RETINOPATHY OF PREMATURITY

The classification of ROP was established by an international committee,[17–19] and includes five stages, three zones, and the presence or absence of "plus" disease (Figure 25.1). Stage 1 consists of a demarcation line that separates avascular from vascularized retina. Stage 2 consists of an elevated ridge that separates avascular from vascularized retina. Stage 3 consists of a ridge with extraretinal fibrovascular proliferation. Stage 4 consists of a retinal detachment; when the macula is not involved, it is called stage 4A, and when the macula is detached, it is called stage 4B. Stage 5 implies a total retinal detachment that may be open or narrow in configuration.

The retinal zones center in the optic disc. Zone I corresponds to a circle with a radius that extends from the disc to twice the disc–fovea distance. Zone II corresponds to a circle that extends from the limits of zone I to the nasal ora serrata. Zone III corresponds to the remaining crescent-shaped area temporally between zone II and the ora serrata. The extent of the disease is expressed in clock hours. "Plus" disease is characterized by posterior venous and arterial tortuosity and dilation. "Threshold" ROP is defined as 5 or more contiguous or 8 cumulative clock hours of stage 3 ROP in the presence of "plus" disease. It is called "threshold" because it is predicted that, at this point, approximately 50% of patients will have an unfavorable outcome.

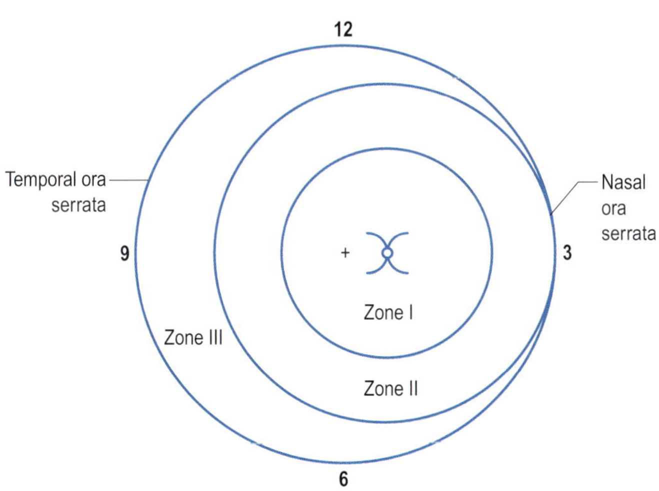

Figure 25.1 Diagram of zones of the retina and clock hours used to describe the location and extent of retinopathy of prematurity.

Aggressive posterior (AP) ROP consists of posterior location (usually zone I), "plus" disease without prominent ridge proliferation or classic stage 3, low-lying, tangled web of vessel (called flat neovascularization), that typically extends circumferentially. This is an uncommon form of ROP, which is severe and progresses rapidly to stages 4 and 5 if left untreated.

TREATMENT OPTIONS FOR RETINOPATHY OF PREMATURITY

Treatment options for ROP include the following:

- Cryotherapy to ischemic retina for patients with prethreshold and threshold disease with clear media
- Laser therapy to ischemic retina for patients with prethreshold and threshold disease with clear media
- Intravitreal antiangiogenic agents for patients with prethreshold and threshold disease, and some patients with opaque media and/or limited retinal detachment
- Lens-sparing vitrectomy for patients with ROP stage 4A or B
- Vitrectomy without sparing the lens for patients with ROP stage 5.

TREATMENT OUTCOMES AND PROGNOSIS

CRYOTHERAPY AND LASER THERAPY

The Cryotherapy for Retinopathy of Prematurity (CRYO-ROP) study was the first multicenter clinical trial for the treatment of ROP. In patients who developed bilateral threshold ROP, one eye was randomized to receive treatment with cryoablation of the peripheral avascular retina, and the other eye received no treatment. In patients with unilateral threshold ROP, the affected eye was randomized to either cryotherapy or no treatment. At 1-year follow-up, 44.7% of untreated eyes and 25.1% of treated eyes had an unfavorable structural outcome (defined as a retinal fold in the macula or the presence of retrolental tissue).[20] At 15 years of follow-up, an unfavorable structural outcome was seen in 51.9% of untreated eyes and 30% of treated eyes.[21]

Several years later, the Early Treatment for Retinopathy of Prematurity (ET-ROP) study was designed in order to compare laser treatment for threshold disease (conventional treatment) with laser treatment for eyes with high-risk "prethreshold" disease (defined as zone I, any stage ROP, less than threshold; zone II, stage 2, with plus disease or stage 3 without plus disease; zone II, stage 3 with plus disease, but less than the threshold; the "high-risk" was calculated according to the retinal status and other risk factors about the infant, based on a theoretical model created with CRYO-ROP study data). The study showed that, at 9 months of postmenstrual age of follow-up, early treatment reduced unfavorable visual outcomes from 19.5% to 14.5% and reduced unfavorable structural outcome from 15.6% to 9.1%.[22]

INTRAVITREAL ANTI-VEGF THERAPY FOR ROP

Rationale for Treatment

The fact that VEGF levels are markedly increased in intraocular fluids of patients with ROP raises the question whether treatment directed to block VEGF and its effects would be helpful for the treatment of ROP or to avoid its complications. To date, only intravitreal bevacizumab

(Avastin, Genentech) has been used for the treatment of ROP. The first cases were treated by our group in September 2005,[23,24] and included patients in whom neither cryotherapy nor laser could be applied because of poor pupil dilation or vitreous hemorrhage, with very good results, which led to a larger series.[25]

Injection Technique

Treatment can be administered under sedation or general anesthesia. Intravitreal bevacizumab injection is performed as follows. The patient must be prepped with sterile povidone-iodine solution around the eye to be injected. A lid speculum is used to retract the lids, and 2–3 drops of 5% povidone-iodine are placed on the eye to be injected. Using a caliper, 2 mm are measured posterior to the limbus in the inferotemporal quadrant, and 0.05 ml (1.25 mg) of bevacizumab are then injected at this location with a 27 or 30-gauge needle. Anterior-chamber paracentesis must be performed in order to achieve appropriate intraocular pressure.

Patients

Patients to be treated with intravitreal bevacizumab for ROP were divided into three groups. Group I (n = 4 eyes) consisted of ROP stage 4A or 4B that did not respond to conventional treatment. Group II (n = 5 eyes) consisted of threshold disease which was difficult to treat because of vitreous hemorrhage or poor pupil dilation. Group III consisted of high-risk prethreshold or threshold disease (n = 9 eyes). In addition to complete ophthalmologic evaluation, patients underwent complete pediatric evaluation at baseline, 1 day after injection, and in weeks 1, 2, 4, 12, 24, and 38.

Results

Of the four eyes in group I, two of them required vitrectomy, and remained with the retina attached at 38 weeks follow-up. The other two eyes (both of the same patient) had complete regression of neovascularization with spontaneous reattachment of the retina (Figure 25.2).

Of the five eyes in group II, all of them presented regression of neovascularization in the retina and/or the tunica vasculosa lentis at 38-week follow-up, without the need for further treatment (Figure 25.3).

Of the nine eyes in group III, all of them presented complete regression of neovascularization at 38-week follow-up, without the need for further treatment.

There were no adverse ocular or systemic side-effects after intravitreal bevacizumab injection.

Other Reported Results

Travassos et al.[26] reported treatment with 0.75 mg intravitreal bevacizumab in three eyes of three patients with AP ROP. Two of the eyes received bevacizumab as the sole treatment for ROP, while one eye also received laser treatment. In the three eyes, complete regression of anterior- and posterior-segment neovascularization was seen, without any ocular or systemic side-effects.

Chung et al.[27] reported a case of bilateral aggressive zone I ROP treated with indirect laser and intravitreal bevacizumab as an adjuvant. After 3 months, treatment resulted in ROP regression, prompt resolution of plus signs, and neovascular proliferation in both eyes, without apparent systemic or ocular adverse events.

Concerns with Intravitreal Anti-VEGF Therapy for ROP

Ocular complications

Intravitreal injection of any substance carries the risk for ocular complications, which are more thoroughly discussed in Section 4 of this book. Patients with ROP have ocular pathology that may increase the risk of complications: (1) the injection must be via pars plicata, with increased risk of touching the lens; and (2) if the patient has retrolental tissue, it can be damaged with the needle, and a vitreous hemorrhage or rhegmatogenous retinal detachment may be induced. Special care must be taken to place the injection site in a meridian where there is no evidence of retrolental tissue or peripheral traction.

Another theoretic ocular complication of intravitreal bevacizumab in patients with ROP is failure of normal peripheral retinal vascularization to complete properly, since VEGF is required for this process. On one hand, this complication has not been described in any of the series or case reports published so far. On the other hand, it has been described as the most common vascular sequela in patients with regressed ROP, even without treatment.[28] However, more experience is needed with this treatment to evaluate possible ocular complications.

Systemic Complications

Great attention has been paid to the possible systemic absorption and consequent side-effects of intravitreal bevacizumab in newborns with ROP. Systemic side-effects described in adult patients who have received intravitreal injections of bevacizumab include acute elevation of systemic blood pressure (0.59%), cerebrovascular accidents (0.5%), myocardial infarctions (0.4%), or even death (0.4%).[24] Additional questions have been raised in the case of premature infants, because in animal models, VEGF is crucial for normal organ development.[29]

Evaluating systemic side-effects in preterm newborns becomes very difficult because prematurity itself may be the cause of multiple-organ dysfunction, neurodevelopmental, behavioural, or other sequelae.[30] To date, no systemic complication has been reported in published series or case reports. However, there is a need for more solid evidence regarding this treatment, to assess possible systemic side-effects.

Vitrectomy

The technique, outcome, and prognosis of surgical treatment for ROP are beyond the scope of this chapter and may be reviewed elsewhere.[31]

SUMMARY

ROP is one of the most important causes of preventable blindness among children. Treatment with cryotherapy or laser therapy dramatically modifies the natural history of the disease, but results are far from optimal. Since VEGF plays a prominent role in the pathogenesis of ROP, intravitreal injection of bevacizumab is a promising alternative for the treatment of patients with this disease. Studies so far have yielded encouraging results with very few short-term complications. However, further studies need to be performed to determine the timing, safety, and long-term efficacy and safety of intravitreal bevacizumab for the treatment of ROP, either as first-line therapy with or without laser or after failure of conventional therapy.

Key points

- ROP is among the leading causes of blindness in children.
- Main risk factors for ROP are birth weight less than 1500 g, gestational age at birth of 32 weeks or less, and prolonged exposure to high concentrations of oxygen after birth.
- VEGF plays a key role in the development of the normal retinal vasculature, but in excess may lead to ROP.
- Conventional treatment for prethreshold and threshold ROP includes laser therapy and cryotherapy.
- Intravitreal antiangiogenic drugs have proven to be beneficial for the treatment of ROP, alone or in conjunction with conventional treatment.
- As our understanding of the pathophysiology of ROP becomes clearer, better treatments can be designed to avoid the disastrous consequences in the eyes afflicted with this disease.

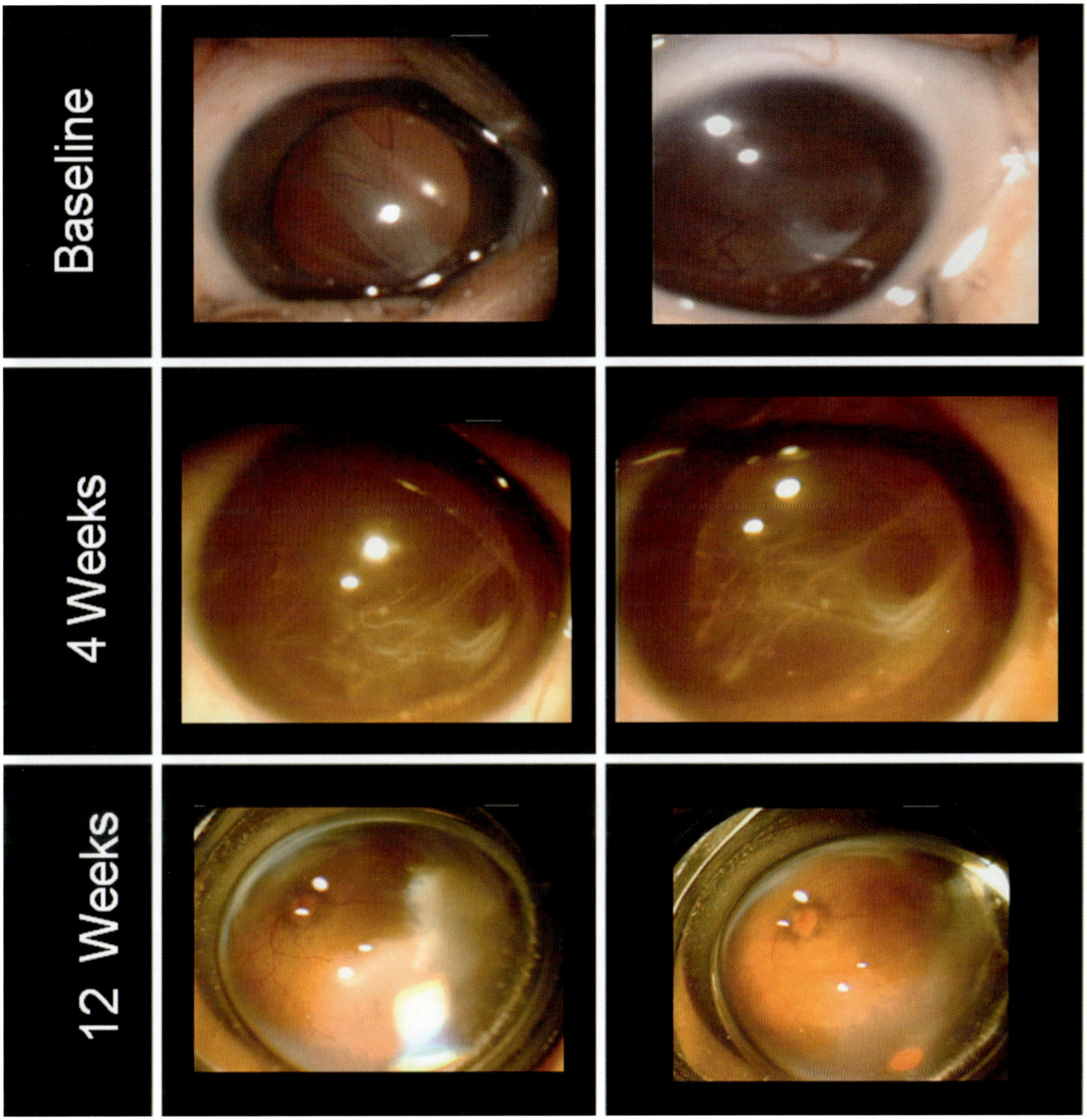

Figure 25.2 At baseline, a retrolental fibrovascular membrane was present, associated to a retinal detachment (top row). Four weeks after injection with bevacizumab, retrolental fibrosis remained, without active vessels (middle row). Twelve weeks after treatment, there was spontaneous reattachment of the retina, and regression of neovascularization (bottom row).

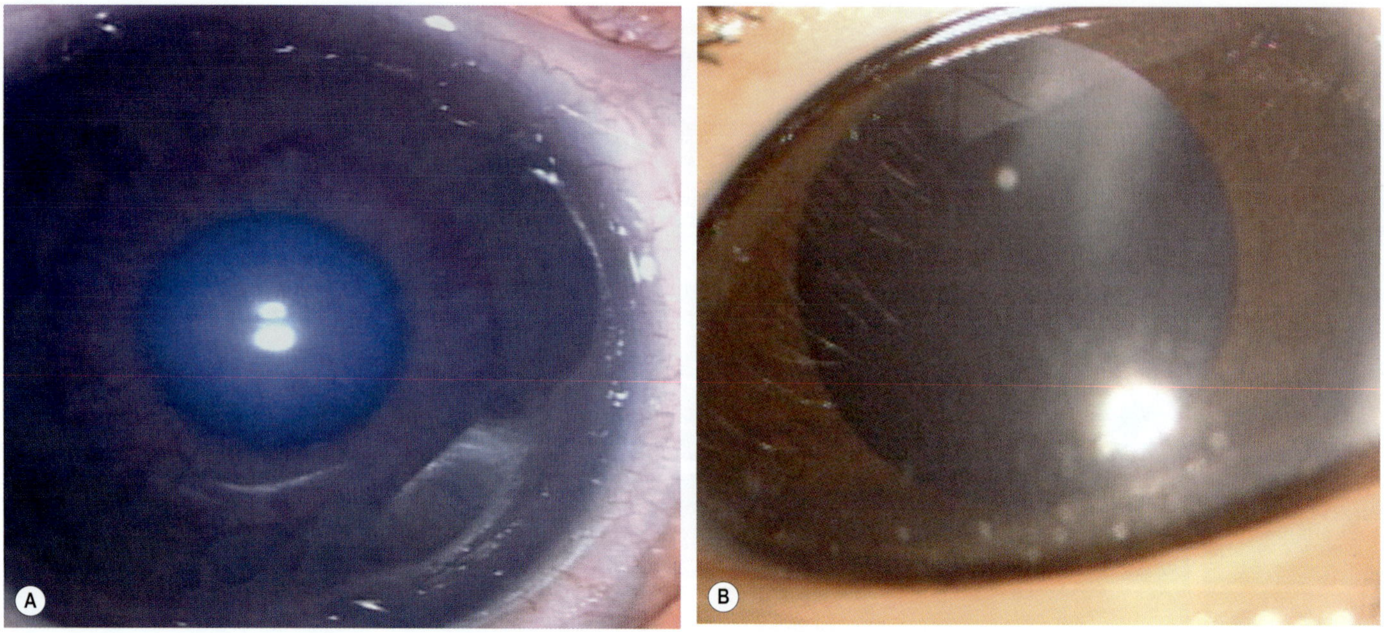

Figure 25.3 (A) At baseline, poor pupil dilation was observed, with extensive iris neovascularization. (B) Two weeks after treatment, complete regression of iris neovascularization was observed, with improved pupil dilation.

REFERENCES

1. Hatton DD, Schwietz E, Boyer B, et al. Babies Count: the national registry for children with visual impairments, birth to 3 years. J AAPOS 2007;11(4):351–355.
2. Gilbert C, Rahi J, Eckstein M, et al. Retinopathy of prematurity in middle-income countries. Lancet 1997;350:12–14.
3. Palmer EA, Flynn JT, Hardy RJ, et al. Incidence and early course of retinopathy of prematurity. The Cryotherapy for Retinopathy of Prematurity Cooperative Group. Ophthalmology 1991;98(11):1628–1640.
4. Hughes S, Yang H, Chan-Ling T. Vascularisation of the human fetal retina: roles of vasculogenesis and angiogenesis. Invest Ophthalmol Vis Sci 2000;41:1217–1228.
5. Fleck BW, McIntosh N. Pathogenesis of retinopathy of prematurity and possible preventive strategies. Early Human Development 2008;84:83–88.
6. Flynn JT, Chan-Ling T. Retinopathy of prematurity: two distinct mechanisms that underlie zone 1 and zone 2 disease. Am J Ophthalmol 2006;142:46–59.
7. Pierce EA, Foley ED, Smith LE. Regulation of vascular endothelial growth factor by oxygen in a model of retinopathy of prematurity. Arch Ophthalmol 1996;114:1219–1228.
8. Robbins SG, Conaway JR, Ford BL, et al. Detection of vascular endothelial growth factor (VEGF) protein in vascular and non-vascular cells of the normal and oxygen-injured rat retina. Growth Factors 1997;14:229–241.
9. Pierce EA, Avery RL, Foley ED, et al. Vascular endothelial growth factor/vascular permeability factor expression in a mouse model of retinal neovascularization. Proc Natl Acad Sci USA 1995;92:905–909.
10. Dorey CK, Aouididi S, Reynaud X, et al. Correlation of vascular permeability factor/vascular endothelial growth factor with extraretinal neovascularization in the rat. Arch Ophthalmol 1996;114:1210–1217.
11. Sonmez K, Drenser KA, Capone A, et al. Vitreous levels of stromal cell-derived factor 1 and vascular endothelial growth factor in patients with retinopathy of prematurity. Ophthalmology 2008;115:1065–1070.
12. Ruiz-García H, Velez-Montoya R, Ustariz-Gonzalez O, et al. Vascular endothelial growth factor levels in aqueous, vitreous, blood and subretinal fluid in patients with stage V retinopathy of prematurity. ARVO 2008, Abstract no. 3877.
13. Smith L. Pathogenesis of retinopathy of prematurity. Growth Horm IGF Res 2004;14(Suppl A):S140–S144.
14. Chen J, Smith LE. Retinopathy of prematurity. Angiogenesis 2007;10:133–140.
15. Dueñas Z, Rivera JC, Quiroz-Mercado H, et al. Prolactin in eyes of patients with retinopathy of prematurity: implications for vascular regression. Invest Ophthalmol Vis Sci 2004;45:2049–2055.
16. Wilkinson AR, Haines L, Head K, et al. U.K. Retinopathy of prematurity guideline. Early Hum Dev 2008;84:71–74.
17. The International Committee for the Classification of Retinopathy of Prematurity. An international classification of retinopathy of prematurity. Arch Ophthalmol 1984;102:1130–1134.
18. The International Committee for the Classification of the Late Stages of Retinopathy of Prematurity. An international classification of retinopathy of prematurity. Arch Ophthalmol 1987;105:906–912.
19. An International Committee for the Classification of Retinopathy of Prematurity. The international classification of retinopathy of prematurity revisited. Arch Ophthalmol 2005;123:991–999.
20. Cryotherapy for Retinopathy of Prematurity Group. Multicenter trial of cryotherapy for retinopathy of prematurity:one year outcome – structure and function. Arch Ophthalmol 1990;108:1408–1413.
21. Cryotherapy for Retinopathy of Prematurity Cooperative Group. 15-year outcomes following threshold retinopathy of prematurity: final results from the multicenter trial of cryotherapy for retinopathy of prematurity. Arch Ophthalmol 2005;123:311–318.
22. Early Treatment for Retinopathy of Prematurity Cooperative Group. Revised indications for the treatment of retinopathy of prematurity – results of the early treatment for retinopathy of prematurity randomized trial. Arch Ophthalmol 2003;121:1684–1694.
23. Quiroz-Mercado H, Ustariz-González O, Martinez-Castellanos MA, et al. Our experience after 1765 intravitreal injections of bevacizumab: the importance of being part of a developing story. Semin Ophthalmol 2007;22:109–125.
24. Quiroz-Mercado H. Antiangiogenic Therapy with intravitreal bevacizumab for the treatment of retinopathy of prematurity. Presented at the Retina Subspecialty Day, American Academy of Ophthalmology Meeting 2007.
25. Quiroz-Mercado H, Martinez-Castellanos MA, Hernandez-Rojas M, et al. Antiangiogenic therapy with intravitreal bevacizumab for retinopathy of prematurity. Retina 2008;28:S19–S25.
26. Travassos A, Teixeira S, Ferreira P, et al. Intravitreal bevacizumab in aggressive posterior retinopathy of prematurity. Ophthalmic Surg Lasers Imaging 2007;38:233–237.
27. Chung EJ, Kim JH, Ahn HS, et al. Combination of laser photocoagulation and intravitreal bevacizumab (Avastin) for aggressive zone I retinopathy of prematurity. Graefes Arch Clin Exp Ophthalmol 2007;245:1727–1730.
28. Preslan MW, Butler J. Regression pattern in retinopathy of prematurity. J Pediatr Ophthalmol Strabismus 1994;31:172–176.
29. Gerber HP, Hillan KJ, Ryan AM, et al. VEGF is required for growth and survival in neonatal mice. Development 1999;126:1149–1159.
30. Saigal S, Doyle LW. An overview of mortality and sequelae of preterm birth from infancy to adulthood. Lancet 2008;371:261–269.
31. Trese M. Retinopathy of Prematurity. In Ryan SJ, Hinton DR, Schachat AP, Wilkinson P, editors. Retina, 4th edn. St. Louis: Mosby; 2005.

CHAPTER

26 Idiopathic macular telangiectasia

Peter Charbel Issa, MD, FEBO, Robert P. Finger, MD, MIH, Carsten H. Meyer, MD, Hendrik P.N. Scholl, MD, MA, and Frank G. Holz, MD

INTRODUCTION

Idiopathic macular telangiectasia (IMT) was first classified as a group as idiopathic juxtafoveolar retinal telangiectasis. In 1993, Gass and Blodi modified the description of this condition, and today, it remains the most commonly used classification.[1] It encompasses three different groups (or types) of rare disease entities with the common feature of telangiectasia of juxtafoveolar small vessels that predominantly occur temporally to the foveola. Data on the prevalence of any of the types of IMT are lacking. The term "idiopathic" distinguishes the incoherent group of diseases from other similar secondary vascular alterations such as after retinal vein occlusion, vasculitis, diabetes, carotid occlusive disease, or radiation therapy.[1,2]

According to Gass and Blodi, type 1 has a male predominance and occurs unilaterally with a marked exudative component. Type 2 occurs more frequently than type 1 and usually presents bilaterally with atrophic neuroretinal changes and no gender predilection. Further functional deterioration may occur through the development of secondary neovascular membranes or macular holes. The very rare type 3 presents with angiographically visible obliteration of the perifoveal capillary network and may occur with an associated vasculopathy of the central nervous system. Further subclassifications for each type were suggested.[1] Due to the rarity of type 3 IMT and the lack of clinical treatment studies, therapy of this subtype is not further addressed in this chapter.

TYPE 1 IDIOPATHIC MACULAR TELANGIECTASIA

Mean age of type 1 IMT was reported to be 37–56 years (range 7–74 years), with a male predominance of 61–70%.[2] The disease is thought to be a developmental anomaly. The clinical hallmarks are visible aneurysmatic telangiectatic changes with cystoid retinal edema and surrounding exudates. Mean visual acuity in the affected eye was reported to be 20/40 (range 20/20–1/200) if the disease encompasses more than 2 clock-hours parafoveally.[1] Deterioration of visual acuity usually occurs once the cystoid edema affects the fovea. Both, functional improvement and deterioration may occur in the long-term follow-up.

Studies to characterize the disease further using new imaging methods are lacking. Type 1 IMT may encompass a spectrum with only minimal affection of capillaries in the very vicinity to the foveal avascular zone on the one end and pronounced vascular alterations with strong exudation at the temporal posterior pole on the other end. Possibly, type 1 IMT encompasses different disease entities.

DIAGNOSTIC APPROACH AND CLINICAL FINDINGS

Patients usually complain about a unilateral loss of visual acuity and/or metamorphopsia. On clinical examination, ophthalmoscopy shows retinal aneurysmatic telangiectasia temporal to the foveola with surrounding retinal edema and retinal lipid exudates. The vascular changes typically involve an irregular or oval zone centered temporal to the fovea. The affected area is typically 1–2 disc diameters in size but may also encompass larger extramacular areas and rarely even involves areas in the peripheral fundus. Larger aneurysms may be associated with retinal hemorrhage. Microaneurysms and hard exudates may appear in the early disease stages. The disease manifestations may slowly progress but may also regress after years. Early-phase fluorescein angiography reveals aneurysmatic abnormalities with a diffuse leakage in late-phase angiography. The aneurysms involve the deep and superficial capillary network and some patients have minimal capillary ischemia.[3] Optical coherence tomography (OCT) shows retinal thickening in the presence of cystoid macular edema. Localized neurosensory detachment may also occur.[3] OCT imaging may be useful for documentation and for the evaluation of treatment effects.

THERAPY

Focal laser photocoagulation of the affected area may lead to a decrease of macular edema and improvement of visual acuity.[1,4–6] Li and co-workers reported the effect using intravitreal administration of triamcinolone in a single patient in whom prior laser treatment was not successful.[7] The macular edema regressed but showed a rebound effect 6 months after treatment. A similar experience was reported by our group.[2] Recently, Gamulescu and co-workers presented a patient with type 1 IMT whose macular edema and visual acuity improved after a single intravitreal injection of bevacizumab,[8] suggesting that vascular endothelial growth factor (VEGF) is involved in the pathogenesis of the disease. The effect remained stable within a follow-up period of 10 months.

The natural history of type 1 IMT and long-term treatment effects have not been investigated in larger trials. It should be noted that spontaneous resolution of the pathology has been reported in individual cases.[1,9] Currently, no treatment recommendations based on a high level of evidence can be provided. Due to the rarity of the disease, prospective multicenter studies to elucidate the natural history of the disease further (as for type 2 IMT; see below) would be a helpful basis for future prospective interventional trials. Besides focal laser coagulation, pharmacological interventions such as VEGF antagonization might be a promising therapeutic approach. However, patients suffering from type 1 IMT are relatively young and therefore the perspective of long-term intravitreal drug application is unfavorable. With the development of safer and longer-lasting therapeutic strategies, these obstacles may be overcome.

TYPE 2 IDIOPATHIC MACULAR TELANGIECTASIA

In this most common form of IMT, subtle telangiectasia are only visible in a subgroup of patients and often are rather ectatic appearing parafoveolar capillaries. The altered capillaries can be visualized on early-phase fluorescein angiography whereas leakage from these altered vessels becomes apparent in late angiographic phases.

Gass and Blodi[1] proposed five consecutive stages. Stage 1 is characterized by a diffuse juxtafoveolar hyperfluorescence in late-phase fluorescein angiography. In stage 2, a reduced parafoveolar retinal transparency becomes evident ophthalmoscopically. The hallmark of stage 3 is dilated right-angled venules and of stage 4 intraretinal proliferation of pigment epithelial cells typically along right-angled vessels. Stage 5 is characterized by secondary retinal neovascularizations. The predilection site for all these pathological changes is temporal to the foveola. Further sequels of type 2 IMT may be lamellar or full-thickness macular holes, presumably due to progressive degeneration and atrophy of neurosensory retina.[10] A series of recent publications described characteristic findings on OCT imaging, which suggests this new imaging technique as an objective measure of therapeutic effects complementing angiography.

NONPROLIFERATIVE STAGE

In disease stages without neovascular membranes (i.e., stages 1–4 following the classification of Gass and Blodi), argon laser photocoagulation,[1,4,11–13] photodynamic therapy (PDT),[14] intravitreal injection of steroids alone,[15–17] or in combination with indocyanine green (ICG)-mediated photothrombosis[18] and posterior juxtascleral administration of steroids[19] have been tried. As in type 1 IMT, the effect of intravitreal injections of VEGF inhibitors[8,20–23] has recently suggested a pathophysiological involvement of VEGF in type 2 IMT.

Hutton and co-workers, who were the first to describe type 2 IMT as a distinct disease entity with a possible genetic background, reported the successful treatment of two patients by focal argon laser photocoagulation.[13] In four eyes of three patients, the treatment resulted in a reduction of metamorphopsia and improvement of visual acuity within a follow-up period between 6 months and 3.5 years. Park and co-workers retrospectively analyzed the long-term outcome (median follow up time 73 months) in 10 eyes of eight patients after argon laser photocoagulation.[11] Visual acuity did not change significantly and a reduction of macular edema was only achieved in 20% of treatments. Previous laser photocoagulation was associated with an increased distortion of retinal vessels, new fibrovascular tissue, increased changes of the retinal pigment epithelium, new draining venules, and retinal hemorrhages. The authors concluded that patients with type 2 IMT did not benefit from argon laser photocoagulation within the area of leakage. In a series by Gass and Blodi,[1] 10 eyes of 10 patients received laser treatment. Of eight eyes with long-term follow-up (mean 43 months, range 33–52 months), visual acuity remained unchanged in four eyes and worsened by 2 or more lines in four eyes. Of the untreated fellow eyes, four worsened, three remained unchanged and one improved. Overall, there may be an increased risk of the development of new fibrovascular membranes after argon laser photocoagulation in type 2 IMT.[1,11,24,25]

PDT (using the standard parameters adopted from treatment of wet age-related macular degeneration) was applied in two eyes of two patients with nonproliferative type 2 IMT.[14] In both patients, the authors did not observe significant changes in visual acuity, fluorescein angiographic leakage, or findings in OCT imaging. It was therefore concluded that PDT does not have beneficial effects in this disease.

The clinical course of individual patients after intravitreal injection of triamcinolone was reported by several authors.[15–17] A reduction of the late-phase hyperfluorescence in fluorescein angiography with[17] or without[15,16] significant improvement (i.e., more than 2 lines) in visual acuity was reported. However, Smithen and Spaide found no changes after intravitreal injection of 4 mg triamcinolone in a nonproliferative eye, neither functionally nor angiographically.[26] The eye of the patient presented by Martinez showed an increase in visual acuity from initially 20/63 to 20/30 after 6 weeks and 20/25 after 6 months.[17] Cakir and co-workers documented a reduction in retinal thickness after intravitreal injection of triamcinolone and a waning effect of the therapy at a follow-up 9 months after treatment.[16] Fernando Arevalo and co-workers suggested a combined therapy of intravitreal injection of triamcinolone with ICG-mediated photothrombosis to be more effective.[18] ICG-mediated photothrombosis is thought to produce a selective endothelium-bound intraluminal photothrombosis following an intravenous injection of a highly concentrated ICG solution and focal activation with a low-irradiance, 810-nm laser light. It is thought that this technique largely preserves the retinal architecture with minimal loss of visual cells. However, confirmatory evidence of this pilot study is lacking.

A recent study reported the effect of posterior juxtascleral administration of 15 mg anecortave acetate, an angiostatic synthetic cortisol derivative with negligible corticosteroid bioactivity.[19] In the two nonproliferative eyes of this study, visual acuity was stabilized over a period of 24 months. However, no data were provided with regard to the natural history in the fellow eye for comparison, the angiographic effects, or alterations on OCT imaging.

A new pharmacological approach in nonproliferative type 2 IMT, the intravitreal inhibition of VEGF, was first proposed by our group. In an initial report, we showed that intravitreal application of 1.5 mg of the VEGF antagonist bevacizumab resulted in a marked decrease of juxtafoveolar leakage without an apparent increase in visual acuity.[20] Short-term effects on angiography and retinal thickness in six nonproliferative eyes were subsequently analyzed.[21] Two injections were performed with an interval of 4 weeks. Four weeks after the second treatment, there was a decrease in retinal thickness within the central 3 mm of the retina in all eyes. Assessment of fluorescein angiography revealed a reduction of ectatic capillaries seen in the early phase as well as of late-phase leakage (Figure 26.1). Visual acuity improved in a subset of patients. An increase of more than 15 ETDRS letters was observed in one eye and of 10–15 ETDRS letters in two eyes, while the other four eyes remained stable. Gamulescu and co-workers observed decreased leakage on angiography and a stable visual acuity in two patients after three initial injections in monthly intervals over a follow-up period of 11 and 12 months.[8] Retinal thickness did not decrease; however, they only reported measurements at baseline and the end of follow-up. A further study of our group reported the long-term effects of intravitreal

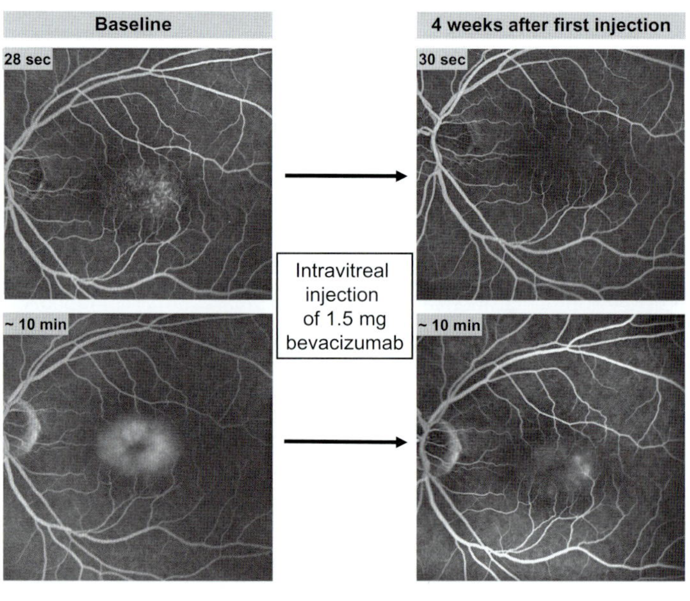

Figure 26.1 Early (top) and late (bottom) fluorescein angiography of the left eye of a patient with nonproliferative type 2 idiopathic macular telangiectasia before (left column) and after (right column) intravitreal application of 1.5 mg bevacizumab. The telangiectatic capillaries in early- as well as the late-phase leakage in late-phase angiography show a marked reduction after therapy. At the same time, retinal thickness decreased within the corresponding area. Visual acuity did not change significantly. (Eye number 5 from reference 21.)

bevacizumab injections after a mean follow-up period of 18 months.[22] The effect of the anti-VEGF treatment, monitored by fluorescein angiography and OCT imaging, decreased after 3–4 months. Further treatments showed similar effects within the follow-up period. Maia Junior and co-workers published an observation after intravitreal bevacizumab injection (1.25 mg) in three nonproliferative eyes with foveal detachment on OCT analysis.[23] The foveal anatomy regained a normal configuration and visual acuity significantly increased after a single intravitreal injection of bevacizumab.

In conclusion, there is as yet insufficient information on potential treatment benefits for nonproliferative type 2 IMT to make any general recommendation. Generally, visual deficits seem to evolve very slowly early in the course of the disease. Therefore, short-term observations after therapeutic interventions might not be sufficient to evaluate potential treatments for this chronic disease. Moreover, the functional parameters to monitor treatment effects have to be chosen carefully. For instance, the development or changes of characteristic paracentral scotomata appear to be a functional outcome measure which might respond differently to therapeutic interventions than visual acuity.[2,22] It was suggested that therapeutic strategies such as intravitreal inhibition of VEGF might be most effective in a temporary "active" disease stage with marked vascular alterations.[22] However, confirmation of such an active disease is lacking. In this regard, results from a large international multicenter natural history study (www.mactelresearch.org) may provide further insights. A progressive neurosensory atrophy with secondary involvement of retinal vessels was suggested to underlie the disease. In this case, the long-term success of treatments targeting altered retinal capillaries may be limited and antagonization of the neuroprotective properties of VEGF may even be unfavorable. Regardless of the underlying pathophysiology, the potential gain of function might be limited by the atrophic neurosensory changes before therapy and therefore, initial phenotypic and functional characterization is most important.

PROLIFERATIVE STAGE

Development of secondary neovascularizations represents a major cause of severe vision loss in type 2 IMT[1,25] and various therapeutic approaches have been tried to limit the consequences of this disease stage. Park and co-workers found little change in the size of the fibrovascular tissue over time and consequently questioned the usefulness for treatment in stage 5 eyes.[24] Therefore, interventions appear to be most beneficial in early and active proliferative disease stages (i.e., while a neovascular membrane grows) before the development of fibrotic membranes.

Several approaches to treat proliferative type 2 IMT have been reported: focal laser photocoagulation,[27,28] PDT alone[29–34] or combined with intravitreal injection of triamcinolone,[26] transpupillary thermotherapy,[35] posterior juxtascleral administration of steroids[19] and, recently, intravitreal injection of VEGF inhibitors.[21,23,36–38]

Visual stabilization as well as deterioration has been reported after argon laser photocoagulation in stage 5 type 2 IMT.[27,28] This treatment approach seems to be relatively safe in terms of recurrence of the membranes. However, large parafoveal scars, as reported in the literature, might severely interfere with, e.g., reading ability. However, this functional outcome measure was not reported.

PDT with verteporfin has been shown to be beneficial for the treatment of subfoveal choroidal neovascularization secondary to age-related macular degeneration or other diseases. PDT was first reported in a patient with recent decrease in visual acuity due to proliferative type 2 IMT by Potter and co-workers.[30] After two treatments in accordance with the standard protocol established for age-related macular degeneration, visual acuity improved 2 lines and remained stable within a follow-up period of 7 months. Interestingly, leakage from the neovascular membrane disappeared whereas parafoveal leakage typical for type 2 IMT continued. The largest series, a retrospective analysis, encompassed seven eyes of six patients.[29] Patients received on average 2.4 treatments and mean follow-up after the last treatment was 21 months. Median initial and final visual acuity was 20/80. More than 2 lines decrease or increase in visual acuity was observed in one eye each while the other five eyes remained stable. Hussain and co-workers treated six eyes of three patients three times with an interval of 2 months.[32] Their patients had a stable visual acuity after a median follow-up of 10 months (range 6–21 months). The researchers noted associated retinal pigment epithelium collateral damage in all six eyes of their study. There is the theoretical concern that the photosensitizing drug may leak out of the retinal vessels in the macula and potentially cause harm.[30,32] Indeed, Shanmugam et al. showed atrophy of the retinal pigment epithelium (along with a decrease in visual acuity) corresponding to the size of the laser spot.[34] However, others did not observe any side-effects.[29,30] Snyers and co-workers reported their results after treating four eyes of four patients with PDT.[33] Within a follow-up period of 9–23 months, three eyes maintained a stable visual acuity after 1–3 treatments. One eye deteriorated significantly within 14 months' follow-up despite four treatment sessions. Based on a single case report, Hershberger and colleagues emphasized that the neovascular membranes in type 2 IMT might tend to reperfuse rapidly.[31] Smithen and Spaide treated a patient with combined PDT and intravitreal injection of triamcinolone (4 mg).[26] They found a regression of the neovascular membrane along with significant improvement of visual acuity. Within a follow-up period of 12 months, a second combined therapy was performed at 9 months due to recurrence of angiographically visible leakage.

In a retrospective report studying the effect of transpupillary thermotherapy, the majority (92%) of 14 eyes showed stabilization or improvement in visual acuity as well as regression of the vascular membrane.[35] Posterior juxtascleral administration of anecortave acetate resulted in stabilization or improvement of lesion size, resolution of leakage, and stabilization of vision in five eyes of four patients.[19]

Intravitreal application of bevacizumab for proliferative type 2 IMT was first described by Jorge and co-workers.[38] A single injection of 1.5 mg in their patient presenting with an extrafoveal membrane resulted in the absence of signs of activity and significant improvement of visual acuity within a follow-up period of 6 months. Later, similar single observations of significant functional and anatomical improvement in a proliferative disease stage were reported in individual patients with[23] or without[36] accompanying foveal detachment. In a patient with a larger subfoveal membrane, no increase in visual acuity despite anatomical improvement was achieved.[21] In a case series including six eyes of six patients with a follow-up of 3–6 months, visual acuity improved by more than 2 lines in all but one patient.[37] A second injection was only necessary in one eye.

There are two reports on subretinal surgery with removal of subfoveal vascular membranes in two eyes with type 2 macular telangiectasia.[39,40] Due to the adherence of the membranes to the neurosensory retina, removal proved to be difficult and visual outcome was poor.

In summary, there is as yet insufficient evidence on treatment benefits and too short follow-up periods to make any general recommendations for the treatment of proliferative type 2 IMT. Moreover, the natural course of neovascular membranes in this disease, once developed, may be less aggressive compared to, e.g., those in age-related macular degeneration. Therefore, stabilization of visual acuity in eyes with neovascular type 2 IMT that have been stable for several months may not be an adequate outcome measure. More information about the natural history of this disease entity will most likely influence treatment recommendations. Until studies with a higher evidence level become available, PDT and intravitreal inhibition of VEGF seem to be the most promising treatment approaches in patients with recent visual loss. Patients with stable visual function and constant size of the neovascular membrane (Figure 26.2) may just be observed rather than treated for the time being.

SUMMARY AND KEY POINTS

In summary, IMT presents in three different types (type 1, 2, and 3), with type 2 being the most common form. Establishing the diagnosis is generally straightforward, but treatment of the condition may be chal-

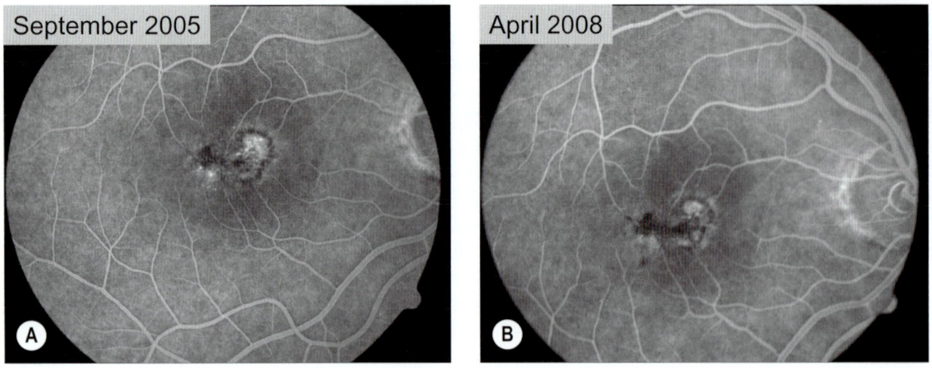

Figure 26.2 (A, B) Right eye of a patient with proliferative type 2 idiopathic macular telangiectasia. The size and activity of the neovascular membrane did not change within the observational period of 2½ years without any therapeutic intervention. The foveal neurosensory retina showed an atrophic aspect in September 2005. Visual acuity remained stable at 20/200.

lenging. The natural history has not been fully elucidated, though hopefully the MacTel project (www.mactelresearch.org) will provide much-needed information in this regard in the near future. In type 2 IMT, visual impairment may occur as part of an atrophic disease process, or may occur secondary to development of associated neovascularization. The various proposed treatment strategies for type 2 IMT should be used with caution since they appear to be beneficial only in selected situations such as in proliferative disease stages. To date, there is no controlled trial to document true proof of treatment benefit. Due to the progressive atrophic retinal alterations in type 2 IMT, future neuroprotective treatments may offer alternative treatment approaches.

REFERENCES

1. Gass JD, Blodi BA. Idiopathic juxtafoveolar retinal telangiectasis. Update of classification and follow-up study. Ophthalmology 1993;100: 1536–1546.
2. Charbel Issa P, Scholl HPN, Helb HM, et al. Idiopathic macular telangiectasia. In: Holz FG, Spaide RF, editors. Medical Retina. Heidelberg: Springer; 2007. p. 183–197.
3. Yannuzzi LA, Bardal AM, Freund KB, et al. Idiopathic macular telangiectasia. Arch Ophthalmol 2006;124:450–460.
4. Chopdar A. Retinal telangiectasis in adults: fluorescein angiographic findings and treatment by argon laser. Br J Ophthalmol 1978;62: 243–250.
5. Lowe MA, Akduman L, Olk RJ. Laser photocoagulation and glucose metabolism in idiopathic juxtafoveolar retinal telangiectasis. Ophthalmic Surg Lasers 1998;29:126–139.
6. Casswell AG, Chaine G, Rush P, et al. Paramacular telangiectasis. Trans Ophthalmol Soc UK 1986;105(Pt 6):683–692.
7. Li KK, Goh TY, Parsons H, et al. Use of intravitreal triamcinolone acetonide injection in unilateral idiopathic juxtafoveal telangiectasis. Clin Exp Ophthalmol 2005;33:542–544.
8. Gamulescu MA, Walter A, Sachs H, et al. Bevacizumab in the treatment of idiopathic macular telangiectasia. Graefes Arch Clin Exp Ophthalmol 2008;246:1189–1193.
9. Gass JD, Oyakawa RT. Idiopathic juxtafoveolar retinal telangiectasis. Arch Ophthalmol 1982;100:769–780.
10. Charbel Issa P, Scholl HP, Gaudric A, et al. Macular full-thickness and lamellar holes in association with type 2 idiopathic macular telangiectasia. Eye 2009;23:435–441.
11. Park DW, Schatz H, McDonald HR, et al. Grid laser photocoagulation for macular edema in bilateral juxtafoveal telangiectasis. Ophthalmology 1997;104:1838–1846.
12. Friedman SM, Mames RN, Stewart MW. Subretinal hemorrhage after grid laser photocoagulation for idiopathic juxtafoveolar retinal telangiectasis. Ophthalmic Surg 1993;24:551–553.
13. Hutton WL, Snyder WB, Fuller D, et al. Focal parafoveal retinal telangiectasis. Arch Ophthalmol 1978;96:1362–1367.
14. De Lahitte GD, Cohen SY, Gaudric A. Lack of apparent short-term benefit of photodynamic therapy in bilateral, acquired, parafoveal telangiectasis without subretinal neovascularization. Am J Ophthalmol 2004;138: 892–894.
15. Alldredge CD, Garretson BR. Intravitreal triamcinolone for the treatment of idiopathic juxtafoveal telangiectasis. Retina 2003;23:113–116.
16. Cakir M, Kapran Z, Basar D, et al. Optical coherence tomography evaluation of macular edema after intravitreal triamcinolone acetonide in patients with parafoveal telangiectasis. Eur J Ophthalmol 2006;16:711–717.
17. Martinez JA. Intravitreal triamcinolone acetonide for bilateral acquired parafoveal telangiectasis. Arch Ophthalmol 2003;121:1658–1659.
18. Arevalo JF, Sanchez JG, Garcia RA, et al. Indocyanine-green-mediated photothrombosis (IMP) with intravitreal triamcinolone acetonide for macular edema secondary to group 2A idiopathic parafoveal telangiectasis without choroidal neovascularization: a pilot study. Graefes Arch Clin Exp Ophthalmol 2007;245:1673–1680.
19. Eandi CM, Ober MD, Freund KB, et al. Anecortave acetate for the treatment of idiopathic perifoveal telangiectasia: a pilot study. Retina 2006;26:780–785.
20. Charbel Issa P, Scholl HPN, Holz FG. Intravitreal bevacizumab for the treatment of type 2 idiopathic macular telangiectasis. Retinal Cases Brief Rep 2007;1:189–191.
21. Charbel Issa P, Holz FG, Scholl HPN. Findings in fluorescein angiography and optical coherence tomography after intravitreal bevacizumab in type 2 idiopathic macular telangiectasia. Ophthalmology 2007;114:1736–1742.
22. Charbel Issa P, Finger RP, Holz FG, et al. Eighteen-month follow-up of intravitreal bevacizumab in type 2 idiopathic macular telangiectasia. British Journal of Ophthalmology 2008;92:941–945.
23. Maia Junior OO, Bonanomi MT, Takahashi WY, et al. Intravitreal bevacizumab for foveal detachment in idiopathic perifoveal telangiectasia. Am J Ophthalmol 2007;144:296–299.
24. Park D, Schatz H, McDonald HR, et al. Fibrovascular tissue in bilateral juxtafoveal telangiectasis. Arch Ophthalmol 1996;114:1092–1096.
25. Engelbrecht NE, Aaberg TM Jr, Sung J, et al. Neovascular membranes associated with idiopathic juxtafoveolar telangiectasis. Arch Ophthalmol 2002;120:320–324.
26. Smithen LM, Spaide RF. Photodynamic therapy and intravitreal triamcinolone for a subretinal neovascularization in bilateral idiopathic juxtafoveal telangiectasis. Am J Ophthalmol 2004;138:884–885.
27. Lee BL. Bilateral subretinal neovascular membrane in idiopathic juxtafoveolar telangiectasis. Retina 1996;16:344–346.
28. Watzke RC, Klein ML, Folk JC, et al. Long-term juxtafoveal retinal telangiectasia. Retina 2005;25:727–735.
29. Potter MJ, Szabo SM, Sarraf D, et al. Photodynamic therapy for subretinal neovascularization in type 2A idiopathic juxtafoveolar telangiectasis. Can J Ophthalmol 2006;41:34–37.
30. Potter MJ, Szabo SM, Chan EY, et al. Photodynamic therapy of a subretinal neovascular membrane in type 2A idiopathic juxtafoveolar retinal telangiectasis. Am J Ophthalmol 2002;133:149–151.
31. Hershberger VS, Hutchins RK, Laber PW. Photodynamic therapy with verteporfin for subretinal neovascularization secondary to bilateral idiopathic acquired juxtafoveolar telangiectasis. Ophthalmic Surg Lasers Imaging 2003;34:318–320.
32. Hussain N, Das T, Sumasri K, et al. Bilateral sequential photodynamic therapy for sub-retinal neovascularization with type 2A parafoveal telangiectasis. Am J Ophthalmol 2005;140:333–335.
33. Snyers B, Verougstraete C, Postelmans L, et al. Photodynamic therapy of subfoveal neovascular membrane in type 2A idiopathic juxtafoveolar retinal telangiectasis. Am J Ophthalmol 2004;137:812–819.
34. Shanmugam MP, Agarwal M. RPE atrophy following photodynamic therapy in type 2A idiopathic parafoveal telangiectasis. Indian J Ophthalmol 2005;53:61–63.
35. Shukla D, Singh J, Kolluru CM, et al. Transpupillary thermotherapy for subfoveal neovascularization secondary to group 2A idiopathic juxtafoveolar telangiectasis. Am J Ophthalmol 2004;138:147–149.
36. Shanmugam MP, Mythri HM, Shetty NS. Intravitreal bevacizumab for parafoveal telangiectasia-associated choroidal neovascular membrane. Indian J Ophthalmol 2007;55:490–491.
37. Mandal S, Venkatesh P, Abbas Z, et al. Intravitreal bevacizumab (Avastin) for subretinal neovascularization secondary to type 2A idiopathic juxtafoveal telangiectasia. Graefes Arch Clin Exp Ophthalmol 2007;245: 1825–1829.
38. Jorge R, Costa RA, Calucci D, et al. Intravitreal bevacizumab (Avastin) associated with the regression of subretinal neovascularization in idiopathic juxtafoveolar retinal telangiectasis. Graefes Arch Clin Exp Ophthalmol 2006;245:1045–1048.
39. Davidorf FH, Pressman MD, Chambers RB. Juxtafoveal telangiectasis – a name change? Retina 2004;24:474–478.
40. Berger AS, McCuen BW, Brown GC, et al. Surgical removal of subfoveal neovascularization in idiopathic juxtafoveolar retinal telangiectasis. Retina 1997;17:94–98.

CHAPTER

27 Neovascular glaucoma

J. Fernando Arévalo, MD, FACS and David G. Zeballos, MD

INTRODUCTION

Neovascular glaucoma (NVG) is classified as a secondary glaucoma. Historically, it has been referred to as hemorrhagic glaucoma, thrombotic glaucoma, congestive glaucoma, rubeotic glaucoma, and diabetic hemorrhagic glaucoma. In 1906 Coats[1] described the histologic finding of new vessels on the irides of eyes with central retinal vein occlusion (CRVO). In 1928, Salus[2] described similar new vessels on the irides of eyes of diabetic patients. Later, after the introduction of clinical gonioscopy, Kurz[3] correlated his clinical observation of fine new vessels in the angle with the histologic finding of connective tissue along these vessels. Weiss et al.[4] proposed the term "neovascular glaucoma," because the glaucoma is due to the new vessels rather than the inconsistently present intraocular bleeding.

The formation of a fibrovascular membrane on the anterior surface of the iris (rubeosis iridis) and extending into the chamber angle leads to irreversible obliteration of the outflow system, with a corresponding rise in intraocular pressure (IOP). NVG may result in a painful blind eye. Numerous secondary ocular and systemic diseases that share one common element, retinal ischemia/hypoxia and subsequent release of an angiogenesis factor, cause NVG. This angiogenesis factor causes new blood vessel growth from preexisting vascular structures. According to the degree of progression, the treatment methods consist of panretinal photocoagulation (PRP), anterior-chamber angle photocoagulation, cryotherapy, filtering surgery, glaucoma implants, cyclophotocoagulation, beta-blockers, carbonic anhydrase inhibitors, and enucleation.[5]

Rubeosis iridis is one of the severest complications of the occlusive diseases of retinal vessels associated with retinal hypoxia. Neovascularization of the anterior-chamber angle then very often results in the development of the prognostically very unfavorable NVG. Data show that the most effective methods of treatment of rubeosis iridis so far are the so-called coagulation techniques – PRP or cryocoagulation. By application of these techniques, we achieve the destruction of the anatomical substrate that is responsible for the production of the vasoproliferative substance, and the result is involution of rubeosis on the iris and in the anterior-chamber angle. Medical therapy is based on the use of topical steroids and atropine, to reduce inflammation and congestion. Drugs reducing aqueous production (β-blockers, carbonic anhydrase inhibitors, α-agonists) are helpful, although ocular hypertension is often refractory. However, there has been a recent interest in the management of rubeosis iridis and NVG with pharmacologic therapy, including steroids and antiangiogenic agents.

The objective of this chapter is to describe the characteristic clinical findings of NVG as well as the current pharmacotherapy options to treat this condition.

DISEASE PREVALENCE AND INFLUENCE

The prevalence of NVG is estimated to affect about 75 000–113 000 persons in the European Union. In the USA the incidence of NVG is rare. However, the treatment and maintaining visual acuity in patients with NVG are difficult. NVG is more prevalent in elderly patients.[6]

In patients with ischemic CRVO, anterior-segment neovascularization with associated NVG develops in more than 60% of cases. This can happen within a few weeks and up to 1–2 years after the onset of CRVO. It has been reported that the fellow eye may develop retinal vein occlusion in about 7% of cases within 2 years.[7] In another report, the 4-year risk of developing second venous occlusion is 2.5% in the same eye and 11.9% in the fellow eye.[8]

Neovascularization of the iris (NVI) in diabetes appears most often after the development of proliferative retinopathy. The onset of glaucoma after the appearance of NVI with diabetes is usually after a period of many years, as compared with only a few months with CRVO.[9] The incidence of NVI in diabetic patients ranges between 1% and 17%.[10] In patients with proliferative diabetic retinopathy (PDR), NVI has been reported at much higher incidence rates, ranging from 33% to 64%.[11] In patients with severe PDR, NVG occurs in 5–8% of cases.[12] In addition, for diabetic patients with NVG in one eye, NVG developed in the second eye in one-third of patients.[13]

RISK FACTORS

The most frequent cause is retinal ischemia resulting either from vascular occlusion or from diabetic alterations. Therefore, some of the risk factors that lead to ischemia in retinal vascular occlusions or in diabetic retinopathy (DR) are common to NVG. An increased risk of CRVO was found in patients with systemic hypertension, diabetes mellitus, and open-angle glaucoma; the risk of CRVO was decreased for patients with increasing levels of physical activity and increasing levels of alcohol consumption. For women, the risk decreased with the use of postmenopausal estrogen and increased with a higher erythrocyte sedimentation rate. The following conditions all showed a significant association with ischemic cases only: cardiovascular disease, electrocardiographic abnormalities, albumin:globulin ratio, history of treatment for diabetes mellitus, and blood glucose level. Both systolic and diastolic blood pressure showed significant associations with both types of CRVO, but the odds ratio is greater for ischemic CRVO. Overall, a stronger cardiovascular risk profile was shown for the ischemic type of CRVO.

The greatest visual threat to patients having both glaucoma and diabetes is the development of NVG. Over 60 years ago, it was hypothesized that ischemic retinal tissue released a diffusable angiogenic substance that stimulated neovascularization.[14] However, only recently was vascular endothelial growth factor (VEGF) found to be an agent that satisfies this description.[15] It has been discovered that significantly higher VEGF levels occur in the ocular fluids of patients with PDR when compared with patients without that disorder. Extremely elevated levels of VEGF were found in the ocular fluids of patients with NVG.

ETIOLOGY/PATHOGENESIS

In 1948, Michaelson[14] proposed that "there exists in the retina a factor or factors affecting the budding of new vessels." Ashton[16] and others later expanded the model to suggest that hypoxia of the retina was the

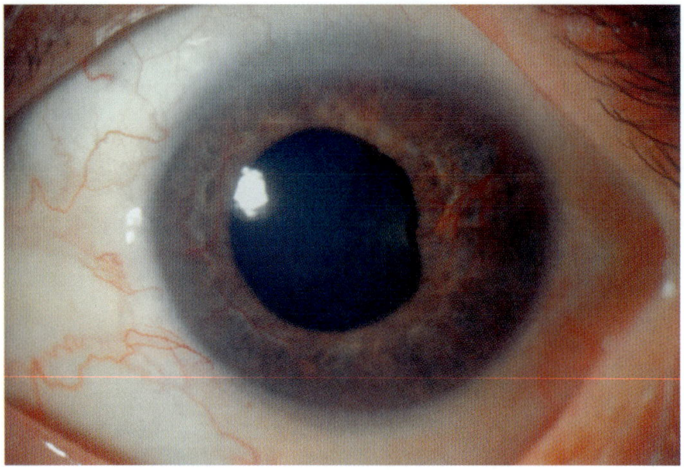

Figure 27.1 Neovascularization of the iris (NVI) appears to progress sequentially from the pupil to the periphery.

primary stimulus of retinal production of angiogenic factors. Leung et al.[17] identified and purified a heparin-binding VEGF from media conditioned by bovine pituitary follicular or folliculostellate cells. VEGF is a potent mitogen for vascular endothelial cells isolated from both small and large vessels, but does not affect the growth of BHK-21 fibroblasts, lens epithelial cells, corneal endothelial cells, keratinocytes, or adrenal cortex cells. The presence of VEGF in high concentrations in the medium conditioned by folliculostellate cells suggested that VEGF is a secreted molecule and that it may be a soluble mediator of endothelial cell growth and angiogenesis. Current reports support that VEGF and its receptors serve an important role in various steps of intraocular angiogenesis by virtue of its ability to be induced by hypoxia and its diffusible nature. However, angiogenesis is a multistep process in which many growth factors and cytokines are involved and have essential roles.[18] Besides VEGF, other molecules that have been demonstrated to be correlated with the development of NVG include basic fibroblast growth factor,[19] platelet-derived growth factor, insulin-like growth factor-1,[20] and interferon-α.[21]

The neovascular process begins as endothelial budding from capillaries of the minor arterial circle at the pupil. Clinically, this NVI appears to progress sequentially from the pupil to the periphery (Figure 27.1). However, histologically, once the process starts at the papillary margin, new endothelial buds may appear from vessels anywhere in the iris, including the major arterial circle in the iris root. These endothelial buds progress to become glomerulus-like vascular tufts. These new vessels are composed of endothelial cells without a muscular layer or much adventitia and supportive tissue. They have a tendency to be thin-walled and to be located toward the surface of the iris, but can be anywhere within the stroma of the iris.[9]

The fibrous component of the fibrovascular membrane in NVG consists of proliferating myofibroblasts, which are fibroblasts with smooth-muscle differentiation. The fibrous portion of the membrane is clinically transparent but produces a flattening of the iris surface architecture. The contractile smooth-muscle components explain the effacement of the iris surface, the development of ectropion uveae, formation of peripheral anterior synechiae (PAS), and ultimately, synechial angle closure.[22]

All conditions associated with diffuse hypoxia of the posterior segment, retinal detachment, and some intraocular tumors may cause NVG. Currently, probably one-third of cases of NVG are attributable to CRVO, one-third to DR, and one-third to other causes, with carotid artery occlusive disease (CAOD) being prominent.

Less frequent causes of NVG include the following: branch retinal vein occlusion, central retinal artery occlusion (CRAO), intraocular tumor, chronic retinal detachment, secondary to intraocular lens (uveitis–glaucoma–hyphema (UGH) syndrome), chronic or severe ocular inflammation, endophthalmitis, sickle-cell retinopathy, retinopathy of prematurity, radiation retinopathy, Eales' disease, Coats' disease, carotid cavernous fistula, ocular ischemic syndrome/carotid insufficiency, Takayasu's disease, giant-cell arteritis, and trauma.

CENTRAL RETINAL VEIN OCCLUSION

Numerous studies have reported that approximately 25% of CRVOs show over 10 disc areas of retinal capillary nonperfusion on fluorescein angiography (defined ischemic) and 75% are nonischemic (Figure 27.2). The natural history of untreated CRVO is that essentially none of the nonischemic eyes progress to NVG, whereas 18–60% of eyes in the ischemic group do.[23] NVG had been thought to appear 2–3 months after the CRVO (hence the term "90-day glaucoma"). However, NVG can occur anywhere from 2 weeks to 2 years after the initial occlusion. Nevertheless, in over 80% of cases, NVI and NVG appear within the first 6 months after CRVO. A fluorescein angiogram is imperative in the diagnosis, and ultimately the treatment, of CRVO. Clinically, it is sometimes impossible to determinate the degree of capillary nonperfusion because retinal hemorrhages block visualization of these areas. The nonischemic type can convert to the ischemic type. The CRVO study showed a 16% conversion rate within 4 months of the occlusion. This has led to the recommendation that the follow-up of nonischemic type should be within 2 months of presentation.[24]

The bilateral occurrence of CRVO has been reported to be around 15%. The CRVO study found 9% of eyes with CRVO had a vascular occlusion, including central retinal artery and branch or central vein occlusion, in the fellow eye.[24]

DIABETIC RETINOPATHY

Diabetes mellitus is a group of metabolic diseases characterized by hyperglycemia resulting from defects in insulin secretion, insulin action, or both. The chronic hyperglycemia of diabetes is associated with long-term damage, dysfunction, and failure of various organs, especially the eyes, kidneys, nerves, heart, and blood vessels.

In adults from about age 20 to 60 years, it is the leading cause of new blindness and one of the major causes of NVG. Most blindness in diabetic patients is due to PDR and only 5% is due to NVG. The overall prevalence of NVG in diabetes mellitus is about 2%, but increases to over 21% in PDR, where the frequency of iris neovascularization is 65%. It is now well accepted that NVI is associated with retinal hypoxia and proliferative retinopathy (Figure 27.3).

The crucial risk factor for the development of DR is the duration of diabetes. Several studies have shown that tight glycemic control (glycohaemoglobin < 7.5%) can delay the onset of the microvascular complications and therefore also NVG.

DIABETIC NEOVASCULAR GLAUCOMA

If a diabetic patient develops NVG in one eye, the disease tends to affect the fellow eye if prophylactic treatment is not provided. Bilateral NVI or NVG in adults is almost exclusively due to DR. The time interval between the onset of NVI and NVG in untreated cases varies from 1 month to over 3 years. Furthermore, it is unpredictable as to which untreated eyes with NVI ultimately progress to NVG. In eyes with early changes (microaneurysms and hemorrhages), 45% were found to return to retinopathy-free status at least once during regular annual ophthalmic examinations, and NVI can undergo spontaneous regression in over 26% of cases.[25]

Capillary dropout and retinal hypoxia make the eye with DR vulnerable to further insult. Surgical procedures such as cataract extraction may aggravate DR and precipitate NVG. All procedures that interrupt the integrity of the anterior hyaloid or posterior capsule constitute a risk, since these structures probably act as a barrier against the diffusion of angiogenic factors. Therefore, before surgery, the fundus should be carefully evaluated, performing PRP if necessary. Close postoperative control must be scheduled and first or further PRP carried out if NVI appears.

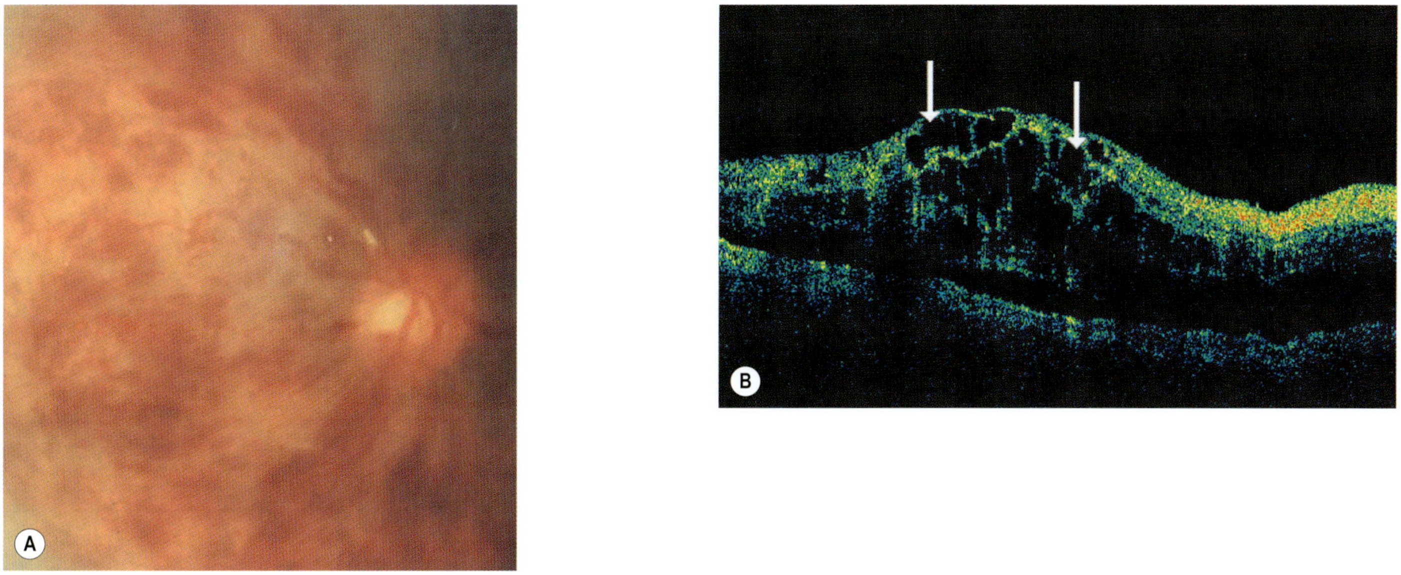

Figure 27.2 Acute central retinal vein occlusion. (A) Fundus photograph. Notice the venous dilatation, tortuousity, swollen optic nerve, and the scattered intraretinal hemorrhages in all four quadrants. (B) Optical coherence tomography scan showed a thickened elevated macula with numerous low reflective cystic spaces representing fluid accumulation (arrows). A detachment of the neurosensory retina with subretinal fluid accumulation is observed underneath the fovea.

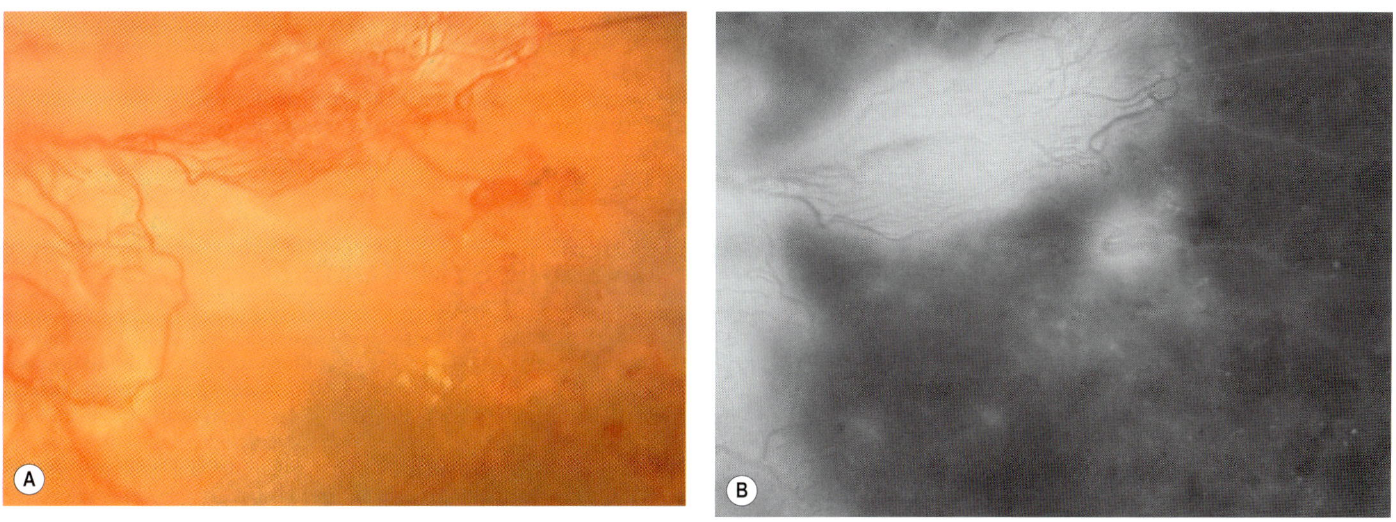

Figure 27.3 Proliferative diabetic retinopathy. Neovascularization elsewhere (NVE). (A) Color photograph. (B) Fluorescein angiography.

CAROTID ARTERY OCCLUSIVE DISEASE

CAOD is currently recognized as the third most common cause of NVG, accounting for at least 13% of cases. NVG represents only one manifestation of CAOD. The spectrum ranges from transient ischemic attack, to hypoperfusion retinopathy, to ocular ischemic syndrome. It has been estimated that evidence of chronic ocular ischemia will be found in 4–18% of patients with CAOD.

There are several unique aspects of NVG from CAOD. Decreased perfusion of the ciliary body following ligation of the carotid artery or from CAOD decreases aqueous humor production. Thus, despite extensive synechial angle closure, IOP may be normal or even low. Possible CAOD must always be considered in the event of NVI with no apparent ocular cause, if the patient shows a marked asymmetry of DR in the two eyes or if NVI does not regress after PRP.

Diagnostic examinations include carotid Doppler imaging, carotid arteriography, if required, but particularly retrobulbar vessel color Doppler imaging. This show greatly reduced peak systolic velocity and increased resistance in the central retinal artery and posterior ciliary arteries, associated with reversal of blood flow in the ophthalmic artery.

The prognosis of CAOD appears to be strongly correlated with the presence of NVI, which indicates a deeper ocular hypoxia.

CENTRAL RETINAL ARTERY OCCLUSION

The incidence of NVG due to CRAO alone is between 5% and 10%. With CRAO there is destruction of the inner retinal layer and capillary endothelium. This explains why retinal neovascularization is extremely rare in CRAO and BRAO. Neovascularization of the disc occurs after CRAO very rarely. Hayreh and Podhajsky[26] have proposed that preexisting CAOD causes ocular ischemia, leading to NVI and secondary NVG. At the same time, the decreased perfusion of the central retinal artery makes it susceptible to occlusion, especially if there is increased IOP from the existing NVG. The time interval between the onset of CRAO and NVG was generally between 1 week and 5 months.

INTRAOCULAR TUMORS

Malignant melanoma

The incidence of NVG with malignant melanoma is not high, and malignant melanoma as a cause of NVG is relatively low on the list of differential diagnosis. Nevertheless, in an eye with NVG in which the posterior segment is not visible because of opaque media, malignant melanoma must be considered, especially in the absence of DR in the contralateral eye or a history of CRVO in the ipsilateral eye.

Retinoblastoma

Walton and Grant[27] found 38 of 56 children with NVI to have retinoblastomas and that the duration of the tumor was associated with the development of NVI. They also reviewed 88 eyes enucleated for retinoblastoma and found that 39 (44%) had histologically confirmed NVI, with a significant association between the presence of NVI and choroidal involvement by the tumor.

Ultrasound, computed tomography, magnetic resonance imaging, and other appropriate studies must be performed. Iris neovascularization has also been described in eyes with metastatic tumors and reticulum cell sarcoma. In these cases the direct effect of tumor-secreted angiogenesis factor may be the cause of the new vessels.[28]

MISCELLANEOUS CAUSES

There are several common pathways, such as chronic retinal detachment and extensive capillary nonperfusion with resultant retinal hypoxia. These include Stickler's syndrome, Wagner–Stickler's syndrome, autosomal-dominant neovascular inflammatory vitreoretinopathy, and retinopathy of prematurity. More localized anterior-segment perfusion compromise has been shown to be the cause of NVI in Fuchs' heterochromic iridocyclitis and exfoliation syndrome. The association between scleritis and NVG is also probably due to secondary vascular occlusion. Other miscellaneous retinal conditions that may be associated with the development of NVG include Coat's disease, Eales' disease, giant-cell astrocytoma of the retina, and X-linked retinoschisis.

DIAGNOSIS AND ANCILLARY TESTING

The key aim in the treatment of NVG is early diagnosis so that the optimal treatment regimen can be instituted. Every patient with NVG should undergo a comprehensive medical and ocular evaluation with particular attention to the pupil, slit-lamp, gonioscopic, and dilated fundus examinations. The IOP should be measured if at all possible by applanation tonometry. A nondilated slit-lamp examination including gonioscopy is vitally important to detect early angle neovascularization and early anterior synechiae. Sometimes a few cells may be seen in the anterior chamber, which may erroneously be diagnosed as a sign of uveitis. Other methods, including angiography and electroretinography, have been described to detect subclinical anterior-segment neovascularization in patients at risk for rubeosis. Angiographic examinations of the iris, angle, and retina have been used in an attempt to predict the development of rubeosis. Iris fluorescein angiography shows a leakage of fluorescein from NVI (Figure 27.4). The electroretinogram measures a mass electrical response of the retina, allowing for assessment of the retinal periphery, which cannot be seen with fluorescein angiography. The electroretinogram can measure the degree of retinal ischemia, and its reading can then be correlated to the likelihood of rubeosis developing.

DIFFERENTIAL DIAGNOSIS

Iris and angle neovascularization (sometimes with hyphema) is occasionally present in Fuchs' heterochromic cyclitis, but progression to

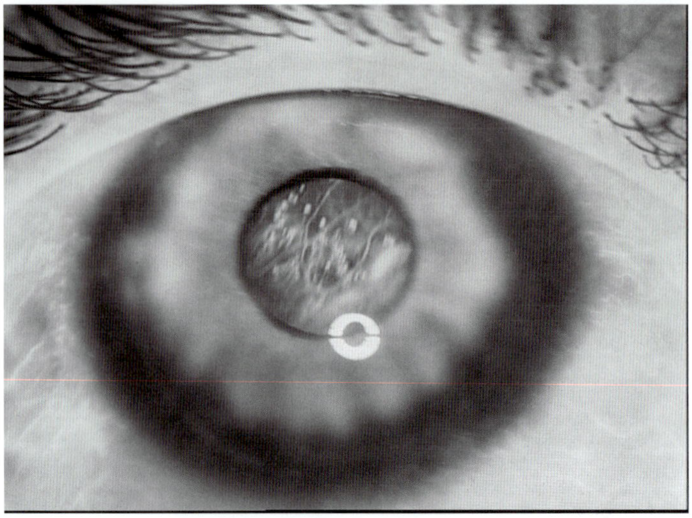

Figure 27.4 Iris fluorescein angiography demonstrates leakage of fluorescein from neovascularization of the iris in a case with Coats' disease and neovascular glaucoma.

NVG is extremely rare. Very thin nonprogressive iris neovascularization can be observed at the pupillary margin in pseudoexfoliation syndrome, myotonic dystrophy, abnormal insulin secretion, and in elderly normal subjects. In acute iridocyclitis and after ocular surgery (particularly in diabetic patients), the engorgement of iris vessels can mimic fulminant NVG, but this rapidly resolves with topical steroids. Advanced NVG may be confused with acute angle closure glaucoma, but gonioscopy of the fellow eye generally shows a nonoccludible angle. Other causes of hyphema and ghost-cell glaucoma should be excluded.

SIGNS AND SYMPTOMS

The first visible signs of incipient NVG are tiny tufts of new vessels at the pupillary margin, site of the maximum turnover of aqueous containing specific growth factors. As NVI progresses, new vessels extend from the peripupillary tufts in an irregular, meandering manner. New vessels, at least clinically, characteristically appear on the surface of the iris. When new vessels reach the iris collarette, the collarette vessel, which is often normally present but not visible, may become engorged and appear as part of the NVI. In the more advanced stages, it is common to see effacement of the normal iris surface architecture, resulting in a relatively smooth iris. When these new vessels reach the angle, they cross the ciliary body band and scleral spur to arborize on the trabecular meshwork. At the angle, the larger vessels, after crossing the scleral spur, arborize with very fine capillaries over several clock-hours of the trabecular meshwork.

Until angle neovascularization covers a signicant portion of the trabecular meshwork, the IOP may be normal. The angle neovascularization is associated with fibrous tissue, and the fibrovascular membrane, which is invisible on gonioscopy, may block enough of the trabecular meshwork to cause open-angle glaucoma.

The fibrovascular membrane contracts, pulls the new vessels taut, and draws the iris root near the trabecular meshwork, determining mydriasis and focal and subsequently diffuse PAS. The new vessels can also spread over the anterior lens surface, with rapid cataract formation.

The eye is painful and photophobic. Vision is usually at the counting fingers to hand motion level, and the IOP may be as high as 60 mmHg or greater. There is a moderate to marked conjunctival congestion frequently associated with a steamy cornea, through which NVI and ectropion uveae are often visible. There are variable degrees of synechial angle closure observed gonioscopically.

Advanced stage is characterized by some or all of the following: acute severe pain, headache, nausea, and/or vomiting, photophobia, reduced visual acuity (counting fingers to hand motion), elevated IOP (60 mmHg), conjunctival injection, corneal edema, synechial angle closure, severe rubeosis, distorted, fixed, mid dilated pupil and ectropion uveae, retinal neovascularization, and/or hemorrhage.

TREATMENT OPTIONS

The management of NVG is highly unpredictable, difficult, and controversial. There are two key aspects to the management of NVG: treatment of the underlying disease process responsible for rubeosis and treatment of the increased IOP. Treatment of rubeosis is directed at the ischemic retina in most cases. PRP is considered the treatment of choice (Figure 27.5). However, other modalities such as panretinal cryotherapy, transscleral diode laser retinopexy, and panretinal diathermy have been described. Goniophotocoagulation has been used to directly treat the new vessels in the angle in an effort to prevent synechial closure.

TREATMENT OF THE UNDERLYING DISEASE ASSOCIATED WITH NVG

Central retinal vein occlusion

NVG is the most dreaded and blinding complication of ischemic CRVO. If CRVO is of the ischemic type, PRP should be performed as soon as possible. Patients with nonischemic CRVO should be followed up carefully because 16% can become ischemic within 4 months. Without PRP, approximately 40% of CRVO of the ischemic type proceed to NVG.[6]

Diabetic retinopathy

For NVG to develop in diabetes mellitus there must be retinal hypoxia associated with proliferative retinopathy. The major factor in the onset of proliferative retinopathy is the duration of diabetes. Once PDR is present, there is strong evidence that PRP is the treatment of choice for prevention of development of NVG and has shown the beneficial effects in causing regression of NVI.

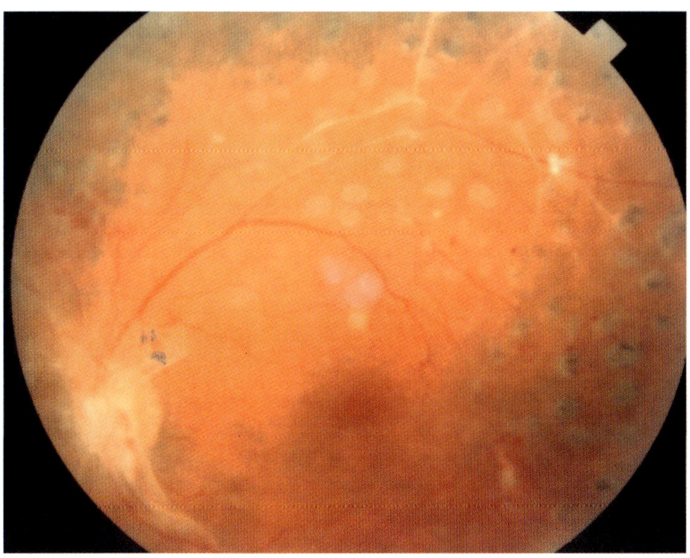

Figure 27.5 Panphotocoagulation in an eye with neovascularization of the disc (NVD). Notice the chorioretinal scars outside the arcades.

Carotid artery occlusive disease

In neurologically symptomatic patients with carotid disease, endarterectomy is recommended, and resolution of NVI and NVG has been reported after this procedure.[29] For asymptomatic patients, endarterectomy is not recommended,[30] even if NVI or NVG is present.

Central retinal artery occlusion

Since NVG has been reported to occur anywhere from 1 week to 5 months after CRAO, patients with CRAO should be followed up carefully for at least 6 months and PRP instituted when NVI is first noted.

PHARMACOLOGIC THERAPIES

Medical treatment to control high IOP

Pilocarpine and other anticholinergic agents are generally contraindicated, because they may increase inflammation, cause miosis, worsen synechial angle closure, and decrease uveoscleral outflow. Medications that decrease aqueous humor production, such as topical β-blockers and topical and systemic carbonic anhydrase inhibitors, are beneficial but do not usually lower the IOP to a normal range in eyes with a closed angle. Topical apraclonidine, an α-adrenergic agonist, may be used short-term (days to weeks). Prostaglandins may not be of much help because they work by increasing the uveal outflow, which may be covered by a membrane. Hyperosmotic agents can be used intermittently.

The most important medications remain topical atropine and topical corticosteroids to decrease congestion and inflammation, and often provide adequate symptomatic relief despite pressures as high as 60 mmHg.

Anti-VEGF therapy

There is evidence now that VEGF is an important factor in the pathogenesis of ocular neovascularization and NVG.[31] Several case studies have attempted to ascertain the value of intraocular anti-VEGF therapy with bevacizumab as an adjunctive treatment for NVI associated with glaucoma. A single application of the drug caused a dramatic reduction of leakage from rubeotic vessels. Oshima et al.[32] reported a case series of seven eyes with NVI secondary to PDR. The NVI regressed in all patients at 1 week, and repeated injections stabilized the recurrence (in two eyes) that was seen 2 months after the initial injection (Figure 27.6). In another report, Krzystolik et al.[33] reported one patient with complicated neovascular DR, who received an intravitreal injection of 0.3 mg pegaptanib sodium in his right eye. Within 9 days, the iris vessels resolved. Despite an initial favorable response, the patient developed postoperative vitreous hemorrhage and recurrent rubeosis on postoperative day 7. The patient received repeated injections and has stabilized the recurrence seen 4 months after the initial injection.

Corticosteroid therapy

One of the most important still unsolved problems in clinical ophthalmology is the proliferation of vascular cells in eyes with intraocular neovascular disease. The new vessels on the iris surface and anterior-chamber angle are secondary to ischemic and, to a lesser degree, to inflammatory retinal diseases. For many years, corticosteroids have been known to reduce intraocular inflammation and, depending on the concentration, to suppress cell proliferation. Jonas et al.[34] proposed the intravitreal injection of crystalline cortisone as an adjunctive therapy to manage NVG. They reported using a single injection of approximately 20 mg triamcinolone acetonide with little vehicle in patients with established NVG. After a follow-up period of 3.10 ± 2.4 months, they showed a significant decrease of the degree of rubeosis iridis, improvement in IOP, and no significant changes in visual acuity.

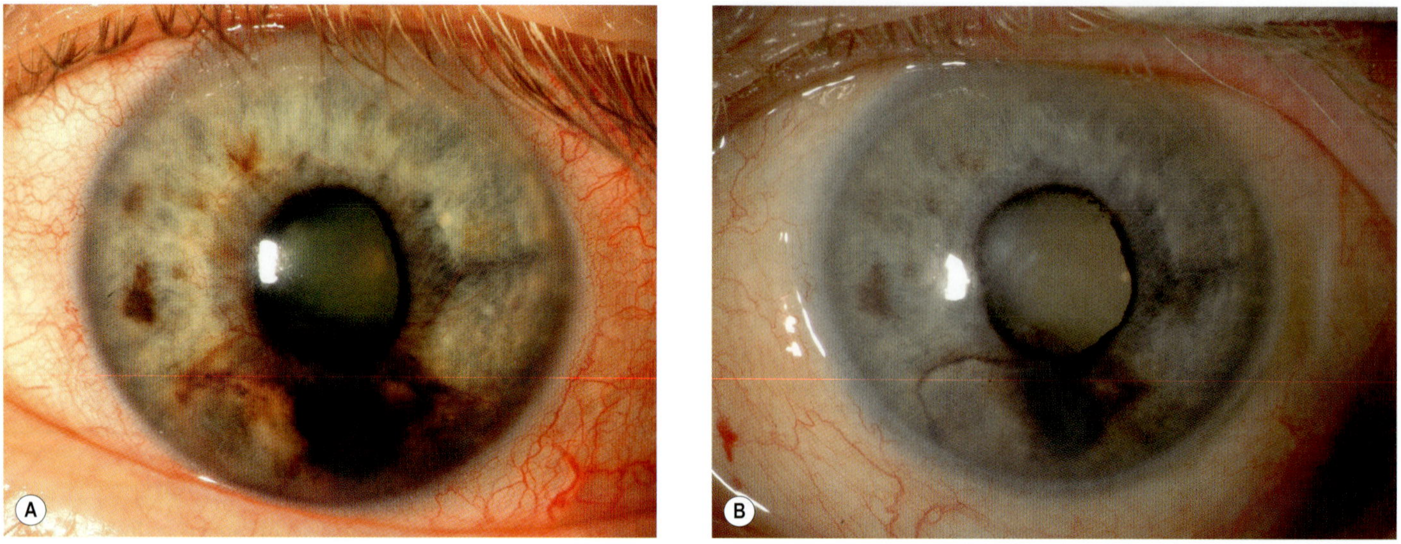

Figure 27.6 A patient with iris melanoma in his only seeing eye: the melanoma grew quite large and neovascular glaucoma developed. The patient was then treated with plaque radiotherapy. A single application of intraocular antivascular endothelial growth factor therapy with bevacizumab caused a dramatic reduction of leakage from rubeotic vessels. (A) Color photograph before bevacizumab. (B) Color photograph after bevacizumab. (Courtesy of Carol L. Shields, MD.)

Photodynamic therapy

In 1984, in an experimental study in rhesus monkeys with iris neovascularization, Packer et al.[35] reported marked reduction of leakage from NVI on fluorescein angiography after photodynamic therapy, but the effect was temporary and required repeated application to control NVI. Parodi and Iacono[36] reported that photodynamic therapy might be a promising approach for NVG. In their series of 16 NVG eyes, there was a 39% decrease in IOP overall and treatment did not control IOP satisfactorily in 31%.

TREATMENT OUTCOMES AND PROGNOSIS

Despite the many advances in the treatment of NVG, visual prognosis remains poor. The key to improving patient outcomes is early detection of angle neovascularization and initiation of treatment of the underlying disease responsible for the rubeosis. Once IOP becomes elevated, successful management of the disease may be extremely difficult.

In the management strategy, the first priority should be to try to prevent its development by appropriate management of the causative diseases. Currently, there is no satisfactory means of treating NVG and preventing visual loss in the majority, in spite of multiple modes of medical and surgical options advocated over the years and claims made.

Adjuvant bevacizumab for NVG may offer a more causal treatment of the neovascular trigger, might be able to prevent further PAS formation and secondary angle damage, and is likely to open a therapeutic window for PRP. The intravitreal application of triamcinolone acetonide helps to reduce the NVI temporarily. With the normalization of IOP and clearing of the corneal edema, laser application to the retina is possible through clear media.

SUMMARY AND KEY POINTS

In the management strategy, the first priority should be to try to prevent its development by appropriate management of the causative diseases. The most common diseases responsible for development of NVG are ischemic CRVO, DR, and ocular ischemic syndrome. Although PRP is considered the standard treatment of retinal ischemia, the best alternative method is still undetermined. Currently, there is considerable interest in the anti-VEGF drugs for the management of ocular neovascularization in age-related macular degeneration, but, so far, we have little long-term worthwhile information in a large series of patients about its effectiveness in prevention or control of NVG or ocular neovascularization elsewhere. The explanation of the signal transduction pathway in ocular angiogenesis may lead to the development of new antivasoproliferative pharmacologic agents. The ideal modalities for early detection of angle neovascularization remain to be defined.

REFERENCES

1. Coats G. Further cases of thrombosis of the central vein. Royal London Ophthalmic Hospital Report 1906;16:516.
2. Salus R. Rubeosis iridis diabetic, eine bischer unbekannte diabetische Irisveranderung. Med Klin 1928;24,256.
3. Kurz O. Zur Rubeosis iridis diabetic. Arch Augenheilkd 1937;10:284.
4. Weiss DI, Shaffer RN, Nehrenberg TR. Neovascular glaucoma complicating carotid-cavernous fistula. Arch Ophthalmol 1963;69:304–307.
5. Sivak-Callcott JA, O'Day DM, Gass JD, et al. Evidence-based recommendations for the diagnosis and treatment of neovascular glaucoma. Ophthalmology 2001;108:1767–1776.
6. Hayreh SS, Rojas P, Podhajsky P, et al. Ocular neovascularization with retinal vascular occlusion – III. Incidence of ocular neovascularization with retinal vein occlusion. Ophthalmology 1983;90:488–506.
7. Magargal LE, Brown GC, Augsburger JJ, et al. Neovascular glaucoma following central retinal vein obstruction. Ophthalmology 1981;88:1095–1101.
8. Pollack A, Dottan S, Oliver M. The fellow eye in retinal vein occlusive disease. Ophthalmology 1989;96:842–845.
9. Gartner S, Henkind P. Neovascularization of the iris (rubeosis iridis). Surv Ophthalmol 1978;22:291–312.
10. Brodell LP, Olk RJ, Arribas NP, et al. Neovascular glaucoma: a retrospective analysis of treatment with peripheral panretinal cryotherapy. Ophthalmic Surg 1987;18:200–206.
11. Tasman W, Magargal LE, Augsburger JJ. Effects of argon laser photocoagulation on rubeosis iridis and angle neovascularization. Ophthalmology 1980;87:400–402.
12. Sinclair SH, Aaberg TM, Meredith TA. A pars plana filtering procedure combined with lensectomy and vitrectomy for neovascular glaucoma. Am J Ophthalmol 1982;93:185–191.
13. Ohrt V. The frequency of rubeosis iridis in diabetic patients. Acta Ophthalmol 1971;49:301–307.
14. Michaelson IC. The mode of development of the vascular system of the retina, with some observations on its significance for certain retinal disease. Trans Ophthalmol Soc UK 1948;68:137–180.

15. Aiello LP, Avery RL, Arrigg PG, et al. Vascular endothelial growth factor in ocular fluid of patients with diabetic retinopathy and other retinal disorders. N Engl J Med 1994;331:1480–1487.
16. Ashton N. Retinal vascularization in health and disease. Am J Ophthalmol 1957;44:7–24.
17. Leung DW, Cachianes G, Kuang WJ, et al. Vascular endothelial growth factor is a secreted angiogenic mitogen. Science 1989;246:1306–1309.
18. Cohen T, Nahari D, Cerem LW, et al. Interleukin-6 induces the expression of vascular endothelial growth factor. J Biol Chem 1996;271:736–741.
19. Hanneken A, de Juan Jr E, Lutty GA, et al. Altered distribution of basic fibroblast growth factor in diabetic retinopathy. Arch Ophthalmol 1991;109:1005–1011.
20. Meyer-Schwickerath R, Pfeiffer A, Blum WF, et al. Vitreous levels of the insulin-like growth factors I and II, and the insulin-like growth factor binding proteins 2 and 3, increase in neovascular eye disease. Studies in nondiabetic and diabetic subjects. J Clin Invest 1993;92:2620–2625.
21. Ayaki M. Development of neovascular glaucoma in the course of interferon alpha therapy for hepatitis type C. Br J Ophthalmol 1994;78:238.
22. John T, Sassani JW, Eagle Jr RC. The myofibroblastic component of rubeosis iridis. Ophthalmology 1983;90:721–728.
23. Laatikainen L, Kohner EM, Khoury D, et al. Panretinal photocoagulation in central retinal vein occlusion: a randomised controlled clinical study. Br J Ophthalmol 1977;61:741–753.
24. Baseline and early natural history report. The Central Vein Occlusion Study. Arch Ophthalmol 1993;111:1087–1095.
25. Madsen PH. Rubeosis of the iris and hemorrhagic glaucoma in patients with proliferative diabetic retinopathy. Br J Ophthalmol 1971;55:368–371.
26. Hayreh SS, Podhajsky P. Ocular neovascularization with retinal vascular occlusion. II. Occurrence in central and branch retinal artery occlusion. Arch Ophthalmol 1982;100:1585–1596.
27. Walton DS, Grant WM. Retinoblastoma and iris neovascularization. Am J Ophthalmol 1968;65:598–599.
28. Shields MB, Proia AD. Neovascular glaucoma associated with an iris melanoma. A clinicopathologic report. Arch Ophthalmol 1987;105:672–674.
29. Neupert JR, Brubaker RF, Kearns TP, et al. Rapid resolution of venous stasis retinopathy after carotid endarterectomy. Am J Ophthalmol 1976;81:600–602.
30. Barnett HJ, Haines SJ. Carotid endarterectomy for asymptomatic carotid stenosis. N Engl J Med 1993;328:276–279.
31. Tripathi RC, Li J, Tripathi BJ, et al. Increased level of vascular endothelial growth factor in aqueous humor of patients with neovascular glaucoma. Ophthalmology 1998;105:232–237.
32. Oshima Y, Sakaguchi H, Gomi F, et al. Regression of iris neovascularization after intravitreal injection of bevacizumab in patients with proliferative diabetic retinopathy. Am J Ophthalmol 2006;142:155–158.
33. Krzystolik MG, Filippopoulos T, Ducharme JF, et al. Pegaptanib as an adjunctive treatment for complicated neovascular diabetic retinopathy. Arch Ophthalmol 2006;124:920–921.
34. Jonas JB, Hayler JK, Söfker A, et al. Regression of neovascular iris vessels by intravitreal injection of crystalline cortisone. J Glaucoma 2001;10:284–287.
35. Packer AJ, Tse DT, Gu XQ, et al. Hematoporphyrin photoradiation therapy for iris neovascularization. A preliminary report. Arch Ophthalmol 1984;102:1193–1197.
36. Parodi MB, Iacono P. Photodynamic therapy with verteporfin for anterior segment neovascularizations in neovascular glaucoma. Am J Ophthalmol 2004;138:157–158.

CHAPTER 28

Retinal hereditary and degenerative/dystrophic diseases (non-AMD)

Sandeep Grover, MD and Ravi Keshavamurthy, MD

INTRODUCTION

Hereditary retinal diseases are a group of diseases that are slowly progressive and may lead to severe visual disability. These are orphan diseases, which, in the USA, are defined as conditions affecting fewer than 200,000 people. A majority of these conditions have no proven means of treatment. However, more and more genetic mutations are being identified, which provides a better understanding of the pathophysiology of these diseases. Thus, the past decade has seen a tremendous growth in therapeutic research in these diseases.

The retina, retinal pigment epithelium (RPE), and choroid form an important complex and are functionally interdependent. Even though the mutant gene may be expressed in only one of these layers and cause apoptosis, the other two layers degenerate in the corresponding areas as well. Treatment for these conditions can be in the form of replacing the gene (as in Leber's congenital amaurosis (LCA)), providing growth factors to sustain the degenerating photoreceptors (ciliary neurotrophic factors (CNTF) in retinitis pigmentosa (RP)), or dietary restriction of a toxic protein that is not being metabolized in the retina (phytanic acid in Refsum disease). Some of these degenerative diseases that have a therapeutic valence are discussed in this chapter.

SPECIFIC DISEASES

RETINITIS PIGMENTOSA

RP is a group of inherited retinal diseases that affects approximately 1 in 4000 people. The mode of inheritance can be autosomal-recessive, autosomal-dominant, or X-linked recessive. Symptoms of RP include problems with night vision and peripheral vision. The central vision is also affected. Fundus examination shows a pale-appearing optic nerve, attenuated arterioles, and bone-spicule pigmentary changes in the mid peripheral retina (Figure 28.1). Visual field testing shows a concentric restriction or ring scotoma, eventually leading to "tunnel vision." Electroretinography (ERG) shows reduced or absent rod function with subsequent reduction of cone function. RP can be associated with cystoid macular changes and atrophic lesions in the fovea.

Nutrients and retinitis pigmentosa

RP has no treatment yet. A report in 1993 concluded that an oral supplement of high-dose vitamin A palmitate (15,000 IU/day) is helpful in slowing down the progress of disease.[1] Although this was a well-planned, randomized, controlled, and double-masked study, the interpretation was considered controversial.[2,3] The results of the study concluded that patients who were on this high dose of vitamin A had less decline of cone ERG amplitudes. However, none of the other retinal function tests, including visual acuity and visual field, were significantly affected. Moreover, there was concern that this high dose of vitamin A is teratogenic and when taken over years may be hepatotoxic and possibly cause osteoporosis. The same study also reported possible accelerated course of the disease with vitamin E supplementation. Hence, vitamin E is not recommended in patients with RP.

Docosahexaenoic acid (DHA) is a long-chain, omega-3 fatty acid that is normally found in red blood cell (RBC) membranes and outer segments of rod photoreceptors. Significant correlation between the DHA levels in RBCs and ERG amplitudes has been reported. A phase I trial with supplementation of 400 mg/day of DHA in patients with X-linked RP for a period of 4 years did not show any adverse toxic effects.[4] Furthermore, there was no statistically significant difference in the rate of loss of cone ERG amplitudes between the treated and untreated groups. Also, there was no change in visual function between the two groups. Another study investigated the effect of 15 000 IU vitamin A with or without 1200 mg/day DHA in patients with RP. No significant difference was reported in the ERG amplitudes between the two groups – hence, DHA is not yet recommended as a treatment.[5]

Cystoid Macular Edema (CME) associated with RP

CME is present in 15–20% of patients with RP. With the advent of optical coherence tomography (OCT), the incidence is even higher.[6] Macular edema may be evident on clinical examination, fluorescein angiography, and/or OCT. Although the mechanism of CME is not clear, the assumption is that the RPE cells are unable to pump out the fluid from the outer retina. Treatment of CME consists of carbonic anhydrase inhibitors (CAIs). Systemic CAIs like acetazolamide[7] and methazolamide[8] can lead to resolution of macular edema with improvement in visual function in some patients. However, they can cause side-effects like fatigue, tinnitus, "tingling" sensation in the extremities, loss of appetite, and renal stones. Rarely, more serious problems like aplastic anemia and agranulocytosis have been reported. Topical dorzolamide (used three times a day) is also effective in some patients in reducing the CME with improvement in visual acuity.[9] However, the CME should be monitored with OCT at regular intervals as both systemic and topical CAIs can cause a "rebound phenomenon," whereby the CME can get worse while still on treatment.[9–11]

Ciliary Neurotrophic Factor and retinitis pigmentosa

Neurotrophic factors like basic fibroblast growth factor and CNTF have been shown to have a neuroprotective role on degenerating photoreceptors in animal models, CNTF being the most common. Although this has been known for several years, the mode of drug delivery was difficult. It could not be given orally or intravenously because of relative impermeability of the blood–retina barrier. Since CNTF was found to be neurotoxic in large doses, leading to decrease in ERG amplitudes,[12,13] it could not be injected intravitreally.

Based on the fact that CNTF may be useful in optimal concentrations only, a drug delivery device (NT-501, Neurotech, USA) was developed using encapsulated cell technology. This is a 6-mm long semipermeable intravitreal implant that consists of a hollow fiber membrane containing genetically modified human cells secreting CNTF at a fixed concentration (Figure 28.2A). The fiber membrane is designed so that it permits

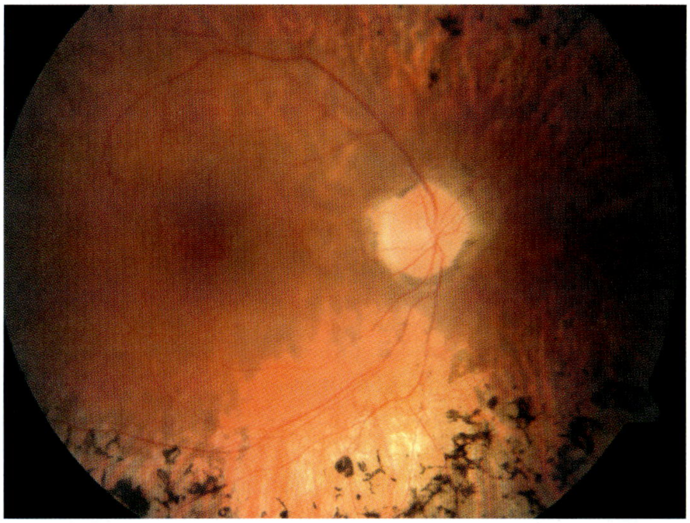

Figure 28.1 Fundus photograph of the right eye from a patient with retinitis pigmentosa showing attenuated arterioles and mid peripheral bone-spicule pigmentary retinopathy.

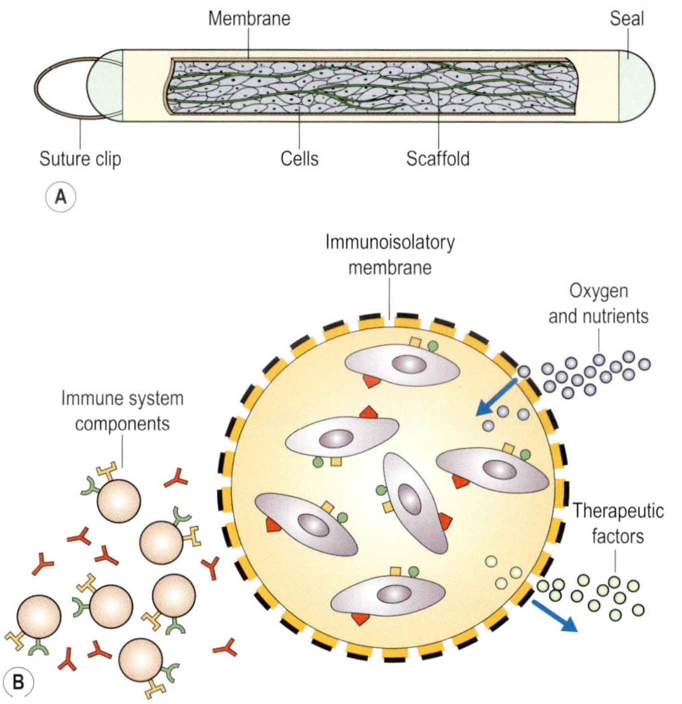

Figure 28.2 Depiction of encapsulated cell technology showing the structure of the intravitreal implant (A) containing the cells secreting a known concentration of ciliary neurotrophic factor (CNTF). The implant is also shown in cross-section (B).

egress of CNTF into the vitreous cavity, allows influx of various nutrients and oxygen, but prevents the entry of immune antibodies (Figure 28.2B). This device allows for long-term sustained delivery of constant levels of CNTF in the vitreous cavity close to the retina (Figure 28.3). Another advantage of this technology is that it can be retrieved, if needed. It was implanted in dog and rabbit models of RP with no deleterious effects on ERG. Based on several prior animal studies, a phase I human clinical trial was completed in 10 patients with RP, which showed that the implant was relatively safe for a period of at

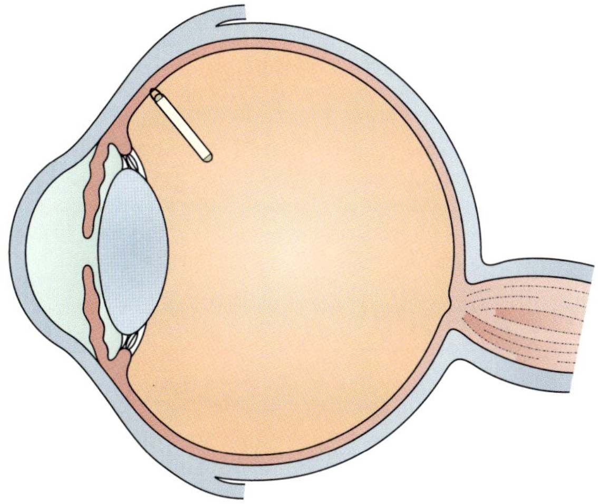

Figure 28.3 Depiction of surgical placement of the intravitreal implant in the eye with secretion of ciliary neurotrophic factor into the vitreous.

least 6 months.[14] Two randomized, double-masked, multicentered, sham-controlled phase II/III trials are now under way in patients with early and late stages of RP to establish the effectiveness of CNTF.

REFSUM'S DISEASE

Refsum's disease is a rare autosomal-recessive disorder caused by defective alpha-oxidation of phytanic acid (3,7,11,15 tetramethylhexadecanoic acid), a branched-chain fatty acid. The source of phytanic acid is all exogenous and comes from a wide range of food products, including dairy products, some meats, and fish.[15] The physiological role of phytanic acid in the body is unknown and is normally metabolized by an enzyme phytanoyl-CoA hydroxylase, which converts it to pristanic acid.[16] Deficiency of this enzyme results in accumulation of phytanic acid, with elevated levels in blood, cerebrospinal fluid, and other tissues, including fat and neurons.[17,18] In the eye, accumulation of phytanic acid in the RPE is postulated to interfere with vitamin A esterification and progressive visual function loss.

Clinically, there is RP-like retinal degeneration associated with cerebellar ataxia, polyneuropathy, elevated levels of proteins in cerebrospinal fluid with normal cell count, nerve deafness, and ichthyosis. Plasma phytanic acid concentration of more than 200 μmol/l is diagnostic for Refsum's disease. It is now considered to be a peroxisomal disorder with mutations having been identified in two genes: PHYH, the gene encoding phytanoyl-CoA hydroxylase and PEX7, the gene that encodes the type 2 peroxisome-targeting signal receptor.

Treatment

Dietary restriction

Since the source of phytanic acid is almost exclusively dietary, the key factor in the treatment of Refsum's disease is dietary restriction.[19] An average diet consists of 50–100 mg/day of phytanic acid. Fish, lamb, beef, and dairy products are rich sources of phytanic acid.[20] Restriction of dietary consumption to 10–20 mg/day is required to decrease serum levels. Obviously, the sooner the restriction starts in life, the less the pathological damage. Improvement in ataxia, polyneuropathy, motor nerve conduction velocity, and cerebrospinal fluid protein levels after initiation of treatment has been reported. However, the factors that negatively affect patient compliance are that the effect of diet restriction is not seen immediately as phytanic acid has to be mobilized from the body lipids,[18,19] and diets low in phytanic acid are extremely unpalatable.

Plasmapheresis

Plasma exchange (PE) in Refsum disease can be helpful if the disease is severe or rapidly worsening. Lundberg et al. in 1972 first described the use of PE in two siblings who were resistant to treatment with dietary restriction alone.[21] Since then PE has mainly been used in patients with Refsum's disease whose serum phytanic acid levels are above 900 μmol/l, or patients not complying with the diet, or in cases where diet control is ineffective.[22] However, PE can lead to complications including ventricular ectopic beats and urticarial rash.

GYRATE ATROPHY

Gyrate atrophy is a progressive chorioretinal dystrophy, characterized by well-demarcated scalloped areas of RPE and choroidal atrophy. It initially begins in the mid peripheral retina but extends both peripherally and centrally to become more diffuse later on. Inherited as an autosomal-recessive condition, it manifests by late childhood and is associated with hyperornithinemia. High ornithine levels are detectable in urine, plasma, aqueous humor, and cerebrospinal fluid. Ornithine, an intermediate compound in the formation of urea, is reportedly 10–15 times the normal levels in gyrate atrophy. Ornithine is normally converted to glutamic γ-semialdehyde and subsequently to proline by ornithine ketoacid aminotransferase,[23] also known as ornithine aminotransferase (OAT). It is the deficiency of this enzyme, OAT, that causes the hyperornithinemia. OAT is a mitochondrial matrix enzyme that utilizes vitamin B_6 (pyridoxal phosphate) as a cofactor.

This is a night-blinding disorder: symptoms usually start around the second decade of life. Visual fields show mid peripheral scotomas that coalesce to form a ring scotoma, extending both peripherally and centrally, consistent with the RPE and choroidal atrophy. The ERG is subnormal to nondetectable, depending on the extent of atrophy. Abnormalities in electromyogram have been reported in a majority of patients and muscle biopsy shows atrophic type 2 muscle fibers with tubular aggregates on electron microscopy.

Treatment

Treatment of gyrate atrophy consists of either reducing the substrate arginine, from which ornithine is formed, or increasing the activity of OAT enzyme by providing more cofactor vitamin B_6.

Arginine-restricted diet

Since ornithine is produced from arginine, a low-protein diet with arginine restriction is recommended in lowering serum ornithine levels in patients with gyrate atrophy.[24] Although there is no short-term advantage, the long-term lowering of serum ornithine level slows the progression of chorioretinal degeneration in these patients. When six pairs of siblings, all 10 years or younger, were placed on an arginine-restricted diet and observed over a period of 16–17 years, the younger sibling in two of six pairs, who had received the diet at an earlier age, showed slower progression of the chorioretinal lesions than older siblings.[25] In adults, who already have the full-blown manifestation of the disease, as long as the plasma ornithine levels can be maintained below an average of 5.29–6.61 mg/dl (about six times the normal range), it may slow the progression of disease as measured by sequential ERG.[26]

Vitamin B_6 supplementation

Vitamin B_6 supplementation has been found to be effective in reducing serum ornithine levels in a subset of patients with gyrate atrophy. There are two categories of patients – responders and nonresponders to B_6 supplementation. "Responders" have been shown to manifest a milder form of the disease as compared to "nonresponders." Dosage of 15–20 mg/day of vitamin B_6 was found to be effective in responders.[27] Certain genetic mutations have been identified in vitamin B_6 responders and nonresponders that may account for this difference in response to vitamin B_6.

ABETALIPOPROTEINEMIA (BASSEN–KORNZWEIG SYNDROME)

Abetalipoproteinemia, an autosomal-recessive disorder, is characterized by retinal degeneration similar to RP associated with spinocerebellar ataxia, peripheral neuropathy, lipid malabsorption, absence or severe reduction of serum cholesterol and acanthocytosis.[28,29]

The basic defect is the deficiency of microsomal triglyceride transfer protein activity leading to failure of synthesis of beta-apolipoproteins. This then disrupts the transmembrane transport of fat-soluble vitamins in the intestines, leading to deficiency of vitamins A, E, and K. The manifestations of this disease are mainly due to hypovitaminosis. Due to a lack of vitamins A and E, there is photoreceptor degeneration resembling RP.

Treatment

Supplementing vitamin A, E, and K with essential fatty acids for life may help to forestall the progress of neurological and retinal degeneration. The recommended treatment schedule is to administer vitamin A 300 units/kg/day; vitamin E 100 units/kg/day; vitamin K 0.15 mg/kg/day; and omega-3 fatty acids 0.19 mg/kg/day.[30]

LEBER CONGENITAL AMAUROSIS

LCA is probably the most severe form of retinal degeneration. Inherited in an autosomal-recessive manner, it consists of a group of retinal diseases characterized by severe and early visual impairment, sensory nystagmus, amaurotic pupils, and nonrecordable electrical signals on ERG.[31] Manifesting in early infancy, the symptoms include poor vision, photoaversion, nyctalopia, and the presence of oculodigital phenomenon. LCA has a wide phenotypic variability – features described are normal-appearing retina with attenuated arterioles, macular coloboma-like lesions, and pigmentary retinopathy that can vary from bone spicule pattern to salt and pepper pigmentation or preserved para-arteriolar RPE.[31,32] Visual acuity in LCA patients ranges widely, usually from 20/200 to light perception or even no light perception.[32] High refractive errors, typically hyperopia, keratoconus, and cataracts, are commonly associated with LCA.

LCA is a heterogeneous disease with the underlying disease genes identified in up to an estimated 60–70% of the cases. To date, mutations in 14 different genes have been identified. Mutations in the genes involve phototransduction pathways (AIPL1, GUCY2D), the retinoid cycle (RDH12, LRAT, RPE65), photoreceptor development and structure (CRX, CRB1), transport across photoreceptor connecting cilium (TULP1, RPGRIP1, CEP290, Lebercilin) and some others (IMPDH1, MERTK, RD3).[31] Some of these genes have very specific genotype–phenotype correlations.[33] RPE65 (RPE-specific 65-kDa) gene is an important component of the retinoid cycle and isomerizes the conversion of all-*trans*-retinal ester to 11-*cis*-retinol in the RPE cells. This leads to decreased formation of rhodopsin, thereby causing severe retinal degeneration.

Treatment

RPE65 gene therapy

The main impetus for gene therapy in LCA secondary to RPE65 mutations came after successful treatment in a canine model of human LCA (Briard dogs). These dogs are born blind and have a more severe disease than human LCA. The RPE65 gene was transferred through an adeno-associated virus injected into the subretinal space to provide the gene to the RPE cells. ERG and qualitative improvement were noted in these treated dogs.[34] A lentiviral-mediated RPE65 gene therapy in a mouse model also showed substantial improvement.[35] Results from both these studies formed the basis of human treatment trials.

The results of recently reported phase I trials have shown that gene therapy is safe, at least in the short term.[36–38] Although these studies were designed to be safety studies, some improvement of visual function was also reported. However, further studies are needed to establish long-term efficacy and safety.

X-LINKED JUVENILE RETINOSCHISIS

X-linked juvenile retinoschisis is one of the juvenile-onset macular dystrophies that is characterized by decreased central vision, cystic changes in the macula, peripheral retinal schisis in 50% of patients, and selective reduction of ERG b-wave amplitude. The foveal cystic changes are usually apparent very early after birth, due to splitting within inner retinal layers. However, visual acuity is not severely reduced until the fifth or sixth decade of life. Other clinical features include vitreous veils, vitreous hemorrhage, pigmentary retinopathy, and dendritiform lesions of the retina. The gene XLRS1 encodes for the protein retinoschisin that is responsible for cell-to-cell adhesion; mutation in this gene causes splitting of the retina and development of cystic spaces in the inner nuclear and outer plexiform layers of the retina.

Treatment

Although there is no treatment available for the disease itself, a recent study reported improvement in visual acuity and retinal thickness on OCT in a substantial number of patients (n = 8) treated with topical dorzolamide.[39] Similar to patients with RP and CME, the recommendation is that these patients on topical dorzolamide should be monitored with an OCT at regular intervals.

SUMMARY AND KEY POINTS

In summary, this is an era when clinicians, basic scientists, molecular biologists, pharmaceutical companies, and funding agencies have all teamed up to identify more genes, provide phenotype–genotype correlations, and prepare animal models of various diseases in an attempt to understand better the pathogenesis of some of these yet untreatable conditions. There are several ongoing treatment trials in various phases which provide a reason for optimism in the future.

REFERENCES

1. Berson EL, Rosner B, Sandberg MA, et al. A randomized trial of vitamin A and vitamin E supplementation for retinitis pigmentosa. Arch Ophthalmol 1993;111:761–772.
2. Massof RW, Finkelstein D. Supplemental vitamin A retards loss of ERG amplitude in retinitis pigmentosa [editorial]. Arch Ophthalmol 1993;111:751–754.
3. Massof RW, Finkelstein D. Vitamin supplementation for retinitis pigmentosa [letter]. Arch Ophthalmol 1993;111:1458–1459.
4. Wheaton DH, Hoffman DR, Locke KG, et al. Biological safety assessment of docosahexaenoic acid supplementation in a randomized clinical trial for X-linked retinitis pigmentosa. Arch Ophthalmol 2003;121:1269–1278.
5. Berson EL, Rosner B, Sandberg MA, et al. Clinical trial of docosahexaenoic acid in patients with retinitis pigmentosa receiving vitamin A treatment. Arch Ophthalmol 2004;122:1297–1305.
6. Hajali M, Fishman GA, Anderson RJ. The prevalence of cystoid macular edema in retinitis pigmentosa patients determined by optical coherence tomography. Br J Ophthalmol 2008;92:1065–1068.
7. Cox SN, Hay E, Bird AC. Treatment of chronic macular edema with acetazolamide. Arch Ophthalmol 1988;106:1190–1195.
8. Fishman GA, Gilbert LD, Anderson RJ, et al. Effect of methazolamide on chronic macular edema in patients with retinitis pigmentosa. Ophthalmology 1994;101:687–693.
9. Grover S, Apushkin MA, Fishman GA. Topical dorzolamide for the treatment of cystoid macular edema in patients with retinitis pigmentosa. Am J Ophthalmol 2006;141:850–858.
10. Fishman GA, Glenn AM, Gilbert LD. Rebound of macular edema with continued use of methazolamide in patients with retinitis pigmentosa. Arch Ophthalmol 1993;111:1640–1646.
11. Apushkin MA, Fishman GA, Grover S, et al. Rebound of cystoid macular edema with continued use of acetazolamide in patients with retinitis pigmentosa. Retina 2007;27:1112–1118.
12. Liang FQ, Dejneka NS, Cohen DR, et al. AAV-mediated delivery of ciliary neurotrophic factor prolongs photoreceptor survival in the rhodopsin knockout mice. Mol Ther 2001;3:241–248.
13. Bok D, Yasumura D, Matthes MT, et al. Effects of adeno-associated virus-vectored ciliary neurotrophic factor on retinal structure and function in mice with a P216L rds/peripherin mutation. Exp Eye Res 2002. 74:719–735.
14. Sieving PA, Caruso RC, Tao W, et al. Ciliary neurotrophic factor (CNTF) for human retinal degeneration: phase I trial of CNTF delivered by encapsulated cell intraocular implants. Proc Natl Acad Sci USA 2006; 103:3896–3901.
15. Verhoeven NM, Wanders RJ, Poll BT, et al. The metabolism of phytanic acid and pristanic acid in man: a review. J Inherit Metab Dis 1998:21:697–728.
16. Jansen GA, Wanders RJ, Watkins PA, et al. Phytanoyl-coenzyme A hydroxylase deficiency – the enzyme defect in Refsum's disease. N Engl J Med 1997;337:133–134.
17. Wills AJ, Manning NJ, Reilly MM. Refsum's disease. Q J Med 2001;94:403–406.
18. Wierzbicki AS, Lloyd MD, Schofield CJ, et al. Refsum's disease: a peroxisomal disorder affecting phytanic acid α-oxidation. J Neurochem 2002;80:727–735.
19. Steinberg D, Mize CE, Herndon Jr JH. Phytanic acid in patients with Refsum's syndrome and response to dietary treatment. Arch Intern Med 1970;125:75–87.
20. Brown PJ, Mei G, Gibberd FB, et al. Diet and Refsum's disease. J Hum Nutr Dietet 1993;6:295–305.
21. Lundberg A, Lilja LG, Lundberg PO, et al. Heredopathia atactica polyneuritiformis (Refsum's disease): experiences of dietary treatment and plasmapheresis. Eur Neurol 1972;8:309–324.
22. Harari D, Gibberd FB, Dick JP, et al. Plasma exchange in the treatment of Refsum's disease (heredopathia atactica polyneuritiformis). J Neurol Neurosurg Psychiatry 1991;54:614–617.
23. Simell O, Takki K. Raised plasma-ornithine and gyrate atrophy of the choroid and retina. Lancet 1973;1:1031–1033.
24. McInnes RR, Arshinoff SA, Bell L, et al. Hyperornithinemia and gyrate atrophy of the retina: improvement of vision during treatment with a low-arginine diet. Lancet 1981;1:513–516.
25. Kaiser-Kupfer MI, Caruso RC, Valle D. Gyrate atrophy of the choroid and retina: further experience with long-term reduction of ornithine levels in children. Arch Ophthalmol 2002;120:146–153.
26. Kaiser-Kupfer MI, Caruso RC, Valle D, et al. Use of an arginine-restricted diet to slow progression of visual loss in patients with gyrate atrophy. Arch Ophthalmol 2004;122:982–984.
27. Weleber RG, Kennaway NG. Clinical trial of vitamin B_6 for gyrate atrophy of the choroid and retina. Ophthalmology 1981;88:316–324.
28. Atchaneeyasakul L, Weleber RG, Illingworth DR. Abetalipoproteinemia (Bassen-Kornzweig syndrome) and homozygous familial hypobetalipoproteinemia. In: Fraunfelder FT, Roy FH, editors. Current Ocular Therapy, 5th edn. Philadelphia: W.B. Saunders; 2000. p. 595–597.
29. Kane JP, Havel RJ. Disorders of the biogenesis and secretion of lipoproteins containing the B apolipoproteins. In: Scriver CR, Beaudet AL, Sly WS, et al. editors. The metabolic and molecular bases of inherited disease, vol. 2, 8th edn. New York: McGraw-Hill; 2001. p. 2717–2752.
30. Grant CA, Berson EL. Treatable forms of retinitis pigmentosa associated with systemic neurological disorders. Int Ophthalmol Clin 2001;41:103–110.
31. den Hollander AI, Roepman R, Koenekoop RK, et al. Leber congenital amaurosis: genes, proteins and disease mechanisms. Prog Retin Eye Res 2008;27:391–419.
32. Fulton AB, Hansen RM, Mayer DL. Vision in Leber congenital amaurosis. Arch Ophthalmol 1996;114:698–703.
33. Dharmaraj SR, Silva ER, Pina AL, et al. Mutational analysis and clinical correlation in Leber congenital amaurosis. Ophthalmic Genet 2000;21:135–150.
34. Acland GM, Aguirre GD, Ray J, et al. Gene therapy restores vision in a canine model of childhood blindness. Nat Genet 2001;28:92–95.
35. Bemelmans AP, Kostic C, Crippa SV, et al. Lentiviral gene transfer of RPE65 rescues survival and function of cones in a mouse model of Leber congenital amaurosis. PLoS Med 2006;3:e347.
36. Maguire AM, Simonelli F, Pierce EA, et al. Safety and efficacy of gene transfer for Leber's congenital amaurosis. N Engl J Med 2008;358: 2240–2248.
37. Bainbridge JW, Smith AJ, Barker SS, et al. Effect of gene therapy on visual function in Leber's congenital amaurosis. N Engl J Med 2008;358: 2231–2239.
38. Hauswirth W, Aleman TS, Kaushal S, et al. Treatment of Leber congenital amaurosis due to RPE65 mutations by ocular subretinal injection of adeno-associated virus gene vector: short-term results of a phase I trial. Hum Gene Ther 2008;19:979–990.
39. Apushkin MA, Fishman GA. Use of dorzolamide for patients with X-linked retinoschisis. Retina 2006;26:741–745.

CHAPTER 29

Nonsteroidal anti-inflammatory drugs (NSAIDs) in the treatment of retinal diseases

Eduardo Büchele Rodrigues, MD, Michel Eid Farah, MD, Juliana Mantovani Bottós, MD, and Fabio Bom Aggio, MD

KEY FEATURES

Retinal pharmacotherapy has evolved vastly in recent years. Retinal diseases such as choroidal neovascularization (CNV) or macular edema (ME) can be currently managed with local or systemic application of drugs such as corticosteroids or monoclonal antibodies. However, such agents have major side-effects, including glaucoma, cataract, and inflammation. As a result, nonsteroidal anti-inflammatory drugs (NSAIDs) have arisen as great alternative pharmacologic agents. Nevanac, diclofenac, ketorolac and bromfenac are some notable NSAID candidates which should be investigated intravitreally or topically for retinal pharmacotherapy (Figure 29.1).

INTRODUCTION AND HISTORY

In ophthalmology, NSAIDs were initially used for the prevention of intraoperative miosis. However, they were later found to have a modulating effect on ocular inflammation and pain through the prevention of prostaglandin (PG) synthesis via cyclooxygenase (COX) inhibition. More importantly, NSAIDs have also been found to be effective in the prevention and treatment of cystoid macular edema (CME) secondary to cataract surgery.[1–3]

The use of NSAIDs for various vitreoretinal conditions has become a reasonable therapeutic approach in recent years. For retinal pharmacotherapy, the ideal drug would penetrate target intraocular tissues at therapeutic levels, thereby reaching high concentrations in both the uveal tract and posterior segment. In this way, desired effects such as pain reduction as well as the prevention and treatment of anterior- and posterior-segment inflammation or edema could be achieved. COX inhibitors are potent anti-inflammatory agents that have shown a quite safe profile when applied to the ocular surface. Some COX inhibitors that have been proposed for retinal diseases in the recent past include nepafenac, diclofenac, and ketorolac.[3]

PHARMACOLOGY, DRUG MECHANISM, AND EFFECTS

DICLOFENAC

Diclofenac sodium (Voltaren Ophthalmic, Novartis), 0.1% ophthalmic solution, is a sterile topical NSAID product for ophthalmic use. Diclofenac sodium is designated chemically as 2-[(2,6-ichlorophenyl) amino] benzeneacetic acid, monosodium salt, with an empirical formula of $C_{14}H_{10}C_{12}NO_2Na$, molecular weight of 318, and osmolarity of 300 mOsmol/ml. Diclofenac sodium is a faintly yellow-white to light-beige, slightly hygroscopic crystalline powder. It is freely soluble in methanol and sparingly soluble in water. An oily solution has been formulated in an attempt to overcome the poor water solubility of diclofenac. Results from a bioavailability study established that plasma levels of diclofenac following ocular instillation of two drops of Voltaren Ophthalmic to each eye were below the limit of detection (10 ng/ml) over a 4-hour period. This study suggests that limited, if any, systemic absorption occurs with Voltaren Ophthalmic.[1,3,4] Apart from the commercially available conventional dosage form, various other delivery systems such as novel polydisperse carrier solution (Sophisen), ophthalmic gels, ocular inserts, and liposomes of diclofenac have been evaluated. Polydisperse carrier solutions of diclofenac were reported to provide better tolerance and sustained release of diclofenac. In addition, precorneal retention of diclofenac sodium has been reported to be increased by the use of liposomes.[1,2]

KETOROLAC

Ketorolac tromethamine is a member of the pyrrolo-pyrrole group of NSAIDs for ophthalmic use as 0.5% solution (Acular, Allergan, USA). The chemical name for ketorolac is benzoyl-2,3-dihydro-1H-pyrrolizine-1-carboxylic acid, and its chemical formula is $C_{19}H_{24}N_2O_6$. In its commercial formula, ketorolac tromethamine 0.4% contains a preservative, 0.006% benzalkonium chloride, and it is supplied as a sterile isotonic solution with a pH of approximately 7.4. Among all the formulations, ketorolac tromethamine ophthalmic solution containing benzalkonium chloride and ethylenediamine tetraacetic acid (EDTA) provided more extensive corneal penetration. The osmolarity of Acular ophthalmic solution is approximately 290 mOsmol/kg.

It has been observed that unbuffered ketorolac tromethamine drops of pH 6.5–8.5 provided enhanced chemical stability. Ketorolac tromethamine may exist in three crystal forms, all of which are equally soluble in water. Acular is commercially available as a tromethamine salt and has higher water solubility compared to ketorolac. Acular ophthalmic solution is a racemic mixture of R-(+) and S-(–)- ketorolac tromethamine. As with other NSAIDs, the mechanism of the drug is associated with the chiral S form, as conversion of the R enantiomer into the S enantiomer has been shown to occur in its metabolism. Thus, the chemical form and physical state of the drug could affect ocular permeation.[2,5]

Investigations on the *in vitro* corneal penetration of ketorolac revealed that reducing the pH of the formulation increased the corneal penetration of ketorolac. Both ketorolac free acid and ketorolac tromethamine have also been formulated as ointment dosage forms. *In vivo* comparison of the aqueous, oil, and ointment formulations of ketorolac for ocular availability in rabbits revealed that the ketorolac drops formulated in oil provided prolonged precorneal residence and sustained effect. The mechanism of action for ketorolac's anti-inflammatory, antipyretic and analgesic effects refers to the specific biochemical interaction through inhibition of PG synthesis by competitive blocking of the enzyme, and, like most NSAIDs, it is a nonselective COX inhibitor.[6,7]

NEVANAC

Nepafenac (Nevanac, Alcon Labs, USA) is a prodrug with low inherent COX-inhibiting activity. The active NSAID compound of nepafenac is

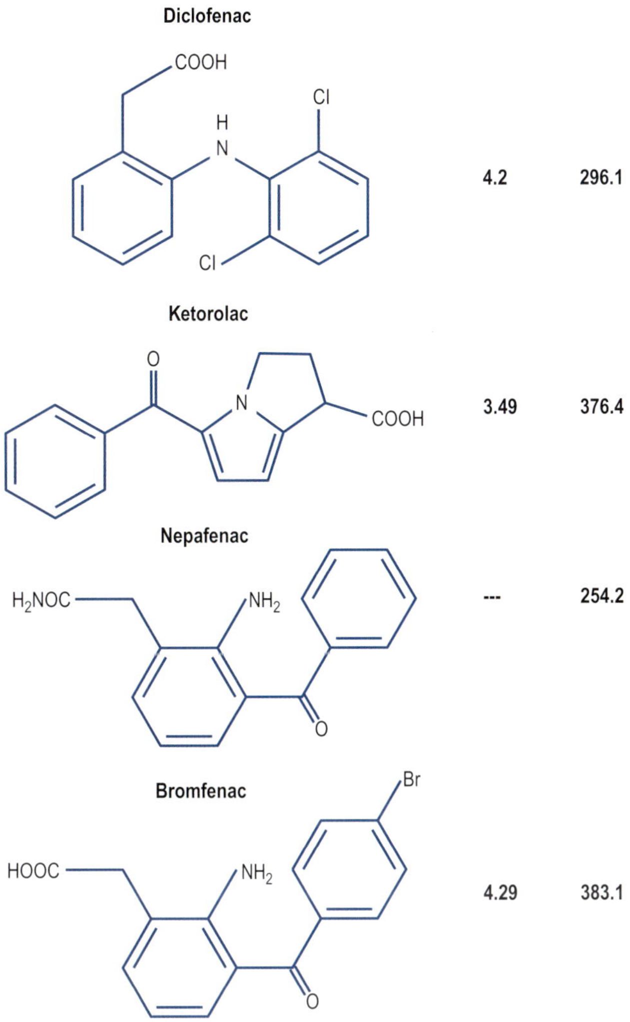

Figure 29.1 Physicochemical characteristics of various nonsteroidal anti-inflammatory drugs used in ocular and retinal pharmacotherapy. The two columns to the right of the chemical structures show the pKa and molecular weight of the drugs.

called amfenac (2-amino-3-benzoylbenzeneacetic acid) which is an NSAID with an arylacetic acid structure exhibiting potent antipyretic and analgesic properties (Figure 29.2). Nepafenac is designated chemically as 2-amino-3-benzoylbenzeneacetamide with an empirical formula of $C_{15}H_{14}N_2O_2$ and molecular weight of 254.28 g/mol. Nepafenac ophthalmic suspension 0.1% was recently made available for ophthalmic use and supplied as a sterile drug with a pH of approximately 7.4 and an osmolality of 305 mOsmol/kg.[8] As a prodrug, nepafenac is a less active form of the drug, which is converted to the more active form, amfenac, after metabolic conversion through intraocular enzymatic hydrolysis. Nepafenac is a member of the new class of NSAID prodrugs for ophthalmic use, providing a novel drug delivery mechanism. The analgesic and anti-inflammatory effect of nepafenac is the result of its fast penetration through the cornea in addition to conversion to amfenac. The superior corneal permeability of nepafenac is likely due to its molecular structure; it is an uncharged molecule whereas the other NSAIDs have acidic structures.[9]

The conversion of nepafenac to amfenac occurs predominantly in the intraocular vascular tissues, especially in the retina and choroid. The nepafenac conversion rates are higher in more posterior sites within the eye because of the higher hydrolase activity in these tissues. It is twice as high in the ciliary body when compared with that in the cornea and 20 times higher in the retina and choroid than in the cornea.

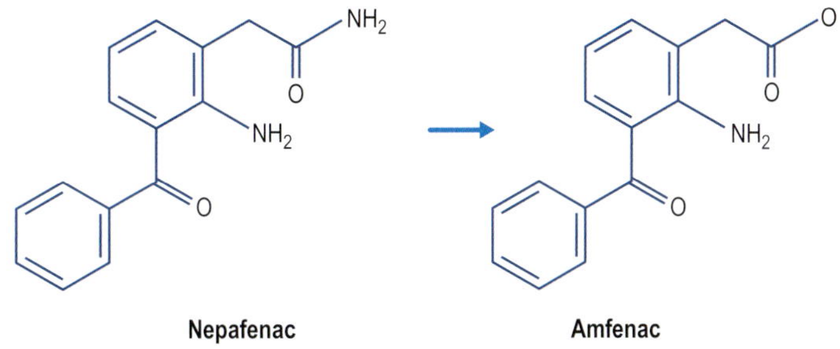

Figure 29.2 Nepafenac is converted to a potent cyclooxygenase inhibitor, amfenac, by intraocular hydrolases.

While nepafenac exhibits some COX inhibition, the activated form, amfenac, is a potent inhibitor of both COX-1 and COX-2 activities. The analgesic action of NSAIDs has also been attributed both to the reduction of PG synthesis and to a direct effect on the excitability of ocular nociceptor sensory nerve terminals by nepafenac. The rapid onset of nepafenac analgesic action is probably due to an inherent analgesic activity and a rapid saturation of the corneal epithelial layer, highly innervated by nociceptors.

Corneal epithelial concentrations of nepafenac may be initially sufficient to attenuate corneal nociceptor PG formation without invoking an immediate conversion to amfenac. Nepafenac has been shown to inhibit PG synthesis in both the anterior and posterior portions of the eye following a single topical ocular application in animal models.[2,9] Following a single dose of Nevanac in 25 cataract surgery patients, aqueous humor concentrations were measured at 15–60 minutes postdose. The maximum mean aqueous humor concentrations were observed at the 1-hour time point (nepafenac, 177 ng/ml; amfenac, 44.8 ng/ml), indicating rapid corneal penetration. Following a three-times-daily dosing of nepafenac eye drops in both eyes, low but quantifiable plasma concentrations of nepafenac and amfenac were observed in the majority of subjects 2 and 3 hours postdose. The mean steady-state plasma concentration (C_{max}) for nepafenac and for amfenac were 0.310 ± 0.104 and 0.422 ± 0.121 ng/ml respectively following ocular administration.

BROMFENAC

Bromfenac ophthalmic solution 0.09% (Xibrom, Senju Pharmaceuticals, Japan) is a sterile topical NSAID for ophthalmic use. Each milliliter of Xibrom contains 1.035 mg bromfenac sodium (equivalent to 0.9 mg bromfenac free acid). Bromfenac sodium is designated chemically as sodium 2-amino-3-(4-bromobenzoyl) phenylacetate sesquihydrate, with an empirical formula of $C_{15}H_{11}BrNNaO_3$ and molecular weight of 383.17. The osmolality of Xibrom ophthalmic solution is approximately 300 mOsmol/kg. The commercially available formulation is buffered to pH 8.3 and contains polysorbate 80 as solubilizer and benzalkonium chloride (0.005%) as preservative.[10] It shows good ocular penetration, and significant amounts are also absorbed systemically after topical administration.

The introduction of bromine in bromfenac makes it more lipophilic, facilitating corneal penetration, increased duration of action, and enhanced COX-2 inhibitory activity. Bromfenac has been found to be 3.7, 6.5, and 18 times more potent in inhibiting COX-2 than diclofenac, amfenac, and ketorolac, respectively. Aqueous drops of the sodium salt (containing an equivalent of 0.09% wt/vol bromfenac) have been used in the management of postoperative ocular inflammation and pain in patients after undergoing cataract extraction. The plasma concentration of bromfenac following ocular administration of 0.09% Xibrom in humans has not been thoroughly studied so far. Based on the maximum proposed dose of one drop to each eye (0.09 mg) and pharmacokinetics data from other routes of administration, the systemic concentration of bromfenac is estimated to be below the limit of detection (50 ng/ml).[2,10]

DRUG USE IN OCULAR AND RETINAL DISEASES

DICLOFENAC

Diclofenac sodium 0.1% solution has been shown to be effective as a prophylactic treatment against the development of CME after cataract surgery, and it has also been approved for inflammation after cataract surgery. Effects of topically applied NSAIDs in eyes undergoing cataract surgery have been demonstrated in many randomized prospective controlled clinical studies. Diclofenac 0.1% seems to be one of the most effective NSAIDs, where the decrease in inflammatory response has been over 30% in eyes treated with diclofenac sodium compared to other NSAID ophthalmic solutions.[1,11] Moreover, the inflammatory response can be quite enhanced with a combination of diclofenac 0.1% and dexamethasone 0.1%. In addition, diclofenac may be applied topically in the eye for the management of pain in corneal epithelial defects following surgery or accidental trauma, treatment of postoperative ocular inflammations, chronic noninfectious inflammations, prevention of intraoperative miosis during cataract surgery, and for symptomatic relief of seasonal allergic conjunctivitis. Some studies could also demonstrate positive effects in managing symptoms of acute allergic conjunctivitis with topical diclofenac sodium 0.1% and treating contact lens-associated giant papillary conjunctivitis or venereal conjunctivitis with suprofen. Diclofenac 0.1% is also approved by the Food and Drug Administration (FDA) to reduce photophobia and pain after refractive surgery. Recently topical diclofenac has been proposed as useful adjuvant therapy to photodynamic therapy in the treatment of CNV.[12]

KETOROLAC

Pharmacodynamic evaluation of aqueous, oily, and ointment formulations of ketorolac in PGE_2-induced ocular inflammation in animals established the efficacy of ketorolac formulations in inhibiting many inflammatory cytokines. Ketorolac 0.5% is FDA-approved to reduce photophobia and pain after refractive surgery. Kaiser et al. compared corneal healing time after contact lens-unrelated traumatic corneal abrasion (less than 10 mm in diameter) in patients with patching and patients who received ketorolac 0.5% without patching.[13] In this study, ketorolac tromethamine 0.5% ophthalmic solution promoted enhanced comfort without clinical adverse effects when used as adjunctive therapy in the treatment of noninfected, noncontact lens-related, traumatic corneal abrasions.

Ketorolac has been also applied topically in the management of seasonal allergic conjunctivitis. Of the topical NSAIDs, ketorolac tromethamine 0.5% ophthalmic solution has been shown to be effective in the treatment of established chronic aphakic and pseudophakic CME. Subsequent studies of the prophylactic use of topical NSAIDs including ketorolac demonstrated a reduction in angiographic CME, but a statistically significant reduction has been difficult to establish. A systematic review of the literature for randomized controlled trials that evaluated the effects of NSAIDs in the treatment of CME following cataract surgery was done according to the Cochrane Collaboration methodology; treatment with topical 0.5% ketorolac for chronic CME was found to be effective in two trials.[14]

NEPAFENAC

The effectiveness of nepafenac was initially examined in experimental studies using animal models. Nepafenac's inhibitory efficacy and longer duration of action were demonstrated by assessing protein and PGE_2 accumulation in aqueous humor in a trauma-induced rabbit model of acute ocular inflammation. The preclinical pharmacodynamic profile exhibited by nepafenac indicates the potential to suppress PG-mediated inflammation in both anterior-segment tissues and retinal tissue following topical ocular administration. In rabbit tissue, the greater corneal permeability of nepafenac was demonstrated by a permeability coefficient that was approximately 4 times greater than that of diclofenac, 19 times greater than that of bromfenac, and 28 times greater than that of ketorolac.[15] Nepafenac has also exhibited superior pharmacodynamic properties in the posterior segment following topical ocular dosing, suggesting a unique therapeutic potential for a variety of conditions associated with retinal edema, subretinal fluid, or exudation. Topical nepafenac reaches the retina of rats in sufficient concentrations to inhibit multiple biochemical and morphologic abnormalities of the early stages of diabetic retinopathy in animals. Topical nepafenac also seems to inhibit CNV and ischemia-induced retinal neovascularization in mice, by decreasing the production of vascular endothelial growth factor.[16] Nepafenac 0.1% also prevented the development of induced panretinal edema following topical ocular application in the rabbit.

Nepafenac has been shown to be well tolerated and effective in the prevention and treatment of inflammation and ocular pain associated with cataract surgery and pseudophakic CME (Figure 29.3). The preoperative administration of topical NSAIDs prevents inflammation by inhibiting the COX pathway before surgical trauma induces the activation of PG production. Used after surgery, NSAIDs inhibit the continued PG formation that persists for days after cataract surgery.[2] In August 2005, the US FDA approved nepafenac for the treatment of pain and inflammation after cataract surgery. The approved dosing regimen is one drop 3 times daily, starting 1 day before surgery and continuing for 14 days after surgery. Five unpublished clinical trials supported the efficacy and safety of nepafenac ophthalmic suspension for its approval.[17,18] The cataract surgery studies consisted of one pivotal trial, one efficacy and safety study, two dose–response studies, and one trial comparing nepafenac with diclofenac regarding safety and tolerability. A placebo-controlled dose study (C-02-53) was conducted on 212 patients to determine the efficacy of QD, BID, and TID nepafenac 0.1%. Both QD and BID dosing produced significantly less anterior-segment inflammation and less ocular pain than placebo. In a randomized, placebo-controlled trial of 476 patients undergoing cataract surgery (C-03-32), nepafenac 0.1% was statistically superior to placebo in pain-free rate and reducing anterior-segment inflammation. The two dose–response studies C-95-93 and C-97-30 compared nepafenac suspension concentrations ranging from 0.003% to 0.3%. All the concentrations were shown to be efficacious in the treatment of inflammation due to cataract surgery.

In more recent years, numerous studies of case series have been conducted in humans to analyze the safety and efficacy of nepafenac and to understand better the ability of topical NSAIDs to reach various tissues in the eye. Nepafenac concentrations in the aqueous humor peaked at the first time point (30 minutes) and declined steadily thereafter, in contrast to the low levels of amfenac. These observations are consistent with the hypothesis that nepafenac serves as a source for continued amfenac production; the early rise, then decline in prodrug concentration and concomitant increase in amfenac concentration can be explained by the conversion of the former drug into the latter. Recent reports indicated that nepafenac may be useful in the therapy of other forms of ME (Figure 29.4).[2]

BROMFENAC

Bromfenac (Xibrom, ISTA Pharmaceuticals, Irvine, USA; Bronuck, Senju Pharmaceutical, Osaka, Japan) is indicated for the treatment of postoperative inflammation and the reduction of ocular pain in patients after undergoing cataract extraction. For this task, one drop of Xibrom may be applied to the affected eye twice daily beginning 24 hours after cataract surgery and continuing for the first 2 weeks of the postoperative period. The clinical safety and efficacy of bromfenac have been extensively studied in diverse comparative investigations, including the treatment of external or anterior ocular inflammatory diseases, allergic conjunctivitis, scleritis, and postoperative inflammation.[10] The results of two phase III multicenter, randomized double-masked placebo-controlled clinical trials showed that bromfenac ophthalmic solution 0.09% was effective in the rapid resolution of ocular pain after cataract surgery, and there was a statistically significant difference

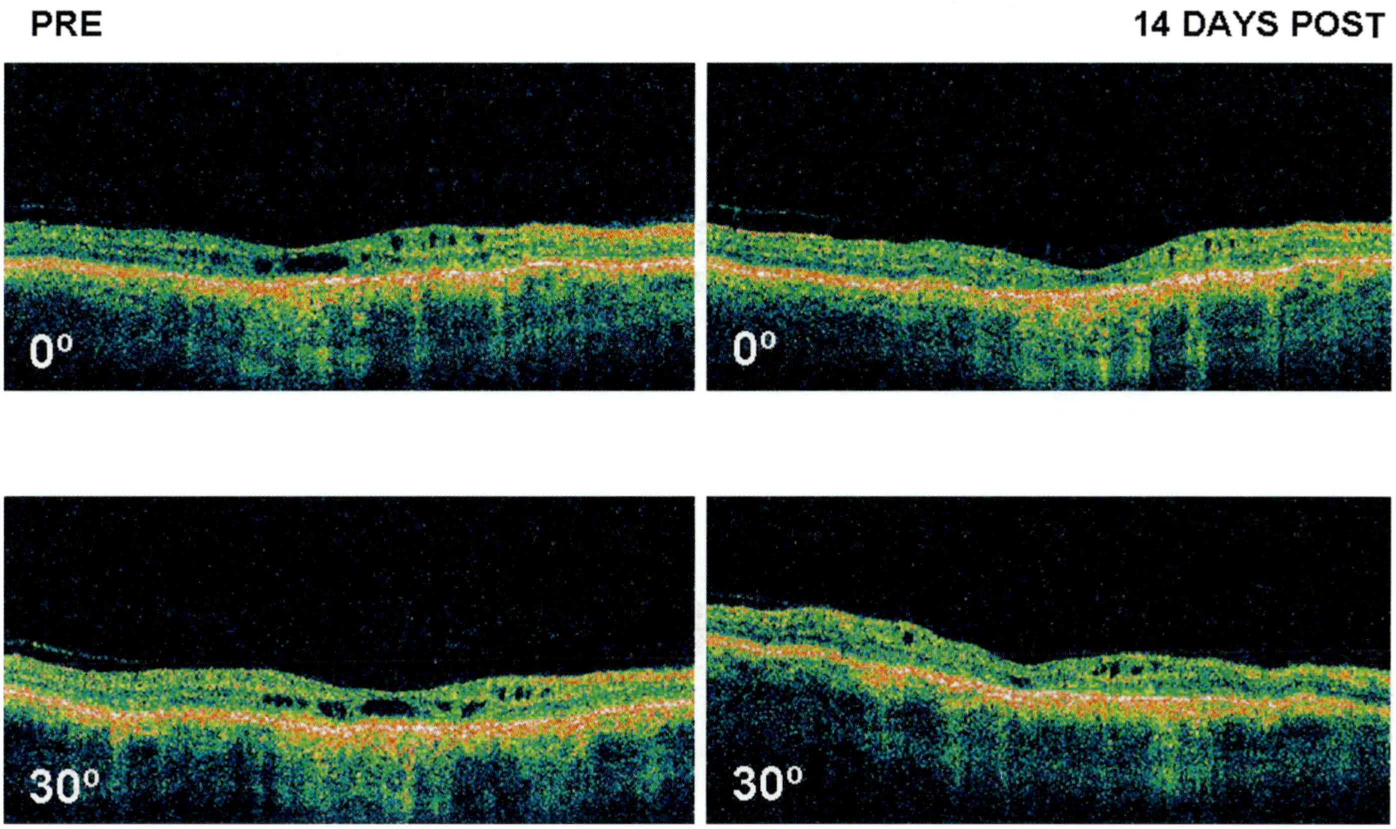

Figure 29.3 Optical coherence tomography demonstrates improvement of cystoid macular edema after the use of nepafenac TID for 14 days.

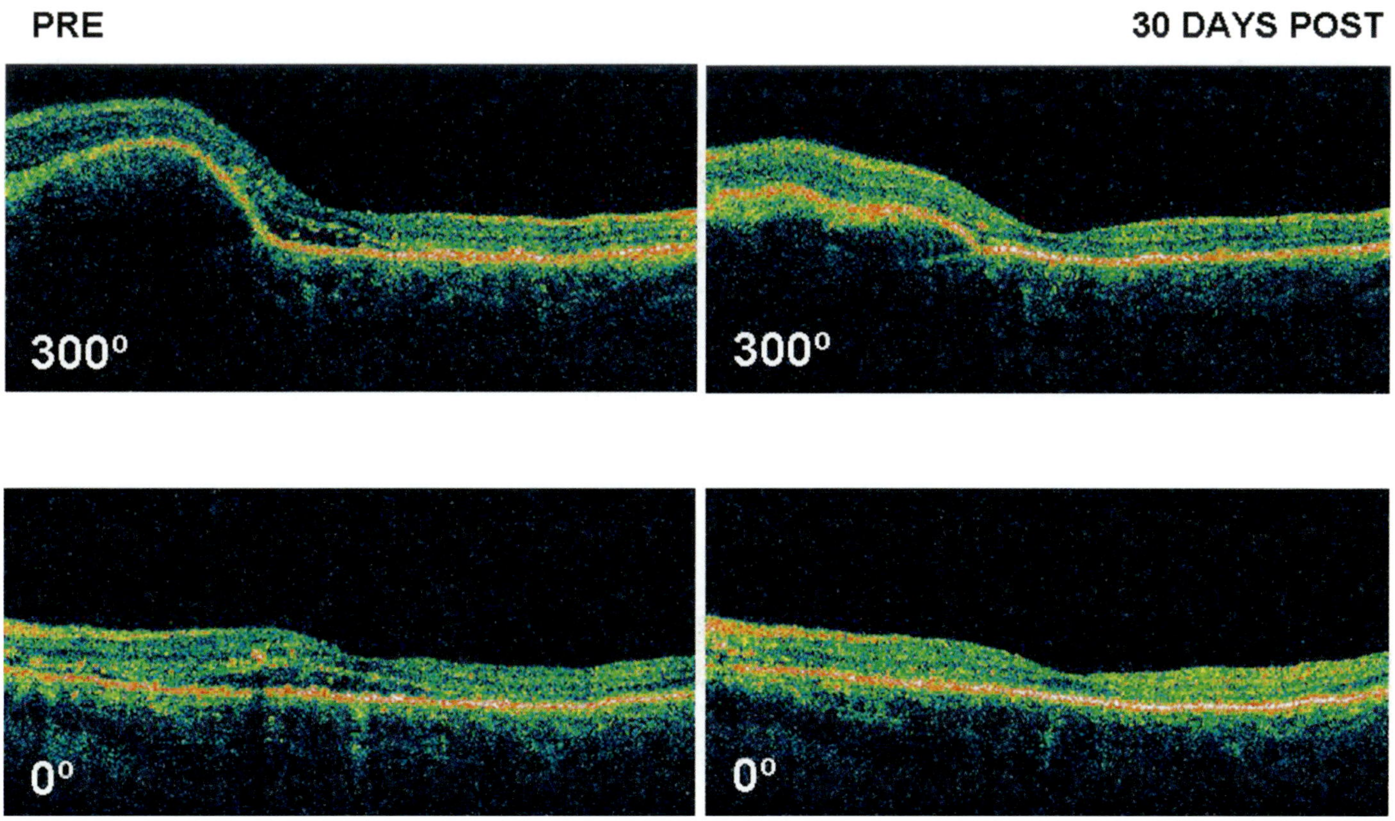

Figure 29.4 Optical coherence tomography showing the use and effect of nepafenac as adjuvant therapy in a case of pigment epithelium detachment associated with age-related macular degeneration. Anatomical improvement was observed after 30 days using nepafenac TID.

between the bromfenac and placebo groups demonstrated in these phase III clinical trials.

CONTRAINDICATIONS, COMPLICATIONS, AND TOXICITY

While NSAIDs used in ophthalmology possess a quite heterogeneous chemical constitution, these agents share similar therapeutic properties and adverse effects. Topical NSAIDs reduce the systemic absorption of the medication and thereby diminish the potential for systemic side-effects such as renal dysfunction or gastric ulcer. Nevertheless, absorption of topical ophthalmic NSAIDs in the nasal mucosa promotes systemic exposure and the occurrence of adverse systemic events, for instance exacerbation of bronchial asthma. Local consequences of topical ophthalmic NSAIDs include conjunctival hyperemia, burning, stinging, and corneal anesthesia.[19,20] A more serious complication with topical ophthalmic NSAIDs is indolent corneal ulceration and full-thickness corneal melts.

The analysis of NSAID-associated corneal events suggests that diclofenac sodium ophthalmic solution may be the primary most frequent agent. An elucidation of possible pharmacodynamic explanations of NSAID-induced corneal injury refers to the initiation of severe epithelial hypoxia. Moreover, the use of NSAIDs under conditions of corneal hypoxia may therefore cause worsening of the therapeutic response, but it may also induce a paradoxical inflammatory exacerbation.[19,20] Other potential mechanisms include the relationship between NSAIDs and corneal matrix metalloproteinase and direct toxicity due to cytotoxic excipients such as surfactants, solubilizers, and preservatives found in topical NSAID ophthalmic preparations. The concurrent use of NSAIDs with topical corticosteroids in the face of significant preexisting corneal inflammation has been identified as a risk factor in precipitating corneal erosions and melts. Until clinical evidence dictates otherwise, care should be taken to prevent NSAID toxicity after ophthalmic NSAID use.

SUMMARY AND KEY POINTS

NSAIDs act primarily as COX inhibitors and thus reduce the formation of endogenous PGs. Several NSAIDs have been commercially available for many years: diclofenac, flurbiprofen, indomethacin, ketorolac, and suprofen. Despite their controversial history, topical NSAIDs offer various advantages after intraocular and refractive surgery. For intraocular surgery NSAIDs can promote the prevention of intraoperative miosis, reduction of ocular pain, decrease of postoperative inflammation, and prevention of CME. Indeed, topical NSAIDs have been proven to be efficacious as prophylactic treatment to reduce the incidence of angiographic aphakic and pseudophakic CME. In refractive surgery, some NSAIDs provide an analgesic effect and again diminish postoperative discomfort. However, a number of past generations of NSAIDs have been associated with problems that varied from corneal stinging to corneal melt, and their use has subsequently declined.

Newer-generation NSAIDs have arisen in recent years for the treatment of ocular pain and inflammation. Nepafenac ophthalmic suspension 0.1% is a new topical NSAID prodrug that has been approved by the FDA for the treatment of pain and inflammation after cataract surgery. Preliminary data suggest nepafenac may also provide unique efficacy in the posterior segment, since its corneal permeability characteristics are superior to those of other NSAIDs. The FDA recently approved Xibrom as a topical twice-daily NSAID solution for the treatment of ocular inflammation following cataract surgery. The company asserts that Xibrom is one of the most selective and potent COX-2 inhibitors known. The distinct clinical difference between the two new-generation NSAIDs, nepafenac and bromfenac, in treating retinal diseases including ME has yet to be determined. Several retinal, choroidal, and vitreous diseases may be the target for future nepafenac studies, either as monotherapy or as concomitant treatments.

ACKNOWLEDGMENTS

We are grateful to Fundação de Amparo a Pesquisa do Estado de Sao Paulo (FAPESP) and to Pan-American Association of Ophthalmology (PAAO)/Pan-American Ophthalmological Foundation (PAOF) for their support.

REFERENCES

1. Schalnus R. Topical nonsteroidal anti-inflammatory therapy in ophthalmology. Ophthalmologica 2003;217:89–98.
2. Ahuja M, Dhake AS, Sharma SK, et al. Topical ocular delivery of NSAIDs. AAPS J 2008;10:229–241.
3. Jampol LM. Pharmacologic therapy of aphakic and pseudophakic cystoid macular edema. 1985 update. Ophthalmology 1985;92:807–810.
4. Italian Diclofenac Study Group. Efficacy of diclofenac eyedrops in preventing postoperative inflammation and long-term cystoid macular edema. J Cataract Refract Surg 1997:1183–1189.
5. Donnenfeld ED, Perry HD, Wittpenn JR, et al. Preoperative ketorolac tromethamine 0.4% in phacoemulsification outcomes: pharmacokinetic–response curve. J Cataract Refract Surg 2006;32:1474–1482.
6. Heier J, Cheetham JK, DeGryse R, et al. Ketorolac tromethamine 0.5% ophthalmic solution in the treatment of moderate to severe ocular inflammation after cataract surgery: a randomized, vehicle-controlled clinical trial, Am J Ophthalmol 1999;127:253–259.
7. Flach AJ, Dolan BJ, Irvine AR. Effectiveness of ketorolac tromethamine 0.5% ophthalmic solution for chronic aphakic and pseudophakic cystoid macular edema. Am J Ophthalmol 1987;103:479–486.
8. Lane SS. Nepafenac: a unique nonsteroidal prodrug. Int Ophthalmol Clin 2006;46:13–20.
9. Lindstrom R, Kim T. Ocular permeation and inhibition of retinal inflammation: an examination of data and expert opinion on the clinical utility of nepafenac. Curr Med Res Opin 2006;22:397–404.
10. Donnenfeld ED, Donnenfeld A. Global experience with Xibrom (bromfenac ophthalmic solution) 0.09%: the first twice-daily ophthalmic nonsteroidal anti-inflammatory drug. Int Ophthalmol Clin 2006;46:21–40.
11. Colin J, Paquette B. Comparison of the analgesic efficacy and safety of nepafenac ophthalmic suspension compared with diclofenac ophthalmic solution for ocular pain and photophobia after excimer laser surgery: a phase II, randomized, double-masked trial. Clin Ther 2006;28:527–536.
12. Adjunctive Diclofenac with Verteporfin (ADD-V) Study Group. Effect of adjunctive diclofenac with verteporfin therapy to treat choroidal neovascularization due to age-related macular degeneration: phase II study. Retina 2007;27:693–700.
13. Kaiser PK, Pineda 2nd R. A study of topical nonsteroidal anti-inflammatory drops and no pressure patching in the treatment of corneal abrasions. Corneal Abrasion Patching Study Group. Ophthalmology 1997;104:1353–1359.
14. Sivaprasad S, Bunce C, Patel N. Non-steroidal anti-inflammatory agents for treating cystoid macular oedema following cataract surgery. Cochrane Database Syst Rev 2005;1.
15. Kapin MA, Yanni JM, Brady MT, et al. Inflammation-mediated retinal edema in the rabbit is inhibited by topical nepafenac. Inflammation 2003;27:281–291.
16. Takahashi K, Saishin Y, Saishin Y, et al. Topical nepafenac inhibits ocular neovascularization. Invest Ophthalmol Vis Sci 2003;44:409–415.
17. Trattler W, McDonald M. Double-masked comparison of ketorolac tromethamine 0.4% versus nepafenac sodium 0.1% for postoperative healing rates and pain control in eyes undergoing surface ablation. Cornea 2007;26:665–669.
18. Duong HV, Westfield KC, Chalkley TH. Ketorolac tromethamine LS 0.4% versus nepafenac 0.1% in patients having cataract surgery. Prospective randomized double-masked clinical trial. J Cataract Refract Surg 2007;33:1925–1929.
19. Flach AJ. Corneal melts associated with topically applied nonsteroidal anti-inflammatory drugs. Trans Am Ophthalmol Soc 2001;99:205–210.
20. Acosta MC, Luna C, Graff G, et al. Comparative effects of the nonsteroidal anti-inflammatory drug nepafenac on corneal sensory nerve fibers responding to chemical irritation. Invest Ophthalmol Vis Sci 2007;48: 182–188.

CHAPTER

30 Corticosteroids: triamcinolone, dexamethasone, fluocinolone, and others

Raja Narayanan, MD and Baruch D. Kuppermann, MD, PhD

KEY FEATURES

Steroids have been extensively used to treat macular edema due to diabetic retinopathy, venous occlusive disease, ocular inflammation, and also in cases of choroidal neovascularization (CNV). The various intraocular steroids that have been used include dexamethasone, triamcinolone, and fluocinolone. This chapter provides an extensive description of the pathophysiology of macular edema as well as the pharmacology, efficacy, and adverse effects associated with the use of steroids in various retinal diseases. At the end of the chapter, a section is devoted to ongoing clinical trials for the treatment of macular edema secondary to retinal vascular diseases, and also to the development of new and exciting drug delivery systems for long-term delivery of steroids.

INTRODUCTION

Macular edema occurs when a variety of disease states induce changes to retinal capillaries, resulting in a breakdown of the tight junctions that form the blood–retinal barrier, and subsequent increased retinal vascular permeability.[1] Chronic, low-grade inflammation of the retinal microvasculature appears to be a significant contributor to this process. As such, the goals of therapy for macular edema should be to reduce inflammation, restore blood–retinal barrier patency, and interfere with the production or action of vascular endothelial growth factor (VEGF) and other proinflammatory cytokines. Several agents have the potential to achieve one or more of these goals. However, corticosteroids are unique in that they are the one class of agents that acts upon most of the multiple processes in the pathophysiology of macular edema (Figure 30.1). For example, corticosteroids are capable of inhibiting prostaglandin and leukotriene synthesis as well as interfering with intercellular adhesion molecule-1 (ICAM-1), interleukin-6, VEGF-α, and stromal cell derived factor-1 pathways[2–5] Corticosteroids also have been shown to decrease paracellular permeability and increase tight junction integrity both by directly restoring tight junctional proteins to their proper location at the cell border and by increasing the gene expression of those proteins.[6–9]

Corticosteroid usage in ophthalmology dates back to the early 1950s. Periocular and intraocular usage of corticosteroids, after a period of disrepute due to its side-effects, is in a phase of renaissance with the advent of long-acting steroids such as triamcinolone acetonide. Over the last two decades there has been an extensive increase in usage of steroids to treat macular edema due to diabetic retinopathy,[10,11] venous occlusive disease,[11] ocular inflammation,[12,13] and also in cases of CNV.[14,15] Triamcinolone acetonide is especially being used for conditions requiring long-term administration such as uveitis, macular edema secondary to retinal vascular disease, diabetic macular edema, and CNV. Dexamethasone is also used clinically to reduce intraocular inflammation, but since it is only available in a soluble form, its duration of action is much less than that of triamcinolone acetonide. Fluocinolone acetonide is currently utilized in a drug delivery implant placed in the vitreous cavity (Retisert, Bausch & Lomb), and additional intravitreal drug delivery implants are being developed using dexamethasone (Ozurdex, Allergan), triamcinolone acetonide (I-vation, Surmodics), and fluocinolone acetonide (Medidur/Iluvien, Alimera). The ongoing clinical trials on the use of various steroids in retinal diseases will be discussed briefly at the end of this chapter.

PHARMACOLOGY

STRUCTURE

Triamcinolone acetonide is designated chemically as 9-fluoro-11β,16α,17,21-tetrahydroxypregna-1,4-diene-3,20-dione cyclic 16,17-acetal with acetone. The empirical formula is $C_{24}H_{31}FO_6$ and the molecular weight is 434.50 Da (Figure 30.2).

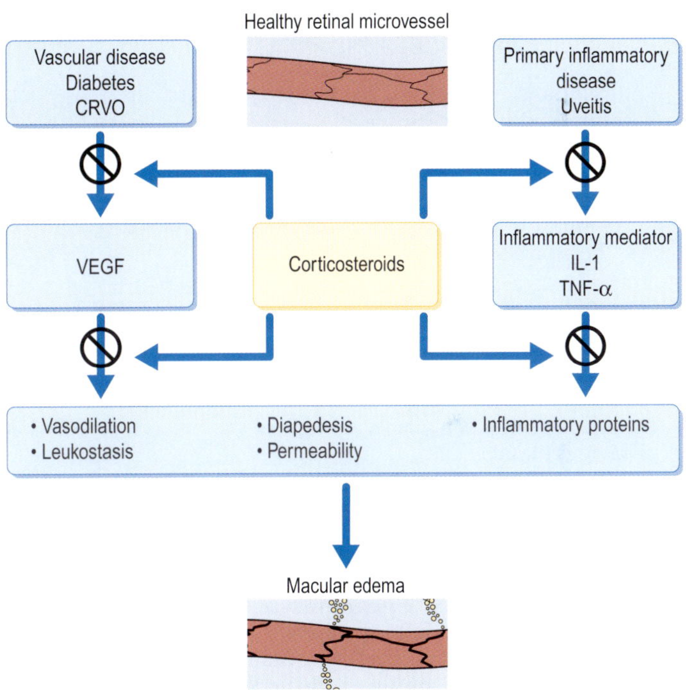

Figure 30.1 Targets of corticosteriod-based therapies. CRVO, central retinal vein occlusion; IL-1, interleukin-1; TNF-α, tumor necrosis factor-α.

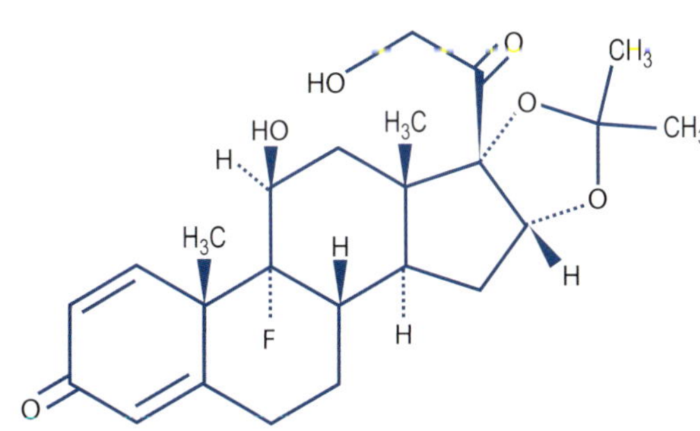

Figure 30.2 Triamcinolone acetonide is designated chemically as 9-fluoro-11β,16α,17,21-tetrahydroxypregna-1,4-diene-3,20-dione cyclic 16,17-acetal with acetone. The empirical formula is $C_{24}H_{31}FO_6$ and the molecular weight is 434.50 Da.

Table 30.1 Relative anti-inflammatory strength of various corticosteroids

Steroid	Relative potency
Hydrocortisone	1.0
Prednisolone	4.0
Methylprednisolone	5
Triamcinolone	5
Dexamethasone	26
Betamethasone	33

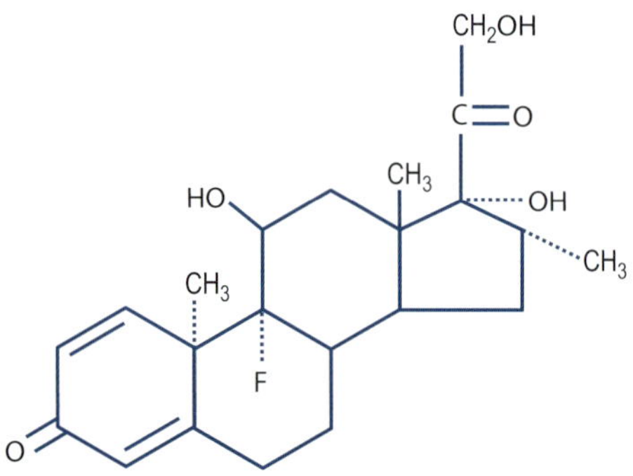

Figure 30.3 Dexamethasone. The molecular weight for dexamethasone is 392.47 Da. It is designated chemically as 9-fluoro-11β,17,21-trihydroxy-16α-methylpregna-1,4-diene-3,20-dione. The empirical formula is $C_{22}H_{29}FO_5$.

The prolonged duration of action of triamcinolone acetonide is due to the fact that it is an insoluble form and therefore, it acts as a depot injection when injected into a sequestered body cavity such as in the vitreous.

The relative anti-inflammatory strength of various corticosteroids is as given in Table 30.1.[16]

METABOLISM

In ophthalmic practice triamcinolone acetonide is used in its injectable form. The biologic half-life of parenterally administered triamcinolone acetonide is 18–36 hours. The most commonly used intravitreal dosages include 4 and 20 mg. Serum levels after intravitreal injection of triamcinolone acetonide 20–25 mg are mostly undetectable.

Clearance of intravitreal triamcinolone acetonide in a rabbit model showed that normal eyes had the longest retention of 41 days. Eyes that were post vitrectomy cleared the steroid in an average of 17 days. Eyes that were post lensectomy and vitrectomy cleared the steroid fastest, in an average 6.5 days.[17]

Beer and colleagues[18] examined the pharmacokinetics of triamcinolone acetonide after a 4-mg intravitreal injection for macular edema in nonvitrectomized eyes. The mean elimination half-life was 18.6 days, suggesting that triamcinolone acetonide would be present in measurable concentrations in nonvitrectomized eyes for approximately 3 months. The peak aqueous humor concentration ranged from 2.15 to 7.20 μg/ml.

Dexamethasone

The molecular weight for dexamethasone (Figure 30.3) is 392.47 Da. It is designated chemically as 9-fluoro-11β,17,21-trihydroxy-16α-methylpregna-1,4-diene-3,20-dione. The empirical formula is $C_{22}H_{29}FO_5$.

The plasma half-life of parenterally administered dexamethasone is 3–4 hours. The intravitreal dose is typically 350–400 μg.

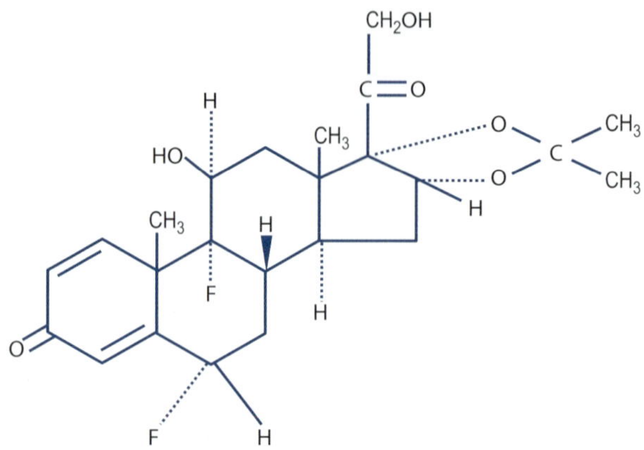

Figure 30.4 Fluocinolone acetonide has an empirical formula of $C_{24}H_{30}F_2O_6$ and a molecular weight of 452.49 Da.

Fluocinolone

Fluocinolone acetonide (Figure 30.4) has an empirical formula of $C_{24}H_{30}F_2O_6$ and a molecular weight of 452.49 Da. In a study of pigmented rabbits, 0.59 mg fluocinolone acetonide intravitreal implant (Retisert) was inserted and the vitreous concentration of the drug was determined at various time points. The concentration of fluocinolone acetonide[19] was found to be relatively constant from the first time point, 2 hours, through 1 year. Concentrations of fluocinolone acetonide were generally higher in the vitreous (11–18 ng/g) and retina (42–87 ng/g) than in the aqueous humor (0.21–1.1 ng/g). Urine and plasma values were below the lower limit of quantitation (200 pg/ml) for all observations.

USAGE OF STEROIDS IN OCULAR DISEASES

CYSTOID MACULAR EDEMA

Intravitreal injection of triamcinolone acetonide for refractory cystoid macular edema after cataract extraction improves visual acuity and central macular thickness (CMT) by optical coherence tomography (OCT).[20] The doses used have ranged from 1 to 25 mg. However, the effects may be transient and patients may require reinjection, typically after 4 months.[21]

DIABETIC MACULAR EDEMA

Intravitreal triamcinolone acetonide is a useful treatment modality for diabetic macular edema. However, the high risk of secondary glaucoma and cataract has made it somewhat less popular, especially with the advent of anti-VEGF agents. Pharmacologic attenuation of the effects of VEGF is one of the rationales for the use of corticosteroids in the treatment of macular edema associated with diabetic retinopathy. Corticosteroids, a class of substances with anti-inflammatory properties, have been demonstrated to inhibit the expression of the VEGF gene. Initial studies focused on the use of corticosteroids for macular edema that failed to respond to conventional laser photocoagulation.[10,11,22] More recent studies have included using triamcinolone acetonide as primary therapy.[23]

Martidis et al.[11] studied 16 eyes with clinically significant diabetic macular edema that failed to respond to at least two previous sessions of laser photocoagulation and observed a decrease in the CMT by OCT[24] of 55%, 57.5%, and 38%, at the 1-, 3-, and 6-month follow-up intervals after a 0.1-ml intravitreal injection of 4 mg triamcinolone acetonide. Intravitreal triamcinolone acetonide was effective in improving vision, reducing macular thickness, and inducing reabsorption of hard exudates in diffuse diabetic macular edema.

However, there can be recurrence of macular edema once the effect of triamcinolone wanes. Reports of time to recurrence range from 8 to 36 weeks.[23,25]

Audren et al.[25] studied diffuse diabetic macular edema refractory to laser photocoagulation in 17 patients. Each patient had bilateral disease so one eye received a single 4-mg injection of triamcinolone acetonide and the second eye was used as control. The main outcome measure was CMT measured by OCT (preinjection, 4, 12, and 24 weeks). The mean CMT prior to injection was 566.4 in injected eyes. The mean CMT at follow-up week 24 was 358.5. The measured outcome, ETDRS vision, was significantly improved at all visits.

In another prospective, placebo-controlled, randomized, interventional study which included 40 eyes (38 patients) with diabetic macular edema, 28 (70%) eyes were randomized to treatment and 12 (30%) eyes randomized to receive a placebo injection. The treatment group received an intravitreal injection of approximately 20 mg triamcinolone acetonide. Visual acuity increased significantly in the study group by 3.4 lines. Difference in change of best visual acuity was significant ($P < 0.001$) between both groups. At 6 months after baseline, 11 (11/23; 48%) eyes and 9 (9/23; 39%) eyes, respectively, improved by at least 2 and 3 lines, respectively, in the study group, versus 0 (0%) eyes improved in the control group.[26]

The results of a large, multicenter, randomized controlled study comparing triamcinolone acetonide and laser photocoagulation for diabetic macular edema has recently been published by the Diabetic Retinopathy Clinical Research network (DRCRnet). The study showed that, over a 2-year period, focal/grid laser photocoagulation was more effective and had fewer adverse effects than preservative-free intravitreal triamcinolone.[27] The study enrolled 840 eyes (693 subjects) at 88 clinical sites. Patients were randomized in a 1:1:1 ratio into one of three treatment groups: laser (n = 330); intravitreal triamcinolone acetonide 1 mg (n = 256); and intravitreal triamcinolone acetonide 4 mg (n = 254). Patients were retreated every 4 months as needed and followed for 2 years. Initially, groups treated with intravitreal triamcinolone acetonide, particularly the 4-mg group, appeared to have better visual outcomes at 4 (statistically significant) and 8 months (no longer statistically significant), but by 1 year there were no differences between groups. By 16 months onward, laser was statistically superior to 4 mg intravitreal triamcinolone acetonide in terms of visual outcomes. At the primary endpoint of 2 years, eyes treated with laser had a mean best corrected visual acuity (BCVA) improvement of 1 letter, whereas eyes treated with 1 mg intravitreal triamcinolone acetonide had a mean vision loss of 2 letters and eyes treated with 4 mg intravitreal triamcinolone acetonide had a mean loss of 3 letters. Decreases in macular thickness as assessed by OCT thickness followed this same pattern, with a mean decrease in central foveal subfield thickness at 2 years of 139 µm in the laser group, 86 µm in the 1-mg intravitreal triamcinolone acetonide group, and 77 µm in the 4-mg intravitreal triamcinolone acetonide group. Additionally, the incidence of cataracts and increased intraocular pressure (IOP) was significantly greater in the intravitreal triamcinolone acetonide groups than in the laser groups. By 2 years, the percentage of eyes with increase of at least 10 mmHg from baseline was 4% in the laser group, 16% in the 1-mg intravitreal triamcinolone acetonide group, and 33% in the 4-mg intravitreal triamcinolone acetonide group. Cataract extraction was performed by 2 years in 13% of the eyes in the laser group, 23% of eyes in the 1-mg intravitreal triamcinolone acetonide group, and 51% of eyes in the 4-mg intravitreal triamcinolone acetonide group.

RETINAL VEIN OCCLUSION

Intravitreal triamcinolone acetonide has been shown to improve visual acuity, reduce angiographic leakage, and decrease CMT in the management of persistent macular edema as a result of nonischemic central retinal vein occlusion (CRVO).

Park et al.[28] studied 10 eyes of 9 patients with perfused CRVO with visual acuity of 20/50 or worse. Triamcinolone acetonide (4 mg in 0.1 ml) was injected intravitreally. The study outcomes included measuring BCVA, IOP, fluorescein angiography, and OCT. The mean duration from the time of diagnosis to the intravitreal injection was 15.4 months. The study demonstrated biomicroscopic improvement in cystoid macular edema in all 10 eyes with corresponding improvement in volumetric OCT measurements from a mean of 4.2 mm^3 preinjection to a mean of 2.6 mm^3 at last follow-up ($P < 0.001$). In addition, the mean BCVA improved from 58 letters (range, 37–72) at baseline to 78 letters (range, 50–100 letters) at last follow-up (average, 4.8 months, $P = 0.01$). Three eyes (30%) without previous history of glaucoma required initiation of topical aqueous suppressant therapy for IOP elevation at last follow-up and one eye with a previous history of open-angle glaucoma required a trabeculectomy.

Ip et al.[29] studied 13 eyes with macular edema associated with CRVO treated with an injection of intravitreal triamcinolone acetonide (4 mg). They found that eyes with nonischemic CRVO (n = 5) demonstrated a significant improvement in visual acuity, whereas eyes with ischemic CRVO (n = 8) demonstrated a nonsignificant visual acuity improvement. During the follow-up no patient had a decrease in visual acuity. OCT analysis showed mean baseline foveal thickness of 590 µm. At the 6-month follow-up examination, mean foveal thickness as measured by OCT for 13 patients was 281 µm. Four patients developed a recurrence of macular edema between months 4 and 6 of follow-up. Three of the 4 patients were retreated with a second injection of triamcinolone acetonide and 2 of these patients experienced an improvement in visual acuity following retreatment.

Bashshur et al.[30] studied 20 patients with a 3–4-month history of persistent macular edema resulting from CRVO. According to the authors, 75% of patients treated with intravitreal triamcinolone acetonide (4 mg) had complete resolution of macular edema on clinical exam using Goldmann contact lens at 10–12 months of follow-up. In addition, at the final follow-up examination the treated group had a mean visual acuity of 20/37 versus 20/110 in the observation group.

A study assessing the Ozurdex implant for the treatment of retinal vein occlusion was recently completed (ClinicalTrials.gov identifier NCT00168298). The primary efficacy endpoint of the study was visual acuity at 6 months with safety and secondary efficacy endpoints out to 12 months. The exact number of patients enrolled has not been announced. Patients were randomly assigned to observation, 350 µg Ozurdex, or 700 µg Ozurdex in a 1:1:1 allocation. Allergan recently completed the initial analysis of data for this trial, but to date has only released the following top-line data from the Allergan website, accessed March 22, 2009:

Patients receiving either the 350 microgram or the 700 microgram dose of OZURDEX® had a statistically significant increase in vision based on a 3-line or better improvement in visual acuity compared to a sham treatment. In addition, both doses of OZURDEX® were well tolerated in the studies. Less than 7% of patients receiving 700 or 350 micrograms of OZURDEX® experienced an elevation of intraocular pressure (IOP) greater than 35 mmHg at any time during the 6 month study, and at 6 months less than 1% of patients had an IOP above 25 mmHg. In the fourth quarter, Allergan completed filing the last module of its new drug application (NDA) with the US Food and Drug Administration (FDA) for the approval of OZURDEX® to treat macular edema associated with RVO.

The Standard of Care vs. Corticosteroid for Retinal Vein Occlusion (SCORE) study – the National Eye Institute-sponsored study of triamcinolone for macular edema secondary to central or branch retinal vein occlusion (BRVO) – will be discussed later in the chapter.

EXUDATIVE AGE-RELATED MACULAR DEGENERATION (AMD)

The antiangiogenic property of triamcinolone acetonide has been studied in the treatment of exudative AMD.[31,32] Various uncontrolled studies have been conducted.

In a prospective, comparative nonrandomized clinical interventional study by Jonas et al., all patients had shown an increase or stabilization of visual acuity after a first intravitreal injection of 25 mg triamcinolone acetonide.[32] In the study, the mean visual acuity increased significantly ($P = 0.005$ and $P = 0.003$, respectively) from 0.17 to 0.32 and from 0.15 to 0.23, respectively, after the first and second injections. An increase in visual acuity was found for 10 patients (77%) after the first and second injections. In the control group, visual acuity did not vary significantly during follow-up ($P = 0.81$). The peak in visual acuity and, in a chronologically parallel manner, the peak in IOP elevation occurred 2–5 months after each injection.

In another study, 67 patients (71 eyes) who presented with exudative AMD of predominantly or total occult type ($n = 68$) or classic type ($n = 3$) received intravitreal injection of 25 mg crystalline triamcinolone acetonide. Visual acuity increased significantly ($P < 0.001$) from 0.16 to a mean maximum of 0.23. Postinjection visual acuity was highest 1–3 months after the injection. Forty-seven (66.2%) eyes gained in maximal visual acuity and 11 (15.5%) eyes lost in visual acuity. IOP increased significantly ($P < 0.001$) from 15.1 mmHg at baseline to a maximal value of 23.0 mmHg. Owing to a decrease in visual acuity after an initial increase, 6 patients received a second intravitreal triamcinolone acetonide injection, after which visual acuity increased again in three eyes.[33]

A randomized clinical trial of a single injection of 4 mg triamcinolone acetonide was performed in 27 patients followed up for 6 months. The study by Danis et al.[14] included exudative AMD with subfoveal or occult CNV, and visual acuity between 20/40 and 20/400. Visual acuity was significantly better in the treated group compared with control subjects at both 3 and 6 months ($P < 0.005$). IOP elevation was seen in 25% of treated patients, but was controlled with topical medications. Progression of cataract was more frequently seen in the treated group.

A double-masked, placebo-controlled, randomized clinical trial was performed by Gillies et al.[34] on patients with CNV for less than 1 year, and a visual acuity of 20/200 or better. A single 4-mg intravitreal injection was administered. A total of 151 eyes were randomized into the study, and follow-up data were obtained for 73 (97%) of the 75 eyes in the treated group and for 70 (92%) of the 76 eyes in the control group. Using severe vision loss (30 letters) as the main outcome measure, Gillies et al. found that there was no difference between the two groups during the first year of the study. In addition, although the change in size of the neovascular membranes was significantly less in eyes receiving triamcinolone acetonide than in those receiving placebo 3 months after treatment ($P = 0.01$), no difference was noted after 12 months. After 12 months, treated eyes had a significantly higher risk of an elevated IOP determined by increase of 5 mmHg or more (31/75 (41%) versus 3/76 (4%); $P < 0.001$), but not of cataract progression ($P = 0.29$).[34] Currently, corticosteroids have a very limited primary role in the management of neovascular AMD. Prior to the advent of anti-VEGF agents for neovascular AMD, intravitreal triamcinolone was frequently used in combination with photodynamic therapy (PDT) for the treatment of CNV associated with AMD.[35–38] More recently, Augustin and others[39,40] have proposed the use of intravitreal dexamethasone in combination with PDT and anti-VEGF therapy to provide so-called "triple therapy" for CNV/AMD. Additionally, studies looking at steroid-based drug delivery implants such as Ozurdex in combination with anti-VEGF therapy are under way. However, steroids as sole therapy for CNV/AMD are not currently considered a viable option.

COMPLICATIONS OF OCULAR STEROID THERAPY

The common adverse effects of ocular steroid therapy are glaucoma and cataract.[41–43] Additionally, given that the commonly used formulation of triamcinolone acetonide, Kenalog, is not formulated for the eye, there is a known risk of pseudoendophthalmitis and a hypothethical potential for clinical retinal toxicity from the vehicle when injected intravitreally.[44–46] There have been reports of toxicity of triamcinolone acetonide on retinal pigment epithelial cells *in vitro*[47,48] whereas ex vivo[49] and *in vivo*[50] studies have failed to show any significant toxicity on the retina. Triamcinolone acetonide also causes phototoxicity of erythrocytes *in vitro* and may also have weak photosensitizing properties *in vivo*.[19]

Raised intraocular pressure

Corticosteroid-induced IOP elevation is a common occurrence that resembles open-angle glaucoma. Patient selection is an important factor when considering the possibility of steroid-induced glaucoma, especially in the setting of a long-acting steroid such as triamcinolone acetonide. A history of chronic open-angle glaucoma or family history of glaucoma is a significant risk factor for the development of steroid-induced elevation of IOP. Other patients at risk for developing steroid-induced IOP elevation are high myopes, diabetics, and patients with connective tissue diseases.[51,52]

Elevated IOP in association with intravitreal triamcinolone acetonide has been reported in several recent studies.[53] One study reported an increase in IOP to over 21 mmHg in 52% of eyes 2 months after a 25-mg injection.[41] However, two other studies of 4-mg injections showed similar incidences of IOP increase over different time periods. One study by Bakri and Beer retrospectively reviewed cases receiving a single dosage of 4 mg. Their study showed over a 4-week period an incidence of 48.8% of eyes demonstrating an IOP increase of 5 mmHg or greater, and 27.9% showing an increase in IOP of 10 mmHg or greater at a mean time of 6.6 weeks. The study concluded with a follow-up time of 12 weeks.[43]

The second study by Smithen and colleagues followed patients for a mean of 40 weeks and defined a pressure elevation as an IOP of 24 mmHg or greater. In this study, 40.6% of eyes experienced a pressure elevation at a mean time of 14 weeks with the longest duration of pressure elevation present at 42 weeks. In nonglaucomatous patients with a baseline IOP of 15 mmHg or greater, 60% experienced a pressure elevation compared to only 22.7% of patients with baseline pressures below 15 mmHg. Pressure elevation in both studies was controllable with topical glaucoma medications. In rare instances surgical glaucoma intervention has been necessary with vitrectomy to remove the residual triamcinolone acetonide for intractable cases or glaucoma fistulization procedure.[54]

The increase in IOP following intravitreal steroid injection is higher than those reported for topical and posterior sub-Tenon steroids. In a retrospective study of 202 consecutive posterior sub-Tenon steroid injections in 63 eyes of 55 patients, the highest reported IOP was 27 mmHg.[55] That study showed no statistical difference between pre- and postinjection IOP measurements. Anterior sub-Tenon steroids are much more likely to increase IOP and cases have been reported necessitating surgical removal of the steroid depot secondary to intractable IOP elevation.

Infectious, sterile, and pseudoendophthalmitis associated with triamcinolone acetonide

Infectious, sterile, and pseudoendophthalmitis may all be seen following intravitreal triamcinolone acetonide. Two specific areas of concern after intravitreal triamcinolone acetonide are the potential for decreased local immunity induced by the corticosteroid that may increase infection risk and the anti-inflammatory action of the steroid masking the symptoms of endophthalmitis.

Moshfeghi and coworkers reported a retrospective multicenter study in which 8 of 922 eyes (0.87%) developed infectious endophthalmitis following intravitreal triamcinolone acetonide. The median time of diagnosis was 7.5 days postinjection. All 8 patients presented with iritis, vitritis, and hypopyon. Five of the 8 experienced decreased vision as an initial complaint. One eye had no culture growth but demonstrated intracellular Gram-positive cocci with polymorphonuclear cells on Gram stain. The remaining cases were culture-positive with coagulase-negative staphylococcus ($n = 2$), *Streptobacillus parasanguis* ($n = 2$), *Mycobacterium chelonae* ($n = 1$), *Streptobacillus* species ($n = 1$) and *Streptobacillus intermedius* ($n = 1$). Despite aggressive intervention with vitreal tap and injection of antibiotics (6 of 8 patients) or pars plana vitrectomy with intravitreal antibiotics (2 of 8 patients), 3 patients deteriorated to no light perception vision and 1 patient required enucleation.[56,57]

Noninfectious (sterile) endophthalmitis following intravitreal triamcinolone acetonide injection has been described in several studies. This sterile inflammatory reaction could be secondary to a component of the drug formulation or to bacterial toxins that could be present even in sterile solutions.[44] Additionally, the triamcinolone acetonide crystals themselves may migrate into the anterior chamber, creating a picture of pseudoendophthalmitis.

Cataract

Intravitreal triamcinolone acetonide has been associated with posterior subcapsular cataract formation. A study by Gillies et al.[58] has demonstrated that steroid-related cataracts are more likely to form in patients who are steroid responders. These authors reported a strong association between the mechanism responsible for the development of steroid-induced posterior subcapsular cataract and raised IOP.

Thompson studied by linear regression analysis lens scores from lens opacity standards in evaluating 93 eyes with intravitreal injection of 4 mg triamcinolone acetonide. Lens opacities were graded using the Lens Opacity Classification System II (LOCS II) scale. Thompson found that nuclear sclerosis increased at a rate of 0.175 U/year, posterior subcapsular cataracts at 0.423 U/year, and cortical cataracts at 0.045 U/year.[59]

Retinal detachment

Although traumatic retinal holes with resultant detachment are theoretical risks associated with intravitreal injection, no case reports could be found in the peer-reviewed literature. The risk of retinal tears and retinal detachment associated with intravitreal injection of steroids has not been shown to be common.

FUTURE CONSIDERATIONS AND ONGOING STUDIES

THE SCORE STUDY

The SCORE study is a multicenter, randomized, phase III trial to compare the effectiveness and safety of standard care versus triamcinolone acetonide injection for the treatment of macular edema associated with CRVO and BRVO. Standard care is defined as observation of macular edema in CRVO and for BRVO immediate observation of eye with dense macular hemorrhage and then grid photocoagulation when clearing of hemorrhage permits or immediate grid photocoagulation in eyes without dense macular hemorrhage.

The primary outcome is improvement by 15 or more letters from baseline in best corrected ETDRS visual acuity score at the 12-month visit. Secondary outcomes include changes from baseline in best corrected ETDRS visual acuity score, changes in retinal thickness as assessed by stereoscopic color fundus photography and OCT, and adverse ocular outcomes. The SCORE study has completed its subject recruitment and is expected to report results when all patients have completed primary endpoints.

STEROID-SUSTAINED RELEASE DEVICES

The STRIDE study

The prospective, randomized, double-masked Sustained Triamcinolone Release for Inhibition of Diabetic Macular Edema (STRIDE) trial is assessing the safety and tolerability of the I-vation triamcinolone acetonide (SurModics, Irvine, CA) in 30 patients. In the study, patients are randomized to either a slow-release or fast-release implant, each containing 925 µg triamcinolone. They also were stratified by baseline visual acuity and by presence or absence of prior laser treatment.

From screening to 6 months, the proportion of patients with visual acuity of at least 70 ETDRS letters (in the study eye) increased from 14% to 46% in the slow group and from 18% to 41% in the fast group. A gain of more than 15 letters occurred in 8% of patients in the slow group and 18% in the fast group. Both implant formulations were associated with improvements in macular thickness. Further studies with I-vation triamcinolone acetonide have been suspended as the roles of triamcinolone are being evaluated by the sponsors.

FLUOCINOLONE ACETONIDE DEVICE

In 2005, the Food and Drug Administration approved a fluocinolone acetonide-containing intraocular implant (Retisert, Bausch & Lomb, Rochester, NY) for the treatment of chronic noninfectious uveitis, affecting the posterior segment of the eye. The Retisert is implanted into the eye via a surgical procedure entailing a 3.5-mm circumferential incision through the pars plana and the implant is sutured to the eye wall.

The fluocinolone implant investigated in the uveitis study has also been studied in a multicenter, randomized, controlled clinical trial for the treatment of diabetic macular edema. Patients in the study were randomized 2:1 to receive either a 0.59-mg fluocinolone implant or standard of care, defined as repeat laser treatment or observation.

Pearson and colleagues reported that, at 36 months, the implant resolved edema at the center of the macula and produced a 3-line or more improvement in visual acuity in a significant proportion of eyes studied ($n = 197$).[60] At 36 months, no evidence of edema was present in 58% of implanted eyes compared with 30% of eyes that received the standard of care ($P < 0.001$). Visual acuity improvements of 3 lines or more occurred more frequently in implanted eyes (28% versus 15%, $P < 0.05$).

The most common serious adverse events in the implanted eyes were cataract development, requiring extraction, and increase in IOP. Ninety-five percent of phakic implanted eyes required cataract surgery, and 35% of implanted eyes experienced increased IOP. A filtering procedure was necessary in 28% of implanted eyes, and explantation was performed in 5% of eyes to manage IOP.

NEW-GENERATION FLUOCINOLONE DEVICE

A second fluocinolone acetonide sustained-delivery device has been developed. The injectable Medidur/Iluvien FA (Alimera Sciences Inc., Alpharetta, Ga./pSivida, Watertown, MA) does not require sutures and can be inserted in a physician's office (Figure 30.5).

Enrollment in the phase III Fluocinolone Acetonide in diabetic Macular Edema (FAME) trial, which is evaluating a daily dose of 0.2 µg

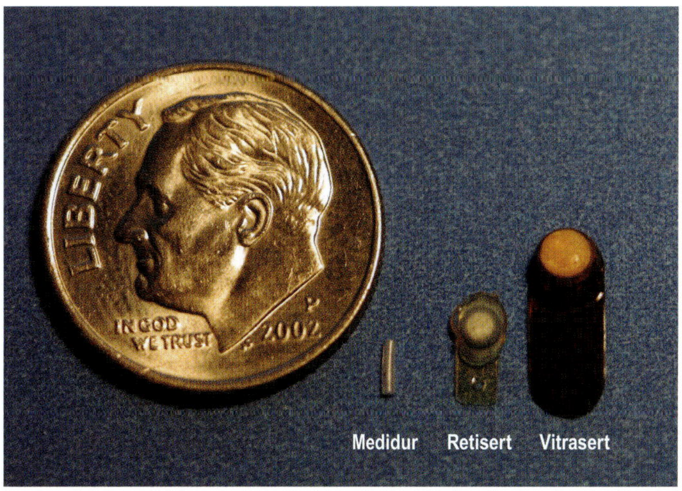

Figure 30.5 Comparative sizes of Medidur, Retisert, and Vitrasert.

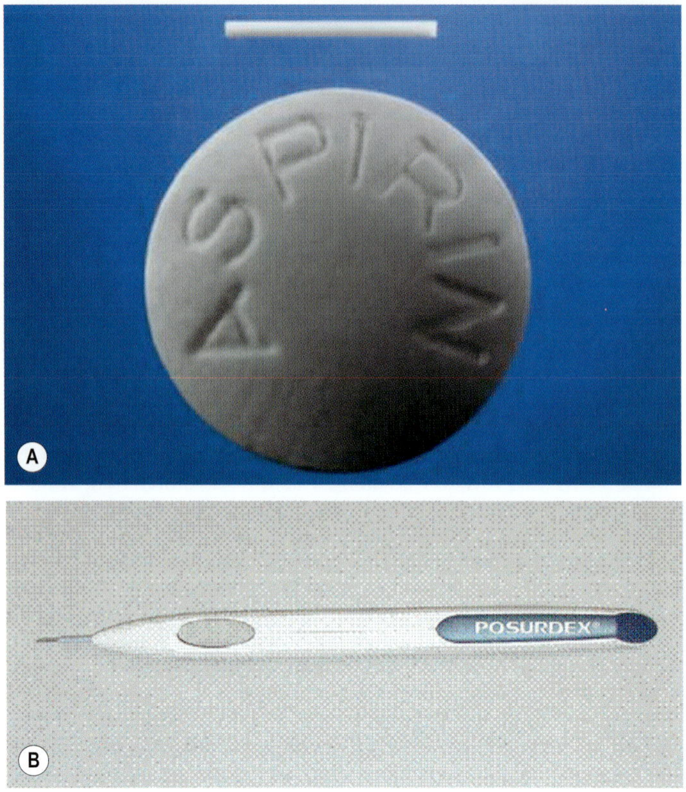

Figure 30.6 (A, B) Dexamethasone (Ozurdex, Allergan, Irvine, CA), currently in phase III clinical trials for the treatment of macular edema delivery system.

and 0.5 μg of fluocinolone to the retina, is complete. The FAME study is a double-masked, randomized, multicenter clinical trial involving more than 900 patients in the USA, Canada, Europe, and India. Safety and efficacy will be assessed at 2 years, and patients will be followed for 3 years. Results from the FAME study will help to determine if Medidur FA is effective and capable of reducing the steroid-induced side-effects seen in the Retisert trial.

DEXAMETHASONE DRUG DELIVERY SYSTEM

A sustained-delivery formulation of dexamethasone (Ozurdex, Allergan, Irvine, CA) is in phase III clinical trials for the treatment of macular edema. The phase III trial employs the new applicator, allowing placement of an extruded, rather than pelleted, form of the dexamethasone delivery system through a small self-sealing puncture (Figure 30.6).

Two doses of dexamethasone were evaluated in a 6-month, phase II, multicenter, randomized clinical trial.[61] The 315 patients in the trial had persistent macular edema due to diabetic retinopathy ($n = 172$), retinal vein occlusion ($n = 102$), Irvine–Gass syndrome ($n = 27$), or uveitis ($n = 14$). In each patient, one eye was randomized to treatment with a 350-μg dose of Ozurdex, a 700-μg dose of Ozurdex (both inserted into the vitreal cavity via a small pars plana incision) or observation.

Implantation with Ozurdex resulted in a statistically significant increase in patients gaining 2 and 3 lines or more of visual acuity in a dose-dependent fashion at 90 and 180 days compared with observation ($P < 0.025$). The percentages of patients who gained 2 lines or more of visual acuity 180 days after implantation were 32.4% in the 700-μg group, 24.3% in the 350-μg group, and 21% in the observation group ($P = 0.06$). The percentages of patients who gained 3 lines or more of visual acuity 180 days after implantation were 18.1% in the 700-μg group, 14.6% in the 350-μg group, and 7.6% in the observation group ($P = 0.02$). The visual acuity improvements achieved with the 700-μg implant were consistent across all subgroups at day 90.

In addition, at the primary endpoint, 2% of the patients who were implanted with the 350-μg and 700-μg dose of Ozurdex had an increase in IOP of 10 mmHg or more from baseline, compared with 1% of patients in the observation arm. All were successfully managed with either observation or topical IOP-lowering medication. Cataracts were present in 15% of the 350-μg group, 17.8% of the 700-μg group, and 12.4% of the observation group ($P < 0.001$ versus observation).

SUMMARY AND KEY POINTS

In summary, macular edema occurs when a variety of disease states induce changes to retinal capillaries resulting in a breakdown of the tight junctions that form the blood–retinal barrier, with subsequent increased retinal vascular permeability.[1,62] Chronic, low-grade, inflammation of the retinal microvasculature appears to be a significant contributor to this process. The goals of therapy should be to reduce inflammation, restore blood–retinal barrier patency, and interfere with the production or action of VEGF and other proinflammatory cytokines. Corticosteroids are the one class of agents that acts upon most of the multiple processes in the pathophysiology of macular edema. However, despite their significant benefits, the primary ocular adverse effects associated with the use of steroids – IOP rise and cataract – are important issues which may limit their use in certain situations. The need for repeated injections may be offset by the use of long-term sustained-release implants, most of which are in advanced stages of clinical trials. Once approved, the steroid implants may be extremely beneficial in the management of serious retinal diseases.

REFERENCES

1. Ferris FL 3rd, Patz A. Macular edema. A complication of diabetic retinopathy. Surv Ophthalmol 1984;28(Suppl):452–461.
2. Felinski EA, Nauck M, Karakiulakis G, et al. Corticosteroids inhibit the expression of the vascular endothelial growth factor gene in human vascular smooth muscle cells. Eur J Pharmacol 1998;341(2–3):309–315.
3. Tamura H, Miyamoto K, Kiryu J, et al. Intravitreal injection of corticosteroid attenuates leukostasis and vascular leakage in experimental diabetic retina. Invest Ophthalmol Vis Sci 2005;46(4):1440–1444.
4. Felinski EA, Nauck M, Karakiulakis G, et al. Corticosteroids inhibit the expression of the vascular endothelial growth factor gene in human vascular smooth muscle cells. Eur J Pharmacol 1998;341(2–3):309–315.
5. Tamura H, Miyamoto K, Kiryu J, et al. Intravitreal injection of corticosteroid attenuates leukostasis and vascular leakage in experimental diabetic retina. Invest Ophthalmol Vis Sci 2005;46(4):1440–1444.
6. Felinski EA, Antonetti DA. Glucocorticoid regulation of endothelial cell tight junction gene expression: novel treatments for diabetic retinopathy. Curr Eye Res 2005;30(11):949–957.
7. Antonetti DA, Wolpert EB, DeMaio L, et al. Hydrocortisone decreases retinal endothelial cell water and solute flux coincident with increased content and decreased phosphorylation of occludin. J Neurochem 2002;80(4):667–677.
8. Antonetti DA. Glucocorticoid regulation of endothelial cell tight junction gene expression: novel treatments for diabetic retinopathy. Curr Eye Res 2005;30(11):949–957.
9. Antonetti DA, Wolpert EB, DeMaio L, et al. Hydrocortisone decreases retinal endothelial cell water and solute flux coincident with increased content and decreased phosphorylation of occludin. J Neurochem 2002;80(4):667–677.
10. Jonas JB, Hayler JK, Sofker A, et al. Intravitreal injection of crystalline cortisone as adjunctive treatment of proliferative diabetic retinopathy. Am J Ophthalmol 2001;131(4):468–471.
11. Martidis A, Duker JS, Greenberg PB, et al. Intravitreal triamcinolone for refractory diabetic macular edema. Ophthalmology 2002;109(5):920–927.
12. Antcliff RJ, Spalton DJ, Stanford MR, et al. Intravitreal triamcinolone for uveitic cystoid macular edema: an optical coherence tomography study. Ophthalmology 2001;108(4):765–772.
13. Young S, Larkin G, Branley M, et al. Safety and efficacy of intravitreal triamcinolone for cystoid macular oedema in uveitis. Clin Exp Ophthalmol 2001;29(1):2–6.
14. Danis RP, Ciulla TA, Pratt LM, et al. Intravitreal triamcinolone acetonide in exudative age-related macular degeneration. Retina 2000;20(3):244–250.
15. Ciulla TA, Criswell MH, Danis RP, et al. Intravitreal triamcinolone acetonide inhibits choroidal neovascularization in a laser-treated rat model. Arch Ophthalmol 2001;119(3):399–404.
16. Zimmerman T, Kooner K, Sharir M, et al. Textbook of Ocular Pharmacology. Philadelphia: Lippincott-Raven; 1997. p. 683–684.

17. Schindler RH, Chandler D, Thresher R, et al. The clearance of intravitreal triamcinolone acetonide. Am J Ophthalmol 1982;93(4):415–417.
18. Beer PM, Bakri SJ, Singh RJ, et al. Intraocular concentration and pharmacokinetics of triamcinolone acetonide after a single intravitreal injection. Ophthalmology 2003;110(4):681–686.
19. Miolo G, Ricci A, Caffieri S, et al. *In vitro* phototoxic properties of triamcinolone 16,17-acetonide and its main photoproducts. Photochem Photobiol 2003;78(5):425–430.
20. Jonas JB, Kreissig I, Degenring RF. Intravitreal triamcinolone acetonide for pseudophakic cystoid macular edema. Am J Ophthalmol 2003;136(2):384–386.
21. Conway MD, Canakis C, Livir-Rallatos C, et al. Intravitreal triamcinolone acetonide for refractory chronic pseudophakic cystoid macular edema. J Cataract Refract Surg 2003;29(1):27–33.
22. Ciardella AP, Klancnik J, Schiff W, et al. Intravitreal triamcinolone for the treatment of refractory diabetic macular oedema with hard exudates: an optical coherence tomography study. Br J Ophthalmol 2004;88(9):1131–1136.
23. Jonas JB, Degenring RF, Kamppeter BA, et al. Duration of the effect of intravitreal triamcinolone acetonide as treatment for diffuse diabetic macular edema. Am J Ophthalmol 2004;138(1):158–160.
24. Audren F, Erginay A, Haouchine B, et al. Intravitreal triamcinolone acetonide for diffuse diabetic macular oedema: 6-month results of a prospective controlled trial. Acta Ophthalmol Scand 2006;84(5):624–630.
25. Audren F, Tod M, Massin P, et al. Pharmacokinetic-pharmacodynamic modeling of the effect of triamcinolone acetonide on central macular thickness in patients with diabetic macular edema. Invest Ophthalmol Vis Sci 2004;45(10):3435–3441.
26. Jonas JB, Kamppeter BA, Harder B, et al. Intravitreal triamcinolone acetonide for diabetic macular edema: a prospective, randomized study. J Ocul Pharmacol Ther 2006;22(3):200–207.
27. A randomized trial comparing intravitreal triamcinolone acetonide and focal/grid photocoagulation for diabetic macular edema. Ophthalmology 2008;115(9):1447–1449, 1449 e1–e10.
28. Park CH, Jaffe GJ, Fekrat S. Intravitreal triamcinolone acetonide in eyes with cystoid macular edema associated with central retinal vein occlusion. Am J Ophthalmol 2003;136(3):419–425.
29. Ip MS, Gottlieb JL, Kahana A, et al. Intravitreal triamcinolone for the treatment of macular edema associated with central retinal vein occlusion. Arch Ophthalmol 2004;122(8):1131–1136.
30. Bashshur ZF, Ma'luf RN, Allam S, et al. Intravitreal triamcinolone for the management of macular edema due to nonischemic central retinal vein occlusion. Arch Ophthalmol 2004;122(8):1137–1140.
31. Jonas JB, Kreissig I, Degenring RF. Factors influencing visual acuity after intravitreal triamcinolone acetonide as treatment of exudative age related macular degeneration. Br J Ophthalmol 2004;88(12):1557–1562.
32. Jonas JB, Akkoyun I, Budde WM, et al. Intravitreal reinjection of triamcinolone for exudative age-related macular degeneration. Arch Ophthalmol 2004;122(2):218–222.
33. Jonas JB, Kreissig I, Hugger P, et al. Intravitreal triamcinolone acetonide for exudative age related macular degeneration. Br J Ophthalmol 2003;87(4):462–468.
34. Gillies MC, Simpson JM, Luo W, et al. A randomized clinical trial of a single dose of intravitreal triamcinolone acetonide for neovascular age-related macular degeneration: one-year results. Arch Ophthalmol 2003;121(5):667–673.
35. Spaide RF, Sorenson J, Maranan L. Photodynamic therapy with verteporfin combined with intravitreal injection of triamcinolone acetonide for choroidal neovascularization. Ophthalmology 2005 Feb;112(2 #0):301–304.
36. Augustin AJ, Schmidt-Erfurth U. Verteporfin and intravitreal triamcinolone acetonide combination therapy for occult choroidal neovascularization in age-related macular degeneration. Am J Ophthalmol 2006 Apr;141(4):638–645.
37. Spaide RF, Sorenson J, Maranan L. Photodynamic therapy with verteporfin combined with intravitreal injection of triamcinolone acetonide for choroidal neovascularization. Ophthalmology 2005;112(2):301–304.
38. Augustin AJ, Schmidt-Erfurth U. Verteporfin and intravitreal triamcinolone acetonide combination therapy for occult choroidal neovascularization in age-related macular degeneration. Am J Ophthalmol 2006;141(4):638–645.
39. Augustin AJ, Puls S, Offermann I. Triple therapy for choroidal neovascularization due to age-related macular degeneration: verteporfin PDT, bevacizumab, and dexamethasone. Retina 2007;27(2):133–140.
40. Augustin AJ, Puls S, Offermann I. Triple therapy for choroidal neovascularization due to age-related macular degeneration: verteporfin PDT, bevacizumab, and dexamethasone. Retina. 2007;27:133–140.
41. Jonas JB, Kreissig I, Degenring R. Intraocular pressure after intravitreal injection of triamcinolone acetonide. Br J Ophthalmol 2003;87(1):24–27.
42. Wingate RJ, Beaumont PE. Intravitreal triamcinolone and elevated intraocular pressure. Aust N Z J Ophthalmol 1999;27(6):431–432.
43. Bakri SJ, Beer PM. The effect of intravitreal triamcinolone acetonide on intraocular pressure. Ophthalmic Surg Lasers Imaging 2003;34(5):386–390.
44. Moshfeghi AA, Scott IU, Flynn HW, et al. Pseudohypopyon after intravitreal triamcinolone acetonide injection for cystoid macular edema. Am J Ophthalmol 2004;138(3):489–492.
45. Nelson ML, Tennant MT, Sivalingam A, et al. Infectious and presumed noninfectious endophthalmitis after intravitreal triamcinolone acetonide injection. Retina 2003;23(5):686–691.
46. Benz MS, Murray TG, Dubovy SR, et al. Endophthalmitis caused by *Mycobacterium chelonae abscessus* after intravitreal injection of triamcinolone. Arch Ophthalmol 2003;121(2):271–273.
47. Yeung CK, Chan KP, Chan CK, et al. Cytotoxicity of triamcinolone on cultured human retinal pigment epithelial cells: comparison with dexamethasone and hydrocortisone. Jpn J Ophthalmol 2004;48(3):236–242.
48. Narayanan R, Mungcal JK, Kenney MC, et al. Toxicity of triamcinolone acetonide on retinal neurosensory and pigment epithelial cells. Invest Ophthalmol Vis Sci 2006;47(2):722–728.
49. Tokuda K, Tsukamoto T, Fujisawa S, et al. Evaluation of toxicity due to vital stains in isolated rat retinas. Acta Ophthalmol Scand 2004;82(2):189–194.
50. Kivilcim M, Peyman GA, El-Dessouky ES, et al. Retinal toxicity of triamcinolone acetonide in silicone-filled eyes. Ophthalmic Surg Lasers 2000;31(6):474–478.
51. Gaston H, Absolon MJ, Thurtle OA, et al. Steroid responsiveness in connective tissue diseases. Br J Ophthalmol 1983;67(7):487–490.
52. Podos SM, Becker B, Morton WR. High myopia and primary open-angle glaucoma. Am J Ophthalmol 1966;62(6):1038–1043.
53. Jonas JB. Intravitreal triamcinolone acetonide: a change in a paradigm. Ophthalmic Res 2006;38(4):218–245.
54. Smithen LM, Ober MD, Maranan L, et al. Intravitreal triamcinolone acetonide and intraocular pressure. Am J Ophthalmol 2004;138(5):740–743.
55. Mueller AJ, Jian G, Banker AS, et al. The effect of deep posterior subtenon injection of corticosteroids on intraocular pressure. Am J Ophthalmol 1998;125(2):158–163.
56. Moshfeghi AA, Flynn HJ. Complications of intravitreal triamcinolone injection. Rev Ophthalmol 2004;4:64–67.
57. Moshfeghi DM, Kaiser PK. Acute endophthalmitis following intravitreal triamcinolone acetonide injection. Am J Ophthalmol 2003;136(5):791–796.
58. Gillies MC, Kuzniarz M, Craig J, et al. Intravitreal triamcinolone-induced elevated intraocular pressure is associated with the development of posterior subcapsular cataract. Ophthalmology 2005;112(1):139–143.
59. Thompson JT. Cataract formation and other complications of intravitreal triamcinolone for macular edema. Am J Ophthalmol 2006;141(4):629–637.
60. Pearson P, Levy B, Comstock T. Fluocinolone Acetonide Implant Study Group. Fluocinolone Acetonide Intravitreal Implant to Treat Diabetic Macular Edema: 3-Year Results of a Multi–Center Clinical Trial. Invest Ophthalmol Vis Sci 2006;47:E-Abstract 5442.
61. Kuppermann BD, Blumenkranz MS, Haller JA, et al. Randomized controlled study of an intravitreous dexamethasone drug delivery system in patients with persistent macular edema. Arch Ophthalmol 2007;125(3):309–317.
62. Ferris 3rd FL, Patz A. Macular edema. A complication of diabetic retinopathy. Surv Ophthalmol 1984;28(Suppl):452–461.

CHAPTER 31

Anecortave acetate

Hajir Dadgostar, MD and Peter K. Kaiser, MD

KEY FEATURES

Anecortave acetate is a member of a novel class of steroid analogues known as angiostatic cortisenes. It is similar in structure to cortisol and displays many of the antiangiogenic properties of glucocorticoids but lacks their anti-inflammatory and immunosuppressive effects. It also does not exhibit the common ocular side-effects associated with glucocorticoids, including cataract formation and intraocular pressure (IOP) elevation. It is administered as a posterior juxtascleral depot (PJD) adjacent to the macula using a specially designed, blunt-tipped cannula, and it is well tolerated systemically and from an ocular standpoint. Anecortave acetate has demonstrated efficacy in the treatment of exudative age-related macular degeneration (AMD) and is currently being evaluated as means of reducing the risk of progression in high-risk nonexduative AMD.

INTRODUCTION AND HISTORY

Glucocorticoids have been widely used in the treatment of retina disease because of their angiostatic properties.[1] Although their beneficial effect on retinal edema is well recognized, the use of this class of agents has been limited by their known association with ocular complications such as elevated IOP and cataract formation.[2] Other steroid compounds, including the estrogen derivative 2-methoxyestradiol, the progesterone derivative 17α-medroxyprogesterone, and squalamine, have also been found to have angiostatic activity in various systems,[3–6] suggesting that the angiostatic properties of steroid compounds may be distinct from other activities characteristic of glucocorticoids. In 1985, Crum and colleagues demonstrated the angiostatic properties of a new class of steroids that lack conventional glucocorticoid activity but were able to inhibit neovascularization in the presence of cofactors such as heparin or cyclodextran.[7]

Based on such data, efforts were made to design a steroid derivative with good ocular bioavailability which lacked conventional glucocorticoid activity but retained angiostatic activity. After testing over 100 compounds in a chicken embryo model and further testing 15 compounds in a rabbit corneal neovascularization model, two compounds were found to have potent angiostatic activity.[8] These molecules, anecortave acetate (Retaane, Alcon Laboratories, Fort Worth, TX) and anecortave desacetate define a novel class of angiostatic nonglucocorticoid steroid derivatives known as cortisenes.

As shown in Figure 31.1, both anecortave acetate and anecortave desacetate are derived from cortisol and both lack the 11β-hydroxyl group. Removal of hydroxyl group at this position is believed to eliminate glucocorticoid activity. Instead a double bond was introduced at the C9–11 position, and this conversion of a hydroxyl group to a double bond is reflected in the nomenclature of this class of molecules (cortisol versus cortisene). The only structural difference between anecortave desacetate and anecortave acetate is that the latter contains an additional 21-acetate group which is believed to enhance ocular penetration and prolong treatment duration when the drug is delivered as a local depot (see below).

The initial screening tests for angiostatic activity were performed using the chick embryo chorioallantoic membrane (CAM) system, an extensively used model of angiogenesis.[9,10] In this system, embryos are carefully removed from fertilized chicken eggs and grown in a sterile Petri dish for 3 days and then exposed to a lipid suspension containing 10 μl agarose pellets impregnated with the compound of interest. Growth of capillaries around the pellet site is scored after 2 days of further incubation. As mentioned above, after the screening of many steroid derivatives, the C9–11 cortisenes were found to be the most potent inhibitors of vascular growth in this assay.[11]

Anecortave acetate behaves similarly in a rabbit corneal neovascularization model. This model involves the implantation of bacterial lipopolysaccharide (LPS)-containing pellets in a stromal pocket near the limbus, after which the extent of neovascular growth into the cornea is measured. Anecortave acetate was shown to inhibit corneal neovascularization in this system when implanted in pellet form and also when administered as 0.1% and 1% topical suspensions (Figure 31.2).[11,12] Studies using topical administration showed dose-dependent suppression of neovascular growth even when treatment was initiated several days after the implantation of LPS pellets.[12]

PHARMACOLOGY

Based on dose titration studies in various *in vitro* models, it was determined that the effective concentration of anecortave acetate required to achieve effective angiostasis in target tissues is above 0.01 μm.[13] Thus, this concentration was used as the target for animal studies evaluating pharmacokinetics and delivery routes.

Topical and systemic administration in animals resulted in insufficient drug concentrations in the retina and choroid; however, intravitreal injections of a 5-mg dose as well as sub-Tenon's injections of either a 10-mg or 50-mg dose resulted in adequate drug concentrations for about 6 months.[13] In the case of sub-Tenon's injections, adequate drug concentrations were maintained only when the depot was deposited directly in contact with the sclera, but this delivery route was still considered more appealing than the intravitreal route because of its more favorable safety profile. For this reason, a specially designed, curved, blunt-tipped posterior juxtascleral cannula was designed so that depot doses of anecortave acetate could be delivered directly adjacent to the sclera in the macular region. Briefly, the recommended injection procedure in humans, which is described in detail elsewhere,[14,15] involves making a small radial conjunctival incision 8 mm posterior to the limbus in the superotemporal quadrant after application of topical anesthetic. As shown in Figure 31.3, a specially designed curved blunt cannula is then advanced through this incision within the sub-Tenon's space and the drug is slowly delivered as a PJD. A counterpressure device is held over the conjunctiva with the cannula in place to minimize drug reflux and thus improve the reproducibility of the dose delivered.

Using this delivery method, human pharmacokinetic studies were performed as part of a randomized, multicenter, placebo-controlled phase II trial in subjects with exudative AMD.[13] Subjects received one of three doses of PJD anecortave acetate (3, 15, or 30 mg) or placebo at

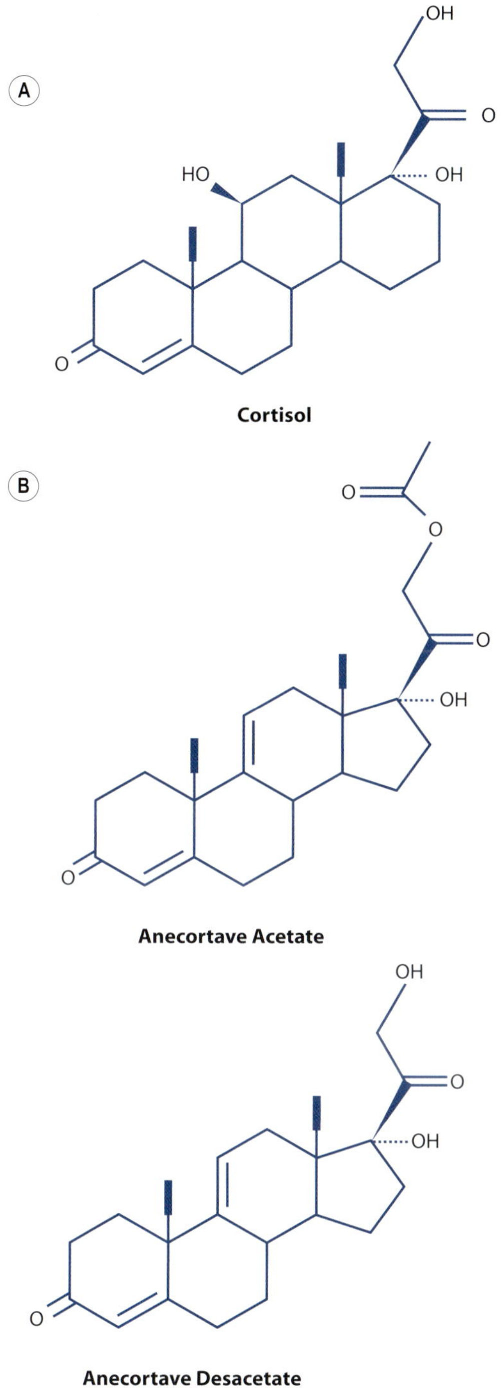

Figure 31.1 The molecular structures of (A) cortisol, and (B) the angiostatic cortisenes, anecortave acetate and anecortave desacetate.

6-month intervals. In this study, plasma concentrations of anecortave desacetate reached maximal concentrations at 1–2 days after injection, but were minimally detectable at 2 weeks. The proportionality of the maximal plasma dose with the depot dose suggested linear pharmacokinetics.

The observed plasma half-life of anecortave desacetate in humans, based on this and similar studies, was about 3–5 days; however, in preclinical studies, the half-life of the juxtascleral depot was about 2 weeks. Further, after disappearance of the visible drug depot, effective drug concentrations were maintained in the choroid and retina for 6 months in animals (Figure 31.4).[13] Consistent with these data, plasma concentrations on repeat dosing in humans were similar to those after

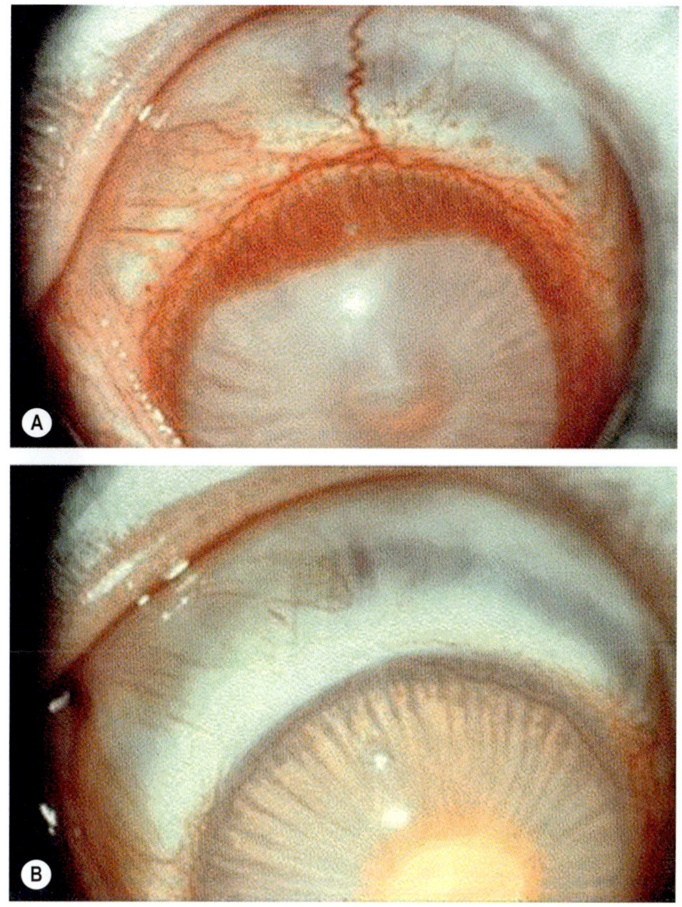

Figure 31.2 Neovascularization in a rabbit cornea model after stromal lipopolysaccharide implantation followed by topical treatment three times daily for 3 weeks with vehicle (A) or 1% anecortave acetate (B). (Reprinted from BenEzra D, Griffin BW, Maftzir G, et al. Topical formulations of novel angiostatic steroids inhibit rabbit corneal neovascularization. Invest Ophthalmol Vis Sci 1997;38:1954–1962, with permission from *Investigative Ophthalmology and Visual Science*.)

the original injection, indicating that the drug did not accumulate systemically when injected at 6-month intervals. Pharmacokinetic parameters such as maximal plasma concentration and half-life were not affected by verteporfin photodynamic therapy (PDT) administered at least 5 days prior to injection. Gender also had no effect on pharmacokinetics.

Anecortave acetate is hydrolyzed *in vivo* to anecortave desacetate, which is 93.5% plasma protein-bound.[13] Anecortave desacetate, like cortisol, undergoes hepatic metabolism via NADPH-dependent reductases and these metabolites circulate as glucuronide conjugates until they are eliminated. Based on C^{14}-labeling studies, the major metabolite in humans (representing about 80% of the total) was a compound termed AL-38508, which has a saturated A-ring with a 3-hydroxyl group as a result of reduction of the C-4/C-5 double bond and 3-ketone (Figure 31.5). After a 15-mg subcutaneous dose, subjects with Child–Pugh class C hepatic impairment (severe deficiency) had a slightly higher maximal plasma concentration of anecortave desacetate compared to healthy subjects, but otherwise displayed similar pharmacokinetics for the drug and its major metabolite.[13] Pharmacokinetic parameters in subjects with milder levels of hepatic impairment were reported to be comparable to those in healthy subjects, and no drug was detected in plasma after 5 weeks, even in those with severe impairment. Finally, anecortave desacetate is not metabolized through the cytochrome P-450 pathway, and accordingly, *in vitro* testing on a number of human isozymes revealed no inhibitory effect.

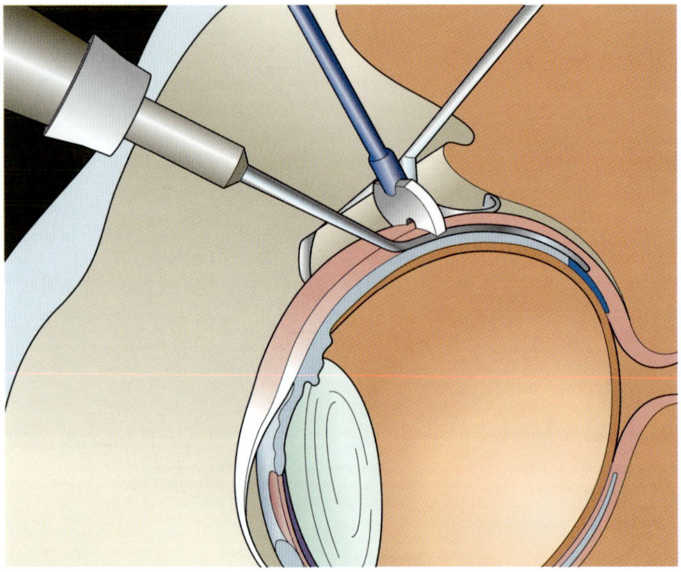

Figure 31.3 The posterior juxtascleral depot injection technique. (Reprinted from Slakter JS. Anecortave acetate for treating or preventing choroidal neovascularization. Ophthalmol Clin North Am 2006;19:373–380, with permission from *Ophthalmology Clinics of North America*.)

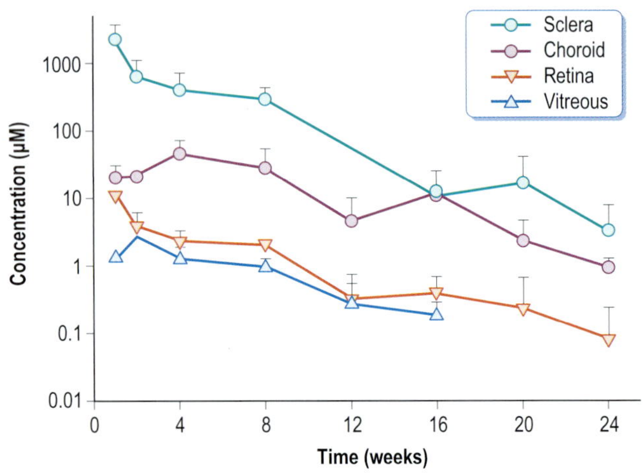

Figure 31.4 Mean concentrations of anecortave desacetate over 24 weeks in ocular tissues of cynomolgus monkeys after posterior juxtascleral injection of 15 mg anecortave acetate. Error bars represent standard deviation. (Reprinted from Dahlin DC, Rahimy MH. Pharmacokinetics and metabolism of anecortave acetate in animals and humans. Surv Ophthalmol 2007;52(Suppl. 1):S49–S61 with permission from *Survey of Ophthalmology*.)

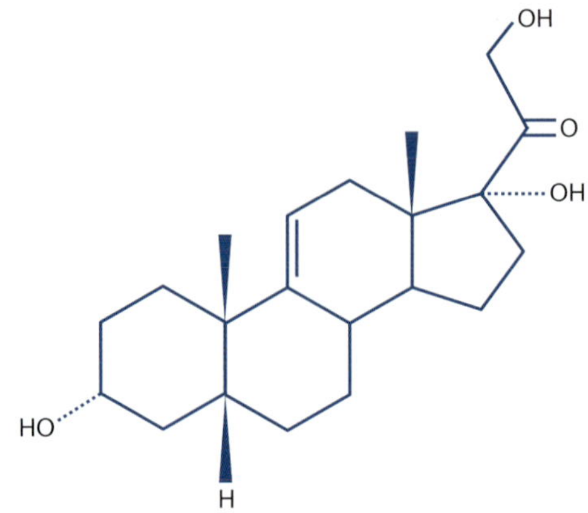

Figure 31.5 The major metabolite of anecortave desacetate, AL-38508, circulates in plasma as a glucuronide conjugate.

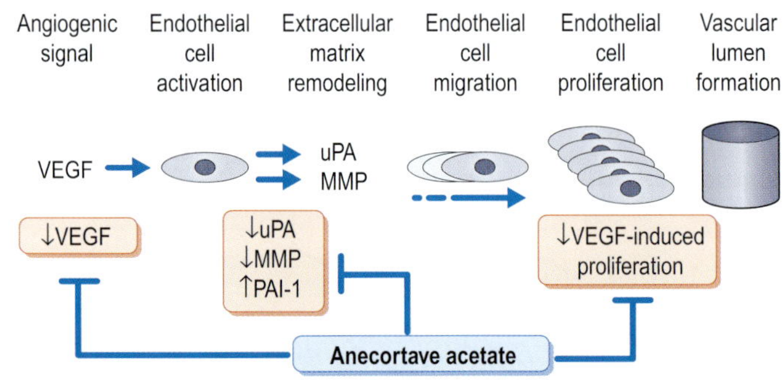

Figure 31.6 Schematic representation of the major steps in the angiogenesis cascade, highlighting the points at which anecortave acetate may regulate the process. VEGF, vascular endothelial growth factor; MMP, matrix metalloproteinase; PAI-1, plasminogen activator inhibitor-1.

DRUG MECHANISM

The endogenous receptor for anecortave desacetate is unknown. Importantly, however, it does not appear to be a receptor in the glucocorticoid pathway based on data from a number of experimental models. The production of interleukin-1β by cultured human U937 cells after stimulation with LPS can be inhibited by a variety of glucocorticoids, but treatment with anecortave acetate and anecortave desacetate had no inhibitory effect on this inflammatory response.[8] Similarly, *in vivo* studies on LPS-mediated uveitis in rabbits and rats revealed no anti-inflammatory effect. In the same models, adding angiostatic cortisenes did not inhibit the anti-inflammatory effect of glucocorticoids, suggesting these agents also do not act as competitive inhibitors of glucocorticoid function. If the angiostatic cortisenes do not exhibit glucocorticoid activity, then it is expected that they would also not produce ocular side-effects typical of glucocorticoids, such as cataract and elevated IOP.

Anecortave acetate does inhibit the production of urokinase plasminogen activator and pro-matrix metalloproteinase (MMP) in cultured human vascular endothelial cells.[16] The elaboration of both of these molecules is important for the initiation of the proteolytic cascade that allows endothelial cells to migrate and establish new vessels in the angiogenic process, as summarized in Figure 31.6. Other *in vitro* studies have revealed a dose-dependent inhibitory effect of anecortave acetate on vascular endothelial growth factor (VEGF)-stimulated endothelial cell proliferation, suggesting an additional step in the neovascularization process that may be blocked by this drug (reviewed in Clark[8]).

Data from *in vivo* studies support this mechanism of action as well. In a rat model of retinopathy of prematurity (ROP), intravitreal anecortave acetate stimulated the production of plasminogen activator inhibitor-1,[17] which is able to inhibit urokinase plasminogen activator activity.[18] Also, in a mouse retinoblastoma model, this drug was able to regulate the production of MMP-2 and MMP-9 and even suppress retinal expression of VEGF (reviewed in Clark[8]). Thus, based on these data, it is believed that anecortave acetate can inhibit neovascularization both upstream and downstream of VEGF and, through its inhibitory effect on the proteolytic cascade, may also inhibit neovascularization induced by growth factors other than VEGF (Figure 31.6).

DRUG EFFECTS IN RETINAL DISEASES

PRECLINICAL STUDIES

Retinopathy of prematurity

ROP is the leading cause of blindness associated with premature birth. Its incidence is correlated with birth weight and gestational age, with 84% of those born at <28 weeks' gestational age being affected. The majority of cases are mild and regress spontaneously; however, threshold ROP occurs in 7–8% of infants with a birth weight of <1251 g.[19,20] The pathogenesis of this disease is believed to be related to incomplete peripheral retinal vascularization combined with exposure to high oxygen levels in the neonatal intensive care unit setting. Upon return to normal oxygen concentrations, the avascular peripheral retina becomes ischemic, giving rise to a neovascular response with devastating potential consequences, including vitreous hemorrhage and tractional partial or total retinal detachment. The current standard of care in the treatment of prethreshold to threshold ROP is laser photocoagulation delivered to all avascular areas of the retina in order to induce regression of neovascularization.

Anecortave acetate has been evaluated in two animal models of ROP. One of these is a rat model in which retinal neovascularization is induced in newborn rats exposed to alternating oxygen concentrations of 10% and 50% shortly after birth and then returned to room air 14 days later. Intravitreal anecortave acetate injected at various timepoints inhibited pathologic retinal neovascularization in this model by 50% or more compared to vehicle.[17] In another model of ROP, newborn kittens were exposed to 80% oxygen for 80 hours and then returned to room air.[21] In this model, intravitreal anecortave desacetate dose-dependently reduced pathologic neovascularization with a 50% reduction at the highest dose (reviewed in Clark[11]).

Intraocular tumors

Uveal melanoma and retinoblastoma are the most common primary intraocular malignancies in adults and children, respectively, and both can display aggressive spread with life-threatening complications. A fundamental principle in the pathophysiology of most malignant tumors is the fact that as a tumor outgrows its blood supply; it must elaborate growth factors to induce further angiogenesis in order to sustain its growth.[22,23]

Anecortave acetate has been used to target tumor angiogenesis in two ocular tumor models. When 99E3 uveal melanoma cells are transplanted into the eyes of nude mice, they grow rapidly and become highly vascularized. Topical application of 1% anecortave acetate at various timepoints posttransplantation significantly inhibited tumor growth by 40–70% compared to vehicle.[24] Since there was no effect on the *in vitro* growth of tumor cells, it was presumed that the inhibitory effect *in vivo* was a result of reduced angiogenesis, although this was not directly demonstrated. In a mouse retinoblastoma model developed by transgenic expression of SV40 T-antigen under a retina-specific promoter, subconjunctival anecortave acetate was able to inhibit tumor growth and vascularity in a dose-dependent fashion.[25]

Choroidal neovascularization

When defects in Bruch's membrane allow a network of choroidal vessels to grow beneath the retinal pigment epithelium (RPE) and/or retina, vision loss can occur as a result of exudation, hemorrhage, or fibrosis. Although the most common cause of choroidal neovascularization (CNV) among the elderly is AMD,[26] there is a large list of other diagnoses where CNV can occur, including presumed ocular histoplasmosis syndrome, pathologic myopia, angioid streaks, choroidal rupture, trauma, and a variety of inflammatory chorioretinopathies.

It is believed that angiogenic growth factors are needed to sustain the growth of CNV, and a rabbit model of CNV has been developed by implanting a sustained-release depot of basic fibroblast growth factor (FGF) in the subretinal space.[27] In this model, a single posterior juxtascleral administration of 0.5 mg anecortave acetate immediately after FGF depot implantation resulted in no detectable leakage on fluorescein angiography at 8 weeks in 6/8 animals compared to 2/10 animals receiving vehicle after FGF implant ($P < 0.025$). In a mouse model using laser damage to disrupt Bruch's membrane and induce CNV, intravitreal anecortave acetate resulted in a 58% inhibition of CNV ($P < 0.001$; reviewed in Clark[11]).

CLINICAL STUDIES

Exudative AMD

Until recently, the only available treatments for exudative AMD, the leading cause of blindness among the aging population in developed countries, were laser photocoagulation and verteporfin PDT.[26] In recent years a number of pharmacotherapeutic agents targeting various steps in the angiogenesis pathway have been and are being investigated as treatments for exudative AMD.[28] Among these are the VEGF inhibitors pegaptanib (Macugen, OSI-Eyetech, New York, NY), ranibizumab (Lucentis, Genentech, South San Francisco, CA), and bevacizumab (Avastin, Genentech, South San Francisco, CA), which have shown great promise in this context (discussed elsewhere). Because the broad mechanism of anecortave acetate is believed to target multiple points in the neovascularization process, possibly including VEGF-independent pathways as well (see above), and because the PJD delivery route requires less frequent dosing and is less invasive than intravitreal administration, anecortave acetate has been evaluated in clinical trials for the treatment of exudative AMD (Table 31.1).

The Anecortave Acetate Clinical Study Group reported the 12-month results of a randomized, placebo-controlled clinical safety and efficacy trial comparing three different doses of anecortave acetate (3, 15, and 30 mg) with placebo.[29] This monotherapy trial enrolled 128 subjects with subfoveal CNV, 80% of which were predominantly classic lesions at baseline. Subjects were randomized to either placebo treatment or one of the three doses of anecortave acetate delivered using the specially designed PJD cannula at 6-month intervals. As shown in Figure 31.7, the most beneficial effect was derived from the intermediate (15-mg) dose, which resulted in significantly better visual acuity at 12 months than placebo (visual acuity difference of 1.8 logMAR lines; $P = 0.0131$). The percentage of subjects losing <3 lines of visual acuity at 12 months was 79% in the 15-mg anecortave acetate group compared to 53% in the placebo group ($P = 0.0323$). Severe vision loss (6 lines) occurred in 1/33 eyes (3%) in the 15-mg group compared to 7/30 eyes (23%) in the placebo group ($P = 0.0224$). A subgroup analysis of the patients with predominantly classic CNV revealed similar data, with 84% in the 15-mg group losing <3 lines compared to 50% in the placebo group ($P = 0.01$) and none with severe vision loss in the 15-mg group compared to 23% in the placebo group ($P = 0.0299$). Thus, anecortave acetate was shown to be superior to placebo for the stabilization of visual acuity in the setting of subfoveal CNV in this clinical trial.

A separate combination treatment trial randomized 136 subjects to PDT followed within 8 days by a single dose of anecortave acetate (either 15 or 30 mg) or vehicle (reviewed in Russell et al.[30]). In this 6-month study, subjects in the PDT-only group lost 1.5 lines of visual acuity, whereas subjects in the PDT–anecortave acetate 15-mg group lost 1 line of visual acuity. Overall, there was a trend toward less vision loss in the combination groups; however, these differences were not statistically significant.

In a pivotal phase III trial, the efficacy of anecortave acetate was compared directly to that of PDT.[31] This was a noninferiority study enrolling 530 subjects with predominantly classic subfoveal CNV who were randomized to anecortave acetate 15 mg after sham PDT or stan-

Table 31.1 Summary of major clinical trials investigating the efficacy and safety of anecortave acetate in the treatment of exudative age-related macular deneration

Study	Treatment	No. of eyes	Follow-up	Outcome
C-98-03[29,42]	Anecortave acetate 3 mg Anecortave acetate 15 mg Anecortave acetate 30 mg Vehicle (all at 6-month intervals)	128	24 months	Mean VA at 12 months 1.8 lines greater with anecortave acetate 15 mg (n = 33) than vehicle (n = 3, P = 0.0131); loss of <3 lines was 79% in 15-mg group and 53% in vehicle group (P = 0.0323); these differences were greater in the predominantly classic subgroup; 15 mg appeared superior to other doses; similar data at 24 months
C-00-07	PDT + anecortave acetate 15 mg PDT + anecortave acetate 30 mg PDT + vehicle	136	6 months	Mean VA loss at 6 months was 1.5 lines with PDT + vehicle and 1.0 lines with PDT + anecortave acetate 15 mg; maintenance of VA was 78% in the combination therapy groups and 67% in the PDT + vehicle group; the difference was not statistically significant
C-01-99[31]	Anecortave acetate 15 mg PDT	530	12 months	Loss of <3 lines was 45% with anecortave acetate 15 mg and 49% with PDT (P = 0.43); noninferiority criteria not met with 7% CI limit, but were met with 14% CI limit; drug reflux and treatment intervals >6 months seemed to impact responder rates in anecortave acetate group

VA, visual acuity; PDT, photodynamic therapy; CI, confidence interval.

dard PDT followed by a sham PJD injection. At 12 months, the percentage of subjects in the anecortave acetate group losing <3 lines of visual acuity was 45% compared to 49% in the PDT group (P = 0.43); however, the confidence interval was greater than the 7 percentage point limit required by the study protocol, and thus the prospectively defined, noninferiority criteria were not met (Figure 31.8). The study authors argued that a 14 percentage point confidence interval limit was more clinically relevant to prove noninferiority to PDT based on the pivotal PDT phase III studies. Had this confidence interval been used instead of the more stringent limit employed by this study, the noninferiority criteria would have been met. The authors also suggest that documented drug reflux from the injection tract and repeat treatments outside the 6-month window required for anecortave acetate may have contributed to reduced effective drug dosage for some of the subjects in the treatment groups. Indeed, in retrospective analyses, removing subjects with documented drug reflux or reinjection >6 months after the initial treatment from the anecortave acetate group increased the percentage with <3 lines vision loss to 57% compared to 49% for the PDT group (P = 0.193).

The issue of reflux deserves special mention in this context. At the time that this study was being performed, counterpressure was maintained at the injection site using sterile cotton swabs held over the shaft of the PJD cannula. The manufacturer has since developed a specialized counterpressure device that fits tightly over the cannula, minimizing drug reflux (Figure 31.9). Thus, with special attention to avoiding reflux and performing treatments within a 6-month window, it is probable that anecortave acetate is at least as effective as PDT for the maintenance of visual acuity in the setting of subfoveal CNV. Anecortave acetate has gained regulatory approval in Australia for the treatment of exdudative AMD.

Dry AMD

Because of its 6-month dosing interval as well as the relatively low risk of PJD injections compared to intravitreal injections, anecortave acetate is being considered as a prophylactic treatment in subjects with high-risk dry AMD to prevent progression to wet AMD. The Anecortave Acetate Risk Reduction Trial (AART) is a 48-month randomized, placebo-controlled phase III safety and efficacy trial that is currently investigating the use of anecortave acetate in subjects with high-risk dry AMD in the study eye and wet AMD in the fellow eye. About 2500 subjects have been randomized in a 2:1 ratio to anecortave acetate (either 15 or 30 mg) or placebo, with the primary endpoint being prevention of sight-threatening CNV in the study eye. The above-mentioned protocol issues have been addressed in this study. Recently, the study was halted by the Data Safety Monitoring Board when it was found that there did not appear to be a treatment effect. Full details of the clinical study have not been released publicly.

Other diseases

Retinal angiomatous proliferation (RAP) is a specific, often difficult-to-treat, variant of neovascularization accounting for 12–15% of exudative AMD. In a small uncontrolled pilot study, 34 subjects with RAP lesions were administered one of three doses of anecortave acetate and followed for 12 months.[32] There was a reduction in the amount of fluid accumulation, but subjects continued to lose visual acuity, suggesting anecortave acetate at the studied doses is likely not adequate as monotherapy for this condition. Idiopathic perifoveal telangiectasia is a distinct condition characterized by capillary dilation and leakage adjacent to the fovea. In a small uncontrolled pilot study on 7 eyes of 6 subjects with this condition, anecortave acetate treatment resulted in stabilization of visual acuity for as long as 24 months.[33]

More recently, anecortave acetate using an anterior juxtascleral injection has been tested to lower IOP in patients with primary open-angle glaucoma (POAG). A pilot proof-of-concept study in 89 patients with POAG confirmed visual field changes with IOP between 24 and 36 mmHg. The patients were randomly assigned in a 1:1:1:1 ratio between 7.5, 15, and 30 mg/ml anecortave acetate or 0.5 ml control vehicle (presented at American Glaucoma Society, Washington, DC 2008). All patients received an injection of drug or vehicle at baseline and IOP was assessed at 2, 6, and 12 weeks. Retreatment with the original treatment was allowed if more than 42 days had passed since the last administration and the IOP was >18 mmHg at two consecutive

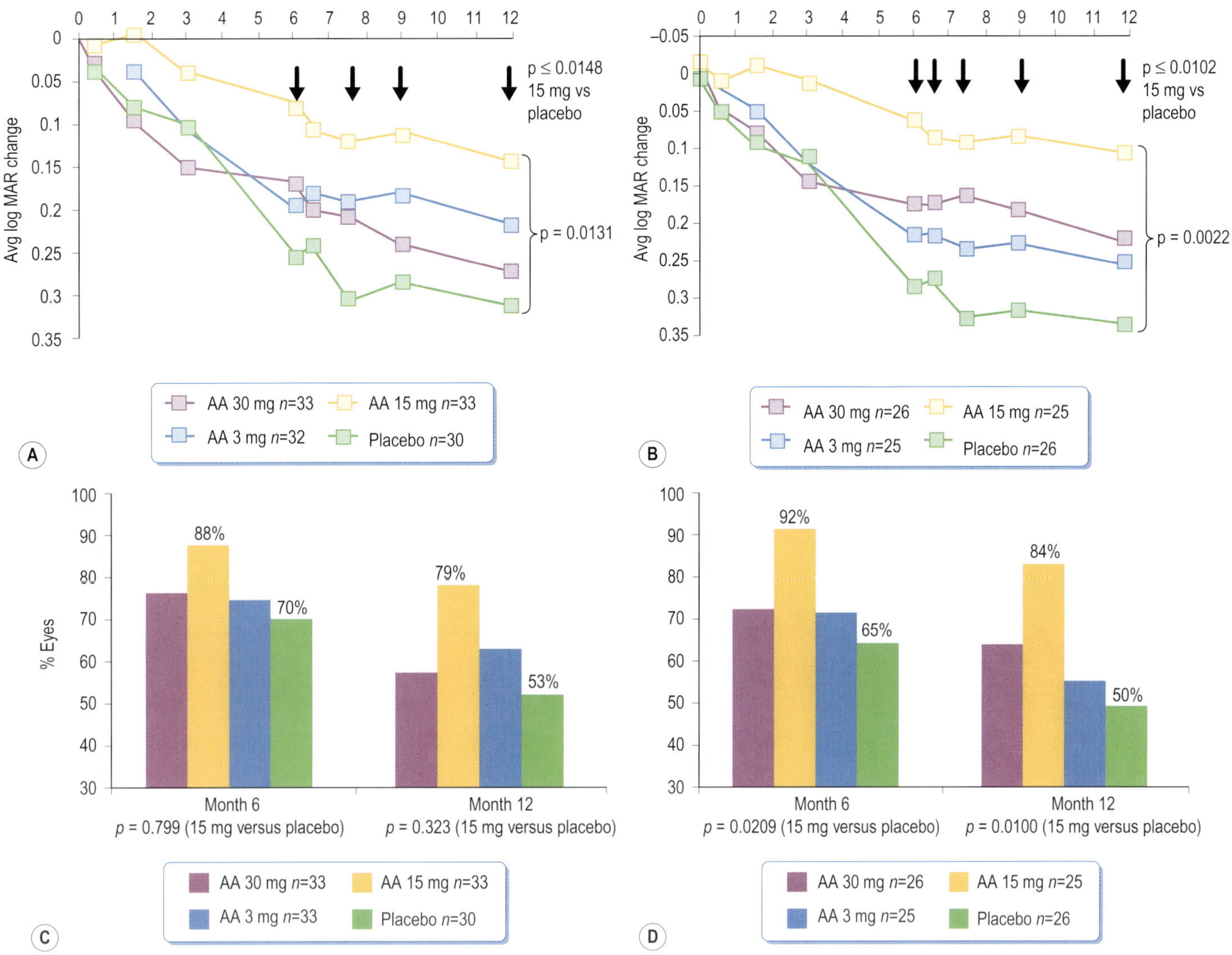

Figure 31.7 Twelve-month results of the anecortave acetate (AA) monotherapy trial. Average visual acuity change by treatment group over 12 months in all study subjects (A) and the subgroup of subjects with predominantly classic lesions (B); arrows represent time points at which there was a statistically significant difference in visual acuity change between anecortave acetate 15 mg and placebo. Percentage of eyes avoiding moderate vision loss (<3 logMAR lines) in all subjects (C) and those with predominantly classic lesions (D). (Reprinted from D'Amico DJ, Goldberg MF, Hudson H, et al. Anecortave acetate as monotherapy for treatment of subfoveal neovascularization in age-related macular degeneration: twelve-month clinical outcomes. Ophthalmology 2003;110:2372–2383; discussion 2384–2385, with permission from *Ophthalmology*.)

visits scheduled 1 week apart. The safety was excellent: mild eye pain, foreign-body sensation, hyperemia, and blurred vision were reported in 5–15% of patients. In addition, the 7.5- and 15-mg anecortave acetate doses had statistically significant lower mean IOP than vehicle at the 12-week primary efficacy endpoint ($P < 0.05$). Another way to look at the data is to define treatment success as maintenance of IOP at 21 mmHg. Approximately 55% of patients in the 7.5- and 15-mg arms treated with anecortave acetate had treatment success at week 12. In contrast, in the vehicle control group approximately 50% of patients were treatment failures by week 2 and only 2 patients (6.4%) were treatment successes at 12 weeks.

EFFICACY AND COMPARISON WITH OTHER AGENTS

The only treatment modality for exudative AMD that has been compared head to head with anecortave acetate to date is PDT.[31] As discussed above, these two treatments may be comparable in efficacy; however, anecortave acetate has the advantage that treatments need only be repeated once every 6 months. Also, PDT carries the small but significant risk of acute severe vision loss as well as the possible risk of delayed RPE atrophy,[34–37] both of which would be unlikely with anecortave acetate (see below).

In the past few years, intravitreal VEGF inhibitors, such as pegaptanib, ranibizumab, and bevacizumab, have largely replaced other treatment modalities as the first-line monotherapy for subfoveal CNV in the setting of wet AMD.[28,38] Ranibizumab and bevacizumab are currently the most commonly used agents in this setting and both have been shown to be very effective in the treatment of exudative AMD (discussed elsewhere). Although none of these agents has been compared directly with anecortave acetate, indirect evidence from comparisons of studies enrolling similar subject populations suggests that ranibizumab (and likely bevacizumab) is superior to anecortave acetate in this setting. Similar to the anecortave acetate phase III wet AMD trial, the Anti-VEGF Antibody for the Treatment of Predominantly Classic Choroidal Neovascularization in AMD (ANCHOR) trial, a 2-year, prospective, randomized, placebo-controlled trial, compared ranibizumab with PDT in subjects with predominantly classic CNV.[39] In this trial, the percentage of subjects in the 0.5-mg ranibizumab group losing <3 lines of visual acuity and those gaining 3 lines at 12 months were 96.4%

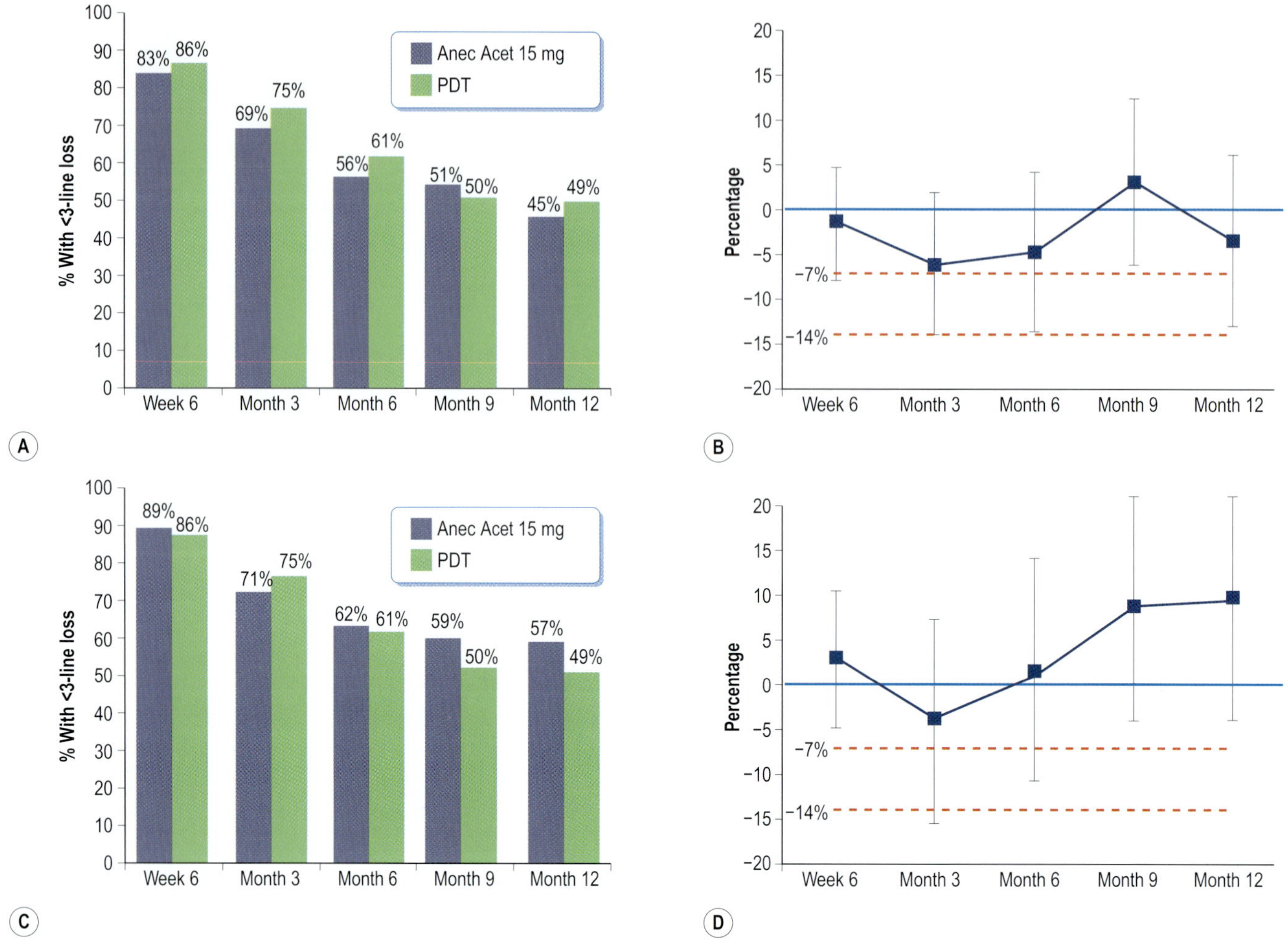

Figure 31.8 Results of the anecortave acetate (AA) versus photodynamic therapy (PDT) comparison trial. Percentage of eyes avoiding moderate (3 lines) visual acuity loss (left) and difference between groups over time with 95% confidence intervals (right) with dashed lines representing 7% (planned noninferiority criteria for this study) and 14% confidence limits. Results shown are for all subjects (A and B) and a retrospective subgroup excluding eyes with reflux and those with >6 months between injections (C and D). (Reprinted from Slakter JS, Bochow TW, D'Amico DJ, et al. Anecortave acetate (15 milligrams) versus photodynamic therapy for treatment of subfoveal neovascularization in age-related macular degeneration. Ophthalmology 2006;113:3–13, with permission from *Ophthalmology*.)

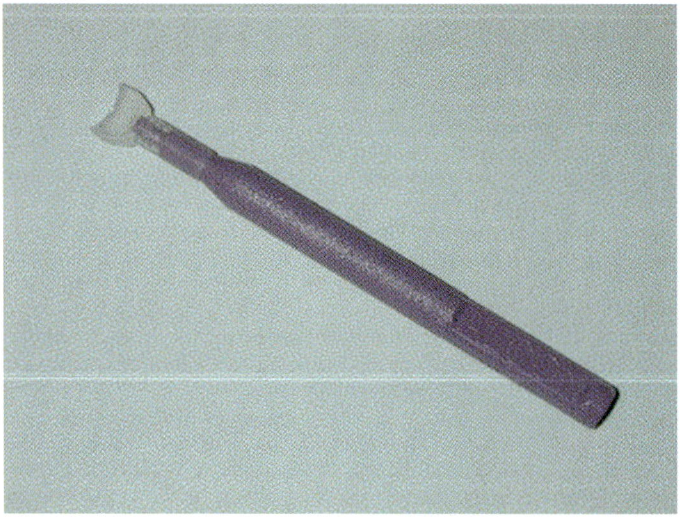

Figure 31.9 Counterpressure device for minimizing drug reflux during posterior juxtascleral depot injection.

and 40.3%, respectively, compared to 64.3% ($P < 0.001$) and 5.6% ($P < 0.001$), respectively, in the PDT group. Even accounting for reflux and missed dosing windows, a side-by-side comparison of the ANCHOR data with those from the anecortave acetate versus PDT comparison trial would seem to suggest that ranibizumab is a more effective treatment (Figure 31.10). This comparison is, however, provided only for illustrative purposes, and it is difficult to make firm conclusions based on such comparisons across trials owing to probable differences between study populations and other baseline conditions. Of note, the PDT group also fared better in the ANCHOR trial than in the anecortave acetate comparison trial, highlighting the probable existence of such differences.

CONTRAINDICATIONS

OCULAR COMPLICATIONS AND TOXICITY

Preclinical safety studies performed on rabbits and monkeys revealed a transient mild episcleral inflammation at the PJD site in some eyes.[40]

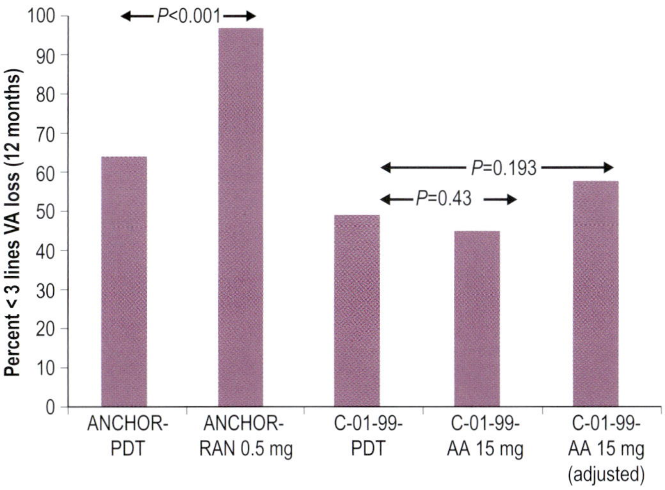

Figure 31.10 Side-by-side comparison of the percentage of eyes avoiding moderate (3 lines) visual acuity loss in a trial of photodynamic therapy (PDT) versus ranibizumab (ANCHOR[39]) and a trial of PDT versus anecortave acetate (AA) (C-01-99[31]). For the latter, data on the AA group are shown for all subjects and for the subgroup (adjusted), excluding those eyes with reflux and/or >6-month treatment interval.

Otherwise slit-lamp biomicroscopy, indirect ophthalmoscopy, IOP measurement and electroretinogram testing revealed no ocular toxicity with various doses and at various timepoints.

Pooled safety data from the major clinical trials of anecortave acetate were reported by Regillo et al.[41] With respect to ocular complications, the most frequent adverse events when anecortave acetate was used as either primary therapy (Table 31.2) or adjunctive therapy (Table 31.3) included visual acuity decrease, cataract, and eye pain, among others. None of these ocular adverse events differed significantly in frequency between the anecortave acetate and placebo groups. Particular attention was paid to the incidence of cataract and IOP increase, as both of these are known ocular complication of glucocorticoid therapy. The incidence of cataract was less frequent among 313 subjects receiving anecortave acetate (15%) than among 267 subjects receiving PDT (18%) or 30 subjects receiving vehicle (40%). The incidence of IOP increase was 5.4%, 6.7%, and 0% among those receiving anecortave acetate, PDT, and vehicle, respectively. The most frequent adverse events related to the PJD procedure when anecortave acetate was given as primary therapy included eye pain (8.9%), eye discomfort (4.8%), eye hyperemia (3.2%), and subconjunctival hemorrhage (3.2%). The only serious ocular adverse event reported was retinal detachment in one subject receiving a PJD injection. Based on these data, it was concluded that anecortave acetate does not exhibit glucocorticoid-mediated side-effects and is well tolerated from an ocular standpoint.

SYSTEMIC COMPLICATIONS AND TOXICITY

Preclinical safety studies in a number of *in vitro* and *in vivo* models revealed no toxicity in any organ system, no genotoxicity, no carcinogenicity, and no reproductive toxicity or teratogenicity.[40]

Table 31.2 Most frequent ocular adverse events in subjects receiving anecortave acetate as primary therapy. Listed are all reported adverse events (top) and treatment-related adverse events (bottom)

Adverse event	Anecortave acetate 15 mg (*n* = 313)	PDT (*n* = 267)	*P* (15 mg versus PDT)	Vehicle (*n* = 30)	*P* (15 mg versus vehicle)
All ocular					
Visual acuity decrease	108 (34.5%)	92 (34.5%)	0.9904	13 (43.3%)	0.3337
Cataract	47 (15%)	48 (18%)	0.3368	12 (40%)	0.0005
Ocular pain	38 (12.1%)	25 (9.4%)	0.2840	5 (16.7%)	0.5606
Vitreous detachment	27 (8.6%)	1 (0.4%)	<0.0001	3 (10%)	0.7363
Foreign-body sensation	23 (7.3%)	15 (5.6%)	0.4013	3 (10%)	0.4864
Abnormal vision	21 (6.7%)	21 (7.9%)	0.5924	1 (3.3%)	0.7069
Pupil disorder	20 (6.4%)	18 (6.7%)	0.8645	4 (13.3%)	0.1461
IOP increase	17 (5.4%)	18 (6.7%)	0.5089	0 (0%)	0.3805
Treatment-related ocular					
Visual acuity decrease	17 (5.4%)	7 (2.6%)	0.0904	0 (0%)	0.3805
Eye pain	8 (2.6%)	6 (2.2%)	0.8092	1 (3.3%)	0.5657
Cataract	6 (1.9%)	6 (2.2%)	0.7806	2 (6.7)	0.1488
IOP decrease	4 (1.3%)	0 (0%)	0.1284	0 (0%)	1.0000
Foreign-body sensation	3 (1%)	4 (1.5%)	0.7087	1 (3.3%)	0.3077
Eye hyperemia	3 (1%)	2 (0.7%)	1.0000	0 (0%)	1.0000
Ptosis	3 (1%)	1 (0.4%)	0.6284	2 (6.7%)	0.0627
Conjunctival cicatrix	3 (1%)	0 (0%)	0.2534	0 (0%)	1.0000

Adapted from data reported in Regillo CD, D'Amico DJ, Mieler WF, et al. Clinical safety profile of posterior juxtascleral depot administration of anecortave acetate 15 mg suspension as primary therapy or adjunctive therapy with photodynamic therapy for treatment of wet age-related macular degeneration. Surv Ophthalmol 2007;52(Suppl. 1):S70–S78.

PDT, photodynamic therapy; IOP, intraocular pressure.

Table 31.3 Most frequent ocular adverse events in subjects receiving anecortave acetate as adjunctive therapy

Adverse event	Anecortave acetate 15 mg + PDT (*n* = 45)	Vehicle + PDT (*n* = 46)	*P*
All ocular			
Cataract	14 (31.1%)	8 (17.4%)	0.1264
Eye pain	10 (22.2%)	4 (8.7%)	0.0738
Eye hyperemia	9 (20%)	11 (23.9%)	0.6522
Visual acuity decrease	8 (17.8%)	10 (21.7%)	0.6353
Foreign-body sensation	3 (6.7%)	8 (17.4%)	0.1166
Ptosis	3 (6.7%)	1 (2.2%)	0.3610
Eye pruritus	3 (6.7%)	1 (2.2%)	0.3610
Anisocoria	3 (6.7%)	1 (2.2%)	0.3610
IOP decrease	3 (6.7%)	0 (0%)	0.1168

Adapted from data reported in Regillo CD, D'Amico DJ, Mieler WF, et al. Clinical safety profile of posterior juxtascleral depot administration of anecortave acetate 15 mg suspension as primary therapy or adjunctive therapy with photodynamic therapy for treatment of wet age-related macular degeneration. Surv Ophthalmol 2007;52(Suppl. 1):S70–S78.

PDT, photodynamic therapy; IOP, intraocular pressure.

Table 31.4 Most frequent systemic adverse events in subjects receiving anecortave acetate as primary therapy

Adverse event	Anecortave acetate 15 mg (*n* = 313)	PDT (*n* = 267)	*P* (15 mg versus PDT)	Vehicle (*n* = 30)	*P* (15 mg versus vehicle)
All systemic					
Hypertension	56 (17.9%)	46 (17.2%)	0.8344	4 (13.3%)	0.5302
Arthritis	31 (9.9%)	22 (8.2%)	0.4881	5 (16.7%)	0.2241
Infection	29 (9.3%)	14 (5.2%)	0.0654	1 (3.3%)	0.4953
Hypercholesterolemia	29 (9.3%)	20 (7.5%)	0.4437	2 (6.7%)	1.0000
Accidental injury	25 (8%)	21 (7.9%)	0.9568	1 (3.3%)	0.7142
Gastrointestinal disorder	25 (8%)	20 (7.5%)	0.8237	3 (10%)	0.7238
Lung disorder	22 (7%)	18 (6.7%)	0.8918	0 (0%)	0.2387
Hyperlipemia	21 (6.7%)	6 (2.2%)	0.0110	1 (3.3%)	0.7069
Depression	20 (6.4%)	19 (7.1%)	0.7277	1 (3.3%)	1.0000
Nausea	19 (6.1%)	16 (6%)	0.9687	2 (6.7%)	0.7041
Diabetes mellitus	19 (6.1%)	14 (5.2%)	0.6683	0 (0%)	0.3921

Adapted from data reported in Regillo CD, D'Amico DJ, Mieler WF, et al. Clinical safety profile of posterior juxtascleral depot administration of anecortave acetate 15 mg suspension as primary therapy or adjunctive therapy with photodynamic therapy for treatment of wet age-related macular degeneration. Surv Ophthalmol 2007;52(Suppl. 1):S70–S78.

PDT, photodynamic therapy.

Based on clinical trial data, frequent systemic adverse events in subjects receiving anecortave acetate as either primary therapy (Table 31.4) or adjunctive therapy (Table 31.5) included hypertension, peripheral edema, arthritis, and depression among others.[41] There was no statistically significant difference between subjects receiving the treatment drug and those receiving vehicle with respect to the incidence of any of these systemic adverse events. No treatment-related deaths were reported.

DRUG INTERACTIONS

To date, there have been no reported drug interactions with anecortave acetate.

SUMMARY AND KEY POINTS

Anecortave acetate represents a novel class of steroid compounds, the angiostatic cortisenes, which lack the anti-inflammatory properties and ocular complications associated with glucocorticoids but retain their antiangiogenic effects. Its receptor is not known, and its molecular mechanism of action is only partially understood; however, it appears to regulate the process of neovascularization at multiple levels. It inhibits the production of VEGF and the proliferation of endothelial cells in response to VEGF. It also inhibits the production of extracellular proteinases, which play in important role in the migration of endothelial cells during the angiogenic process.

Studies in preclinical models support the ability of anecortave acetate to inhibit neovascularization in a variety of settings. In clinical

Table 31.5 Most frequent systemic adverse events in subjects receiving anecortave acetate as adjunctive therapy

Adverse event	Anecortave acetate 15 mg + PDT (*n* = 45)	Vehicle + PDT (*n* = 46)	*P*
All systemic			
Peripheral edema	5 (11.1%)	4 (8.7%)	0.7394
Arthritis	4 (8.9%)	2 (4.3%)	0.4345
Depression	4 (8.9%)	2 (4.3%)	0.4345
Hypertension	3 (6.7%)	1 (2.2%)	0.3610
Alopecia	3 (6.7%)	0 (0%)	0.1168
Bradycardia	3 (6.7%)	0 (0%)	0.1168

Adapted from data reported in Regillo CD, D'Amico DJ, Mieler WF, et al. Clinical safety profile of posterior juxtascleral depot administration of anecortave acetate 15 mg suspension as primary therapy or adjunctive therapy with photodynamic therapy for treatment of wet age-related macular degeneration. Surv Ophthalmol 2007;52(Suppl. 1):S70–S78.

PDT, photodynamic therapy.

trials, it has been shown to reduce vision loss associated with exudative AMD. Although no direct comparison has been made in a clinical trial, anecortave acetate may not be as effective as monthly intravitreal VEGF inhibitors, such as ranibizumab, to treat exudative AMD as monotherapy. Nevertheless, its 6-month dosing interval and the relative safety of the PJD injection procedure make anecortave acetate an appealing potential adjuvant treatment which may augment and prolong the effect of other therapeutic modalities in combined regimens. As more pharmacologic inhibitors of neovascularization emerge in the coming years, the study of combination regimens in the treatment of AMD as well as other ocular diseases in which pathologic angiogenesis plays a role will become increasingly important. An even greater impact, however, will be made in the future by pharmacologic prevention of neovascularization by intervention during the preproliferative stages of disease. The AART trial was testing this theory by evaluating the use of anecortave acetate in patients with high-risk dry AMD to prevent progression to wet AMD, but the delivery may not have been optimal to obtain a positive result and the study was terminated early due to lack of efficacy. As the molecular pathogenesis of these diseases is further elucidated, more emphasis may be placed in the future on arresting the disease process before the onset of vision loss. Finally, other diseases, such as glaucoma, may also benefit from anecortave acetate. Only time will tell.

ACKNOWLEDGMENTS

Dr. Kaiser has received honoraria for serving on Alcon's Scientific Advisory Board that has been disclosed to the Conflict of Interest Committee of the Cleveland Clinic. The Cole Eye Institute, Dr. Kaiser's employer, has received research grant support on his behalf from Alcon.

REFERENCES

1. Ciulla TA, Walker JD, Fong DS, et al. Corticosteroids in posterior segment disease: an update on new delivery systems and new indications. Curr Opin Ophthalmol 2004;15:211–220.
2. Gillies MC, Kuzniarz M, Craig J, et al. Intravitreal triamcinolone-induced elevated intraocular pressure is associated with the development of posterior subcapsular cataract. Ophthalmology 2005;112:139–143.
3. Ciulla TA, Criswell MH, Danis RP, et al. Squalamine lactate reduces choroidal neovascularization in a laser-injury model in the rat. Retina 2003;23:808–814.
4. Fotsis T, Zhang Y, Pepper MS, et al. The endogenous oestrogen metabolite 2-methoxyoestradiol inhibits angiogenesis and suppresses tumour growth. Nature 1994;368:237–239.
5. Robinson MR, Baffi J, Yuan P, et al. Safety and pharmacokinetics of intravitreal 2-methoxyestradiol implants in normal rabbit and pharmacodynamics in a rat model of choroidal neovascularization. Exp Eye Res 2002;74:309–317.
6. Yamamoto T, Terada N, Nishizawa Y, et al. Angiostatic activities of medroxyprogesterone acetate and its analogues. Int J Cancer 1994;56:393–399.
7. Crum R, Szabo S, Folkman J. A new class of steroids inhibits angiogenesis in the presence of heparin or a heparin fragment. Science 1985;230:1375–1378.
8. Clark AF. Mechanism of action of the angiostatic cortisene anecortave acetate. Surv Ophthalmol 2007;52(Suppl. 1):S26–S34.
9. McNatt LG, Lane D, Clark AF. Angiostatic activity and metabolism of cortisol in the chorioallantoic membrane (CAM) of the chick embryo. J Steroid Biochem Mol Biol 1992;42:687–693.
10. McNatt LG, Weimer L, Yanni J, et al. Angiostatic activity of steroids in the chick embryo CAM and rabbit cornea models of neovascularization. J Ocul Pharmacol Ther 1999;15:413–423.
11. Clark AF. Preclinical efficacy of anecortave acetate. Surv Ophthalmol 2007;52(Suppl. 1):S41–S48.
12. BenEzra D, Griffin BW, Maftzir G, et al. Topical formulations of novel angiostatic steroids inhibit rabbit corneal neovascularization. Invest Ophthalmol Vis Sci 1997;38:1954–1962.
13. Dahlin DC, Rahimy MH. Pharmacokinetics and metabolism of anecortave acetate in animals and humans. Surv Ophthalmol 2007;52(Suppl. 1):S49–S61.
14. Kaiser PK, Goldberg MF, Davis AA. Posterior juxtascleral depot administration of anecortave acetate. Surv Ophthalmol 2007;52(Suppl. 1):S62–S69.
15. Slakter JS. Anecortave acetate for treating or preventing choroidal neovascularization. Ophthalmol Clin North Am 2006;19:373–380.
16. Taylor HR. Pterygium. The Hague, Monroe, NY: Kugler; 2000. p. vi, 181.
17. Penn JS, Rajaratnam VS, Collier RJ, et al. The effect of an angiostatic steroid on neovascularization in a rat model of retinopathy of prematurity. Invest Ophthalmol Vis Sci 2001;42:283–290.
18. Penn JS, Rajaratnam VS. Inhibition of retinal neovascularization by intravitreal injection of human rPAI-1 in a rat model of retinopathy of prematurity. Invest Ophthalmol Vis Sci 2003;44:5423–5429.
19. The natural ocular outcome of premature birth and retinopathy. Status at 1 year. Cryotherapy for Retinopathy of Prematurity Cooperative Group. Arch Ophthalmol 1994;112:903–912.
20. Palmer EA, Flynn JT, Hardy RJ, et al. Incidence and early course of retinopathy of prematurity. The Cryotherapy for Retinopathy of Prematurity Cooperative Group. Ophthalmology 1991;98:1628–1640.
21. Phelps DL, Rosenbaum AL. Vitamin E in kitten oxygen-induced retinopathy. II. Blockage of vitreal neovascularization. Arch Ophthalmol 1979;97:1522–1526.
22. Folkman J. Angiogenesis inhibitors: a new class of drugs. Cancer Biol Ther 2003;2:S127–S133.
23. Folkman J. A novel anti-vascular therapy for cancer. Cancer Biol Ther 2004;3:338–339.
24. Clark AF, Mellon J, Li XY, et al. Inhibition of intraocular tumor growth by topical application of the angiostatic steroid anecortave acetate. Invest Ophthalmol Vis Sci 1999;40:2158–2162.
25. Jockovich ME, Murray TG, Escalona-Benz E, et al. Anecortave acetate as single and adjuvant therapy in the treatment of retinal tumors of LH(BETA) T(AG) mice. Invest Ophthalmol Vis Sci 2006;47:1264–1268.
26. Bressler NM. Age-related macular degeneration is the leading cause of blindness. JAMA 2004;291:1900–1901.
27. Kimura H, Sakamoto T, Hinton DR, et al. A new model of subretinal neovascularization in the rabbit. Invest Ophthalmol Vis Sci 1995;36:2110–2119.

28. Kaiser PK. Antivascular endothelial growth factor agents and their development: therapeutic implications in ocular diseases. Am J Ophthalmol 2006;142:660–668.
29. D'Amico DJ, Goldberg MF, Hudson H, et al. Anecortave acetate as monotherapy for treatment of subfoveal neovascularization in age-related macular degeneration: twelve-month clinical outcomes. Ophthalmology 2003;110:2372–2383; discussion 2384–2385.
30. Russell SR, Hudson HL, Jerdan JA. Anecortave acetate for the treatment of exudative age-related macular degeneration – a review of clinical outcomes. Surv Ophthalmol 2007;52(Suppl. 1):S79–S90.
31. Slakter JS, Bochow TW, D'Amico DJ, et al. Anecortave acetate (15 milligrams) versus photodynamic therapy for treatment of subfoveal neovascularization in age-related macular degeneration. Ophthalmology 2006;113:3–13.
32. Klais CM, Eandi CM, Ober MD, et al. Anecortave acetate treatment for retinal angiomatous proliferation: a pilot study. Retina 2006;26:773–779.
33. Eandi CM, Ober MD, Freund KB, et al. Anecortave acetate for the treatment of idiopathic perifoveal telangiectasia: a pilot study. Retina 2006;26:780–785.
34. Bressler NM. Verteporfin therapy in age-related macular degeneration (VAM): an open-label multicenter photodynamic therapy study of 4,435 patients. Retina 2004;24:512–520.
35. Postelmans L, Pasteels B, Coquelet P, et al. Severe pigment epithelial alterations in the treatment area following photodynamic therapy for classic choroidal neovascularization in young females. Am J Ophthalmol 2004;138:803–808.
36. Schlotzer-Schrehardt U, Viestenz A, Naumann GO, et al. Dose-related structural effects of photodynamic therapy on choroidal and retinal structures of human eyes. Graefes Arch Clin Exp Ophthalmol 2002;240:748–757.
37. Wachtlin J, Behme T, Heimann H, et al. Concentric retinal pigment epithelium atrophy after a single photodynamic therapy. Graefes Arch Clin Exp Ophthalmol 2003;241:518–521.
38. Rosenfeld PJ, Rich RM, Lalwani GA. Ranibizumab: Phase III clinical trial results. Ophthalmol Clin North Am 2006;19:361–372.
39. Brown DM, Kaiser PK, Michels M, et al. Ranibizumab versus verteporfin for neovascular age-related macular degeneration. N Engl J Med 2006;355:1432–1444.
40. Heaton J, Kastner P, Hackett R. Preclinical safety of anecortave acetate. Surv Ophthalmol 2007;52(Suppl. 1):S35–S40.
41. Regillo CD, D'Amico DJ, Mieler WF, et al. Clinical safety profile of posterior juxtascleral depot administration of anecortave acetate 15 mg suspension as primary therapy or adjunctive therapy with photodynamic therapy for treatment of wet age-related macular degeneration. Surv Ophthalmol 2007;52(Suppl. 1):S70–S78.
42. D'Amico DJ, Goldberg MF, Hudson H, et al. Anecortave acetate as monotherapy for the treatment of subfoveal lesions in patients with exudative age-related macular degeneration (AMD): interim (month 6) analysis of clinical safety and efficacy. Retina 2003;23:14–23.

CHAPTER

32 Therapeutic monoclonal antibodies and fragments: bevacizumab

Ainat Klein, MD and Anat Loewenstein, MD

KEY FEATURES

Vascular endothelial growth factor-A (VEGF-A) has become a frequent target for the treatment of ocular diseases in which angiogenesis plays a role as a result of the growing body of evidence that it is an important regulator of angiogenesis, vascular development and differentiation, and vascular permeability. Several anti-VEGF therapies have become available for clinical use. This chapter will discuss the pharmacokinetics of bevacizumab, an anti-VEGF antibody.

INTRODUCTION AND HISTORY

The development of a vascular supply is essential for tissue repair and reproductive functions; thus, normal angiogenesis is vital for proper functioning of the human body. Angiogenesis is also implicated in the pathogenesis of a variety of systemic disorders, such as autoimmune diseases (e.g., rheumatoid arthritis, psoriasis), as well as in tumor growth and metastasis. It is also involved in the pathogenesis of ocular diseases, such as proliferative retinopathies, age-related macular degeneration (AMD), and others. Vascularization plays a unique role in the exchange of secretory products between the interstitial fluid surrounding the parenchymal cells and the plasma.[1,2]

A breakthrough in the understanding of normal and pathological angiogenesis occurred in 1948. Michaelson proposed that the existence of a diffusible angiogenic, "factor X," produced by the retina is responsible for retinal and iritic neovascularization that occurs in proliferative diabetic retinopathy (PDR) and other retinal disorders, such as central retinal vein occlusion (CRVO).[3]

It took another 20 years until another breakthrough was achieved from a different direction. In 1968, the first experiments to test the hypothesis directly that tumors produce angiogenic factors were performed. Greenblatt and Shubik[4] and Ehrmann and Knoth[5] demonstrated that transplantation of melanoma cells or choriocarcinoma cells promoted blood vessel proliferation even when a millipore filter was interposed between the tumor and the host, providing evidence that tumor angiogenesis was mediated by diffusible factors produced by the tumor cells. In 1971, Folkman et al.[6] proposed that antiangiogenesis may be an effective approach in treating human cancer. Folkman et al.[6] initiated the first efforts aimed at isolating a "tumor angiogenesis factor" from human and animal tumors. In 1985, the purification to homogeneity and sequencing of both acidic (aFGF) and basic fibroblast growth factors (bFGF) were reported, and in the subsequent year their cDNAs were cloned. It also became clear that these molecules are not efficiently secreted and are mostly cell-associated.[7]

Independent and unrelated lines of research converged toward the identification of VEGF. In 1983, Senger et al.[8] described the partial purification of a protein capable of inducing vascular leakage in the skin from the conditioned medium of a guinea pig tumor cell line and named the protein "tumor vascular permeability factor" (VPF). The authors proposed that VPF could be a mediator of the high permeability of tumor blood vessels. In a later publication, they reported the purification and NH_2-terminal amino acid sequencing of guinea pig VPF.[8] In 1989, Ferrara and Henzel reported the isolation of a diffusible endothelial cell-specific mitogen from medium conditioned by bovine pituitary follicular cells, which they named "vascular endothelial growth factor" to reflect the restricted target cell specificity of this molecule. NH_2-terminal amino acid sequencing of purified VEGF proved that this protein was distinct from the known endothelial cell mitogens, such as aFGF or bFGF, and that they did not match any known protein in available databases.[9] Connolly et al.[10] continued the work by Senger et al. and independently reported the isolation and sequencing of human VPF from U937 cells. cDNA cloning of VEGF and VPF, also reported in 1989, demonstrated that VEGF and VPF were the same molecule. The finding that VEGF is potent, diffusible, and specific for vascular endothelial cells led to the hypothesis that this molecule might play a role in the regulation of physiological and pathological growth of blood vessels.[11]

It emerged that this hypothesis was correct, with VEGF having been proven able to promote growth of vascular endothelial cells derived from arteries, veins, and lymphatics. VEGF is also a survival factor for endothelial cells and prevents endothelial apoptosis. It plays a role in the enhancement of vascular permeability and hemodynamic effects. Although endothelial cells are the primary targets of VEGF, several studies have reported mitogenic effects also on certain nonendothelial cell types, such as retinal pigment epithelial cells, pancreatic duct cells, Schwann cells, alveolar type II cells and other cells. VEGF has the ability to promote monocyte chemotaxis and was reported to have hematopoietic effects, inducing colony formation.[7]

From the ocular point of view, angiogenesis is a basic and critical part in the pathogenesis of many ocular neovascular syndromes and their complications. VEGF-A is believed to play a significant role in the formation of blood vessels that grow abnormally and leak. These blood vessels are fragile and can bleed, and potentially cause distortion of the retina, leading to deterioration of central vision.

Several strategies to inhibit the action of VEGF have been explored, including neutralizing anti-VEGF antibodies, receptor antagonists, soluble receptors, antagonistic VEGF mutants, inhibitors of VEGF receptor function, and upstream inhibitors of VEGF regulators such as protein kinase C. Bevacizumab (Avastin) is a recombinant humanized monoclonal immunoglobulin antibody that inhibits the activity of VEGF (see section on drug mechanism, below). It was designed as antitumor treatment in order to treat advanced carcinoma patients. Ranibizumab (Lucentis) is also a humanized antibody fragment against VEGF which was specifically designed for intraocular use as a smaller antibody fragment to penetrate through the retina better. The Food and Drug Administration (FDA) approved ranibizumab for treatment of subfoveal neovascular AMD in June, 2006. It was the first treatment for AMD shown to improve visual acuity (VA) in a substantial percentage of patients as opposed to slowing visual loss. A number of prospective, double-blind, placebo-controlled studies have proven its efficacy in treating minimally classic or occult choroidal neovascularization (CNV) secondary to AMD[12] as well as predominantly classic CNV.[13] Bevacizumab has a similar action and is related to the ranibizumab compound with respect to its structure. Bevacizumab was first approved by the FDA for the treatment of metastatic colorectal cancer in 2004, but it has not gained approval for intravitreal use. It has, however, recently been reported to treat patients successfully with a number of ocular diseases with off-label use.

PHARMACOLOGY

Bevacizumab is produced in a Chinese hamster ovary mammalian cell expression system in a nutrient medium containing the antibiotic gentamicin; it has a molecular weight of approximately 149 kDa. Bevacizumab is clear to slightly opalescent, colorless to pale brown, sterile, and has a pH of 6.2 in solution for intravenous infusion.[14] Bevacizumab is degraded by the reticuloendothelial system. When administered intravenously, usually at a dose of 1–20 mg/kg, it has an estimated clearance of 0.207 l/day and a central compartment volume of distribution of 2.39 l for a typical female, while being 26% faster in men. The estimated terminal half-life is approximately 20 days for both men and women. Body weight and gender are the most significant covariates for explaining interpatient variability. The clearance is also dependent upon tumor burden. The clearance is faster in patients with low serum albumin and high serum alkaline phosphatase.[15] In the pediatric population, the median clearance of bevacizumab was 4.1 ml/day/kg (range, 3.1–15.5 mL/day/kg), and the median half-life was 11.8 days (range, 4.4–14.6 days). Those values are consistent with the available adult data.[16]

The intravitreal pharmacokinetics of bevacizumab was mainly studied using experimental rabbit models. Vitreous concentrations of bevacizumab were found to decline in a monoexponential fashion with a half-life of 4.32 days. When 1.25 mg was injected, concentrations of over 10 μg/ml bevacizumab were maintained in the vitreous humor for 30 days. Bevacizumab concentrations in the aqueous humor of the injected eye reached a peak of 37.7 μg/ml 3 days after drug administration. A maximum serum concentration of 3.3 μg/ml was achieved 8 days after intravitreal injection, with the concentration falling below 1 μg/ml 29 days after injection. Very low concentrations of bevacizumab could be detected in the fellow uninjected eye.[17] One human study reported that the half-life of intravitreal bevacizumab was approximately 3 days, and also showed that a single dose of intravitreal bevacizumab was likely to provide complete intravitreal VEGF blockade for a minimum of 4 weeks.[18]

Dib et al.[19] recently evaluated subretinal detection of bevacizumab after an intravitreous injection in rabbit eyes. They detected bevacizumab molecules in the subretinal space of all six eyes studied 2 hours after an intravitreous bevacizumab injection of 0.05 ml (1.25 mg), possibly as the result of diffusion through the retina.

DRUG MECHANISM

The human VEGF-A gene is organized in eight exons separated by seven introns and is localized in chromosome 6p21.3. VEGF is a heparin-binding homodimeric glycoprotein of 45 kDa. VEGF binds two highly related receptor tyrosine kinases, VEGFR-1 and VEGFR-2. Both receptors have seven Ig-like domains in the extracellular domain, a single-transmembrane region, and a consensus tyrosine kinase sequence that is interrupted by a kinase-insert domain.[20]

Bevacizumab is a recombinant humanized monoclonal IgG_1 antibody that binds to and inhibits the biologic activity of human VEGF in *in vitro* and *in vivo* assay systems. Bevacizumab contains human framework regions and the complementary-determining regions of a murine antibody (anti-VEGF monoclonal antibody A.4.6.1) that binds to VEGF. It binds VEGF-A with a similar affinity as the native antibody. Bevacizumab has two antigen-binding domains (ranibizumab has only one) and blocks all active forms of VEGF-A (in contrast to, for example, pegaptanib which blocks only isoform $VEGF_{165}$).

Bevacizumab binds to VEGF with high affinity, minimizing the amount of circulating VEGF available to bind to the receptors and activate the angiogenesis process. Researchers using preclinical models have shown that anti-VEGF agents such as bevacizumab may work by causing a number of changes in blood vessels. Besides inhibiting vessel growth and neovascularization, they promote regression of existing microvessels and induce "normalization" of surviving mature vasculature, stabilize the vessel, and prevent leakage.[11]

DRUG EFFECTS IN HUMAN NONOCULAR DISEASES

In situ hybridization studies have demonstrated that the VEGF mRNA is expressed in the vast majority of human tumors thus far examined, including carcinoma of the lung, breast, gastrointestinal tract, kidney, bladder, ovary, endometrium, and several intracranial tumors, including glioblastoma multiforme and sporadic as well as von Hippel–Lindau syndrome-associated capillary hemangioblastoma.

VEGF blockade using an anti-VEGF monoclonal antibody decreased tumor perfusion, vascular volume, microvascular density, interstitial fluid pressure, and the number of viable, circulating endothelial and progenitor cells in colorectal cancer patients.[21] Several studies have shown that combining anti-VEGF treatment with chemotherapy or radiation therapy resulted in greater antitumor effects than either treatment alone.

The activity of bevacizumab in patients with metastatic colorectal cancer that progressed or after receiving both irinotecan-based and oxiliplatin-based chemotherapy regimens was evaluated in an open-access trial in combination with intravenous 5-fluorouracil-based chemotherapy. In all those studies the combination with bevacizumab yielded better response to treatment, longer overall survival, and longer disease-free survival. Bevacizumab showed significantly improved overall and progression-free survival when used in combination with standard first-line chemotherapy in patients with advanced nonsmall cell lung cancer (NSCLC). The FDA granted approval to the combination regimen of bevacizumab/carboplatin/paclitaxel, and it is considered the standard of care as the first-line treatment of advanced NSCLC.[22]

A large phase III trial in previously untreated patients with locally recurrent or metastatic breast cancer showed a significant and clinically relevant increase in progression-free survival in patients receiving intravenous bevacizumab plus paclitaxel compared to paclitaxel monothery.[23]

DRUG USE IN RETINAL DISEASES

Diabetes mellitus, CRVO, and retinopathy of prematurity (ROP) can all be associated with retinal ischemia and intraocular neovascularization, which may result in vitreous hemorrhages, retinal detachment, neovascular glaucoma (NVG), and blindness. As mentioned earlier, Michaelson[3] had postulated the existence of a diffusible angiogenic factor released by the ischemic retina in diseases such as diabetes mellitus and occlusion of the central retinal vein, and prematurity. Given its ability to induce hypoxia, VEGF became an attractive candidate as a mediator of pathological intraocular neovascularization. VEGF-A expression was increased in human pigment epithelial cells during the early stages of AMD, and high concentrations of VEGF-A have been observed in excised choroidal neovascular membranes and in the vitreous humor of patients with subretinal CNV.[24] A positive correlation between intraocular VEGF-A levels and the formation of ocular blood vessels was also observed in patients with diabetic retinopathy and ischemic CRVO.[25] This has led to the hypothesis that blockage of VEGF activity can act as a treatment for those and other ischemic ocular diseases.

AGE-RELATED MACULAR DEGENERATION

AMD is the most common disease that results in CNVs and the most exhaustively studied with anti-VEGF therapy. As noted above, ranibizumab was proven effective in a number of large, multicenter, prospective, and placebo-controlled studies. There are no similar studies on bevacizumab to date, but the clinical experience published in many small retrospective and a few prospective clinical studies confirms its beneficial use in treating the same indications.

Systemic bevacizumab therapy for neovascular AMD was well tolerated and effective in an open-label, single-center, uncontrolled clinical study on patients treated with an intravenous infusion of bevacizumab (5 mg/kg) followed by one or two additional doses given at

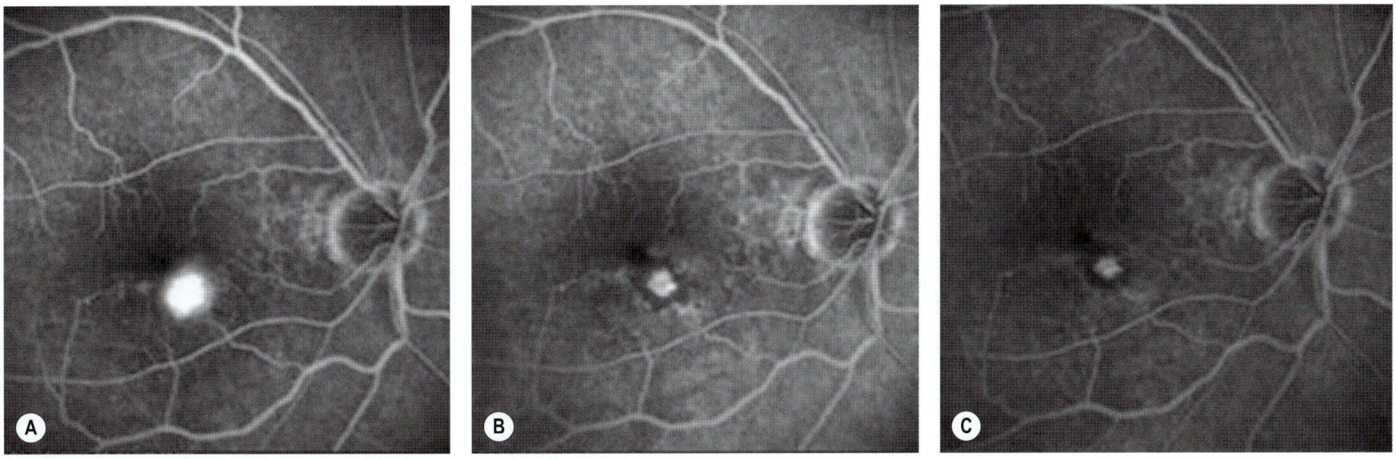

Figure 32.1 (A) Late fluorescein angiography photograph (8 minutes) of the right eye of a 60-year-old male with neovascular age-related macular degeneration; a choroidal neovascular lesion near inferotemporal arcade is illustrated. (B) Same lesion 1 month after intravitreal injection of bevacizumab. (C) Same lesion after second injection, 3 months apart. Size of lesion and leakage had decreased.

2-week intervals. No serious ocular or systemic adverse events were identified throughout 24 weeks of follow-up, with the exception of a mild elevation of mean systolic and diastolic blood pressure measurements. By 24 weeks, the mean VA letter score increased by 14 letters in the study eyes and the mean central retinal thickness (CCT) as measured by optical coherence tomography (OCT) decreased by 112 μm.[26]

Cleary et al.[27] conducted a large, retrospective study involving 112 eyes of patients with neovascular AMD, including choroidal neovascular membranes, pigment epithelial detachment, and macular hemorrhage. The median follow-up was 5 months. Intravitreal bevacizumab was found to be an effective treatment, resulting in improved vision and foveal anatomy at 6 months and even lasting up to 9 months of follow-up. The authors emphasized that 60% of patients who received only one injection maintained improved or stable vision at 6 months.

In another retrospective review of 118 eyes with neovascular AMD, VA improved by more than 15 ETDRS letters in 22.8% of eyes and stabilized in a further 65.2%. Only 11.9% lost 15 letters or more of vision. The mean VA improved from a Snellen equivalent of 6/30 to 6/24 at 1 month, and this improvement was maintained at 6 months. The mean macular thickness decreased by 87 μm, with a reduction in intraretinal and subretinal fluid and pigment epithelial detachment. Classic and predominantly classic CNV groups showed a greater improvement in vision, whereas the occult CNV group showed the least visual improvement after treatment.[28]

A prospective, open-label, nonrandomized clinical study of 60 eyes with subfoveal CNV that were treated with intravitreal bevacizumab with over 12 months of follow-up showed significant anatomical and functional improvement. The mean VA improved from 45.7 letters at baseline to 53.1 letters at 12 months, and 92.2% of eyes lost fewer than 15 letters. The mean CRT decreased from 327.4 μm at baseline to 227.8 μm.[29] Examples of the employment of bevacizumab in the management of neovascular AMD are illustrated in Figures 32.1 and 32.2.

One study compared visual outcomes and macular thickness changes associated with primary and secondary bevacizumab therapy for CNV. Eighteen eyes received primary bevacizumab treatment and 20 eyes received pegaptanib (Macugen) as initial treatment followed by bevacizumab therapy. The mean VA improvement and mean decrease in retinal thickness in the primary bevacizumab treatment cohort were better than the secondary bevacizumab treatment group. Primary bevacizumab therapy resulted in significantly greater visual improvement and a larger mean decrease in retinal thickness than secondary bevacizumab treatment at 3 and 6 months.[30] The change in retinal thickness is often best demonstrated on OCT, as illustrated in Figure 32.3.

DIABETIC RETINOPATHY

The chronic hyperglycemia of diabetes mellitus and wide areas of ischemic retina results in activation of VEGF and increases its synthesis. The upregulation in VEGF is associated with neovascularization in PDR as well as with diabetic macular edema (DME). Studies show that intravitreal bevacizumab resulted in marked regression of retinal neovascularization in patients with PDR and previous panretinal phototherapy, and rapid resolution of vitreous hemorrhage. It also achieved short-term reduction of fluorescein leakage from persistent active neovascularization and improved vision in patients with diabetic retinopathy.[31] Pretreatment of bevacizumab before vitrectomy is also effective in preventing bleeding during surgical dissection of fibrovascular membrane. The optimal time for preoperative injection is apparently 48–72 hours, and vitrectomy after 7 days can be associated with strong fibrosis and adhesion of fibrovascular membrane, resulting in some surgical complications.[32]

Primary intravitreal bevacizumab at doses of 1.25–2.5 mg seems to provide stability or improvement in patients with DME. An interventional retrospective multicenter study demonstrated that 41.1% eyes remained stable, 55.1% improved ≥2 ETDRS lines of best corrected VA (BCVA), and 3.8% decreased ≥2 ETDRS lines of BCVA. Mean central macular thickness (CMT) at baseline as measured by OCT was 387.0 ± 182.8 μm and it decreased to a mean of 275.7 ± 108.3 after 6 months of follow-up.[33]

A randomized phase II clinical trial comparing photocoagulation and intravitreal injection of 1.25–2.5 mg in the treatment of DME demonstrated that bevacizumab can reduce DME in some eyes. It was found to achieve a greater reduction in central subfield thickness (CST) at 3 weeks and about 1 line better median VA over 12 weeks. There were no meaningful differences between the two doses.[34]

RETINAL VEIN OCCLUSION (RVO)

Currently, increasing data support the role of intravitreal bevacizumab as an effective treatment for patients with macular edema secondary to RVO. Multiple injections seem to be necessary in order to achieve visual stabilization and macular changes. The effect of a single injection seems to last 6–8 weeks. The most common treatment protocol is two to three injections over the first 5–6 months. Patients who had minimal or no response to laser therapy appeared to benefit from bevacizumab.[35] A prospective study in patients with branch RVO (BRVO) found that intravitreal injections of bevacizumab 1.25 or 2.5 mg improved BCVA by 5.1 and 4.8 lines, respectively, after 6 months of repeated injections. There was also a decrease in CMT.[36] A combined (BRVO and CRVO) prospective study followed 29 eyes. Three intravitreal injections of 1 mg bevacizumab (0.04 ml) were administered at 4-week intervals; further

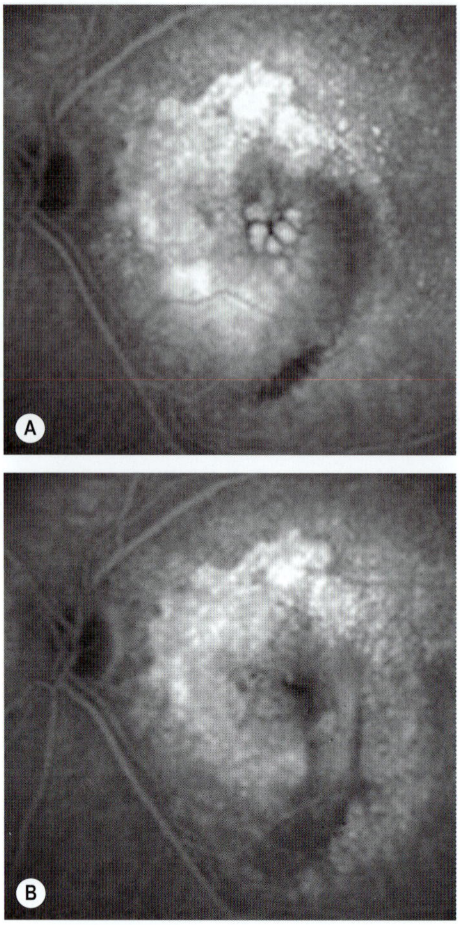

Figure 32.2 (A) Late fluorescein angiography photograph (13 minutes) of an 85-year-old female with age-related macular degeneration. A large juxtrafoveal choroidal neovascularization lesion is illustrated with petaloid macular edema. (B) Same lesion 2 months after two bevacizumab injections. The leakage has decreased dramatically.

retreatment was based on OCT findings. CRT significantly decreased 1 day after the first injection, and three injections reduced macular edema to 328 μm CRT from an average baseline of 558 μm (range 353–928 μm) and improved BCVA to 20/50 (from a baseline of 20/100). Fluorescein angiography (FA) showed no evidence of increased avascular zones.[37]

Another prospective study on patients with CRVO revealed a mean ETDRS letter gain 13.92 letters ± SD of 14.4 from baseline to 6 months. The mean CRT decreased from 535 ± SD of 148 μm at baseline to 323 ± 116 μm at 6-month follow-up. Ischemic CRVO was associated with significantly lower VA than nonischemic CRVO, although the VA gain was similar in both groups.[38]

UVEITIC CYSTOID MACULAR EDEMA (CME)

Intravitreal bevacizumab seems to be an effective treatment in the management of refractory inflammatory CME. One study demonstrated a reduction in CRT with a mean foveal thickness reduction of 127.2 μm at 4 weeks: 4 out of 10 patients had concurrent improvement in VA, which was unchanged in the other 6. The authors noted that the effect is transient and that reinjections may be necessary.[39]

CHOROIDAL NEOVASCULARIZATION SECONDARY TO MYOPIA

Intravitreal injection of bevacizumab seems to be an effective treatment for myopic CNV. One nonrandomized, interventional case series reported that the BCVA improved by 2 lines or more in 75% of

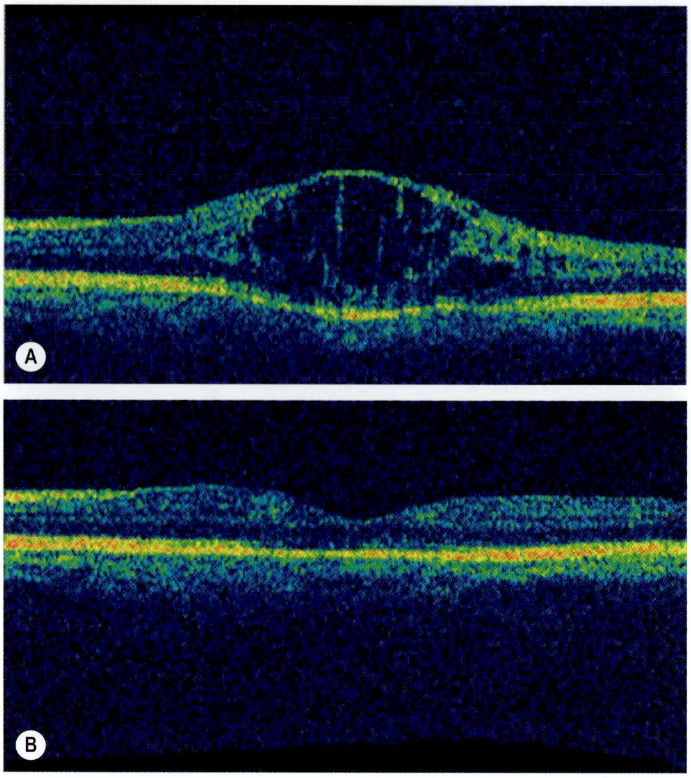

Figure 32.3 (A) Optical coherence tomography of a 72-year-old male with advanced (neovascular) age-related macular degeneration in the left eye with severe cystic macular edema. (B) Same section after two bevacizumab intravitreal injections. Complete resolution of the edema is illustrated. There was also improvement in visual acuity of 6 ETDRS letters.

eyes and remained the same in 25%. Leakage from the myopic CNV on FA decreased in 87.5% of eyes while the CNV area on FA and the foveal thickness on OCT images decreased significantly after the treatment.[40]

RETINOPATHY OF PREMATURITY (ROP)

Retinopathy of prematurity is a disease characterized by incomplete vascularization of the peripheral retina leading to retinal neovascularization. Standard therapy has consisted of ablation of the peripheral retina once threshold disease is reached.

There are no controlled studies on treatment of ROP with bevacizumab and data are limited to a number of case reports in which intravitreal bevacizumab (0.4–0.75 mg) was used in combination with indirect laser photocoagulation treatment in severe cases of ROP with zone 1 involvement with or without plus disease. Treatment resulted in ROP regression, prompt resolution of plus signs, and neovascular proliferation with regression of the vascular component of the fibrovascular membrane and acute fibrosis. There is currently an open-label phase I/II trial for babies with stage III–V ROP who are otherwise untreatable with laser or cryotherapy. Notably, due to bevacizumab's potential side-effects in this young age, this treatment should first be evaluated in well-controlled studies and after careful consideration.[41–43]

RETINAL TELANGIECTASIAS

Short-term results indicate that inhibition of VEGF by intravitreal bevacizumab is associated with a decrease in retinal thickness and a reduction in angiographic leakage in type 2 idiopathic macular telangiectasia (IMT). Furthermore, it may improve VA in affected patients.[44] It was also reported as a treatment of foveal detachment in idiopathic perifoveal telangiectasia (IPT). The OCT images showed marked reversal of the foveal detachment after the injection, with restoration of foveal depression in all eyes. The vision of all treated eyes improved and remained unchanged up until the last follow-up visit.[45]

NEOVASCULAR GLAUCOMA (NVG)

NVG is a condition that results from iris rubeosis in response to ischemia of the posterior retina. It can be the expression of advanced diabetic retinopathy, RVO, ocular ischemic syndrome, and other ischemic disease of the retina.

Intravitreal bevacizumab effectively stabilized iris neovascularization activity (with regression following one injection) and controlled intraocular pressure (IOP) in patients with iris neovascularization alone and early-stage NVG without angle closure (71% had normalization of IOP 21 mmHg). Intravitreal bevacizumab cannot control IOP in advanced NVG, but may be used adjunctively to improve subsequent surgical results.[46] Bevacizumab was also reported to give similar results by intracameral injection. In this study patients with iritic neovascularization secondary to proliferative retinal vasculopathies received 1.25 mg bevacizumab intracamerally. All 15 patients with neovascularization demonstrated reduction in leakage of the neovascularization within 3 weeks of the injection, as observed on slit-lamp photography and FA. IOP was controlled with maximum medical therapy in 8 of 9 eyes, thereby reducing the need for glaucoma surgery. VA improved from a median of hand motions to 20/200.[47]

OTHERS

Intravitreal bevacizumab was found to improve or maintain vision and reduce hemorrhage and retinal edema in cases of radiation retinopathy related to plaque radiation therapy.[48,49]

Intravitreal injection of bevacizumab, although safe, is still controversial in its efficacy in patients with postoperative CME.[50,51]

The use of bevacizumab (by intravitreal injection and by local application to the conjunctiva or cornea) is also being investigated for a number of other ocular diseases. There are several small studies and case reports on the use of bevacizumab as an adjuvant treatment during pterygium and glaucoma surgery and in severe cases of corneal neovascularization, especially before corneal transplantation. The efficacy of this regimen is still controversial.

EFFICACY AND COMPARISON WITH OTHER AGENTS

In a prospective, randomized, controlled clinical study that compared intravitreal bevacizumab therapy versus photodynamic therapy (PDT) plus intravitreal triamcinolone for neovascular AMD, treatment with bevacizumab was found to be more beneficial. Patients treated with bevacizumab improved by 2.2 ETDRS lines at 6 months of follow-up. Eyes treated in the PDT plus intravitreal triamcinolone arm had a stable mean VA at month 6 compared with baseline. It should be noted that the reduction in CRT was not significantly different between both groups (as demonstrated on OCT).[52]

A prospective randomized study compared verteporfin PDT with intravitreal bevacizumab for the management of predominantly classic CNV associated with AMD in 62 eyes. At the 6-month follow-up, the mean BCVA and greatest linear dimension were significantly better in the bevacizumab group compared to the standard PDT group.[53] Currently, the phase III study, Comparison of AMD Treatment Trial (CATT), supported by the National Eye Institute of the National Institutes of Health (USA), is being conducted to compare the efficacy of bevacizumab with ranibizumab in the management of neovascular AMD.

Intravitreal bevacizumab injection was found more beneficial than focal photocoagulation in cases of DME. There was a CST reduction of >11% at 3 weeks in 43% of bevacizumab-treated eyes and in 28% of eyes treated with laser alone, and in 50% and 37% of eyes, respectively, at 6 weeks. Combining focal photocoagulation with bevacizumab resulted in no apparent short-term benefit or adverse outcomes.[33] In a second study, intravitreal bevacizumab treatment of patients with DME yielded better visual outcome than laser photocoagulation. No further beneficial effect of intravitreal triamcinolone could be demonstrated. Finally, intravitreal bevacizumab remarkably augmented the short-term response to scatter panretinal laser photocoagulation.[54]

As mentioned above, the use of bevacizumab is adjuvant to the laser photocoagulation in cases of RVO. Patients who had minimal or no response to laser therapy appeared to benefit more from bevacizumab.[35]

In severe cases of NVG, the use of bevacizumab as adjuvant to antiglaucomatotic agents or as previtrectomy treatment (in cases of vitreous hemorrhage) was found beneficial and achieved better results.[46]

The use of bevacizumab for the rest of the above-mentioned indications is currently reserved as a last resort in severe cases where other approved, standard therapy failed to yield results.

CONTRAINDICATIONS

There are no absolute contraindications to local treatment with bevacizumab given as intravitreal injection. Due to its related side-effects, however, there are some relative contraindications. For instance, it is wise to withhold treatment in patients who had suffered a cardiovascular event or cerebrovascular event during the previous year.[55]

Bevacizumab has been shown to be teratogenic in rabbits when administered in doses that approximate the human dose on an mg/kg basis. For that reason, it is not recommended during pregnancy. It is not known whether bevacizumab is secreted in human milk. Because human IgG_1 is secreted into human milk, the potential for absorption and harm to the infant after ingestion is unknown. Women should be advised to discontinue nursing during treatment with bevacizumab. Because physeal dysplasia was observed in juvenile cynomolgus monkeys with open growth plates (although this effect was found to be partially reversible upon cessation of treatment) it is less favored in treating children.

Systemic use of bevacizumab is also contraindicated around major surgery (because of impairing wound healing), or if severe systemic side-effects appear (e.g., significant increase in blood pressure).[14]

OCULAR COMPLICATIONS AND TOXICITY

Reports in the literature indicate that repeated intravitreal injections of either 1.25 or 2.5 mg bevacizumab are reasonably safe and well tolerated. Ocular complications include transient corneal abrasion (0.2%), chemosis (0.2%), subconjunctival hemorrhage (0.03%), lens injury (0.1%), bacterial endophthalmitis (0.01–0.16%), tractional retinal detachments (0.04–0.16%), uveitis (0.09%), rhegmatogenous retinal detachment (0.02%), and vitreous hemorrhage (0.02%). Notably, these adverse events are related to the injection procedure and are in the expected range for any intravitreal injections.[56,57]

Ocular adverse events possibly related to bevacizumab include episodes of inflammation (0.14%), cataract progression (0.01%), acute vision loss (0.07%), central retinal artery occlusion (0.01%), new or progressive subretinal hemorrhages (0.06%), and tears of the retinal pigment epithelium (0.06%). Inflammation usually occurs 2–7 days after the injection, and lasts no longer than 1 week. Cataract progression usually occurs in a patient with a pre-existing mature cataract.[55] It should be borne in mind that bevacizumab injections cause a predictable, probably volume-related, rise in IOP of about 20 mmHg during the first 3 minutes after injection (from a baseline mean IOP of 15.17 mmHg to a mean of 36.27 mmHg). This is followed by a spontaneous decrease to a mean of 24.56 mmHg at 10 minutes after the injection. Occlusion of the central retinal artery has not been reported.[58]

SYSTEMIC COMPLICATION AND TOXICITY

Most of the systemic adverse events probably relate to the antiangiogenic effect of bevacizumab. Those effects are rare and occur at different rates among different studies (written in brackets). Systemic adverse events that could possibly be related to bevacizumab include facial skin redness (0.1%), itchy diffuse rash (0.1%), mild blood pressure increase (0.2–0.5%), iliac artery aneurysm (0.17%), toe amputation (0.17%), myocardial infarctions (0.4%), transient ischemic attack (0.01%), cerebrovascular accident (0.07–0.5%), deep venous thrombosis (0.01%), and death (0.03%). Notably, the patients who suffered severe adverse affects were at high risk of cardiovascular and cerebrovascular disease prior to the intravitreal administration of bevacizumab. In addition, the incidence of those events was not increased from that of the general population at large.[56–58]

Systemic administration of bevacizumab is known to have a higher incidence of the above-mentioned side-effects. A rare but severe side-effect is gastrointestinal perforation complicated by intra-abdominal abscesses or fistula formation. This complication has an increased incidence in patients receiving bevacizumab compared to controls. It also increases the rate of hemorrhages, especially hemoptysis in patients with nonsmall cell lung cancer. It can also worsen proteinuria and increase the rate of heart failure related to treatment with chemotherapy. Reversible posterior leukoencephalopathy syndrome (RPLS) has been reported in clinical studies (with an incidence of <0.1%) and in postmarketing experience. RPLS is a neurological disorder which can present with headache, seizure, lethargy, confusion, blindness, and other visual and neurological disturbances. No carcinogenicity data are available for bevacizumab in animals or humans.[14]

DRUG INTERACTIONS

A study performed on monkeys indicates that the combination of bevacizumab with the chemotherapeutic agents paclitaxel and cisplatin does not result in a pharmacokinetic interaction.[59] Concentrations of SN38, the active metabolite of irinotecan, were on average 33% higher in patients receiving a bolus combination treatment of intravenous irinotecan, 5-fluorouracil, and leucovorin (IFL, a common treatment for colorectal carcinoma) in combination with bevacizumab when compared with bolus IFL alone. There are still no data on other drug interactions when administered systemically.[14]

As mentioned above, there is an additive efficacy during intravitreal administration, although there is no information available about changes in drug levels.

SUMMARY AND KEY POINTS

The pathogenesis of many retinal disorders is based on neovascularization and increased permeability of blood vessels. VEGF is a basic factor mediating those processes. Bevacizumab, a humanized monoclonal antibody that blocks VEGF activity, has been proved *in vitro* to inhibit vessel growth and neovascularization, promote regression of existing microvessels, and decrease leakage. This enables it to be a considerable treatment for retinal neovascular disease. It has had wide off-label use in ophthalmology during the last decade. Its efficacy was proven in small retrospective and prospective studies in the treatment of cases of AMD, DME, and NVG, and there are many case reports demonstrating its beneficial use in other neovascular retinal disease, as detailed above. Large, prospective, double-blind, placebo-controlled trails are warranted in order to determine the exact role of bevacizumab in the long-term treatment of ocular diseases in which angiogenesis plays a role.

REFERENCES

1. Folkman J. Angiogenesis in cancer, vascular, rheumatoid and other disease. Nat Med 1995;1:27–31.
2. Garner A. Vascular diseases. In: Garner A, Klintworth GK, editors. Pathobiology of ocular disease. New York: Marcel Dekker; 1994. p. 1625–1710.
3. Michaelson IC. The mode of development of the vascular system of the retina with some observations on its significance for certain retinal disorders. Trans Ophthalmol Soc UK 1948;68:137–180.
4. Greenblatt M, Shubik P. Tumor angiogenesis: transfilter diffusion studies in the hamster by the transparent chamber technique. J Natl Cancer Inst 1968;41:111–124.
5. Ehrmann RL, Knoth M. Choriocarcinoma. Transfilter stimulation of vasoproliferation in the hamster cheek pouch. Studied by light and electron microscopy. J Natl Cancer Inst 1968;41:1329–1341.
6. Folkman J, Merler E, Abernathy C, et al. Isolation of a tumor factor responsible for angiogenesis. J Exp Med 1971;133:275–288.
7. Ferrara N. Vascular endothelial growth factor: basic science and clinical progress. Endocr Rev 2004 Aug;25(4):581–611.
8. Senger DR, Galli SJ, Dvorak AM, et al. Tumor cells secrete a vascular permeability factor that promotes accumulation of ascites fluid. Science 1983;219:983–985.
9. Ferrara N, Henzel WJ. Pituitary follicular cells secrete a novel heparin-binding growth factor specific for vascular endothelial cells. Biochem Biophys Res Commun 1989;161:851–858.
10. Connolly DT, Olander JV, Heuvelman D, et al. Human vascular permeability factor. Isolation from U937 cells. J Biol Chem 1989;264: 20017–20024.
11. Ferrara N, Houck KA, Jakeman LB, et al. The vascular endothelial growth factor family of polypeptides. J Cell Biochem 1991;47:211–218.
12. Brown DM, Kaiser PK, Michels M, et al. Ranibizumab versus verteporfin for neovascular age-related macular degeneration. N Engl J Med 2006 Oct 5;355(14):1432–1444.
13. Brown DM, Kaiser PK, Michels M, et al. Ranibizumab versus verteporfin for neovascular age-related macular degeneration. N Engl J Med 2006 Oct 5;355(14):1432–1444.
14. http://www.gene.com/gene/products/information/pdf/avastin-prescribing.pdf.
15. Lu JF, Bruno R, Eppler S, et al. Clinical pharmacokinetics of bevacizumab in patients with solid tumors. Cancer Chemother Pharmacol 2008 Jan 19.
16. Bender JL, Adamson PC, Reid JM, et al. Phase I trial and pharmacokinetic study of bevacizumab in pediatric patients with refractory solid tumors: a Children's Oncology Group Study. J Clin Oncol 2008 Jan 20;26(3):399–405.
17. Bakri SJ, Snyder MR, Reid JM, et al. Pharmacokinetics of intravitreal bevacizumab (Avastin). Ophthalmology 2007 May;114(5):855–859.
18. Beer PM, Wong SJ, Hammad AM, et al. Vitreous levels of unbound bevacizumab and unbound vascular endothelial growth factor in two patients. Retina 2006 Oct;26(8):871–876.
19. Dib E, Maia M, Longo-Maugeri IM, et al. Subretinal bevacizumab detection after intravitreous injection in rabbits. Invest Ophthalmol Vis Sci 2008 Mar;49(3):1097–1100.
20. Youssoufian H, Hicklin DJ, Rowinsky EK. Review: monoclonal antibodies to the vascular endothelial growth factor receptor-2 in cancer therapy. Clin Cancer Res 2007 Sep 15;13(18 Pt 2):5544s-5548s.
21. Willett CG, Boucher Y, Di Tomaso E, et al. Direct evidence that the VEGF-specific antibody bevacizumab has antivascular effects in human rectal cancer. Nat Med 2004;10:145–147.
22. Gutierrez M, Giaccone G. Antiangiogenic therapy in nonsmall cell lung cancer. Curr Opin Oncol 2008 Mar;20(2):176–182.
23. Scott LJ. Bevacizumab: in first-line treatment of metastatic breast cancer, Drugs 2007;67(12):1793–1799.
24. Wells JA, Murthy R, Chibber R, et al: Levels of vascular endothelial growth factor are elevated in the vitreous of patients with subretinal neovascularisation. Br J Ophthalmol 1996;80:363–366.
25. Aiello LP, Avery RL, Arrigg PG, et al. Vascular endothelial growth factor in ocular fluid of patients with diabetic retinopathy and other retinal disorders. N Engl J Med 1994;331:1480–1487.
26. Moshfeghi AA, Rosenfeld PJ, Puliafito CA, et al. Systemic bevacizumab (Avastin) therapy for neovascular age-related macular degeneration: twenty-four-week results of an uncontrolled open-label clinical study. Ophthalmology 2006 Nov;113(11):2002.e1–2002.e12. Epub 2006 Oct 5.
27. Cleary CA, Jungkim S, Ravikumar K, et al. Intravitreal bevacizumab in the treatment of neovascular age-related macular degeneration, 6- and 9-month results. Eye 2008 Jan;22(1):82–86.
28. Madhusudhana KC, Hannan SR, Williams CP, et al. Intravitreal bevacizumab (Avastin) for the treatment of choroidal neovascularization in age-related macular degeneration: results from 118 cases. Br J Ophthalmol 2007 Dec;91(12):1716–1717.
29. Bashshur ZF, Haddad ZA, Schakal A, et al. Intravitreal bevacizumab for treatment of neovascular age-related macular degeneration: a one-year prospective study. Am J Ophthalmol 2008 Feb;145(2):249–256. Epub 2007 Dec 11.
30. Falkenstein IA, Cheng L, Morrison VL, et al. Standardized visual acuity results associated with primary versus secondary bevacizumab (Avastin) treatment for choroidal neovascularization in age-related macular degenerationm. Retina 2007 Jul–Aug;27(6):701.

31. Jorge R, Costa RA, Calucci D, et al. Intravitreal bevacizumab (Avastin) for persistent new vessels in diabetic retinopathy (IBEPE study). Retina 2006 Nov–Dec;26(9):1006–1013.
32. Ishikawa K, Honda S, Tsukahara Y, et al. Preferable use of intravitreal bevacizumab as a pretreatment of vitrectomy for severe proliferative diabetic retinopathy. Eye 2009;23:108–111.
33. Arevalo JF, Fromow-Guerra J, Quiroz-Mercado H, et al. Primary intravitreal bevacizumab (Avastin) for diabetic macular edema: results from the Pan-American Collaborative Retina Study Group at 6-month follow-up. Ophthalmology 2007 Apr;114(4):743–750.
34. Scott IU, Edwards AR, Beck RW, et al. A phase II randomized clinical trial of intravitreal bevacizumab for diabetic macular edema, Ophthalmology 2007 Oct;114(10):1860–1867.
35. Badalà F. The treatment of branch retinal vein occlusion with bevacizumab. Curr Opin Ophthalmol 2008 May;19(3):234–238.
36. Wu L, Arevalo JF, Roca JA, et al. Comparison of two doses of intravitreal bevacizumab (Avastin) for treatment of macular edema secondary to branch retinal vein occlusion: results from the Pan-American Collaborative Retina Study Group at 6 months of follow-up. Retina 2008 Feb;28(2): 212–219.
37. Kriechbaum K, Michels S, Prager F, et al. Intravitreal Avastin for macular oedema secondary to retinal vein occlusion: a prospective study. Br J Ophthalmol 2008 Apr;92(4):518–522.
38. Priglinger SG, Wolf AH, Kreutzer TC, et al. Intravitreal bevacizumab injections for treatment of central retinal vein occlusion: six-month results of a prospective trial. Retina 2007 Oct;27(8):1004–1012.
39. Mackensen F, Heinz C, Becker MD, et al. Intravitreal bevacizumab (Avastin) as a treatment for refractory macular edema in patients with uveitis: a pilot study. Retina 2008 Jan;28(1):41–45.
40. Sakaguchi H, Ikuno Y, Gomi F, et al. Intravitreal injection of bevacizumab for choroidal neovascularisation associated with pathological myopia. Br J Ophthalmol 2007 Feb;91(2):161–165.
41. Travassos A, Teixeira S, Ferreira P, et al. Intravitreal bevacizumab in aggressive posterior retinopathy of prematurity. Ophthalmic Surg Lasers Imaging 2007 May–Jun;38(3):233–237.
42. Chung EJ, Kim JH, Ahn HS, et al. Combination of laser photocoagulation and intravitreal bevacizumab (Avastin) for aggressive zone I retinopathy of prematurity. Graefes Arch Clin Exp Ophthalmol 2007 Nov;245(11):1727–1730.
43. Dell'omo R, Kulkarni A, Franks WA. Intravitreal and intracameral bevacizumab to treat neovascular complications of retinopathy of prematurity. Acta Ophthalmol 2008;86:698–700.
44. Charbel Issa P, Holz FG, Scholl HP. Findings in fluorescein angiography and optical coherence tomography after intravitreal bevacizumab in type 2 idiopathic macular telangiectasia. Ophthalmology 2007 Sep;114(9): 1736–1742.
45. Maia Júnior OO, Bonanomi MT, Takahashi WY, et al. Intravitreal bevacizumab for foveal detachment in idiopathic perifoveal telangiectasia. Am J Ophthalmol 2007 Aug;144(2):296–299.
46. Wakabayashi T, Oshima Y, Sakaguchi H, et al. Intravitreal bevacizumab to treat iris neovascularization and neovascular glaucoma secondary to ischemic retinal diseases in 41 consecutive cases. Ophthalmology 2008;115:1571–1580.
47. Chalam KV, Gupta SK, Grover S, et al. Intracameral Avastin dramatically resolves iris neovascularization and reverses neovascular glaucoma. Eur J Ophthalmol 2008 Mar–Apr;18(2):255–262.
48. Mason 3rd JO, Vail RS, Albert Jr MA, et al. Intravitreal bevacizumab treatment for radiation macular edema after plaque radiotherapy for choroidal melanoma. Retina 2007 Sep;27(7):903–907.
49. Finger PT, Chin K, Anti-vascular endothelial growth factor bevacizumab (avastin) for radiation retinopathy. Arch Ophthalmol 2007 Jun;125(6):751–756.
50. Arevalo JF, Garcia-Amaris RA, Roca JA, et al. Primary intravitreal bevacizumab for the management of pseudophakic cystoid macular edema: pilot study of the Pan-American Collaborative Retina Study Group. J Cataract Refract Surg 2007 Dec;33(12):2098–2105.
51. Spitzer MS, Ziemssen F, Yoeruek E, et al. Efficacy of intravitreal bevacizumab in treating postoperative pseudophakic cystoid macular edema. J Cataract Refract Surg 2008 Jan;34(1):70–75.
52. Weigert G, Michels S, Sacu S, et al. Intravitreal bevacizumab (Avastin) therapy versus photodynamic therapy plus intravitreal triamcinolone for neovascular age-related macular degeneration: 6-month results of a prospective, randomized, controlled clinical study. Br J Ophthalmol 2008 Mar;92(3):356–360.
53. Bashshur ZF, Schakal A, Hamam RN, et al. Intravitreal bevacizumab vs verteporfin photodynamic therapy for neovascular age-related macular degeneration. Arch Ophthalmol 2007 Oct;125(10):1357–1361.
54. Soheilian M, Ramezani A, Bijanzadeh B, et al. Intravitreal bevacizumab (avastin) injection alone or combined with triamcinolone versus macular photocoagulation as primary treatment of diabetic macular edema. Retina 2007 Nov–Dec;27(9):1187–1195.
55. Fung AE, Rosenfeld PJ, Reichel E. The International Intravitreal Bevacizumab Safety Survey: using the internet to assess drug safety worldwide. Br J Ophthalmol 2006 Nov;90(11):1344–1349.
56. Wu L, Martínez-Castellanos MA, Quiroz-Mercado H, et al. Twelve-month safety of intravitreal injections of bevacizumab (Avastin(R)): results of the Pan-American Collaborative Retina Study Group (PACORES). Graefes Arch Clin Exp Ophthalmol 2008 Jan;246(1):81–87.
57. Shima C, Sakaguchi H, Gomi F, et al. Complications in patients after intravitreal injection of bevacizumab. Acta Ophthalmol Scand 2008;886:372–376.
58. Falkenstein IA, Cheng L, Freeman WR Changes of intraocular pressure after intravitreal injection of bevacizumab (Avastin). Retina 2007 Oct;27(8):1044–1047.
59. Xu L, Zuch CL, Lin YS, et al. Pharmacokinetics and safety of bevacizumab administered in combination with cisplatin and paclitaxel in cynomolgus monkeys. Cancer Chemother Pharmacol 2008 Apr;61(4):607–614.

CHAPTER 33

Therapeutic monoclonal antibodies and fragments: ranibizumab

Ursula Schmidt-Erfurth, MD

KEY FEATURES

Ranibizumab (Lucentis, Genentech, South San Francisco, CA; Novartis Pharma, Basel, Switzerland) is a recombinant, humanized, monoclonal antibody Fab fragment against vascular endothelial growth factor A (VEGF-A), which was developed specifically for intraocular use. Ranibizumab has been extensively investigated in clinical trials in neovascular age-related macular degeneration (AMD), and is also being studied in other retinal diseases.

Ranibizumab was the first therapeutic agent to demonstrate improvements in visual acuity (VA) and patient-reported visual function for patients with neovascular AMD, and has been licensed for this indication. Ranibizumab has demonstrated a good tolerability profile in clinical trials, with a low incidence of ocular and systemic serious adverse events (AEs).

INTRODUCTION AND HISTORY

The VEGF family of growth factors, of which VEGF-A is the prototype member, plays an important role in a variety of *in vitro* processes, including angiogenesis, microvascular permeability, and endothelial cell survival. Whilst these activities are all essential to survival, VEGF has been linked to a number of pathogenic conditions, including neovascular AMD, diabetic retinopathy, and cancer.[1,2]

The first monoclonal antibody developed to target VEGF-A was bevacizumab, a humanized murine monoclonal antibody.[3] Bevacizumab was initially investigated as a cancer treatment, and received approval as a first-line therapy for widespread colorectal cancer from the US Food and Drugs Administration in 2004. Bevacizumab has subsequently been approved for use in nonsmall-cell lung cancer and breast cancer.

The successful development of VEGF as an oncology target led to interest in the potential of anti-VEGF treatment for other therapeutic indications, including ocular neovascular disorders.

VEGF-A has been identified as the primary angiogenesis mediator in the eye. It is implicated in ocular neovascularization through its promotion of blood vessel formation and permeability.[2,4] A role for VEGF-A in neovascular AMD is suggested by immunohistochemistry localization in human choroidal neovascular (CNV) lesions and extrapolation from other disease models.[5] New blood vessel formation and leakage are important facets of the neovascular form of AMD, and clinical trials of agents that block VEGF-A activity have produced more evidence that VEGF-A is important in the development of this disease.[6,7]

PHARMACOLOGY

PHARMACOLOGICAL DESIGN

Systemic administration of an anti-VEGF agent was initially considered for the treatment of CNV lesions; however, the possibility of AEs, and toxicity data from clinical trials of bevacizumab in cancer patients, indicated that a more targeted therapy was warranted. Consequently, ranibizumab was designed specifically for ocular use.

Ranibizumab was generated from a Fab fragment of humanized murine anti-VEGF monoclonal antibody. The use of a Fab fragment, rather than full-length IgG, was indicated by their enhanced retinal penetration and diffusibility. In addition, the absence of the Fc portion of IgG eliminates the possibility of complement-mediated or cell-dependent cytotoxicity, and the decreased half-life of Fab in comparison with IgG minimizes the extent of systemic exposure.[5]

Ranibizumab was selected through a combination of phage display technology and engineering of the Fab framework based on previous studies. The resulting construct neutralized the biologic activities of all VEGF-A isoforms and the proteolytic cleavage product $VEGF_{110}$, and displayed 5–10-fold greater potency than bevacizumab in bioassays measuring human VEGF-induced mitogenesis.[5] Furthermore, as ranibizumab is a humanized antibody fragment and is produced in a bacterial vector, such that it does not undergo mammalian glycosylation, the potential for immunogenicity is minimized.

PHARMACOKINETICS

Intraocular pharmacokinetic data derived from studies in monkeys demonstrated that intravitreal doses of ranibizumab (500 or 2000 μg/eye) distributed rapidly to the retina and had a vitreous half-life of 2.6–4.0 days.[8] In those animals receiving ranibizumab 500 μg/eye, approximately 50% of the intravitreally injected ranibizumab reached the serum after 2 days. However, serum concentrations were negligible and tissue concentrations were undetectable.[8]

Pharmacokinetic analysis in humans has indicated that circulating ranibizumab does not reach concentrations at which the normal physiological roles of VEGF will be affected. One hour after a 300 μg/eye intravitreal injection, mean serum ranibizumab levels were below the level of quantification (<0.3 ng/ml) in 73% of participants (n = 120). Moreover, when ranibizumab 300 or 500 μg/eye was administered monthly, ranibizumab concentrations were lower than the Kd of ranibizumab for VEGF-A.[9]

PHARMACODYNAMICS

Studies in several animal models have confirmed that ranibizumab displays rapid retinal penetration.[8,10] This rapid diffusion of the ranibizumab Fab fragment is in stark contrast to full-length recombinant humanized IgG which does not penetrate to the retinal layer.[11]

In a phase III study, ranibizumab (0.3 or 0.5 mg) monthly intravitreal injections resulted in a stabilization of the size of the area of CNV and a decrease in the area of vascular leakage as measured by fluorescein angiography.[12] In addition, in patients receiving ranibizumab treatment, optical coherence tomography (OCT) measurements revealed a mean decrease in center point thickness of 123 μm; this compared favorably with an average outcome of no change in thickness in sham-treated patients.

DRUG MECHANISM

Alternative splicing of the VEGF-A gene results in four main VEGF-A isoforms, of 121, 165, 189, and 206 amino acids. Several minor splice variants have also been described.[1] The most abundant isoform is $VEGF\text{-}A_{165}$; this and the longer isoforms are bound to the extracellular matrix but may be released into a soluble form by plasmin cleavage, generating $VEGF\text{-}A_{110}$.

Ranibizumab binds to the VEGF receptor-binding domain that is common to all isoforms and proteolytic cleavage products of VEGF-A. Ranibizumab binding to VEGF-A inhibits VEGF-A binding to its receptor on the surface of endothelial cells. Consequently, the signaling cascade which results in endothelial cell proliferation, vascular leakage, and angiogenesis is not initiated.

DRUG USE IN RETINAL DISEASES

VEGF-A levels are increased in many ocular neovascular diseases. Intraocular levels of VEGF have been shown to be significantly greater in patients with neovascular disease and VEGF has been implicated as playing a major role in active intraocular neovascularization.[13]

In addition to AMD, elevated VEGF levels have been identified in the aqueous humor of diabetic patients with macular edema,[14] in patients with iris neovascularization,[13] and in patients with central retinal vein occlusion (CRVO).[15] In patients with diabetic macular edema, VEGF is implicated in the breakdown of the blood–retinal barrier, leading to a vascular permeability imbalance.[16] VEGF has been shown to stimulate neovascularization of the anterior and posterior segment of the eye, and capillary leakage, leading to macular edema associated with CRVO.[15] Furthermore, in an animal model, VEGF is sufficient to induce iris neovascularization in a nonhuman primate.[17]

In light of the integral part played by VEGF in retinal neovascular disease, there is a strong scientific rationale to support the investigation of treatment of these disorders with ranibizumab. Such treatment would aim to reduce hyperpermeability and inhibit neovascularization.

EFFICACY

EFFICACY IN AMD

Ranibizumab was the first therapeutic agent to demonstrate an improvement in VA and patient-reported outcomes for patients with neovascular AMD. Data from two pivotal 2-year, randomized, controlled phase II trials, ANCHOR (n = 423)[18] and MARINA (n = 716),[7] led to the licensing of ranibizumab for AMD treatment (Table 1). The ANCHOR trial compared monthly injections of two ranibizumab doses (0.3 and 0.5 mg) with verteporfin photodynamic therapy (PDT), while the MARINA trial compared monthly doses of ranibizumab (0.3 and 0.5 mg) with monthly sham injections. In the two trials, 90% of patients receiving ranibizumab 0.5 mg experienced stabilization of VA (loss of <15 letters from baseline) at 24 months, and 33–41% of patients gained VA (experienced improvements of 15 letters from baseline). At 24 months, the mean increase in VA from baseline with ranibizumab 0.5 mg was 10.7 and 6.6 letters in ANCHOR and MARINA, respectively. These outcomes were significantly better ($P < 0.001$) than those achieved by the control groups. In both trials, a biphasic treatment effect was observed, with the majority of the visual gain achieved in the first 3 months of treatment (the loading phase) followed by stabilization of the gain (the maintenance phase).

Patient-reported outcomes were also assessed in the ANCHOR and MARINA trials, using the National Eye Institute Visual Function Questionnaire, to measure the influence of the ranibizumab-mediated

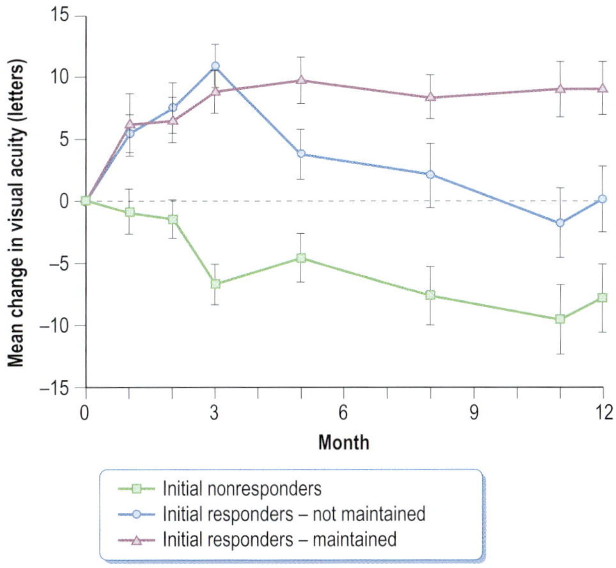

Figure 33.1 Subgroup analysis of visual acuity gain in PIER.

improvements in VA on quality of life. The data demonstrated that patients treated with ranibizumab were more likely to report improvements in near activities, distance activities, and vision-specific dependency which were maintained over the 2-year duration of the trial.[19,20] These data demonstrate that the clinical improvements seen with ranibizumab treatment translate into meaningful benefits for the patient.

The observed biphasic treatment effect raised the possibility that, after the initial 3-month loading phase, maintenance of the VA gain may be achieved with less frequent treatments. A third phase III trial, PIER (n = 184),[21,22] evaluated ranibizumab administered monthly for 3 months, followed by quarterly injections, and compared this with sham treatment. Under this administration schedule, ranibizumab did provide a significant VA benefit; a significantly greater number of patients achieved VA stabilization at 24 months compared with patients receiving sham treatment. However, subgroup analysis revealed that VA gains observed during the first 3 months of treatment were only maintained in 40% of patients over the duration of the trial, and for the remaining 60% quarterly dosing was not suitable (Figure 33.1).

Subsequent to the PIER trial, further investigation of a flexible dosing approach was carried out. The phase IIIb EXCITE trial (n = 353) directly compared a maintenance phase of quarterly injections against the monthly regimen. Consistent with previous observations, an initial gain was made in the first 3 months, after which patients receiving monthly injections continued to gain VA, whilst those receiving quarterly injections showed a decrease from their month 3 VA levels.[23]

The SUSTAIN trial (n = 531) is a 12-month, open-label, nonrandomized trial in which patients received three consecutive monthly loading doses of ranibizumab, followed by a maintenance phase of monthly visits and treatment guided by either VA (>5-letter decrease from the highest VA score at any previous visit) or OCT measurements (>100 μm increase in central retinal thickness (CRT) from the thinnest measurement at any previous visit). The results of an interim analysis of 69 patients show that, at 12 months, the initial VA gain is maintained with a mean VA gain of 6.7 letters and an average of 2.3 injections during the maintenance phase. This suggests that good efficacy outcomes can be achieved with a lower than monthly average number of treatments.[24]

Trials of ranibizumab in different patient populations have also been undertaken or are planned (Table 2). The EXTEND-I trial (n = 88) in Japanese patients has reported results consistent with previous phase III trials of ranibizumab and demonstrated that ranibizumab is safe and effective in the Japanese population.[25]

EFFICACY IN OTHER RETINAL DISEASES

Preliminary results from clinical trials of ranibizumab in ocular neovascular diseases other than AMD have been promising. Interim results from the RESOLVE phase I/II trial ($n = 150$) of ranibizumab in diabetic macular edema show that patients who received ranibizumab (0.3 or 0.5 mg) achieved, on average, a decrease in macular thickness and an increase in VA; this was in contrast to sham-treated patients in whom there was a slight increase in macular thickness and a decrease in VA (Novartis; data on file). Phase III trials of ranibizumab as monotherapy (RISE/RIDE) or as adjunctive therapy, when added to laser photocoagulation (RESTORE), for diabetic macular edema are currently in progress. Furthermore, phase III trials of ranibizumab in CRVO and branch retinal vein occlusion (BRVO) are under way (BRAVO and CRUISE).

CONTRAINDICATIONS

Ranibizumab is contraindicated in patients with ocular or periocular infections. Ranibizumab is also contraindicated in patients with known hypersensitivity to ranibizumab or any of the known excipients in the drug formulation. Hypersensitivity reactions may manifest as severe intraocular inflammation.[26]

OCULAR COMPLICATIONS AND TOXICITY

There is now a significant body of evidence from pre- and postlicensing trials to show that ranibizumab is generally safe and well tolerated.[7,18,21] The most frequently reported ocular AEs in the three trials, occurring more often in ranibizumab treatment groups compared with control groups, are conjunctival hemorrhage (43–77%), eye pain (17–37%), vitreous floaters (3–32%), and increased intraocular pressure (8–25%).[26]

The incidence of serious ocular AEs is low (<1.5% of patients): in the MARINA and ANCHOR trials, the most common were endophthalmitis (0–1.4%) and uveitis (0–1.3%). Other serious ocular AEs reported were retinal detachment, retinal tear, retinal hemorrhage, and vitreous hemorrhage. In the PIER trial, there were no serious ocular AEs.[21,22]

SYSTEMIC COMPLICATIONS AND TOXICITY

Systemic VEGF inhibition is suspected to be associated with an increased risk of hypertension and arterial thromboembolic events (ATEs). Given the average age of patients requiring treatment for AMD, it is important that their treatment does not significantly increase the risk of these events. In phase III trials of ranibizumab, the incidence of Antiplatelet Trialists Collaboration[27] ATEs and hypertension was low. Over the 24-month trial period, the rate of ATEs in the ranibizumab 0.5-mg treatment group of the ANCHOR, MARINA, and PIER trials was 5.0%, 4.6%, and 0%, respectively, compared with 4.2%, 3.8%, and 0% in the control arms.[7,18,21]

Interim analysis of safety data from a further phase III trial, SAILOR ($n = 2378$), which is designed to investigate further the safety of a quarterly monitoring regimen and ranibizumab injections based on VA (>5-letter loss from the previous highest VA score during the first 3 months) or OCT (>100 μm increase in CRT from the previous lowest measurement), indicates that there is a higher incidence of stroke in patients with pre-existing risk factors, particularly a previous history of stroke (data on file). The incidence of stroke continues to be monitored in phase IV trials; however, the risk should be taken into account, particularly in patients with a history of stroke.

The most frequently occurring nonocular AEs, for which the incidence is greater than in the control groups, are nasopharyngitis (5–25%), headache (2–15%), and upper respiratory tract infection (4–12%).[26]

DRUG INTERACTIONS

Drug interaction studies have not been conducted with ranibizumab.

Combined therapy with ranibizumab and verteporfin PDT has been investigated in patients with predominantly classic CNV secondary to AMD. At 12 months, combination therapy resulted in a greater proportion of patients losing fewer than 15 letters than with PDT alone (90.5% and 67.9%, respectively).[28] This VA benefit persisted at 24 months; on average, patients receiving ranibizumab plus PDT exhibited less lesion growth and greater reduction of CNV leakage, and required fewer PDT treatments than patients receiving PDT alone.[29] Ranibizumab treatment did increase the incidence of serious ocular inflammation and endophthalmitis; however, affected patients, on average, still experienced a VA gain.[28–30]

SUMMARY AND KEY POINTS

Ranibizumab is the first treatment for neovascular AMD to show an improvement in VA and patient-reported outcomes. There is now a significant body of evidence, from several large clinical trials, to support the use of ranibizumab in patients with neovascular AMD.

Table 33.1 Summary table of controlled (multicenter, randomized) ranibizumab clinical trials

Study design	MARINA ($n = 716$)	ANCHOR ($n = 423$)	PIER ($n = 184$)	EXCITE ($n = 353$)
Study masking	Double	Double	Double	Single
Study duration	24 months	24 months	24 months	12 months
Lesion type	Minimally classic and occult (with no classic) CNV	Predominantly classic CNV	All CNV types	All CNV types
Visit regimen in maintenance phase	Monthly	Monthly	Quarterly	Monthly for control arm Quarterly for study arms
Ranibizumab regimen in maintenance phase	Monthly	Monthly	Quarterly	Monthly for control arm Quarterly for study arms
No. of ranibizumab injections in maintenance phase (over first 12-month period)	9	9	3	9 for control arm 3 for study arms

CNV, choroidal neovascularization.

Table 33.2 Summary table of uncontrolled ranibizumab clinical trials

Study design	PrONTO (n = 40)	SUSTAIN (n = 531)	SAILOR (n = 2378)
Study type	Open-label, single-center, nonrandomized, investigator-sponsored	Open-label, multicenter, nonrandomized	Single-masked, multicenter, randomized
Study duration	24 months	12 months	12 months
Lesion type	All CNV types	All CNV types	All CNV types
Visit regimen in maintenance phase	Monthly	Monthly	Quarterly
Ranibizumab regimen in maintenance phase	Individualized	Individualized	Individualized
Mean no. of ranibizumab injections in maintenance phase	2.6	2.3	1.6

CNV, choroidal neovascularization.

The clinical data support the use of a 3-month loading phase of consecutive monthly injections. For optimal outcomes, this should be followed by continued monthly injections or, if this is not possible, monthly monitoring and treatment as required.

Overall, ranibizumab has been well tolerated in the clinical trials completed to date, with a low incidence of ocular and systemic serious AEs. The safety profile continues to be monitored in postmarketing trials.

In conclusion, ranibizumab has demonstrated significant benefits to patients with neovascular AMD, not only in terms of VA gains but also in terms of improved quality of life. As such, it represents a valuable therapeutic option for ophthalmologists treating neovascular AMD.

REFERENCES

1. Ferrara N, Gerber HP, LeCouter J. The biology of VEGF and its receptors. Nat Med 2003;9:669–676.
2. Rosen LS. VEGF-targeted therapy: therapeutic potential and recent advances. Oncologist 2005;10:382–391.
3. Presta LG, Chen H, O'Connor SJ, et al. Humanization of an anti-vascular endothelial growth factor monoclonal antibody for the therapy of solid tumors and other disorders. Cancer Res 1997;57:4593–4599.
4. van Wijngaarden P, Coster DJ, Williams KA. Inhibitors of ocular neovascularization: promises and potential problems. JAMA 2005;293:1509–1513.
5. Ferrara N, Damico L, Shams N, et al. Development of ranibizumab, an anti-vascular endothelial growth factor antigen binding fragment, as therapy for neovascular age-related macular degeneration. Retina 2006;26:859–870.
6. Gragoudas ES, Adamis AP, Cunningham ET Jr, et al. Pegaptanib for neovascular age-related macular degeneration. N Engl J Med 2004;351: 2805–2816.
7. Rosenfeld PJ, Brown DM, Heier JS, et al. Ranibizumab for neovascular age-related macular degeneration. N Engl J Med 2006;355:1419–1431.
8. Gaudreault J, Fei D, Rusit J, et al. Preclinical pharmacokinetics of ranibizumab (rhuFabV2) after a single intravitreal administration. Invest Ophthalmol Vis Sci 2005;46:726–733.
9. Haughney PC, Lowe J, Kearns A, et al. Clinical pharmacokinetics of ranibizumab (Lucentis) in subjects with AMD. Invest Ophthalmol Vis Sci 2005;46:E-Abstract 1383.
10. Mordenti J, Thomsen K, Licko V, et al. Efficacy and concentration-response of murine anti-VEGF monoclonal antibody in tumor-bearing mice and extrapolation to humans. Toxicol Pathol 1999;27:14–21.
11. Mordenti J, Cuthbertson RA, Ferrara N, et al. Comparisons of the intraocular tissue distribution, pharmacokinetics, and safety of ^{125}I-labeled full-length and Fab antibodies in rhesus monkeys following intravitreal administration. Toxicol Pathol 1999;27:536–544.
12. Kaiser PK, Blodi BA, Shapiro H, et al. Angiographic and optical coherence tomographic results of the MARINA study of ranibizumab in neovascular age-related macular degeneration. Ophthalmology 2007;114:1868–1875.
13. Aiello LP, Avery RL, Arrigg PG, et al. Vascular endothelial growth factor in ocular fluid of patients with diabetic retinopathy and other retinal disorders. N Engl J Med 1994;331:1480–1487.
14. Funatsu H, Yamashita H, Noma H, et al. Increased levels of vascular endothelial growth factor and interleukin-6 in the aqueous humor of diabetics with macular edema. Am J Ophthalmol 2002;133:70–77.
15. Boyd SR, Zachary I, Chakravarthy U, et al. Correlation of increased vascular endothelial growth factor with neovascularization and permeability in ischemic central vein occlusion. Arch Ophthalmol 2002;120:1644–1650.
16. Qaum T, Xu Q, Joussen AM, et al. VEGF-initiated blood–retinal barrier breakdown in early diabetes. Invest Ophthalmol Vis Sci 2001;42: 2408–2413.
17. Tolentino MJ, Miller JW, Gragoudas ES, et al. Vascular endothelial growth factor is sufficient to produce iris neovascularization and neovascular glaucoma in a nonhuman primate. Arch Ophthalmol 1996;114:964–970.
18. Brown DM, Kaiser PK, Michels M, et al. Ranibizumab versus verteporfin for neovascular age-related macular degeneration. N Engl J Med 2006;355:1432–1444.
19. Chang TS, Bressler NM, Fine JT, et al. Improved vision-related function after ranibizumab treatment of neovascular age-related macular degeneration: results of a randomized clinical trial. Arch Ophthalmol 2007;125:1460–1469.
20. Korobelnik JF. Ranibizumab therapy in patients with neovascular age-related macular degeneration: patient-reported outcomes in the ANCHOR and PIER trials. Presented at EURETINA, 2008.
21. Regillo CD, Brown DM, Abraham P, et al. Randomized, double-masked, sham-controlled trial of ranibizumab for neovascular age-related macular degeneration: PIER study year 1. Am J Ophthalmol 2008;145:239–248.
22. Regillo CD, Yue H, Shams N. Ranibizumab (Lucentis) in treatment of neovascular age-related macular degeneration (AMD): 2-year results of PIER study. Poster PO459 presented at the AAO, 2007.
23. Schmidt-Erfurth UM. Ranibizumab treatment effects in patients with neovascular age-related macular degeneration: 12-month results from the EXCITE trial. Presented at World Ophthalmology Congress, 2008.
24. Meyer CH, Eter N, Holz FG, SUSTAIN study group. Ranibizumab in patients with subfoveal choroidal neovascularization secondary to age-related macular degeneration. Interim results from the SUSTAIN trial. Invest Ophthalmol Vis Sci 2008;49:E-Abstract 273.
25. Tano Y. The safety and efficacy of ranibizumab in Japanese patients with subfoveal choroidal neovascularization secondary to age-related macular degeneration: 12-month results from the phase I/II EXTEND-I study. Invest Ophthalmol Vis Sci 2008;49:E-Abstract 272.
26. Novartis Pharma AG. Lucentis – Full Prescribing Information. Novartis Pharma AG. 2008.
27. Antiplatelet Trialists' Collaboration. Collaborative overview of randomised trials of antiplatelet therapy – I: Prevention of death, myocardial infarction, and stroke by prolonged antiplatelet therapy in various categories of patients. BMJ 1994;308:81–106.
28. Heier JS, Boyer DS, Ciulla TA, et al. Ranibizumab combined with verteporfin photodynamic therapy in neovascular age-related macular degeneration: year 1 results of the FOCUS Study. Arch Ophthalmol 2006;124:1532–1542.
29. Antoszyk AN, Tuomi L, Chung CY, et al. Ranibizumab combined with verteporfin photodynamic therapy in neovascular age-related macular degeneration (FOCUS): year 2 results. Am J Ophthalmol 2008;145: 862–874.
30. Heier JS, Boyer DS, Ciulla TA, et al. Ranibizumab combined with verteporfin photodynamic therapy in neovascular age-related macular degeneration: year 1 results of the FOCUS Study. Arch Ophthalmol 2006;124:1532–1542.

CHAPTER 34

Pathophysiology of vascular endothelial growth factor and other angiogenic molecules

Napoleone Ferrara, MD and Yongping Crawford, MD, PhD

KEY FEATURES

Vascular endothelial growth factor (VEGF) has been demonstrated through multiple studies to play an important role in angiogenesis and in the pathophysiology of various types of tumors, and ocular diseases such as neovascular age-related macular degeneration (AMD) and diabetic retinopathy. Inhibitors and antagonists of VEGF have demonstrated their abilities to interfere with angiogenesis, halt disease progression, and restore functional loss, such as visual gain. In addition, fibroblast growth factor (FGF), placental growth factor (PlGF), and delta-like ligand 4 (Dll4) are among other factors that also play a role in angiogenesis. Comprehension of VEGF and other factors, and their interrelationship, will enable clinician scientists to understand better antiangiogenic approaches to managing related diseases.

INTRODUCTION

Angiogenesis is important for a variety of physiological processes, including embryonic and postnatal development, reproductive functions, and wound healing.[1] Research performed in recent decades has established that angiogenesis is a complex and coordinated process which requires a series of signaling steps in endothelial and in mural cells elicited by numerous families of ligands (reviewed by Yancopoulos et al.[2]). Moreover, a variety of endogenous inhibitors of angiogenesis have been identified, including endostatin, tumstatin, and vasostatin.[3] However, despite such complexity and potential redundancy, VEGF-A appears to be necessary for growth of blood vessels in a variety of normal and pathological circumstances.[4–7] *VEGF-A* is the prototype member of a gene family that also includes PlGF, VEGF-B, VEGF-C, VEGF-D, and the orf-virus-encoded VEGF-E (reviewed by Ferrara et al.,[8,9] and Alitalo et al.[10]). In normal adult tissues, with the exception of the female reproductive system, VEGF expression is relatively low. However, in human tumors, overexpression of VEGF has been frequently observed.[11] In fact, increased VEGF expression was found to correlate frequently with tumor progression, recurrence, and survival.[12,13]

Definitive clinical studies, resulting in approval by the US Food and Drug Administration (FDA) of several drugs, have established that VEGF-A is an important therapeutic target for cancer and neovascular AMD (reviewed by Ferrara et al.[14]).

While the main emphasis of this chapter is on the pathophysiology of VEGF-A, other proangiogenic molecules will also be discussed.

BIOLOGICAL EFFECTS OF VEGF-A

VEGF-A promotes growth of vascular endothelial cells[15,16] and also induces angiogenesis in a variety of *in vivo* models.[16] Administration of VEGF also induces increases in microvascular permeability in several experimental model systems (reviewed by Dvorak[11]).

Inactivation of a single VEGF-A allele results in early embryonic lethality in mice, indicating that during early development there is a critical VEGF-A gene dosage requirement.[9] VEGF-A plays an important role also in early postnatal life.[17,18] VEGF is important for endochondral bone formation and growth plate angiogenesis and morphogenesis.[19] Another key function of VEGF-A is the regulation of the cyclical angiogenesis that occurs in the female reproductive tract.[20] VEGF-A is also a survival factor for endothelial cells, both *in vitro* and *in vivo*.[21–24] VEGF induces expression of the antiapoptotic proteins Bcl-2, A1,[22] and survivin[25] in endothelial cells. *In vivo*, VEGF's prosurvival effects are dependent on the stage of development since VEGF inhibition results in apoptotic changes and regression of the vasculature of neonatal, but not of adult, mice.[17]

VEGF-A ISOFORMS

Alternative exon splicing results in the generation of four main VEGF-A isoforms, which have respectively 121, 165, 189, and 206 amino acids after the signal sequence is cleaved ($VEGF_{121}$, $VEGF_{165}$, $VEGF_{189}$, and $VEGF_{206}$).[26,27]

Like $VEGF_{165}$, native VEGF is a heparin-binding homodimeric glycoprotein of 45 kDa.[28,29] In contrast, $VEGF_{121}$ lacks heparin-binding properties.[30] $VEGF_{189}$ and $VEGF_{206}$ bind to heparin with affinity comparable to that of basic FGF.[30] Whereas $VEGF_{121}$ is a freely diffusible protein, $VEGF_{189}$ and $VEGF_{206}$ are almost completely bound to heparin-like moieties in the cell surface or in the extracellular matrix. $VEGF_{165}$ has intermediate properties in terms of heparin affinity and bioavailability.[31] Heparin-binding isoforms may be released in a diffusible form by proteolytic cleavage. Early studies showed that plasmin is able to cleave $VEGF_{165}$ at the COOH terminus, generating $VEGF_{110}$, a bioactive fragment consisting of the first 110 NH_2-terminal amino acids.[30,32] Interestingly, recent studies have shown that various matrix metalloproteinases (MMPs), especially MMP-3, may also cleave $VEGF_{165}$ to generate diffusible, nonheparin-binding fragments.[33] Proteolytic processing of $VEGF_{165}$ by MMP-3 occurs in steps, with sequential cleavage at residues 135, 120, and finally at residue 113.[33] Thus, the final product of MMP-3 processing, $VEGF_{113}$, is expected to be biologically and biochemically very similar to the plasmin-generated VEGF fragment.

VEGF RECEPTORS

VEGF-A binds two receptor tyrosine kinases (RTK), VEGFR-1[34] and VEGFR-2.[35] Both VEGFR-1 and VEGFR-2 have seven immunoglobulin (Ig)-like domains in the extracellular portion. VEGFR-1 was the first RTK to be identified as a VEGF receptor more than 15 years ago.[36] It binds VEGF with very high affinity (Kd ~ 10–20 pM). Early studies demonstrated that the second Ig-like domain is essential for ligand binding.[37] This structural information was important for the design of high-affinity soluble receptors currently undergoing clinical testing.[38] The functions and signaling properties of VEGFR-1 appear to vary with the developmental stage and the cell type, e.g., endothelial versus nonendothelial cells. VEGFR-1 binds not only VEGF-A but also PlGF and VEGF-B and fails to mediate a strong mitogenic signal in endothelial cells.[39,40] Nonmitogenic functions mediated by VEGFR-1 in the vascular endothelium include the release of growth factors[41] and the induction of MMP-9.[42] Furthermore, VEGFR-1 mediates hematopoiesis[43] and monocyte chemotaxis[44] in response to VEGF-A or PlGF.

VEGFR-2 also has a high-affinity binding interaction with VEGF-A.[35,45] VEGF-C and VEGF-D may also bind and activate VEGFR-2, following their proteolytic cleavage.[9] The role of VEGFR-2 in developmental angiogenesis and hematopoiesis is underscored by lack of vasculogenesis and failure of blood island development in Flk-1 null mice.[46] There is now agreement that VEGFR-2 is the major mediator of the proangiogenic and permeability-enhancing effects of VEGF-A. VEGFR-2 undergoes dimerization and strong ligand-dependent tyrosine phosphorylation in intact cells and results in a mitogenic, chemotactic and prosurvival signal. Several tyrosine residues have been shown to be phosphorylated (for review, see Olsson et al.[47]). In 1998 Neuropilin-1 was identified as a receptor for isoforms of VEGF-A containing the exon 7-encoded heparin-binding domain.[48]

ROLE OF VEGF-A IN TUMOR ANGIOGENESIS

Many tumor cell lines secrete VEGF-A *in vitro* (reviewed by Ferrara[16]). *In situ* hybridization studies have demonstrated that the VEGF mRNA is expressed in many human tumors.[11] A variety of transforming events also lead to induction of VEGF gene expression. Oncogenic mutations or amplification of ras lead to VEGF up-regulation.[49] Renal cell carcinomas have a particularly high level of VEGF-A expression, consistent with the notion that inactivating mutation in the von Hippel–Lindau tumor suppressor gene, resulting in high transcription of the hypoxia-inducible factor (HIF) target genes under normoxic conditions, occur in ~50% of such tumors.[50]

In 1993, monoclonal antibodies targeting VEGF-A were reported to inhibit the growth of several tumor cell lines in nude mice.[51] Inhibition of tumor growth has also been achieved with other anti-VEGF-A treatments, including small-molecule inhibitors of VEGFR-2 signaling (reviewed by Manley et al.[52]), anti-VEGFR-2 antibodies,[53] and soluble VEGF receptors.[38,54]

Although tumor cells frequently represent the major source of VEGF-A, tumor-associated stroma is also an important site of VEGF production.[54] Studies have shown that tumor-derived platelet-derived growth factor-A (PDGF-A) may be especially important for the recruitment of an angiogenic stroma that produces VEGF-A and potentially other angiogenic factors.[55,56]

Combining anti-VEGF treatment with chemotherapy[57] or radiation therapy[58] results in a greater antitumor effect than either of these therapies alone. The mechanism of such potentiation is complex. One possibility is that antiangiogenic agents normalize the tumor vasculature, improving delivery of chemotherapy to tumor cells.[59] Alternatively, chemotherapy-induced damege to tumor endothelial cells may be amplified by blockade of a key prosurvival factor like VEGF.[57]

Several VEGF inhibitors have been developed as anticancer agents. These include a humanized anti-VEGF-A monoclonal antibody (bevacizumab; Avastin),[60,61] an anti-VEGFR-2 antibody,[53] various small molecules inhibiting VEGFR-2 signal transduction,[52] and a VEGF receptor chimeric protein.[38] For recent reviews, see Gasparini et al.,[62] Ferrara and Kerbel,[63] and Jain et al.[64]

ROLE OF VEGF-A IN INTRAOCULAR NEOVASCULAR SYNDROMES

Earlier studies indicated that expression of VEGF-A mRNA is spatially and temporally correlated with neovascularization in several animal models of retinal ischemia.[21,65] This is consistent with the notion that VEGF-A gene expression is regulated by oxygen tension, via HIF-dependent transcriptional activation.[66] In 1994 it was reported that levels of VEGF-A are elevated in the aqueous and vitreous humor of human eyes with proliferative retinopathy secondary to diabetes and other conditions.[67,68] Subsequently, animal studies using various VEGF inhibitors, including soluble VEGF receptors,[69] anti-VEGF-A monoclonal antibodies,[70] and small-molecule VEGF RTK inhibitors,[71] have conclusively demonstrated the role of VEGF as a key mediator of ischemia-induced intraocular neovascularization.

AMD is the most common cause of severe, irreversible vision loss in the elderly.[72] AMD is classified as nonexudative (dry) or exudative (wet or neovascular) disease. Although the exudative form accounts for ~10–20% of cases, it is responsible for 80–90% of the visual loss associated with AMD.[73] Three pharmacologic therapies for neovascular AMD have been approved by the FDA. One is verteporfin (Visudyne) photodynamic therapy (PDT)[74] for only predominantly classic lesions, in which 50% or more of the lesion consists of classic choroidal neovascularization (CNV). The other is pegaptanib sodium (Macugen),[75] approved in December 2004 for all angiographic subtypes of neovascular AMD. Although both treatments can slow the progression of vision loss, only a small percentage of treated patients experience any improvement in visual acuity. The third is ranibizumab, which was approved by the FDA for the treatment of all subtypes of neovascular AMD in June 2006.[76]

INTRAVITREAL ANTI-VEGF THERAPY FOR NEOVASCULAR AMD: PEGAPTANIB, RANIBIZUMAB AND BEVACIZUMAB

Pegaptanib sodium injection (Macugen) and ranibizumab (Lucentis) are the first ocular anti-VEGF treatments evaluated in large, randomized, controlled clinical trials for the treatment of neovascular AMD (for recent reviews, see Andreoli and Miller,[77] Jager et al.,[78] and Pieramici and Rabena[79]). Both are administered locally by intravitreal injection. Pegaptanib sodium is a pegylated oligonucelotide aptamer that binds to and inactivates $VEGF_{165}$.[80] In a combined analysis of the VISION trials – two identical, large, controlled, double-masked, randomized, multicenter clinical trials involving patients with all CNV lesion types – pegaptinib sodium prevented moderate vision loss (the primary endpoint, which was defined as loss < than 15 letters of vision) in 70% of subjects compared with 55% for the control group at 1 year ($P < 0.001$).[75] However, on average, patients in the pegaptinib sodium group lost ~8 letters at 1 year, compared with a loss of ~15 letters in the sham injection group ($P < 0.002$). The proportion of subjects who experienced a moderate gain in vision (defined as a change of 15 letters at 1 year from baseline) was 6% in the pegaptinib sodium group compared to 2% in the sham injection group ($P = 0.04$). Key adverse events observed in the pegaptinib sodium groups were uncommon and included endophthalmitis in 1.3%, traumatic lens injury in 0.7%, and retinal detachment in 0.6% of patients.

Ranibizumab (Lucentis) is a recombinant, humanized Fab that binds to and potently neutralizes the biological activities of all known human VEGF-A isoforms, as well as the proteolytic cleavage product $VEGF_{110}$.[76,81] Ranibizumab has been evaluated in two large, phase III, multicenter, randomized, double-masked, controlled pivotal trials in different neovascular AMD patient populations.

The MARINA trial randomized subjects with minimally classic (less than 50% of the lesion consisting of classic CNV) or occult without classic CNV to monthly sham injections or monthly intravitreal injections of one of two doses of ranibizumab (0.3 or 0.5 mg).[82] At both 1-year and 2-year analysis, the study met its primary endpoint, with a significantly greater proportion of ranibizumab subjects avoiding moderate vision loss than sham-injected subjects. Moreover, on average, ranibizumab-treated subjects gained vision at 1 year compared with baseline while sham-injection subjects lost vision. A significantly larger percentage of subjects treated with ranibizumab gained 15 letters at 1 year than did the sham-injection group. Key serious ocular adverse events occurring in ranibizumab-treated subjects included uveitis and endophthalmitis and were uncommon.

The ANCHOR trial randomized subjects with predominantly classic CNV to verteporfin PDT with monthly sham ocular injections or to monthly intravitreal injections of one of two doses of ranibizumab with a sham PDT procedure. In the primary analysis at 1 year – the study met its primary endpoint – there was a significantly greater proportion of ranibizumab subjects avoiding moderate vision loss compared with subjects treated with verteporfin through PDT.[83] In addition, on average, ranibizumab-treated subjects gained vision at 1 year compared with baseline while verteporfin PDT subjects lost vision, and a significantly larger percentage of subjects treated with ranibizumab gained 15 letters at 1 year than did the verteporfin PDT group. Most recently, a 2-year analysis of the ANCHOR trial has been published and shows that ranibizumab provided greater clinical benefit than verteporfin PDT in patients with AMD with new-onset, predominantly classic CNV.[84]

Encouraging ranibizumab (Lucentis) preliminary phase III clinical trial results have led to growing interest in the possibility of off-label use of bevacizumab (Avastin) as a therapeutic option for the treatment of neovascular AMD[85–87] (for recent reviews, see Andreoli and Miller,[77] Jager et al.,[78] and Pieramici and Rabena[79]). Systemic bevacizumab has been the subject of numerous open-label uncontrolled trials showing short-term benefits. These reports are difficult to compare with rigorous, double-masked, controlled phase III data reported for verteporfin PDT, pegaptanib, and ranibizumab.[88] Nevetheless, bevacizumab is widely used worldwide. A phase III study comparing ranibizumab and bevacizumab is ongoing.

OTHER ANTI-VEGF THERAPIES IN CLINICAL DEVELOPMENT FOR AMD

A number of other molecules targeting VEGF and its signaling pathway are in early stages of clinical development for the treatment of neovascular AMD. The VEGF-Trap[38] was initially tested by the systemic route of administration, but the occurrence of hypertension and proteinuria led to discontinuation of these studies[89,90] The VEGF-Trap is currently administered intravitreally and is being investigated in phase III clinical trials for neovascular AMD and phase II for diabetic macular edema. Cand5 and Sirna-027 are short interfering RNA molecules that inhibit the expression of genes encoding VEGF and VEGF receptor 1, respectively.[91,92] While not being developed for neovascular AMD, ruboxistaurin (LY333531) is an oral protein kinase C-beta inhibitor that is being developed for diabetic retinopathy.[93]

OTHER ANGIOGENIC FACTORS

FIBROBLAST GROWTH FACTOR FAMILY

The FGF family has been implicated in a wide variety of important processes such as neurogenesis, organ development, and angiogenesis and includes 18 ligands interacting with four receptors.[94] While the prototype members, FGF-1 and FGF-2, are devoid of a signal peptide and thus are poorly secreted proteins,[95] most members of the family are efficiently secreted.[94] Using the Rip-Tag model, Casanovas et al. found that FGF-1 and FGF-2 are up-regulated in tumors that relapsed following anti-VEGFR antibody (DC101) treatment.[96] Moreover, their expression correlated with the restoration of tumor vasculature that initially regressed during the responsive phase to anti-VEGFR therapy. To assess the functional importance of FGF in the regrowth of tumor vessels and relapse of tumor growth, the authors treated mice with a FGF-trap (FGFR-Fc fusion peptide) when tumors were in a maximum response phase to VEGFR inhibitors.[96] The combinatorial treatment resulted in slowed tumor growth and attenuated tumor angiogenesis, indicating that FGF signaling is required for tumor regrowth in the presence of VEGFR inhibitors. Similarly, FGF-2 increases were also found in the blood of patients relapsed from treatment using VEGFR inhibitors,[97] suggesting that FGF-2 may be responsible for the acquired resistance observed in patients. Conceivably, tumor cells that express high levels of FGF-2 prior to treatment are likely to be intrinsically resistant to VEGF or VEGFR inhibitors.

PLACENTAL GROWTH FACTOR

PlGF is a member of the VEGF family that binds specifically to VEGFR1.[39,98] While PlGF null mice are viable and fertile, they have been reported to have reduced angiogenesis during pathological conditions.[99] Up-regulation of both VEGF and PlGF has been reported in patients treated with agents targeting the VEGF–VEGFR2 pathway.[97,100] This observation led to the speculation that PlGF may be involved in providing an escape pathway when VEGF-A is inhibited. Using an anti-PlGF neutralizing antibody, Fischer et al. reported that inhibition of PlGF signaling slows tumor growth and inhibits metastasis in multiple murine models.[101] However, the role of PlGF in tumor angiogenesis and growth remains controversial. In a preclinical study employing sunitinib, a VEGFR2 small-molecule inhibitor, Ebos et al.[102] found that PlGF was up-regulated in nontumor-bearing mice, suggesting a non-tumor-specific host response to the treatment. Moreover, a high-affinity chimeric soluble VEGFR1 variant, mFlt (1-3)-IgG, which simultaneously blocks VEGF-A, B, and PlGF, performed comparably to an anti-VEGF-A antibody alone in inhibiting tumor growth.[103] Similarly, an anti-VEGFR1 antibody did not inhibit tumor angiogenesis or tumor growth in the Rip-Tag model, nor did it add benefits when combined with anti-VEGFR2 antibodies.[96] Further studies are necessary to investigate the role of PlGF in tumor and other types of pathological angiogenesis.

DELTA-LIKE LIGAND 4

Dll4 belongs to the Delta/Jagged family of transmembrane ligands that binds to Notch receptors.[104] Delta-Notch signaling mediates cell–cell communication and regulates cell fate determination. Like the VEGF pathway, Delta/Notch signaling is also critically important for proper vascular development.[104] One particular endothelial cell notch ligand, Dll4, was required for properly regulating tip cell formation during angiogenesis.[105] Activation of Dll/Notch pathway decreased tip cell numbers. Conversely, reduced Dll4 signaling increased tip cell formation. Up-regulation of Dll4 was also found in tumor vessels.[106] Two groups demonstrated independently that inhibiting Dll4 with an antibody or a Dll4-fc inhibits tumor growth by deregulating angiogenesis, resulting in increased, but nonfunctional, vessels.[107,108]

SUMMARY AND KEYPOINTS

Research conducted for almost two decades has demonstrated that VEGF-A is important for the regulation of the normal angiogenesis processes. Moreover, VEGF inhibition has been shown to suppress pathological angiogenesis in a variety of cancer models, leading to the clinical development of a variety of VEGF inhibitors. Definitive clinical studies have proved that VEGF inhibition, by means of bevacizumab in combination with chemotherapy, provides a significant clinical benefit in patients with metastatic colorectal cancer, nonsmall-cell lung carcinoma, and metastatic breast cancer, in combination with cytotoxic chemotherapy.[109–112] Furthermore, two small molecule tyrosine kinase inhibitors, sunitinib[113] and sorafenib,[114] have been approved by the FDA for metastatic renal cell carcinoma and their mechanism of tumor suppression consists, at least partly, in inhibition of VEGF signaling.[62–64]

A particularly active area of research concerns the elucidation of the mechanisms of refractoriness or resistance to anti-VEGF therapies. Tumor cell-intrinsic or treatment-induced expression of angiogenic factors may be implicated.[96,115] Recent studies have provided evidence that, at least in some murine models, refractoriness to anti-VEGF therapy is related to the ability of the tumor to recruit CD11b+Gr1+ myeloid cells, which in turn promotes angiogenesis.[103] Subsequent studies indicated that a secreted protein called Bv8 or prokineticin-2 is a mediator of myeloid cell-dependent angiogenesis.[116–118] It remains to be established whether these findings also apply to human tumors and other pathological conditions. In this context, it is noteworthy that myeloid cell infiltration has also been implicated in CNV.[119]

Reliable markers are needed to monitor the activity of antiangiogenic drugs. Circulating endothelial cells and their progenitor subset are a potential candidate, as is magnetic resonance imaging dynamic measurement of vascular permeability/flow in response to angiogenesis inhibitors, but neither has been clinically validated.[63] Emphasizing the difficulty of identifying predictive markers, a recent study found that

VEGF-A and thrombospondin expression or microvessel density in tumor sections does not correlate with clinical response to bevacizumab in patients with metastatic colorectal cancer and patients showed a survival benefit from the treatment, irrespective of these parameters.[120]

VEGF inhibitors have demonstrated a marked clinical benefit also in neovascular AMD. Blockade of all VEGF-A isoforms and bioactive fragmemts with ranibizumab not only slowed down vision loss, but, unexpectedly, appears to have the potential to enable many AMD patients to obtain a meaningful and sustained gain of vision. Current work is testing the hypothesis that VEGF blockade may be beneficial for other conditions such as macular edema associated with diabetic retinopathy and retinal vein occlusion.[121,122] Furthermore, ongoing work is attempting to identify strategies to augment the efficacy of VEGF pathway inhibitors. In this context, recent studies suggest that blocking PDGF-β may have the added benefit of inhibiting fibrosis.[123]

REFERENCES

1. Folkman J, Klagsbrun M. Angiogenic factors. Science 1987;235:442–447.
2. Yancopoulos GD, Davis S, Gale NW, et al. Vascular-specific growth factors and blood vessel formation. Nature 2000;407(6801):242–248.
3. Sund M, Hamano Y, Sugimoto H, et al. Function of endogenous inhibitors of angiogenesis as endothelium-specific tumor suppressors. Proc Natl Acad Sci USA 2005;102(8):2934–2939.
4. Ferrara N. VEGF and the quest for tumour angiogenesis factors. Nat Rev Cancer 2002;2(10):795–803.
5. Coultas L, Chawengsaksophak K, Rossant J. Endothelial cells and VEGF in vascular development. Nature 2005;438(7070):937–945.
6. Ellis LM, Hicklin DJ. VEGF-targeted therapy: mechanisms of anti-tumour activity. Nat Rev Cancer 2008;8(8):579–591.
7. Kerbel RS. Tumor angiogenesis. N Engl J Med 2008;358(19):2039–2049.
8. Ferrara N, Gerber HP, LeCouter J. The biology of VEGF and its receptors. Nature Med 2003;9:669–676.
9. Ferrara N, Carver Moore K, Chen H, et al. Heterozygous embryonic lethality induced by targeted inactivation of the VEGF gene. Nature 1996;380(6573):439–442.
10. Alitalo K, Tammela T, Petrova TV. Lymphangiogenesis in development and human disease. Nature 2005;438:946–953.
11. Dvorak HF. Vascular permeability factor/vascular endothelial growth factor: a critical cytokine in tumor angiogenesis and a potential target for diagnosis and therapy. J Clin Oncol 2002;20(21):4368–4380.
12. Poon RT, Fan ST, Wong J. Clinical implications of circulating angiogenic factors in cancer patients. J Clin Oncol 2001;19(4):1207–1225.
13. Zhang J, Jia Z, Li Q, et al. Elevated expression of vascular endothelial growth factor correlates with increased angiogenesis and decreased progression-free survival among patients with low-grade neuroendocrine tumors. Cancer 2007;109(8):1478–1486.
14. Ferrara N, Mass RD, Campa C, et al. Targeting VEGF-A to treat cancer and age-related macular degeneration. Annu Rev Med 2007;58:491–504.
15. Leung DW, Cachianes G, Kuang WJ, et al. Vascular endothelial growth factor is a secreted angiogenic mitogen. Science 1989;246(4935):1306–1309.
16. Ferrara N. Vascular endothelial growth factor: basic science and clinical progress. Endocr Rev 2004;25:581–611.
17. Gerber HP, Hillan KJ, Ryan AM, et al. VEGF is required for growth and survival in neonatal mice. Development 1999;126:1149–1159.
18. Malik AK, Baldwin ME, Peale F, et al. Redundant roles of VEGF-B and PlGF during selective VEGF-A blockade in mice. Blood 2006;107:550–557.
19. Gerber HP, Vu TH, Ryan AM, et al. VEGF couples hypertrophic cartilage remodeling, ossification and angiogenesis during endochondral bone formation. Nature Med 1999;5:623–628.
20. Ferrara N, Chen H, Davis-Smyth T, et al. Vascular endothelial growth factor is essential for corpus luteum angiogenesis. Nature Medicine 1998;4:336–340.
21. Alon T, Hemo I, Itin A, et al. Vascular endothelial growth factor acts as a survival factor for newly formed retinal vessels and has implications for retinopathy of prematurity. Nat-Med 1995;1(10):1024–1028.
22. Gerber HP, Dixit V, Ferrara N. Vascular endothelial growth factor induces expression of the antiapoptotic proteins Bcl-2 and A1 in vascular endothelial cells. The Journal of Biological Chemistry 1998;273: 13313–13316.
23. Gerber HP, McMurtrey A, Kowalski J, et al. VEGF regulates endothelial cell survival by the PI3-kinase/Akt signal transduction pathway. Requirement for Flk-1/KDR activation. J Biol Chem 1998;273: 30336–30343.
24. Benjamin LE, Golijanin D, Itin A, et al. Selective ablation of immature blood vessels in established human tumors follows vascular endothelial growth factor withdrawal [see comments]. Journal of Clinical Investigation 1999;103(2):159–165.
25. Tran J, Master Z, Yu JL, et al. A role for survivin in chemoresistance of endothelial cells mediated by VEGF. Proc Natl Acad Sci USA 2002;99(7):4349–4354.
26. Houck KA, Ferrara N, Winer J, et al. The vascular endothelial growth factor family: identification of a fourth molecular species and characterization of alternative splicing of RNA. Molecular Endocrinology 1991;5(12):1806–1814.
27. Tischer E, Mitchell R, Hartman T, et al. The human gene for vascular endothelial growth factor. Multiple protein forms are encoded through alternative exon splicing. Journal of Biological Chemistry 1991;266(18): 11947–11954.
28. Ferrara N, Henzel WJ. Pituitary follicular cells secrete a novel heparin-binding growth factor specific for vascular endothelial cells. Biochemical & Biophysical Research Communications 1989;161(2):851–858.
29. Plouet J, Schilling J, Gospodarowicz D. Isolation and characterization of a newly identified endothelial cell mitogen produced by AtT20 cells. EMBO Journal 1989;8:3801–3808.
30. Houck KA, Leung DW, Rowland AM, et al. Dual regulation of vascular endothelial growth factor bioavailability by genetic and proteolytic mechanisms. J Biol Chem 1992;267(36):26031–26037.
31. Park JE, Keller G-A, Ferrara N. The vascular endothelial growth factor isoforms (VEGF): Differential deposition into the subepithelial extracellular matrix and bioactivity of extracellular matrix-bound VEGF. Molecular Biology of the Cell 1993;4:1317–1326.
32. Keyt BA, Berleau LT, Nguyen HV, et al. The carboxyl-terminal domain (111–165) of vascular endothelial growth factor is critical for its mitogenic potency. Journal of Biological Chemistry 1996;271(13):7788–7795.
33. Lee S, Jilani SM, Nikolova GV, et al. Processing of VEGF-A by matrix metalloproteinases regulates bioavailability and vascular patterning in tumors. J Cell Biol 2005;169(4):681–691.
34. Shibuya M, Yamaguchi S, Yamane A, et al. Nucleotide sequence and expression of a novel human receptor-type tyrosine kinase (flt) closely related to the fms family. Oncogene 1990;8:519–527.
35. Terman BI, Dougher-Vermazen M, Carrion ME, et al. Identification of the KDR tyrosine kinase as a receptor for vascular endothelial cell growth factor. Biochemical & Biophysical Research Communications 1992;187(3):1579–1586.
36. de Vries C, Escobedo JA, Ueno H, et al. The fms-like tyrosine kinase, a receptor for vascular endothelial growth factor. Science 1992;255(5047): 989–991.
37. Davis-Smyth T, Chen H, Park J, et al. The second immunoglobulin-like domain of the VEGF tyrosine kinase receptor Flt-1 determines ligand binding and may initiate a signal transduction cascade. EMBO Journal 1996;15(18):4919–4927.
38. Holash J, Davis S, Papadopoulos N, et al. VEGF-Trap: a VEGF blocker with potent antitumor effects. Proc Natl Acad Sci USA 2002;99(17): 11393–11398.
39. Park JE, Chen HH, Winer J, et al. Placenta growth factor. Potentiation of vascular endothelial growth factor bioactivity, *in vitro* and *in vivo*, and high affinity binding to Flt-1 but not to Flk-1/KDR. J Biol Chem 1994;269(41):25646–25654 issn: 0021–9258.
40. Olofsson B, Korpelainen E, Pepper MS, et al. Vascular endothelial growth factor B (VEGF-B) binds to VEGF receptor-1 and regulates plasminogen activator activity in endothelial cells. Proc Natl Acad Sci USA 1998;95(20):11709–11714.
41. LeCouter J, Moritz DR, Li B, et al. Angiogenesis-independent endothelial protection of liver: role of VEGFR-1. Science 2003;299: 890–893.
42. Hiratsuka S, Nakamura K, Iwai S, et al. MMP9 induction by vascular endothelial growth factor receptor-1 is involved in lung-specific metastasis. Cancer Cell 2002;2(4):289–300.
43. Hattori K, Heissig B, Wu Y, et al. Placental growth factor reconstitutes hematopoiesis by recruiting VEGFR1(+) stem cells from bone-marrow microenvironment. Nat Med 2002;8(8):841–849.
44. Barleon B, Sozzani S, Zhou D, et al. Migration of human monocytes in response to vascular endothelial growth factor (VEGF) is mediated via the VEGF receptor flt-1. Blood 1996;87(8):3336–3343.
45. Quinn TP, Peters KG, De Vries C, et al. Fetal liver kinase 1 is a receptor for vascular endothelial growth factor and is selectively expressed in vascular endothelium. Proc Natl Acad Sci USA 1993;90(16): 7533–7537.
46. Shalaby F, Rossant J, Yamaguchi TP, et al. Failure of blood-island formation and vasculogenesis in Flk-1-deficient mice. Nature 1995;376(6535):62–66.
47. Olsson AK, Dimberg A, Kreuger J, et al. VEGF receptor signalling – in control of vascular function. Nat Rev Mol Cell Biol 2006;7(5): 359–371.
48. Soker S, Takashima S, Miao HQ, et al. Neuropilin-1 is expressed by endothelial and tumor cells as an isoform-specific receptor for vascular endothelial growth factor. Cell 1998;92(6):735–745.
49. Okada F, Rak JW, Croix BS, et al. Impact of oncogenes in tumor angiogenesis: mutant K-ras up-regulation of vascular endothelial growth factor/vascular permeability factor is necessary, but not sufficient for tumorigenicity of human colorectal carcinoma cells. Proc Natl Acad Sci USA 1998;95(7):3609–3614.
50. Lonser RR, Glenn GM, Walther M, et al. von Hippel–Lindau disease. Lancet 2003;361(9374):2059–2067.
51. Kim KJ, Li B, Winer J, et al. Inhibition of vascular endothelial growth factor-induced angiogenesis suppresses tumor growth *in vivo*. Nature 1993;362:841–844.

52. Manley PW, Martiny-Baron G, Schlaeppi JM, et al. Therapies directed at vascular endothelial growth factor. Expert Opin Investig Drugs 2002;11(12):1715–1736.
53. Prewett M, Huber J, Li Y, et al. Antivascular endothelial growth factor receptor (fetal liver kinase 1) monoclonal antibody inhibits tumor angiogenesis. Cancer Res 1999;59:5209–5218.
54. Gerber HP, Kowalski J, Sherman D, et al. Complete inhibition of rhabdomyosarcoma xenograft growth and neovascularization requires blockade of both tumor and host vascular endothelial growth factor. Cancer Res 2000;60:6253–6258.
55. Dong J, Grunstein J, Tejada M, et al. VEGF-null cells require PDGFR alpha signaling-mediated stromal fibroblast recruitment for tumorigenesis. EMBO J 2004;23:2800–2810.
56. Tejada M, Yu L, Dong J, et al. Tumor-driven paracrine PDGF receptor-a signaling is a key determinant of stromal cell recruitment in a model of human lung carcinoma. Clin Cancer Res 2006;12:2676–2688.
57. Klement G, Baruchel S, Rak J, et al. Continuous low-dose therapy with vinblastine and VEGF receptor-2 antibody induces sustained tumor regression without overt toxicity [see comments]. Journal of Clinical Investigation 2000;105(8):R15–R24.
58. Lee CG, Heijn M, di Tomaso E, et al. Anti-vascular endothelial growth factor treatment augments tumor radiation response under normoxic or hypoxic conditions. Cancer Res 2000;60:5565–5570.
59. Jain RK. Normalization of tumor vasculature: an emerging concept in antiangiogenic therapy. Science 2005;307(5706):58–62.
60. Presta LG, Chen H, O'Connor SJ, et al. Humanization of an anti-VEGF monoclonal antibody for the therapy of solid tumors and other disorders. Cancer Res 1997;57:4593–4599.
61. Ferrara N, Hillan KJ, Gerber HP, et al. Discovery and development of bevacizumab, an anti-VEGF antibody for treating cancer. Nat Rev Drug Discov 2004;3(5):391–400.
62. Gasparini G, Longo R, Toi M, et al. Angiogenic inhibitors: a new therapeutic strategy in oncology. Nat Clin Pract Oncol 2005;2(11): 562–577.
63. Ferrara N, Kerbel RS. Angiogenesis as a therapeutic target. Nature 2005;438:967–974.
64. Jain RK, Duda DG, Clark JW, et al. Lessons from phase III clinical trials on anti-VEGF therapy for cancer. Nat Clin Pract Oncol 2006;3(1):24–40.
65. Miller JW, Adamis AP, Shima DT, et al. Vascular endothelial growth factor/vascular permeability factor is temporally and spatially correlated with ocular angiogenesis in a primate model. Am J Pathol 1994;145(3): 574–584.
66. Safran M, Kaelin WJ Jr. HIF hydroxylation and the mammalian oxygen-sensing pathway. J Clin Invest 2003;111:779–783.
67. Aiello LP, Avery RL, Arrigg PG, et al. Vascular endothelial growth factor in ocular fluid of patients with diabetic retinopathy and other retinal disorders [see comments]. New England Journal of Medicine 1994;331(22): 1480–1487.
68. Malecaze F, Clemens S, Simorer-Pinotel V, et al. Detection of vascular endothelial growth factor mRNA and vascular endothelial growth factor-like activity in proliferative diabetic retinopathy. Archives of Ophthalmology 1994;112:1476–1482.
69. Aiello LP, Pierce EA, Foley ED, et al. Suppression of retinal neovascularization *in vivo* by inhibition of vascular endothelial growth factor (VEGF) using soluble VEGF-receptor chimeric proteins. Proc Natl Acad Sci USA 1995;92(23):10457–10461.
70. Adamis AP, Shima DT, Tolentino MJ, et al. Inhibition of vascular endothelial growth factor prevents retinal ischemia-associated iris neovascularization in a nonhuman primate. Arch Ophthalmol 1996;114(1):66–71.
71. Ozaki H, Seo MS, Ozaki K, et al. Blockade of vascular endothelial cell growth factor receptor signaling is sufficient to completely prevent retinal neovascularization. American Journal of Pathology 2000;156(2):697–707.
72. Congdon N, O'Colmain B, Klaver CC, et al. Causes and prevalence of visual impairment among adults in the United States. Arch Ophthalmol 2004;122(4):477–485.
73. Ferris FL 3rd, Fine SL, Hyman L. Age-related macular degeneration and blindness due to neovascular maculopathy. Arch Ophthalmol 1984;102(11):1640–1642.
74. Photodynamic therapy of subfoveal choroidal neovascularization in age-related macular degeneration with verteporfin. One-year results of 2 randomized clinical trials – TAP report 1. Arch Ophthalmol 1999;117:1329–1345.
75. Gragoudas ES, Adamis AP, Cunningham ET Jr, et al. Pegaptanib for neovascular age-related macular degeneration. N Engl J Med 2004;351(27):2805–2816.
76. Ferrara N, Damico L, Shams N, et al. Developmemt of ranibizumab, an anti-vascular endothelial growth factor antigen binding fragment, as therapy for neovascular age-related macular degeneration. Retina 2006;26:859–870.
77. Andreoli CM, Miller JW. Anti-vascular endothelial growth factor therapy for ocular neovascular disease. Curr Opin Ophthalmol 2007;18(6): 502–508.
78. Jager RD, Mieler WF, Miller JW. Age-related macular degeneration. N Engl J Med 2008;358(24):2606–2617.
79. Pieramici DJ, Rabena MD. Anti-VEGF therapy: comparison of current and future agents. Eye 2008.
80. Ng EW, Sima DT, Calias P, et al. Pegaptanib, a targeted anti-VEGF aptamer for ocular vascular disease. Nat Rev Drug Discov 2006;5:123–132.
81. Chen Y, Wiesmann C, Fuh G, et al. Selection and analysis of an optimized anti-VEGF antibody: crystal structure of an affinity-matured Fab in complex with antigen. Journal of Molecular Biology 1999;293(4): 865–881.
82. Rosenfeld PJ, Brown DM, Heier JS, et al. Ranibizumab for neovascular age-related macular degeneration. N Engl J Med 2006;355:1419–1431.
83. Brown DM, Kaiser PK, Michels M, et al. Ranibizumab versus verteporfin for neovascular age-related macular degeneration. N Engl J Med 2006;355(14):1432–1444.
84. Brown DM, Michels M, Kaiser PK, et al. Ranibizumab versus verteporfin photodynamic therapy for neovascular age-related macular degeneration: two-year results of the ANCHOR study. Ophthalmology 2009;116(1):57–65 e5.
85. Michels S, Rosenfeld PJ, Puliafito CA, et al. Systemic bevacizumab (Avastin) therapy for neovascular age-related macular degeneration: twelve-week results of an uncontrolled open-label clinical study. Ophthalmology 2005;112(6):1035–1047.
86. Rosenfeld PJ, Moshfeghi AA, Puliafito CA. Optical coherence tomography findings after an intravitreal injection of bevacizumab (Avastin) for neovascular age-related macular degeneration. Ophthalmic Surg Lasers Imaging 2005;36(4):331–335.
87. Avery RL, Pieramici DJ, Rabena MD, et al. Intravitreal bevacizumab (Avastin) for neovascular age-related macular degeneration. Ophthalmology 2006;113:363–372.
88. la Cour M. Intravitreal VEGF-inhibitors: is Avastin a generic substitute for Lucentis? Acta Ophthalmol Scand 2007;85(1):2–4.
89. Michels S, Schmidt-Erfurth U, Rosenfeld PJ. Promising new treatments for neovascular age-related macular degeneration. Expert Opin Investig Drugs 2006;15(7):779–793.
90. Nguyen QD, Shah SM, Hafiz G, et al. A phase I trial of an IV-administered vascular endothelial growth factor trap for treatment in patients with choroidal neovascularization due to age-related macular degeneration. Ophthalmology 2006;113:1522.e1–1522.e14.
91. Tolentino MJ, Brucker AJ, Fosnot J, et al. Intravitreal injection of vascular endothelial growth factor small interfering RNA inhibits growth and leakage in a nonhuman primate, laser-induced model of choroidal neovascularization. Retina 2004;24(4):660.
92. Shen J, Samul R, Silva RL, et al. Suppression of ocular neovascularization with siRNA targeting VEGF receptor 1. Gene Ther 2006;13:225–234.
93. The effect of ruboxistaurin on visual loss in patients with moderately severe to very severe nonproliferative diabetic retinopathy initial results of the Protein Kinase C β inhibitor Diabetic Retinopathy Study (PKC-DRS) multicenter randomized clinical trial. The PKC-DRS Study Group. Diabetes 2005;54:2188–2197.
94. Beenken A, Mohammadi M. The FGF family: biology, pathophysiology and therapy. Nat Rev Drug Discov 2009;8(3):235–253.
95. Bikfalvi A, Klein S, Pintucci G, et al. Biological roles of fibroblast growth factor-2. Endocrine Reviews 1997;18(1):26–45.
96. Casanovas O, Hicklin DJ, Bergers G, et al. Drug resistance by evasion of antiangiogenic targeting of VEGF signaling in late-stage pancreatic islet tumors. Cancer Cell 2005;8(4):299–309.
97. Batchelor TT, Sorensen AG, di Tomaso E, et al. AZD2171, a pan-VEGF receptor tyrosine kinase inhibitor, normalizes tumor vasculature and alleviates edema in glioblastoma patients. Cancer Cell 2007;11(1): 83–95.
98. Maglione D, Guerriero V, Viglietto G, et al. Isolation of a human placenta cDNA coding for a protein related to the vascular permeability factor. Proc Natl Acad Sci USA 1991;88(20):9267–9271.
99. Carmeliet P, Moons L, Luttun A, et al. Synergism between vascular endothelial growth factor and placental growth factor contributes to angiogenesis and plasma extravasation in pathological conditions. Nat Med 2001;7(5):575–583.
100. Motzer RJ, Dror Michaelson M, Redman BG, et al. Activity of SU11248, a multitargeted inhibitor of vascular endothelial growth factor receptor and platelet-derived growth factor receptor, in patients with metastatic renal cell carcinoma. J Clin Oncol 2006;24:16–24.
101. Fischer C, Jonckx B, Mazzone M, et al. Anti-PlGF inhibits growth of VEGF(R)-inhibitor-resistant tumors without affecting healthy vessels. Cell 2007;131(3):463–475.
102. Ebos JM, Lee CR, Christensen JG, et al. Multiple circulating proangiogenic factors induced by sunitinib malate are tumor-independent and correlate with antitumor efficacy. Proc Natl Acad Sci USA 2007;104: 17069–17074.
103. Shojaei F, Wu X, Malik AK, et al. Tumor refractoriness to anti-VEGF treatment is mediated by CD11b+Gr1+ myeloid cells. Nature Biotechnology 2007;25:911–920.
104. Dufraine J, Funahashi Y, Kitajewski J. Notch signaling regulates tumor angiogenesis by diverse mechanisms. Oncogene 2008;27(38):5132–5137.
105. Hellstrom M, Phng LK, Hofmann JJ, et al. Dll4 signalling through Notch1 regulates formation of tip cells during angiogenesis. Nature 2007;445: 776–780.
106. Mailhos C, Modlich U, Lewis J, et al. Delta4, an endothelial specific notch ligand expressed at sites of physiological and tumor angiogenesis. Differentiation; research in biological diversity 2001;69(2–3):135–144.

107. Noguera-Troise I, Daly C, Papadopoulos NJ, et al. Blockade of Dll4 inhibits tumour growth by promoting non-productive angiogenesis. Nature 2006;444(7122):1032–1037.
108. Ridgway J, Zhang G, Wu Y, et al. Inhibition of Dll4 signalling inhibits tumour growth by deregulating angiogenesis. Nature 2006;444(7122):1083–1087.
109. Hurwitz H, Fehrenbacher L, Novotny W, et al. Bevacizumab plus irinotecan, fluorouracil, and leucovorin for metastatic colorectal cancer. N Engl J Med 2004;350:2335–2342.
110. Giantonio BJ, Catalano PJ, Meropol NJ, et al. Bevacizumab in combination with oxaliplatin, fluorouracil, and leucovorin (FOLFOX4) for previously treated metastatic colorectal cancer: results from the Eastern Cooperative Oncology Group Study E3200. J Clin Oncol 2007;25(12):1539–1544.
111. Sandler A, Gray R, Perry MC, et al. Paclitaxel-carboplatin alone or with bevacizumab for non-small-cell-lung cancer. N Engl J Med 2006;355:2542–2550.
112. Miller K, Wang M, Gralow J, et al. Paclitaxel plus bevacizumab versus paclitaxel alone for metastatic breast cancer. N Engl J Med 2007;357(26):2666–2676.
113. Faivre S, Demetri G, Sargent W, et al. Molecular basis for sunitinib efficacy and future clinical development. Nat Rev Drug Discov 2007;6(9):734–745.
114. Escudier B, Eisen T, Stadler WM, et al. Sorafenib in advanced clear-cell renal-cell carcinoma. N Engl J Med 2007;356(2):125–134.
115. Kerbel RS, Yu J, Tran J, et al. Possible mechanisms of acquired resistance to anti-angiogenic drugs: implications for the use of combination therapy approaches. Cancer Metastasis Rev 2001;20(1–2):79–86.
116. Shojaei F, Wu X, Zhong C, et al. Bv8 regulates myeloid cell-dependent tumour angiogenesis. Nature 2007;450:825–831.
117. Shojaei F, Singh M, Thompson JD, et al. Role of Bv8 in neutrophil-dependent angiogenesis in a transgenic model of cancer progression. Proc Natl Acad Sci USA 2008 105:2640–2645.
118. Shojaei F, Zhong C, Wu X, et al. Role of myeloid cells in tumor angiogenesis and growth. Trends Cell Biology 2008 18:372–378.
119. Zhou J, Pham L, Zhang N, et al. Neutrophils promote experimental choroidal neovascularization. Mol Vis 2005;11:414–424.
120. Jubb AM, Hurwitz HI, Bai W, et al. Impact of vascular endothelial growth factor-A expression, thrombospondin-2 expression, and microvessel density on the treatment effect of bevacizumab in metastatic colorectal cancer. J Clin Oncol 2006;24:217–227.
121. Nguyen QD, Tatlipinar S, Shah SM, et al. Vascular endothelial growth factor is a critical stimulus for diabetic macular edema. Am J Ophthalmol 2006;142:961–969.
122. Campochiaro PA, Hafiz G, Shah SM, et al. Ranibizumab for macular edema due to retinal vein occlusions; implication of VEGF as a critical stimulator. Mol Ther 2008;16:791–799.
123. Akiyama H, Kachi S, Silva RL, et al. Intraocular injection of an aptamer that binds PDGF-B: a potential treatment for proliferative retinopathies. J Cell Physiol 2006;207(2):407–412.

CHAPTER 35

Biologic therapies: infliximab, adalimumab, etanercept, daclizumab, and others

Steven Yeh, MD and Robert B. Nussenblatt, MD, MPH

KEY FEATURES

The biologic agents, a group of therapeutic agents targeting mediators of inflammation including soluble factors (e.g., cytokines, chemokines), cytokine/chemokine receptors, and immune cell surface markers, have been increasingly used in the treatment of ocular inflammatory diseases. As the pathogenic mechanisms underlying uveitis and ocular inflammation continue to be uncovered, the indications for specific immunomodulatory agents such as the biologic agents will likely continue to expand.

INTRODUCTION

The development of experimental models of uveitis, particularly experimental autoimmune uveitis (EAU), has been particularly helpful in the study of the mechanisms underlying uveitis and in novel therapeutic agents. Clinical studies evaluating the aqueous, vitreous, and serum factors of patients have also provided valuable information about the various soluble and cellular mediators of inflammation in specific disease entities. Several agents have been designed to antagonize the action of tumor necrosis factor-α (TNF-α), and have been used for the treatment of ocular inflammatory diseases. These agents include infliximab, adalimumab, and etanercept. The interleukin-2 (IL-2) receptor antagonist daclizumab has also been utilized for the successful treatment of endogenous uveitis. Several other biologic agents, including alemtuzumab and anakinra, have also been reported in some series for ocular inflammatory diseases. This chapter will focus on the pharmacology, indications, contraindications, and side-effects associated with the TNF-α antagonists, IL-2 receptor antagonist daclizumab, and other biologic agents, which have been used for the treatment of uveitis.

TUMOR NECROSIS FACTOR-ALPHA ANTAGONISTS

In EAU, histologic studies have demonstrated a uveal infiltration of macrophages and T cells, resulting in an inflammatory cytokine and cellular milieu with subsequent loss of tissue architecture and function. TNF-α appears to be a key inflammatory cytokine involved in EAU[1] and its presence has also been detected in the aqueous humor of uveitis patients.[2] Thus, TNF-α inhibition is an attractive target for therapy. Three TNF-α inhibitors – infliximab, adalimumab, and etanercept – have been approved by the Food and Drug Administration (FDA) for systemic autoimmune indications, and all of these agents have been used for the treatment of ocular inflammatory diseases.

INFLIXIMAB (REMICADE)

Pharmacology and mechanism

Infliximab is a mouse-derived chimeric monoclonal antibody, which antagonizes TNF-α. Its inhibition is mediated via interference of TNF binding to two known receptors – TNFr1, which binds to soluble TNF, and TNFr2, which binds to membrane-bound TNF.

A mean terminal half-life between 9 and 12 days has been reported at doses between 5 and 20 mg/kg. Following its administration, infliximab has been detected in most patient sera from 8 to 12 weeks after infusion.[3] Interestingly, in a study of infliximab for rheumatoid arthritis (RA), patients with shorter elimination half-lives of infliximab were less responsive to the medication than those patients with longer elimination half-lives, which may explain, in part, the differential efficacy of this medication amongst patients.[4]

Infliximab is administered via intravenous infusion in doses ranging from 3 to 20 mg/kg for both systemic and ophthalmic indications. Most studies in systemic autoimmune diseases have reported dosing intervals varying from 4- to 8-week dosing intervals. In the ophthalmic literature, doses vary from 3 to 10 mg/kg/dose; however, higher doses of infliximab have been reported for the treatment of refractory pediatric uveitis.

Systemic indications for infliximab

Initially reported in a group of patients with RA,[5] the efficacy of infliximab has been reported for a number of rheumatic diseases, including additional randomized controlled clinical trials for RA,[6,7] Crohn's disease,[8,9] ulcerative colitis,[10] ankylosing spondylitis,[11] and psoriatic arthritis.[12] In pediatric patients, the use of infliximab has been investigated in Crohn's disease[13] and polyarticular juvenile RA.[14] In one study comparing the efficacy of infliximab versus etanercept for RA patients who had responded incompletely to etanercept, a numerical response towards efficacy with infliximab was observed, although this study was underpowered to detect a significant difference between groups.[15]

Ophthalmic indications for infliximab

The efficacy of infliximab has been evaluated for a number of ophthalmic inflammatory diseases (Table 35.1). A paucity of prospective clinical trial data is available for infliximab use in ocular disease; however, its efficacy has been demonstrated for select conditions in a number of case reports and small case series. Conditions for which infliximab has been used include Behçet's disease-associated panuveitis[16] and retinal vasculitis (as illustrated in Figure 35.1), juvenile idiopathic arthritis (JIA)-associated uveitis, human leukocyte antigen (HLA)-B27-associated uveitis, scleritis, and peripheral ulcerative keratitis.

Suhler et al.[17] reported their experience in a prospective, phase II, open-label study of infliximab for refractory autoimmune uveitis. The various diagnoses from their series included pars planitis, sarcoidosis, Crohn's disease, and Behçet's disease. Infliximab was administered in 3- or 5-mg/kg doses via intravenous infusion at weeks 0, 2, and 6 with clinical assessment at week-10 follow-up. A total of 18 (78%) of 23 patients treated with infliximab met clinical criteria for success at the week-10 visit (i.e., improved visual acuity, two-step decrease in intraocular inflammation, ability to taper immunosuppression, or decrease in inflammatory signs by optical coherence tomography or fluorescein angiography). Of the 14 patients maintained on infliximab therapy for a full year, 7 (50%) patients maintained successful grades. However, the number of adverse events observed in their series was concerning and

Table 35.1 **Selected reports on infliximab for uveitis**

Authors	No. of patients	Diagnoses	Dosage	Efficacy outcomes	Follow-up	Adverse events
Sfikakis et al.[114]	5	BD (5)	5 mg/kg × 1 dose	5/5 remissions at 1 week	28 days	None reported
Joseph et al.[26]	5	BD (3), idiopathic PU (2)	5 mg/kg at week 0, 2, and 6	4/5 remissions at 6 months	6–7 months	Ocular and systemic TB
Abu El-Asrar et al.[19]	6	BD (6)	5 mg/kg at week 0, 2, 6, then q 8 weeks	6/6 remissions at 2 months; 3/6 sustained remission; 3/6 relapsed requiring more infusions or more frequent dosing	23 months (mean)	ANA positivity (2)
Lindstedt et al.[24]	13	BD (6), idiopathic PU (5), sarcoidosis (1), BRC (1)	200 mg (~3 mg/kg)	13/13 effective VA ↑ in 5/6 BD	2 years or greater	Rash, atopic dermatitis
Tugal-Tutkun et al.[20]	13	BD (13)	5 mg/kg at week 0, 2, 6 and 14	Fewer attacks and lower prednisone dose during infusion period (weeks 0–22) versus observation period (weeks 23–54)	12 months	URI, infusion reaction, no serious adverse events
Suhler et al.[17]	23	Idiopathic IU (6), pars planitis/IU (2), idiopathic PU (3), sarcoidosis PU (3), BRC (3), MFC (1), Crohn's PU (1), BD (4)	3–5 mg/kg at week 0, 2, and 6	18 (78%) clinical success at week 10 (i.e., improved VA, decreased inflammation, decreased IMT, improved FA); 7/14 (50%) clinical success at 12-month endpoint	12 months	Pulmonary embolus, CHF, lupus-like reaction (2), VH (2), ANA positivity (15/20)
Accorinti et al.[21]	12	BD (12)	5 mg/kg at week 0, 2, then q month for 4–6 months	11/12 (92%) showed reduction in relapses; 11/11 reduced IMT	15 months (median)	Pulmonary TB, HSV keratitis, nonocular HSV infection, recurrent UTIs
Niccoli et al.[18]	12	BD (12)	1 mg/kg prednisolone, 5 mg/kg × 9 infusions over 12 months	9/12 CR (12 months) 7/9 CR (24 months)	12 months (12 patients) 24 months (9 patients)	Headache, mild hypotension, URI (4)
Kahn et al.[31]	17	JIA (10), VKH (2), sarcoidosis (2), idiopathic (3)	10–20 mg/kg	13/17 patients with no inflammation after second infusion; remaining 4 patients in remission after 3–7 infusions; all patients decreased IMT	3–34 months	ANA-positive (2)

BD, Behçet's disease; PU, posterior uveitis; TB, tuberculosis; ANA, antinuclear antibodies; PU, panuveitis; BRC, birdshot retinochoroidopathy; VA, visual acuity; URI, upper respiratory infection; IU, intermediate uveitis; MFC, multifocal choroiditis; VA, visual acuity; IMT, immunomodulatory therapy; FA, fluorescein angiogram; CHF, congestive heart failure; VH, vitreous hemorrhage; HSV, herpes simplex virus; UTI, urinary tract infection; CR, complete remission; JIA, juvenile idiopathic arthritis; VKH, Vogt Koyanagi Harada syndrome.

included congestive heart failure, pulmonary embolus, lupus-like reaction, and vitreous hemorrhage in 2 patients. Antinuclear antibodies were also identified in 15 (75%) of 20 patients who received more than three infusions. Based on this study, the authors recommended additional long-term studies to assess further the safety and efficacy of infliximab for ophthalmic inflammatory diseases.

Niccoli et al.[18] prospectively evaluated the efficacy of infliximab for Behçet's disease-associated posterior uveitis, which had failed therapy with at least one immunosuppressive medication prior to enrollment. In their series of 12 Behçet's disease patients, results were encouraging, with 9 (75%) patients demonstrating a complete remission at 12-month follow-up. The total number of ocular attacks across all patients decreased from 40 in the year prior to infliximab therapy to five attacks in the year following cessation of infliximab.[18] Abu El-Asrar et al.[19] reported their experience with infliximab for refractory Behçet's disease-associated uveitis in 6 patients who had each failed at least one

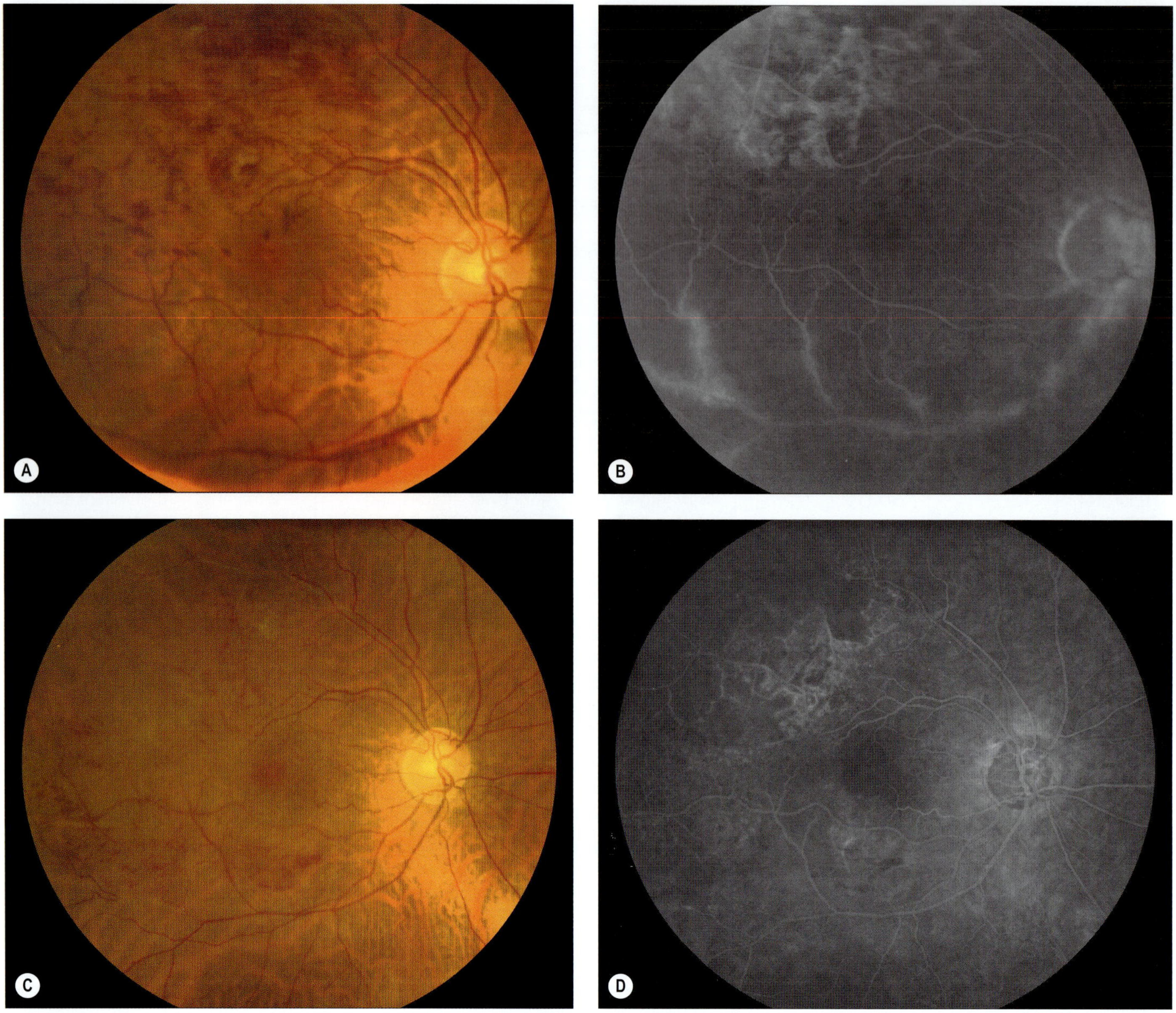

Figure 35.1 Fundus photograph of patient with idiopathic retinal vasculitis and a history of bilateral, consecutive branch retinal vein occlusions (A). Fluorescein angiogram shows segmental hyperfluorescence of inferotemporal arcade (B). Following infliximab therapy, most retinal hemorrhages have resolved (C), as well as retinal vasculitis along inferotemporal arcade (D). The sequelae of branch retinal vein occlusions are observed inferotemporally.

other immunosuppressive medication. In this small prospective trial, patients were treated with infliximab at a dosage of 5 mg/kg infusions at weeks 0, 2, 6, and every 8 weeks thereafter. All 6 patients achieved remission by the 2-month time period and 3 patients remained relapse-free during the follow-up period (range, 16–36 months, mean, 23.6 months). From their study, it appeared that long-term remission could be maintained by repeated infusions.[19]

Tugal-Tutkun et al.[20] reported encouraging results from a prospective trial of infliximab for Behçet's disease-associated uveitis resistant to azathioprine, cyclosporine, and corticosteroids. Thirteen male patients were treated with infliximab (5 mg/kg) at weeks 0, 2, 6, and 14 in this trial, and uveitis exacerbations were documented during an infusion period (weeks 0–22) and observation period (weeks 23–54). One patient demonstrated a sustained remission with no ocular attacks during both infusion and observation periods, and 4 patients (30.8%) demonstrated remission during the infusion period. During the observation period, 36 attacks of uveitis in 12 patients were documented, and the treatment protocol was amended to allow the reinstitution of infliximab infusions because of the severity of sight-threatening ocular attacks. Three of the 12 patients required the reinstitution of infliximab therapy. Of note, the mean daily corticosteroid requirement and mean number of uveitis attacks were lower in the infusion period compared to the observation period (weeks 23–54). No serious adverse events were reported in this study.

Accorinti et al.[21] also described their experience with infliximab in 12 patients with Behçet's disease-associated ocular inflammatory disease. Of the 12 patients in their series, 11 patients demonstrated a decrease in the number of ocular relapses per month in the follow-up period. In addition, all 11 patients on corticosteroids prior to therapy were able to decrease their daily corticosteroid requirement. Significant side-effects observed included tuberculosis, herpetic keratitis, severe nonocular herpetic infection, and recurrent urinary tract infections. Two of these 4 patients experienced uveitic exacerbations when infliximab infusions were delayed because of these side-effects. Thus, while infliximab appeared to benefit some patients, infectious complications possibly related to the medication in this series were concerning.[21]

Other retrospective studies have supported the efficacy of infliximab for Behçet's disease-associated panuveitis and retinal vasculitis.[22–26] Outcome measures have differed between these retrospective case series, making comparisons between studies difficult. Improvement in visual acuity, decreased intraocular inflammation, and reduction of daily corticosteroid requirements have been reported. However, the development of ocular and systemic tuberculosis in 1 patient[26] and an episode of thoracic herpes zoster in another patient[25] required systemic antimicrobial therapy.

Besides Behçet's disease-associated uveitis, sarcoid-associated uveitis has also been treated successfully with infliximab therapy. Cruz et al.[27] reported the successful use of infliximab (3 mg/kg infusions given at day 0, week 2, and week 6) in 2 patients with retinal vasculitis and multisystem sarcoidosis. Other patients with sarcoid-associated uveitis have also experienced therapeutic benefit with infliximab.[17,24,28]

Other retrospective case series have reported a therapeutic benefit of infliximab for JIA-associated uveitis.[29,30] Richards et al.[30] reported improved control of intraocular inflammation in 6 of 6 patients treated with infliximab and maintenance low-dose immunosuppression. This study suggested a role for infliximab as adjunctive therapy in JIA-associated uveitis. Rajaraman et al.[29] also evaluated infliximab for pediatric uveitis due to a variety of etiologies, including JIA-associated uveitis (3 patients), pars planitis (1 patient), retinal vasculitis (1 patient), and idiopathic uveitis (1 patient). All patients demonstrated improvements in intraocular inflammation while on infliximab and 5 of 6 patients were able to wean completely off corticosteroid therapy by the end of the study period evaluated (mean follow-up 48 weeks). Vitreous hemorrhage developed in 1 patient while another patient experienced a transient upper respiratory infusion reaction.

The use of high-dose infliximab (10–20 mg/kg) for pediatric patients with refractory uveitis was reported by Kahn et al.[31] In 17 patients evaluated, 13 individuals demonstrated quiescence of inflammation following two infliximab infusions, and the remaining 4 patients achieved this outcome after three to seven infusions. All patients receiving oral steroids before therapy discontinued steroid treatment over a period varying between 2 weeks and 2 years, and 15 of 17 patients were tapered off topical corticosteroids. No significant adverse events were noted, although 2 patients developed autoantibody formation (i.e., positive antinuclear antibody or anti-dsDNA), although no features of lupus were noted in either patient.[31]

One prospective noncomparative case series of infliximab as monotherapy for HLA-B27-associated anterior uveitis demonstrated a rapid decrease in anterior-chamber inflammation in 7 patients treated with infliximab (10 mg/kg) infusions.[32] However, 1 patient required a second infusion after 3 weeks because of a flare-up, and median time to relapse in the 4 patients was 5 ± 6.4 months.

Besides these reports of its efficacy for intraocular inflammation, infliximab has also been successfully utilized for the treatment of scleritis and peripheral ulcerative keratitis due to a variety of etiologies, including Wegener's granulomatosis, RA, and relapsing polychondritis.[33–37] The efficacy of infliximab for posterior scleritis in a pediatric patient has also been reported.[30]

Contraindications

Infliximab is contraindicated in patients with known hypersensitivity to known murine proteins or any component of infliximab.[39] Infliximab is also contraindicated in patients with New York Heart Association class III or IV congestive heart failure.

Ocular complications and toxicity

Ocular complications attributed to infliximab therapy have rarely been reported in the literature; however, recurrence of disease following infliximab cessation has been reported and should be discussed with patients prior to discontinuation of medication.[20,32] Herpetic keratitis,[21] vitreous hemorrhage,[17,29] optic neuritis,[40] and ocular tuberculosis[26] have been reported during infliximab therapy.

Systemic complications and toxicity

A number of systemic complications have been associated with infliximab therapy, the most concerning of which include reactivation of latent tuberculosis, exacerbation of congestive heart failure, unmasking of demyelinating disease, the development of autoantibody formation (i.e., antinuclear antibodies, anti-dsDNA antibodies), and the formation of anti-infliximab antibodies.[41] In the pediatric population, reports of hepatosplenic T-cell lymphoma following infliximab therapy for Crohn's disease have been extremely concerning.[42] The possible contribution of anti-TNF therapy to increased lymphoma risk in RA patients is unclear at this time. Increased risk of lymphoma has been associated with RA independent of anti-TNF therapy, but further studies are needed.[43–46] Severe hepatotoxicity complicating infliximab therapy has also been reported both with and without concomitant use of other medications with known hepatotoxicity.[47] Thoracic herpes zoster, herpetic keratitis, nonocular herpetic infection, and optic neuritis have also been reported rarely following infliximab therapy for ophthalmic disease.

Drug interactions

Specific drug interactions, including interactions of infliximab with methotrexate, have not been studied extensively. However, many patients with RA or Crohn's disease have been on other immunosuppressive medications in combination with infliximab. RA patients have been treated with infliximab and methotrexate whereas Crohn's disease patients have been treated with infliximab while concomitantly using a number of other medications, including antibiotics, antivirals, corticosteroids, 6-mercaptopurine, azathioprine, and aminosalicylates.[39]

Summary

Infliximab, a mouse–human chimeric monoclonal antibody targeting TNF-α, has been utilized successfully for the treatment of a number of systemic autoimmune conditions, including RA, Crohn's disease, Behçet's disease, and psoriatic arthritis. The efficacy of infliximab for a number of uveitic syndromes, including Behçet's disease-associated panuveitis and retinal vasculitis, JIA-associated anterior uveitis, and HLA-B27-associated uveitis, is supported by limited prospective studies and a number of retrospective case series and interventional case reports. The utility of infliximab for scleritis and peripheral ulcerative keratitis due to a number of etiologies has also been described in several retrospective case series. Currently, doses used by ocular inflammatory specialists range from 3 to 10 mg/kg intravenous infusion, although higher doses of infliximab have been rarely reported. While the efficacy of infliximab for a number of sight-threatening ocular inflammatory syndromes appears promising, a thorough medical workup and caution are advisable because of serious adverse events reported in the literature, including reactivation of latent tuberculosis, unmasking of demyelinating disease, hepatosplenic lymphoma in pediatric patients, lupus-like syndrome, congestive heart failure exacerbations, and the possible association of infliximab with an increased risk of lymphoma in RA patients.

ADALIMUMAB (HUMIRA)

Pharmacology and mechanism

Adalimumab is a fully human, anti-TNF-α IgG_1 monoclonal antibody, which blocks the interaction of TNF-α with p55 and p75 cell surface receptors.

Adalimumab is typically administered as a 20- or 40-mg dose via subcutaneous injection either weekly or every other week. The subcutaneous route of administration may be favorable to infliximab, which requires an intravenous infusion.

The terminal half-life of adalimumab ranges from 15 to 19 days and early phase I trials demonstrated no significant pharmacokinetic advantage to weight-based dosing strategies.[48]

Systemic indications

Adalimumab has been evaluated in a number of clinical trials for RA,[49,50] Crohn's disease,[10,51] ankylosing spondylitis,[52] and psoriatic arthritis.[53,54] Initially evaluated as adjunctive therapy to RA patients on methotrexate, adalimumab demonstrated rapid improvement in American College of Rheumatology 20 scores at 1 week of administration. The PREMIER trial compared combination adalimumab plus methotrexate therapy with either medication given alone and found that the combination of adalimumab plus methotrexate was superior to adalimumab or methotrexate monotherapy.[55]

Ophthalmic indications

The efficacy of adalimumab for uveitis has been reported in several retrospective series for adults and pediatric patients. Its efficacy for Behçet's disease-associated uveitis was reported in two retrospective reports.[56,57] Mushtaq et al. reported 3 patients with Behçet's disease-associated uveitis who were successfully switched from infliximab to adalimumab while in clinical remission. Follow-up was variable in this series, varying from 11 to 24 months; however, intraocular inflammation remained well controlled during the follow-up period. Administration of adalimumab for severe Vogt–Koyanagi–Harada syndrome allowed the successful tapering of corticosteroid and cyclosporine in one case report.[58]

Vazquez-Cobian et al.[59] reported the successful treatment of pediatric uveitis (9 JIA-associated and 5 idiopathic) with adalimumab. In their series, adalimumab was well tolerated with no reports of serious adverse events. A total of 21 of 26 (80%) eyes with inflammation at baseline experienced a decrease in intraocular inflammation while 4 (15%) eyes remained stable and 1 (4%) eye worsened. A decrease in topical corticosteroid use was observed in 11 of 14 patients (79%) while 4 of 14 patients (29%) completely discontinued topical medications. In addition, other corticosteroid-sparing medications were decreased in a number of patients during the period of adalimumab therapy. Another retrospective series by Biester et al.[60] described the efficacy of adalimumab for uveitis in 18 pediatric patients. Seventeen patients were JIA-associated while 1 was idiopathic. Ophthalmic efficacy was demonstrated in 16 of 18 patients (88%). Adalimumab also appeared effective or mildly effective for JIA-associated arthritis in 13 of 16 patients (81%) during the follow-up period.

Contraindications

Adalimumab is contraindicated in patients with known hypersensitivity to the medication or any of its components and in patients at risk for sepsis. In addition, the medication should be avoided in patients with a history of multiple sclerosis, active infection, or malignancy.

Ocular toxicity

Herpes simplex keratitis has been reported in one 5-year-old female patient treated with adalimumab for pauciarticular JIA-assoicated uveitis.[60]

Systemic toxicity

Injection site reactions appear to be the most commonly reported adverse event and occur in up to 10% of patients treated. In an efficacy and safety study of adalimumab for ankylosing spondylitis, the number of adverse events was higher in patients receiving subcutaneous adalimumab 40 every other week than in those receiving placebo. The percentage of patients who experienced infectious complications was higher in the patients receiving adalimumab, but this finding was not statistically significant. No occurrences of latent tuberculosis reactivation, lupus-like syndromes, congestive heart failure, or secondary malignancies were reported.[61] In a postmarketing surveillance study of RA patients, Schiff et al.[62] reported that adalimumab appeared to be relatively safe and well tolerated. In their study, safety data from randomized clinical trials, open-label extensions, phase IIIb trials, and postmarketing reporting of adverse events in the USA were collected. Reported adverse events included serious infections (5.1 events/100 patient-years (PYs)), lymphoma (0.12/100 PYs), tuberculosis (0.27/100 PYs), opportunistic infections (0.08 events/100 PYs), demyelinating diseases (0.08/100 PYs), systemic lupus erythematosis/lupus-like syndrome (0.10/100 PYs), and congestive heart failure (0.28/100 PYs). The incidence of lymphoma did not appear to be significantly higher in patients treated with adalimumab than in RA patients who were naïve to anti-TNF-α therapy; however, the rate of lymphoma may be higher in RA patients compared to the general population, particularly in patients with severe RA. Adverse events reported in patients with ophthalmic inflammatory disease treated with adalimumab have included injection site reactions, herpes simplex keratitis, and elevation of liver enzymes requiring cessation of therapy.[60]

Drug interactions

Adalimumab is currently approved for RA and psoriatic arthritis in combination with methotrexate and low-dose prednisone. Live viruses should be avoided in patients on adalimumab and its use may decrease the immunologic protection conferred by live attenuated vaccines. No clear data are available for its use in combination with other biologic agents, so this combination should be avoided until further studies have demonstrated efficacy and safety.

Summary

Like infliximab, adalimumab has been used successfully in clinical trials for the treatment of RA, Crohn's disease, ankylosing spondylitis, and psoriatic arthritis. Ophthalmic studies are limited, but suggest that this agent may be effective for pediatric uveitis, Behçet's disease-associated uveitis, and other uveitic entities in which TNF-α may play a role. Because it is fully human (cf. chimeric structure of infliximab), it is likely that this medication is less immunogenic than infliximab. The subcutaneous route of administration offers advantages over the intravenous route of infliximab with the inherent risks of intravenous medication administration, as well as the higher costs associated with hospitalization. Further studies are needed to determine its relative efficacy and safety compared to infliximab therapy for ophthalmic inflammatory diseases.

ETANERCEPT (ENBREL)

Pharmacology and mechanism

The third FDA-approved TNF antagonist is etanercept, which differs structurally from the monoclonal antibody structure of infliximab and adalimumab. Etanercept is a recombinant TNF-α receptor fusion protein composed of the constant (Fc) portion of human IgG1 and two copies of the extracellular ligand-binding portion of TNF receptor p75.

Etanercept is given via subcutaneous injection at a dose of 25–50 mg twice weekly. Its elimination half-life is 102 hours following a single subcutaneous dose of 25 mg.[63]

Systemic indications

Etanercept has demonstrated efficacy for a number of systemic autoimmune conditions, including RA,[64,65] JIA,[66] ankylosing spondylitis,[67] and psoriatic arthritis.[68] However, its efficacy in the treatment of ocular inflammatory disease has been variable in limited series.

Ophthalmic indications

Smith et al.[69] reported the results of a randomized, controlled, masked trial of etanercept for JIA-associated anterior uveitis. In their study, no apparent difference in anterior-segment inflammation was observed between etanercept and placebo.[70] Another prospective study of etanercept for pediatric uveitis, including 7 juvenile RA patients, reported a decrease in anterior-chamber inflammation in 10 of 16 affected eyes (63%).[71] Patients in this study were treated with 0.4 mg/kg subcutaneous injection twice weekly for 12 weeks, and the dose was increased to 25 mg twice weekly for patients with an incomplete response. While the majority of eyes experienced an improvement in anterior-chamber cellular reaction at 12 weeks, 7 responses were incomplete at 3-month follow-up, and no further improvement was demonstrated after 6 months of therapy. Mild injection reactions were observed, but no other significant adverse events were reported in their series. The successful use of etanercept for sight-threatening scleritis and sterile corneal ulceration has also been previously reported.[72]

A retrospective study by Guignard et al.[73] evaluated the efficacy of anti-TNF agents for the prevention of uveitic flares. Their study found a decrease in the risk of a uveitic exacerbation in ankylosing spondylitis patients treated with monoclonal antibodies (i.e., infliximab, adalimumab) targeting TNF-α, but no such benefit was observed in patients treated with etanercept. A retrospective comparison of etanercept and infliximab for the treatment of uveitis by Galor et al.[74] was consistent with these findings. In their report, 17 of 18 (94%) patients on infliximab showed a reduction in intraocular inflammation at their final follow-up, whereas 0 of 4 patients on etanercept experienced a reduction in intraocular inflammation. Findings from questionnaires from pediatric rheumatologists regarding the differential efficacy of the TNF-α inhibitors for JIA-associated uveitis therapy and the prevention of uveitic exacerbations have reported greater efficacy of infliximab when compared to etanercept.[75] In addition, although arthritis appeared to respond to therapy in 87% of patients, etanercept did not appear to influence the frequency or severity of uveitis episodes.[76]

Contraindications

Etanercept is contraindicated in patients allergic to the medication or its ingredients. Patients with active infections (chronic or acute), risk of sepsis, medical conditions predisposing patients to infection (e.g., poorly controlled diabetes mellitus), patients less than 4 years old, pregnant women, and nursing mothers should not receive etanercept therapy.[39]

Ocular toxicity

New-onset uveitis and acute exacerbations of ocular inflammatory disease (i.e., scleritis, uveitis, myositis) have been observed in patients treated with etanercept.[77] In one report, flare-ups of ankylosing spondylitis-associated uveitis were temporally associated with etanercept therapy.[78] Four patients receiving etanercept injections have also developed optic neuritis; 3 patients discontinued therapy because of optic neuritis.[79] Tuberculous panuveitis has also been observed in 1 patient treated with etanercept.[80] The question of etanercept-associated eye disease was studied in a retrospective review of 70 patients by Saurenmann et al.[81] In this study, no increased risk of the development of new onset uveitis was found; however, etanercept therapy was unable to prevent the onset of uveitis in 2 patients from their cohort.

Systemic toxicity

The most commonly observed adverse effects in both children and adults have been injection site reactions, infection, headache, rhinitis, and dizziness.[63] Serious infections and tuberculosis have been reported in patients receiving etanercept in postmarketing surveillance. The development of antibodies to etanercept is infrequent (less than 5%); however, reports of the development of autoantibodies and symptoms consistent with lupus-like syndromes have been observed in postmarketing experience. Neurologic events (i.e., new-onset central nervous system demyelinating disorders, seizures) and hematologic toxicities have rarely been reported.[63] Bathon et al.[82] reviewed the serious adverse events and infectious episodes in elderly and younger RA patients from four randomized clinical trials of etanercept for RA. In their report, serious adverse events and infectious episodes tended to be higher in elderly patients than younger patients; however, no difference was observed between patients treated with etanercept and controls (treated with placebo or methotrexate). Of 5815 PYs of etanercept exposure, 4 cases of opportunistic infection (in patients younger than 65 years) and no cases of tuberculosis were observed.

Drug interactions

The efficacy of etanercept combined with methotrexate has been previously demonstrated in patients with RA and psoriasis. Clinical information regarding dosage adjustment in patients with hepatic or renal dysfunction is limited.[47]

Summary

There is currently a paucity of clinical trial data supporting the efficacy of etanercept for intraocular inflammatory disease. While limited retrospective series have described some success in the use of etanercept for scleritis, prospective trials have not demonstrated long-term benefit of etanercept therapy for conditions such as JIA-associated anterior uveitis. While the medication appears to be well tolerated in both adult and pediatric populations, limited efficacy data do not support the use of etanercept as first-line therapy for uveitis at this time.

INTERLEUKIN-2 RECEPTOR ANTAGONIST

DACLIZUMAB (ZENAPAX)

Pharmacology and mechanism

Daclizumab is a humanized monoclonal recombinant IgG_1 antibody targeting Tac, a 55-kDa IL-2α receptor subunit expressed by most T, B, and natural killer (NK) cells following activation by interaction with an antigen or with IL-2. The IL-2 receptor (IL-2R) system is a lymphokine receptor system composed of three subunits (α, β, and γ) and plays a central role in the induction of the immune response. IL-2 binding to its receptor system facilitates antibody formation, cell-mediated immune responses, and NK cell responses. The association of the Tac subunit with IL-2R β and γ subunits forms a high-affinity IL-2R complex, which is a critical step in the activation of all T cells, which are major contributors to autoimmune disease and allograft rejection.

In experimental models of uveoretinitis, IL-2 appears to play a critical role in the pathogenesis of T-cell-mediated intraocular inflammation.[83,84] In a nonhuman primate model of uveitis, administration of humanized anti-Tac[85] markedly reduced intraocular inflammation *in vivo* and reduced T-cell proliferation *in vitro* as well.[86] Greater levels of soluble IL-2 receptor have also been observed in serum and aqueous from uveitis patients when compared to controls.[87,88]

Doses of daclizumab 1 mg/kg in 2–4-week intervals have been reported in published studies to date for ocular inflammatory diseases, as 6-week intervals led to uveitis recurrences. Doses of 2 mg/kg given in 4–5-week intervals via intravenous infusion or subcutaneous injection have been utilized for maintenance immunosuppression in a number of patients.[85]

Systemic indication

Originally approved for the prevention of renal allograft rejection,[89,90] daclizumab has since been used for the prevention of a number of different solid-organ transplant rejection protocols, including pancreatic,[91] cardiac,[92] and liver transplantation.[93,94] Daclizumab has also demonstrated efficacy for the treatment of lymphoma patients with increased IL-2 receptor alpha chain on T cells, including human T-cell lymphotrophic virus (HTLV)-associated adult T-cell leukemia/lymphoma and hairy-cell leukemia. Several case series have demonstrated a benefit of daclizumab for graft-versus-host disease as well.

Ophthalmic indications

Several prospective studies and retrospective case series have reported the use of daclizumab for the successful treatment of intermediate, posterior, and panuveitis (Table 35.2). In the initial nonrandomized, open-label pilot study of daclizumab for uveitis, intravenous daclizumab therapy in up to 4-week intervals allowed the successful tapering of immunosuppressive medication (i.e., corticosteroids, cyclosporine) in 8 of 10 patients enrolled during the first 8 weeks of therapy. Of note, daclizumab prevented the expression of sight-threatening inflammatory disease in these patients treated over a 12-month follow-up period. Uveitic syndromes treated with daclizumab included sarcoidosis, Vogt–Koyanagi–Harada's disease, idiopathic intermediate uveitis, idiopathic panuveitis, and multifocal choroiditis.[70]

A longer-term (>4-year) phase I/II interventional study of intravenous daclizumab and a short-term phase II study using subcutaneous

Table 35.2 Selected reports on interleukin-2 receptor antagonist daclizumab for uveitis

Authors	No. of patients	Diagnoses	Dosage	Efficacy outcomes	Follow-up (months)	Adverse events
Nussenblatt et al.[70]	10	Sarcoidosis (3), idiopathic IU (1), VKH (2), idiopathic PU (1), MFC (1)	1 mg/kg IV q 2 weeks, increasing to q 4 weeks after 24 weeks	IMT tapered in 8/10 patients; VA improved in majority of patients (significant in worse eye)	12	Cutaneous lesions, herpes zoster, peripheral edema
Nussenblatt et al.[85]	10* 5†	Phase I/II: sarcoidosis (3), idiopathic IU (1), VKH (2), idiopathic PU (1), MFC (1) Phase II : idiopathic PU idiopathic IU	**Phase I/II**: 1 mg/kg IV q 2 weeks, increasing to q 4 or q 6 weeks **Phase II:** 2 mg/kg SC × 2 doses q 2 weeks, then 1 mg/kg q 2 weeks	**Phase I/II**: 7/10 patients continued therapy for >4 years; 3 of 4 patients on q 6-week dosing intervals experienced recurrences **Phase II:** 4/5 patients on SC therapy tapered ≥50% of IMT after 12 weeks; 5/5 patients tapered ≥50% of IMT after 26 weeks	>4 year in phase I/II study; 26 weeks in SC phase II trial	Renal cell carcinoma, cutaneous lesions, elevated liver enzymes, rashes, peripheral edema
Papaliodis et al.[97]	14	Scleritis, PU, keratouveitis, uveitis (unspecified, 7 patients), OCP	1 mg/kg IV q 2 weeks until 12 weeks, then q 3 weeks until 24 weeks	VA improved in 12/27 eyes; inflammation improved in 16/27 eyes (59%)	Mean 45 weeks (range 14–74 weeks)	Fatigue, transient leucopenia, no medication-related SAEs
Nussenblatt et al.[115]	15	IU (3), idiopathic posterior (2), PU (6), MFC, RV, BRC, unspecified granulomatous	2 mg/kg IV × 2 doses q 2 weeks, then 1 mg/kg q 2 weeks for 6 months	10/15 patients (67%) reduced IMT by 50% while maintaining VA	26 weeks	Rash, URI, UTI, elevated liver enzymes, no SAEs requiring therapy discontinuation
Kiss et al.[98]	2	BRC	1 mg/kg IV q 2 weeks, increasing to q 6 weeks	LogMAR VA range from –0.10 to 0.20 change during follow-up	18–33 months	None reported
Buggage et al.[95]	17‡	BD-associated uveitis (9)	1 mg/kg × 2 weeks for 6 weeks, then 1 mg/kg q 4 weeks	No difference in ocular attacks between daclizumab and placebo or reduction in IMT	Median 15 months (range 1–34 months)	No safety endpoints reported
Sobrin et al.[33]	8	BRC	1 mg/kg IV q 2 weeks	VA stabilized or improved in 7/8 eyes and resolution of vitreous inflammation; retinal vasculitis resolved in 6/6 eyes; IMT discontinued in 4 patients	Mean 26 months	Elevated liver enzymes, transient leukopenia

IU, intermediate uveitis; VKH, Vogt–Koyanagi–Harada syndrome; PU, panuveitis; MFC, multifocal choroiditis; IV, intravenous; IMT, immunomodulatory therapy; VA, visual acuity; SC, subcutaneous; OCP, ocular cicatricial pemphigoid; SAE, serious adverse event; RV, retinal vasculitis; BRC, birdshot retinochoroidopathy; URI, upper respiratory tract infection; UTI, urinary tract infection.

**10 patients received IV therapy (long-term >4-year follow-up from previous daclizumab study[68]).*

†5 patients received SC therapy.

‡Randomized, placebo-controlled, double-masked clinical trial.

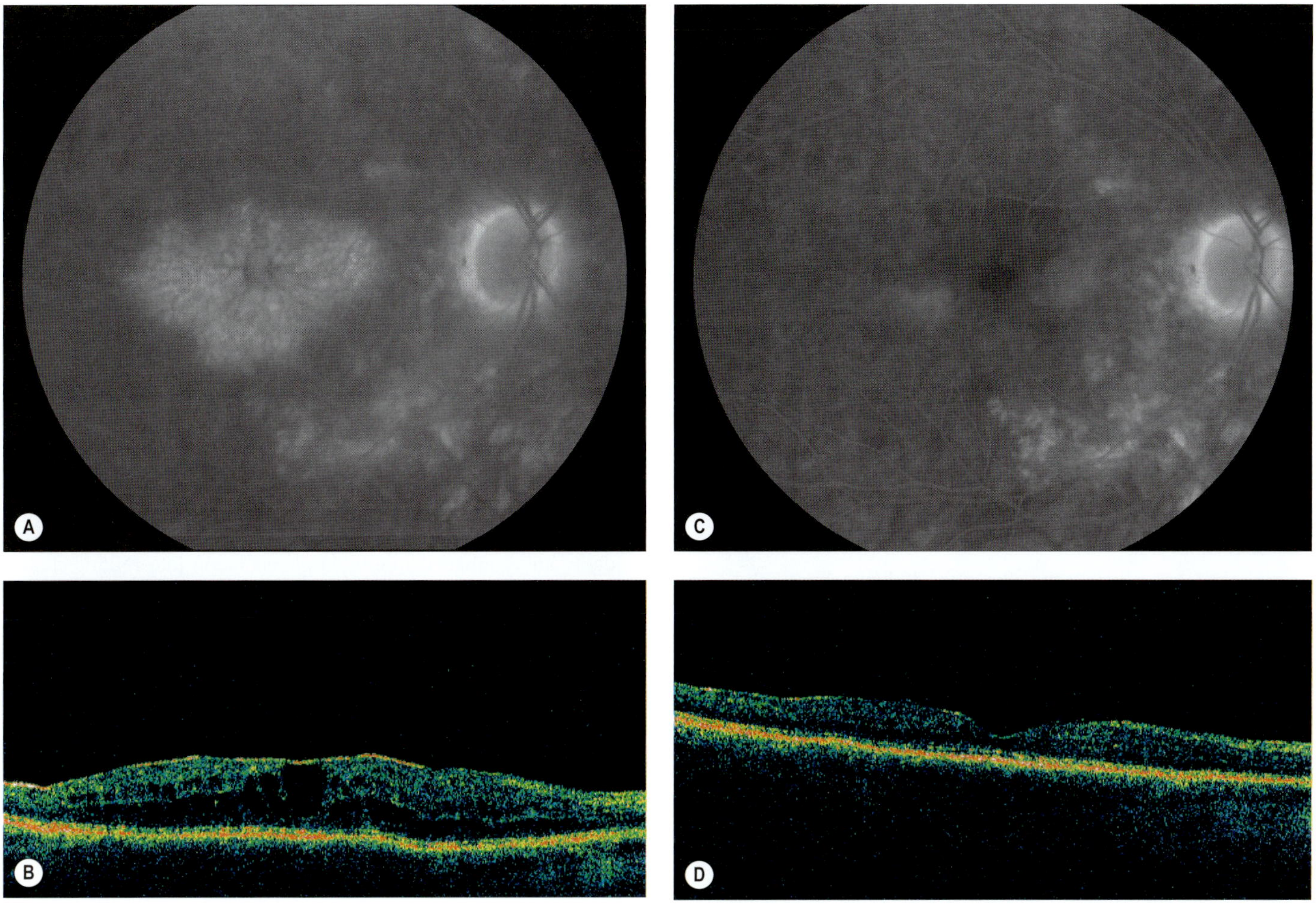

Figure 35.2 Fluorescein angiogram and optical coherence tomography of patient with birdshot retinochoroidopathy (top left, bottom left) and history of bilateral, recurrent, cystoid macular edema despite multiple periocular corticosteroid injections. Following repeat sub-Tenon's triamcinolone and monthly daclizumab infusions at a dosage of 2 mg/kg, the cystoid macular edema has resolved without recurrence (upper right) with restoration of the foveal contour (lower right) and moderate retinal thinning from photoreceptor damage.

daclizumab further supported the efficacy of daclizumab for the long-term control of uveitis. Of the 10 patients enrolled in this study, 7 patients were able to taper off all other immunosuppressive medications and were maintained exclusively on daclizumab for over 4 years.[85] In the long-term study, a dosing interval of 6 weeks resulted in recurrent uveitis, whereas 2–4-week intervals did not. In the short-term phase II study evaluating the preliminary safety and activity of subcutaneous daclizumab, 4 of 5 patients enrolled met their primary study endpoint for success by 12 weeks of therapy (i.e., 50% reduction in immunosuppressive medication and maintenance of visual acuity within 5 letters), and all 5 patients met this endpoint by week 26. None of the patients in the long-term study stopped daclizumab due to adverse events attributable to daclizumab.

In a randomized, double-masked, placebo-controlled trial evaluating the efficacy of daclizumab for Behçet's disease, there was no suggestion that daclizumab was beneficial in comparison with placebo. Specifically, efficacy outcomes (i.e., number of ocular attacks per year, visual acuity change from baseline, and immunosuppressive medication load) were comparable between the daclizumab and placebo arms.[95]

Several other retrospective studies have reported the use of daclizumab for a variety of ocular inflammatory diseases in both children and adults.[96,97] Papaliodis et al.[97] described the use of daclizumab for 14 patients with a variety of inflammatory conditions, including scleritis, ocular cicatricial pemphigoid, and panuveitis. An improvement in visual acuity was seen in 12 of 27 eyes (44%) and in 5 of 14 (36%) patients. Intraocular inflammation improved in 16 of 27 eyes (59%), remained stable in 3 of 27 (11%) eyes, and worsened in 8 of 27 (30%) eyes. A decrease in ocular inflammation was observed in 59% of eyes in their series. Efficacy of daclizumab has also been observed for birdshot retinochoroidopathy (as illustrated in Figure 35.2), leading to improvements in visual acuity and resolution in vitreous inflammation in the majority of patients treated.[33,98]

Gallagher et al.[96] described the use of biologic response modifier therapy in 23 pediatric patients with uveitis: 5 patients in this series were treated with daclizumab. Conditions treated with daclizumab in this series included sarcoidosis, panuveitis, keratouveitis, and uveitis. Of these 5 patients, 4 of 10 eyes demonstrated improvements in visual acuity and 8 of 10 eyes showed improvements in ocular inflammatory grade.

Contraindications

Daclizumab should not be administered to patients with known hypersensitivity to daclizumab or any of its components. Daclizumab is considered pregnancy category C and should not be used in pregnant women unless the potential benefit outweighs the potential risk to the fetus.

Ocular toxicity

No known ocular toxicities have been reported in patients on daclizumab therapy.

Systemic toxicity

In several studies of daclizumab for the prevention of renal allograft rejection, no difference in serious infectious complications or cancer has been observed when comparing patients receiving daclizumab or placebo. The formation of antidaclizumab antibodies has been reported in up to 15% of adult patients and on this medication, but its relationship to the medication's efficacy has not been clearly defined.[99]

Of the patients treated at the National Eye Institute, one case of renal cell carcinoma was diagnosed and daclizumab was stopped. Following successful treatment of the tumor with a partial nephrectomy, the patient required prednisone, mycophenolate mofetil, and cyclosporine to treat a uveitis recurrence with cystoid macular edema (CME). Because of the severe side-effects that subsequently developed from these medications (i.e., weight gain, cushingoid body habitus, hypertension) and the equal potential risk of secondary malignancy from this immunosuppressive regimen, daclizumab infusions were reinstated without any further untoward effects.[85]

Drug interactions

In clinical trials evaluating the efficacy of daclizumab for solid-organ transplants, daclizumab has been used with cyclosporine, mycophenolate mofetil, ganciclovir, acyclovir, azathioprine, and corticosteroids with no incremental increase in adverse reactions. In renal allograft recipients treated with daclizumab and mycophenolate mofetil concomitantly, an interaction of daclizumab with the active metabolite of mycophenolate mofetil was not observed.

Summary

Prospective phase I and phase I/II trials for daclizumab for uveitis have demonstrated its efficacy for the treatment of intermediate, posterior, and panuveitis syndromes, particularly those conditions in which Th1-mediated processes are thought to be instrumental. However, one randomized trial was not supportive of its use in treatment of Behçet's disease-associated uveitis. Several retrospective trials have supported its use for the treatment of birdshot retinochoroidopathy and some cases of pediatric uveitis. The safety of daclizumab has been established in larger trials for the prevention of renal allograft rejection and the treatment of HTLV-associated T-cell lymphoma/leukemia. Further studies will be needed to determine the disease-specific efficacy of daclizumab for ophthalmic inflammatory conditions and optimal dosing strategies.

OTHER BIOLOGIC AGENTS

Other biologic agents, which have been used in several retrospective series and case reports for the treatment of uveitis, include anakinra, alemtuzumab, and interferon-α (IFN-α). Rituximab, an anti-CD20 monoclonal antibody targeting B cells, has been reported for the treatment of primary intraocular lymphoma.

Anakinra (Kineret) a is recombinant human IL-1 receptor antagonist that binds to IL-1 type 1 receptors, down-regulating the proinflammatory effects of IL-1. Its efficacy for the treatment of ocular inflammation has been demonstrated in murine models of uveitis.[100] Recently, several reports have described the efficacy of anakinra for the treatment of specific uveitic syndromes thought to be IL-1-mediated. Specifically, pediatric patients with uveitis associated with chronic infantile neurologic, cutaneous, and articular (CINCA) syndrome[101] and the NOD2 gene-associated pediatric granulomatous arthritis were treated successfully with anakinra therapy.[102]

Alemtuzumab (Campath-1H), the anti-CD52 monoclonal antibody that targets T and B lymphocytes, has been used for a variety of hematologic indications, including myelodysplastic syndrome, aplastic anemia, chronic lymphocytic leukemia, and a number of T-cell leukemias/lymphomas.[103–105] Dick et al.[106] reported the use of alemtuzumab for severe, recalcitrant ocular inflammation in 10 patients with a variety of ophthalmic inflammatory diseases, which included Wegener's granulomatosis-associated peripheral ulcerative keratitis and pseudotumor, retinal vasculitis, sympathetic ophthalmia, and Behçet's disease.[106] All patients showed an initial improvement following Campath-1H administration; however 2 of 10 patients required retreatment. Remission was observed in 8 patients who received Campath-1H, and no opportunistic infections or malignancies were observed at short-term follow-up.[106]

IFN-α has been utilized for its antineoplastic and antiviral effects; however its precise mechanism of action is unknown. Its use in the prevention of ocular relapses, as well as in the treatment of Behçet's disease-associated ocular inflammation,[16] has been reported previously.[21,107] Kotter et al.[107] reported that IFN-2α in combination with low-dose steroid led to remission of ocular disease in 7 patients with Behçet's disease-associated panuveitis. A more recent report suggested a potential benefit of IFN-2α for treatment-resistant CME, with 6 of 8 patients responding to IFN-2α with resolution of CME during the first 6 months of therapy.[108] Further studies into IFN-2α as a therapeutic modality are required before its implementation into routine clinical practice, however.

Rituximab, a monoclonal anti-CD20 antibody targeting B cells, has been used systemically for the treatment of a number of hematologic malignancies and lymphoproliferative disease processes, including primary central nervous system lymphoma.[109,110] Recent studies have supported its use for ocular adnexal lymphomas,[111,112] and limited case series have also reported its benefit for the treatment of primary intraocular lymphoma.[113] While the use of rituximab has been advocated for the treatment of primary intraocular lymphoma recurrences, vigilant central nervous system surveillance, management, and treatment with a neuro-oncologist for systemic chemotherapy are highly recommended.

SUMMARY AND KEY POINTS

As the disease mechanisms underlying specific uveitic syndromes are uncovered, precisely targeted therapies will become more viable as a treatment strategy. The current biologic agents used in clinical practice include the TNF-α antagonists infliximab, adalimumab, and etanercept and the IL-2 receptor antagonist daclizumab (Table 35.3). Infliximab and adalimumab have demonstrated efficacy for uveitic syndromes in a number of retrospective case series and few prospective trials, whereas the role of etanercept for uveitis is less clear. The efficacy of daclizumab as a corticosteroid-sparing and cyclosporine-sparing agent for intermediate, posterior, and panuveitis has been established in several controlled, prospective trials, as well as in several retrospective case series. Experience with other agents, including anakinra, alemtuzumab, IFN-α, and rituximab, is limited at this time.

Because the long-term side-effects of these agents are largely unknown (i.e., theoretical increased risk of malignancy, possible increase in opportunistic infection), a thorough medical evaluation and full understanding of the potential risks of each of these therapies by the patient and provider are recommended prior to their administration. These risks must be weighed against the potential benefits of biologic therapy, including improved visual acuity, better quality of life, and ability to work, and a decrease in the side-effects associated with other traditionally used immunosuppressive medications (e.g., osteoporosis, hyperglycemia associated with corticosteroid use). Thus, while judicious use of the biologics is certainly warranted, tailored therapy with these agents has tremendous promise, and the number of ophthalmic indications for which biologic therapy may be used will likely expand in the future.

Table 35.3 Biologic agents reported for the treatment for ocular inflammatory disease

Biologic agent (trade name)	Mechanism of action	Clinical indications	Ophthalmic indications*	Major toxicities	Dosage §
TNF-α inhibitors					
Infliximab (Remicade)	Chimeric human murine IgG_1 monoclonal antibody. Binds to soluble and transmembrane forms of TNF-α, inhibiting binding of TNF-α with its receptors	RA, Crohn's disease, ankylosing spondylitis	JIA-associated uveitis, Behçet's disease, HLA-B27-associated uveitis, scleritis, intermediate uveitis	Reactivation of latent TB, lupus-like syndrome, unmasking of demyelinating disease, hepatosplenic lymphoma	3, 5, or 10 mg/kg infusion at weeks 0, 2, and 6, then q 4–8 weeks
Etanercept (Enbrel)	Binds TNF-α and blocks interaction with p55 and p75 cell surface TNF receptors	RA, polyarticular JIA, psoriasis, psoriatic arthritis, ankylosing spondylitis	One report of panuveitis, peripheral ulcerative keratitis/scleritis	TB, infection, injection site reactions, optic neuropathy	25 mg twice per week (full dose) or once per week (half-dose) SQ
Adalimumab (Humira)	Recombinant human monoclonal IgG_1 antibody to TNF-α	RA, psoriatic arthritis, ankylosing spondylitis, Crohn's disease	JIA-associated uveitis, Behçet's disease	Tuberculosis, headache, minor infections (URI, UTI), thrombocytopenia, aplastic anemia	20 mg or 40 mg SQ every week or every other week
Daclizumab (Zenapax)	Humanized anti-T-cell IL-2 receptor; prevents T-cell activation	Kidney, liver, and cardiac transplants	Sarcoidosis, idiopathic intermediate uveitis, idiopathic panuveitis, VKH	Cutaneous lesions, herpes zoster eruption, edema, upper-extremity neuralgia, renal cell carcinoma (one report)‡	1–2 mg/kg IV†
Anakinra (Kineret)	IL-1 receptor antagonist	JIA, CINCA, adult-onset Still's disease	CINCA, RA-associated scleritis	Serious infection, injection site reaction	1–2 mg/kg day SQ (100 mg/day SQ)

TNF-α, tumor necrosis factor-α; RA, rheumatoid arthritis; JIA, juvenile idiopathic arthritis; HLA, human leukocyte antigen; TB, tuberculosis; SQ, subcutaneous; URI, upper respiratory tract infection; UTI, urinary tract infection; IL-2, interleukin-2; VKH, Vogt–Koyanagi–Harada disease; CINCA, chronic infantile neurological cutaneous and articular syndrome.

**Ophthalmic indications listed include those conditions in which complete or partial response reported in literature*

†Current studies are under way evaluating higher-dose daclizumab (8 mg/kg intravenously) for induction therapy.

‡One report of low-grade renal cell carcinoma in National Eye Institute study; surgically resected and patient restarted on daclizumab following treatment.

§Dosing reported in ophthalmic literature; treatment regimens for neoplastic and autoimmune conditions may differ from ophthalmic literature.

Reproduced with permission from Yeh S, Nussenblatt RB, Levy-Clarke GA. Emerging biologics in the treatment of uveitis. Exp Rev Clin Immunol 2007;3:781–796.

REFERENCES

1. Foxman EF, Zhang M, Hurst SD, et al. Inflammatory mediators in uveitis: differential induction of cytokines and chemokines in Th1- versus Th2-mediated ocular inflammation. J Immunol 2002;168(5):2483–2492.
2. Santos Lacomba M, Marcos Martín C, Gallardo Galera JM, et al. Aqueous humor and serum tumor necrosis factor-alpha in clinical uveitis. Ophthalmic Res 2001;33(5):251–255.
3. Kavanaugh A, St Clair EW, McCune WJ, et al. Chimeric anti-tumor necrosis factor-alpha monoclonal antibody treatment of patients with rheumatoid arthritis receiving methotrexate therapy. J Rheumatol 2000;27(4):841–850.
4. Mori S. A relationship between pharmacokinetics (PK) and the efficacy of infliximab for patients with rheumatoid arthritis: characterization of infliximab-resistant cases and PK-based modified therapy. Mod Rheumatol 2007;17(2):83–91.
5. Elliott MJ, Maini RN, Feldmann M, et al. Randomised double-blind comparison of chimeric monoclonal antibody to tumour necrosis factor alpha (cA2) versus placebo in rheumatoid arthritis. Lancet 1994;344(8930):1105–1110.
6. Maini RN, Breedveld FC, Kalden JR, et al. Therapeutic efficacy of multiple intravenous infusions of anti-tumor necrosis factor alpha monoclonal antibody combined with low-dose weekly methotrexate in rheumatoid arthritis. Arthritis Rheum 1998;41(9):1552–1563.
7. Lipsky PE, van der Heijde DM, St Clair EW, et al. Infliximab and methotrexate in the treatment of rheumatoid arthritis. Anti-Tumor Necrosis Factor Trial in Rheumatoid Arthritis with Concomitant Therapy Study Group. N Engl J Med 2000;343(22):1594–1602.
8. Targan SR, Hanauer SB, van Deventer SJ, et al. A short-term study of chimeric monoclonal antibody cA2 to tumor necrosis factor alpha for Crohn's disease. Crohn's Disease cA2 Study Group. N Engl J Med 1997;337(15):1029–1035.
9. Rutgeerts P, D'Haens G, Targan S, et al. Efficacy and safety of retreatment with anti-tumor necrosis factor antibody (infliximab) to maintain remission in Crohn's disease. Gastroenterology 1999;117(4):761–769.
10. Rutgeerts P, Sandborn WJ, Feagan BG, et al. Infliximab for induction and maintenance therapy for ulcerative colitis. N Engl J Med 2005;353(23):2462–2476.
11. van der Heijde D, Dijkmans B, Geusens P, et al. Efficacy and safety of infliximab in patients with ankylosing spondylitis: results of a randomized, placebo-controlled trial (ASSERT). Arthritis Rheum 2005;52(2):582–591.
12. Antoni C, Krueger GG, de Vlam K, et al. Infliximab improves signs and symptoms of psoriatic arthritis: results of the IMPACT 2 trial. Ann Rheum Dis 2005;64(8):1150–1157.

13. Baldassano R, Braegger CP, Escher JC, et al. Infliximab (REMICADE) therapy in the treatment of pediatric Crohn's disease. Am J Gastroenterol 2003;98(4):833–838.
14. Ruperto N, Lovell DJ, Cuttica R, et al. A randomized, placebo-controlled trial of infliximab plus methotrexate for the treatment of polyarticular-course juvenile rheumatoid arthritis. Arthritis Rheum 2007;56(9): 3096–3106.
15. Furst DE, Gaylis N, Bray V, et al. Open-label, pilot protocol of patients with rheumatoid arthritis who switch to infliximab after an incomplete response to etanercept: the opposite study. Ann Rheum Dis 2007;66(7): 893–899.
16. Gottlieb AB, Masud S, Ramamurthi R, et al. Pharmacodynamic and pharmacokinetic response to anti-tumor necrosis factor-alpha monoclonal antibody (infliximab) treatment of moderate to severe psoriasis vulgaris. J Am Acad Dermatol 2003;48(1):68–75.
17. Suhler EB, Smith JR, Wertheim MS, et al. A prospective trial of infliximab therapy for refractory uveitis: preliminary safety and efficacy outcomes. Arch Ophthalmol 2005;123(7):903–912.
18. Niccoli L, Nannini C, Benucci M, et al. Long-term efficacy of infliximab in refractory posterior uveitis of Behçet's disease: a 24-month follow-up study. Rheumatology (Oxford) 2007;46(7):1161–1164.
19. Abu El-Asrar AM, Abboud EB, Aldibhi H, et al. Long-term safety and efficacy of infliximab therapy in refractory uveitis due to Behçet's disease. Int Ophthalmol 2005;26(3):83–92.
20. Tugal-Tutkun I, Mudun A, Urgancioglu M, et al. Efficacy of infliximab in the treatment of uveitis that is resistant to treatment with the combination of azathioprine, cyclosporine, and corticosteroids in Behçet's disease: an open-label trial. Arthritis Rheum 2005;52(8):2478–2484.
21. Accorinti M, Pirraglia MP, Paroli MP, et al. Infliximab treatment for ocular and extraocular manifestations of Behçet's disease. Jpn J Ophthalmol 2007;51(3):191–196.
22. Wechsler B, Sablé-Fourtassou R, Bodaghi B, et al. Infliximab in refractory uveitis due to Behçet's disease. Clin Exp Rheumatol 2004;22(4 Suppl 34):S14–S16.
23. Tognon S, Graziani G, Marcolongo R. Anti-TNF-alpha therapy in seven patients with Behçet's uveitis: advantages and controversial aspects. Ann N Y Acad Sci 2007;1110:474–484.
24. Lindstedt EW, Baarsma GS, Kuijpers RW, et al. Anti-TNF-alpha therapy for sight threatening uveitis. Br J Ophthalmol 2005;89(5):533–536.
25. Lanthier N, Parc C, Scavennec R, et al. Infliximab in the treatment of posterior uveitis in Behçet's disease. Long term follow up in four patients. Presse Med 2005;34(13):916–918.
26. Joseph A, Raj D, Dua HS, et al. Infliximab in the treatment of refractory posterior uveitis. Ophthalmology 2003;110(7):1449–1453.
27. Cruz BA, Reis DD, Araujo CA. Refractory retinal vasculitis due to sarcoidosis successfully treated with infliximab. Rheumatol Int 2007;27(12):1181–1183.
28. Benitez-del-Castillo JM, Martinez-de-la-Casa JM, Pato-Cour E, et al. Long-term treatment of refractory posterior uveitis with anti-TNFalpha (infliximab). Eye 2005;19(8):841–845.
29. Rajaraman RT, Kimura Y, Li S, et al. Retrospective case review of pediatric patients with uveitis treated with infliximab. Ophthalmology 2006;113(2): 308–314.
30. Richards JC, Tay-Kearney ML, Murray K, et al. Infliximab for juvenile idiopathic arthritis-associated uveitis. Clin Experiment Ophthalmol 2005;33(5):461–468.
31. Kahn P, Weiss M, Imundo LF, et al. Favorable response to high-dose infliximab for refractory childhood uveitis. Ophthalmology 2006;113(5):860–864 e2.
32. El-Shabrawi Y, Hermann J. Anti-tumor necrosis factor-alpha therapy with infliximab as an alternative to corticosteroids in the treatment of human leukocyte antigen B27-associated acute anterior uveitis. Ophthalmology 2002;109(12):2342–2346.
33. Sobrin L, Huang JJ, Christen W, et al. Daclizumab for treatment of birdshot chorioretinopathy. Arch Ophthalmol 2008;126(2):186–191.
34. Murphy CC, Ayliffe WH, Booth A, et al. Tumor necrosis factor alpha blockade with infliximab for refractory uveitis and scleritis. Ophthalmology 2004;111(2):352–356.
35. El-Shabrawi Y, Hermann J. Anti-TNF alpha therapy in chronic necrotizing scleritis resistant to standard immunomodulatory therapy in a patient with Wegener's granulomatosis. Eye 2005;19(9):1017–1018.
36. Cazabon S, Over K, Butcher J. The successful use of infliximab in resistant relapsing polychondritis and associated scleritis. Eye 2005;19(2):222–224.
37. Thomas JW, Pflugfelder SC. Therapy of progressive rheumatoid arthritis-associated corneal ulceration with infliximab. Cornea 2005;24(6):742–744.
38. Weiss K, Rieger R, Keitzer R, et al. Successful infliximab treatment of posterior scleritis in a 13-year-old child refractory to other immunosuppressive therapy. Graefes Arch Clin Exp Ophthalmol 2007;245(11):1735–1737.
39. Luong BT, Chong BS, Lowder DM. Treatment options for rheumatoid arthritis: celecoxib, leflunomide, etanercept, and infliximab. Ann Pharmacother 2000;34(6):743–760.
40. Tran TH, Milea D, Cassoux N, et al. Optic neuritis associated with infliximab. J Fr Ophtalmol 2005;28(2):201–204.
41. Nahar IK, Shojania K, Marra CA, et al. Infliximab treatment of rheumatoid arthritis and Crohn's disease. Ann Pharmacother 2003;37(9):1256–1265.
42. Mackey AC, Green L, Liang LC, et al. Hepatosplenic T cell lymphoma associated with infliximab use in young patients treated for inflammatory bowel disease. J Pediatr Gastroenterol Nutr 2007;44(2):265–267.
43. Wolfe F, Michaud K. Lymphoma in rheumatoid arthritis: the effect of methotrexate and anti-tumor necrosis factor therapy in 18,572 patients. Arthritis Rheum 2004;50(6):1740–1751.
44. Geborek P, Bladström A, Turesson C, et al. Tumour necrosis factor blockers do not increase overall tumour risk in patients with rheumatoid arthritis, but may be associated with an increased risk of lymphomas. Ann Rheum Dis 2005;64(5):699–703.
45. Baecklund E, Askling J, Rosenquist R, et al. Rheumatoid arthritis and malignant lymphomas. Curr Opin Rheumatol 2004;16(3):254–261.
46. Wolfe F, Michaud K. The effect of methotrexate and anti-tumor necrosis factor therapy on the risk of lymphoma in rheumatoid arthritis in 19,562 patients during 89,710 person-years of observation. Arthritis Rheum 2007;56(5):1433–1439.
47. Callen JP. Complications and adverse reactions in the use of newer biologic agents. Semin Cutan Med Surg 2007;26(1):6–14.
48. Weisman MH, Moreland LW, Furst DE, et al. Efficacy, pharmacokinetic, and safety assessment of adalimumab, a fully human anti-tumor necrosis factor-alpha monoclonal antibody, in adults with rheumatoid arthritis receiving concomitant methotrexate: a pilot study. Clin Ther 2003;25(6):1700–1721.
49. den Broeder AA, Assmann KJ, van Riel PL, et al. Nephrotic syndrome as a complication of anti-TNFalpha in a patient with rheumatoid arthritis. Neth J Med 2003;61(4):137–141.
50. Weinblatt ME, Keystone EC, Furst DE, et al. Adalimumab, a fully human anti-tumor necrosis factor alpha monoclonal antibody, for the treatment of rheumatoid arthritis in patients taking concomitant methotrexate: the ARMADA trial. Arthritis Rheum 2003;48(1):35–45.
51. Sandborn WJ, Hanauer S, Loftus EV Jr, et al. An open-label study of the human anti-TNF monoclonal antibody adalimumab in subjects with prior loss of response or intolerance to infliximab for Crohn's disease. Am J Gastroenterol 2004;99(10):1984–1989.
52. Haibel H, Rudwaleit M, Brandt HC, et al. Adalimumab reduces spinal symptoms in active ankylosing spondylitis: clinical and magnetic resonance imaging results of a fifty-two-week open-label trial. Arthritis Rheum 2006;54(2):678–681.
53. Gladman DD, Mease PJ, Ritchlin CT, et al. Adalimumab for long-term treatment of psoriatic arthritis: forty-eight week data from the adalimumab effectiveness in psoriatic arthritis trial. Arthritis Rheum 2007;56(2): 476–488.
54. Mease PJ, Gladman DD, Ritchlin CT, et al. Adalimumab for the treatment of patients with moderately to severely active psoriatic arthritis: results of a double-blind, randomized, placebo-controlled trial. Arthritis Rheum 2005;52(10):3279–3289.
55. Breedveld FC, Weisman MH, Kavanaugh AF, et al. The PREMIER study: A multicenter, randomized, double-blind clinical trial of combination therapy with adalimumab plus methotrexate versus methotrexate alone or adalimumab alone in patients with early, aggressive rheumatoid arthritis who had not had previous methotrexate treatment. Arthritis Rheum 2006;54(1):26–37.
56. van Laar JA, Missotten T, van Daele PL, et al. Adalimumab: a new modality for Behçet's disease? Ann Rheum Dis 2007;66(4):565–566.
57. Mushtaq B, Saeed T, Situnayake RD, et al. Adalimumab for sight-threatening uveitis in Behçet's disease. Eye 2007;21(6):824–825.
58. Diaz Llopis M, Amselem L, Romero FJ, et al. Adalimumab therapy for Vogt–Koyanagi–Harada syndrome. Arch Soc Esp Oftalmol 2007;82(3):131–132.
59. Vazquez-Cobian LB, Flynn T, Lehman TJ. Adalimumab therapy for childhood uveitis. J Pediatr 2006;149(4):572–575.
60. Biester S, Deuter C, Michels H, et al. Adalimumab in the therapy of uveitis in childhood. Br J Ophthalmol 2007;91(3):319–324.
61. van der Heijde D, Pangan AL, Schiff MH, et al. Adalimumab effectively reduces the signs and symptoms of active ankylosing spondylitis in patients with total spinal ankylosis. Ann Rheum Dis 2008;67:1218–1221.
62. Schiff MH, Burmester GR, Kent JD, et al. Safety analyses of adalimumab (HUMIRA) in global clinical trials and US postmarketing surveillance of patients with rheumatoid arthritis. Ann Rheum Dis 2006 Jul;65(7): 889–894.
63. Culy CR, Keating GM. Spotlight on etanercept in rheumatoid arthritis, psoriatic arthritis and juvenile rheumatoid arthritis. BioDrugs 2003;17(2):139–145.
64. Moreland LW, Schiff MH, Baumgartner SW, et al. Etanercept therapy in rheumatoid arthritis. A randomized, controlled trial. Ann Intern Med 1999;130(6):478–486.
65. Weinblatt ME, Kremer JM, Bankhurst AD, et al. A trial of etanercept, a recombinant tumor necrosis factor receptor:Fc fusion protein, in patients with rheumatoid arthritis receiving methotrexate. N Engl J Med 1999;340(4):253–259.
66. Lovell DJ, Giannini EH, Reiff A, et al. Etanercept in children with polyarticular juvenile rheumatoid arthritis. Pediatric Rheumatology Collaborative Study Group. N Engl J Med 2000;342(11):763–769.
67. Davis Jr JC, Van Der Heijde D, Braun J, et al. Recombinant human tumor necrosis factor receptor (etanercept) for treating ankylosing spondylitis: a randomized, controlled trial. Arthritis Rheum 2003;48(11): 3230–3236.

68. Mease PJ, Van Der Heijde D, Braun J, et al. Etanercept in the treatment of psoriatic arthritis and psoriasis: a randomised trial. Lancet 2000;356(9227):385–390.
69. Smith JA, Thompson DJ, Whitcup SM, et al. A randomized, placebo-controlled, double-masked clinical trial of etanercept for the treatment of uveitis associated with juvenile idiopathic arthritis. Arthritis Rheum 2005 Feb 15;53(1):18–23.
70. Nussenblatt RB, Fortin E, Schiffman R, et al. Treatment of noninfectious intermediate and posterior uveitis with the humanized anti-Tac mAb: a phase I/II clinical trial. Proc Natl Acad Sci USA 1999;96(13): 7462–7466.
71. Reiff A, Takei S, Sadeghi S, et al. Etanercept therapy in children with treatment-resistant uveitis. Arthritis Rheum 2001;44(6):1411–1415.
72. Hernandez-Illas M, Tozman E, Fulcher SF, et al. Recombinant human tumor necrosis factor receptor Fc fusion protein (Etanercept): experience as a therapy for sight-threatening scleritis and sterile corneal ulceration. Eye Contact Lens 2004;30(1):2–5.
73. Guignard S, Gossec L, Salliot C, et al. Efficacy of tumour necrosis factor blockers in reducing uveitis flares in patients with spondylarthropathy: a retrospective study. Ann Rheum Dis 2006;65(12):1631–1634.
74. Galor A, Perez VL, Hammel JP, et al. Differential effectiveness of etanercept and infliximab in the treatment of ocular inflammation. Ophthalmology 2006;113(12):2317–2323.
75. Foeldvari I, Nielsen S, Kümmerle-Deschner J, et al. Tumor necrosis factor-alpha blocker in treatment of juvenile idiopathic arthritis-associated uveitis refractory to second-line agents: results of a multinational survey. J Rheumatol 2007;34(5):1146–1150.
76. Schmeling H, Horneff G. Etanercept and uveitis in patients with juvenile idiopathic arthritis. Rheumatology (Oxford) 2005;44(8):1008–1011.
77. Reddy AR, Backhouse OC. Does etanercept induce uveitis? Br J Ophthalmol 2003;87(7):925.
78. Taban M, Dupps WJ, Mandell B, et al. Etanercept (enbrel)-associated inflammatory eye disease: case report and review of the literature. Ocul Immunol Inflamm 2006;14(3):145–150.
79. Tauber T, Turetz J, Barash J, et al. Optic neuritis associated with etanercept therapy for juvenile arthritis. J AAPOS 2006;10(1):26–29.
80. Fonollosa A, Segura A, Giralt J, et al. Tuberculous uveitis after treatment with etanercept. Graefes Arch Clin Exp Ophthalmol 2007;245(9): 1397–1399.
81. Saurenmann RK, Levin AV, Feldman BM, et al. Risk of new-onset uveitis in patients with juvenile idiopathic arthritis treated with anti-TNFalpha agents. J Pediatr 2006;149(6):833–836.
82. Bathon JM, Fleischmann RM, Van der Heijde D, et al. Safety and efficacy of etanercept treatment in elderly subjects with rheumatoid arthritis. J Rheumatol 2006;33(2):234–243.
83. Caspi RR, Roberge FG, McAllister CG, et al. T cell lines mediating experimental autoimmune uveoretinitis (EAU) in the rat. J Immunol 1986;136(3):928–933.
84. Rozenszajn LA, Muellenberg-Coulombre C, Gery I, et al. Induction of experimental autoimmune uveoretinitis by T-cell lines. Immunology 1986;57(4):559–565.
85. Nussenblatt RB, Thompson DJ, Li Z, et al. Humanized anti-interleukin-2 (IL-2) receptor alpha therapy: long-term results in uveitis patients and preliminary safety and activity data for establishing parameters for subcutaneous administration. J Autoimmun 2003;21(3):283–293.
86. Guex-Crosier Y, Raber J, Chan CC, et al. Humanized antibodies against the alpha-chain of the IL-2 receptor and against the beta-chain shared by the IL-2 and IL-15 receptors in a monkey uveitis model of autoimmune diseases. J Immunol 1997;158(1):452–458.
87. Torun N, Callizo J, Orlic N, et al. Serum cytokine receptor levels in noninfectious uveitis. Ophthalmic Res 2005;37(2):112–116.
88. Martin CM, Lacomba MS, Molina CI, et al. Levels of soluble ICAM-1 and soluble IL-2R in the serum and aqueous humor of uveitis patients. Curr Eye Res 2000;20(4):287–292.
89. Nashan B, Light S, Hardie IR, et al. Reduction of acute renal allograft rejection by daclizumab. Daclizumab Double Therapy Study Group. Transplantation 1999;67(1):110–115.
90. Ekberg H, Bäckman L, Tufveson G, et al. Daclizumab prevents acute rejection and improves patient survival post transplantation: 1 year pooled analysis. Transpl Int 2000;13(2):151–159.
91. Sutherland DE, Gruessner RW, Dunn DL, et al. Lessons learned from more than 1,000 pancreas transplants at a single institution. Ann Surg 2001;233(4):463–501.
92. Lietz K, John R, Beniaminovitz A, et al. Interleukin-2 receptor blockade in cardiac transplantation: influence of HLA-DR locus incompatibility on treatment efficacy. Transplantation 2003;75(6):781–787.
93. Eckhoff DE, McGuire B, Sellers M, et al. The safety and efficacy of a two-dose daclizumab (zenapax) induction therapy in liver transplant recipients. Transplantation 2000;69(9):1867–1872.
94. Aalamian Z. Reducing adverse effects of immunosuppressive agents in kidney transplant recipients. Prog Transplant 2001;11(4):271–282; quiz 283–4.
95. Buggage RR, Levy-Clarke G, Sen HN, et al. A double-masked, randomized study to investigate the safety and efficacy of daclizumab to treat the ocular complications related to Behçet's disease. Ocul Immunol Inflamm 2007;15(2):63–70.
96. Gallagher M, Quinones K, Cervantes-Castañeda RA, et al. Biological response modifier therapy for refractory childhood uveitis. Br J Ophthalmol 2007;91(10):1341–1344.
97. Papaliodis GN, Chu D, Foster CS. Treatment of ocular inflammatory disorders with daclizumab. Ophthalmology 2003;110(4):786–789.
98. Kiss S, Ahmed M, Letko E, et al. Long-term follow-up of patients with birdshot retinochoroidopathy treated with corticosteroid-sparing systemic immunomodulatory therapy. Ophthalmology 2005;112(6):1066–1071.
99. Daclizumab (Zenapax) package insert. Roche 2003.
100. Li Z, Lim WK, Mahesh SP, et al. Cutting edge: *in vivo* blockade of human IL-2 receptor induces expansion of CD56(bright) regulatory NK cells in patients with active uveitis. J Immunol 2005;174(9):5187–5191.
101. Teoh SC, Sharma S, Hogan A, et al. Tailoring biological treatment: anakinra treatment of posterior uveitis associated with the CINCA syndrome. Br J Ophthalmol 2007;91(2):263–264.
102. Arostegui JI, Arnal C, Merino R, et al. NOD2 gene-associated pediatric granulomatous arthritis: clinical diversity, novel and recurrent mutations, and evidence of clinical improvement with interleukin-1 blockade in a Spanish cohort. Arthritis Rheum 2007;56(11):3805–3813.
103. Nabhan C. The emerging role of alemtuzumab in chronic lymphocytic leukemia. Clin Lymphoma Myeloma 2005;6(2):115–121.
104. Osterborg A, Mellstedt H, Keating M. Clinical effects of alemtuzumab (Campath-1H) in B-cell chronic lymphocytic leukemia. Med Oncol 2002;19(Suppl):S21–S26.
105. Dearden C. The role of alemtuzumab in the management of T-cell malignancies. Semin Oncol 2006;33(2 Suppl 5):S44–S52.
106. Dick AD, Meyer P, James T, et al. Campath-1H therapy in refractory ocular inflammatory disease. Br J Ophthalmol 2000;84(1):107–109.
107. Kotter I, Deuter C, Stubiger N, et al. Interferon-α (IFN-α) application versus tumor necrosis factor-α antagonism for ocular Behçet's disease: focusing more on IFN. J Rheumatol 2005;32(8):1633; author reply 1634.
108. Deuter CM, Koetter I, Guenaydin I, et al. Interferon alfa-2a: a new treatment option for long lasting refractory cystoid macular edema in uveitis? A pilot study. Retina 2006;26(7):786–791.
109. Hoang-Xuan K, Camilleri-Broet S, Soussain C. Recent advances in primary CNS lymphoma. Curr Opin Oncol 2004;16(6):601–606.
110. Bosly A, Keating MJ, Stasi R, et al. Rituximab in B-cell disorders other than non-Hodgkin's lymphoma. Anticancer Drugs 2002;13(Suppl 2):S25–S33.
111. Rigacci L, Nassi L, Puccioni M, et al. Rituximab and chlorambucil as first-line treatment for low-grade ocular adnexal lymphomas. Ann Hematol 2007;86(8):565–568.
112. Ferreri AJ, Ponzoni M, Martinelli G, et al. Rituximab in patients with mucosal-associated lymphoid tissue-type lymphoma of the ocular adnexa. Haematologica 2005;90(11):1578–1579.
113. Kitzmann AS, Pulido JS, Mohney BG, et al. Intraocular use of rituximab. Eye 2007;21(12):1524–1527.
114. Sfikakis PP, Theodossiadis PG, Katsiari CG, et al. Effect of infliximab on sight-threatening panuveitis in Behçet's disease. Lancet 2001;358(9278): 295–296.
115. Nussenblatt RB, Peterson JS, Foster CS, et al. Initial evaluation of subcutaneous daclizumab treatments for noninfectious uveitis: a multicenter noncomparative interventional case series. Ophthalmology 2005;112(5):764–770.

CHAPTER 36

Immunomodulatory therapy in uveitis

Zohar Habot-Wilner, MD and Susan Lightman, PhD, FRCP, FRCOphth

KEY FEATURES

Corticosteroids are the mainstay of therapy for ocular inflammatory diseases and can be given by a variety of routes. However, additional immunosuppressive drug therapy may be necessary in patients with an inflammatory disease which is poorly responsive to corticosteroid treatment, a chronic or relapsing disease that requires the long-term use of systemic corticosteroids at a dose above 7.5 mg/day, which is likely to produce side-effects, or when the corticosteroid side-effects are intolerable and result in the need for a corticosteroid-sparing agent.

For the disease patterns mentioned above, early and aggressive immunosuppressive drug therapy can be invaluable in preventing irreversible visual loss.

Because most of the immunosuppressive drugs take several weeks to have an effect, initial therapy of sight-threatening ocular inflammation is typically with high-dose oral corticosteroids due to their rapid anti-inflammatory effect. Once the disease is quiescent, the corticosteroids can either be tapered to a low level or, if possible, discontinued. Subsequently, the immunosuppressive drugs are tapered down.

CALCINEURIN INHIBITORS

Ciclosporin (CsA) and tacrolimus are termed calcineurin inhibitors due to their ability to bind to the cytosolic protein cyclophilin of immunocompetent T lymphocytes. This complex inhibits calcineurin, which under normal circumstances is responsible for activating the transcription of interleukin-2. It also inhibits product of tumor necrosis factor (TNF)-α, interferon (IFN)-γ, interleukin-3, and interleukin-4 and therefore leads to suppression of effector T-cell function. Table 36.1 summarizes the properties and dosages of the two common calcineurin inhibitors.[1,2]

CICLOSPORIN (CYCLOSPORIN: CsA)

Key features, introduction, and history

CsA is a cyclic peptide of 11 amino acids produced by the fungus *Beauveria nivea*. Its success in preventing organ rejection was first shown in liver transplants in 1980 and it was subsequently approved for use in 1983. The use of this drug in uveitis has been described since 1987.

Pharmacology

Two oral preparations of CsA are available, Neoral and Sandimmune. Neoral, which has greater bioavailability, is used in uveitis. The drug is metabolized in the liver and excreted in the bile, with very little of the parent drug or its metabolites appearing in the urine. The average half-life of CsA is about 8.4 hours (range 5–18 hours). CsA leaves the vasculature readily and has been found in the intraocular fluids of uveitis patients. CsA crosses the placenta and is excreted in human milk.[1]

Drug effects in human nonocular diseases

CsA is approved by the Food and Drug Administration (FDA) for the prevention and treatment of graft rejection, rheumatoid arthritis that is poorly responsive to methotrexate, and plaque psoriasis in adults. It is also used in atopic dermatitis, ulcerative colitis, and a variety of glomerular disorders.

Drug use in retinal diseases

Ozdal et al.[3] evaluated the long-term use of low-dose CsA in 52 patients (104 eyes) with ocular Behçet's disease using CsA for at least 1 year. The initial dose was 5 mg/kg/day and the dose was tapered gradually over 2 months to a maintenance dose of 3 mg/kg/day. Prednisone was added when necessary. Visual acuity improved or stabilized in 72 (69.2%) and deteriorated in 32 (30.8%) of the 104 eyes. No ocular attacks occurred in 50% of the eyes during therapy.

Pediatric case series

Kilmartin et al.[4] treated 14 patients (25 eyes) with refractory noninfectious childhood uveitis, at a maintenance CsA dose of 4.0 mg/kg/day as monotherapy or in combination with prednisolone or azathioprine. Visual acuity improved or was maintained in 23 (92%) eyes and binocular indirect ophthalmoscopy score outcomes improved in 19 (76%) eyes. Height centiles were preserved and the maintenance prednisolone dose was 6.3 mg/day, where required, in 10 (71%) patients.

EFFICACY AND COMPARISON WITH OTHER AGENTS

Ciclosporin versus tacrolimus

Murphy et al.[5] compared, in a prospective randomized study, the treatment of CsA 2.5–5.0 mg/kg/day to tacrolimus 0.03–0.08 mg/kg/day in 37 patients with noninfectious posterior-segment intraocular inflammation. They showed that tacrolimus and CsA were similar with regard to efficacy for posterior-segment intraocular inflammation. However, CsA therapy was associated with a higher incidence of reported adverse effects. Mean arterial pressure and serum cholesterol level were significantly higher at 3 months in the CsA group than in the tacrolimus group.

Drug mechanism, systemic and ocular complications and toxicity, drug interactions, and contraindications are summarized in Table 36.1.[2,6–8]

TACROLIMUS

Key features, introduction, and history

Tacrolimus is a macrolide antibiotic produced from the fermentation broth of a strain of *Streptomyces tsukubaensis*, discovered by a Japanese team in 1987. Its name was derived from *T*sukuba m*acrol*ide

Table 36.1 Summary of calcineurin inhibitors' standard dose administration, mechanism of action, recommended laboratory tests, side-effects, drug interactions, and contraindications

Name	Oral formulation	Dose initial/ maximum	Mechanism	Expected onset	Lab test*	Side-effects	Comments	Contraindications
Ciclosporin (Neoral)	25/100 mg capsule 100 mg/ml oral suspension	2–7.5 mg/kg/ day (equally divided dose) Children: 2–4 mg/kg/ day (equally divided dose)	T-cell inhibitor	2–6 weeks (dose-dependent)	BP RFTs LFTs Lipid profile Electrolytes Glucose CBC Urine dipstick	Serious: Nephrotoxicity HTN Hepatotoxicity Common: Hypercholesterolemia GI upset Gum hyperplasia Hirsutism Electrolyte changes‡ Hyperglycemia Tremor Headache	Reduced by 25–50%: • Creatinine >30% baseline • Diastolic BP>95 mmHg Discontinue if reversibility (within 25% of baseline) of serum creatinine is not achievable after two dosage modifications Chronic nephrotoxicity is irreversible Serum levels increased by grapefruit juice Clarithromycin Erythromycin Fluconazole Ketoconazole Voriconazole Tacrolimus Diltiazem Decreased serum levels by St. John's wort herbal supplement Rifampicin and barbiturates Vaccinations may be less effective CsA in pregnancy: premature birth and low birth weight	Absolute: • Abnormal renal function • Uncontrolled HTN • Uncontrolled infections • Malignancy • Breast-feeding • Concomitant use of tacrolimus and rosuvastatin • Use of live attenuated vaccines should be avoided Relative: • Liver disease • Abnormal CBC • Pregnancy

Table 36.1 Summary of calcineurin inhibitors' standard dose administration, mechanism of action, recommended laboratory tests, side-effects, drug interactions, and contraindications—cont'd

Name	Oral formulation	Dose initial/ maximum	Mechanism	Expected onset	Lab test*	Side-effects	Comments	Contraindications
Tacrolimus (Prograf)	0.5/1/5 mg capsule 5 mg/ml oral suspension	0.15–0.3 mg/ kg/day (equally divided dose) Children: 1½–2 times higher than the adult doses to achieve similar blood levels	T-cell inhibitor	2–6 weeks (dose-dependent	BPRFTs LFTs Lipid profile Electrolytes Glucose CBC Urine dipstick	Serious: Nephrotoxicity Neurotoxicity† Teratogenic Common: Hyperglycemia GI upset Hypercholesterolemia Electrolyte changes‡ Headache HTN Hepatotoxicity Ocular complications: Blurred vision	Administered on an empty stomach, meals with a moderate content of fat reduce absorption rate Serum levels increased by grapefruit juice Clarithromycin Erythromycin Fluconazole Ketoconazole Voriconazole Diltiazem Serum levels decreased by St. John's wort herbal supplement, rifampicin, and barbiturates Vaccinations may be less effective	Absolute: • Hypersensitivity to macrolides • Abnormal renal function • Uncontrolled infections • Malignancy • Avoid concurrent administration with CsA • Pregnancy • Breast-feeding • Use of live attenuated vaccines should be avoided Relative: • Liver disease • Abnormal CBC • Diabetes • Poorly controlled HTN

BP, blood pressure; RFTs, renal function tests; LFTs, liver function tests; (primarily aspartate and alanine aminotransferases) CBC, complete blood count; HTN, hypertension; GI, gastrointestinal; HTN, hypertension; CsA, cyclosporine A; CBC, complete blood count.

**Lab tests: at baseline, every 2 weeks in first month and then every month.*

†Neurotoxic effects include aphasia, seizures, confusion, psychosis, and tremors.

‡Electrolyte changes include: hyperkalemia, hypomagnesemia, hyperuricemia.

immunosuppressant. It was approved by the FDA in 1994 for use in liver transplantation. The drug use in uveitis has been described since 1991.

Pharmacology

Absorption of tacrolimus from the gastrointestinal tract is both incomplete and variable. The plasma protein binding of tacrolimus is approximately 99%. Tacrolimus is primarily metabolized by the cytochrome P-450 system. Fecal elimination accounts for over 90% of elimination. The average half-life of tacrolimus is about 35 hours. Tacrolimus crosses the placenta and is excreted in human milk.[1]

Drug effects in human nonocular diseases

Tacrolimus is FDA-approved to prevent and treat liver, kidney, or heart transplant rejection. It is also used in the treatment of ulcerative colitis and atopic dermatitis.

Drug use in retinal diseases

Sloper et al.[9] demonstrated that tacrolimus has a useful role as an immunosuppressive agent for the treatment of sight-threatening uveitis (3 patients had Behçet's disease, 1 had microscopic polyangiitis, 1 had pars planitis, and 1 had idiopathic retinal vasculitis) in patients who did not respond to CsA either because of lack of therapeutic effect or unacceptable adverse effects. The posterior uveitis remained controlled in all 6 patients while they were taking tacrolimus. Five of the 6 patients showed improvement, defined as improvement of 2 lines or more of Snellen acuity or a decrease in the binocular indirect ophthalmoscopy score.

Hogan et al.[10] showed in a retrospective case series of 62 consecutive patients with noninfectious uveitis that tacrolimus's efficacy is maintained long-term, and its cardiovascular risk profile is excellent. The patients successfully tapered their oral prednisone to 10 mg daily, with an 85% probability of achieving ≤ 10 mg after 1.2 years of treatment. There was no requirement for alternative second-line immunosuppressive therapy and the rate of tacrolimus dose reduction or discontinuation due to side-effects was minimal.

Drug mechanism, systemic and ocular complications and toxicity, drug interactions and contraindications are summarized in Table 36.1.[2,6–8]

Summary and key points

CsA and tacrolimus are effective second-line agents. However, despite the use of low-dose regimens, CsA toxicity (renal toxicity, hypertension) remains an important problem. This forms a major limitation to successful long-term treatment with CsA.

Tacrolimus may cause fewer adverse effects when compared with CsA in part due to its greater immunosuppressive potency and therefore lower dose, but it is used less frequently.

ANTIMETABOLITES

MYCOPHENOLATE MOFETIL (MMF)

Key features, introduction, and history

MMF is a prodrug derived from the fungus *Penicillium stoloniferum*. The drug use in uveitis has been described since 1998.

Pharmacology

MMF has high oral bioavailability and is absorbed within 30 minutes. It is metabolized in the liver to the active compound mycophenolic acid, which is excreted renally.[6]

Drug mechanism

MMF is a selective inhibitor of inosine monophosphate dehydrogenase, the enzyme that controls the rate of synthesis of guanine monophosphate in the de novo pathway of purine synthesis used in the proliferation of B and T lymphocytes. It prevents lymphocyte proliferation, suppresses antibody synthesis, interferes with cellular adhesion to vascular endothelium, and decreases recruitment of leukocytes to sites of inflammation.[6]

Drug effects in human nonocular diseases

MMF is FDA-approved for prevention of renal, cardiac, or hepatic allograft rejection and is also used in systemic lupus erythematosus, Crohn's disease, nephrotic syndrome, and psoriasis.

Drug use in retinal diseases

Thorne et al.[11] evaluated MMF treatment outcomes in 84 patients with inflammatory eye disease. After 1 month of treatment, 96.4% of patients had control of their ocular inflammation. Treatment success, as judged by the ability to control the inflammation and taper the prednisone to <10 mg daily, was achieved in 60 patients (71%). The median time to treatment success after the institution of MMF was 3.5 months. Approximately 18% of patients required the addition of a second immunosuppressive drug, and, of these patients, 71% had control of their disease. MMF starting dose was 2 g. However, 11% of patients required an increase in the dose of MMF to 3 g daily.

Siepmann et al.[12] evaluated the outcomes of 106 patients with different forms of chronic uveitis treated with MMF at a dose of 1 g twice daily. The number of recurrences was 0 or 1 in 92 patients, 2 in 6 cases and 3 or more in 8 patients. In none of the patients had MMF been stopped at the time of data analysis.

Sobrin et al.[13] evaluated the outcomes of treatment with MMF in 85 patients with scleritis and uveitis refractory to or intolerant of methotrexate. They demonstrated that MMF was effective in controlling inflammation in approximately half of the patients who had previously failed with or did not tolerate methotrexate.

Pediatric case series

Doycheva et al.[14] assessed the efficacy of MMF in 17 children (32 eyes) with chronic noninfectious uveitis who received MMF for at least 6 months. The average maintenance dose was 1 g daily (range 750 mg to 2 g daily). A steroid-sparing effect was achieved in 88% of patients. Twenty-four percent of patients remained relapse-free during the treatment, but a reduction in the relapse rate was observed in all other patients except one. Visual acuity was increased or maintained in 13 children (76%).

Drug mechanism, systemic and ocular complications and toxicity, drug interactions, and contraindications are summarized in Table 36.2.[2,6–8]

METHOTREXATE

Key features, introduction, and history

Methotrexate is a folic acid analogue that was originated in the 1940s when folic acid effects were tested on children with acute leukemia. It gained FDA approval as an oncology drug in 1953. The drug use in uveitis has been described since 1966.

Pharmacology

Methotrexate is metabolized by intestinal bacteria and the percentage of oral absorption decreases as the dose increases. It is eliminated primarily through the kidney. The half-life is approximately 3–10 hours.[2,6]

Drug mechanism

Methotrexate is a folic acid analogue and an inhibitor of dihydrofolate reductase, the enzyme responsible for the conversion of dihydrofolate to tetrahydrofolate. This action inhibits the production of thymidylate, which is essential for DNA replication. It inhibits rapidly dividing cells, such as leukocytes, producing an anti-inflammatory effect.[2,6]

Drug effects in human nonocular diseases

Methotrexate is FDA-approved for use in the treatment of neoplastic disorders such as acute lymphoblastic leukemia, non-Hodgkin lymphoma, carcinoma of breast, lung, head, and neck, as well as rheumatoid arthritis, juvenile idiopathic arthritis, and psoriasis. It is also used in systemic lupus erythematosus, ankylosing spondylitis, Crohn's disease, psoriatic arthritis, and Behçet's disease.

Drug use in retinal diseases

Samson et al.[15] evaluated methotrexate treatment among 160 patients with chronic noninfectious uveitis unresponsive to steroid therapy. Control of inflammation was achieved in 76.2% of patients; the average maintenance dosage of these patients was 12.3 mg weekly. Steroid-sparing effect was achieved in 56% of patients. Visual acuity was maintained or improved in 90% of patients. Side-effects requiring discontinuation of medication occurred in 18% of patients. Potentially serious adverse reactions occurred in only 8.1% of patients.

Pediatric case series

Heiligenhaus et al.[16] studied the efficacy of methotrexate in the treatment of 35 patients with severe chronic juvenile idiopathic arthritis-associated iridocyclitis. Methotrexate was given at a dosage of approximately 15 mg weekly/m^2 body surface, either orally or subcutaneously. Quiescence of uveitis was obtained in 21 patients with additional topical steroids and in 4 patients without additional topical steroids. Visual acuity deteriorated in 6, improved in 13, and was stable in the remaining eyes. The data suggest that methotrexate is very effective in controlling inflammation of uveitis in patients with juvenile idiopathic arthritis. However, additional topical steroids or systemic immunosuppressive drugs are often required.

Intravitreal methotrexate injection

Hardwig et al.[17] published a report on intravitreal injection of 400 μg methotrexate as treatment for ocular disease other than primary central nervous system lymphoma. They included 9 patients with uveitis and showed that, among 7 patients, vision improved, in 1 it deteriorated, and in 1 patient it did not change. There was no observed toxicity attributable to methotrexate in any case. The authors concluded that intraocular methotrexate is a reasonable alternative to continued use of corticosteroids in uveitis patients.

Drug mechanism, systemic and ocular complications and toxicity, drug interactions, and contraindications are summarized in Table 36.2.[2,6–8]

Taylor et al.[18] had published recently a prospective study on the use of intravitreal methotrexate for the treatment of uveitis and uveitic cystoid macular edema on 15 patients. They showed that visual acuity improved at all time points and was statistically significant at the 3- and 6-month follow-up examinations. No statistical difference was found between the best visual acuity obtained after MTX injection and after previous corticosteroid treatment. Five patients relapsed after a median of 4 months; however a similar improvement was seen after re-injection. Ocular inflammation scores improved at all time points, and systemic immunosuppressive medication was reduced in 3 of 7 patients taking this at the start of the trial.

AZATHIOPRINE

Key features, introduction, and history

Azathioprine is a prodrug, converted to the active metabolites 6-mercaptopurine and 6-thioinosinic acid. It replaced 6-mercaptopurine as an immunosuppressive treatment for kidney transplants. The drug use in uveitis has been described since 1967.

Pharmacology

Azathioprine is well absorbed orally. Thirty percent of the drug is bound to serum proteins. It is rapidly eliminated from the blood and cannot be detected in urine after 8 hours. The enzyme thiopurine S-methyltransferase (TPMT) deactivates 6-mercaptopurine. Low activity of TPMT can lead to excessive drug toxicity, thus assay of serum TPMT may be useful to prevent this complication.[2]

Drug mechanism

Azathioprine is a purine nucleoside analogue. It interferes with adenine and guanine ribonucleotides by suppression of inosinic acid synthesis, which in turn interferes with DNA replication and RNA transcription. It decreases the numbers of peripheral T and B lymphocytes, and reduces mixed lymphocyte reactivity, interleukin-2 synthesis and IgM production.[6]

Drug effects in human nonocular diseases

Azathioprine is FDA-approved as an adjunct for the prevention of rejection in renal homotransplantations and for the management of active rheumatoid arthritis. It is also used in psoriatic arthritis, Reiter syndrome, and systemic lupus erythematosus.

Drug use in retinal diseases

Yazici et al.[19] conducted a 2-year randomized, placebo-controlled, double-blind trial of azathioprine (2.5 mg/kg/day) in Turkish men with Behçet's syndrome with and without eye disease. Corticosteroid treatment remained available to all the patients. Azathioprine was superior to placebo in the prevention of new eye disease in both groups. There were fewer episodes of hypopyon uveitis, oral ulcers, genital ulcers, and arthritis. There were no serious side-effects attributable to azathioprine.

Vianna et al.[20] described the clinical course of 4 patients (5 eyes) with active serpiginous choroiditis treated with azathioprine (1.5–2.0 mg/kg/day) in combination with corticosteroids. Within 3 weeks of treatment, all patients experienced decreased ocular inflammation and improved visual acuity. One patient, however, had a recurrence in both eyes while oral prednisone was being tapered and in another patient serpiginous choroiditis recurred 40 months after the initial treatment. None of the 4 patients presented serious systemic side-effects secondary to treatment.

Kim and Yu[21] evaluated treatment outcomes with low-dose azathioprine (1.0–2.5 mg/kg/day) in 16 patients with Vogt–Koyanagi–Harada disease. Six patients received azathioprine in the acute uveitic phase and 10 patients in the chronic recurrent phase. A corticosteroid-sparing effect was achieved in 86.5% of patients given azathioprine in the acute uveitic phase and 90.0% of patients given in the chronic recurrent phase. Median time to corticosteroid-sparing effect was 3.5 months. Twelve of 16 patients showed improved activity in 1 month after initiation of azathioprine therapy.

Pediatric case series

Schatz et al.[22] review, with respect to etiology, the efficacy and complications of different immunosuppressants used in a steroid-sparing strategy in 40 children with uveitis. Uveitis was anterior in 55% of cases, intermediate in 2.5%, posterior in 42.5%, and bilateral in 62.5%. Where corticosteroid use was combined with azathioprine, a 61% improvement in visual acuity was achieved. However, corticosteroid therapy associated with MMF resulted in a 94% improvement.

Drug mechanism, systemic and ocular complications and toxicity, drug interactions, and contraindications are summarized in Table 36.2.[2,6–8]

Summary and key points

The antimetabolite agents are effective as corticosteroid-sparing drugs in the treatment of ocular inflammatory disease. The properties, dosing, and most common adverse events of the three commonly used antimetabolites are summarized in Table 36.2. MMF is effective for controlling diseases that had been refractory to treatment with other immunosuppressive agents among adults and children; it is well tolerated and has few side-effects. Methotrexate is the most common

Table 36.2 Summary of antimetabolites' standard dose administration, mechanism of action, recommended laboratory tests, side-effects, drug interactions, and contraindications

Name	Oral formulation	Dose initial/ maximum	Mechanism	Expected onset	Lab test*	Side-effects	Comments	Contraindications
Mycophenolate mofetil (Cellcept)	250/500 mg capsule 200 mg/ml oral suspension	1–3 g/day (equally divided dose) Children: 750 mg–2 g/day (equally divided dose)	Selective IMP dehydrogenase inhibitor (purine synthesis inhibitor)	4–6 weeks (dose-dependent)	LFTs CBC Lipid profile	Serious: Hepatotoxicity Bone marrow suppression Teratogenic Opportunistic infections(CMV, HSV) Secondary malignancy: Nonmelanoma skin cancers Lymphoma Common: GI upset Less common: Fatigue Dizziness Eczema Hair loss Fever Headache	Should be ingested on an empty stomach Increased serum levels by aciclovir or ganciclovir Decreased serum levels by antacids and cholestyramine Decreased effectiveness of vaccinations	Absolute: • Pregnancy • Breast-feeding • Avoid live vaccines • Avoid concomitant use with clozapine • Avoid concomitant use with azathioprine or methotrexate because of the potential to cause bone marrow suppression Relative: GI disorders due to risk of hemorrhage, ulceration, and perforation
Methotrexate (Rheumatrex)	2.5 mg tablet	10–25 mg/week (a single undivided dose) • Most common: 15 mg/week Children: 7.5–15 mg/week (10–25 mg/m^2) • Given with folic acid (1 mg/day) to minimize toxicity	DHFR inhibitor (DNA replication inhibition)	6–8 weeks (dose-dependent)	LFTs RFTs CBC Chest X-ray • At baseline: Hepatitis BsAg Hepatitis C Ab	Serious: Hepatoxicity Nephrotoxicity Bone marrow suppression Interstitial pneumonia Teratogenic Opportunistic infections (PCP) Secondary malignancy: Nonmelanoma skin cancers Lymphoma Common: GI upset† Less common: Alopecia Rash	If ALT or AST is > two times normal on two separate occasions, the dose should be reduced Liver biopsy if LFTs are abnormal after drug discontinuation Abstain from alcohol consumption After discontinuation of methotrexate contraception should be continued in men for 3 months and in women for at least one ovulatory cycle Decreased absorption by food and oral nonabsorbable antibiotics: vancomycin, neomycin, bacitracin	Absolute: • Pregnancy • Breast-feeding • Liver disease • Avoid concomitant use with clozapine, nitrous oxide, azathioprine, mycophenolate mofetil

Table 36.2 Summary of antimetabolites' standard dose administration, mechanism of action, recommended laboratory tests, side-effects, drug interactions, and contraindications—cont'd

Name	Oral formulation	Dose initial/ maximum	Mechanism	Expected onset	Lab test*	Side-effects	Comments	Contraindications
Azathioprine (Imuran)	50 mg tablet	1–4 mg/kg/day • Most effective: 2 mg/kg/day Children: 1–2 mg/kg/day (30–60 mg/m^2)	Purine nucleoside analog (DNA replication and RNA transcription suppression)	4–6 weeks (dose-dependent)	CBC LFTs	Serious: Severe bone marrow suppression Hepatoxicity Teratogenic Opportunistic infections Secondary malignancy: Nonmelanoma skin cancers Lymphoma Common: GI upset† Less common: Alopecia Rash Fever Arthralgia	Serum TPMT assay before starting treatment If ALT or AST is > 1.5 times normal on two separate occasions, the dose should be reduced by 25–50 mg/day, and the liver enzyme level reevaluated after 2 weeks If there is marked enzyme elevation the drug should be stopped Dosage should be decreased when given with allopurinol Concomitant use with ACE inhibitors has been reported to induce anemia and severe leukopenia	Absolute: • Liver disease • Pregnancy • Breast-feeding • Avoid concomitant use with clozapine

IMP, inosine monophosphate; DHFR, dihydrofolate reductase; LFTs, liver function tests (primarily aspartate and alanine aminotransferases); CBC, complete blood count; RFTs, renal function tests; CMV, cytomegalovirus; HSV, herpes simplex virus; GI, gastrointestinal; PCP, Pneumocystis carinii *pneumonia; ALT, alanine aminotransferase; AST, aspartate aminotransferase; TPMT, thiopurine S-methyltransferase; ACE, angiotensin-converting enzyme.*

**Lab tests: at baseline, every 2 weeks in first month, and then every month.*

†Gatrointestinal upset: abdominal pain, nausea, vomiting, diarrhea, stomatitis, and anorexia.

immunosuppressive agent used in children and has been reported to be an effective treatment for the uveitis associated with juvenile idiopathic arthritis. Azathioprine is associated with more severe side-effects compared to other antimetabolite agents, which limits its use.

ALKYLATING AGENTS

Cyclophosphamide and chlorambucil are termed alkylating agents due to their ability to alkylate nucleic acids. As a result, DNA to DNA intrastrand crosslinking and DNA to protein crosslinking occur, which lead to interference in DNA and RNA replication and transcription. This process results in cell death, because the cells are unable to replicate. They are cytotoxic to both resting and dividing lymphocytes. So the number of activated T and B lymphocytes decreases, and T-helper lymphocyte function and cytokine production are suppressed.

CYCLOPHOSPHAMIDE

Key features, introduction, and history

Cyclophosphamide is a nitrogen mustard-alkylating agent, a prodrug of several alkylating agents which are formed as hepatic metabolites. The first drug clinical trials were published at the end of the 1950s. The drug use in uveitis has been described since 1969.

Pharmacology

Cyclophosphamide is well absorbed and is enzymatically converted by the hepatic enzymes to multiple metabolites. It is extensively metabolized before excretion, primarily by the kidney, with less than 25% remaining unchanged in the urine. One of these metabolites, acrolein, is thought to be responsible for the urologic toxicity. The use of 2-mercaptoethane sulfonate may detoxify acrolein and reduce bladder toxicity. Cyclophosphamide reaches its peak plasma level within 1 hour and has a plasma half-life of 4–10 hours.[6]

Drug effects in human nonocular diseases

Cyclophosphamide is FDA-approved as an adjunct for the treatment of lymphomas, some forms of leukemia, some solid tumors, and "minimal-change" nephrotic syndrome in children. It is also used in systemic lupus erythematosus and Wegener granulomatosis.

Drug use in retinal diseases

Akpek et al.[23] reported on 9 patients with active, vision-threatening serpiginous choroiditis who had progressive inflammation while on steroids and/or immunosuppressive agents other than alkylating agents, who were treated with either chlorambucil or cyclophosphamide. During a follow-up time of between 15 and 96 months, no patients had recurrences while on therapy and no further visual loss was encountered after starting the therapy. Six of the patients regained vision. All but 2 patients achieved prolonged drug-free remissions. Side-effects included transient bone marrow suppression, nausea, and fatigue. Secondary malignancy was encountered in 1 patient, whose carcinoma of the urinary bladder was treated successfully.

Durrani et al.[24] assess the efficacy and short-term safety of pulse intravenous cyclophosphamide therapy in the treatment of 38 patients with severe or treatment-resistant autoimmune ocular inflammatory disease. Improvement of ocular inflammation occurred in 68% of patients, with 55% achieving complete quiescence. A steroid-sparing effect was achieved in all patients previously on systemic steroid, allowing successful discontinuation of the drug in 41%. Visual acuity was maintained in 66% and improved in 21% of involved eyes. Panuveitis with concurrent retinal vasculitis and ocular cicatricial pemphigoid were the most common disease entities treated. Scleritis seemed to be the most responsive to treatment, followed by panuveitis with retinal vasculitis and ocular cicatricial pemphigoid. The most common side-effects observed were fatigue (63%), nausea (32%), and headache (22%). None required permanent discontinuation of therapy.

Efficacy and comparison with other agents

Ozyazgan et al.[25] conducted a single masked trial of CsA, 5 mg/kg/day, versus monthly 1 g intravenous boluses of cyclophosphamide in 23 patients with Behçet's syndrome and active, potentially reversible uveitis. During the initial 6 months the visual acuity significantly improved in the CsA group whereas this was not observed in the cyclophosphamide group. The subsequent follow-up of patients up to 24 months suggested that the initial improvement in visual acuity with CsA was not sustained.

Drug mechanism, systemic and ocular complications and toxicity, drug interactions, and contraindications are summarized in Table 36.3.[2,6,8]

CHLORAMBUCIL

Key features, introduction, and history

Chlorambucil is a nitrogen mustard alkylating agent which substitutes an alkyl group for hydrogen ions in organic compounds. The drug use in uveitis has been described since 1970.

Pharmacology

Chlorambucil is rapidly and completely absorbed from the gastrointestinal tract and food increases its bioavailability. Peak plasma levels are reached within 1 hour and estimated half-life is 1.5 hours. Chlorambucil undergoes rapid metabolism to phenylacetic acid mustard, the major metabolite. The combined urinary excretion of chlorambucil and phenylacetic acid mustard is extremely low – less than 1% in 24 hours.[6]

Drug effects in human nonocular diseases

Chlorambucil is FDA-approved for the treatment of chronic lymphocytic leukemia, Hodgkin and non-Hodgkin lymphoma. It is also used in rheumatic diseases but less frequently than cyclophosphamide, and in Behçet's disease.

Drug use in retinal diseases

Tessler et al.[26] treated 5 patients with intractable sympathetic ophthalmia and 6 patients with severe Behçet's disease by high-dose, short-term chlorambucil therapy. Among the Behçet's disease group the average duration was 23 weeks and the average total dose was 2.2 g. Among the sympathetic ophthalmia group the average duration was 11 weeks and the total average dose was 0.9 g. After termination of therapy all 11 patients had a sustained remission of their eye disease. Unless subretinal neovascularization was present, all had a final visual acuity of 20/50 or better. In addition concomitant systemic corticosteroids were discontinued within 6–8 weeks. Malignancy has not developed in any of the cases, with a follow-up ranging from 6 months to 12 years (mean, 4.5 years).

Mudun et al.[27] evaluated the effects of short-term chlorambucil therapy (23 weeks) in the management of 44 patients with refractory uveitis associated with Behçet's disease. The therapy was judged to be effective if the patient had ≤1 attack a year and/or ≥1 year between the attacks. The mean follow-up time was 51.4 ± 32.5 months (range, 13–122 months). Following the therapy, the mean frequency of attacks per year had significantly decreased from 4.9 ± 2.3 to 0.9 ± 1.4 and the mean longest period between the attacks was significantly prolonged from 4.4 ± 2.3 to 25.7 ± 23.1 months. The ratio of severe attacks had decreased from 74.1 ± 34% to 51.3 ± 36.6%. New attacks were seen in 56.8% of patients and another immunosuppressive agent or agents was given to 40.9% of the patients 1–8 months after treatment. No serious side-effects

Table 36.3 Summary of alkylating agents' standard dose administration, mechanism of action, recommended laboratory tests, side-effects, drug interactions, and contraindications

Name	Oral formulation	Dose initial/ maximum	Mechanism	Expected onset	Lab test	Side-effects	Comments	Contraindications
Cyclophosphamide (Cytoxan)	25/50 mg tablet	1–3 mg/kg/day (equally divided dose) Children: 1–2 mg/kg/day (equally divided dose) • Intravenous administration: 1 g/m² body surface area infused over a 2-hour period Repeated every 3–4 weeks, depending on the clinical response and leukocyte count	DNA cross-linking (inhibition of cell replication and protein synthesis)	2–6 weeks (dose-dependent)	CBC Urinalysis	Serious: Bone marrow suppression Opportunistic infections Hemorrhagic cystitis Hematuria Secondary malignancy: Bladder and hematological malignancies Teratogenicity Ovarian suppression Testicular atrophy Azoospermia Common: GI upset† Reversible alopecia	The goal is to maintain a WBC of 3500–5000 cells/ml Neutrophil counts > 1500 cells/ml platelet counts >75 000 cells/ml For WBC of 2500–3500 cells/ml reduce drug by 25–50 mg/day Stop treatment when WBC <2500 cells/ml or bladder toxicity. If hematuria persists after 3–4 weeks, a urologist should be consulted Hemorrhagic cystitis is common with bladder stasis-patients should drink at least 2 liters of fluid/day	Absolute: • Pregnancy • Breast-feeding • Infection • Neoplasm • Avoid concomitant use with clozapine, pentostatin

							Cryopreservation of eggs or sperm before beginning of treatment When given concomitantly with allopurinol or cimetidine dose should be reduced by 30–50%	
Chlorambucil (Leukeran)	2 mg tablet	0.1–0.2 mg/kg/day (6–12 mg/day) (as a single dose) • Short-term, high-dose therapy: initial dose of 2 mg/day for 1 week, followed by escalation by 2 mg/day each week. The dose escalation is continued until inflammation is completely suppressed. Treatment lasts 3–6 months Children: As adults	DNA cross- linking (inhibition of cell replication and protein synthesis)	4–12 weeks (dose-dependent)	CBC	Serious: Bone marrow suppression Opportunistic infections Hematological malignancies Teratogenicity Irreversible azoospermia and amenorrhea Seizures Common: GI upset†	Drug should be taken with food Therapy is given for 1 year after quiescence of the disease to induce a long-term drug-free remission Malignancies can occur years after the cessation of the drug – long-term follow-up of patients is needed	Absolute: • Pregnancy • Breast-feeding • Infection • Neoplasm

DNA, deoxyribonucleic acid; CBC, complete blood count; GI, gastrointestinal; WBC, white blood cells.

**Lab tests at baseline, every week, when dosing is stable every month.*

†Gastrointestinal upset: abdominal pain, nausea, vomiting, diarrhea, stomatitis. and anorexia.

were observed during the chlorambucil therapy. In summary, short-term chlorambucil therapy for refractory uveitis in Behçet's disease was found effective in controlling the disease in two-thirds of patients.

Miserocchi et al.[28] reported their experience with chlorambucil in 56 eyes of 28 patients with various uveitides (Behçet's disease, juvenile idiopathic arthritis, pars planitis, sympathetic ophthalmia, idiopathic uveitis, Crohn's disease, and human leukocyte antigen (HLA)-B27-associated uveitis) unresponsive to oral corticosteroids and other immunosuppressive therapy. The median duration of treatment was 12 months (range, 4–50 months); the median daily dosage was 8 mg (range, 4–22 mg). Median follow-up period was 46 months (range, 4–166 months). Vision improved or stabilized in 82% of patients, prednisone was successfully discontinued in 68% of patients, and 50% of patients had inactive disease without systemic therapy at the end of follow-up. However, 25% of patients had to discontinue therapy because of side-effects (temporary amenorrhea, unacceptable gastrointestinal intolerance, and progressive leucopenia).

Goldstein et al.[29] treated 53 patients with intractable sight-threatening uveitis with short-term (average 16 weeks) high-dose chlorambucil (average 20 mg/day). Seventy-seven percent of patients treated were in remission with an average follow-up of 4 years. Forty-seven percent had at least 2 lines of improvement in Snellen visual acuity after treatment, with an average gain of 3.5 lines. By the time the chlorambucil regimen was stopped, 78% of patients had discontinued oral corticosteroids. Adverse effects include secondary amenorrhea (26% of females), nonophthalmic herpes zoster (12%), testicular atrophy, and erectile dysfunction. None of the patients had developed any malignancy as of their last follow-up.

Efficacy and comparison with other agents

O'Duffy et al.[30] assessed the results of various treatments among 21 patients with Behçet's disease. Treatment with chlorambucil, 0.1 mg/kg daily, compared favorably with corticosteroids. Uveitis and visual acuities improved in 5 of 7 eyes when the patients were treated with chlorambucil, whereas improvement was observed in only 4 of 13 eyes when treatment consisted of corticosteroids. Toxicity from chlorambucil included leukopenia (2 patients), thrombocytopenia (1), bronchopneumonia (1), and amenorrhea (1). The duration of chlorambucil therapy averaged 1.8 years.

Drug mechanism, systemic and ocular complications and toxicity, drug interactions, and contraindications are summarized in Table 36.3.[2,6,8]

Summary and key points

Alkylating agents, in view of their potential toxicity, can be a reasonable choice for patients with ocular inflammatory disease resistant to other forms of second-line immunosuppressive agents. The common properties of alkylating agents are summarized in Table 36.3. Chlorambucil therapy can be associated with unpredictable and sudden pancytopenia, and for that reason many clinicians prefer to use cyclophosphamide. However, cyclophosphamide can be associated with hemorrhagic cystitis and an increased risk of bladder cancer but is most effective in Wegener granulomatosis and mucous membrane pemphigoid.

SUMMARY

Comparison outcome studies have shown unequivocally that immunomodulatory therapy, such as the calcineurin inhibitors, the antimetabolites, and the alkylating agents, should have a much more important role to play today in the care of patients with ocular inflammation. Clinician scientists caring for patients with uveitis and ocular inflammatory diseases should aim toward the goal of no tolerance to any degree of inflammation. When employed properly and monitored appropriately, the potential adverse events of immunomodulatory therapy are manageable and may be acceptable when benefits to patients can be demonstrated.

REFERENCES

1. Kapturczak MH, Meier-Kriesche HU, Kaplan B. Pharmacology of calcineurin antagonists. Transplantation Proc 2004;36(2 Suppl):25S-32S.
2. Kurup SK, Chan CC. Immunotherapeutic approaches in ocular inflammatory diseases. Arch Immunol Ther Exp 2005;53:484–496.
3. Ozdal PC, Ortac S, Taskintuna I, et al. Long-term therapy with low dose cyclosporin A in ocular Behçet's disease. Doc Ophthalmol 2002;105:301–312.
4. Kilmartin DJ, Forrester JV, Dick AD. Cyclosporin A therapy in refractory non-infectious childhood uveitis. Br J Ophthalmol 1998;82:737–742.
5. Murphy CC, Greiner K, Plskova J, et al. Cyclosporine vs tacrolimus therapy for posterior and intermediate uveitis. Arch Ophthalmol 2005;123:634–641.
6. Jabs DA, Rosenbaum JT, Foster CS, et al. Guidelines for the use of immunosuppressive drugs in patients with ocular inflammatory disorders: recommendations of an expert panel. Am J Ophthalmol 2000;130:492–513.
7. Gerber DA, Bonham CA, Thomson AW. Immunosuppressive agents: recent developments in molecular action and clinical application. Transplant Proc 1998;30:1573–1579.
8. Becker MD, Smith JR, Max R, et al. Management of sight-threatening uveitis: new therapeutic options. Drugs 2005;65:497–519.
9. Sloper CM, Powell RJ, Dua HS. Tacrolimus (FK506) in the treatment of posterior uveitis refractory to cyclosporine. Ophthalmology 1999;106:723–728.
10. Hogan AC, McAvoy CE, Dick AD, et al. Long-term efficacy and tolerance of tacrolimus for the treatment of uveitis. Ophthalmology 2007;114:1000–1006.
11. Thorne JE, Jabs DA, Qazi FA, et al. Mycophenolate mofetil therapy for inflammatory eye disease. Ophthalmology 2005;112:1472–1477.
12. Siepmann K, Huber M, Stübiger N, et al. Mycophenolate mofetil is a highly effective and safe immunosuppressive agent for the treatment of uveitis: a retrospective analysis of 106 patients. Graefes Arch Clin Exp Ophthalmol 2006;244:788–794.
13. Sobrin L, Christen W, Foster CS. Mycophenolate mofetil after methotrexate failure or intolerance in the treatment of scleritis and uveitis. Ophthalmology 2008;115:1416–1421.
14. Doycheva D, Deuter C, Stuebiger N, et al. Mycophenolate mofetil in the treatment of uveitis in children. Br J Ophthalmol 2007;91:180–184.
15. Samson CM, Waheed N, Baltatzis S, et al. Methotrexate therapy for chronic noninfectious uveitis: analysis of a case series of 160 patients. Ophthalmology 2001;108:1134–1139.
16. Heiligenhaus A, Mingels A, Heinz C, et al. Methotrexate for uveitis associated with juvenile idiopathic arthritis: value and requirement for additional anti-inflammatory medication. Eur J Ophthalmol 2007;17:743–748.
17. Hardwig PW, Pulido JS, Erie JC, et al. Intraocular methotrexate in ocular diseases other than primary central nervous system lymphoma. Am J Ophthalmol 2006;142:883–885.
18. Taylor SR, Habot-Wilner Z, Pacheco P, et al. Intraocular methotrexate in the treatment of uveitis and uveitic cystoid macular edema. Ophthalmology 2009;116:797–801.
19. Yazici H, Pazarli H, Barnes CG, et al. A controlled trial of azathioprine in Behçet's syndrome. N Engl J Med 1990;322:281–285.
20. Vianna RN, Ozdal PC, Deschênes J, et al. Combination of azathioprine and corticosteroids in the treatment of serpiginous choroiditis. Can J Ophthalmol 2006;41:183–189.
21. Kim SJ, Yu HG. The use of low-dose azathioprine in patients with Vogt–Koyanagi–Harada disease. Ocul Immunol Inflamm 2007;15:381–387.
22. Schatz CS, Uzel JL, Leininger L, et al. Immunosuppressants used in a steroid-sparing strategy for childhood uveitis. J Pediatr Ophthalmol Strabismus 2007;44:28–34.
23. Akpek EK, Jabs DA, Tessler HH, et al. Successful treatment of serpiginous choroiditis with alkylating agents. Ophthalmology 2002;109:1506–1513.
24. Durrani K, Papaliodis GN, Foster CS. Pulse IV cyclophosphamide in ocular inflammatory disease: efficacy and short-term safety. Ophthalmology 2004;111:960–965.
25. Ozyazgan Y, Yurdakul S, Yazici H, et al. Low dose cyclosporin A versus pulsed cyclophosphamide in Behçet's syndrome: a single masked trial. Br J Ophthalmol 1992;76:241–243.
26. Tessler HH, Jennings T. High-dose short-term chlorambucil for intractable sympathetic ophthalmia and Behçet's disease. Br J Ophthalmol 1990;74:353–357.
27. Mudun BA, Ergen A, Ipcioglu SU, et al. Short-term chlorambucil for refractory uveitis in Behçet's disease. Ocul Immunol Inflamm 2001;9:219–229.
28. Miserocchi E, Baltatzis S, Ekong A, et al. Efficacy and safety of chlorambucil in intractable noninfectious uveitis: the Massachusetts Eye and Ear Infirmary experience. Ophthalmology 2002;109:137–142.
29. Goldstein DA, Fontanilla FA, Kaul S, et al. Long-term follow-up of patients treated with short-term high-dose chlorambucil for sight-threatening ocular inflammation. Ophthalmology 2002;109:370–377.
30. O'Duffy JD, Robertson DM, Goldstein NP. Chlorambucil in the treatment of uveitis and meningoencephalitis of Behçet's disease. Am J Med 1984;76:75–84.

CHAPTER

37 Fusion proteins: VEGF-Trap

Diana V. Do, MD, Shawn Wilker, MD, Syed Mahmood Shah, MBBS, Mohamed Ibrahim, MD, and Quan Dong Nguyen, MD, MSc

KEY FEATURES

Vascular endothelial growth factor (VEGF) blockers currently used to treat eye diseases have included monoclonal antibodies, antibody fragments, and an aptamer. A different method of achieving VEGF blockade in retinal diseases includes the concept of a cytokine trap. Cytokine traps are being evaluated for the treatment of various diseases that are driven by excessive cytokine levels. Traps consist of two extracellular cytokine receptor domains fused together to form a human immunoglobulin G (IgG).[1] VEGF Trap-Eye is a soluble fusion protein which combines ligand-binding elements taken from the extracellular components of VEGF receptors 1 and 2 fused to the Fc portion of IgG_1.[2] This protein contains all human amino acid sequences, which minimizes the potential for immunogenicity in human patients (Figure 37.1).[2]

VEGF has two main receptors in normal biological systems: VEGFR1 and VEGFR2. VEGFR2 is responsible for most of the endothelial cell-proliferating activity of VEGF,[3,4] whereas VEGFR1 mediates other activities of VEGF, such as its chemoattractant properties.[4] Both receptors are important for the angiogenic-promoting properties of VEGF.[3,4] Due to the more recent discovery of other VEGF family members, the original VEGF molecule is now often referred to as VEGF-A. Although several VEGF family members have now been identified, VEGF-A and placental growth factor (PlGF) are the forms believed to be most involved in angiogenesis.[2,5] Other family members that exist in mammals include VEGF-B, VEGF-C, and VEGF-D.[3,4]

VEGF-A is important for vascular permeability, which is important for normal physiological processes such as wound healing but can potentially increase leakage in pathological disease states, such as neovascular age-related macular degeneration (AMD).[3,4] VEGF-A also appears to promote the survival of hematopoietic stem cells; the migration of these cells appears to be promoted via interactions with VEGFR1.[4] It has been suggested VEGF-A is a critical factor for the recruitment of monocytes and macrophages in inflammatory neovascularization.[6]

VEGF-B may be particularly important for cardiovascular development and cardiovascular angiogenesis. Although the role of VEGF-B in angiogenesis is not completely understood, there is evidence that it may be involved in inflammatory angiogenesis in various disease states, and may also modulate endothelial proliferation and vessel growth.[7] VEGF-C and -D appear to be involved in the development of the lymphatic system.[4]

A large body of recent research indicates that PlGF may be another factor important for promotion of pathological neoangiogenesis.[8,9] There is specific evidence for the involvement of PlGF in neoangiogenesis in eye pathologies. For example, absence of PlGF prevents pathologic angiogenesis and vascular leakage in animal models of cancer, retinal ischemia, and wound healing.[10] In the rabbit cornea and the chick chorioallantoic membrane, PlGF was shown to be as effective as VEGF in inducing angiogenesis.[11] In mice with experimental choroidal neovascularization (CNV), PlGF (as well as VEGF) was upregulated during initial CNV development. In PlGF null mice or in wild-type mice treated with an anti-VEGFR-1 antibody, a significant reduction in the incidence and severity of laser-induced CNV was observed.[12] PlGF was present in the vitreous and in the neovascular membranes in humans with proliferative diabetic retinopathy (PDR).[13,14] It therefore seems that PlGF is a critical factor involved in pathological neoangiogenesis.

Unlike the currently available monoclonal VEGF antibody and the VEGF antibody fragment, VEGF Trap-Eye binds VEGF-A, VEGF-B, and PlGF.[2,5,6,15,16] Figure 37.1 illustrates the characteristics of VEGF Trap-Eye. VEGFR1 and VEGFR2 normally bind VEGF-A with binding affinity of 10–30 and 100–300 pM kD, respectively. VEGF Trap-Eye has a much higher binding affinity of approximately 0.5 pM kD. The currently available VEGF antibody fragment binds VEGF-A with an affinity of ≤99–179 pM kD,[17] which has approximately 10-fold greater affinity than the currently available VEGF monoclonal antibody.[15] The higher binding affinity of VEGF Trap-Eye to VEGF-A, as well as binding to VEGF-B and PlGF, may confer a differential antiangiogenic activity relative to currently available anti-VEGF agents.[2,5,6,15,16] The clinical development of VEGF Trap-Eye is intended to explore the potential relevance of these pharmacologic differences.

INTRODUCTION AND HISTORY

Early studies demonstrated that treatment with a truncated, soluble VEGFR1 molecule almost completely suppressed VEGF bioactivity and thereby virtually halted corpus luteum angiogenesis in a rat ovulation model.[18] A soluble VEGFR chimeric protein exhibited greater VEGF inhibition than inducible VEGF gene ablation in newborn mice. The VEGF receptor chimera almost completely halted VEGF-mediated growth and was lethal in these animals.[19] Several other studies have similarly demonstrated that decoy receptors provide an effective means of blocking VEGF and its angiogenic effects.[20–22]

The current VEGF Trap-Eye evolved from a parental VEGF-Trap.[2,5,23,24] In this initial trap, the first three Ig domains of VEGFR1 were fused to the Fc region of human IgG_1. Three additional VEGF traps were then engineered based on that initial molecule; these were called VEGF TrapΔB1 (in which a highly basic 10-amino-acid sequence was removed from the third Ig domain of the parental trap), VEGF TrapΔB2 (in which the entire first Ig domain from VEGF TrapΔB1 was removed), and VEGF-Trap R1R2. VEGF-Trap R1R2 was created via the fusion of the second Ig domain of VEGFR1 with the third domain of VEGFR2.[2] These modifications enhanced VEGF-A affinity for the R1R2 trap relative to the other traps constructed and improved the pharmacokinetic properties of the VEGF-Trap R1R2. The initial parental VEGF-Trap had very high affinity for VEGF-A and binding affinity for PlGF, but was a strongly positively charged molecule that bound the extracellular matrix in addition to VEGF-A and PlGF. Modifications resulted in a less positively charged molecule that retained high affinity for VEGF-A and VEGF-B as well as PlGF, but did not nonspecifically bind the extracellular matrix.[2,16]

Different formulations of VEGF-Trap are currently being developed for oncology and ophthalmologic indications. VEGF-Trap for oncology (aflibercept) has been designed to be administered via intravenous infusion. VEGF Trap-Eye is intended to be delivered via intravitreal injection. Therefore, the molecule itself undergoes additional purification steps to avoid irritation of the eye. Therefore, VEGF Trap-Eye is formulated as an iso-osmotic formulation consisting of buffers used at

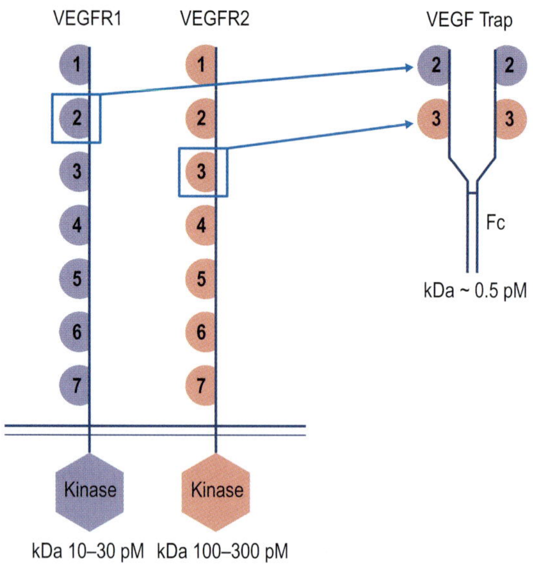

Figure 37.1 Vascular endothelial growth factor (VEGF) Trap-Eye (R1R2) combines the second domain of VEGF receptors 1 (seen in blue) and the third domain of VEGF receptor 2 (seen in red) fused to the Fc portion of IgG_1. VEGFR1 and VEGFR2 bind VEGF with affinity of 10–30 and 100–300 kD, respectively. Both are normally linked to a kinase, which mediates intracellular signal transduction. VEGF Trap-Eye has a binding affinity of approximately 0.5 pM.

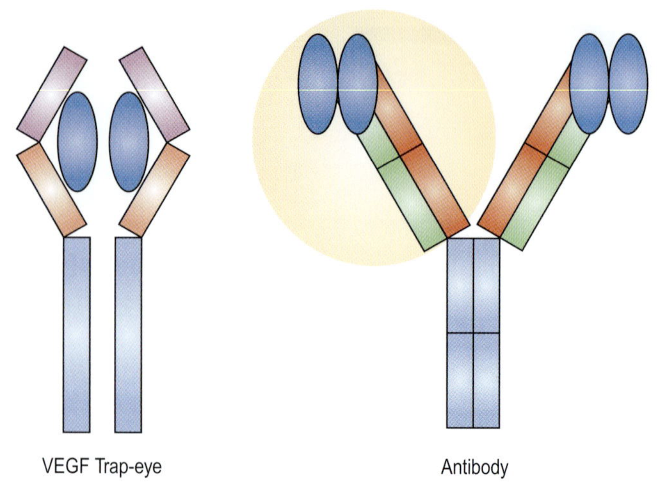

Figure 37.2 Vascular endothelial growth factor (VEGF)-Trap binds VEGF dimers (seen as two blue ovals) as a decoy receptor, in a different manner than the way in which VEGF antibodies bind VEGF dimers. VEGF-Trap binds the VEGF dimer on both sides of the dimer "like two hands on a football." The trap prevents VEGF from activating its cell surface receptor. In contrast, anti-VEGF antibodies bind in a manner that allows the VEGF dimer to interact further with other molecules.

different concentrations as well as a different concentration of buffers than in the oncology formulation.

PHARMACOLOGY

The pharmacokinetics and ocular distribution of 500 µg intravitreal VEGF Trap-Eye were studied in rabbits. Maximum vitreous concentrations of free VEGF Trap-Eye were approximately 500 µg/ml 0.25–6 hours following the 500-µg injection, and the VEGF Trap-Eye vitreous elimination half-life was about 4.5 days. VEGF Trap-Eye was detected in both retina and choroid, from which it was eliminated with a similar half-life. Ten days after the injection, maximal plasma total VEGF Trap-Eye levels were 1.6 µg/ml. At week 4, vitreous free VEGF Trap-Eye was 10-fold greater than levels of excess bound VEGF Trap-Eye. Therefore, ocular VEGF production would likely be completely suppressed for greater than 6 weeks following an intravitreal injection based on these results.[25]

In early experiments, modifications led to improved binding affinity for VEGF-Trap R1R2 relative to the parental VEGF-Trap, since parental VEGF-Trap had a binding affinity (kD) of about 5 pM, whereas VEGF Trap-R1R2 had a kD of approximately 1 pM.[2] Furthermore, its VEGF receptor-binding domains have a high affinity for PlGF – about 45 pM. A large body of recent research indicates that PlGF may be another factor that is important for promoting pathological neoangiogenesis.[8,9] Based on initial studies demonstrating high-affinity and improved pharmacokinetics, the development of this molecule has advanced to human clinical trials, including for the treatment of wet AMD and diabetic macular edema (DME). Experimental studies with intravitreal injections indicate that VEGF Trap-Eye should penetrate all layers of the retina (molecular weight ~110 000) with minimal systemic exposure.[26] In an animal model (diabetic rats), an intravitreal injection of VEGF Trap-Eye was distributed to all retinal layers, with little, if any, systemic exposure.[27] The agent also displays an extended half-life, allowing for long-term blockade.[5]

A recent modeling study predicted that the VEGF-binding activity of VEGF Trap-Eye would far exceed that of the anti-VEGF monoclonal antibody ranibizumab, based on the higher binding affinity and longer intravitreal half-life of VEGF Trap-Eye. Approximately 1.15 mg VEGF Trap-Eye is an equimolar concentration to 0.5 mg ranibizumab. This concentration of VEGF Trap-Eye (1.15 mg) would have binding activity at 79 days, comparable to 0.5 mg ranibizumab binding activity at 30 days. According to this study 0.5, 2, and 4 mg VEGF Trap-Eye injected intravitreally would have binding activity at 73, 83, and 87 days respectively, comparable to ranibizumab 0.5 binding activity at 30 days.[28] A similar study predicted that binding activity for the monoclonal antibody ranibizumab would be roughly comparable to that of the anti-VEGF monoclonal antibody bevacizumab, implying that VEGF Trap-Eye should have more extended binding activity than either anti-VEGF monoclonal antibody.[29] This study hypothesizes that VEGF Trap-Eye should have more durable effects than currently available treatments, which would likely result in longer intervals between doses.

VEGF Trap-Eye theoretically binds VEGF more tightly than native receptors or monoclonal antibodies. This suggests that a much lower dose of VEGF Trap-Eye may be used versus anti-VEGF monoclonal antibodies.[2] VEGF TRAP-Eye (R1R2) blocks all VEGF-A isoforms and PlGF.[2,5,6] It also blocks all isoforms of VEGF-B.[16] Consistent with this comprehensive receptor-blocking effect, VEGF Trap-Eye was shown *in vitro* to block several biological effects of VEGF, including potent blockade of the activation of VEGFR by VEGF, complete blockade of VEGFR2-induced phosphorylation in cultured human umbilical vein endothelial cells, and blockade of VEGF-induced proliferation of NIH/3T3 cells transfected with a VEGFR2/TrkB chimeric receptor.[2]

DRUG MECHANISM

The VEGF-Trap forms a stable and inert complex with VEGF.[30] Figure 37.2 illustrates differences in how VEGF-Trap binds VEGF dimers as a decoy receptor, in contrast to the manner in which VEGF antibodies bind VEGF dimers. VEGF normally binds its receptors as homo- or heterodimers.[3] VEGF-Trap binds the VEGF dimer on both sides of the dimer "like two hands on a football." The trap binds VEGF very tightly and prevents it from activating its cell surface receptor. In contrast, anti-VEGF antibodies bind in a manner that allows the VEGF dimer to interact further with other molecules. Since, in contrast to antibody complexes, the VEGF-Trap forms inert complexes with VEGF,[30] this minimizes the potential for VEGF-Trap to interact with more than one VEGF-Trap molecule, for example, thus multimeric complexes will not be formed as a consequence of VEGF Trap-Eye binding VEGF. Multimeric complexes could potentially aggregate in bodily tissues, causing immunogenic responses.

DRUG EFFECTS IN PRECLINICAL MODELS

Preclinical animal studies have evaluated the efficacy of VEGF Trap-Eye (R1R2) in several models of neovascularization in the eye, including the suppression of CNV in mice, and suppression of VEGF-induced breakdown of the blood–retinal barrier. Subcutaneous injections or a single intravitreal injection of VEGF Trap-Eye (R1R2) strongly suppressed CNV in mice with laser-induced rupture of Bruch's membrane.[31] Subcutaneous injection of VEGF Trap-Eye (R1R2) also significantly inhibited subretinal neovascularization in transgenic mice that express VEGF in photoreceptors.[31] VEGF Trap-Eye blocked angiogenesis in a mouse model of suture-induced inflammatory corneal neovascularization.[6] Intravitreal administration of VEGF Trap-Eye prevents the development of grade 4 choroidal neovascular lesions in primates, and markedly reduced proliferative responses of the retina to laser injury in adult cynomolgus monkeys.[32] VEGF Trap-Eye administration every 4 weeks via intravitreal injection was also demonstrated to be safe in cynomolgus monkeys after 13 weeks of administration.[33]

SYSTEMIC AND OCULAR COMPLICATIONS AND TOXICITY

In phase I and II studies, intravitreal injections of VEGF Trap-Eye caused no drug-related systemic adverse events.[34,35] In the phase II AMD study there were no drug-related serious adverse events and no systemic adverse events were classified by the investigators as being related to study drug administration.[36] There was one reported case of culture-negative endophthalmitis/uveitis in the study eye and one arterial thrombotic event, neither of which was deemed to be drug-related. The most common adverse events were those typically associated with intravitreal injections.

BIOACTIVITY IN HUMAN EYE DISEASES

NEOVASCULAR AMD PHASE I

VEGF Trap-Eye is currently being evaluated for two eye diseases: neovascular (wet) AMD and DME. VEGF Trap-Eye has undergone phase I and II clinical trials in wet AMD, and is presently in phase III clinical testing. The phase I study, known as CLEAR-IT 1 (CLinical Evaluation of Anti-angiogenesis in the Retina Intravitreal Trial), consisted of two parts. It was designed to evaluate the safety, tolerability, and biological effects of intravitreal VEGF-Trap in patients with neovascular AMD. The primary bioactivity measure was the change from baseline in central retinal lesion thickness. Patients were also monitored for ocular and systemic safety. Effects of VEGF Trap-Eye on disease status were followed with best-corrected ETDRS visual acuity (BCVA) using the electronic visual acuity system. Fluorescein angiography assessments were also conducted.

Part 1 was a single, ascending-dose study comprising 21 patients with 6 weeks of observation. VEGF Trap-Eye was injected intravitreally once, with groups of 3–6 patients each receiving single doses of 0.05, 0.15, 0.5, 1, 2, or 4 mg VEGF Trap-Eye.[34,35] Inclusion criteria were BCVA of 20/40 (73 letters) or worse. Following a 6-week observation period, patients were redosed at a frequency determined at the discretion of the treating physician under an extension protocol.

For the combined cohorts, a sustained reduction in retinal thickness and an improvement in visual acuity were reported with VEGF Trap-Eye at the 6-week primary endpoint. BCVA letters improved by a mean of 4.4 letters and central retinal lesion thickness decreased by −78.8 µm. Furthermore, a potential durability of effect with VEGF Trap-Eye was demonstrated, with patients averaging more than 5 months to the first retreatment in an extension study. The mean time to retreatment was 166 days (median, 127 days; range, 42–470 days) (Table 37.1).[34,35]

Part 2 of the CLEAR-IT 1 trial was a parallel-group, randomized trial comprising 28 patients who received a single intravitreal dose of 0.15 or 4 mg VEGF Trap-Eye (the range of doses demonstrating clinical activity in part 1) followed by 8 weeks of observation. Patients enrolled and treated in the CLEAR-IT 1 part 2 study had to satisfy the criteria for entry. After 8 weeks postdose, patients were reassessed for retreatment using established criteria.[34,35]

For part 2 of the CLEAR-IT 1 trial, results have been presented for the first 24 of 28 patients enrolled.[34] Both doses reduced retinal thickness at 2 weeks, but the duration of effect was longer in the 4-mg group than in the 0.15-mg group, as evidenced by a significantly greater reduction in retinal thickness in the 4-mg dose group than the 0.15-mg dose group at weeks 4 and 8. Reductions for the 4-mg dose and the 0.15-mg dose were −200 and −72.9 µm at 4 weeks, respectively. Reductions for the 4-mg dose and the 0.15-mg dose were −175 and −67.3 µm at 8 weeks, respectively ($P < 0.05$ for the 4-mg versus the 0.15-mg group).[34] Visual acuity improvements were sustained within the 4-mg dose group through 8 weeks (Figure 37.3).

Fewer patients in the high-dose group required retreatment based on objective criteria at the study's 8-week endpoint visit. In an extension study, the time to second dose in days for the 0.15-mg group was a

Table 37.1 Decreased retinal thickness and improvement in best corrected visual acuity (BCVA) at 6 weeks

Change to week 6	VEGF-TRAP (All Cohorts Combined) *n*	*Mean*	*SD*
BCVA (letters)	21	4.4	11.8
CRLT (µm)	17	−78.8	204.9

VEGF, vascular endothelial growth factor; CRLT, Central Retinal Lesion Thickness.

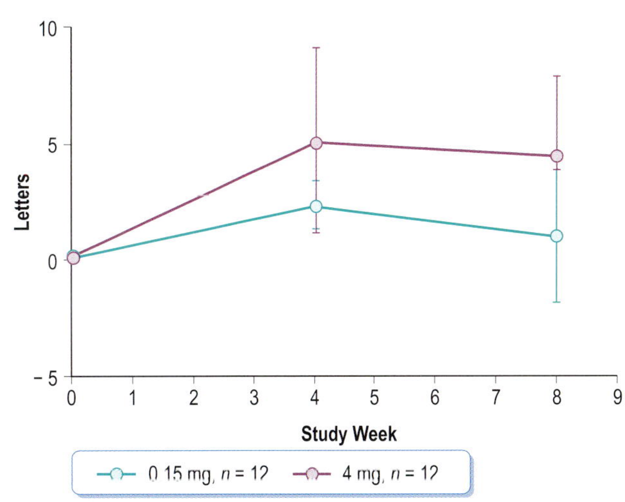

Figure 37.3 A greater sustained improvement in best corrected visual acuity was seen in the 4 mg dose compared to the 0.15 mg dose.

mean of 78 days (median, 64 days; range, 57–141 days), whereas the mean time to retreatment in the 4-mg group was 109 days (median, 69 days; range, 57–242 days). The most common indication for retreatment was new or persistent fluid on optical coherence tomography (OCT: 9/14 patients retreated).[34]

Overall, in the CLEAR-IT 1 part 1 and part 2 studies, intravitreal injection of up to 4 mg of VEGF Trap-Eye was well tolerated with no ocular inflammation seen.[34,35] In part 1, no inflammation or endophthalmitis was observed. There were no serious adverse events, ocular adverse events were mild to moderate in severity, and only one ocular adverse event was considered to be related to the study drug.[35] Most adverse events in part 2 were related to the study drug injection procedure. There was no evidence of ocular inflammation. Of the subjects for whom increased intraocular pressure (IOP) was reported, none exceeded 30 mmHg.[34]

NEOVASCULAR AMD PHASE II CLINICAL TRIAL

CLEAR-IT 2 was designed based upon the phase I study results showing clinically meaningful improvement in visual acuity with single doses of 0.5, 2.0, and 4.0 mg and sustained clinical activity beyond 1 month. CLEAR-IT 2 was a randomized, phase II, masked, controlled study designed to explore the safety and efficacy of VEGF Trap-Eye for wet AMD at various doses and dosing regimens (n = 159 randomized; n = 157 treated). Patients were randomized into five groups and treated with VEGF Trap-Eye in the study eye at 0.5 and 2.0 mg q 4 weeks and 0.5, 2.0, and 4.0 mg q 12 weeks for 12 weeks, followed by as-needed (pro re nata: PRN) dosing thereafter until week 52.

Inclusion criteria were: (1) males and females 50 or older with subfoveal CNV secondary to AMD; (2) central retinal lesion thickness of 300 μm or greater as measured by OCT; (3) ETDRS BCVA of 73–34 letters; (4) a loss of 5 or more ETDRS letters or one or more Snellen line in BCVA over the last 6 months (for previously treated patients with minimally classic or occult lesions); and (5) lesion greatest linear diameter of 5400 μm or less (including blood, scars, atrophy, and neovascularization) as assessed by fluorescein angiography, with subretinal hemorrhage making up 50% or less of the total lesion size and sparing the fovea and an area of scar 25% or less of the total lesion.

Patients were monitored for retinal thickness, visual acuity, and safety. The primary endpoint was change in central retinal lesion thickness as determined from a single-line high-resolution posterior-pole OCT scan read at an independent reading center.

A preplanned interim analysis of the first 78 patients who completed 12 weeks of treatment showed that VEGF Trap-Eye met its primary endpoint of a statistically significant mean reduction in retinal thickness after 12 weeks compared with baseline (all groups combined, decrease of 135 μm; $P < 0.0001$). Patients dosed either on a monthly or quarterly schedule achieved significant reductions in retinal thickness as measured by OCT posterior-pole scan versus baseline over the 12-week monitoring period. While results were similar at 8 weeks, monthly dosing was numerically, but not statistically, superior to quarterly dosing at 12 weeks (Figure 37.4).[36]

The mean change from baseline in visual acuity also demonstrated statistically significant improvement (all groups combined, increase of 5.9 letters; $P < 0.0001$). All but one patient maintained or improved vision at 12 weeks. In terms of visual acuity, monthly and quarterly dosing did not result in substantially different results at 8 weeks. Monthly dosing was numerically superior to quarterly dosing at 12 weeks, although not statistically significant. Monthly dosing resulted in continued visual acuity improvement through week 12 (range of means, 8.8–10.4 letters gained). Quarterly dosing resulted in substantial improvements at week 8 (range of means, 4.4–5.4 letters gained) and at week 12 (range of the means, 2.8–5.1 letters gained) (Figure 37.5).[36]

At the interim analysis in the CLEAR-IT 2 study, the most common adverse events were those typically associated with intravitreal injections and appeared to be related to the injection procedure. There was no relationship between VEGF Trap-Eye dose and the occurrence of any particular ocular adverse event. No adverse consequences of increased IOP were reported.[36]

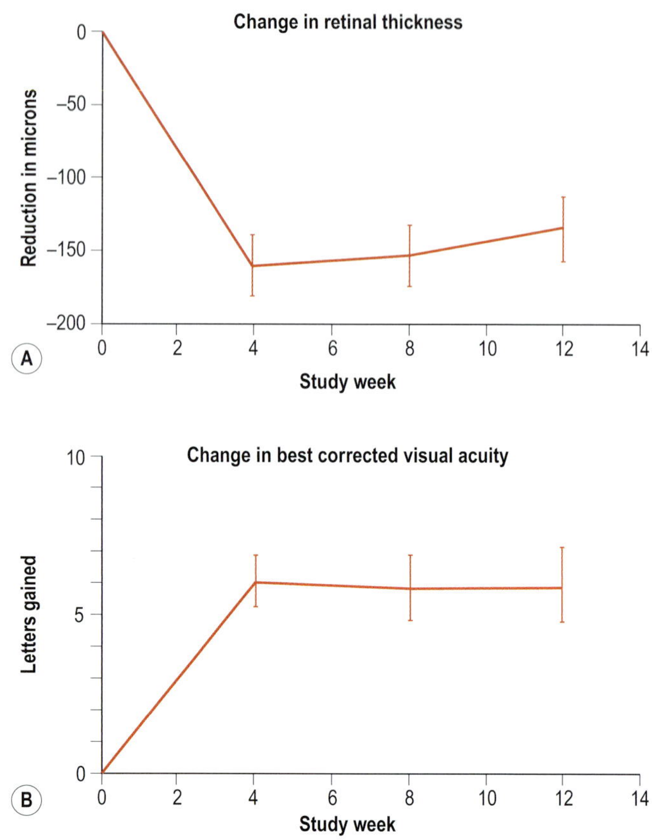

Figure 37.4 These graphs show retinal thickness and visual acuity for all groups combined (mean ± SEM). Vascular endothelial growth factor (VEGF) Trap-Eye met its primary endpoint of statistically significant mean reduction in retinal thickness over 12 weeks compared with baseline (all groups combined, decrease of 135 μm; $P < 0.0001$); 65 patients for whom readings were available and interpretable were included in the analysis. Mean change from baseline in visual acuity for all patients included in the interim analysis (n = 78) also demonstrated statistically significant improvement (all groups combined, increase of 5.9 letters, $P < 0.0001$). All but one patient maintained or improved vision at 12 weeks. CR/LT, BCVA, best corrected visual acuity.

NEOVASCULAR AMD PHASE III PROGRAM

Based upon the preliminary phase II study results which indicated that doses of 0.5 and 2 mg monthly produced substantial gains in visual acuity and a single 2-mg dose had a sustained improvement in visual acuity as compared to 2 mg monthly for at least 8 weeks, the phase III program was designed to evaluate these dosing schedules as compared to the standard dosing schedule for ranibizumab 0.5 mg monthly. Two identical, noninferiority phase III studies are currently under way to evaluate VEGF Trap-Eye for wet AMD, known as VIEW (VEGF Trap-Eye: Investigation of Efficacy and Safety in Wet AMD) 1 and VIEW 2. Both will compare VEGF Trap-Eye with the monoclonal antibody fragment ranibizumab using a noninferiority design. Both are randomized, double-masked, active-controlled, efficacy and safety studies with a primary endpoint of the proportion of patients treated with VEGF Trap-Eye who maintain vision at the end of one year, compared to ranibizumab patients. Visual acuity will be measured via the total number of letters read correctly on the ETDRS chart (2-year study).[16]

Both studies are double-masked, randomized, controlled-dose and interval-ranging studies of repeated intravitreal VEGF Trap-Eye

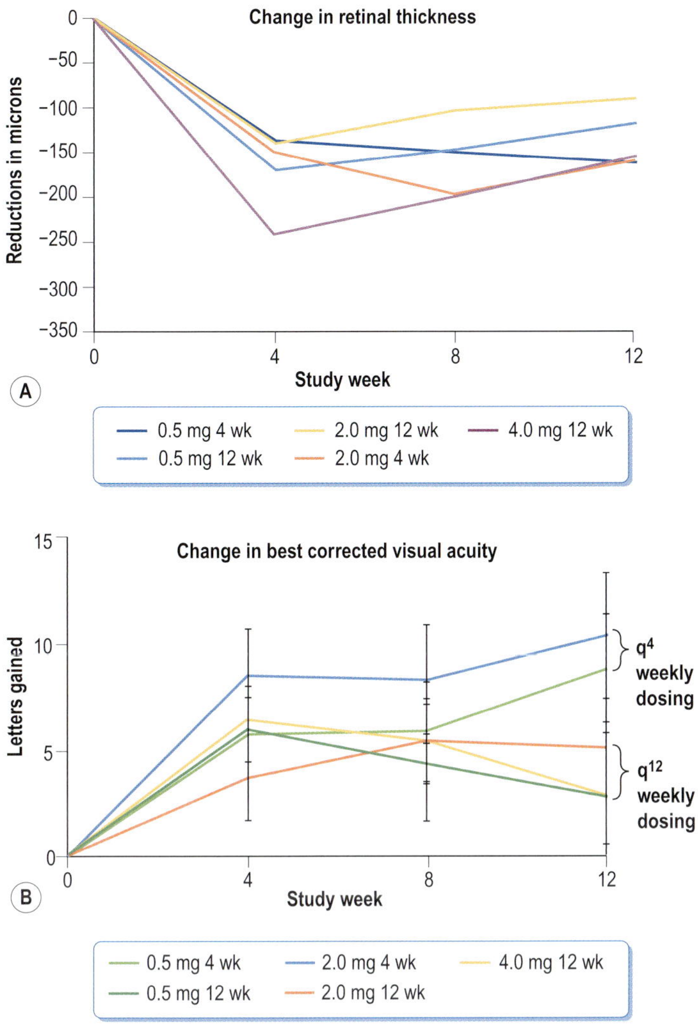

Figure 37.5 Retinal thickness and visual acuity in individual groups are shown separately (mean ± SEM). Monthly and quarterly dosing did not result in substantially different results at 8 weeks. Even quarterly dosing resulted in substantial improvements at week 8 (range of means, 4.4–5.4 letters gained), and at week 12 (range of means, 2.8–5.1 letters gained). Monthly dosing was numerically superior at 12 weeks, though not statistically significant. Monthly dosing resulted in continued best corrected visual acuity (BCVA) improvement through week 12 (range of means at week 12, 8.8–10.4 letters gained).

administration versus monthly dosing of ranibizumab in patients with neovascular AMD. Four equal treatment groups will be followed for a 52-week primary endpoint. Three VEGF Trap-Eye treatment groups, 0.5 mg q 4 weeks, 2.0 mg q 4 weeks, and 2.0 mg q 8 weeks, will be compared with ranibizumab 0.5 mg q 4 weeks. A 3-monthly loading dose of VEGF Trap-Eye will be administered to all VEGF Trap-Eye subgroups. All VEGF Trap-Eye and ranibizumab patients will be treated on a PRN basis in year 2, with reinjection required at least once every 3 months. Men and women 50 years of age or older with subfoveal CNV due to neovascular AMD will be included who meet the inclusion criteria of: (1) active primary subfoveal CNV lesions secondary to AMD (including juxtafoveal lesions that affect the fovea); (2) ≥50% active CNV; and (3) best corrected ETDRS protocol visual acuity of ≤20/40–20/320 (letter score of 73–25) in the study eye.

During the second year of study, patients will be evaluated every 4 weeks and will receive an intravitreal injection at least every 12 weeks. During this period, injections may be given as frequently as every 4 weeks, but no less frequently than every 12 weeks, based on specific retreatment criteria.[16]

The primary objective will be to assess the efficacy of intravitreally administered VEGF Trap-Eye compared to ranibizumab in a noninferiority paradigm in preventing moderate vision loss in subjects with all subtypes of neovascular AMD. One secondary objective will be to assess the safety and tolerability of repeated intravitreal administration of VEGF Trap-Eye in patients with all subtypes of neovascular AMD for periods up to 2 years. Another secondary objective will be to assess the effect of repeated intravitreal administrations of VEGF Trap-Eye on vision-related quality of life (QOL) in subjects with all subtypes of neovascular AMD, as assessed using the National Eye Institute VFQ-25 questionnaire.[16]

DIABETIC MACULAR EDEMA PHASE I CLINICAL STUDY

The initial phase I study of VEGF Trap-Eye in DME, CLEAR-IT DME, was an exploratory study of the safety, tolerability, and biological effect of a single intravitreal administration of VEGF Trap-Eye in patients with DME.[37] The study was conducted at two centers involving 5 patients. It was an open-label study evaluating a single intravitreal injection of 4 mg VEGF Trap-Eye. Patients were followed for 6 weeks for safety, BCVA, centerpoint thickness, and macular volume by OCT.

The maximum change from baseline in key outcome measures at 6 weeks included reductions in centerpoint retinal thickness, with a mean reduction of –115.4 μm and a median reduction of –118 μm ($P < 0.03$). Macular volume was reduced by a mean of –1 μm^3 and a median of –0.6 μm^3 ($P < 0.04$). ETDRS BCVA letters improved by a mean of 6.8 and a median of 9 ($P < 0.03$).[37]

Intravitreal injection of VEGF Trap-Eye for DME in a phase I study showed only mild ocular adverse events that were related to the injection procedure. No serious ocular adverse events were reported.[37]

A phase II dose-ranging study comparing various doses of VEGF Trap-Eye administered at various dosing intervals to focal laser treatment is currently in development.

SUMMARY AND KEY POINTS

Existing anti-VEGF therapies have transformed the treatment of wet AMD into a disease in which improvement of vision may be expected by both patients and physicians. However, medications that allow for greater efficacy, or efficacy for more patients, and/or a longer dosing interval are still desired by physicians and patients, reflecting a continuing medical need for better treatments.

VEGF Trap-Eye, a fusion protein of VEGF receptors 1 and 2, is a promising treatment currently in development. It is fully human and has high affinity, binding VEGF more tightly than native receptors or monoclonal antibodies. It blocks all VEGF-A isoforms, VEGF-B, and PlGF, and, based on its molecular weight, should penetrate all retinal layers. Unlike antibody complexes, VEGF-Trap forms inert complexes that do not interact further with the VEGF receptor.

VEGF Trap-Eye has thus far demonstrated clinical activity with an acceptable safety profile in clinical trials. The CLEAR-IT DME study demonstrated reduced retinal thickness and improved vision in this common visual disease associated with diabetes. In CLEAR-IT 1 and 2 AMD studies, improved visual acuity and reduced retinal thickness were demonstrated. VEGF Trap-Eye was also generally safe and well tolerated. The two current phase III studies for neovascular AMD, VIEW 1 (USA and Canada) and VIEW 2 (Europe, Asia Pacific, Japan, and Latin America), will help to determine whether VEGF Trap-Eye can offer differential efficacy and/or longer dosing intervals relative to currently available agents.

It is hoped that future armamentaria for managing retinal vascular diseases will include VEGF Trap-Eye as one of their therapeutic agents.

REFERENCES

1. Economides AN, Carpenter LR, Rudge JS, et al. Cytokine traps: multi-component, high-affinity blockers of cytokine action. Nat Med 2003;9:47–52.
2. Holash J, Davis S, Papadopoulos N, et al. VEGF-Trap: a VEGF blocker with potent antitumor effects. Proc Natl Acad Sci USA 2002;99:11393–11398.
3. Breen EC. VEGF in biological control. J Cell Biochem 2007;102:1358–1367.
4. Olsson AK, Dimberg A, Kreuger J, et al. VEGF receptor signalling – in control of vascular function. Nat Rev Mol Cell Biol 2006;7:359–371.
5. Rudge JS, Thurston G, Davis S, et al. VEGF trap as a novel antiangiogenic treatment currently in clinical trials for cancer and eye diseases, and VelociGene- based discovery of the next generation of angiogenesis targets. Cold Spring Harb Symp Quant Biol 2005;70:411–418.
6. Cursiefen C, Chen L, Borges LP, et al. VEGF-A stimulates lymphangiogenesis and hemangiogenesis in inflammatory neovascularization via macrophage recruitment. J Clin Invest 2004;113:1040–1050.
7. Otrock ZK, Makarem JA, Shamseddine AI. Vascular endothelial growth factor family of ligands and receptors: review. Blood Cells Mol Dis 2007;38:258–268.
8. Jain RK, Xu L. alphaPlGF: a new kid on the antiangiogenesis block. Cell 2007;131:443–445.
9. Odorisio T, Cianfarani F, Failla CM, et al. The placenta growth factor in skin angiogenesis. J Dermatol Sci 2006;41:11–19.
10. Carmeliet P, Moons L, Luttun A, et al. Synergism between vascular endothelial growth factor and placental growth factor contributes to angiogenesis and plasma extravasation in pathological conditions. Nat Med 2001;7:575–583.
11. Ziche M, Maglione D, Ribatti D, et al. Placenta growth factor-1 is chemotactic, mitogenic, and angiogenic. Lab Invest 1997;76:517–531.
12. Rakic JM, Lambert V, Devy L, et al. Placental growth factor, a member of the VEGF family, contributes to the development of choroidal neovascularization. Invest Ophthalmol Vis Sci 2003;44:3186–3193.
13. Khaliq A, Foreman D, Ahmed A, et al. Increased expression of placenta growth factor in proliferative diabetic retinopathy. Lab Invest 1998;78:109–116.
14. Mitamura Y, Tashimo A, Ohtsuka K, et al. Placenta growth factor and vascular endothelial growth factor in the vitreous of patients with proliferative vitreoretinopathy. Clin Experiment Ophthalmol 2005;33: 226–227.
15. Chappelow AV, Kaiser PK. Neovascular age-related macular degeneration: potential therapies. Drugs 2008;68:1029–1036.
16. Regeneron. 2008. Data on file.
17. Lowe J, Araujo J, Yang J, et al. Ranibizumab inhibits multiple forms of biologically active vascular endothelial growth factor *in vitro* and *in vivo*. Exp Eye Res 2007;85:425–430.
18. Ferrara N, Chen H, Davis-Smyth T, et al. Vascular endothelial growth factor is essential for corpus luteum angiogenesis. Nat Med 1998;4: 336–340.
19. Gerber HP, Hillan KJ, Ryan AM, et al. VEGF is required for growth and survival in neonatal mice. Development 1999a;126:1149–1159.
20. Gerber HP, Vu TH, Ryan AM, et al. VEGF couples hypertrophic cartilage remodeling, ossification and angiogenesis during endochondral bone formation. Nat Med 1999b;5:623–628.
21. Goldman CK, Kendall RL, Cabrera G, et al. Paracrine expression of a native soluble vascular endothelial growth factor receptor inhibits tumor growth, metastasis, and mortality rate. Proc Natl Acad Sci USA 1998;95: 8795–8800.
22. Millauer B, Longhi MP, Plate KH, et al. Dominant-negative inhibition of Flk-1 suppresses the growth of many tumor types *in vivo*. Cancer Res 1996;56:1615–1620.
23. Kaiser PK. Antivascular endothelial growth factor agents and their development: therapeutic implications in ocular diseases. Am J Ophthalmol 2006;142:660–668.
24. Konner J, Dupont J. Use of soluble recombinant decoy receptor vascular endothelial growth factor trap (VEGF Trap) to inhibit vascular endothelial growth factor activity. Clin Colorectal Cancer 2004;4(Suppl. 2):S81–S85.
25. Furfine E, Coppi A, Koehler-Stec EM, et al. Pharmacokinetics and ocular tissue penetration of VEGF Trap after intravitreal injections in rabbits. Annual Meeting of The Association for Research in Vision and Ophthalmology (ARVO); 2006 April 30-May 4; Fort Lauderdale, FL.
26. Pieramici DJ, Rabena MD. Anti-VEGF therapy: comparison of current and future agents. Eye 2008;22:1330–1336.
27. Cao J, Song H, Renard RA, et al. Systemic or intravitreal administration of VEGF Trap suppresses vascular leak and leukostasis in the retinas of diabetic rats. Invest Ophthalmol Vis Sci 2006;47:e-abstract 1745.
28. Stewart MW, Rosenfeld PJ. Predicted biological activity of intravitreal VEGF Trap. Br J Ophthalmol 2008;92:667–668.
29. Stewart MW. Predicted biologic activity of intravitreal bevacizumab. Retina 2007;27:1196–1200.
30. Rudge JS, Holash J, Hylton D, et al. Inaugural article: VEGF Trap complex formation measures production rates of VEGF, providing a biomarker for predicting efficacious angiogenic blockade. Proc Natl Acad Sci USA 2007;104:18363–18370.
31. Saishin Y, Saishin Y, Takahashi K, et al. VEGF-TRAP(R1R2) suppresses choroidal neovascularization and VEGF-induced breakdown of the blood–retinal barrier. J Cell Physiol 2003;195:241–248.
32. Wiegand SJ, Zimmer E, Nork TM, et al. VEGF Trap both prevents experimental choroidal neovascularization and causes regression of established lesions in non-human primates. Invest Ophthalmol Vis Sci 2005;46:e-abstract 1411.
33. Zimmer E, Christian BJ, Miller PE. Safety evaluation of intravitreal administration of VEGF Trap in cynomolgus monkeys for 13 weeks. Annual Meeting of The Association for Research in Vision and Ophthalmology (ARVO); 2006 April 30-May 4; Fort Lauderdale.
34. Nguyen QD, Hariprasad S, Browning DJ, et al. Interim results from a phase 1, safety, tolerability, and bioactivity study of intravitreal VEGF trap in patients with neovascular age-related macular degeneration: the CLEAR-IT 1 study. Annual Meeting of The Association for Research in Vision and Ophthalmology (ARVO); 2007 May 6–10; Fort Lauderdale.
35. Nguyen QD, Shah SM, Browning DJ, et al. Results of a phase I, dose-escalation, safety, tolerability, and bioactivity study of intravitreous VEGF Trap in patients with neovascular age-related macular degeneration. Annual Meeting of The Association for Research in Vision and Ophthalmology (ARVO); 2006 April 30-May 4; Fort Lauderdale.
36. Benz MS, Nguyen QD, Chu K, et al. Interim results of the Phase II, randomized, controlled dose- and interval-ranging study of repeated intravitreal VEGF trap administration in patients with neovascular age-related macular degeneration (AMD). Annual Meeting of The Association for Research in Vision and Ophthalmology (ARVO); 2007 May 6–10; Fort Lauderdale.
37. Do DV, Nguyen QD, Shah SM, et al. An exploratory study of the safety, tolerability and bioactivity of a single intravitreal injection of vascular endothelial growth factor Trap-Eye in patients with diabetic macular oedema. Br J Ophthalmol 2009 Feb;93(2):144–149.

CHAPTER

38 Aptamers and intramers: pegaptanib

Mauro Goldbaum, MD and Emmett T. Cunningham, Jr, MD, PhD, MPH

KEY FEATURES

Aptamers are chemically synthesized nucleic acid or peptide oligomers that bind a specific target molecule, thus acting like "chemical antibodies." The first and only aptamer therapeutic to be approved by the Food and Drug Administration (FDA) was pegaptanib sodium (Macugen, Eyetech Inc., Palm Beach Gardens, FL), which was approved in December, 2004, and is indicated for the treatment of all angiographic subtypes of neovascular age-related macular degeneration (AMD). Pegaptanib's pharmacologic characteristics as well as its development for the treatment of vascular diseases of the eye are described in this chapter.

INTRODUCTION AND HISTORY

Pegaptanib is a selective anti-vascular endothelial growth factor (VEGF) aptamer that acts in the extracellular space to inhibit the 165 isoform ($VEGF_{165}$), while sparing $VEGF_{121}$.[1] Aptamers (from the Latin *aptus*, meaning "to fit") are oligonucleic acid or peptide molecules that bind a specific target molecule.[2] Intramers are aptamers that act on intracellular targets.[3] Aptamers with a high specificity for virtually any protein target can be selected using the *in vitro* selection process known as systematic evolution of ligands by exponential enrichment (SELEX), in which a population of randomized RNA or DNA oligonucleotides (typically 20–40 nucleotides long) is incubated with the protein target of interest.[4] Aptamers that bind to the target are selected, amplified by reverse transcriptase-polymerase chain reaction, and then reselected in an iterative process repeated as needed to achieve desired affinity and specificity. Selected aptamers can then be sequenced and chemically synthesized.

Using the SELEX process, aptamers blocking VEGF *in vitro* were first described in 1994 by scientists at NeXstar Pharmaceuticals, who were the first to demonstrate the feasibility of an aptamer-based approach to inhibiting neovascularization.[5] These experiments were followed in 1995 by the use of NH_2-substituted nucleotides to improve the resistance of anti-VEGF aptamers to nuclease attack[6] and, subsequently, the use of 2′-F-substituted pyrimidines to improve affinity further in 1998.[7] The addition of a 40-kDa polyethylene glycol (PEG) moiety to the 5′ end of this aptamer improved its ability to block VEGF-mediated vascular permeability in a guinea pig assay, probably due to slowed tissue diffusion.[7] Further experiments demonstrated that an optimized anti-VEGF aptamer, subsequently named pegaptanib sodium, inhibited VEGF binding and VEGF-mediated cell signaling in cultured endothelial cells, and that pretreatment of cells with pegaptanib inhibited proliferative responses to $VEGF_{165}$, but not $VEGF_{121}$.[8]

In follow-up work, pegaptanib was found to be stable in human plasma,[9] paving the way for its evaluation in animal models and in clinical studies. Following intravitreous injection, biologically active pegaptanib could be detected in the vitreous humor of monkey eyes for at least 28 days following a single 0.5-mg dose and was determined to be eliminated from the eye through plasma clearance.[10] No toxicities related to pegaptanib were observed following systemic or ocular administration in monkeys.[10] These preclinical studies established the biological and pharmacokinetic properties of pegaptanib, thus providing the groundwork for clinical trials of pegaptanib in patients with neovascular AMD, diabetic retinopathy, and retinal vascular occlusive disease. Pegaptanib sodium (Macugen) was approved by the FDA in December of 2004, and was both the first approved aptamer therapeutic and the first approved pharmacotherapy for neovascular AMD.

PHARMACOLOGY

Pegaptanib sodium injection is a sterile, clear, preservative-free aqueous solution supplied in a single-dose, prefilled syringe and is formulated as a 3.47 mg/ml solution, measured as the free acid form of the oligonucleotide.[11] The active ingredient is 0.3 mg of the free acid form of the oligonucleotide without PEG, in a nominal volume of 90 μl. Pegaptanib is formulated to have an osmolality of 280–360 mOsmol/kg, and a pH of 6–7.

Pegaptanib sodium is a covalent conjugate of an oligonucleotide of 28 nucleotides in length that terminates in a pentylamino linker, to which two 20-kDa monomethoxy PEG units are covalently attached via the two amino groups on a lysine residue. The molecular formula for pegaptanib sodium is $C_{294}H_{342}F_{13}N_{107}Na_{28}O_{188}P_{28}[C_2H_4O]n$ (where n is approximately 900) and the molecular weight is 49 kDa.[11]

PHARMACOKINETICS

Pegaptanib exhibits "flip-flop" kinetics, a phenomenon wherein the drug remains in the eye for a significant amount of time, is slowly cleared into the systemic circulation, and then is relatively rapidly cleared from the circulation.[12] The pharmacokinetics of pegaptanib following intravitreous injection were profiled in a study of 147 subjects with neovascular AMD.[13] Either 1 or 3 mg of pegaptanib sodium per study eye was administered every 6 weeks for 54 weeks. For the 1-mg dose, mean maximal plasma concentrations ranged from 20 to 24 ng/ml, and pegaptanib was measurable (>8 ng/ml) in the plasma for up to 1 week after injection. The mean apparent terminal plasma half-life, determined from the 3-mg group, was 10 (±4) days. There was no plasma accumulation with administration of repeated doses. Additionally, no serum antibodies against pegaptanib were detected.[13]

Regarding ocular distribution, pegaptanib penetrates all retinal layers.[14] Twenty-four hours following intravitreal injection, labeled pegaptanib can be identified in both the outer nuclear layer and photoreceptor layers, with very little staining within the nuclear layers of the retina. Regarding metabolism and excretion, based on preclinical data, pegaptanib is metabolized by endo- and exonucleases and is eliminated as parent drug and metabolites primarily in the urine.[11]

Plasma concentrations do not appear to be affected by age or gender, but have not been studied in patients under the age of 50. Dose adjustment for patients with renal impairment or weighing greater than 39 kg is not needed when administering the 0.3-mg dose. Pegaptanib has not been studied in patients with hepatic impairment or requiring hemodialysis.[11]

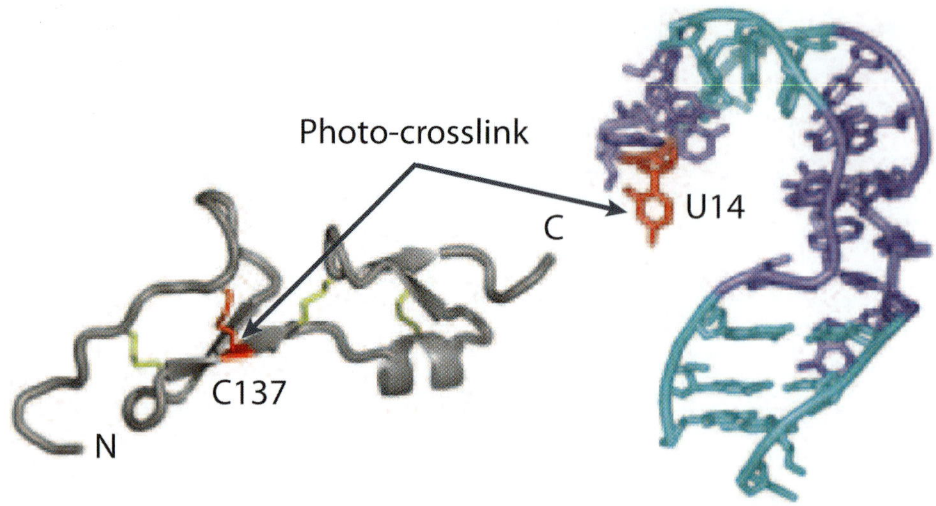

Figure 38.1 Interaction between the 55-amino-acid heparin-binding domain of vascular endothelial growth factor $(VEGF)_{165}$ and pegaptanib. Representation of the nuclear magnetic resonance solution structure of the free heparin-binding domain of $VEGF_{165}$ is shown in gray with disulfide bonds in yellow. The aptamer (blue) is shown as a model based on the secondary structure determined by nuclear magnetic resonance, with the helical stem regions in light blue. The interaction between cysteine-137 (C137) of $VEGF_{165}$ (cysteine-27 of the heparin-binding domain) and uridine-14 (U14) of the aptamer is indicated in red. Reproduced with permission from Ng EW, Shima DT, Calias P, et al. Pegaptanib, a targeted anti-VEGF aptamer for ocular vascular disease. Nat Rev Drug Discov 2006;5:123–132.

DRUG MECHANISM

Pegaptanib therapy is based on its anti-VEGF properties. Pegaptanib selectively inhibits extracellular $VEGF_{165}$ and $VEGF_{188}$, while sparing $VEGF_{121}$.[7,14,15] In preclinical studies, the anti-VEGF aptamer blocked binding of $VEGF_{165}$ to VEGF receptors 1 and 2 (VEGFR-1 and VEGFR-2) and inhibited a variety of $VEGF_{165}$-mediated biological effects, including VEGFR-2 and phospholipase C phosphorylation, calcium mobilization, and cellular proliferation.[1] The selectivity of pegaptanib derives from its interaction with cysteine-137, an amino acid that is contained within the 55-amino-acid heparin-binding domain of VEGF[1,16] and that is not present in $VEGF_{121}$[16–18] (Figure 38.1).

The importance of blocking VEGF in ocular neovascular diseases derives from its key properties as a regulator of physiological and pathological angiogenesis and a potent promoter of vascular permeability.[19,20] However, $VEGF_{165}$ appears to be the main isoform involved in pathologic conditions. It is upregulated in ischemic neovascularization, in retina vascular diseases involving hyperpermeability, and presents more potent proinflammatory properties than $VEGF_{121}$ including chemoattraction of monocytes and upregulation of intercellular cell adhesion molecule-1.[1,21,22]

In addition, selectively blocking $VEGF_{165}$ may preserve a wide range of physiological processes, both in the eye, where it is important in maintenance of retinal neurons and the choriocapillaris, and in the nervous system, kidney, bone, and liver.[21,23–26] Animal studies have shown that sparing $VEGF_{120}$ is sufficient to maintain a neuroprotective effect after an ischemia–reperfusion injury to the retina which disappears after inhibition of both $VEGF_{120}$ and $VEGF_{164}$ (rodent counterparts of human $VEGF_{121}$ and $VEGF_{165}$, respectively).[23]

DRUG EFFECTS IN HUMAN NONOCULAR DISEASES

Aptamers and intramers have been involved in clinical and preclinical studies for the treatment of different disease entities, including oncologic, cardiovascular, and infectious diseases. The most advanced therapeutic aptamer in development for cancer is AS1411, which is being tested in clinical trials. The mechanism underlying its antiproliferative effects in cancer cells seems to involve initial binding to cell surface nucleolin, followed by internalization and inhibition of DNA replication. In a dose escalation phase I study in patients with advanced solid tumors, promising signs of activity have been reported in the absence of any significant adverse effects. Further trials are ongoing in renal and nonsmall-cell lung cancers.[27] Studies with anticoagulant and antithrombotic aptamers have been reported supporting a potential role in cardiovascular disorders like acute coronary disease.[28,29] A phase I study with ARC1779, an anti-von Willebrand factor aptamer, produced dose- and concentration-dependent inhibition of von Willebrand factor activity and platelet function.[29] Preclinical studies have suggested a possible use of aptamers in the treatment of viral diseases, including infections by the human immunodeficiency virus (HIV) and hepatitis C virus.[30,31]

DRUG USE IN RETINAL DISEASES

NEOVASCULAR AGE-RELATED MACULAR DEGENERATION

Pegaptanib sodium is approved for the treatment of all angiographic types of neovascular AMD. Phase I/II clinical trials providing preliminary safety data for pegaptanib in patients with neovascular AMD were soon followed by the results of two large-scale, randomized, double-masked, phase II/III trials collectively known as the VEGF Inhibition Study in Ocular Neovascularization (V.I.S.I.O.N.) trials.[32–34] These concurrent multicenter, dose-ranging trials enrolled a broad range of subjects with neovascular AMD, including all angiographic subtypes, lesions up to 12 disc areas in size (including blood, scar, or atrophy, and neovascularization) and best corrected visual acuity of 20/40 to 20/320 in the study eye. Subjects received sham injection or intravitreous pegaptanib sodium (0.3, 1, or 3 mg) every 6 weeks for 54 weeks for the first year of the study. Photodynamic therapy (PDT) with verteporfin was permitted at the investigator's discretion within 5–10 days prior to each treatment for subjects with predominantly classic lesions. The primary, prespecified efficacy endpoint was the proportion of subjects losing <15 letters of visual acuity between baseline and week 54 (responders). Secondary endpoints included mean changes in visual acuity the proportions gaining 0, 5, 10, or 15 letters of visual acuity,

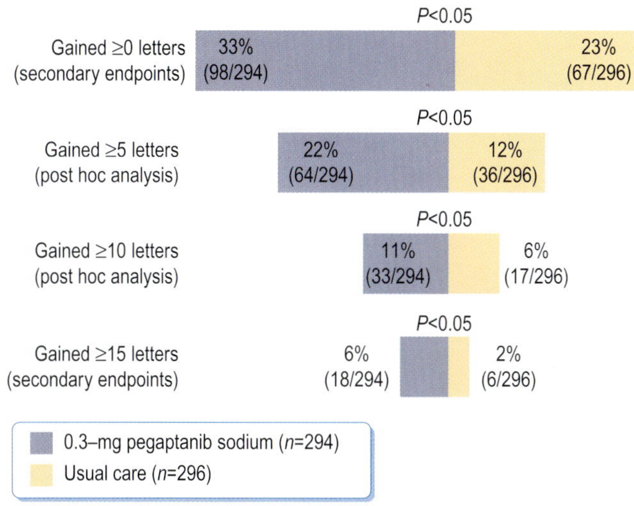

Figure 38.2 Proportion of subjects in the VEGF Inhibition Study in Ocular Neovascularization (V.I.S.I.O.N.) trials who maintained or gained visual acuity at 54 weeks. Reproduced with permission from Ng EW, Adamis AP. Targeting angiogenesis, the underlying disorder in neovascular age-related macular degeneration. Can J Ophthalmol 2005;40:352–368.

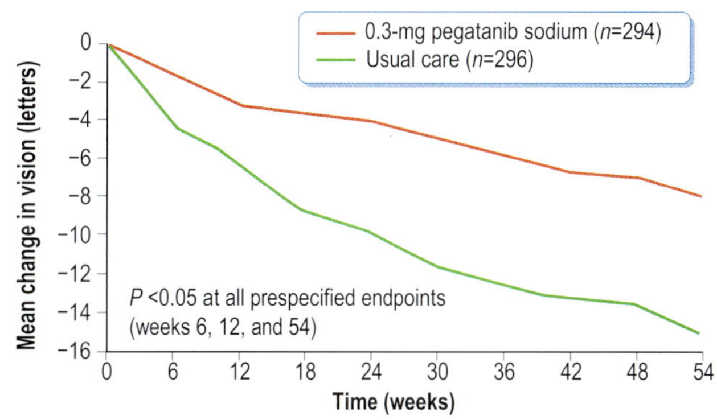

Figure 38.3 Mean change in visual acuity at week 54 in subjects in the VEGF Inhibition Study in Ocular Neovascularization (V.I.S.I.O.N.) trials who received 0.3-mg pegaptanib sodium or sham. Reproduced with permission from Ng EW, Adamis AP. Targeting angiogenesis, the underlying disorder in neovascular age-related macular degeneration. Can J Ophthalmol 2005;40:352–368.

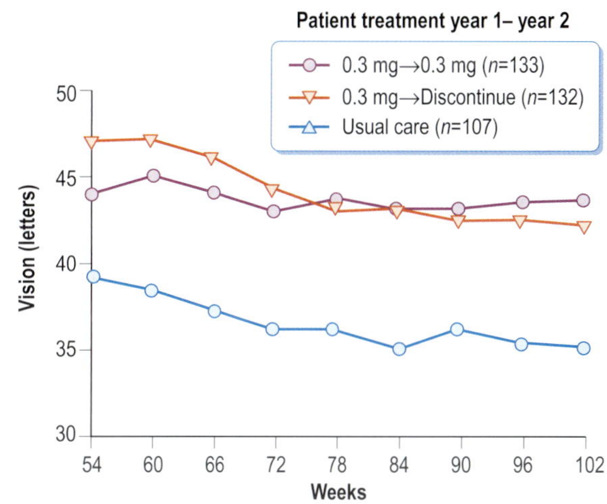

Figure 38.4 Mean visual acuity from week 54 to week 102 in the year-2 extension of the VEGF Inhibition Study in Ocular Neovascularization (V.I.S.I.O.N.) trials. Reproduced with permission from Chakravarthy U, Adamis AP, Cunningham ET Jr et al. Year 2 efficacy results of two randomized controlled clinical trials of pegaptanib for neovascular age-related macular degeneration. Ophthalmology 2006;113(9):1508.e1–25.

losing 30 letters or proceeding to legal blindness (visual acuity 20/200). Treatment efficacy was also assessed anatomically through fluorescein angiography and fundus photography.[34]

In the combined trials, 1186 subjects received at least one study treatment and were included in subsequent analyses.[34] Subjects received an average of 8.5 of 9 possible injections. All three pegaptanib doses were superior to sham for the principal endpoint with 70%, 71%, and 65% of responders in the 0.3-mg ($P < 0.001$), 1-mg ($P < 0.001$), and 3-mg ($P < 0.03$) groups respectively compared to 55% assigned to sham. Similar results were obtained using last observation carried forward or observed data. The approved 0.3-mg dose was the lowest effective dose, therefore, further discussion is limited to that dose. Pegaptanib was superior to sham in the proportion of subjects maintaining or gaining 5, 10, or 15 lines of vision (Figure 38.2).[35] Furthermore, subjects receiving pegaptanib were less likely to have severe vision loss, defined as 30 letters (10 versus 22%, $P < 0.001$), or progress to legal blindness in the treated eye (38% versus 56%, $P < 0.001$). The effectiveness of pegaptanib was evident as early as the first study visit after the first injection (week 6), and it increased over time up to week 54, as measured by the mean loss of visual acuity from baseline to each study visit as compared with that in the sham group ($P < 0.002$). The mean loss in visual acuity at week 54 was −7.95 letters for the pegaptanib 0.3-mg group compared to −15.05 letters for sham-treated subjects ($P < 0.05$), representing a 47% relative difference (Figure 38.3).[35] The treatment effect was independent of angiographic subtype, sex, age, baseline visual acuity, race, or iris color and was present despite the higher rate of use of PDT among patients receiving sham injections.[35] In multivariate analyses based on the inclusion of these factors, as well as prior PDT usage, smoking status, presence of subretinal hemorrhage, lipid, visual acuity better in the fellow eye than study eye, and >3 lines of previous visual acuity loss, only treatment with 0.3-mg pegaptanib significantly affected treatment response ($P = 0.0003$).[35]

After the first year of the V.I.S.I.O.N. trials, subjects who elected to remain in the study were re-randomized for an additional 48 weeks.[36] Those already receiving pegaptanib were randomized either to continue their respective pegaptanib dose or to receive sham injections. Subjects initially receiving sham injections were re-randomized to sham or one of the three pegaptanib doses. Overall, 1053 subjects were re-randomized; 941 subjects (89%) were assessed at week 102, having received an average of 15.7 injections (92% of a possible 17) over 2 years. Of those subjects receiving 0.3 mg pegaptanib during the second year, 59% (78/133) lost <15 letters while the mean loss in visual acuity was 9.4 letters. For those receiving sham injections over 2 years or randomized to discontinue sham in the second year, 45% (48/107) lost <15 letters, and mean visual acuity loss was 17 letters ($P < 0.05$ for both comparisons). (Figure 38.4) There were 21 cases of 3-line loss among subjects continuing pegaptanib 0.3 mg for 2 years versus 35 cases in those randomized to sham after 1 year of therapy ($P < 0.05$).[36] Ten percent of pegaptanib-treated patients gained 3 lines of vision after 2 years. The percentage of patients gaining vision was higher for patients who received 2 years of treatment with 0.3-mg pegaptanib than for patients receiving usual care[36] (Figure 38.5).

Subgroup analyses of the V.I.S.I.O.N. trials as well as case-series reports have suggested that providing treatment with pegaptanib early in the course of neovascular AMD may allow for better outcomes.[37–39]

DIABETIC RETINOPATHY

A randomized, sham-controlled, double-masked, dose-finding, phase II trial was performed to evaluate the efficacy and safety of pegaptanib for treatment of diabetic macular edema (DME).[40] This trial enrolled 172

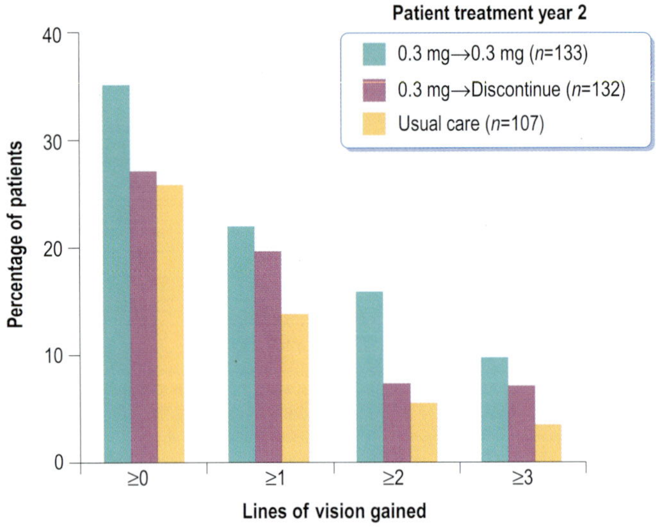

Figure 38.5 Vision gains in the year-2 extension of the VEGF Inhibition Study in Ocular Neovascularization (V.I.S.I.O.N.) trials. Reproduced with permission from Chakravarthy U, Adamis AP, Cunningham ET Jr, et al. Year 2 efficacy results of two randomized, controlled clinical trials of pegaptanib, an anti-VEGF aptamer, for neovascular age-related macular degeneration. Ophthalmology 2006;113:1508.

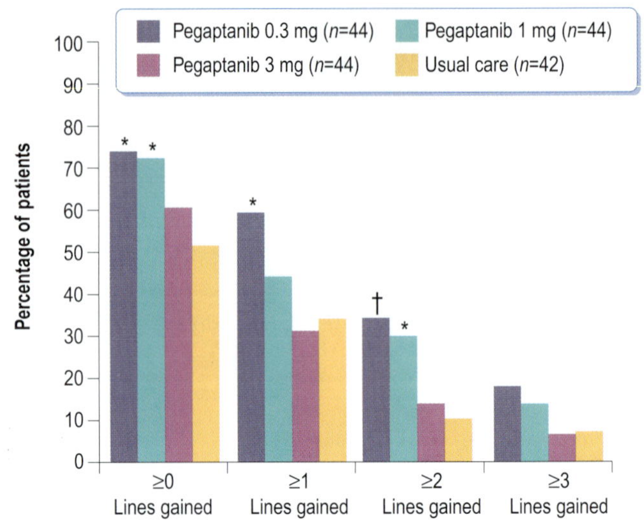

Figure 38.6 Percentage of subjects maintaining or gaining visual acuity from baseline to week 36 in the Macugen for DME phase II trial (intention-to-treat population, *n* = 172 (missing data for one patient each in the 1-mg and sham groups)). **P* < 0.05; †*P* < 0.01. Reproduced with permission from Cunningham ET Jr, Adamis AP, Altaweel M, et al. A phase II randomized double-masked trial of pegaptanib, an anti-vascular endothelial growth factor aptamer, for diabetic macular edema. Ophthalmology 2005;112:1747–1757.

subjects 18 years and older with type 1 or type 2 diabetes. Entry criteria included best corrected visual acuity in the study eye from 20/50 to 20/320 and macular edema in the study eye involving the center of the macula, as confirmed by optical coherence tomography (OCT), together with leakage from microaneurysms, retinal telangiectasis, or both, demonstrable on fluorescein angiography. Subjects with a history of panretinal or focal photocoagulation or other retinal treatments within the previous 6 months were excluded.[40]

Subjects were randomized to three different doses of pegaptanib (0.3, 1, or 3 mg) or sham injections, stratified by study site, size of the thickened retina area (2.5 disc areas versus >2.5 disc areas) and baseline visual acuity (letter score 58 versus <58).[40] Injections were given at baseline, week 6, and week 12 for a minimum of three injections, followed by additional injections given every 6 weeks up to week 30 (for a maximum of six injections) at the discretion of the investigators. In all, 169 subjects received at least one study treatment, with more than 90% of subjects completing the study; 49% of the pegaptanib-treated subjects received the maximal number of injections.[40]

At week 36, the mean change in visual acuity from baseline was +4.7, +4.7, and +1.1 for 0.3-, 1-, and 3-mg groups, respectively, versus –0.4 letters for the sham group (*P* = 0.04, 0.05, and 0.55, respectively). As in the V.I.S.I.O.N. trials for neovascular AMD the 0.3-mg dose was the lowest efficacious dose. The median visual acuity was significantly better in the 0.3-mg group compared with sham (20/50 versus 20/63, *P* = 0.04), as was the percentage of subjects maintaining or gaining vision (Figure 38.6).[40] Pegaptanib treatment was also associated with improvements in macular edema as determined by mean changes in retinal thickness of the center point from baseline to week 36 (Table 38.1).[40] Although there was some improvement in all three pegaptanib groups, only the 0.3-mg group was significantly better when compared with sham (–68.0 μm versus +3.7 μm, *P* = 0.02). In addition, more subjects in the pegaptanib-treated groups had absolute decreases of 75 μm, 100 μm, and 200 μm in macular edema when compared with sham. Benefits in the 0.3-mg group were particularly evident, with 49% showing a decrease of 75 μm in the center point of the central subfield compared with 19% in the sham group (*P* = 0.008) and 42% showing a decrease of 100 μm compared with 16% in the sham arm (*P* = 0.02). (Table 38.1). Both visual and anatomical benefits were achieved with less need for laser photocoagulation. Twenty-five percent of subjects receiving 0.3 mg pegaptanib required intervention with photocoagulation compared to 48% of those receiving sham (*P* = 0.042).[40]

Regarding proliferative diabetic retinopathy, a retrospective analysis of subjects enrolled in the phase II DME trial was conducted to evaluate the effects of pegaptanib on diabetic retinal neovascularization based on evidence that VEGF plays a prominent role in the pathogenesis of this condition.[41,42] A review of all subjects identified 19 of 172 who had retinal neovascularization in the study eye at study baseline; 4 subjects also had retinal neovascularization in the fellow eye.[43] Of these 19 subjects, there was 1 exclusion due to recent scatter photocoagulation therapy and 2 exclusions for incomplete follow-up. In the remaining cohort of 16 subjects, 8 had prior photocoagulation more than 6 months prior to the study and 1 had photocoagulation during the study.[43] Thirteen of these subjects had received pegaptanib, while the remaining 3 subjects received sham injections.[43] Eight of 13 (61%) subjects in the pegaptanib group, including the subject receiving photocoagulation in follow-up, had regression of neovascularization demonstrated by fundus photography and/or angiography at 36 weeks. In contrast, there was no neovascular regression in any of the 3 eyes in the sham group or in the 4 fellow eyes of subjects receiving pegaptanib. After the discontinuation of pegaptanib, there was recurrence of neovascularization between weeks 36 and 52 in 3 of the 8 subjects who originally responded to pegaptanib, including the subject receiving photocoagulation (Figure 38.7).[43] These results were not only supportive of a therapeutic benefit for pegaptanib in the treatment of proliferative diabetic retinopathy, but suggested further that such benefit can be sustained following discontinuation of therapy in a sizable proportion of subjects.

These findings were later supported by an independent randomized small study comparing pegaptanib injections every 6 weeks to panretinal photocoagulation in which more eyes submitted to anti-VEGF therapy responded with complete neovascularization regression.[44]

RETINAL VEIN OCCLUSION

To study the effect of pegaptanib in another major retinal vascular disease involving ischemic-induced hyperpermeability and neovascularization, a randomized, multicenter, double-masked, sham-controlled, phase II trial was conducted with subjects presenting recent vision loss from macular edema secondary to central retinal vein occlusion.[45] In the trial, 98 subjects were randomized to receive pegaptanib

Table 38.1 Changes from baseline to week 36 in retinal thickness of the center point of the central subfield (intention-to-treat population, n = 172*)

	PEGAPTANIB			
Retinal thickness	**0.3 mg (*n* = 44)**	**1 mg (*n* = 44)**	**3 mg (*n* = 42)**	**Sham (*n* = 42)**
Mean at baseline, μm	476.0	451.7	424.7	423.2
Mean change at week 36, μm (95% CI)	–68.0 (–118.9, –9.88)	–22.7 (–76.9, 33.8)	–5.3 (–63.0, 49.5)	+3.7
P-value versus sham†	0.02	0.44	0.81	
≥75 μm decrease from baseline				
Number (%) at week 36	21 (49)	11 (28)	9 (25)	7 (19)
Odds ratio (95% CI)	4.1 (1.5, 11.3)	1.7 (0.6, 5.0)	1.4 (0.5, 4.4)	
P-value versus sham‡	0.008	0.283	0.596	
≥100 μm decrease from baseline				
Number (%) at week 36	18 (42)	10 (26)	7 (19)	6 (16)
Odds ratio (95% CI)	3.7 (1.3, 10.8)	1.8 (0.6, 5.5)	1.3 (0.4, 4.2)	
P-value versus sham‡	0.021	0.303	0.829	
≥200 μm decrease from baseline				
Number (%) at week 36	5 (12)	3 (8)	2 (6)	1 (3)
Odds ratio (95% CI)	4.7 (0.5, 42.5)	3.0 (0.3, 0.2)	2.1 (0.2, 4.4)	
P-value versus sham‡	0.126	0.304	0.678	

CI, confidence interval.

The P-value *is for difference in odds ratios between each dose group and sham.*

**For missing baseline data, day 0 data were used for the analysis. For missing data at week 36, the last observation was carried forward. Missing relevant data for 1 patient in the 0.3-mg group, 5 patients in the 1-mg group, 6 patients in the 3-mg group, and 5 patients in the sham group.*

†Analysis of covariance model adjusted for baseline retinal thickening area, baseline vision, and baseline retinal thickness; P-value *for difference in least-square means between each dose group and sham.*

‡Cochran–Mantel–Haenszel test adjusted for baseline retinal thickening area and baseline vision.

Adapted from: Cunningham ET Jr, Adamis AP, Altaweel M, et al. A phase II randomized double-masked trial of pegaptanib, an anti-vascular endothelial growth factor aptamer, for diabetic macular edema. Ophthalmology 2005;112:1747–1757.

sodium (1.0 or 0.3 mg) or sham injections once every 6 weeks for 24 weeks. The totality of the data analyzed at week 30 suggests that selective VEGF inhibition as provided by pegaptanib intravitreal injections may be a promising therapeutic option in the treatment of this disease.[45] More subjects on pegaptanib gained 15 letters from baseline to week 30, 12/33 (36%) and 13/33 (39%) for pegaptanib 0.3 mg and 1 mg, respectively, versus 9/32 (28%) for sham; $P = 0.48$ and $P = 0.35$ versus sham, respectively. Both doses of pegaptanib had an early and sustained effect on visual acuity. At week 30, subjects receiving 0.3 and 1 mg pegaptanib had gained an average of 7.1 and 9.9 letters, respectively, while those treated with sham had lost an average of 3.2 letters ($P = 0.09$ and $P = 0.02$ for 0.3 and 1 mg pegaptanib versus sham, respectively). Fewer than 10% of those receiving either dose of pegaptanib, but nearly one-third of subjects treated with sham, lost 15 letters of visual acuity by week 30 ($P = 0.03$ and $P = 0.01$ for 0.3 and 1 mg pegaptanib versus sham). Approximately 90% (59/66) of subjects receiving pegaptanib had visual acuities 20/200 at week 30 compared to 63% (20/32) of those treated with sham ($P = 0.02$ and $P = 0.01$ for 0.3 and 1 mg pegaptanib versus sham, respectively). OCT center point thickness assessment revealed progressive reduction of macular edema in all study groups, more so in pegaptanib-treated eyes, although not statistically significant. The same assessment at week 1 showed a mean 250-μm decrease in foveal thickness in both pegaptanib groups ($P < 0.01$) compared to no change in the sham group, supporting an early pharmacodynamic effect of pegaptanib in this disease.[45] Results of a small randomized study on pegaptanib for macular edema secondary to branch retinal vein occlusion were also promising, with 35% and 55% of patients gaining 3 lines of ETDRS visual acuity after 12 and 54 weeks, respectively.[46] The combined results of these studies in diabetic retinopathy and retinal venous occlusive disease suggest a potential role for selective VEGF inhibition in the future management of these disorders.

OTHERS

Results of a pilot study of 5 subjects with advanced von Hippel–Lindau angiomas suggest that intravitreal pegaptanib may have had a small effect on decreasing retinal thickening and reducing retinal hard exudates in some patients.[47] Anecdotal reports of the use of pegaptanib in other retinal disorders include studies in patients with myopic choroidal neovascularization,[48] neovascular glaucoma,[49] retinopathy of prematurity,[50] familial exudative vitreoretinopathy,[51] Coats' disease,[52] and macular edema associated with Irvine–Gass syndrome,[53] retinitis pigmentosa,[54] and tamoxifen therapy.[55]

CONTRAINDICATIONS

The only contraindication to the administration of pegaptanib would be a known, pre-existing drug hypersensitivity to pegaptanib sodium or any other excipient in the product. As with any intravitreal drug, administration is also contraindicated in the presence of ocular or periocular infections because of the increased risk of endophthalmitis.[11]

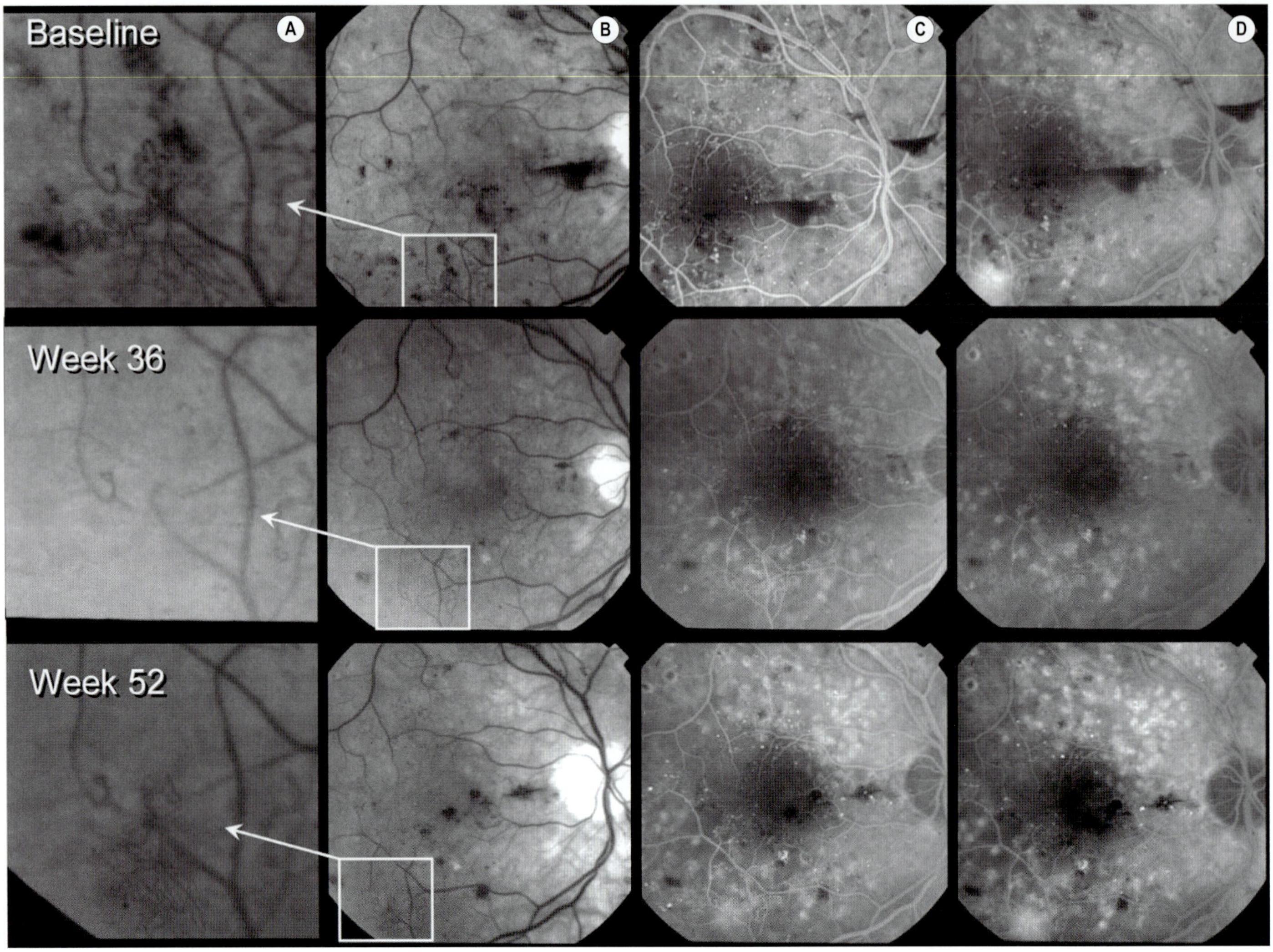

Figure 38.7 Regression of retinal vascularization following pegaptanib treatment in a subject with diabetic retinopathy. First row: Baseline visit shows: (A) magnification of retinal neovascularization elsewhere (NVE); (B) the location of the neovascularization along the inferotemporal arcade (red-free photograph); (C) areas of capillary nonperfusion in the early-phase frame (fluorescein angiogram); and (D) leakage from the NVE in the late-phase frame (fluorescein angiogram). Second row: At week 36, after six periodic pegaptanib injections and 6 weeks since the most recent injection, there is seen regression of NVE on red-free photographs (A, B), less apparent microaneurysms in the early phase (C), and regression of leakage from NVE in the late phase (D). Third row: 52 weeks after study entry and 22 weeks since the last pegaptanib injection, there is seen a reappearance of NVE on red-free photographs (A, B) and a reappearance of leakage from NVE in early- and late-phase frames (C, D). Reproduced with permission from Adamis AP, Altaweel M, Bressler NM, et al. Changes in retinal neovascularization after pegaptanib (Macugen) therapy in diabetic individuals. Ophthalmology 2006;113:23–28.

OCULAR COMPLICATIONS AND TOXICITY

Ocular adverse events observed in pegaptanib clinical studies were generally transient, mild to moderate, and were attributed by the investigators to the injection procedure, rather than to the study drug.[13,34,40] In the first year of V.I.S.I.O.N. trials, common ocular adverse events that occurred more frequently in the study eyes of patients treated with pegaptanib than in those receiving sham injection were eye pain (34 versus 28%), vitreous floaters (33 versus 8%, $P < 0.001$), punctate keratitis (32 versus 27%), cataracts (20 versus 18%), vitreous opacities (18 versus 10%, $P < 0.001$) and anterior-chamber inflammation (14 versus 6%, $P = 0.001$). These events were more common in the study eyes than in the other eyes among patients in the sham injection group, suggesting that the events were in part a result of the preparation procedure for injection, as opposed to the study drug. There was no evidence of a sustained elevation in intraocular pressure or cataract development. A masked review by the reading center at the University of Wisconsin of all angiograms obtained at baseline and at weeks 30 and 54 revealed no evidence of retinal or choroidal vascular toxicity.[34]

Serious ocular adverse events occurring in the first year were mainly injection-related, consisting of endophthalmitis, retinal detachment, and traumatic cataract. The per-injection rates of endophthalmitis (0.16%), retinal detachment (0.08%), and traumatic lens injury (0.07%) in the current trial were similar historical data.[56] In addition the rate of endophthalmitis was significantly decreased after an amendment reinforcing the use of aseptic technique.[57]

The same favorable ocular safety profile was observed after 2 and 3 years of consecutive treatment with pegaptanib.[57,58]

SYSTEMIC COMPLICATIONS AND TOXICITY

No evidence of an increased risk of systemic adverse events was detected in clinical trials and no systemic adverse events were definitively attributed by the independent data management and safety monitoring committee to the study drug. In the V.I.S.I.O.N. trials a comparison of rates of adverse events (for all doses of pegaptanib as compared with sham injection) showed no significant difference in the rates of adverse events associated with systemic administration of nonselective VEGF inhibitors,[34] including vascular hypertensive disorders, nonocular hemorrhagic events, thromboembolic events, and gastrointestinal perforations. The baseline laboratory values were similar in all groups, and median changes in all laboratory values from baseline were small and not clinically meaningful. The death rate was similar to that seen in previous studies of neovascular AMD in this population.[59] Systemic safety data after 3 years of pegaptanib use were consistent with the results reported after 1 and 2 years.[58] No antibodies against pegaptanib were detected in patients receiving intravitreal pegaptanib.[13]

Ocular and systemic safety findings in clinical trials were also consistent with toxicity studies in animals.[60] Rare cases of systemic hypersensitivity have been reported, although an independent review of these cases could not attribute definitive causality to pegaptanib.[61,62] No other ocular or systemic safety concerns have been detected in clinical use after pegaptanib approval.

DRUG INTERACTIONS

Pegaptanib is metabolized by nucleases and is generally not affected by the cytochrome P450 system. However, drug interaction studies have not been conducted.[11] Phase II studies conducted in patients who received pegaptanib after application of PDT with verteporfin revealed no apparent difference in the plasma pharmacokinetics of pegaptanib.[36] Preclinical studies in corneal neovascularization model suggest that the administration of pegaptanib before PDT may diminish the efficacy of PDT-induced vessel regression. Such an effect was not seen with simultaneous administration of both therapies.[63]

SUMMARY AND KEY POINTS

Aptamers are an emerging class of therapeutic agents composed of chemically synthesized nucleic acid or peptide oligomers that bind to and either inhibit or activate a given target. Pegaptanib sodium, a selective $VEGF_{165}$ inhibitor, was the first aptamer therapeutic to be approved by the FDA, and is currently indicated for the treatment of all angiographic subtypes of neovascular AMD. The role of pegaptanib in the treatment of other vascular disorders of the eye is the focus of ongoing investigations.

REFERENCES

1. Ishida ST, Usui T, Yamashiro K, et al. VEGF164-mediated inflammation is required for pathological, but not physiological, ischemia-induced retinal neovascularization. J Exp Med 2003;198(3):483–489.
2. Jayasena SD. Aptamers: an emerging class of molecules that rival antibodies in diagnostics. Clin Chem 1999 Sep;45(9):1628–1650.
3. Famulok M, Blind M, Mayer G. Intramers as promising new tools in functional proteomics. Chem Biol 2001 Oct;8(10):931–939.
4. Tuerk C, Gold L. Systematic evolution of ligands by exponential enrichment: RNA ligands to bacteriophage T4 DNA polymerase. Science 1990;249(4968):505–510.
5. Jellinek D, Green LS, Bell C, et al. Inhibition of receptor binding by high-affinity RNA ligands to vascular endothelial growth factor. Biochemistry 1994;33(34):10450–10456.
6. Green LS, Jellinek D, Bell C, et al. Nuclease-resistant nucleic acid ligands to vascular permeability factor/vascular endothelial growth factor. Chem Biol 1995;2(10):683–695.
7. Ruckman J, Green LS, Beeson J, et al. 2′-Fluoropyrimidine RNA-based aptamers to the 165-amino acid form of vascular endothelial growth factor (VEGF165). Inhibition of receptor binding and VEGF-induced vascular permeability through interactions requiring the exon 7-encoded domain. J Biol Chem 1998;273(32):20556–20567.
8. Bell C, Lynam E, Landfair DJ, et al. Oligonucleotide NX1838 inhibits VEGF165-mediated cellular responses *in vitro*. *In Vitro* Cell Dev Biol Anim 1999;35(9):533–542.
9. Tucker CE, Chen LS, Judkins MB, et al. Detection and plasma pharmacokinetics of an anti-vascular endothelial growth factor oligonucleotide-aptamer (NX1838) in rhesus monkeys. J Chromatogr B Biomed Sci Appl 1999;732(1):203–212.
10. Drolet DW, Nelson J, Tucker CE, et al. Pharmacokinetics and safety of an anti-vascular endothelial growth factor aptamer (NX1838) following injection into the vitreous humor of rhesus monkeys. Pharm Res 2000;17(12):1503–1510.
11. Macugen prescribing information. Macugen package insert. Available online at: http://www.macugen.com/macugenUSPI.pdf.
12. Modi M, for the Macugen AMD Study Group. Pegaptanib population pharmacokinetics and pharmacodynamics in patients with neovascular age-related macular degeneration. *Proceedings of the Association for Research in vision and Ophthalmology (annual meeting)*. Ft. Lauderdale, FL, USA; 2006.
13. Apte RS, Modi M, Masonson H, et al. Pegaptanib 1-year systemic safety results from a safety-pharmacokinetic trial in patients with neovascular age-related macular degeneration. Ophthalmology 2007 Sep;114(9):1702–1712.
14. Ng E, Krilleke D, De Erkenez A, et al. VEGF RNA aptamer binding specificity and inhibition of ligand binding to vegf receptors *in vitro*. *Proceedings of the Association for Research in vision and Ophthalmology (annual meeting)*. Ft. Lauderdale, FL, USA; 2004.
15. Lee JH, Canny MD, De Erkenez A, et al. A therapeutic aptamer inhibits angiogenesis by specifically targeting the heparin binding domain of VEGF165. Proc Natl Acad Sci USA 2005;102:18902–18907.
16. Fairbrother WJ, Champe MA, Christinger HW, et al. Solution structure of the heparin-binding domain of vascular endothelial growth factor. Structure 1998;6(5):637–648.
17. Lim JI, Spee C, Hangai M, et al. Neuropilin-1 expression by endothelial cells and retinal pigment epithelial cells in choroidal neovascular membranes. Am J Ophthalmol 2005;140:1044–1050.
18. Ng EW, Shima DT, Calias P, et al. Pegaptanib, a targeted anti-VEGF aptamer for ocular vascular disease. Nat Rev Drug Discov 2006;5(2):123–132.
19. Ferrara N. Vascular endothelial growth factor: basic science and clinical progress. Endocr Rev 2004;25:581–611.
20. Adamis AP, Shima DT. The role of vascular endothelial growth factor in ocular health and disease. Retina 2005;25:111–118.
21. Starita C, Patel M, Katz B, et al. Vascular endothelial growth factor and the potential therapeutic use of pegaptanib (Macugen) in diabetic retinopathy. Dev Ophthalmol 2007;39:122–148.
22. Usui T, Ishida S, Yamashiro K, et al. VEGF164(165) as the pathological isoform: differential leukocyte and endothelial responses through VEGFR1 and VEGFR2. Invest Ophthalmol Vis Sci 2004;45:368–374.
23. Nishijima K, Ng YS, Zhong L, et al. Vascular endothelial growth factor-A is a survival factor for retinal neurons and a critical neuroprotectant during the adaptive response to ischemic injury. Am J Pathol 2007 Jul;171(1):53–67.
24. Blaauwgeers HG, Holtkamp GM, Rutten H, et al. Polarized vascular endothelial growth factor secretion by human retinal pigment epithelium and localization of vascular endothelial growth factor receptors on the inner choriocapillaris. Evidence for a trophic paracrine relation. Am J Pathol 1999;155:421–428.
25. Kamba T, McDonald DM. Mechanisms of adverse effects of anti-VEGF therapy for cancer. Br J Cancer 2007;96:1788–1795.
26. Verheul HM, Pinedo HM. Possible molecular mechanisms involved in the toxicity of angiogenesis inhibition. Nat Rev Cancer 2007;7:475–485.
27. Ireson CR, Kelland LR. Discovery and development of anticancer aptamers. Mol Cancer Ther 2006;5(12):2957–2962.
28. Gopinath SC, Shikamoto Y, Mizuno H, et al. A potent anti-coagulant RNA aptamer inhibits blood coagulation by specifically blocking the extrinsic clotting pathway. Thromb Haemost 2006 May;95(5):767–771.
29. Gilbert JC, DeFeo-Fraulini T, Hutabarat RM, et al. First-in-human evaluation of anti von Willebrand factor therapeutic aptamer ARC1779 in healthy volunteers. Circulation 2007 Dec 4;116(23):2678–2686.
30. Zhou J, Li H, Li S, et al. Novel dual inhibitory function aptamer-siRNA delivery system for HIV-1 therapy. Mol Ther 2008;16:1481–1489.
31. Bellecave P, Cazenave C, Rumi J, et al. Inhibition of hepatitis C virus (HCV) RNA polymerase by DNA aptamers: mechanism of inhibition of *in vitro* RNA synthesis and effect on HCV-infected cells. Antimicrob Agents Chemother 2008 Jun;52(6):2097–2110.
32. Eyetech Study Group. Preclinical and phase 1A clinical evaluation of an anti-VEGF pegylated aptamer (EYE001) for the treatment of exudative age-related macular degeneration. Retina 2002;22(2):143–152.
33. Eyetech Study Group. Anti-vascular endothelial growth factor therapy for subfoveal choroidal neovascularization secondary to age-related macular degeneration: phase II study results. Ophthalmology 2003;110(5):979–986.
34. Gragoudas ES, Adamis AP, Cunningham Jr ET, et al. VEGF inhibition study in Ocular Neovascularization Clinical Trial Group. Pegaptanib for neovascular age-related macular degeneration. N Engl J Med 2004;351(27):2805–2816.
35. Ng EW, Adamis AP. Targeting angiogenesis, the underlying disorder in neovascular age-related macular degeneration. Can J Ophthalmol 2005;40(3):352–368.
36. Chakravarthy U, Adamis AP, Cunningham Jr ET, et al. Year 2 efficacy results of two randomized, controlled clinical trials of pegaptanib, an

anti-VEGF aptamer, for neovascular age-related macular degeneration. Ophthalmology 2006;113(9):1508.e1–25.
37. Gonzales CR, VEGF Inhibition Study in Ocular Neovascularization Clinical Trial Group. Enhanced efficacy associated with early treatment of neovascular age-related macular degeneration with pegaptanib sodium: an exploratory analysis. Retina 2005;25(7):815–827.
38. Quiram PA, Williams GA, Hassan TS. Treatment of naïve lesions in neovascular age-related macular degeneration with pegaptanib. Retina 2007 Sep;27(7):851–856.
39. Kirsch LS, Hairston RJ. Macugen in the treatment of exudative age-related macular degeneration: experience at the Eye Institute of West Florida. Proceedings of the European Retina, Macula, and Vitreous Society. Lisbon, Portugal: Poster; 2006.
40. Cunningham Jr ET, Adamis AP, Altaweel M, et al. A phase II randomized double-masked trial of pegaptanib, an anti-vascular endothelial growth factor aptamer, for diabetic macular edema. Ophthalmology 2005;112(10):1747–1757.
41. Adamis AP, Miller JW, Bernal MT, et al. Increased vascular endothelial growth factor levels in the vitreous of eyes with proliferative diabetic retinopathy. Am J Ophthalmol 1994;118(4):445–450.
42. Aiello LP, Avery RL, Arrigg PG, et al. Vascular endothelial growth factor in ocular fluid of patients with diabetic retinopathy and other retinal disorders. N Engl J Med 1994;331(22):1480–1487.
43. Adamis AP, Altaweel M, Bressler NM, et al. Changes in retinal neovascularization after pegaptanib (Macugen) therapy in diabetic individuals. Ophthalmology 2006;113(1):23–28.
44. Gonzalez VH, Vann VR, Banda RM, et al. VEGF inhibition: effectiveness in modifying the progression of proliferative diabetic retinopathy (PDR). *Proceedings of the 2006 Annual Meeting of the American Academy of Ophthalmology, 9th Annual European Congress.* Las Vegas, NV, USA, P0370, 2007.
45. Wells III JA, the Pegaptanib in Central Vein Occlusion Study Group. Safety and efficacy of pegaptanib sodium in treating macular edema secondary to central vein retinal occlusion (CRVO). *Proceedings of the 2006 Annual Meeting of the American Academy of Ophthalmology, 9th Annual European Congress.* Las Vegas, NV, USA, P0370, 2006.
46. Wroblewski JJ, Wells, JA, Gonzales C. Pegaptanib Sodium for Macular Edema Secondary to Branch Retinal Vein Occlusion (BRVO). *Proceedings of the Association for Research in vision and Ophthalmology (annual meeting).* Ft. Lauderdale: FL, USA; 2008.
47. Dahr SS, Cusick M, Rodriguez-Coleman H, et al. Intravitreal anti-vascular endothelial growth factor therapy with pegaptanib for advanced von Hippel–Lindau disease of the retina. Retina 2007 Feb;27(2):150–158.
48. Bennett MD, Yee W. Pegaptanib for myopic choroidal neovascularization in a young patient. Graefes Arch Clin Exp Ophthalmol 2007 Jun;245(6):903–905.
49. Filippopoulos T, Ducharme JF, Lowenstein JI, et al. Antiangiogenic agents as an adjunctive treatment for complicated neovascular glaucoma. *Proceedings of the Association for Research in vision and Ophthalmology (annual meeting).* Ft. Lauderdale: FL, USA; 2006.
50. Trese MT, Capone Jr A, Drenser K. Macugen in retinopathy of prematurity. Invest Ophthalmol Vis Sci 2006;47:E-abstract 2330.
51. Drenser KA. Macugen therapy for the treatment of familial exudative vitreoretinopathy. *Proceedings of the Association for Research in vision and Ophthalmology (annual meeting).* Ft. Lauderdale, FL, USA; 2006.
52. Sun Y, Jain A, Moshfeghi DM. Elevated vascular endothelial growth factor levels in Coats disease: rapid response to pegaptanib sodium. Graefes Arch Clin Exp Ophthalmol 2007 Sep;245(9):1387–1388.
53. Querques G, Iaculli C, Delle Noci N. Intravitreal pegaptanib sodium for Irvine–Gass syndrome. Eur J Ophthalmol 2008 Jan-Feb;18(1):138–141.
54. Querques G, Prascina F, Iaculli C, et al. Intravitreal pegaptanib sodium (Macugen) for refractory cystoid macular edema in pericentral retinitis pigmentosa. Int Ophthalmol 2008;86:700–701.
55. Bourla DH, Gonzales CR, Mango CW, et al. Intravitreous vascular endothelial growth factor (VEGF) inhibitor therapy for tamoxifen induced macular edema. Semin Ophthalmol 2007 Apr-Jun;22(2):87–88.
56. Jager RD, Aiello LP, Patel SC, et al. Risks of intravitreous injection: a comprehensive review. Retina 2004;24:676–698.
57. D'Amico DJ, Patel M, Adamis AP, et al. Pegaptanib sodium for neovascular age-related macular degeneration: two-year safety results of the two prospective, multicenter, controlled clinical trials. Ophthalmology 2006;113(6):992–1001.
58. Singerman LJ, Masonson H, Patel M, et al. Pegaptanib sodium for neovascular age-related macular degeneration: third-year safety results of the V.I.S.I.O.N. trial. Br J Ophthalmol 2008;92:1606–1611.
59. Photodynamic therapy of subfoveal choroidal neovascularization in age-related macular degeneration with verteporfin: one-year results of 2 randomized clinical trials – TAP report. Arch Ophthalmol 1999;117:1329–1345.
60. Foy JW, Rittenhouse K, Modi M, et al. Local tolerance and systemic safety of pegaptanib sodium in the dog and rabbit. J Ocul Pharmacol Ther 2007 Oct;23(5):452–466.
61. Steffensmeier AC, Azar AE, Fuller JJ, et al. Vitreous injections of pegaptanib sodium triggering allergic reactions. Am J Ophthalmol 2007 Mar;143(3):512–513.
62. Data on file, Pfizer, Inc.
63. Ju M, Mailhos C, Bradley J, et al. Simultaneous but not prior inhibition of VEGF165 enhances the efficacy of photodynamic therapy in multiple models of ocular neovascularization. Invest Ophthalmol Vis Sci 2008 Feb;49(2):662–670.

CHAPTER

39 Protein kinase C inhibitor: ruboxistaurin

Heidrun L Deissler, Dipl-Chem and Gabriele E Lang, MD

KEY FEATURES

Early events in the development of diabetic retinopathy include the loss of retinal pericytes, thickening of the capillary basement membrane, and increased leukocyte adhesion to retinal endothelial cells. Elevated permeability of retinal endothelial cells leading to macular edema is caused by increased expression of vascular endothelial growth factor (VEGF), which has been found in the vitreous fluid of patients with diabetic retinopathy even at the early stages of the disease.[1–3] Proliferative diabetic retinopathy is associated with neovascularization, which is most likely the result of deregulated proliferation and migration of retinal endothelial cells induced by growth factors like VEGF, basic fibroblast growth factor, or other stimulators.[2,4] At least some of these processes are directly or indirectly associated with the activation of serine/threonine-specific protein kinase C (PKC) and its isoenzymes.[5–9] PKC is therefore considered a valuable target molecule for therapeutic intervention (Figure 39.1).[5–7,10–12]

INTRODUCTION TO PROTEIN KINASE C

PROTEIN KINASE C FAMILY

Protein kinases transfer phosphate groups to either serine/threonine residues (e.g., protein kinase A, PKC, mitogen-activated protein kinases) or to tyrosine residues (e.g., growth factor receptor kinases) of the target protein, leading to its activation or in some cases to its inactivation. The PKC family comprises several different members (PKCα, βI and II, γ, δ, ε, η, θ, ζ, ι/λ) which differ in their structure, cofactor requirement, and substrate specificity[7,11] (Table 39.1 and Figure 39.2). These kinases, of which some are tissue-specifically expressed, are usually located in the cytoplasm. Activation of PKC isoenzymes (α, βI and II, δ, and ε) is usually accompanied by translocalization of the kinase activity from the cytosol to the plasma membrane within minutes in microvascular (retinal) and macrovascular endothelial cells after stimulation with high glucose, VEGF, or phorbol-12-myristate-13-acetate (PMA).[13,14] Whether this short-term effect becomes permanent after long-term treatment of the cells with PMA or VEGF remains to be shown. Each PKC consists of a single polypeptide chain derived from a single gene, except for PKCβ I and II, which are alternative splice variants. PKC members which function as intracellular signal transduction systems for several cytokines and hormones, can be divided into three subgroups (Table 39.1 and Figure 39.2):

1. Activation of **conventional or classical PKCs** (cPKC: α, βI and II, γ) depends on Ca^{2+} ions and adenosine triphosphate (ATP). They can be activated by diacylglycerol or phorbol esters like PMA.
2. **Novel PKCs** (nPKC: δ, ε, θ), which can also be activated by diacylglycerol or PMA, are independent of Ca^{2+} ions.
3. PKCζ and PKCι/λ belong to the group of **atypical PKCs** (aPKCs) which are insensitive to diacylglycerol or PMA but can be activated by phosphatidylserine.

PKCη (PKD1) and PKCμ (PKD3) form a fourth subgroup of PKC isoenzymes, also known as the protein kinase D family, and are not discussed in this chapter.

EFFECTS OF ACTIVATED PKC

It is well known that hyperglycemia leads to elevated levels of diacylglycerol, which is a potent activator of PKC.[15–17] It also results in the deregulation of several cellular processes in which PKC isoenzymes are involved, including those which lead to inhibition of Na-K ATPase, increasing permeability, and stimulation of proliferation in different cell types.[9,18,19] Expression of several genes (cytokines, growth factors, nitric oxide synthase, extracellular matrix proteins) regulated by PKC depends on stimulation of mitogen-activated protein kinase and is mainly mediated through the transcription factors NFκb and AP-1 in retinal and other cells. PKC stimulation by PMA in macrovascular endothelial cells leads directly to synthesis of VEGF mRNA.[20] Whether VEGF expression can be directly induced by activated PKC in retinal endothelial cells remains to be demonstrated, but at least in retinal pericytes expression of VEGF can be activated by stimulation of PKC.[9,21]

In vitro studies using cell culture models indicate that activation of PKC by PMA or high glucose also increases the permeability of various cell types, including (retinal) endothelial cells.[19] The pathway of paracellular signaling in both endothelial and epithelial cells is regulated at tight junctions which consist of transmembrane proteins like occludin and claudins as well as membrane-associated proteins like zonula occludens-1.[22] The composition of complexes containing these proteins determines the rate of transition of molecules through tight junctions, and their reorganization, including delocalization of its components, most likely causes the alteration of endothelial permeability in diabetic retinopathy. There is some evidence that phosphorylation of the tight junction protein occludin by PKCβ and/or PKCδ within 15 minutes of $VEGF_{165}$ treatment influences its reversible translocalization from the plasma membrane to the cytoplasm in retinal endothelial cells, although this seems to be only a temporary effect.[23,24] Expression of endothelin, which controls retinal blood flow, is also induced by PKCβ in the retina of diabetic animals as well as in retinal pericytes after cultivation in medium containing high glucose.[25,26]

PHARMACOLOGY OF RUBOXISTAURIN

Inhibition of PKC, especially of the β-isoform, seems to be a promising approach to treat diabetes-associated microvascular complications. This chapter discusses primarily the characteristics of ruboxistaurin, which specifically inhibits PKCβ, since the nonspecific PKC-inhibitor PKC412 showed severe adverse effects in treated individuals and is no longer under investigation.[27] Ruboxistaurin mesylate (compound identifier LY333531, Eli Lilly, Figure 39.3) is a macrocyclic bisindolylmaleimide compound that specifically inhibits the β-isoform of PKC.[28,29] As a competitive inhibitor for ATP, LY333531 inhibited isolated enzymes PKCβI and βII with a half-maximal inhibitory constant of 4.5 nM and 5.9 nM, respectively, whereas inhibition of other PKC isoforms required 250 times higher concentrations.[29] There is strong evidence that CYP3A4 is the primary cytochrome P450 enzyme responsible for the metabolism of ruboxistaurin to its main equipotent metabolite, *N*-desmethyl ruboxistaurin (LY333522; Figure 39.3).[30] The half-life of ruboxistaurin which can be orally administered is approximately 9 hours and that of its metabolite 16 hours, therefore allowing once-daily dosing. Studies showed that the primary excretion route in humans for these substances was fecal with renal elimination playing a minor role.[31]

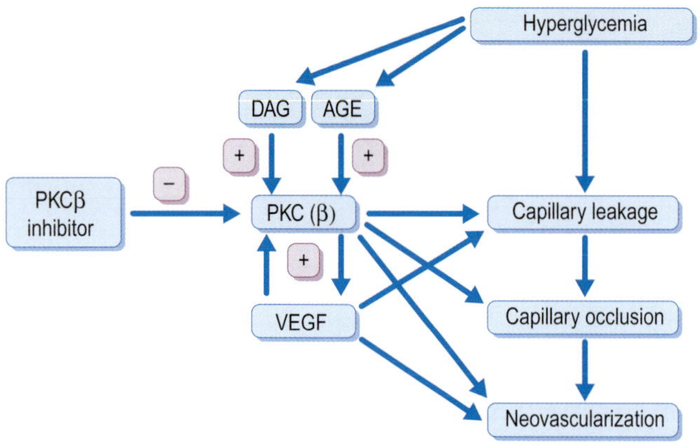

Figure 39.1 Proposed central role of protein kinase Cβ (PKCβ) in the pathogenesis of diabetic retinopathy. Inhibition of PKCβ can affect the progression of diabetic retinopathy at different stages. Synthesis of diacylglycerol (DAG) and advanced glycation endproducts (AGE) is stimulated by hyperglycemia, resulting in the activation of PKC(β). As a consequence, vascular endothelial growth factor (VEGF) expression is stimulated in some cells, which in turn also activates PKC, leading to vascular leakage and neovascularization seen in diabetic retinopathy. These processes may be influenced by PKCβ inhibition. + stimulation of the process by PKC (activation); – inhibition of the process by PKC inhibition.

MECHANISM OF ACTION OF PKC INHIBITORS

Several studies using animal models have indeed shown that PKC inhibitors can counteract cellular processes activated by PKC: Intravitreal injection of VEGF at clinically observed concentrations rapidly activated PKC in the retina in an animal model and led to a more than threefold increase in retinal vasopermeability. Intravitreal or oral administration of a PKCβ inhibitor almost completely reverted this VEGF-induced permeability.[32] In addition, LY333531 prevented diabetes-induced retinal vascular leakage and retinal neovascularization in a mouse model for diabetes type 2.[33] Treatment of diabetic rats with ruboxistaurin resulted in an amelioration of the retinal blood flow in a dose-responsive manner in parallel with inhibition of the retinal PKC activity.[28] Ruboxistaurin also reduced the VEGF-induced blood–retinal barrier breakdown and neovascularization in an animal model. Thereby, the inhibitor abolished both VEGF-induced PKC activation and endothelial cell proliferation, with VEGF's mitogenic effect being inhibited by ruboxistaurin in a concentration-dependent manner.[32] This inhibitor also effectively inhibited preretinal and optic nerve head neovascularization in a porcine model of branch retinal vein occlusion without any apparent systemic toxicity.[34] In this case, the ameliorative effect seemed to be a result of the disruption of the intracellular signal cascade activated by VEGF and other angiogenic growth factors by targeting one of its key components.

EFFECT OF RUBOXISTAURIN IN HUMAN NONOCULAR DISEASES

Since hypergylcemia results in disordered skin microvascular blood flow – possibly through overactivation of PKCβ – the effect of ruboxistaurin on neurovascular function was tested in patients with diabetic peripheral neuropathy. In a double-masked, placebo-controlled study a small number of patients (20 per group) were treated with placebo or 32 mg/day ruboxistaurin over 6 months.[35] A significant increase of the endothelium-dependent and C-fiber-mediated skin microvascular blood flow at the distal calf as well as reduced sensory symptoms were observed in the ruboxstaurin-treated group. In another clinical trial, 250 patients with diabetic peripheral neuropathy were treated with placebo, 32 or 64 mg/day ruboxistaurin over 1 year. However, no significant improvement in abnormal measurable vibration detection threshold was seen in the two groups treated with ruboxistaurin compared to the placebo group.[36] Inhibition of PKCβ by ruboxistaurin also improved kidney disease in animal models.[28,33] Therefore, patients with diabetes type 2-associated nephropathy were treated with 32 mg/day ruboxistaurin in a placebo-controlled pilot study over 1 year. However, no statistically significant changes were observed between the ruboxistaurin- and the placebo-treated group with regard to albuminuria and estimated glomerular filtration rate, which might be due to the small number of individuals.[37]

USE OF PKC INHIBITORS IN THE TREATMENT OF DIABETIC MACULAR EDEMA AND DIABETIC RETINOPATHY

Treatment of DME patients for 3 months with a multitargeting kinase inhibitor PKC412, which also acts as a nonspecific PKC inhibitor, led to a reduction of retinal thickening as evaluated by optical coherence tomography. However the systemic applicability of this nonselective compound was limited by substantial gastrointestinal side-effects and other dose-related signs of low tolerability, e.g., disturbed glycemic control and liver toxicity.[27] On the other hand, treatment with ruboxistaurin mesylate (4 and 32 mg/day), which selectively inhibits the PKCβ isoform, can reduce the retinal vascular leakage in eyes that have DME and markedly elevated leakage, suggesting that this treatment may be most effective in patients with severe forms of macular edema.[38] In patients receiving 16 mg ruboxistaurin twice daily, the diabetes-induced increase in retinal circulation time was improved. A linear correlation between the dose of ruboxistaurin and its effect on retinal circulation time was observed as well as with retinal blood flow.[39]

EFFICACY OF RUBOXISTAURIN IN THE TREATMENT OF DIABETIC RETINOPATHY

In a multicenter, double-masked, randomized, and placebo-controlled study (PKC-DRS study) the safety and efficacy of orally administered ruboxistaurin were evaluated in subjects with moderately severe to very severe nonproliferative diabetic retinopathy.[40] A total of 252 subjects received placebo or ruboxistaurin (8, 16, or 32 mg/day) for 36–46 months. Patients had an ETDRS retinopathy severity level between 47B and 53E inclusive, an ETDRS visual acuity of 20/125 or better, and no history of scatter photocoagulation. Efficacy measurements included progression of diabetic retinopathy, moderate visual loss, and sustained moderate visual loss. Compared with placebo, 32 mg/day ruboxistaurin was weakly associated with a delayed occurrence of moderate visual loss ($P = 0.038$) and sustained moderate visual loss ($P = 0.226$). This was evident only in eyes with definite DME at baseline ($P = 0.017$). As a result of a multivariable Cox proportional hazard analysis, 32 mg/day ruboxistaurin significantly reduced the risk of moderate visual loss compared with placebo ($P = 0.012$).[40] The beneficial effect of ruboxistaurin on moderate visual loss might be due to improved retinal cell viability resulting from PKCβ inhibition, leading to a greater resistance of retinal vascular and neural cells to pathologic stress of hyperglycemia and changes in the hemodynamics of blood flow. Further multicenter trials (e.g., PKC-DMES study) investigated whether ruboxistaurin can reduce the progression of DME and diabetic retinopathy: In a multicenter, double-masked, randomized, placebo-controlled study 686 patients who had DME farther than 300 μm from the center of the macula at baseline were treated with either ruboxistaurin (4, 16, or 32 mg/day) or placebo for 30 months. The primary outcome was progression to sight-threatening DME or application of focal/grid photocoagulation for DME. Although the progression to this primary

Table 39.1 Classification and expression of different isoenzymes of protein kinase C (PKC)[7,11] (list is not complete)

	Activation by	Isoenzyme	Expression in:	Activated in diabetes
Group A: classical, conventional PKC (cPKC)	Diacylglycerol, phosphatidylserine, phorbol ester Ca^{2+}-dependent	α	Aorta, aortic SMC, aortic EC; heart; kidney, glomeruli; retina, cultured retinal EC; monocytes; epithelial cells; RPE	√
		βI	Aortic SMC, aortic EC; heart; kidney, glomeruli; retina, cultured retinal EC, retinal pericytes; RPE; monocytes	√
		βII	Aorta, aortic SMC, aortic EC; heart; kidney, glomeruli; retina, cultured retinal EC, retinal pericytes; RPE; monocytes	√
		γ	RPE; heart	
Group B: novel PKC (nPKC)	Diacylglycerol, phosphatidylserine, phorbol ester Ca^{2+}-independent	δ	Aortic SMC, aortic EC; heart; kidney, glomeruli; retina, cultured retinal EC; RPE; monocytes; fibroblasts	√
		ε	Aortic EC; heart; kidney, glomeruli; retina, cultured retinal EC; RPE; monocytes, lens epithelial cells; cardiomyocytes	√
		θ	Lymphocytes	
Group C: atypical PKC (aPKC)	Phosphatidylserine	ζ	Heart; cultured retinal EC; monocytes, cultured keratinocytes	
		ι/λ	Cultured keratinocytes; RPE	

SMC, smooth-muscle cells; EC, endothelial cells, RPE, retinal pigment epithelial cells.

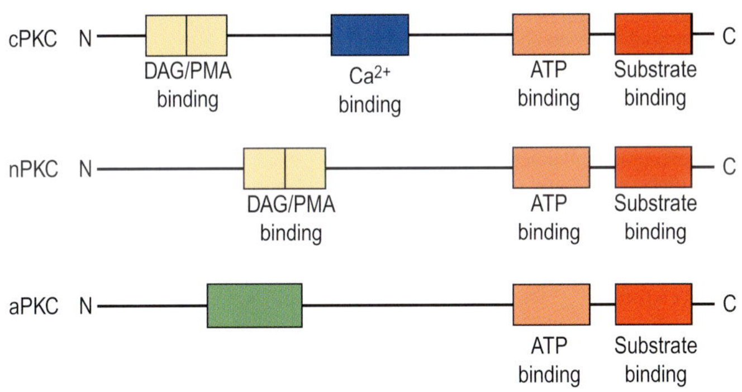

Figure 39.2 Simplified domain structure of the protein kinase C (PKC) family members. The different classes of different PKC isoenzymes are shown[7,11] (Table 39.1). DAG, diacylglycerol; PMA, phorbol-12-myristate-13-acetate; ATP, adenosine triphosphate.

outcome was not delayed, daily oral administration of ruboxistaurin may delay progression of DME to the sight-threatening stage.[41]

CONTRAINDICATIONS OF RUBOXISTAURIN

Aside from obvious contraindications like pregnancy, there are no special contraindications known for ruboxistaurin.

OCULAR AND SYSTEMIC COMPLICATIONS AND TOXICITY OF RUBOXISTAURIN

When considering systemic therapy, the safety profile of a compound is most important. This is a critical aspect, especially when a key signaling enzyme such as PKC is inhibited and substantial toxicity might be due to interference with important processes not related to disease. Whereas treatment with a nonspecific inhibitor of different kinases and PKC isoenzymes resulted in elevated blood concentrations of liver enzymes, nausea, vomiting, and diarrhea, the PKCβ-selective inhibitor ruboxistaurin was very well tolerated without significant adverse events over 52 months of treatment.[27,40,41] The frequency of nonserious adverse events (diarrhea, flatulence, nephropathy, proteinuria, and coronary artery disease) was highest in the group of patients receiving 16 mg/day, but this appeared not to be a ruboxistaurin dose-dependent effect. Patients recieving the highest ruboxistaurin dose of 32 mg/day did not experience these events more often than patients in the placebo group. To date, over 1400 patients have been exposed to ruboxistaurin, and clinically significant adverse effects associated with this drug have not been observed.[40,41]

INTERACTION OF RUBOXISTAURIN WITH OTHER DRUGS

Co-administration of ruboxistaurin with known CYP3A4-inducing agents (rifampicin, carbamazepine, phenobarbital) may decrease the concentrations of ruboxistaurin and its metabolite *N*-desmethyl ruboxistaurin.[42]

SUMMARY AND KEY POINTS

In view of the limited therapeutic potential of the currently available options in the treatment of diabetic retinopathy, novel approaches are urgently needed. Since *in vitro* studies suggested that PKC is involved in several processes which are deregulated in different cell types by hyperglycemia, this protein family could be considered a valuable target for therapeutic intervention. The isoenzyme-specific PKC inhibi-

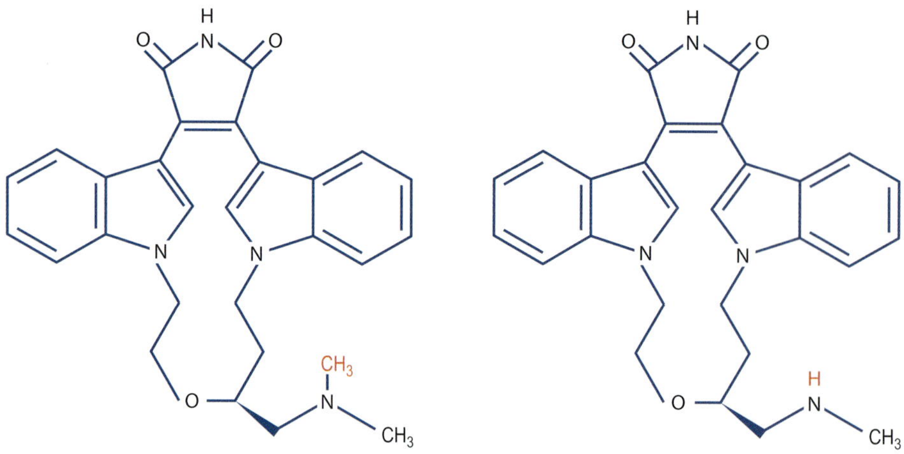

Ruboxistaurin
LY333531
(1)

N-desmethyl ruboxistaurin
LY333522
(2)

Figure 39.3 Structure of ruboxistaurin (LY333531) and its active metabolite, *N*-desmethyl ruboxistaurin (LY333522). LY333531 (1) is metabolized to the equipotent LY333522 (2): the change in structure is highlighted in red.

tor ruboxistaurin provides some blockade of hyperglycemia-induced vascular injury and can be safely administered to humans. First studies indicated that ruboxistaurin treatment may reduce visual loss in patients with moderately severe to very severe nonproliferative diabetic retinopathy, but the potential of this approach in clinical practice will have to be further evaluated in subsequent studies.

REFERENCES

1. Aiello LP, Avery RL, Arrigg PG, et al. Vascular endothelial growth factor in ocular fluid of patients with diabetic retinopathy and other retinal disorders. N Eng J Med 1994;331:1480–1487.
2. Caldwell RB, Bartoli M, Behzadian MA, et al. Vascular endothelial growth factor and diabetic retinopathy: pathophysiological mechanisms and treatment perspectives. Diabetes Metab Res Rev 2003;19:442–455.
3. Nguyen QD, Tatlipinar S, Shah SM, et al. Vascular endothelial growth factor is a critical stimulus for diabetic macular edema. Am J Ophthalmol 2006;142:961–969.
4. Way KJ, Katai N, King GL. Protein kinase C and the development of diabetic vascular complications. Diabet Med 2001;18:945–959.
5. Aiello LP. The potential role of PKCβ in diabetic retinopathy and macular edema. Surv Ophthalmol 2002;47(Suppl 2):S263–S269.
6. Clarke M, Dodson PM. PKC inhibition and diabetic microvascular complications. Best Pract Res Clin Endocrinol Metab 2007;21:573–586.
7. Evicmen ND, King GL. The role of protein kinase C activation and the vascular complications of diabetes. Pharmocol Res 2007;55:498–510.
8. Lang GE, Kampmeier J. Die Bedeutung der Proteinkinase C in der Pathophysiologie der diabetischen Retinopathie. Klin Monatsbl Augenheilkd 2002;219:769–776.
9. Suzuma K, Takahara N, Suzuma I, et al. Characterization of protein kinase C β isoform's action on retinoblastoma protein phosphorylation, vascular endothelial growth factor-induced cell proliferation, and retinal neovascularization. Proc Natl Acad Sci 2002;99:721–726.
10. Idris I, Donelly R. Protein kinase Cβ inhibition: a novel therapeutic strategy for diabetic microangiopathy. Diabetes Vasc Dis Res 2006;3:172–178.
11. Meier M, King GL. Protein kinase C activation and its pharmalogical inhibition in vascular disease. Vasc Med 2000;5:173–185.
12. Taulien CA, Joy SV. Ruboxistaurin. Drugs Today 2006;42:577–585.
13. Rask-Madsen C, King GL. Differential regulation of VEGF signaling by PKCα and PKCε in endothelial cells. Arterioscler Thromb Vasc Biol 2008;28:919–924.
14. Xia P, Aiello LP, Ishii H, et al. Characterization of vascular endothelial growth factor's effect on the activation of protein kinase C, its isoforms, and endothelial cell growth. J Clin Invest 1996;98:2018–2026.
15. Craven PA, Davidson CM, DeRubertis FR. Increase in diacylglycerol mass in isolated glomeruli by glucose from de novo synthesis of glycerolipids. Diabetes 1990;39:667–674.
16. Kishimoto A, Takai Y, Mori T, et al. Activation of calcium and phospholipid-dependent protein kinase by diacylglycerol, its possible relation to phosphatidylinositol turnover. J Biol Chem 1980;255: 2273–2276.
17. Xia P, Inoguchi T, Kern TS, et al. Characterization of the mechanism for the chronic activation of diacylglycerol-protein kinase C pathway in diabetes and hypergalactosemia. Diabetes 1994;43:1122–1129.
18. Crider JY, Yorio T, Sharif NA, et al. The effects of elevated glucose on Na^+/K^+-ATPase of cultured bovine retinal pigment epithelial cells measured by a new nonradioactive rubidium uptake assay. J Ocul Pharmacol Ther 1997;13:337–352.
19. Hempel A, Maasch C, Heintze U, et al. High glucose concentrations increase endothelial cell permeability via activation of protein kinase Cα. Circ Res 1997;81:363–371.
20. Xu H, Czerwinski P, Hortmann M, et al. Protein kinase Cα promotes angiogenic activity of human endothelial cells via induction of vascular endothelial growth factor. Cardiovas Res 2008;78:349–355.
21. Amadio M, Scapagnini G, Lupo G, et al. PKCβII/HuR/VEGF: A new molecular cascade in retinal pericytes for the regulation of VEGF gene expression. Pharmacol Res 2008;57:60–66.
22. Bazzoni G. Endothelial tight junctions: permeable barriers of the vessel wall. Thromb Haemost 2006;95:36–42.
23. Deissler H, Deissler H, Lang S, et al. VEGF-induced effects on proliferation, migration and tight junctions are restored by ranibizumab (Lucentis®) in microvascular retinal endothelial cells. Br J Ophthalmol 2008;92: 839–843.
24. Harhaj NS, Felinski EA, Wolpert EB, et al. VEGF activation of protein kinase C stimulates occludin phosphorylation and contributes to endothelial permeability. Invest Ophthalmol Vis Sci 2006,47: 5106–5115.
25. Park JY, Takahara N, Gabariele A, et al. Induction of endothelin-1 expression by glucose. Diabetes 2000;49:1239–1248.
26. Yokota T, Ma RC, Park JY, et al. Role of protein kinase C on the expression of platelet-derived growth factor and endothelin-1 in the retina of diabetic rats and cultured retinal capillary pericytes. Diabetes 2003;52:838–845.
27. Campochiaro PA, C99-PKC412-003 Study Group. Reduction of diabetic macular edema by oral administration of the kinase inhibitor PKC412. Invest Ophthalmol Vis Sci 2004;45:922–931.
28. Ishii H, Jirousek MR, Koya D, et al. Amelioration of vascular dysfunctions in diabetic rats by an oral PKC-β inhibitor. Science 1996;272: 728–731.
29. Jirousek MR, Gillig JR, Gonzalez CM, et al. (S)-13-[(Dimethylamino) methyl]-10,11,14,15-tetrahydro-4,9:16,21-dimetheno-1H,13H-dibenzo[e,k] pyrrolo[3,4-h][1,4,13]oxa-diazacyclohexadecene-1,3(2H)-dione (LY333531) and related analogues: Isozyme selective inhibitors of protein kinase Cβ. J Med Chem 1996;39:2664–2671.
30. Ring BJ, Gillespie JS, Binkley SN, et al. The interactions of a selective protein kinase β inhibitor with the human cytochromes P450. Drug Metab Dispos 2002;30:957–961.
31. Burkey JL, Campanale KM, Barbuch R, et al. Disposition of [14C] ruboxistaurin in humans. Drug Metab Dispos 2006;34:1909–1917.
32. Aiello LP, Bursell SE, Clermont A, et al. Vascular endothelial growth factor-induced retinal permeability is mediated by protein kinase C *in vivo* and suppressed by an orally effective beta-isoform-selective inhibitor. Diabetes 1997;46:1473–1480.
33. Koya D, Haneda M, Nakagawa H, et al. Amelioration of accelerated diabetic mesangial expansion by treatment with a PKC β inhibitor in diabetic db/db mice, a rodent model for type 2 diabetes. FASEB J 2000;14:439–447.
34. Danis RP, Bingaman DP, Jirousek M, et al. Inhibition of intraocular neovascularization caused by retinal ischemia in pigs by PKCβ inhibition with LY333531. Invest Ophthalmol Vis Sci 1998;39:171–179.
35. Casselini CM, Barlow PM, Rice AL, et al. A 6-month, randomized, double-masked, placebo-controlled study evaluating the effects of the protein kinase Cβ inhibitor ruboxistaurin on skin microvascular blood flow and other measures of diabetic peripheral neuropathy. Diabetes Care 2007;30:896–902.
36. Vinik AI, Bril V, Kempler P, et al. Treatment of symptomatic diabetic peripheral neuropathy with the protein kinase C β-inhibitor ruboxistaurin mesylate during a 1-year, randomized, placebo-controlled, double-blind clinical trial. Clin Ther 2005;27:1164–1180.

37. Tuttle KR, Bakris GL, Tot RD, et al. The effect of ruboxistaurin on nephropathy in type 2 diabetes. Diabetes Care 2005;28:2686–2690.
38. Strom C, Sander B, Klemp K, et al. Effect of Ruboxistaurin on blood–retinal barrier permeability in relation to severity of leakage in diabetic macular edema. Invest Ophthalmol Vis Sci 2005;46:3855–3858.
39. Aiello LP, Clermont A, Arora V, et al. Inhibition of PKCβ by oral administration of Ruboxistaurin is well tolerated and ameliorates diabetes-induced retinal hemodynamic abnormalities in patients. Invest Ophthalmol Vis Sci 2006;47:86–92.
40. The PKC-DRS Study Group. The effect of ruboxistaurin on visual loss in patients with moderately severe to very severe nonproliferative diabetic retinopathy. Diabetes 2005;54:2188–2197.
41. The PKC-DMES Study Group. Effect of ruboxistaurin in patients with diabetic macular edema. Arch Ophthalmol 2007;125:318–324.
42. Yeo KP, Lowe SL, Lim MT, et al. Pharmacokinetics of ruboxistaurin are significantly altered by rifampicin-mediated CYP3A4 induction. Br J Clin Pharmacol 2005;61:200–210.

CHAPTER

40

Small-interference RNA technology: SIRNA 027, bevasiranib, and REDD14NP

John T. Thompson, MD and Quan Dong Nguyen, MD, MSc

KEY FEATURES

The treatment of ocular diseases by controlling gene expression is a potentially powerful means of treating any retinal disease where a protein produced by cells is detrimental to the health of the organism. Posttranscriptional gene silencing occurs when the messenger RNA (mRNA) of a particular target gene is destroyed. The destruction of mRNA coding for the injurious protein prevents translation to form an active gene product. This chapter will discuss two new drugs, bevasiranib, which blocks and destroys mRNA coding vascular endothelial growth factor (VEGF) and SIRNA-027, which destroys mRNA coding for VEGF receptor. These two drugs are relatively new, such that efficacy and comparison with other agents, contraindications, ocular/systemic complications, and drug interactions have not been studied; therefore, these data cannot be presented in any detail in this chapter. Relevant safety data will be presented in the description of the phase I and II trials for these two drugs. In addition, the chapter will also briefly discuss a third mRNA inhibitor, REDD 14NP, which is a small-interference RNA (siRNA) that acts via RNA interference to inhibit the expression of the hypoxia-inducible gene, RTP801.

INTRODUCTION AND HISTORY OF SIRNA FOR RETINAL DISEASES

RNA interference (RNAi) is a common mechanism of posttranscriptional gene silencing. It was initially discovered in the segmented worm *Caenorhabditis elegans* by Fire and colleagues.[1] They found that a double-stranded RNA homologous to a specific gene could turn off that gene. The process is initiated when a larger double-stranded RNA is cleaved by a ribonuclease named Dicer into short double-stranded fragments called siRNAs.

siRNAs are typically 21–23 nucleotides in length and will block protein production for specific proteins encoded by mRNAs whose target sequences are homologous to the siRNAs. Proteins are normally synthesized by a process where the DNA coding for a particular protein is transcribed into mRNA. The mRNA is then translated into protein. During the process of RNAi, siRNAs are incorporated into a multi-protein endoribonuclease complex termed the RNA-induced silencing complex (RISC). A helicase within the RISC unwinds the duplex siRNA, allowing its antisense strand to bind mRNA with a high degree of sequence complementarity. An RNase within RISC then degrades the target mRNA by cleavage, which results in silenced gene expression and reduced protein production, as the cleaved target mRNA cannot reassemble. The same activated RISC can then bind to another identical target mRNA and the process may be repeated hundreds or thousands of times to amplify the response (Figure 40.1).

The prevention of protein synthesis has important implications in many diseases where abnormal production of proteins leads to a particular disease. Antibody and aptamer-based drugs are often designed to bind proteins that cause disease and inactivate them. In contrast to this mechanism of action, RNA interference prevents production of the protein by eliminating the mRNA.

There are many potential retinal diseases which can be targeted by siRNA technology. An obvious choice was to investigate the role of inhibition of VEGF for the treatment of choroidal neovascularization (CNV) since other drugs which block VEGF, such as ranibizumab, bevacizumab, and pegaptanib, were being developed.

Age-related macular degeneration (AMD) is a major cause of decreased vision in elderly patients and has two forms: neovascular (exudative or wet) and nonexudative (dry). Approximately 10% of patients develop the exudative form of AMD, characterized by CNV. The prevalence of either form of AMD is 7.9% in persons 75 years or older, and the presence of milder forms at baseline increases the risk of progression to more advanced forms of maculopathy.[2,3]

VEGF is an important stimulus for the development of CNV and inhibition of VEGF has been demonstrated to inhibit CNV in patients with AMD and improve visual outcomes when compared to the natural history of the disease.[4,5] Ranibizumab, bevacizumab, and pegaptanib all require frequent intravitreal injections (every 4–6 weeks) for 1–2 years to obtain the best visual results.[4,6–8] The burden of frequent injections and the desire to achieve more improvements in visual acuity has led to a search for other inhibitors of VEGF which may help in the treatment of CNV.

The application of siRNA technology for the treatment of CNV represents a new strategy to prevent VEGF synthesis. Several approaches for the inhibition of VEGF are under investigation. OPKO Health (formerly Acuity Pharmaceuticals: Miami, FL) has been developing bevasiranib (previously called Cand5), an siRNA targeting VEGF, to treat AMD. SIRNA Therapeutics (San Francisco, CA) has been evaluating SIRNA-027, an siRNA directed against VEGF receptor 1, in partnership with Merck and Allergan. Another siRNA targeting the VEGF pathway from Alnylam Pharmaceuticals was evaluated in preclinical studies but has not progressed to human trials. Quark has partnered with Pfizer to investigate the role of REDD14NP, the siRNA that inhibits the hypoxia-inducible gene, RTP801, which potentially prevents production of VEGF.

PHARMACOLOGY, DRUG MECHANISM, AND DRUG EFFECTS IN NONOCULAR DISEASES

The first report of the use of siRNA directed against VEGF was published by Reich[9] in a model of CNV in mice, but its application to other diseases, specifically oncology, where VEGF plays an important role in the growth of tumors, was rapidly recognized.

siRNA directed against VEGF has shown positive effects in multiple cell culture and animal models of cancer. The cancer cells in which anti-VEGF therapy has shown positive effects include human fibrosarcoma cells, human prostate cancer cells, human gastric cancer cells, cutaneous malignant melanoma cells, human colorectal cancer cells, murine mammary cancer cells, murine squamous cell carcinomas, murine subcutaneous adenocarcinoma tumors, human leukemia cells, human breast cancer cells, human nasopharyngeal cancer cells, human osteosarcoma cells, and murine liver fibrotic cells.[10–29] The exact

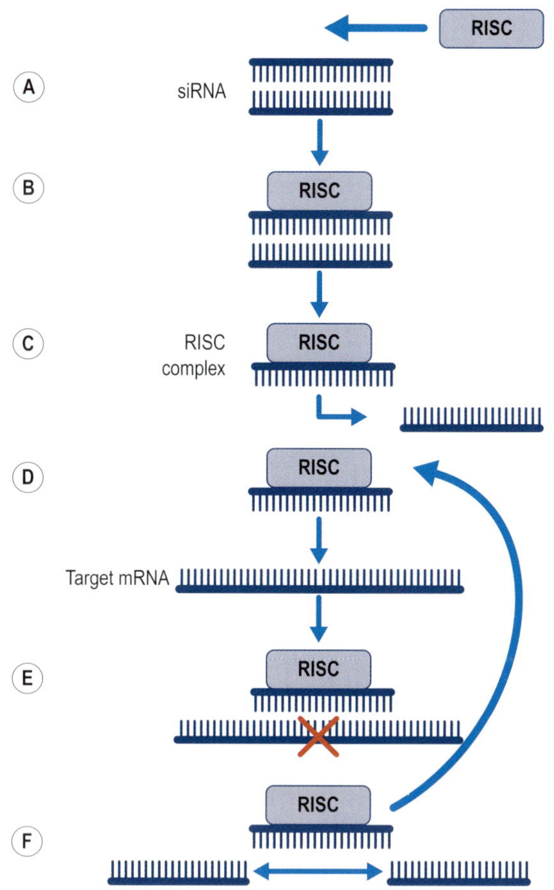

Figure 40.1 (A) Double-stranded small-interference RNAs (siRNAs) are incorporated into a multiprotein endoribonuclease complex (B) termed the RNA-induced silencing complex (RISC). (C) A helicase within the RISC unwinds the duplex siRNA, allowing its antisense strand to bind mRNA with a high degree of sequence complementarity (D). An RNase within RISC then degrades the target mRNA by cleavage (E, F), which results in silenced gene expression and reduced protein. The RISC can then bind with another target mRNA, repeating the process.

mechanism of action for the beneficial effects of siRNAs against VEGF is not known in many of these models, but the studies demonstrate that VEGF inhibition has beneficial effects on a wide variety of tumors.

DRUG USES IN RETINAL DISEASES

BEVASIRANIB FOR SUBFOVEAL CHOROIDAL NEOVASCULARIZATION

RNA interference has also been studied in several animal models of ocular disease. siRNA directed against VEGF was found to inhibit corneal neovascularization.[30–32] siRNA-mediated inhibition of VEGF was also found to decrease tumor growth in a model of retinoblastoma, following subcutaneous delivery.[33]

Bevasiranib is a double-stranded siRNA directed against VEGF and was initially investigated in preclinical studies before progressing to human trials. It was found to inhibit ocular neovascularization in a murine model.[9] It is believed that the siRNA primarily works by silencing VEGF mRNA. Recent work has elucidated another possible mechanism. Kleinman and colleagues demonstrated that CNV inhibition in mice is an siRNA-class effect and is sequence-independent, and that CNV suppression by nontargeted and targeted siRNAs requires activation of Toll-like receptor-3 (TLR3).[34]

Bevasiranib has been investigated in a phase I, open-label, dose escalation study primarily to determine safety and potential dosing. Two injections were given at 6-week intervals, using one of five doses (0.1, 0.33, 1.0, 1.5, 3.0 mg/eye), to 15 eyes. The sample size of 3 eyes per group was too small to make any determination on visual acuity responses. No bevasiranib was detected in the plasma of any patients, suggesting no systemic absorption. Additionally, there were no severe ocular adverse events attributable to the drug. Based on these findings, two phase II trials were initiated. These included the Cand5 Anti-VEGF RNAi Evaluation (CARE) trial for AMD and the RNAi Assessment of Cand5 in diabetic macular Edema (RACE).

BEVASIRANIB FOR NEOVASCULAR MACULAR DEGENERATION: PHASE II STUDY METHODS

The CARE study was a multicenter (28 sites nationwide), randomized, double-masked, placebo-controlled trial of 120 study eyes. Three dose levels of bevasiranib (0.2, 1.5, and 3.0 mg/eye in a 1:1:1 ratio) were administered via intravitreal injection. Two injections of the same dose were given to the study eye, 6 weeks apart. Patients were required to have subfoveal CNV secondary to AMD, which was confirmed by fluorescein angiography, as interpreted by the Digital Angiogram Reading Center (New York, NY). The CARE study was approved by the institutional review board and sponsored by OPKO Health.

The primary inclusion criteria were: (1) patients 50 years of age or greater; (2) the presence of subfoveal classic, predominantly classic, or minimally classic CNV; (3) an Early Treatment Diabetic Retinopathy Study (ETDRS) best corrected visual acuity of 20/50–20/320 (64–24 letters); and (4) subretinal hemorrhage of no more than 50% of the total lesion size with no hemorrhage in the center of the fovea. Minimally classic lesions had to show evidence of lesion activity, defined as the presence of subretinal hemorrhage and/or fluid and/or lipid or loss of one or more lines of visual acuity during the 12 weeks prior to screening visit or fluorescein-documented lesion growth of 10% or greater 12 weeks prior to screening visit.

The exclusion criteria prohibited patients with any of the following characteristics from entering the study: (1) more than two prior intravitreal injections of pegaptanib or administration less than 6 weeks prior to screening visit; (2) more than one prior verteporfin/photodynamic therapy in the study eye or administration less than 12 weeks prior to screening visit; (3) more than one prior intravitreal triamcinolone acetonide treatment or administration less than 24 weeks prior to the screening visit; or (4) periocular steroids less than 24 weeks prior to screening visit. Patients were also excluded if they had other ocular or systemic diseases which could have potentially interfered with the efficacy of bevasiranib or affected the interpretation of study results.

The screening visit was performed within 2 weeks of the initial bevasiranib injection. The intravitreal injection was given at day 0 and patients were examined 3 weeks following injection. An examination and second intravitreal injection of bevasiranib were given at week 6, followed by examinations at weeks 9, 12, 15, 18, 30, 52, and 104. Patients were withdrawn from the study if they withdrew their consent or had intercurrent illness which prevented continuing follow-up visits.

The intravitreal injection consisted of 100 µl bevasiranib (0.2, 1.5, or 3.0 mg/eye) using a 30-gauge needle following sterilization of the eye using iodine scrub and topical antibiotics similar to aseptic techniques used for other intravitreal injections. Bevasiranib was supplied as a colorless solution in vials labeled numerically such that all clinical personnel (refractionist, principal investigator, examining physician, clinical coordinator) were masked to the dose of bevasiranib used. Outcome assessments were made based on refracted ETDRS visual acuity from the refractionist, adverse events from the study coordinator and examining physician, clinical examination data from the examining physician, optical coherence tomography (OCT), and fluorescein angiography.

Rescue therapy was allowed with a treatment approved by the Food and Drug Administration (FDA) for macular degeneration if it was determined that the disease progressed. Initially, verteporfin or pegaptanib was used. Ranibizumab therapy was allowed later in the study once it was FDA-approved. The following criteria indicated disease progression: (1) loss of 6 lines or greater best corrected visual acuity and lesion growth documented by fluorescein angiography less than 12 weeks following the first bevasiranib injection; or (2) loss of 3 lines or greater of best corrected visual acuity and lesion growth documented by fluorescein angiography at 12 weeks or greater following the first bevasiranib injection. Lesion growth was defined for both groups as growth of 300% or more in lesions less than 2 disc areas, 200% or more for lesions of 2–4 disc areas, and 100% or more for lesions greater than 4 disc areas at baseline.

The intent-to-treat population consisted of all subjects who were randomized to a treatment, regardless of whether they received the assigned study drug. The modified intent-to-treat population consisted of all randomized subjects who received at least one dose of intravitreal bevasiranib. The per-protocol population consisted of all randomized subjects who received two intravitreal bevasiranib injections and returned for at least one follow-up efficacy evaluation following the second dose. If subjects missed a study visit, the last observed carried forward (LOCF) was used for missing values. If rescue therapy was initiated, the LOCF for the visit prior to the rescue therapy was carried forward. Results were considered statistically significant if $P < 0.05$.

Positive effects of bevasiranib were defined prior to the initiation of the study by stipulating primary and secondary efficacy endpoints. The primary efficacy endpoint was mean best corrected visual acuity change from baseline to 12-week evaluation for the three dose groups. Another primary efficacy endpoint was the percentage and number of eyes with less than 3 lines decrease in best corrected visual acuity (<15-letter decrease) for each dose group at 12 and 18 weeks posttreatment. Secondary efficacy endpoints were: change in total lesion size; choroidal neovascular membrane size; change in classic component and progression of classic component on fluorescein angiography; change in total lesion thickness (consisting of CNV thickness and pigment epithelial detachment thickness measured by OCT); presence or absence of retinal edema; and presence or absence of other architectural changes such as cysts.

BEVASIRANIB FOR NEOVASCULAR MACULAR DEGENERATION: RESULTS

The intent-to-treat population consisted of 129 eyes, the modified intent-to-treat population consisted of 126 eyes, and the per-protocol analysis consisted of 110 eyes which received both intravitreal bevasiranib injections and at least one follow-up visit. The safety analyses were conducted on the 127 eyes which received at least one bevasiranib injection (one eye was treated with bevasiranib but did not return for required follow-up visits). The efficacy analyses were based on the 110 eyes in the per-protocol analysis. The three groups in the per-protocol analysis were well balanced with respect to visual acuity and lesion type. The numbers of eyes with previous treatment for CNV were also similar between groups. Bevasiranib had an excellent safety profile with no cases of endophthalmitis and only one eye in the 3.0-mg group developed uveitis, which resolved with topical steroids. There were no unexpected systemic adverse events related to the drug and prior pharmacokinetic studies showed no detectable systemic absorption of bevasiranib following intravitreal injection.

The primary efficacy outcomes for change in distance vision are plotted in Figure 40.2. There were no statistically significant differences in visual acuity changes between the three dose groups. The other primary efficacy measure was the number of eyes with <3-line decrease in best corrected visual acuity (Table 40.1).

It is important to recall that bevasiranib blocks the production of VEGF from mRNA, but does not destroy VEGF already produced in the cytoplasm and released into the retina. It became apparent from analysis of this phase II data that treatment of the existing VEGF in the retina prior to injection of bevasiranib using a direct VEGF blocker such as ranibizumab, bevacizumab, or pegaptanib may be important since eyes treated with bevasiranib continued to have decreases in visual acuity, especially following the first intravitreal bevasiranib injection.

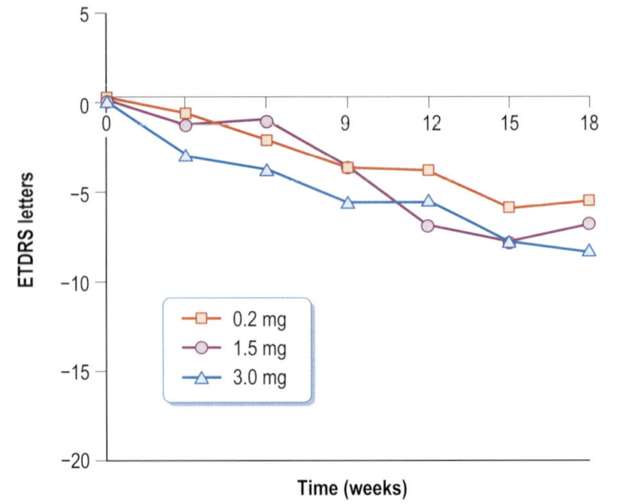

Figure 40.2 The mean distance visual acuity in eyes with choroidal neovascularization declined 1–2 Early Treatment Diabetic Retinopathy Study (ETDRS) lines in all three dose groups after two injections of the small-interference RNA inhibitor bevasiranib at time 0 and 6 weeks, with no statistically significant difference between the three dose groups.

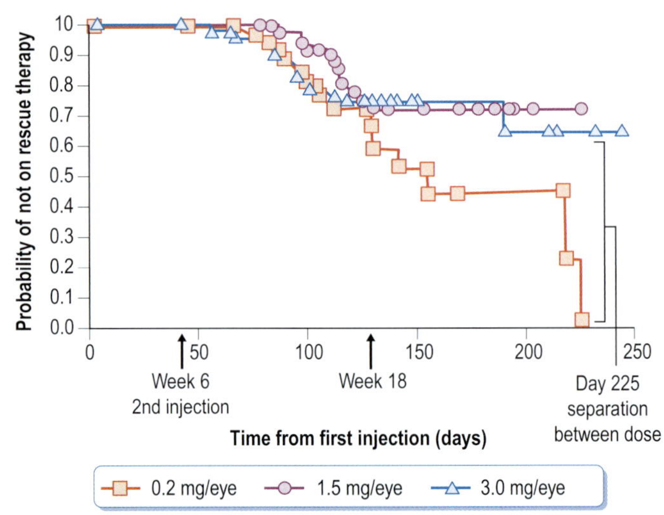

Figure 40.3 The time to rescue therapy which was triggered by vision loss was substantially greater in the higher-dose bevasiranib groups than the lower-dose bevasiranib group, suggesting a longer duration of action at up to 32 weeks following the first bevasiranib injection. This does suggest a dose-related effect of bevasiranib, with higher doses giving more inhibition of vascular endothelial growth factor production.

The time to rescue therapy was shorter (154 days) for eyes treated with the lower-dose (0.2 mg) compared to the higher-dose (1.5 and 3.0 mg) groups, where the median time to rescue therapy was not reached, suggesting that the higher-dose group exhibited more long-term inhibition of CNV (Figure 40.3). This beneficial difference between the higher and lower doses of bevasiranib did not persist when the entire 2-year data set was analyzed.

Bevasiranib was found to be well tolerated with no significant safety concerns up to doses of 3.0 mg/eye at 6-week intervals. The primary endpoints of: (1) mean change in visual acuity; and (2) loss of less than 15 ETDRS letters (3 lines) did not show statistically significant differences between the three groups. There are several explanations for this finding. The first is that the design of the phase II study did not eliminate existing VEGF, which continued to cause vision loss in the early

Table 40.1 Bevasiranib for choroidal neovascularization: distance visual acuity: weeks 3–15 and weeks 3–18				
Best corrected distance visual acuity	**0.2 mg *n* (%)**	**1.5 mg *n* (%)**	**3.0 mg *n* (%)**	**All bevasiranib *n* (%)**
Week 15				
n	34	39	37	110
Acuity gain (≥0 letter gain)	10 (29.4%)	12 (30.8%)	14 (37.8%)	36 (32.7%)
Stable or improved (<15 letters loss)	31 (91.2%)	29 (74.4%)	30 (81.1%)	90 (81.8%)
Week 18				
Acuity gain (≥0 letter gain)	13 (38.2%)	11 (28.2%)	12 (32.4%)	36 (32.7%)
Stable or improved (<15 letters loss)	30 (88.2%)	32 (82.1%)	28 (75.7%)	90 (81.8%)

portions of the study before the biologic effects of bevasiranib could manifest themselves using the study endpoints. Alternatively, the number of bevasiranib injections (2) may have been too small to detect a statistically significant difference. Prior studies with VEGF inhibitors delivered regular intravitreal injections for a minimum of 1 year, rather than two doses 6 weeks apart. Additionally, it is possible that the low-dose group had a biologic effect in inhibiting CNV; consequently, there was no difference between the three groups. Finally, the bevasiranib may not have had any measurable effect on CNV associated with AMD.

A potentially more appropriate study design might be to treat patients initially with direct VEGF inhibitors such as ranibizumab, bevacizumab, or pegaptanib and then to use bevasiranib to help maintain stability of visual acuity and VEGF inhibition. This would eliminate existing VEGF with the potential that bevasiranib would prevent new VEGF from being produced. The phase III Combining Bevasiranib and Lucentis Therapy (COBALT) clinical trial evaluated whether bevasiranib can be used as maintenance therapy for neovascular AMD. In this study, patients were initially treated with three doses of ranibizumab combined with bevasiranib every 8–12 weeks. The study design used ranibizumab to eliminate the VEGF which had already been produced and then used bevasiranib to prevent additional production of VEGF. The control population consisted of eyes treated with ranibizumab every 4 weeks. The Independent Data Safety and Monitoring Committee for the COBALT study recommended termination of the study in early 2009 as the two bevasiranib arms were unlikely to equal the ranibizumab arm in the noninferiority trial study design. There were no significant safety concerns prompting termination of the trial. Details concerning the three treatment arms were not available at the time this manuscript was written.

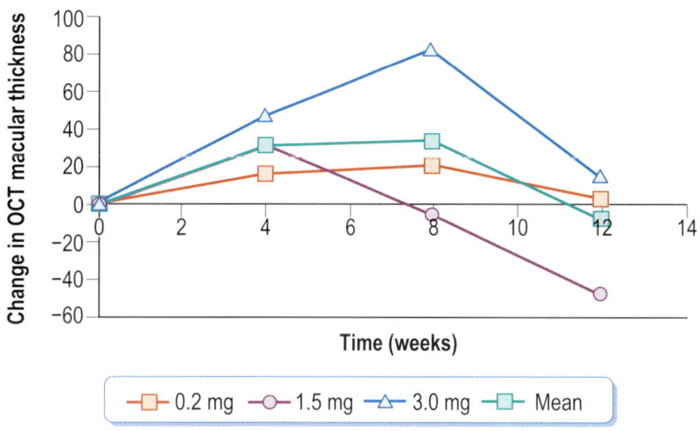

Figure 40.4 Intravitreal bevasiranib was also tested in eyes with diabetic macular edema and only the 1.5-mg treatment group showed a mean decrease in foveal thickness. The differences between groups were not statistically significant. OCT, ocular coherence tomography.

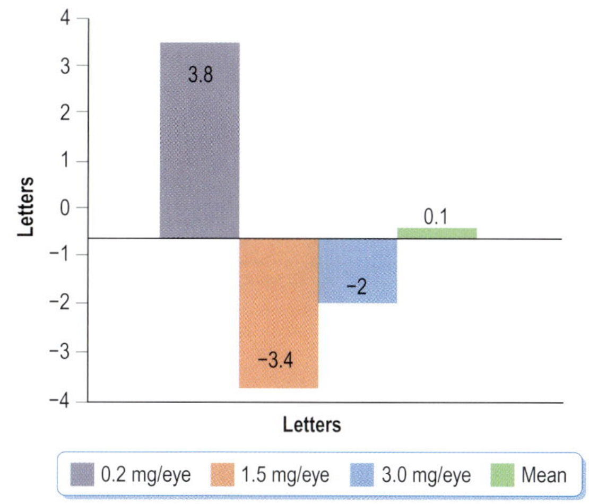

Figure 40.5 The mean visual acuity following bevasiranib for diabetic macular edema showed variable results, with no net change in the mean visual acuity by 12 weeks.

BEVASIRANIB FOR THE TREATMENT OF DIABETIC MACULAR EDEMA (DME)

The RACE trial was a phase II clinical trial which evaluated the short-term treatment of intravitreal bevasiranib for DME. The inclusion criteria consisted of eyes with visual acuities from 20/40 to 20/320 with retinal thickening of 250 μm or greater in the central OCT subfield. Eyes were excluded if patients had panretinal laser or focal laser within 12 weeks of study entry or had any periocular or intravitreal steroids within 6 months. Eyes were given 0.2 mg (18 eyes), 1.5 mg (12 eyes), or 3.0 mg (18 eyes) bevasiranib at baseline, week 4, and week 8. The primary endpoint was mean OCT change at 12 weeks. The modified intent-to-treat population consisted of 18 eyes in the 0.2-mg group, 11 eyes in the 1.5-mg group and 17 eyes in the 3.0-mg group. There was no significant change in OCT at 12 weeks (–8.9 μm) but there was tremendous variability in response, with a mean loss of 548 μm in one eye and a gain of 310 μm in another eye (Figure 40.4). Visual acuity results were parallel, with a mean gain of 0.1 letters (range –39 to + 21 letters; Figure 40.5). There were no significant systemic or ocular safety problems. Iritis was noted in 4/17 eyes in the 3.0-mg group but none of these eyes had vitreous inflammation. The results of this study were likely limited by study design for the same issues identified in the CARE study. The use of bevasiranib in eyes with DME did not eliminate existing VEGF in the retina and vitreous cavity, so any potential effect of the treatment would be delayed until existing VEGF were degraded. Additionally, the injection duration may have been too short to identify a possible latent effect of bevasiranib on DME. At this time, there are no plans to proceed with additional studies to evaluate further the role of bevasiranib in the management of DME. Opko Health is investigating another siRNA compound directed against VEGF which inhibits the angiogenic $VEGFA_{165}$ isoform but does not inhibit the $VEGFA_{165b}$ antiangiogenic isoform. These compounds have not yet progressed to human clinical trials.

SIRNA-027 FOR SUBFOVEAL CHOROIDAL NEOVASCULARIZATION

SIRNA-027 is an siRNA which is directed against VEGF receptor 1 rather than VEGF. It showed promising results in preclinical laboratory studies, reducing CNV in mice.[35] SIRNA-027 was evaluated in a human phase I trial which was an open-label, dose escalation study of a single intravitreal injection of SIRNA-027. The primary objectives were to study the safety and tolerability of intravitreal SIRNA-027 as well as detecting if the drug was systemically absorbed. The primary efficacy endpoints were changes in visual acuity and macular thickness by OCT. Patients were eligible for the study if they were 50 years or older with subfoveal CNV from AMD of 12 disc areas or less. Any subretinal blood or scarring had to occupy less than 50% of the lesion. The retinal thickness on OCT had to be greater than 250 µm. Visual acuity had to be between 20/100 and 20/800 for inclusion. Patients were excluded from the study if CNV was caused by any other ocular or systemic diseases which could interfere with measurements of the efficacy endpoints. Eyes with any standard or experimental therapy for AMD within 3 months of the study were also excluded.

There were 26 eyes divided into five dose groups in the phase I study. The doses of SIRNA-027 varied between 100 and 1600 µg (100, 200, 400, 800, 1200, and 1600 µg). The ocular and systemic safety of SIRNA-027 was excellent, with most ocular problems related to irritation from the intravitreal injection. There were no serious adverse ocular events and no systemic toxicities were noted. The mean change in visual acuity through 12 weeks is summarized in Figure 40.6. Visual acuity improved in all dose groups tested but there was a tendency for visual acuity to regress toward baseline by 12 weeks (there was only one intravitreal injection at time 0). The mean visual acuity for all dose groups combined is summarized in Figure 40.7, which shows that visual acuity increased to a mean improvement of 6.3 letters by 2 weeks following injection. There was a tendency for visual acuity to deteriorate, but the visual acuity had not returned to baseline even by 3 months following injection. Twenty-three percent of eyes gained at least 3 lines or more by 8 weeks following injection and no eyes deteriorated by 3 or more lines. The mean change in foveal thickness by OCT decreased in some groups but not in others, consistent with variability expected in a small sample size of 3–6 eyes per group (Figure 40.8). There was no detectable plasma SIRNA-027, indicating that the drug was not absorbed into the systemic circulation to any measurable degree. Based on the safety data from the phase I study, randomized control studies of SIRNA-027 for neovascular AMD have been conducted by Allergan and Merck. The lack of efficacy and benefits to patients, evaluated through various parameters, has led to discontinuation of further studies with SIRNA-027.

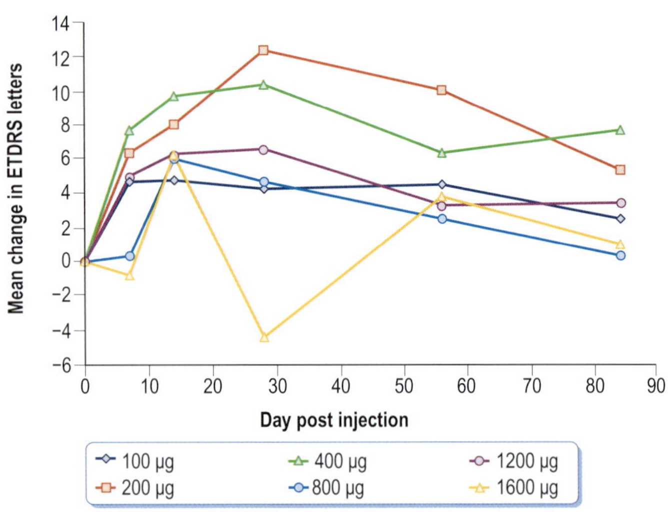

Figure 40.6 SIRNA-027, a small-interference RNA directed against vascular endothelial growth factor receptor 1, showed initial mean visual acuity improvements following one intravitreal injection in a dose-ranging study. Visual acuity improvements tended to decrease toward baseline by 80 days following the single injection. The variability in visual acuity results is not surprising since there were only 3–6 eyes in each dose group.

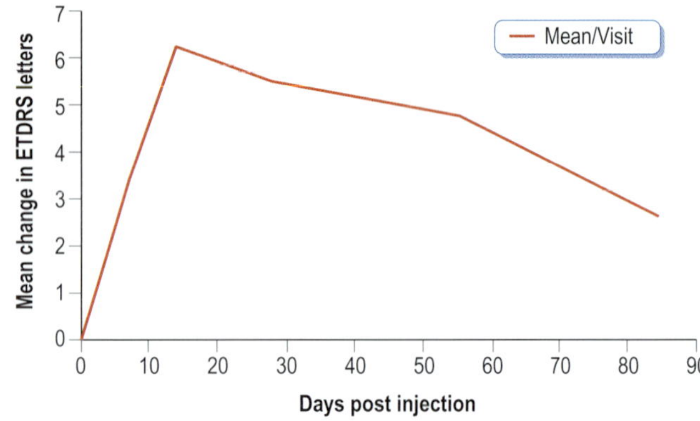

Figure 40.7 The mean visual acuities with SIRNA-027 are plotted, showing the trend toward initial visual acuity improvement by a mean of 6 letters about 2 weeks following injection, followed by decreased vision. There was still a net gain in visual acuity at 80 days.

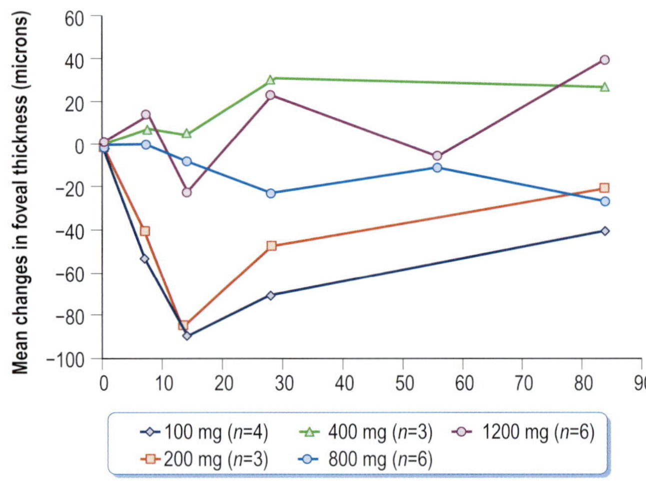

Figure 40.8 Optical coherence tomography measurements of foveal thickness following intravitreal injection of SIRNA-027 also showed decreases in macular thickness with a trend toward increasing thickness by 80 days following a single injection.

REDD14 NP

REDD14NP is an siRNA that acts via RNA interference to inhibit the expression of the hypoxia-inducible gene, RTP801. Expression of the RTP801 gene is dramatically up-regulated in response to hypoxia and/or oxidative stress, which leads to the induction of neuronal cell apoptosis. RTP801 is up-regulated in the retina of mice and rats in a model of retinopathy of prematurity, and RTP801 knockout mice exhibited attenuated pathology.[36] RTP801 knockout mice also exhibited reduced CNV in a laser-induced model of AMD.

In the mouse laser-induced model of AMD, REDD14 was shown to inhibit expression of RTP801 in the retinal pigment epithelium/choroid in a sequence-dependent manner, inhibit neovascularization in a sequence- and dose-dependent manner, inhibit vessel leakage in a sequence- and dose-dependent manner, work in an additive fashion in combination with the antiangiogenic molecules (pegaptanib) and an antimouse VEGF antibody to prevent both neovascularization and vessel leakage, and exhibit anti-inflammatory activity.

The efficacy seen in the mouse model was confirmed in a monkey laser-induced model of AMD.

The data suggest that the different mechanism of action of REDD14NP (i.e., blocking the RTP801 hypoxia/stress pathway) is independent of, and complementary to, the antiangiogenic mechanism of current therapeutic approaches for selected retinal vascular diseases such as neovascular AMD and DME. REDD14NP has also been evaluated in a primate model. Low levels of REDD14NP were detectable in plasma of monkeys up to 22 hours after intravitreal injection (the latest sampling time point), and in the plasma of rabbits up to 6 days after intravitreal injection (the latest sampling time point). The persistence of detectable REDD14NP in plasma likely reflects continued slow egress of the test article from the eye. As such, it attests to the likely persistence of REDD14NP in the eye.

No systemic toxicity or other effects outside the eye were observed with REDD14NP, and there was no indication of any potential for genetic toxicity. Findings in the intravitreal studies that were possibly related to REDD14NP include an increased incidence of cellular infiltration and secondary changes in the eye (e.g., increased intraocular pressure) that occurred at the highest dose level tested in monkeys (i.e., at 3.0 mg/eye); and an increased incidence of hemorrhage that occurred at the highest dose level tested in rats (30 µg/eye). REDD14NP has not been evaluated in human diseases prior to studies in ocular models. Based on the preclinical data demonstrating bioactivity and safety, current clinical trials are being conducted by Pfizer and Quark to evaluate the potential therapeutic role of REDD14NP in neovascular AMD and DME.

SUMMARY AND KEY POINTS

The application of siRNA technology for retinal diseases and other ocular diseases is very early, and the full potential has yet to be determined. The bevasiranib studies have demonstrated safety of intravitreal siRNA in approximately 300 eyes at the time this manuscript was written. SIRNA-027 also appears to be safe based on the smaller study numbers in the phase I trial. The early studies of bevasiranib have also emphasized the importance of eliminating existing target protein before siRNA therapy is initiated, since blocking the synthesis of the target protein does not eliminate existing target protein. Target protein may be degraded at variable rates and can continue to produce damage before the siRNA has a chance to have any biologic effect.

siRNA can be targeted against proteins such as VEGF that contribute to retinal diseases such as CNV and DME. siRNA directed against VEGF and VEGF receptor appear to be well tolerated as intravitreal injections and no systemic absorption or toxicity has been identified to date. In preclinical and phase I studies, bevasiranib and SIRNA-027 showed a possible biologic effect on CNV, but the phase III studies have not confirmed such results. REDD14NP is being evaluated without any definitive results at this time. A detailed analysis of the bevasiranib and SIRNA-027 clinical trial data will help to elucidate why these compounds were not as effective in inhibiting CNV as ranibizumab.

The potential use of siRNAs to treat ocular diseases is exciting, as many conditions are caused by protein overproduction in the eye, and the use of siRNA in human trials to treat ocular diseases will help to clarify the role of mRNA and proteins in causing retinal disease. However, the failure of two siRNA molecules, bevasiranib and SIRNA, to demonstrate efficacy in neovascular AMD, in the era of anti-VEGF therapy, suggests that there are challenges such as targeted delivery of the siRNA molecule that must be overcome before one can consider siRNA in the therapeutic arena for retinal vascular diseases. Further preclinical and clinical studies are needed to define better all the potential uses of siRNA to treat ocular diseases.

ACKNOWLEDGMENT

We wish to thank Sam Reich and his colleagues from OPKO Health, for providing the bevasiranib macular degeneration data, Jonathan Prenner, MD for providing the bevasiranib diabetic macular edema data, and Tuyen Ong, MD and his colleagues at Pfizer for providing information on REDD 14NP, for this chapter prior to the studies' publications.

REFERENCES

1. Fire A, Xu S, Montgomery MK, et al. Potent and specific genetic interference by double-stranded RNA in *Caenorhabditis elegans*. Nature 1998;391:806–811.
2. Gottlieb JL. Age-related macular degeneration. JAMA 2002;288:2233–2236.
3. Klein R, Klein BF, Tomany SC, et al. Ten-year incidence and progression of age-related maculopathy: the Beaver Dam Eye Study. Ophthalmology 2002;109:1767–1779.
4. Gragoudas ES, Adamis AP, Cunningham ET Jr, et al. Pegaptanib for neovascular age-related macular degeneration. N Engl J Med 2004;351: 2805–2816.
5. Heier JS, Antoszyk, AN, Pavan PR, et al. Ranibizumab for treatment of neovascular age-related macular degeneration: a phase I/II multicenter, controlled multidose study. Ophthalmology 2006;113:633–642.
6. Rosenfeld PJ, Brown DM, Heier JS, et al. Ranibizumab for neovascular age-related macular degeneration. N Engl J Med 2006;355:1419–1431.
7. Brown DM, Kaiser PK, Michels M, et al. Ranibizumab versus verteporfin for neovascular age-related macular degeneration. N Engl J Med 2006;355:1432–1444.
8. Rosenfeld PJ, Moshfeghi AA, Puliafito CA. Optical coherence tomography findings after an intravitreal injection of bevacizumab (Avastin) for neovascular age-related macular degeneration. Ophthalmic Surg Lasers Imaging 2005:36:270–271.
9. Reich SJ. Small interfering RNA (siRNA) targeting VEGF effectively inhibits ocular neovascularization in a mouse model. Mol Vis 2003;9:210–216.
10. Filleur S, Courtin A. Ait-Si-Ali S, et al. SiRNA-mediated inhibition of vascular endothelial growth factor severely limits tumore resistance to angiangiogenic thrombospondin-1 and slows tumor vascularization and growth. Cancer Res 2003:63:3919–3922.
11. Takei Y, Kadomatsu K, Yuzawa Y, et al. A small interfering RNA targeting vascular endothelial growth factor as cancer therapeutics. Cancer Res 2004;64:3365–3370.
12. Meng F, Ding J, Liu N, et al. Inhibition of gastric cancer angiogenesis by vector-based RNA interference for Raf-1. Cancer Biol Ther 2005;4:113–117.
13. Detwiller KY, Fernando NT, Segal NH, et al. Analysis of hypoxia-related gene expression in sarcomas and effect of hypoxia on RNA interference of vascular endothelial cell growth factor A. Cancer Res 2005;65:5881–5889.
14. Tao J, Tu YT, Huang CZ, et al. Inhibiting the growth of malignant melanoma by blocking the expression of vascular endothelial growth factor using an RNA interference approach. Br J Dermatol 2005;153:715–724.
15. Chen Z, Varney ML, Backora MW, et al. Down-regulation of vascular endothelial cell growth factor-C expression using small interfering RNA vectors in mammary tumors inhibits tumor lymphangiogenesis and spontaneous metastasis and enhances survival. Cancer Res 2005:65: 9004–9011.
16. Mulkeen AL, Silva T, Yoo PS, et al. Short interfering RNA-medicated gene silencing of vascular endothelial growth factor: effects on cellular proliferation in colon cancer cells. Arch Surg 2006;141:367–374.
17. Matsumoto G, Kushibiki T, Knoshita Y, et al. Cationized gelatin delivery of a plasmid DNA expressing small interference RNA for VEGF inhibits murine squamous cell carcinoma. Cancer Sci 2006;97:313–321.
18. Kim WJ, Christensen LV, Jo S, et al. Cholesteryl oligoarginine delivering vascular endothelial growth factor siRNA effectively inhibits tumor growth in colon carcinoma. Mol Ther 2006;14:343–350.
19. Kim SH, Jeong JH, Lee SH, et al. PEG conjugated VEGF siRNA for anti-angiogenic gene therapy. J Control Release 2006;116:123–129.
20. Shen HL, Xu W, Wu ZY, et al. Vector-based RNAi approach to isoform-specific downregulation of vascular endothelial growth factor (VEGF) 165 expression in human leukemia cells. Leuk Res 2007:31:515–521.
21. Xu WH, Ge YL, Li Q, et al. Inhibitory effect of vascular endothelial growth factors-targeted small interfering RNA on proliferation of gastric cancer cells. World J Gastroenterol 2007;13:2044–2047.
22. Sun P, Gao J, Lin YL, et al. RNA interference (RNAi)-mediated vascular endothelial growth factor-C (VEGF-C) reduction interferes with lymphangiogenesis and enhances Epirubicin sensitivity of breast cancer cells. Mol Cell Biochem 2008;308:161–168.
23. Ly W, Zhang C, Zhou DH, et al. RNAi-mediated gene silencing of vascular endothelial growth factor inhibits growth of colorectal cancer. Cancer Biother Radiopharm 2007;22:841–852.
24. He XW, Lui T, Chen YX, et al. Calcium carbonate nanoparticle delivering vascular endothelial growth factor-C siRNA effectively inhibits

lymphangiogenesis and growth of gastric cancer *in vivo*. Cancer Gene Ther 2008:15:193–202.
25. Chen S, Gao G, Chen W, et al. VEGF-specific siRNAs modified with 2′-deoxy effectively suppress VEGF expression and inhibit growth of nasopharyngeal carcinoma xenograft in a mouse model. Sci China C Life Sci 2008:51:104–110.
26. He XW, Yu X, Liu T, et al. Vector-based RNA interference against vascular endothelial growth factor-C inhibits tumor lymphangiogenesis and growth of colorectal cancer *in vivo* in mice. Chin Med J 2008:121:439–444.
27. Li SD, Chono S, Huang L. Efficient oncogene silencing and metastasis inhibition via systemic delivery of siRNA. Mol Ther 2008:16:942–946.
28. Wang S, Liu H, Ren L, et al. Inhibiting colorectal carcinoma growth and metastasis by blocking the expression of VEGF using RNA interference. Neoplasia 2008;10:399–407.
29. Mei J, Gao Y, Zhang L, et al. VEGF-siRNA silencing induces apoptosis, inhibits proliferation and suppresses vasculogecic micicry in osteosarcoma *in vitro*. Exp Oncol 2008;30:29–34.
30. Kim B, Tang O, Biswas PS, et al. Inhibition of ocular angiogenesis by siRNA targeting vascular endothelial growth factor pathway genes: therapeutic strategy for herpetic stromal keratitis. Am J Pathol 2004:165:2177–2185.
31. Murata M, Takanami T, Shimizu S, et al. Inhibition of ocular angiogenesis by diced small interfering RNAs (siRNAs) specific to vascular endothelial growth factor (VEGF). Curr Eye Res 2006;31:171–180.
32. Singh N, Higgins E, Amin S, et al. Unique homogous siRNA blocks hypoxia-induced VEGF upregulation in human corneal cells and inhibits and regresses murine corneal neovascularization. Cornea 2007;26:65–72.
33. Jia RB, Zhang P, Zhou YX, et al. VEGF-targeted RNA interference suppresses angiogenesis and tumor growth of retinoblastoma. Ophthalmic Res 2007;39:108–115.
34. Kleinman ME, Yamada K, Tadeda A, et al. Sequence- and target-independent angiogenesis suppression by siRNA via TLR3. Nature 2008:45:543–545.
35. Shen J, Samui R, Silva RL, et al. Suppression of ocular neovascularization with siRNA targeting VEGF receptor 1. Gene Ther 2006;13:225–234.
36. Brafman A, Mett I, Shafi M, et al. Inhibition of oxygen-induced retinopathy in RTP801-deficient mice. Invest Ophthalmol Vis Sci 2004; 45:3796–3805.

CHAPTER

41 Ocular gene therapy

Trevor J. McFarland, BS and J. Timothy Stout, MD, PhD, MBA

KEY FEATURES

Gene therapy involves the therapeutic alteration of gene expression to correct an inborn or acquired error, or to modify pathologic cellular behavior. There are two main classes of gene therapy – germline and somatic. Various types of viral vectors are employed in gene therapy. Current diseases being evaluated for therapy include malignancy, inherited retinal disorders, and retinal vascular diseases such as neovascular macular degeneration.

INTRODUCTION TO GENE THERAPY

Germline gene therapy is the replacement of genes in which an offspring would inherit a new trait. This type of gene modification is still in the early stages of human medical intervention but examples do exist, such as in cows modified to have elevated levels of milk production or the capability to secrete human hormones, or "knockin" and "knockout" mouse models, used for decades to elucidate gene function. The second, currently more medically viable and potentially less controversial, is somatic gene therapy. Somatic gene therapy is the introduction of genetic material directly into the body after development. There are three categories of somatic gene transfer: *in vivo*, *in situ*, and ex vivo. *In vivo* is the introduction of genes directly to the body via the blood stream; for example, *in situ* involves targeting a specific organ for gene transfer, such as the eye. By contrast, in ex vivo gene transfer a particular class of cells are removed from a patient, modified, and then replaced back into the patient in order to treat an abnormality or regain a particular function.

The notion of gene therapy arose in the 1960s, and with the advent of stable cell lines and advancing techniques of DNA isolation and manipulation, that idea became more of a reality. Early techniques involved primarily the use of bacteria, such as *Escherichia coli*, and utilized the fact that their genomes are comprised of circular DNA which can be shared with other bacteria in a process known as conjugation. This type of gene transfer is what gives bacteria the ability to share resistance genes among colonies. Microbial molecular biology soon gave rise to advances in techniques such as gene cloning and circular plasmid DNA construction. These techniques offered insights into microbial genetics and in addition led scientists to ponder whether these concepts could be applied to human maladies.

One of the first human diseases to be investigated for gene therapy was the hypoxanthine guanine phosphoribosyl transferase (HPRT) deficiency associated with Lesch–Nyhan syndrome. Researchers studying this disease were able to demonstrate that exogenous DNA was capable of uptake and expression into mammalian cells. Unfortunately, the methods available at the time were unable to produce stable expression efficiently in these cells.[1] It was not until the late 1960s through early 1970s that more viable methods came into development. A major discovery arose when researchers were able to elucidate key events in the ability of polyomavirus to transform cells, integrate, and stably express their DNA.[2–4] This, in addition to chemical transformation methods (i.e., calcium phosphate), enhanced researchers' ability to insert genes into cells.[5] It was at this point that the proof of principle was illustrated with stable introduction of the bacterial HPRT gene analog into deficient mammalian cells.[6] It was also during this period that it was postulated, based on the insight gained regarding polyomaviruses, that it may be possible to manipulate other viruses; amid a genetic revolution this gave way a decade later to the development of retroviral vectors and then to several other viral-mediated gene transfer techniques, several of which are used today and are currently the mainstay of gene therapy applications.

CURRENT VIRAL VECTORS

The viral vectors predominantly in use today fall into two categories: DNA viral-based and RNA viral-based. Each group has various attributes contributing to advantages or disadvantages depending on the desired therapeutic outcome. The two most commonly utilized DNA viruses are the adenovirus and the adeno-associated virus (AAV). The use of adenoviruses for gene transfer purposes was first demonstrated in 1985, by transducing human cells with thymidine kinase (TK) gene.[7] Since then, their application has been documented in numerous gene therapy protocols. Wild-type adenovirus is classified as a nonenveloped iscosahedral viral particle with an average size of 80 nm. Housed within the viral capsid or protein shell is a 36-kb double-stranded DNA genome. Viral replication consists of a two-phase event termed early and late phase. During the early phase, the viral proteins expressed take control of cell cycle machinery, aid in evading immune response signaling, and initiate viral replication. The late-phase viral protein production is associated with viral assembly and packaging, at which point particle buildup and cell lysis occur. Recombinant adenoviral vectors are engineered to be replication-deficient by the removal of the early-phase expressing genes. By manipulating the native viral genome to consist only of *cis*-acting elements such as inverted terminal repeats (ITRs), these vectors are considered to be "gutless" (Figure 41.1). This requires that their assembly be performed in a helper-dependent manner. This is facilitated *in trans* with the use of either co-transfection techniques or packaging cell lines, which provide the key structural components required for full viral particle assembly. Adenoviral vectors are capable of harboring large transgene inserts, can infect cells independent of cell cycle stage, an important consideration of ocular gene therapy due to the G0 state of the eye, and offer a high degree of transgene expression. The main drawback for the use of adenoviral vectors is that in some cases severe immune-mediated responses have been observed. This, and the fact that adenoviruses lack the capability to integrate, makes their transgene expression very transient, usually persisting for 10–50 days on average.

The second class of DNA viral vectors is AAV. The use of AAV for gene transfer has rapidly grown within the last decade and is considered by many to be one of the safest viral-based gene transfer methods available. AAV particles are small single-stranded DNA viruses composed of a 4.7-kb genome. These icosahedral-shaped virions range in size from 20 to 25 nm. Their genome consists of two open reading frames, which code for the Rep and Cap genes, with ITRs on each side of the genome. The Rep genes code for replication-dependent proteins

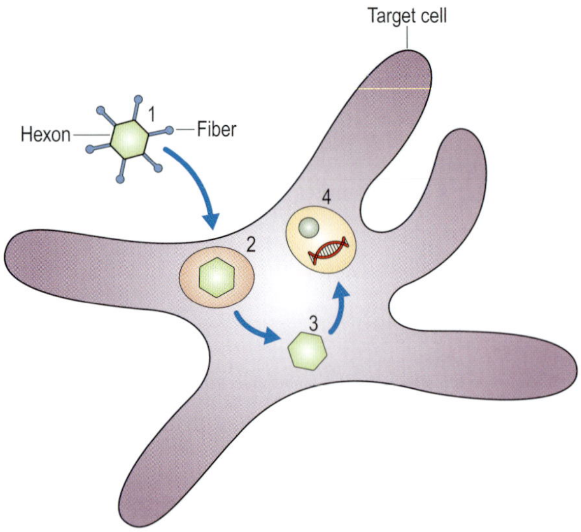

Figure 41.1 Adenoviral vector. 1, Attachment; 2, endosome-mediated entry; 3, capsid breakdown; 4, entry of DNA into the nucleus.

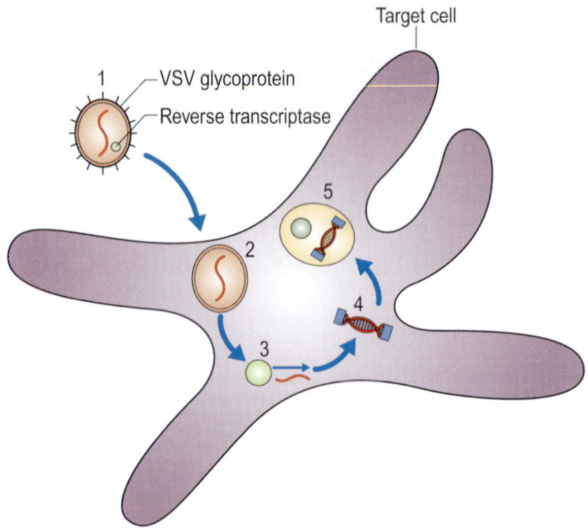

Figure 41.3 Lentiviral vector. 1, Viral attachment and entry; 2, partial uncoating; 3, reverse transcription; 4, double-stranded DNA (dsDNA) with long terminal repeats; 5, genomic integration and expression. VSV, vesicular stomatitis virus.

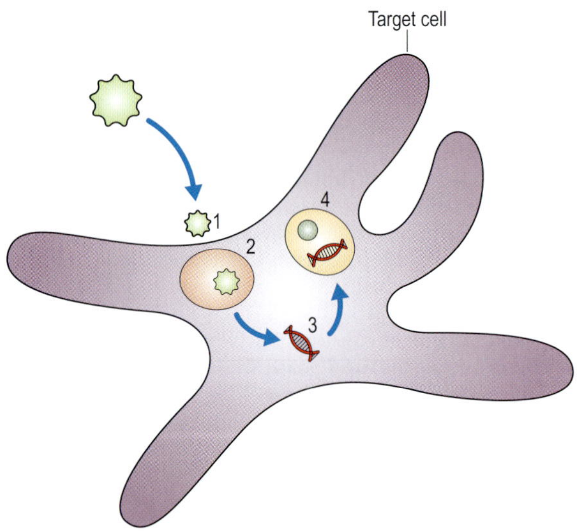

Figure 41.2 Adeno-associated vector. 1, Viral attachment; 2, endosomal-mediated entry; 3, DNA release and translocation to the nucleus; 4, either integrated or episomal gene expression.

and have been shown to be involved in site-specific integration and various cell-specific promoter regulation. The Cap genes code for structural proteins such as the capsid. Similarly to adenovirus, AAV vectors are produced by recombinant methods and are considered to be "gutless," only retaining the ITRs. Modified Rep and Cap genes are supplied *in trans* via co-transfection methods. Wild-type AAV virus is considered to be benign in human cells and thus offers a relatively safe approach to gene transfer. The fact that they are considered to be integrative, although most evidence points to recombinant vectors as being episomal in the nucleus,[8] affords long-term transgene expression. The capability to infect both dividing and nondividing cells makes them an attractive therapeutic vehicle (Figure 41.2). The greatest drawback to their use has been the very small transgene-carrying capacity, with only an insert size of approximately 6 kb, which makes gene selection limited. This, in conjunction with the difficulty producing high titers, makes their use somewhat selective.

RNA viral-based vectors derived namely from retroviruses such as the Moloney murine leukemia virus and the Rous sarcoma virus were first utilized in the 1980s and their efficacy was demonstrated for use by going back to the HPRT-deficiency model, among others.[9–12] These vectors offered the capability of integration but were only proficient at infecting actively dividing cells. It was not until acquired immunodeficiency syndrome (AIDS) research and, more specifically, the study of lentiviruses, that RNA-based viral vectors offered a more viable option for gene transfer, especially for ocular tissue. Human immunodeficiency virus-1 (HIV-1) lentiviral-based vectors offered many advantages to other retroviruses due to the ability to produce high-titer preps, integrative capability, wider cell tropism, and easy purification procedures.

Lentiviruses are large enveloped particles averaging 100 nm in size and are composed of single-stranded RNA genomes 9.2 kb in length. The envelope consists of host cell membrane protein with viral-mediated glycoproteins, which afford it the ability to attach and enter target cells. The viral genome consists of three core proteins: GAG, POL, and ENV. The GAG gene is responsible for the structural matrix, the POL gene codes for a reverse transcriptase enzyme, and the ENV gene provides all of the glycoprotein components. In addition to the core proteins, several accessory proteins involved with replication and viral RNA processing are present. Once the Lentivirus has entered the cell, it is uncoated; the genome is reverse-transcribed into double-stranded DNA, after which it is shuttled to the nucleus for genomic integration. Modern lentiviral vectors are produced to be nonreplicative and are regarded as self-inactivating. This is achieved by deletions to the 3′ long terminal repeat, where the native viral promoters reside. Also, recombinant lentiviral vectors replace the ENV gene with the vesicular stomatitis virus (VSV) gene in order to afford the vector a wider cellular tropism (Figure 41.3). Recently, several modifications have been made to lentiviral vectors – most importantly, the addition of a central polypurine tract and introduction of the woodchuck hepatitis virus post-transcriptional regulatory element. These changes have made transgene nuclear import and expression more robust in targeted cells.[13,14] The fact that lentiviral vectors are integrative makes them highly desirable for gene transfer yet coincidently makes their use a potential risk. Integration allows transgene expression to persist and has been demonstrated for periods greater than 16 months.[15] The drawback is that the site of integration appears to be nonspecific and may vary depending on the cell type in question. Insertion of a transgene into the middle of a native gene could provide deleterious outcomes.

VIRAL VECTOR-ASSOCIATED RISKS

Safety and ethical concerns have always been associated with gene therapy. The potential risks associated with recombinant DNA research prompted the organization of the Asilomar conference of 1975, in which Paul Berg and colleagues laid down the foundation for biosafety with regard to this field of science.[16] A few years later, the National Institutes of Health (NIH) developed guidelines for the use of gene therapy in human subjects. These guidelines later led to the formation of various committees, such as the Recombinant DNA Advisory Committee, in charge of ensuring proper ethics and provisions for human safety. Several events warranted action towards the formation of these committees. One of the earliest experiments to raise public attention was the action by Dr. Martin Cline of UCLA in 1980. In an effort to treat two individuals with the condition beta-thalassemia, a rare hemoglobin disorder, Cline disregarded university internal review and performed the experiments overseas. As a result, he faced harsh criticism by multiple groups, was stripped of all NIH funding and was banned from performing any recombinant DNA experiments.[17,18]

Probably the most notable and publicised complications involved two human clinical trials: one for the treatment of severe combined immunodeficiency (SCID), the other involving a patient being treated for ornithine transcarbamylase (OTC) deficiency. SCID, also referred to as "bubble boy disease," was of interest to gene therapy pioneers as they recognized this disease as a prime candidate for a gene replacement strategy. Since SCID patients lack the T-cell enzyme adenosine deaminase (ADA), a protein crucial to the immune response, replacement of a functional ADA gene was felt likely to be curative.[19] Despite encouraging early results, some patients treated with ADA gene-containing retroviruses developed leukemia. It was later discovered that the integrative viral vector had positioned the ADA gene proximal to a "tumor suppressor" region of the genome in some cells, thus immortalizing those cells.[20] Thus, at least some of the dangers associated with retroviral integration were made clear.

A second complication arose in 1995 when a patient with OTC deficiency was treated with adenoviral particles containing a functional copy of the human OTC gene. OTC deficiency results in an inability to break down ammonia byproducts in the blood formed during protein synthesis. One patient who received a large dose of adenoviral OTC developed an overwhelming immune response and died.[21] This tragedy resulted in an immediate temporary suspension of adenoviral use for gene therapy by the NIH. It also triggered the development of stricter guidelines for gene therapy usage in human subjects.[22]

VIRAL VERSUS NONVIRAL VECTORS

Although viral gene therapy vectors offer the greatest degree of sustained therapeutic gene expression seen to date, several other nonviral gene transfer modalities exist. These consist of two main categories: chemical and physical gene transfer. Chemical gene transfer often employs the use of lipid or polymer-based vehicles to transport DNA to cells where transient expression in these cells is possible. The lipid-based vehicles, or more specifically cationic liposomes, are formed when aqueous plasmid DNA is mixed with hydrophobic phospholipids, similar to eukaryotic cell membranes, to form micelle-like structures with the DNA of interest packaged internally. Cationic polymers are formed from either natural or synthetic small-molecular-weight peptides covalently bound to create complex branching structures. Various chemical functional groups lend charge and physical characteristics enveloping the DNA and thus producing a reliable vector delivery vehicle. Access to the intercellular space is achieved by liposomal or polymer cell fusion and is internalized by endocytosis. Once intercellular, these vehicles are packaged into an endosome where the plasmid DNA is liberated, shuttled to the nucleus, and transcribed. Once transcribed, the message is processed in the cytoplasm and translated to protein as usual.

The second class of nonviral gene transfer involves the physical insertion of DNA into cells. This is achieved by a variety of means, with the end result being the cellular uptake of naked plasmid DNA. The simplest means to this end is by direct injection of DNA systemically, normally via the blood stream, where uptake is somewhat arbitrary but is usually confined to the lymphatic system. Other methods can rely on the delivery of DNA via high-pressure application of either air or fluid. A "bioballistic" approach employs gold nanoparticles that surround the DNA and are shot into an organ or tissue by high air pressure. An analogous approach, termed hydroporation, uses high-pressure fluid, similar to physiological blood pressure, delivered to the site of interest. Although these approaches have demonstrated efficacy, their use for ocular gene therapy is likely limited. Other physical methods of gene transfer exist; these include electroporation, magnetofection, and ultrasound. Electroporation is the use of finely tuned micropulses of electricity which create small pores in a cell's membrane and aid in the absorption of DNA. This method has been demonstrated to achieve efficient and rapid import of DNA into the nuclear region and is a routine choice for *in vitro* gene transfer.[23] Magnetofection is dependent upon magnetic nanoparticles which complex with DNA; these mixtures are then guided by strong magnetic fields to the area of interest. DNA uptake is far greater via this method compared to naked DNA injection alone,[24] yet the implications of long-term exposure to these magnetic particle *in vivo* are not fully understood. Finally, ultrasound is an alternative to increasing cellular permeability. This method has been shown to increase DNA uptake severalfold and appears to be a relatively safe approach. The fact that ultrasound is routinely used for diagnostic imaging by ophthalmologists makes its potential use for gene transfer attractive.

Nonviral gene therapy techniques are intriguing for several reasons. They offer a relatively safe approach to the introduction of foreign DNA to various cell types and can usually be delivered to a specific tissue type. Their application is relatively noninvasive; therefore patient discomfort can be easily managed. The main disadvantage for their use is threefold. First, the expression of the therapeutic gene is completely transient and ranges from a few hours to a few days. Second, the amount of gene product produced via these methods is not uniform. Some techniques are only capable of delivering relatively small amounts of DNA, resulting in the potential of an insufficient dosage. The third disadvantage is the fact that nontargeted cells may also be transfected, which could result in undesired gene expression in bystander cells (Table 41.1).

STRATEGIES FOR RECESSIVE VERSUS DOMINANT DISEASE

The strategies for the treatment of recessive and dominant diseases vary greatly and are constantly evolving. In recessive disease conditions, the underlying pathology is often due to a defect or mutation in both copies of a single gene. The parents of affected individuals are usually phenotypically normal and are heterozygous for disease alleles. Only when their offspring inherit both copies of the abnormal alleles are phenotypic ramifications evident. Some of the most recognizable diseases affecting individuals worldwide are recessive in nature and include cystic fibrosis, hemophilia, albinism, and phenylketonuria. Numerous recessive diseases are theorized to be highly correctable by gene therapy applications. The basic notion is that the insertion of a nonmutated gene copy into appropriate cells or tissue could lead to therapeutic phenotype rescue. One disease that has shown great promise and success, especially from an ophthalmic point of view, has been the genetic treatment of Leber's congenital amaurosis (LCA) in the Briard dog model and recently in human patients. Replacement of the RPE65 gene by an AAV vector to affected animals has been shown repeatedly to restore vision to a state similar to that of control animals.[25] This treatment has displayed such promise that it is currently being tested in multiple multicenter phase I clinical trials.

Dominant disease usually results when one gene allele is mutated and this change is sufficient to cause disease. This can occur because

Table 41.1 Nonviral gene transfer methods

Method	Pros	Cons
Naked DNA	Simple, easy to prepare, pure DNA is nonimmunogenic	Nonspecific transfection, is rapidly cleared from the body, expression is short-term
Cationic liposomes and polymers	Readily available, fair transfection rates, DNA degradation is diminished	Transient expression, use may be limited by cytotoxicity
Bioballistic	Efficient and easy localized delivery	Shear forces and invasiveness unsuitable for some tissues, gold nanoparticles required
Hydroporation	Efficient and easy localized delivery	Low transfection rate, shear force and invasiveness issues
Electroporation	High transfection rate	Transient gene expression, tissue-specific delivery difficult
Magnetoporation	High transfection rate, efficient cellular delivery	Potential long-term metal exposure hazard
Ultrasound	Safe, high transfection rate	Transient gene expression

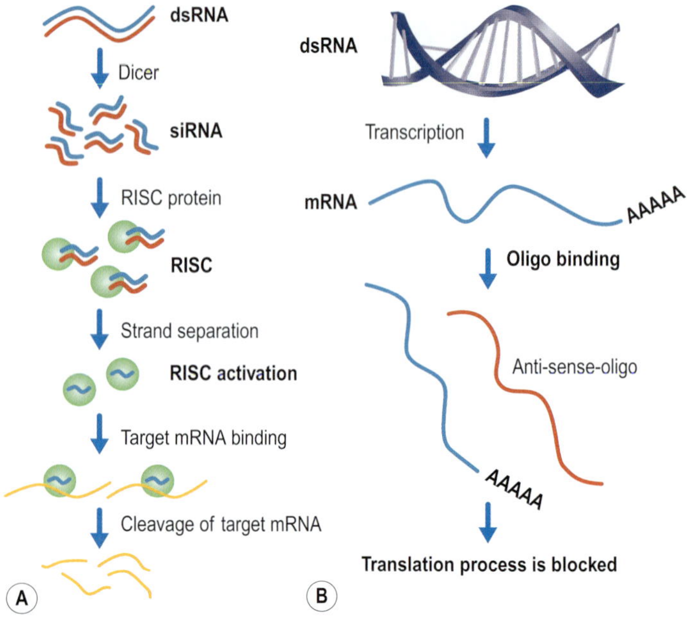

Figure 41.4 Small interfering RNA (siRNA) and antisense therapy. (A) The double-stranded RNA (dsRNA) is introduced into a cell and is cleaved by the dicer enzyme. The fragments are incorporated into the RNA-induced silencing (RISC) complex, binding to a specific complementary messenger RNA (mRNA) sequence. This results in the catalytic cleavage and inactivation of the target mRNA. (B) A specific transcribed mRNA can be inactivated by the introduction of a complementary oligomer that binds to the mRNA, thus inhibiting translation and protein maturation.

a single normal allele is insufficient to maintain health (haploinsufficiency) or because of a deleterious effect of the mutated allele. Usually, if an individual is homozygous for a dominant disorder, the condition is more severe and may be incompatible with life, as is seen in double-dominant achondroplasia. Options for the treatment of these types of inherited diseases is by silencing the mutant transcripts (to prevent translation of the mutant protein) or to silence the mutant protein itself.

Gene silencing is most commonly achieved by one of two methods: RNA interference (RNAi) and antisense therapy. The use of RNAi or small interfering RNA (siRNA) molecules has gained increasing popularity in recent years. The basic principle is simple: double-stranded RNA is produced in the cell, usually facilitated by a viral vector, which is then cleaved into small 21–25 basepair fragments by an enzyme complex known as "dicer." These fragments are then incorporated into the RNA-induced silencing complex (RISC), the complementary complexes bind to a target mRNA at a specific location, and catalytic cleavage of that mRNA is initiated. The end result is the cleavage of the mutant mRNA and thus a failure to produce the defective protein (Figure 41.4). Antisense oligomer therapy works in a similar fashion: small oligos, either DNA or RNA that are complementary to a specific sequence of a target mRNA, are introduced to a cell. These oligos then hybridize to and inactivate the mRNA. These strategies have shown promise, especially in combination with "healthy" gene transfer techniques. One example of this was demonstrated in a murine model for the potential treatment of retinitis pigmentosa.[26] Researchers using siRNA effectively silenced mutant rhodopsin transcripts and simultaneously used a viral vector to introduce wild-type transgenes. The normal transcripts used third-basepair codon wobble in order to evade the siRNAs. This resulted in the elimination of mutant rhodopsin and reintroduction of functional, wild-type transcripts. Due to the complexity of dominant disease, these therapies are still novel and poorly understood. There are potential pitfalls for the use of siRNA and oligos for the treatment of disease and these will need to be elucidated before this type of therapy will be clinically deployed.

STRATEGIES FOR PROLIFERATIVE AND NEOPLASTIC OCULAR DISEASE

Proliferative etiologies account for a large proportion of blinding diseases. Diseases such as age-related macular degeneration (AMD), proliferative diabetic retinopathy, retinopathy of prematurity, posterior capsule opacification, and a myriad of others share an uncontrolled cellular proliferation in pathophysiology. Intense scientific research of cellular signaling pathways has been able to produce numerous targets for gene therapy intervention. One strategy for the treatment of these types of diseases has been through the overproduction of certain factors which cause a shift in the balance to a nonproliferative state. With regard to ocular neovascular diseases such as wet AMD, the majority of treatments have focused on the vascular endothelial growth factor (VEGF) pathway. Current therapies concentrate on inactivating the VEGF protein either by down-regulation or by deactivation by binding the protein before it can activate a cell signaling pathway, and have resulted in a variety of anti-VEGF drugs, although there seems to be variable efficacy among drugs.[27] Gene therapy approaches that involve a variety of VEGF-binding proteins, such as soluble VEGF receptors such as sFLT-1 and sFLK-1, are being studied.[28] Soluble receptors bind extracellular VEGF before it has a chance to interact with these same receptors, which are membrane-bound. Other proteins, like pigment epithelial-derived factor (PEDF), a neuroprotective and antiangiogenic protein, have been shown to blunt the VEGF effect and have been evaluated for use in human clinical trials. A more novel approach which is in development is through the use of transcription factors which regulate gene expression at the DNA promoter level.[29] Genetic modulation at a pretranscriptional level could lead to the treatment of a wide variety of conditions in addition to proliferative ocular disease.

Neoplastic disease and other cancers of the eye, such as retinoblastoma and melanoma, are serious sight- and life-threatening disorders. Given the life-threatening consequences of these diseases, the development of effective treatments that do not require the surgical removal of the eye seems warranted. Current treatment modalities for ocular cancer involve surgery, radiation, chemotherapy, thermochemotherapy, immunotherapy, and photodynamic therapy. The success of these strategies is mixed and depends on the stage and type of cancer in question. These treatments are destructive and often come with severe side-effects. Gene therapy may lead to treatments which effectively target and neutralize malignant cells while preserving ocular function. Two promising strategies employ use of apoptotic-inducing molecules or nonnative suicide genes. Genes that induce apoptosis, such as p53, Bax, and caspase-3, are excellent candidates and their functions are beginning to be understood. By specifically targeting cancerous cells with viral vectors expressing proapoptotic factors, elimination of these cells while avoiding damage to functioning "bystander" tissue may be possible. Another approach to cancer treatment via gene therapy is to target the delivery or expression of molecules with proteolytic activity. Clearly this will require accurate targeting of the malignant cells or the effective control of expression of these toxic genes within the desired cells.

RETINOBLASTOMA GENE THERAPY CLINICAL TRIAL

Retinoblastoma is an intraocular tumor of the retina arising predominantly in pediatric populations and contributes to 6.1% of all cancers in children aged 0–4 years old. The US incidence rate for this age group is approximately 11.8 cases per million children, which correlates well with other reporting countries.[30] The most common form of this cancer arises from a mutation in the RB1 gene, a factor responsible for cell cycle regulation, resulting in aggressive cellular growth that requires swift recognition and therapeutic intervention. Currently the most definitive means of treatment is enucleation; however eyes are now saved by a combination of chemotherapy, radiation, and laser treatments.

The herpes simplex virus synthesizes a form of Thymidine Kinase (TK), which differs significantly from the human form. Ganciclovir has been shown to bind specifically to viral TK, after which it is phosphorylated and competes with guanosine triphosphate binding. This action effectively impedes DNA synthesis and induces apoptosis via a p53-mediated pathway. Thus, cells expressing the viral TK gene are susceptible to killing with ganciclovir, a drug that is innocuous to normal human cells. These data led researchers to investigate a combination therapy strategy for the treatment of various cancers, including retinoblastoma. After tumor shrinkage was observed in rodents receiving adenoviral-delivered herpes simplex thymidine kinase (Ad-TK) with systemic administration of ganciclovir, a human clinical trial was conducted to test whether this vector, when injected into the eyes of children with aggressive retinoblastoma, would reduce the size of tumors.

The phase I trial consisted of 8 children with active bilateral retinoblastoma. In addition, patients must have had the presence of vitreous seeds, had prior treatment failure, and had at least limited remaining visual acuity. The Ad-TK particles were delivered via transcorneal injection in order to minimize tumor spread through the needle tract. The vector was administered in a dose-escalating fashion with the lowest dose being 10^8 particles up to the highest dosage of 10^{11} particles. After 24 postinjection hours, patients began the first of 14 doses of ganciclovir (5 mg/kg) given at 12-hour intervals. If the retinoblastoma was considered to progress, these eyes were to be enucleated, and if no resolution of the tumor occurred with the absence of an adverse reaction, then multiple Ad-TK injections were considered.[31]

The results of this clinical trial were partially encouraging. Of the 8 patients enrolled in the study, 7 demonstrated some vitreous seed resolution. The other patient, who received the lowest dose of 10^8 particles, had tumor resolution around the injection site alone. Minor complications included mild inflammation, corneal edema, and increased intraocular pressure: some of these complications are believed to be the result of prior treatment attempts. There was no evidence of viral vector spread to other organs and viral shedding was not seen. The Ad-TK vector appeared safe but ineffective. All of the patients enrolled in the study did require enucleation at some point after treatment, with best outcome persisting for 38 months postinjection.[31] Whether this lack of efficacy was the result of the transgene or the vector employed remains unclear. Clearly, transgene expression from adenoviral vectors is limited in duration.

THE AdPEDF MACULAR DEGENERATION CLINICAL TRIAL

AMD accounts for the majority of all blindness in people over the age of 50 in industrialized nations.[32] Approximately 90% of vision loss associated with AMD is attributed to choroidal neovascularization (CNV),[33] in which uncontrolled blood vessel growth leads to irreversible scarring and vision loss. Several genetic targets for AMD have been elucidated within the last several years, although VEGF and PEDF have been the most widely investigated to date.

The VGEF isoforms are members of the cysteine-knot growth factor family. VEGF-A is a potent signaling molecule capable of up-regulating migration and mitosis in endothelial cells as well as acting as a chemoattractant for macrophages and granulocytes. PEDF, expressed in the retinal pigment epithelium, is part of the serine protease inhibitor family of molecules. Several groups have shown that the overexpression of PEDF in eyes with CNV results in a significant decrease in neovascularization. In addition, exogenous introduction of PEDF was shown to inhibit laser-induced CNV effectively in various animal models.[34,35]

These data prompted the initiation of a phase I clinical trial of 28 patients to examine the potential of PEDF to treat CNV in patients with AMD. Patients enrolled were at least 50 years of age, had a neovascular AMD diagnosis with active CNV, and visual acuity of 20/200 or poorer. The study was performed in a dose-escalating fashion with doses ranging from 10^6 to $10^{9.5}$ particles.[36]

The trial demonstrated that the intravitreal injection of AdPEDF was well tolerated. There were few complications as a result of the injection aside from mild inflammation, corneal edema, and elevated intraocular pressure in some of the patients, all of which were managed via topical medications. There was no evidence of systemic hematogenous vector spread and patients showed little sign of a systemic immune response to the drug. Although the study was primarily performed to test the safety of the vector, there were some signs of efficacy. Patients who received higher doses had no change in visual acuity as compared to low-dose patients whose acuity appeared to worsen over the course of the study. Vessel hyperpermeability appeared to resolve in some high-dose patients over a 12-week period. Retinal appearance was improved with significantly less hyperfluorescence present in some patients evidenced by fluorescein angiography.[36] The overall success of this trial has lead to the initiation of a second trial to examine the role of AdPEDF.11 on patients with early, less severe AMD.

GENE THERAPY FOR LEBER'S CONGENITAL AMAUROSIS TRIAL

LCA is an inherited blinding retinal disorder which presents typically within the first few months of postnatal life and for which there is no treatment.[37] There are over a dozen known gene mutations that result in LCA; all forms produce a breakdown in the photo transduction cascade. Although the retina in these patients appears normal via fundus and histological examination, there is extreme retinal signaling dysfunction, as measured by electroretinogram (ERG). Current gene therapy trials (three are ongoing and another is planned) are targeted at replacing a defective RPE65 protein. The RPE65 protein is responsible for the conversion of all-*trans*-retinyl ester to 11-*cis*-retinol, a key stage of the visual pathway. The gene transfer vehicle being investigated is the type 2 AAV (AAV2). Recombinant AAV2 has been studied for efficacy in a variety of gene therapy models and has been shown to nontoxic and capable of long-term expression in nondividing cells. Its success for the treatment of LCA has been evaluated in both mouse and dog models of LCA disease. Treatment in the dog model has been documented to persist for over 3 years.[38]

One LCA human study is a combination phase I/II trial, to test both dose toxicity and efficacy in 12 patients. The second and fourth cohort of this trial will include children from 8 to 18 years of age. Participants will be placed into one of four groups and will receive one subretinal injection of the rAAV2-CB-hRPE65 vector at a concentration of either 1.8×10^{11} or 6×10^{11} viral particles. Efficacy will be graded by several parameters, including visual field and acuity changes as well as ERG testing, fundus photography, optical coherence tomography, and quality-of-life surveys.

Current animal data suggest that the overall tolerance to the drug will be well tolerated with little to no side-effects such as edema or intraocular pressure variation.[39] Considering the choice of vector, AAV is not likely to be immunogenic. Based on the fact that LCA is a monogenic disease and the results documented in various animal models, the potential for visual improvement is quite promising.[40,41] Although the incidence of LCA is rare – approximately 3 of every 100 000 births[42] – the success of this treatment could improve the quality of life for a great deal of individuals worldwide as well as advancing the role of gene therapy as a treatment option.

SUMMARY AND KEYPOINTS: THE FUTURE OF GENE THERAPY

As of 2004 there were 613 approved gene therapy trials under way in the USA alone and that number will surely grow in the next several years.[43] As research continues to elucidate the mysteries of the genome, transcriptome, and proteome, our understanding of more complex disease processes will improve. For gene therapy to realize its potential, several key features need to be addressed. Cell-specific targeting, inducible (and repressible) transgene expression, immunogenicity, and minimally invasive delivery techniques will be important features to study.[44] Many advances in vector construction leading to safer more robust systems are under way. The ability to infect specific cell types is being investigated by pseudotyping lentiviral vectors with antibody fragments which bind very specific cellular receptors.[45] Other modifications may eventually lead to site-specific integration, minimizing the risk of random gene silencing or activation, an inherit risk of integrating vectors. One group has demonstrated that, with the use of nonviral recombinase molecules derived from yeast, specific integration is feasible, albeit still in the early stages of discovery.[46] While vectors will continue to improve and treatments become safer, public opinion and concerns will remain. Moral and ethical considerations will always be an important issue. The last two decades have demonstrated incredible progress – the future of gene therapy looks stronger than ever.

REFERENCES

1. Friedmann T. A brief history of gene therapy. Nat Genet 1992;2(2):93–98.
2. Sambrook J. Transformation by polyoma virus and simian virus 40. Adv Cancer Res 1972;16:141–180.
3. Sambrook J, Shatkin AJ. Polynucleotide ligase activity in cells infected with simian virus 40, polyoma virus, or vaccinia virus. J Virol 1969;4(5): 719–726.
4. Sambrook J, Westphal H, Srinivasan PR, et al. The integrated state of viral DNA in SV40-transformed cells. Proc Natl Acad Sci USA 1968;60(4): 1288–1295.
5. Graham FL, van der Eb AJ. A new technique for the assay of infectivity of human adenovirus 5 DNA. Virology 1973;52(2):456–467.
6. Mulligan RC, Berg P. Selection for animal cells that express the *Escherichia coli* gene coding for xanthine-guanine phosphoribosyltransferase. Proc Natl Acad Sci USA 1981;78:2072–2076.
7. Yamada M, Lewis JA, Grodzicker T, et al. Overproduction of the protein product of a nonselected foreign gene carried by an adenovirus vector. Proc Natl Acad Sci USA 1985;82(11):3567–3571.
8. Nakai H, Yant SR, Storm TA, et al. Extrachromosomal recombinant adeno-associated virus vector genomes are primarily responsible for stable liver transduction *in vivo*. J Virol 2001;75(15):6969–6976.
9. Gilboa E, Kolbe M, Noonan K, et al. Construction of a mammalian transducing vector from the genome of Moloney murine leukemia virus. J Virol 1982;44(3):845–851.
10. Feuerman MH, Davis BR, Pattengale PK, et al. Generation of a recombinant Moloney murine leukemia virus carrying the v-src gene of avian sarcoma virus: transformation *in vitro* and pathogenesis *in vivo*. J Virol 1985;54(3):804–816.
11. Miller AD, Jolly DJ, Friedmann T, et al. A transmissible retrovirus expressing human hypoxanthine phosphoribosyltransferase (HPRT): gene transfer into cells obtained from humans deficient in HPRT. Proc Natl Acad Sci USA 1983;80(15):4709–4713.
12. Miller AD, Eckner RJ, Jolly DJ, et al. Expression of a retrovirus encoding human HPRT in mice. Science 1984;225(4662):630–632.
13. Hlavaty J, Schittmayer M, Stracke A, et al. Effect of posttranscriptional regulatory elements on transgene expression and virus production in the context of retrovirus vectors. Virology 2005;341(1):1–11.
14. Van Maele B, De Rijck J, De Clercq E, et al. Impact of the central polypurine tract on the kinetics of human immunodeficiency virus type 1 vector transduction. J Virol 2003;77(8):4685–4694.
15. Loewen N, Leske DA, Cameron JD, et al. Long-term retinal transgene expression with FIV versus adenoviral vectors. Mol Vis 2004;10: 272–280.
16. Berg P, Baltimore D, Brenner S, et al. Summary statement of the Asilomar conference on recombinant DNA molecules. Proc Natl Acad Sci USA 1975;72(6):1981–1984.
17. Dickson D. NIH censure for Dr Martin Cline: tighter rules for future research plans. Nature 1981;291(5814):369.
18. Sun M. Martin Cline loses appeal on NIH grant. Science 1982;218(4567): 37.
19. Blaese RM, Culver KW, Miller AD, et al. T lymphocyte-directed gene therapy for ADA- SCID: initial trial results after 4 years. Science 1995;270(5235):475–480.
20. Hacein-Bey-Abina S, von Kalle C, Schmidt M, et al. A serious adverse event after successful gene therapy for X-linked severe combined immunodeficiency. N Engl J Med 2003;348(3):255–256.
21. Stolberg SG. The biotech death of Jesse Gelsinger. N Y Times Mag 1999;136–140, 149–150.
22. National Institutes of Health. Assessment of adenoviral vector safety and toxicity: report of the National Institutes of Health Recombinant DNA Advisory Committee. Hum Gene Ther 2002;13(1):3–13.
23. Bertling W, Hunger-Bertling K, Cline MJ. Intranuclear uptake and persistence of biologically active DNA after electroporation of mammalian cells. J Biochem Biophys Methods 1987;14(4):223–232.
24. Krotz F, Sohn HY, Gloe T, et al. Magnetofection potentiates gene delivery to cultured endothelial cells. J Vasc Res 2003;40(5):425–434.
25. Le Meur G, Stieger K, Smith AJ, et al. Restoration of vision in RPE65-deficient Briard dogs using an AAV serotype 4 vector that specifically targets the retinal pigmented epithelium. Gene Ther 2007;14(4):292–303.
26. O'Reilly M, Palfi A, Chadderton N, et al. RNA interference-mediated suppression and replacement of human rhodopsin *in vivo*. Am J Hum Genet 2007;81(1):127–135.
27. Klettner A, Roider J. Comparison of bevacizumab, ranibizumab, and pegaptanib *in vitro*: efficiency and possible additional pathways. Invest Ophthalmol Vis Sci 2008;49(10):4523–4527.
28. Sallinen H, Anttila M, Narvainen J, et al. Antiangiogenic gene therapy with soluble VEGFR-1, -2, and -3 reduces the growth of solid human ovarian carcinoma in mice. Mol Ther 2009;(in press).
29. Appukuttan B, McFarland TJ, Davies MH, et al. Identification of novel alternatively spliced isoforms of RTEF-1 within human ocular vascular endothelial cells and murine retina. Invest Ophthalmol Vis Sci 2007;48(8): 3775–3782.
30. Broaddus E, Topham A, Singh AD, et al. Incidence of retinoblastoma in the USA:1975–2004. Br J Ophthalmol 2009;93(1):21–23.
31. Chevez-Barrios P, Chintagumpala M, Mieler W, et al. Response of retinoblastoma with vitreous tumor seeding to adenovirus-mediated delivery of thymidine kinase followed by ganciclovir. J Clin Oncol 2005;23(31): 7927–7935.
32. Korner-Stiefbold U. Age-related macular degeneration (AMD) – therapeutic possibilities and new approaches. Ther Umsch 2001;58(1):28–35.
33. Polito A, Isola M, Lanzetta P, et al. The natural history of occult choroidal neovascularisation associated with age-related macular degeneration. A systematic review. Ann Acad Med Singapore 2006;35(3):145–150.
34. Duh EJ, Yang HS, Suzuma I, et al. Pigment epithelium-derived factor suppresses ischemia-induced retinal neovascularization and VEGF-induced migration and growth. Invest Ophthalmol Vis Sci 2002;43(3):821–829.
35. Mori K, Duh E, Gehlbach P, et al. Pigment epithelium-derived factor inhibits retinal and choroidal neovascularization. J Cell Physiol 2001;188(2):253–263.
36. Campochiaro PA, Nguyen QD, Shah SM, et al. Adenoviral vector-delivered pigment epithelium-derived factor for neovascular age-related macular degeneration: results of a phase I clinical trial. Hum Gene Ther 2006;17(2):167–176.
37. Cremers FP, van den Hurk JA, et al. Molecular genetics of Leber congenital amaurosis. Hum Mol Genet 2002;11(10):1169–1176.
38. Narfstrom K, Vaegan T, Katz M, et al. Assessment of structure and function over a 3-year period after gene transfer in RPE65-/- dogs. Doc Ophthalmol 2005;111(1):39–48.
39. Acland GM, Aguirre GD, Bennett J, et al. Long-term restoration of rod and cone vision by single dose rAAV-mediated gene transfer to the retina in a canine model of childhood blindness. Mol Ther 2005;12(6):1072–1082.

40. Acland GM, Aguirre GD, Ray J, et al. Gene therapy restores vision in a canine model of childhood blindness. Nat Genet 2001;28(1):92–95.
41. Narfstrom K, Katz ML, Bragadottir R, et al. Functional and structural recovery of the retina after gene therapy in the RPE65 null mutation dog. Invest Ophthalmol Vis Sci 2003;44(4):1663–1672.
42. Fazzi E, Signorini SG, Scelsa B, et al. Leber's congenital amaurosis: an update. Eur J Paediatr Neurol 2003;7(1):13–22.
43. Cavazzana-Calvo M, Thrasher A, Mavilio F. The future of gene therapy. Nature 2004;427(6977):779–781.
44. McCain J. The future of gene therapy. Biotechnology Healthcare 2005;53–60.
45. Aires da Silva F, Costa MJ, Corte-Real S, et al. Cell type-specific targeting with sindbis pseudotyped lentiviral vectors displaying anti-CCR5 single-chain antibodies. Hum Gene Ther 2005;16(2):223–234.
46. Moldt B, Staunstrup NH, Jakobsen M, et al. Genomic insertion of lentiviral DNA circles directed by the yeast Flp recombinase. BMC Biotechnol 2008;8:60.

CHAPTER 42

Neuroprotection and retinal diseases

J. Peter Campbell, MD, MPH and Donald J. Zack, MD, PhD

KEY FEATURES

The term "neuroprotection" can be referred to as the process of directly modifying neurons, and/or their surrounding environment, to promote the survival and function of the neurons, especially in environments that normally would be deleterious to their health.

INTRODUCTION

In ophthalmology, although neuroprotection holds great promise, the field in many ways is still in its infancy. This is especially true from the point of view of the clinician. Despite important scientific advances, and some successes in animal models, few therapies have proceeded to clinical trials, and none to overwhelming success. However, over the next 10–20 years, this situation is likely to change significantly. In this chapter we will briefly review some of the scientific background for neuroprotection, but will focus on translational studies that show promise of bringing particular neuroprotective strategies to the clinic. Keeping with the theme of this book, we will emphasize pharmacological studies related to preservation of structure and function of photoreceptors, i.e., those related to retinal degenerative disease, but given the important parallels with retinal ganglion cell (RGC) loss in glaucoma, we will also present studies related to glaucoma where appropriate. Due to space limitations, this chapter is not intended to cover the entire field, but rather will present selected areas in an effort to provide a sense of where retinal neuroprotection is today, and where it is going. For the interested reader, relevant and more comprehensive reviews will be cited.

Over the last 20 years, there has been considerable effort aimed at elucidating the underlying mechanisms of photoreceptor and ganglion cell degeneration and identifying potential neuroprotective strategies.[1–10] There are multiple laboratory models, both cell culture and animal-based, available for the study of both photoreceptor and ganglion cell survival. The retina has a number of advantages as a target for neuroprotection. It is easily accessible, self-contained, and visualizable, thus providing the potential for localized therapy, which minimizes the likelihood of systemic side-effects. Unfortunately, counterbalancing some of these scientific factors favoring the development of retinal neuroprotection have been certain economic issues. With the exception of age-related macular degeneration (AMD) and glaucoma, many of the retinal diseases that would seem the most appropriate for the application of neuroprotection strategies affect relatively small numbers of patients, historically limiting the interest of big pharma. However, the situation has been changing, both because a number of small biotech companies have become interested in retinal neuroprotection, partly due to the attractions of orphan drug legislation, and spin-off from the development of new AMD treatments is also attracting some big pharma interest. Thus, the field may also be poised to move forward from the economic/commercial side.

Before we begin our discussion, we would like first to define more fully our concept of neuroprotection. We will include in our discussion pharmacological agents that act directly on retinal neurons (primarily photoreceptors and ganglion cells) to prevent or delay their premature degeneration and death due to disease.[11] Antihypertensive therapies in glaucoma, for example, though certainly neuroprotective in a general sense, would not necessarily be considered retinal neuroprotectants for the purposes of this discussion. Wheeler et al. provided four general criteria to evaluate pharmacological agents as neuroprotectants, which is helpful as a conceptual framework for the neuroprotective drug discovery process.[12] In order to be a clinically relevant "neuroprotective" agent, the agent must have a molecular target in the retina, achieve therapeutic concentrations in the posterior segment with clinical dosing, and demonstrate neuroprotective properties in laboratory and animal models. Finally, the agent must demonstrate efficacy in clinical trials.[12] There has been much work done that satisfies the first three criteria, but a dearth of therapies have made it to trial, and few therapies have suggested clinical efficacy as retinal neuroprotectants. Our discussion will summarize the clinical work that has been performed and highlight hopeful avenues of research.

Theoretically, neuroprotective agents may be applied in multiple disease states as they act "downstream" of the primary cellular injury due to individual diseases.[8] The mechanism of injury in AMD may differ from retinitis pigmentosa, for example, but a neuroprotective agent targeting downstream processes may slow disease progression in both. Ultimately, apoptosis seems to be the final common mechanism of both RGC and photoreceptor degeneration in multiple disease states.[2] Diabetic retinopathy, traditionally thought of in terms of microvascular disease, is also a neurodegenerative disease, and thus can be considered a potential market for neuroprotective therapies.[13] This review will focus on three broad strategies: antioxidative therapy, neurotrophic support, and antiapoptotic therapy. Many potential pharmacological agents act through multiple mechanisms, and we have tried to emphasize that where possible.

MECHANISM OF PROTECTION: APPROACHES AND CHALLENGES

ANTIOXIDATIVE THERAPY

Oxygen free radicals play an important role in many human diseases, and myriad natural and artificial compounds have been evaluated for their role in protecting both photoreceptors and ganglion cells from oxidative damage. Multiple dietary antioxidants have demonstrated neuroprotective properties in the laboratory, but the three best studied are perhaps vitamin E, vitamin A, and the omega-3 fatty acids, especially docosahexaenoic acid (DHA).[10,14,15] Although still somewhat controversial, a significant advance in antioxidant therapy for retinal disease occurred with the finding from the Age-Related Eye Disease Study (AREDS) that administration of a combination of vitamin A, vitamin E, beta-carotene, and zinc decreased the probability of advancing to end-stage AMD by 25%.[16] The AREDS II study (ongoing) will further evaluate the effects of lutein, zeaxanthin, and two omega-3 fatty acids (DHA and eicosapentanoic acid), all of which have demonstrated neuroprotective properties in preclinical studies.[15]

Vitamin E (α-tocopherol) has demonstrated beneficial effects on photoreceptors and ganglion cells in multiple models. However, clinical trial results in glaucoma have been mixed, with two smaller, open-label studies suggesting an improvement in visual field, but a prospective, large-scale, long-term, study investigating dietary antioxidant intake failing to confirm these findings.[3,17–19] DHA has demonstrated neuroprotective properties in multiple laboratory models and may inhibit photoreceptor apoptosis through modulation of the Bcl-2 family of antiapoptotic proteins in addition to its antioxidant properties. In clinical trials, fish oil (a natural source of DHA) has been studied in AMD with positive results.[15] DHA is currently in phase II/III trials for retinitis pigmentosa.[20] Vitamin A supplementation has also been shown to slow the rate of photoreceptor degeneration in certain forms of retinitis pigmentosa.[21] There are several ongoing clinical trials in retinitis pigmentosa and retinopathy of prematurity.[20]

EXCITOTOXICITY

The role of excitotoxicity in glaucomatous ganglion cell dysfunction, which has been a heavily researched and controversial area, deserves some mention in the context of retinal neuroprotection. Glutamate-mediated excitotoxicity has been hypothesized to be important in RGC damage in glaucoma, and based on this hypothesis efforts have been made to reduce RGC injury by blocking the effect of glutamate. A variety of animal studies with different glutamate antagonists have been reported, but the results have been mixed.[14,22] The best-studied member of this class of drug is memantine, which is approved for the treatment of Alzheimer's disease and is an uncompetitive *N*-methyl-D-aspartic acid (NMDA) receptor antagonist and partial agonist, which allows it to exert its inhibitory effect in the presence of excess glutamate, but have minimal effect in the normal state.[23] The interest in memantine as a retinal neuroprotectant resulted from positive results reported in laboratory and animal models of RGC death.[3] In addition, in monkeys with experimental glaucoma, oral memantine was reported to protect against structural and functional glaucomatous changes, compared with placebo controls.[24,25] However, in a large-scale, randomized, prospective phase III clinical trial, memantine failed to demonstrate a significant improvement over placebo.

In the excitotoxicity paradigm, many common medications modulate cellular neural activity (including glutamate release) and have been explored as potential neuroprotective drugs. Voltage-gated sodium channels begin the process of ionic destabilization by depolarizing the cell, and sodium channel antagonists have been explored to inhibit the influx of sodium during periods of cellular stress.[3] Beta-receptor antagonists have also received attention as potential neuroprotective agents. Betaxolol, which has been reported to have neuroprotective properties in several small clinical trials, appears to have more neuroprotective action than metipranolol, timolol, and nipradilol, though all have shown some benefit in laboratory models, and all may act through different mechanisms.[3,26] Betaxolol modulates sodium and calcium channel activity, upregulates brain-derived neurotrophic factor mRNA, and prevents RGC death in multiple models of retinal injury.[3,26–28] EGb 761, better known as ginkgo biloba and a well-known dietary antioxidant, has been reported to demonstrate neuroprotective activity in rat models of ischemia and ocular hypertension.[3] In a small-scale, prospective, randomized, double-blind, crossover trial, ginkgo biloba improved visual field damage in some patients with normal-tension glaucoma.[29] However, these results are controversial and need to be confirmed in larger studies.

There has been much recent interest in the finding that there is an association between particular complement factor H (CFH) alleles and the risk of developing AMD, which, like many genetic risk factors, appears to be modified by oxidative stress.[30] This association appears to be robust and has been confirmed by a large number of independent studies. As we begin to understand the genetic heterogeneity of risk factors for both rare retinal diseases (e.g., retinitis pigmentosa) and more common diseases (AMD), and their environmental interactions, the efficiency of "downstream" neuroprotective therapy will hopefully become clearer. Persons with high-risk CFH profiles, or perhaps retinitis pigmentosa patients with particular mutations, may one day be able to reduce their disease progression risk by taking prophylactic antioxidative therapy. Better yet, we may find that modification of risk is possible with dietary change alone, a thus far unproven hypothesis.

NEUROTROPHIC FACTORS

Neurotrophic support as a therapeutic paradigm has received much interest in the last decade since basic fibroblast growth factor first demonstrated structural and functional neuroprotective effects on photoreceptor degeneration in a rat model of inherited retinal dystrophy.[21,31] Since then, a number of additional factors have been identified that also demonstrate neuroprotective properties in animal models. To date, human clinical trials have been initiated with two of these factors, pigment epithelium-derived factor (PEDF) and ciliary neutrotrophic factor (CNTF). PEDF acts on multiple pathways in the eye, including modulating glutamate excitotoxicity, protecting against oxidative damage, and inhibiting apoptosis. Intraocular injection of PEDF increased the number of photoreceptors surviving in a light-induced retinal injury model, and slowed degeneration in two mouse models of inherited retinal degeneration.[10] PEDF also demonstrates anti-VEGF activity, and a phase I trial with adenoviral-mediated PEDF administration in wet AMD has been completed, with encouraging results.[32]

CNTF has been one of the most promising molecules in retinal degeneration, demonstrating beneficial effects on both ganglion and photoreceptor cells in multiple laboratory models.[2,3] In a recent phase I safety trial, Sieving and colleagues reported that CNTF-encapsulated retinal implants (NT-501) were well tolerated by 10 patients and provided sustained release of CNTF throughout the trial period, suggesting that encapsulated cell technology might be an effective vehicle for delivering neurotrophic factors to the retina in chronic neurodegenerative diseases.[33] NT-501 is currently in phase II/III trials for retinitis pigmentosa and AMD.[34] In another model, NTC-201, genetically engineered RPE cells designed to overexpress CNTF, has been successfully implanted into rat and canine models of hereditary photoreceptor degeneration.[35] Despite the encouraging results with CNTF, some have raised concerns because in some animal models CNTF can cause dose-dependent adverse effects on ERG and on photoreceptor gene expression.[36] Another promising molecule is glial-derived neurotrophic factor, which has been reported to have impressive antioxidant and antiapoptotic activity in a rat model of oxidative injury without inducing changes in ERG.[37,38] However, it has not yet been tested in clinical trials.

There are several potential delivery mechanisms for neurotrophic factors, some of which are described in more detail elsewhere in this book. As evidenced by the recent demonstration of the apparent safety of RPE-65 gene therapy, adeno-associated viral (AAV) vectors can deliver gene therapy directly to the retina and may represent an ideal treatment vehicle for neurotrophic gene delivery.[39] Alternatively, small interfering RNA molecules (siRNAs) have received much attention for their ability to interfere with specific RNA transcripts, preventing deleterious gene expression. O'Reilly et al. recently reported the ability to suppress disease and wild-type rhodopsin with siRNAs and replace them with mutation-free versions, allowing a single therapy to treat multiple genetically heterogeneous forms of AD retinitis pigmentosa.[40] Polyamide nucleic acids, which are DNA–protein chimeric molecules that can be tailored to maximize cell penetration and RNA specificity, may also prove useful.[41] This is currently a fruitful area of research that may yield answers to some of the practical difficulties with biologic drug delivery to the retina.

ANTIAPOPTOPIC THERAPY

If apoptosis is the final common pathway in neuronal cell death, then pharmacological inhibition of apoptosis could be the ultimate neuroprotective strategy. In reality, many hypothetical and practical obstacles exist to the realization of an effective antiapoptotic therapy in human ocular diseases. Unfortunately, apoptosis is turning out to be a far more complex, and diverse, process than initially thought. In addition, there is some concern that once apoptosis is initiated, the cell may already be too sick to recover fully. Nonetheless, some progress has been made to elucidate the mechanisms of apoptosis and identify possible targets for intervention. These pathways can be interfered with either directly or indirectly to steer the cell away from apoptosis. Brimonidine, for example, has been found to upregulate Bcl-2 and Bcl-X_L, antiapoptotic proteins, and has been associated with RGC survival in experimental models. Brimonidine is currently in clinical trials for AMD and retinitis pigmentosa.[20]

There have been a number of laboratory successes in promoting retinal cell survival through inhibition of apoptotic pathways, including transfer of the Bcl-2 gene to the retina in mouse models of inherited retinal degeneration, calcineurin inhibitors, and caspase inhibitors.[2,24] AAV vector-mediated expression of X-linked inhibitor of apoptosis protein (XIAP) has demonstrated structural and functional improvement in rat model of retinal degeneration and glaucoma.[26,42] Orally tolerated caspase inhibitors have been produced and are in the early phases of clinical trials for other indications. Pralnacasan, from Aventis, is a caspase-1 inhibitor in phase II clinical trial for rheumatoid arthritis.[3] There is also a compound, PF-03491390, a pan-caspase inhibitor, that is in the process of undergoing phase II clinical trials for liver disease.[3] Whether one of these therapies, or another similar drug, will some day

Table 42.1 Currently ongoing clinical trials to investigate the role of retinal neuroprotection

Condition	Title	Phase	Intervention	Sponsors
AMD	Weekly vaccination with copaxone as a potential therapy for dry age-related macular degeneration	I	Copaxone injection	The New York Eye and Ear Infirmary
AMD	Safety and efficacy of brimonidine intravitreal implant in patients with geographic atrophy due to age-related macular degeneration (AMD)	II	Brimonidine tartrate implant	Allergan
AMD	Safety and efficacy of ATG003 in patients with wet age-related macular degeneration (AMD)	II	Mecamylamine	CoMentis
AMD	Copaxone in age related macular degeneration	II/III	Copaxone (glatiramer acetate)	Kaplan Medical Center
AMD	Age-Related Eye Disease Study 2 (AREDS2)	III	Lutein/zeaxanthin	National Eye Institute (NEI) National Heart, Lung, and Blood Institute (NHLBI)
AMD	Safety and efficacy of ATG003 in patients with AMD receiving anti-VEGF	II	Mecamylamine	CoMentis
DR	Evaluation of doxycyline for the treatment of nonproliferative and early proliferative diabetic retinopathy	II	Doxycycline monohydrate	Penn State University Juvenile Diabetes Research Foundation
DR	A safety and efficacy study of Vitreosolve® for non-proliferative diabetic retinopathy subjects	III	Vitreosolve	Vitreoretinal Technologies
LCA	Phase 1 trial of gene vector to patients with retinal disease due to RPE65 mutations	I	rAAV2-CBSB-hRPE65	University of Pennsylvania National Eye Institute (NEI)
LCA	Safety study of RPE65 gene therapy to treat Leber congenital amaurosis	I/II	tgAAG76 (rAAV2/2.hRPE65p.hRPE65)	University College, London Moorfields Eye Hospital Targeted Genetics
RP	Randomized trial for retinitis pigmentosa	III	Vitamin A	National Eye Institute (NEI)
RP	A study of encapsulated cell technology (ECT) implant for participants with early stage retinitis pigmentosa	II/III	NT-501	Neurotech Pharmaceuticals
RP	A study of encapsulated cell technology (ECT) implant for patients with late stage retinitis pigmentosa	II/III	NT-501	Neurotech Pharmaceuticals
RP	An exploratory study to evaluate the safety of brimonidine intravltreal implant in patients with retinitis pigmentosa	I	Brimonidine tartrate implant	Allergan
RP	Investigating the effect of vitamin a supplementation on retinitis pigmentosa	I	Vitamin A	National Eye Institute (NEI)
RP	Randomized clinical trial for retinitis pigmentosa	II/III	Vitamin A	National Eye Institute (NEI)
RP	DHA and X-linked retinitis pigmentosa	II/III	Docosahexaenoic acid	FDA Office of Orphan Products Development Foundation Fighting Blindness Martek Biosciences
ROP	Vitamin A and very low birthweight babies (VitAL)	IV	Aquasol A	Glasgow Royal Infirmary Chief Scientist Office, Scottish Executive
ROP	Single dose intravenous inositol pharmacokinetics in preterm infants	II	Inositol	National Institute of Child Health and Human Development (NICHD) National Eye Institute (NEI)

AMD, age-related macular degeneration; DR, diabetic retinopathy; LCA, Leber's congenital amaurosis; RP, retinitis pigmentosa; ROP, retinopathy of prematurity; FDA, Food and Drug Administration.

prove to be effective and safe for the treatment of retinal disease remains to be seen.

Intracellular calcium concentrations play a pivotal role in cell survival, and abnormalities in calcium homeostasis can lead to loss of cellular integrity and activation of several apoptotic mechanisms. There has been much interest, therefore, in the role of calcium channel modulation in the preservation of neurons. D-diltiazem, nilvadipine, and nicardipine have all demonstrated mixed results in various rat models of inherited retinal degenerations, with some studies suggesting a neuroprotective effect.[10] Flunarizine, flupirtine, lomerizine, and nifedipine have also been reported to promote RGC survival in laboratory and/or animal models, and several calcium channel blockers have been reported to improve visual function in some patients with normal-tension glaucoma. However, these studies have been controversial, and the mechanism is thought by some to involve improved blood flow, rather than direct neuroprotection.[3]

Though not directly antiapoptotic, Schwartz and colleagues have reported a relationship between T-cell function and RGC survival, suggesting that the immune system may play a role in RGC repair after injury, perhaps preventing apoptotic cell death.[3,43,44] In addition to T cells, microglia have also been reported potentially to play a role in both photoreceptor and ganglion cell loss. Therapeutically, this raises the possibility that the immune system might be "primed" for neuroprotection through an immunologic vaccine. Following disappointing results with immunization targeted at myelin-associated protein, attention was turned to glatiramer acetate (copolymer-1), a random oligopeptide that is a low-affinity antigen that cross-reacts with self-reactive T cells, and has been approved by the Food and Drug Administration for the treatment of multiple sclerosis.[3] Immunization with glatiramer acetate has been reported to increase RGC survival in mouse and rat models of RGC injury.[45] Copaxone is currently in phase I, II, and III trials for AMD.

THE FUTURE OF RETINAL NEUROPROTECTION

The field of retinal neuroprotection holds much promise for future clinical advances, but much work clearly remains to be done. Many agents demonstrate neuroprotective properties in some laboratory or animal models, but not others, complicating the decision of which to pursue in clinical trials.[10] Moreover, it is uncertain how well animal models can accurately predict safety and efficacy in humans, as demonstrated by the disappointing results of the memantine clinical trial. In terms of future clinical application, in addition to identifying the most promising agents, development of improved drug delivery approaches for potential therapies will also be of prime importance. This is particularly true because many of the most promising neuroprotective agents that are now being developed are not the traditional small molecules of the past, but rather are large-molecule "biologics," such as proteins and genes, that require special modes of administration.

SUMMARY AND KEY POINTS

Despite the numerous obstacles to ophthalmological drug development in neuroprotection, there are several encouraging reasons to suggest that there will be significant advances in the coming years. The last decade has heralded several fundamental revolutions in eye care delivery. The safety and effectiveness of intravitreal injection proved that medications could be efficiently delivered directly to the retina as needed. The development of implantable steroid devices and encapsulated cell technology for CNTF demonstrated that pharmacologic and biologic therapies could be delivered over long periods of time with tolerable side-effects. Moreover, the ongoing development of small molecules optimized for retinal penetration may further simplify drug delivery and allow more drug development and clinical testing. Finally, at the organizational level, there is increasing infrastructure being established to facilitate the translation from basic science to clinical trials for orphan and other retinal diseases. As one example, the National Eye Evaluation and Research network, established by the National Neurovision Research Institute, was developed to coordinate and facilitate the translation of promising retinal degeneration research from the lab to the clinic. As another indication of the promise that lies ahead, Table 42.1, obtained from the national clinical trials database,[20] summarizes the currently ongoing clinical trials that are relevant to the theories and pharmacologic options described in this chapter. The diversity of treatment approaches and applicable disease states highlights the research interest in (and the potential market of) neuroprotective therapies for retinal diseases. Hopefully, studies such as these, and others that are just being conceived, will some day soon lead to the development of new and more effective neuroprotective approaches for the treatment of disabling retinal diseases that affect millions around the world.

REFERENCES

1. Barkana Y, Belkin M. Neuroprotection in ophthalmology: A review. Brain Res Bull 2004;62:447–453.
2. Chaum E. Retinal neuroprotection by growth factors: A mechanistic perspective. J Cell Biochem 2003;88:57–75.
3. Chidlow G, Wood JP, Casson RJ. Pharmacological neuroprotection for glaucoma. Drugs 2007;67:725–759.
4. Farkas RH, Grosskreutz CL. Apoptosis, neuroprotection, and retinal ganglion cell death: An overview. Int Ophthalmol Clin 2001;41:111–130.
5. Grimm C, Hermann DM, Bogdanova A, et al. Neuroprotection by hypoxic preconditioning: HIF-1 and erythropoietin protect from retinal degeneration. Semin Cell Dev Biol 2005;16:531–538.
6. Isenmann S, Kretz A, Cellerino A. Molecular determinants of retinal ganglion cell development, survival, and regeneration. Prog Retin Eye Res 2003;22:483–543.
7. Isenmann S, Schmeer C, Kretz A. How to keep injured CNS neurons viable – strategies for neuroprotection and gene transfer to retinal ganglion cells. Mol Cell Neurosci 2004;26:1–16.
8. Levin LA. Neuroprotection and regeneration in glaucoma. Ophthalmol Clin North Am 2005;18:585–596, vii.
9. Osborne NN, Chidlow G, Layton CJ, et al. Optic nerve and neuroprotection strategies. Eye 2004;18:1075–1084.
10. Wenzel A, Grimm C, Samardzija M, et al. Molecular mechanisms of light-induced photoreceptor apoptosis and neuroprotection for retinal degeneration. Prog Retin Eye Res 2005;24:275–306.
11. Osborne NN, Chidlow G, Wood JP, et al. Expectations in the treatment of retinal diseases: Neuroprotection. Curr Eye Res 2001;22:321–332.
12. Wheeler L, WoldeMussie E, Lai R. Role of alpha-2 agonists in neuroprotection. Surv Ophthalmol 2003;48(Suppl. 1):S47–S51.
13. Lieth E, Gardner TW, Barber AJ, et al. Retinal neurodegeneration: Early pathology in diabetes. Clin Experiment Ophthalmol 2000;28:3–8.
14. Osborne NN, Casson RJ, Wood JP, et al. Retinal ischemia: Mechanisms of damage and potential therapeutic strategies. Prog Retin Eye Res 2004;23:91–147.
15. Ritch R. Natural compounds: Evidence for a protective role in eye disease. Can J Ophthalmol 2007;42:425–438.
16. Massof RW. Clinical trials with micronutrients and mineral supplements for retinal degenerations: A summary of a breakout session. Retina 2005;25:S50–S51.
17. Birich TV, Birich TA, Marchenko LN, et al. Vitamin E in the complex treatment of patients with primary glaucoma [in Russian]. Vestn Oftalmol 1986;102(2):10–13.
18. Cellini M, Caramazza N, Mangiafico P, et al. Fatty acid use in glaucomatous optic neuropathy treatment. Acta Ophthalmol Scand Suppl 1998;(227):41–42.
19. Kang JH, Pasquale LR, Willett W, et al. Antioxidant intake and primary open-angle glaucoma: a prospective study. Am J Epidemiol 2003;158:(4):337–346.
20. Home – ClinicalTrials.gov. Available at: <http://www.clinicaltrials.gov/>. Accessed 5/16/2008, 2008.
21. Delyfer MN, Leveillard T, Mohand-Said S, et al. Inherited retinal degenerations: Therapeutic prospects. Biol Cell 2004;96:261–269.
22. Levin LA. Axonal loss and neuroprotection in optic neuropathies. Can J Ophthalmol 2007;42:403–408.
23. Chen HS, Lipton SA. The chemical biology of clinically tolerated NMDA receptor antagonists. J Neurochem 2006;97:1611–1626.
24. Hare WA, WoldeMussie E, Lai RK, et al. Efficacy and safety of memantine treatment for reduction of changes associated with experimental glaucoma in monkey, I: Functional measures. Invest Ophthalmol Vis Sci 2004;45:2625–2639.
25. Hare WA, WoldeMussie E, Weinreb RN, et al. Efficacy and safety of memantine treatment for reduction of changes associated with experimental glaucoma in monkey, II: Structural measures. Invest Ophthalmol Vis Sci 2004;45:2640–2651.

26. Chen YN, Yamada H, Mao W, et al. Hypoxia-induced retinal ganglion cell death and the neuroprotective effects of beta-adrenergic antagonists. Brain Res 2007;1148:28–37.
27. Osborne NN, Wood JP, Chidlow G. Invited review: Neuroprotective properties of certain beta-adrenoceptor antagonists used for the treatment of glaucoma. J Ocul Pharmacol Ther 2005;21:175–181.
28. Levin LA, Gordon LK. Retinal ganglion cell disorders: Types and treatments. Prog Retin Eye Res 2002;21:465–484.
29. Quaranta L, Bettelli S, Uva MG, et al. Effect of *Ginkgo biloba* extract on preexisting visual field damage in normal tension glaucoma. Ophthalmology 2003;110(2):359–362.
30. Wu Z, Lauer TW, Sick A, et al. Oxidative stress modulates complement factor H expression in retinal pigmented epithelial cells by acetylation of FOXO3. J Biol Chem 2007;282:22414–22425.
31. Faktorovich EG, Steinberg RH, Yasumura D, et al. Photoreceptor degeneration in inherited retinal dystrophy delayed by basic fibroblast growth factor. Nature 1990;347:83–86.
32. Campochiaro PA, Nguyen QD, Shah SM, et al. Adenoviral vector-delivered pigment epithelium-derived factor for neovascular age-related macular degeneration: Results of a phase I clinical trial. Hum Gene Ther 2006;17:167–176.
33. Sieving PA, Caruso RC, Tao W, et al. Ciliary neurotrophic factor (CNTF) for human retinal degeneration: Phase I trial of CNTF delivered by encapsulated cell intraocular implants. Proc Natl Acad Sci USA 2006;103:3896–3901.
34. Neurotech | News | Press Releases. Available at: <http://www.neurotechusa.com/news_press_041707.asp>. Accessed 5/15/2008, 2008.
35. Tao W. Application of encapsulated cell technology for retinal degenerative diseases. Expert Opin Biol Ther 2006;6:717–726.
36. McGill TJ, Prusky GT, Douglas RM, et al. Intraocular CNTF reduces vision in normal rats in a dose-dependent manner. Invest Ophthalmol Vis Sci 2007;48:5756–5766.
37. Dong A, Shen J, Krause M, et al. Increased expression of glial cell line-derived neurotrophic factor protects against oxidative damage-induced retinal degeneration. J Neurochem 2007;103:1041–1052.
38. Wu WC, Lai CC, Chen SL, et al. Long-term safety of GDNF gene delivery in the retina. Curr Eye Res 2005;30:715–722.
39. Rex TS. Rescue of sight by gene therapy – closer than it may appear. Ophthalmic Genet 2007;28:127–133.
40. O'Reilly M, Palfi A, Chadderton N, et al. RNA interference-mediated suppression and replacement of human rhodopsin *in vivo*. Am J Hum Genet 2007;81:127–135.
41. Shen J, Xie B, Hatara CM, et al. Vegf or EphA2 antisense polyamide-nucleic acids; vascular localization and suppression of retinal neovascularization. Mol Ther 2007;15:1924–1930.
42. Renwick J, Narang MA, Coupland SG, et al. XIAP-mediated neuroprotection in retinal ischemia. Gene Ther 2006;13:339–347.
43. Wax MB. Is there a role for the immune system in glaucomatous optic neuropathy? Curr Opin Ophthalmol 2000;11:145–150.
44. Schwartz M, London A. Glaucoma as a neuropathy amenable to neuroprotection and immune manipulation. Prog Brain Res 2008;173(8):375–384.
45. Bakalash S, Shlomo GB, Aloni E, et al. T-cell-based vaccination for morphological and functional neuroprotection in a rat model of chronically elevated intraocular pressure. J Mol Med 2005;83:904–916.

CHAPTER

43 Photosensitizers and photodynamic therapy: verteporfin

Luis Amselem, MD, Jordi M. Monés, MD, and Lluis Arias, MD

KEY FEATURES

- Verteporfin derives from porphyrin and is also known as the benzoporphyrin monoacid derivative.
- Verteporfin is a light-activated drug used in photodynamic therapy.
- Verteporfin has a peak absorption at a long wavelength that enables the activating nonthermal laser light to penetrate deep into the target tissue.
- Verteporfin selectively damages neovascular endothelial cells.
- The primary mechanism of photodynamic therapy with verteporfin is the immediate occlusion of neovessels within the target.

INTRODUCTION AND HISTORY

Verteporfin is a potent second-generation light-activated drug that selectively damages neovascular endothelial cells, occluding target vessels. It is derived from porphyrin and also known as the benzoporphyrin monoacid derivative. It is a chlorine-type molecule and is a 1:1 mixture of two regioisomers (Figure 43.1). Each of these regioisomers consists of an enantiomeric pair that demonstrates similar pharmacologic activity *in vitro* and *in vivo*.[1] Verteporfin is used in photodynamic therapy (PDT).

PDT is a two-step process that includes the intravenous administration of a pharmacological photosensitizer combined with the physical activation of the substance by a nonthermal diode laser light in the red wavelength. Activation of the drug in the presence of oxygen results in the creation of singlet oxygen and free radicals that are toxic to cells and tissues within the immediate vicinity of the target area.[2]

PDT was first evaluated as a potential diagnostic and therapeutic tool about 25 years ago. It was used for the detection and treatment of skin metastasis in lung cancer and subsequently to evaluate the phototoxic effects in experimental cerebral tumours.[3] Hematoporphyrin derivatives were used as dyes which were laser-activated to achieve the desired clinical effects.

Before the development of PDT with verteporfin, laser photocoagulation was the only treatment proven to be effective for choroidal neovascularization (CNV) secondary to age-related macular degeneration (AMD). However, retinal function was directly damaged by thermal energy, with a high risk of immediate and irreversible vision loss at the site of laser light application. In contrast to laser coagulation, no thermal tissue damage occurs after PDT, and retinal function is maintained.

Verteporfin became available on April 12, 2000, as the first Food and Drug Administration (FDA)-approved drug for patients with subfoveal neovascular AMD, and since 2001, for CNV in pathologic myopia. Thereafter, laser photocoagulation was not considered appropriate for the majority of subfoveal lesions or for poorly demarcated lesions, and its use was limited to a subset of patients with juxtafoveal or extrafoveal lesions in whom it confines vision loss to a smaller area than without treatment.

PHARMACOLOGY

Verteporfin is a chlorine-type molecule and exists as an equal mixture of two regioisomers (Figure 43.1), each of which consists of an enantiomeric pair that demonstrate similar pharmacologic activity *in vitro* and *in vivo*.[1] Verteporfin has a molecular formula of $C_{41}H_{42}N_4O_8$ and a relative molecular weight of 718.81. It is formulated in a lipid-based preparation that augments solubility in the blood.

Verteporfin has a long absorption wavelength with several peaks (Figure 43.2).[1] The strongest absorption peak of verteporfin is at approximately 400 nm (blue light), but this wavelength is not clinically useful for treatment of CNV because it is the same as the absorption peak of oxyhemoglobin.[2] Verteporfin absorbs light efficiently at a wavelength of 689 nm (red light), which can penetrate a thin layer of blood, melanin, or fibrotic tissue.[1] Light at this wavelength is not absorbed strongly by naturally present substances, avoiding thermal damage to retinal tissues[2] (Figure 43.2).

The most suitable light source for use in PDT with verteporfin is a nonthermal diode laser, operating at a wavelength of 689 ± 3 nm.[1] The laser beam is delivered through a slit lamp to the affected area in the retina and the light is targeted to the desired area by means of a low-intensity helium-neon beam through a standard ophthalmologic contact lens. Two laser systems have been specifically designed and approved for use with PDT with verteporfin: the Coherent Opal Photoactivator laser and LaserLink adapter, and the Zeiss Visulas 690s laser and Visulink PDT adapter.

Following intravenous infusion, verteporfin exhibits a biexponential elimination with a terminal elimination half-life of approximately 5–6 hours and is eliminated from the body within approximately 24 hours.[4] The extent of exposure and the maximal plasma concentration are proportional to the dose between 6 and 20 mg/m^2.

Verteporfin is metabolized to a small extent to its diacid metabolite by liver and plasma esterases. NADPH-dependent liver enzyme systems (including the cytochrome P450 isozymes) do not appear to play a role in the metabolism of verteporfin. Elimination is by the fecal route, with less than 0.01% of the dose recovered in urine. At the intended dose of 6 mg/m^2 body surface area, the pharmacokinetic characteristics of verteporfin are not significantly affected by age, gender, race, or mild hepatic or renal impairment, so dose adjustments are not required.[4]

DRUG MECHANISM

The four main stages of the mechanism of action of PDT with verteporfin are described in Figure 43.3.

In vitro studies suggest that lipophilic verteporfin is taken up by a process of receptor-mediated endocytosis via low-density lipoprotein (LDL) receptors.[5] In the blood stream, circulating verteporfin forms complexes with LDL. It selectively accumulates within neovasculature, including neovascular endothelial tissue, probably due to increased uptake of LDL and increased expression of LDL receptors on rapidly proliferating cells.

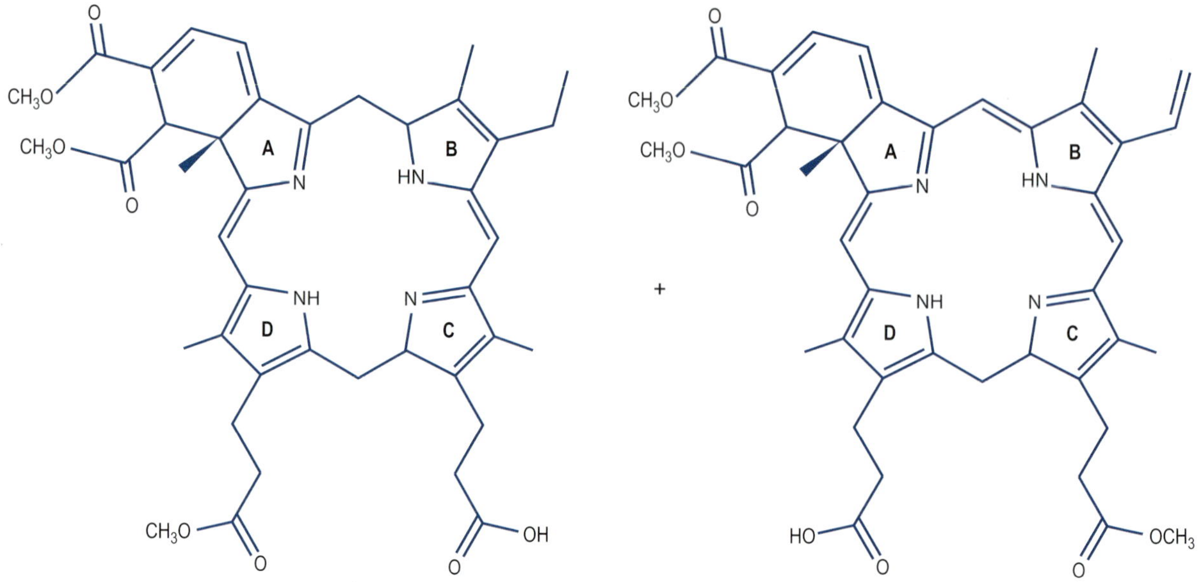

I

O

Figure 43.1 Chemical structures of verteporfin's regioisomers I and II.

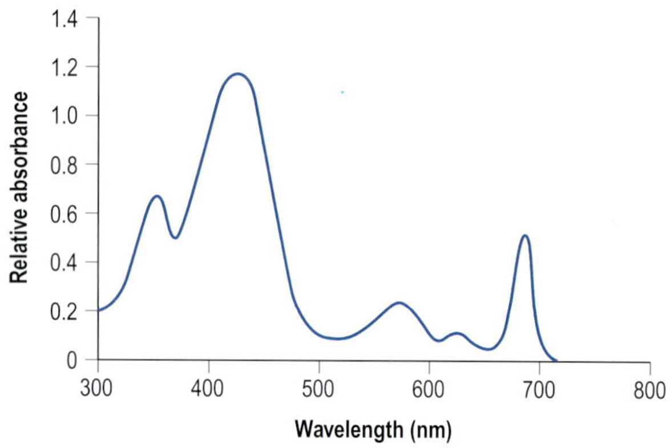

Figure 43.2 Excitation spectrum of verteporfin.

Once verteporfin has bound to surface receptors on endothelial cell membranes, it is taken up into the cell and binds to intracellular or cytoplasmic components.[5]

Application of the nonthermal laser to the target tissue causes verteporfin to transform from a ground singlet state to an excited triplet state.[2]

From its triplet state, verteporfin initiates photochemical reactions either directly via the formation of reactive free radicals (type I mechanism) or indirectly via the transfer of its energy into ground state oxygen ($3O_2$) and highly reactive singlet oxygen ($1O_2$) (type II mechanism).[2] Both photochemical reactions can occur simultaneously and both cause direct and immediate cytotoxicity (Figure 43.3).

Reactive oxygen species can cause lipid and amino acid peroxidation, affecting cell membrane-associated and intracellular targets, and may produce a number of effects on immune cells.[2] The effect is dependent on the doses of both photosensitizer and activating light. Induction of high levels of oxidative stress results in necrotic cell death, while lower-intensity oxidative stress initiates apoptosis. Sublethal doses of PDT may result in the modification of cell surface receptor expression and consequently influence cell activities.

The primary mechanism of action of PDT with verteporfin may be the damage to the fibrovascular tissue through the induction of immediate occlusion of vessels. Red and white blood cells, aggregated platelets, and fibrin can block the lumen of the neovasculature.[2]

Histologically, the endothelial cells lining the vessels are damaged; they are swollen and the nuclear membranes break. Other nearby vessels remain intact, while minimal damage may occur to adjacent retinal structures such as the overlying photoreceptors and retinal pigment epithelium (RPE).[2]

The effects on CNV in humans following PDT with verteporfin have been confirmed by the absence of leakage from CNV on fluorescein angiography after treatment. PDT with verteporfin may subsequently cause selective occlusion of vessels while sparing overlying retinal cells and Bruch's membrane, thereby maintaining function of the retina and helping to reduce the risk of vision loss.[2]

DRUG EFFECTS IN HUMAN NONOCULAR DISEASES

PDT IN ONCOLOGICAL DISORDERS

Mechanisms that have been shown to be involved in the tumoricidal effect of PDT with verteporfin include direct cytotoxicity to tumor cells and selective occlusion of the tumor vasculature, thus starving the tumor of oxygen or nutrients.

Thus, PDT has mostly been considered as a local therapy in which cell and tissue destruction happens primarily in the area that is exposed to light and the immediately surrounding areas. However, mounting evidence suggests that, as opposed to many common cancer therapies that are largely immunosuppressive, PDT can stimulate the immune system. In this respect PDT is similar to adjuvant-enhanced laser immunotherapy that has also been shown to be capable of destroying local tumors, while at the same time sensitizing the immune system to destroy distant metastases.[6]

Furthermore, PDT induces among numerous cell targets membrane damage and alteration in cancer cell adhesiveness, an important parameter in cancer metastasis.[7]

In order to increase its antitumor effects, PDT with verteporfin has been used in combination with other drugs. For example, it has been shown that paclitaxel augments the cytotoxic effect of PDT with verteporfin in gastric and bile duct cancer cells.

PDT has been used alone or in combination with surgery in many oncologic conditions, including gastrointestinal cancers, brain tumors, prostate cancer, skin melanoma, and primary, recurrent, and metastatic

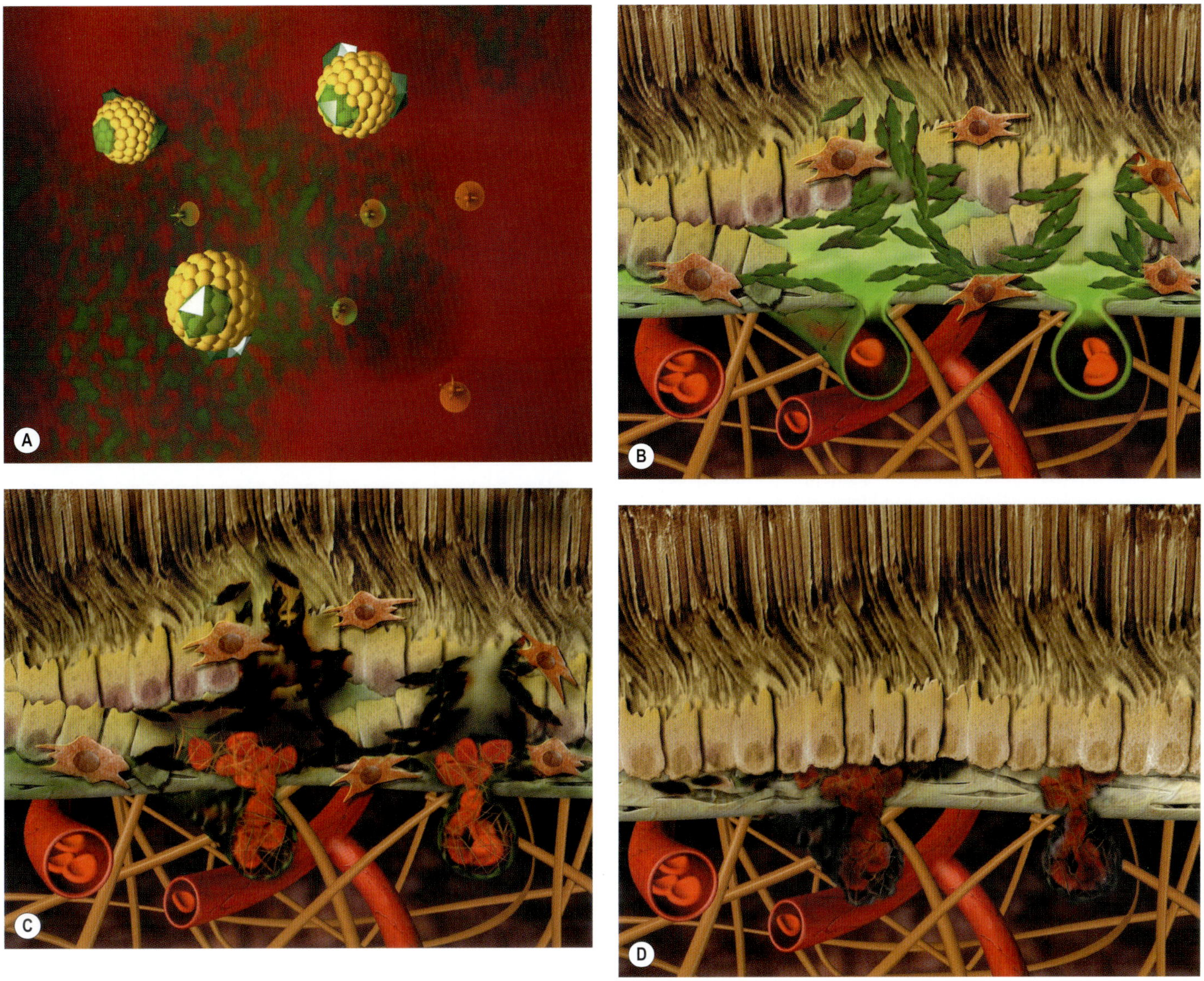

Figure 43.3 Schematic illustration of the rationale and four main stages of the mechanism of action of photodynamic therapy with verteporfin. (A) Circulating verteporfin forms complexes with low-density lipoprotein. (B) Verteporfin selectively accumulates in neovascular tissue, which is rich in low-density lipoprotein receptors. (C) Light-activated verteporfin produces reactive forms of oxygen which cause structural and functional cell damage. (D) Verteporfin selectively occludes neovascular tissue.

nonmelanoma skin cancer, with variable results. Furthermore, PDT has also been used for bone marrow purging prior to bone marrow transplantation in acute leukemia and non-Hodgkin's lymphoma.[8]

However PDT has yet to enter the mainstream of oncology treatments because of its inability to provide results superior to conventional therapies in large randomized controlled trials, and because it has been difficult to find the optimal dose that produces lethal effects on the targeted dysplastic and neoplastic tissues while minimizing damage to adjacent normal tissue.[8]

PDT IN IMMUNE (NONONCOLOGICAL) DISORDERS

Immunomodulatory PDT (IPDT) utilizes mainly apoptotic and sublethal doses. Induction of high levels of oxidative stress results in necrotic cell death, while lower-intensity oxidative stress initiates apoptosis. Sublethal doses may result in the modification of cell surface receptor expression levels and cytokine release. IPDT uses lower doses of both photosensitizer and light, and the light is delivered to a larger area of the body or to the whole body.

IPDT with verteporfin may be effective against inflammation and keratinocyte hyperproliferation of the skin in patients with psoriasis as well as for psoriatic arthitis.[9]

IPDT has also been shown to be effective for the treatment of synovitis in various animal models. These observations support the possibility that PDT could offer a safe clinical option for the management of inflamed joints in rheumatoid arthritis.[10]

DRUG USE IN RETINAL DISEASES

AGE-RELATED MACULAR DEGENERATION

The Treatment of Age-related macular degeneration with Photodynamic therapy (TAP) study,[11,12] and the the Verteporfin in Photodynamic therapy (VIP) study[13,14] demonstrated that PDT with verteporfin is able to prevent further severe visual loss.

In the TAP study, subfoveal lesions up to 5400 μm in diameter and VA ranging from 20/40 to 20/200 were treated with verteporfin

Table 43.1 Stabilization of visual acuity ± 3 lines with different treatments in age-related macular degeneration

Treatment modality	Lesion type	Study	Control	Difference	Study
PDT (quarterly, if lesion activity present)	Predominantly classic CNV	59%	31%	28%	TAP: 24 months
	Minimum classic CNV	48%	44%	3%	TAP: 24 months
	Occult CNV	45%	32%	13%	VIP: 24 months
Pegabtanib 0.3 mg (6-week intervals, fixed regimen)	All CNV subtypes	59%	45%	14%	VISION: 24 months
	Predominantly classic CNV	61%	42%	19%	VISION: 24 months
	Minimum classic CNV	61%	50%	11%	VISION: 24 months
	Occult CNV	56%	41%	15%	VISION: 24 months
Ranibizumab 0.5 mg (4-week intervals, fixed regimen)	Predominantly classic CNV	90%	66%	24%	ANCHOR: 24 months
	Minimum classic + occult CNV	90%	53%	37%	MARINA: 24 months
Ranibizumab 0.5 mg (3-monthly injections then quarterly, fixed regimen)	All CNV types	90%	49%	41%	PIER: 12 months
Combination PDT–ranibizumab (PDT quarterly, if needed; ranibizumab monthly, fixed regimen)	Predominantly classic CNV	91%	68%	23%	FOCUS: 12 months

PDT, photodynamic therapy; CNV, choroidal neovascularization; TAP, treatment of age-related macular degeneration with photodynamic therapy; VIP, Verteporfin in Photodynamic Therapy study; VISION, VEGF Inhibition Study in Ocular Neovascularization; ANCHOR, Anti-VEGF antibody for the treatment of predominantly classic choroidal neovascularization in age-related macular degeneration; MARINA, Minimally classic/occult trial of the anti-VEGF antibody ranibizumab in the treatment of neovascular age-related macular degeneration; PIER, A phase IIIB multicenter, randomized, double-masked, sham injection controlled study of the efficacy and safety of ranibizumab in subjects with subfoveal CNV with or without classic CNV secondary to age-related macular degeneration; FOCUS, A phase I/II, single-masked multicenter study of the safety, tolerability, and efficacy of multiple-dose intravitreal injections of rhuFab V2 I combination with verteporfin (Visudyne) photodynamic therapy in subjects with neovascular age-related macular degeneration.

therapy.[11,12] The primary outcome measure was the proportion of eyes with fewer than 15 letters (approximately 3 lines) of visual acuity loss at the month-24 examination. A benefit was found for the entire population, with 53% of the PDT-treated patients and 38% of the placebo-treated patients. Subgroup analysis revealed that the benefit was largest in predominantly classic lesions (Table 43.1). In this lesion type, 59% of PDT-treated eyes compared with 31% of sham-treated eyes lost fewer than 15 letters. No statistically significant difference was noted for minimally classic lesions.[11,12] Twenty-two per cent of eyes in the PDT group experienced a significant vision loss – defined as VA loss of more than 30 letters – compared to 36% in the sham group. An improvement in vision by 15 letters or more was seen in only 9% of treated patients at the 24 month visit (Figure 43.4).

The VIP study enrolled patients with subfoveal occult CNV with no classic lesions, presumed recent disease progression, larger lesion size (>4 disc areas (DA)), and a BCVA ≥ 20/50 in the affected eye.[13,14] Patients were only eligible if recent disease progression – including vision loss by at least 1 line, new haemorrhage or an enlargement of the CNV by at least 10%, as seen by angiography – was documented. At 2 years, 45% of PDT-treated eyes compared to 32% of sham-treated eyes lost less than 15 letters. Subgroup analysis demonstrated that CNV with a lesion size < 4 DA or worse initial BCVA < 65 letters had a better outcome: 51% of PDT-treated eyes lost fewer than 15 letters versus 25% in the placebo group. A significant loss of 30 letters or more was observed in 29% of eyes in the PDT group versus 47% in the placebo group.

However, the VIO (Visudyne in Occult CNV) study recently demonstrated that, although PDT with Verteporfin was safe and well-tolerated in the treatment of occult with no classic CNV, the differences between PDT treated patients and the placebo group in the primary efficacy variables were not significant.[14] The VIO study included patients with ≥50 years of age with lesion size ≤ 6 disc areas and BCVA of 20/40-20/200. The primary outcome measures were loss of ≥15 and ≥30 letters of VA from baseline at 12 and 24 months. A total of 37% and 47% of verteporfin-treated patients versus 45% and 53% of placebo recipients lost ≥15 letters of VA at month 12 and month 24, respectively; 16% and 23% of verteporfin-treated patients versus 17% and 25% of placebo recipients lost ≥30 letters at month 12 and month 24, respectively. These differences were not statistically significant. Therefore, PDT with Verteporfin may not be recommended for patients with subfoveal occult with no classic CNV.[15]

In summary, these studies demonstrated that, after PDT with verteporfin, the risk for a significant loss in vision is reduced to 50% compared to the spontaneous course of the disease in patients with neovascular AMD with predominantly classic CNV. The mean visual loss ranges between 2 and 4 lines and the proportion of patients showing improvement following verteporfin therapy is very limited. At 24 months, an improvement of ≥1 to <3 lines was seen in 8% and an increase of ≥3 to <6 lines was seen in 5% of patients.[14]

Later demonstration that CNV occlusion after PDT with verteporfin was associated with immediate massive exudation, followed by occlusive effects within the collateral choroid and an enhanced expression of vascular endothelial growth factor (VEGF), VEGFR-3, and pigment epithelium-derived factor, motivated the search for combination treatment strategies.[16]

Combination of PDT with verteporfin and intravitreal triamcinolone showed no visual benefit compared with PDT with verteporfin alone.[17] Combination therapy, however, can reduce the number of treatments required by subjects who have predominantly classic CNV secondary to AMD. This reduced treatment quantity needs to be weighed against potential side effects, such as glaucoma and cataract formation.

Combination of PDT with verteporfin and anti-VEGF agents such as pegaptanib sodium or ranibizumab was safe and effective in predominantly classic lesions and reduced the need for retreatment.[18] However, the prognosis in terms of vision maintenance and improvement appears to be worst in patients treated with PDT with Verteporfin in combination with intravitreal ranibizumab than in patients treated with ranibizumab alone.[19]

PATHOLOGIC MYOPIA

CNV represents the most important complication in pathologic myopia, occurring in a percentage ranging from 5% to 10% of cases, with a positive correlation between risk and degree of myopia.

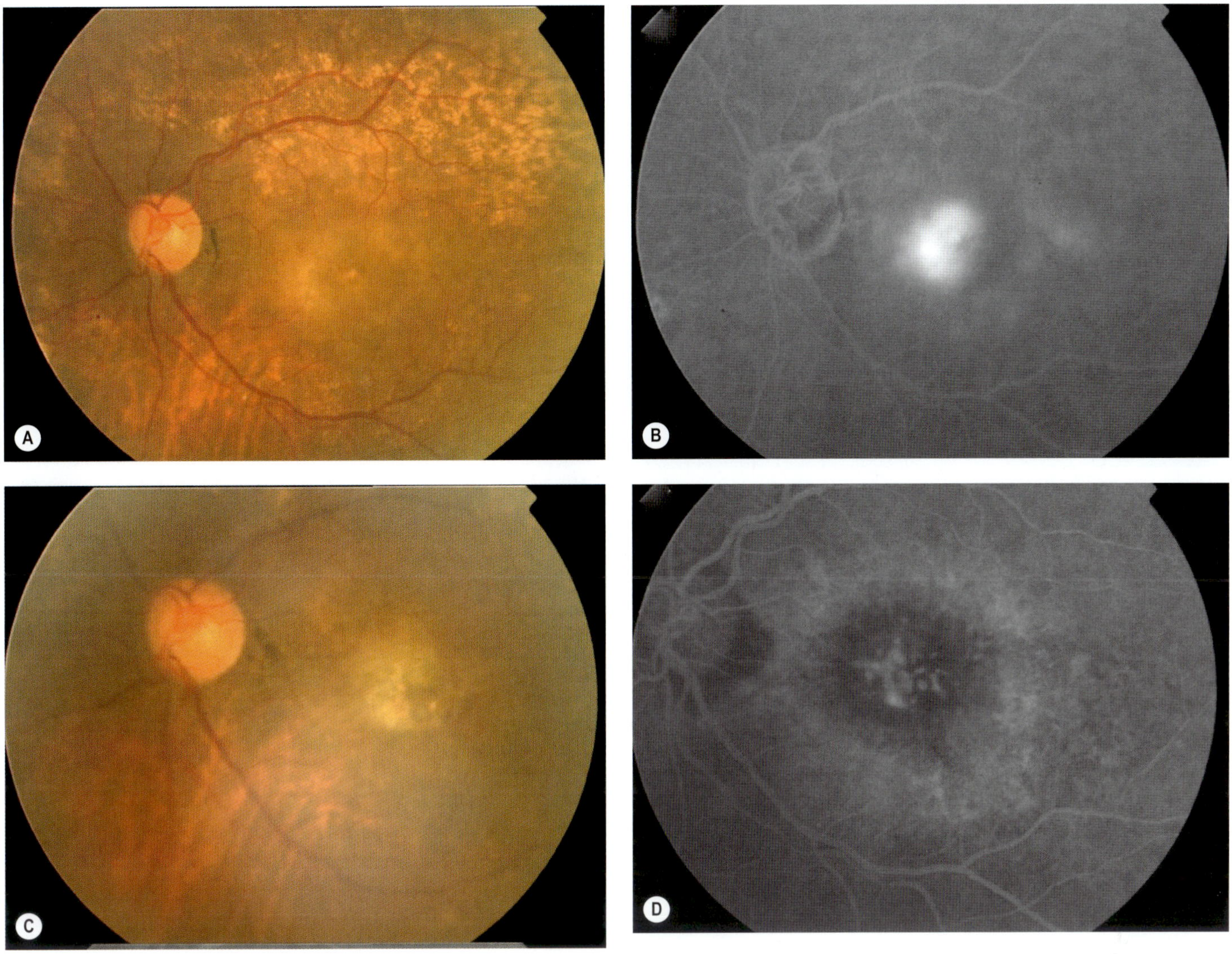

Figure 43.4 Photodynamic therapy (PDT) with verteporfin in age-related macular degeneration. (A) Color fundus photograph and (B) fluorescein angiography of a 76-year-old woman with an active predominantly classic lession and a best corrected visual acuity (BCVA) of 20/400, before treatment. After four courses of PDT with verteporfin, BCVA improved to 20/200 and color fundus photograph (C) and fluorescein angiography (D) showed no subretinal fluid and hyperfluorescent staining with no leakage of fluorescein.

Large-scale, randomized, controlled, double-masked clinical trials have demonstrated that PDT with verteporfin is able to stabilize and, sometime, even to improve the BCVA of patients with subfoveal myopic CNV. At 12-month follow-up, 86% of the verteporfin treated patients lost fewer than 15 letters of BCVA, in comparison to 67% of the placebo-treated patients. At 24-month follow-up, although not statistically significant, the distribution of change in BCVA examination was in favor of the verteporfin-treated group and showed that this group was more likely to have improved BCVA.[20]

OCULAR HISTOPLASMOSIS SYNDROME (OHS)

Median BCVA improved and fluorescein angiographic leakage decreased after PDT with verteporfin for at least 1 year in a small uncontrolled prospective case series of patients with subfoveal CNV caused by OHS. Verteporfin therapy seemed to be safe and well tolerated in these patients. In the prospective 2-year extended study, PDT with verteporfin was associated with maintained or improved BCVA and improved contrast sensitivity in the majority of patients through 48 months of therapy. The low number of treatments required during the extension period demonstrated that the effects of verteporfin therapy on subfoveal CNV in OHS are sustained through at least 4 years.[21]

OTHER SUBFOVEAL AND JUXTAFOVEAL POSTINFLAMMATORY OR IDIOPATHIC CHOROIDAL NEOVASCULARIZATION

PDT with verteporfin has also shown its efficacy in stabilizing BCVA in patients with idiopathic CNV and CNV secondary to postinflammatory conditions, including the following: angioid streaks (Figure 43.5), multifocal choroiditis with panuveitis, punctate inner choroidopathy, sarcoidosis, toxoplasmosis, serpiginous choroiditis, acute posterior pigment placoid epitheliopathy, and sympathetic ophthalmia, among other inflammatory conditions[22] (Figure 43.5).

PDT can also be effective in CNV secondary to central serous chorioretinopathy, macular dystrophy, and parafoveal telangiectasia.

POLYPOIDAL CHOROIDAL VASCULOPATHY

Polypoidal choroidal vasculopathy is characterized by a branching choroidal network with surrounding polypoidal dilatation of the choroidal vessels that causes recurrent serous leakage and hemorrhage.

PDT using verteporfin seems to be the most promising treatment for polypoidal choroidal vasculopathy. At 1-year follow-up, stable or improved vision was achieved in 95% of patients. BCVA improved by

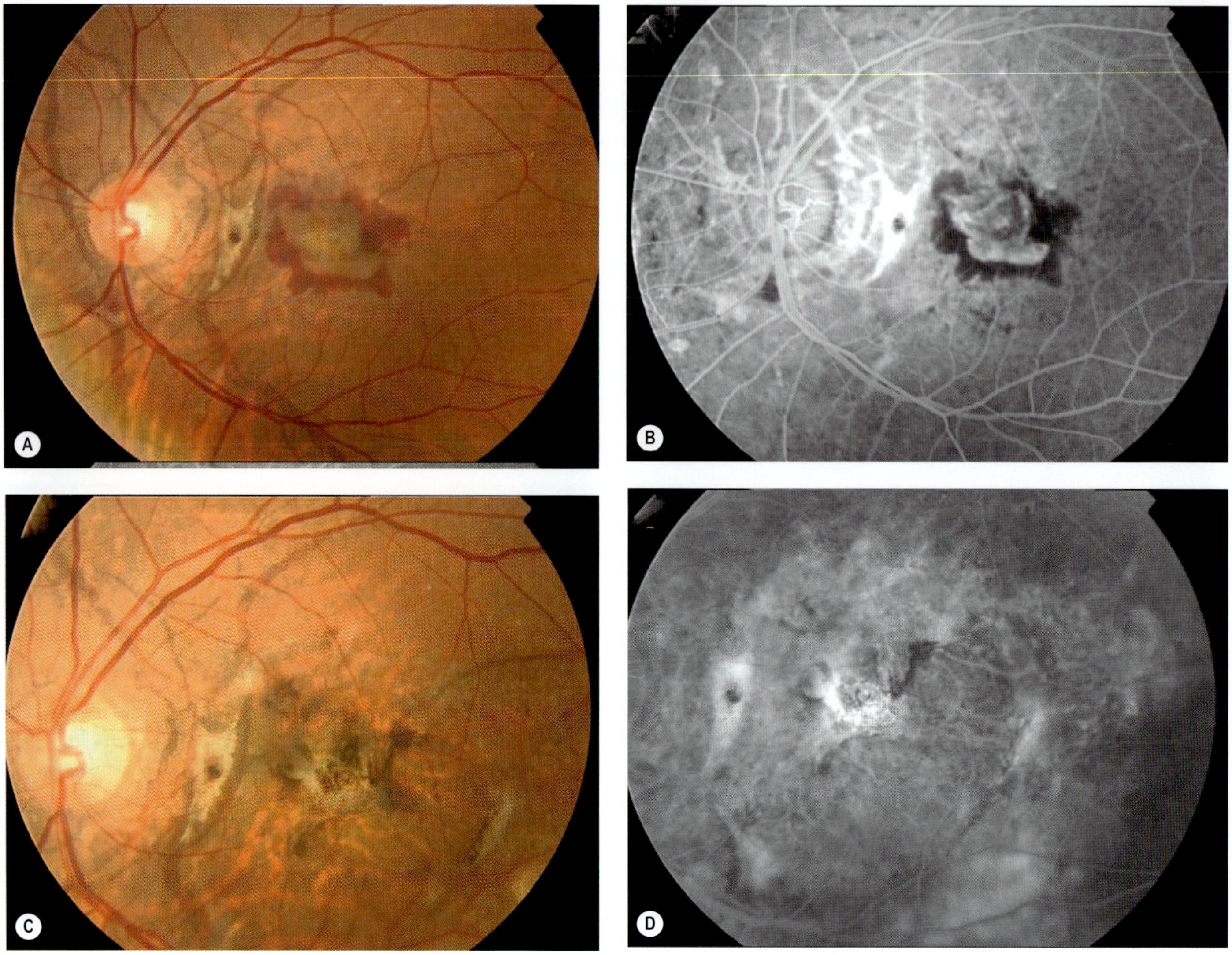

Figure 43.5 Photodynamic therapy (PDT) with verteporfin in choroidal neovascularization secondary to angioid streaks. Color fundus photograph (A) and fluorescein angiography (B) of a 49-year-old woman with active choroidal neovascularization secondary to angioid streaks and a best corrected visual acuity (BCVA) of 20/250, before treatment. After two courses of PDT with verteporfin, BCVA decreased to 20/300 and color fundus photograph (C) and fluorescein angiography (D) showed no subretinal fluid and hyperfluorescent staining with no leakage of fluorescein.

≥3 lines. However, recurrence seriously affects long-term vision during follow-up after PDT.[23] Further studies are needed to determine the efficacy of other treatments besides PDT.

CENTRAL SEROUS CHORIORETINOPATHY

PDT with half-dose verteporfin is effective in treating acute symptomatic central serous chorioretinopathy, resulting in a higher proportion of patients with absence of exudative macular detachment and better BCVA compared with placebo at 12 months.[24]

INTRAOCULAR VASOPROLIFERATIVE TUMORS

Exudative macular changes, such as exudative retinal detachment or cystoid macular edema, may occur in cases of vasoproliferative lesions and may lead to visual function impairment.

Combining PDT with the standard AMD protocol is an effective treatment for choroidal hemangioma in terms of resolution of exudative subretinal fluid and recovery of BCVA.[25]

In patients with idiopathic or secondary vasoproliferative retinal tumors, PDT with verteporfin is also a minimally invasive but effective method of treatment. Retinal tumors showed a marked shrinkage in height and resolution of leakage.[26]

PDT with verteporfin alone or in combination with intravitreal triamcinolone acetonide and/or intravitreal bevacizumab can also cause involution of retinal capillary hemangiomas with reduction in macular edema and improvement in BCVA.[27]

RETINAL ASTROCYTOMA

PDT with verteporfin can induce regression of progressive, vascularized, aggressive retinal astrocytomas and may prevent typical progression to total retinal detachment and enucleation, whether the astrocytoma is associated with tuberous sclerosis or not.[28]

CHOROIDAL OSTEOMA

PDT could be a therapeutic modality for CNV and induction of decalcification of extrafoveal osteoma to prevent tumor growth into the foveola.[29]

CHOROIDAL MELANOMA

PDT with verteporfin has shown promising results in animal studies of choroidal melanoma. However, few patients worldwide have undergone this treatment. In the management of lesions that have failed to respond to brachytherapy and transpupillary thermotherapy, PDT may prevent eyes from undergoing enucleation.[30]

The potential advantage of PDT for lesions close to the macula is a greater potential for preservation of visual acuity. The major disadvantage is the potential for external recurrence despite a normal internal retinal appearance, a complication well described with transpupillary thermotherapy. The role of PDT in this condition, either as primary treatment or as an adjuvant treatment with plaque brachytherapy, remains experimental.

RETINOBLASTOMA

PDT using verteporfin efficiently kills chemotherapy-resistant and non-resistant retinoblastoma cell lines and primary tumor cells *in vitro*, and it warrants further preclinical evaluation as a therapeutic option for the treatment of retinoblastoma.[31]

CONJUNCTIVAL *IN SITU* SQUAMOUS CELL CARCINOMA

There is histopathological evidence that PDT with verteporfin is effective in treating at least *in situ* squamous cell carcinoma. Further studies are required to investigate this proposed modality in order to assess whether cure rates, recurrence rates, and cost-effectiveness are comparable with other treatment modalities.[32]

CORNEAL AND IRIS NEOVASCULARIZATION

PDT with verteporfin may be effective for the treatment of corneal neovascularization secondary to different ocular conditions.[33]

PDT with verteporfin can partially obliterate anterior-segment neovascularizations secondary to ischemic central retinal vein occlusion, preventing the evolution towards advanced stages of neovascular glaucoma, but is not effective in cases with complete angle synechial closure.[34]

PDT has also been effective in recurrent hyphema caused by abnormal intralesional blood vessels after proton beam irradiation of iris melanoma.

EFFICACY AND COMPARISON WITH OTHER AGENTS

Visual outcomes after PDT with verteporfin and other treatment modalities in patients with AMD are shown in Tables 43.1 and 43.2. In terms of general efficacy, PDT with verteporfin is able to prevent further severe visual loss. In AMD, the risk of a significant loss in vision is reduced to 50% compared to the spontaneous course of the disease.[13]

The recent development of anti-VEGF substances for use in clinical routine has markedly improved the prognosis of patients with neovascular AMD. Intravitreal treatment with substances targeting all isotypes of VEGF provide vision maintenance in over 90% and substantial improvement in 25–40% of patients with AMD.[35,36] However, PDT using verteporfin seems to be the most promising treatment for polypoidal choroidal vasculopathy.[23]

Verteporfin may still play an important role in the management of these patients, as the combination with occlusive therapies like PDT with verteporfin may offer a reduction of retreatment frequency and long-term maintenance of the treatment benefit.[16]

CONTRAINDICATIONS

PDT with verteporfin is contraindicated for patients with porphyria or a known hypersensitivity to any component of this preparation.

OCULAR COMPLICATIONS AND TOXICITY

Verteporfin therapy is a particularly safe treatment in terms of ocular safety. In AMD patients, serious adverse events, including acute severe vision loss, arteriolar or venular nonperfusion, retinal capillary nonperfusion, or vitreous hemorrhage, occurred in 3.8% of verteporfin-treated patients and 1.4% of placebo recipients. Severe vision loss (defined as a decrease of at least 4 lines of visual acuity occurring within 7 days of treatment) occurs rarely and is more often seen in the treatment of large occult lesions with a high initial BCVA.[37]

Table 43.2 Improvement of ≥ 3 lines with different treatments in age-related macular degeneration

Treatment modality	Lesion type	Study	Control	Difference	Study
PDT	Predominantly + minimum classic CNV	9%	4%	5%	TAP: 24 months
	Occult CNV	5%	1%	4%	VIP: 24 months
Pegabtanib 0.3 mg	All CNV subtypes	6%	2%	4%	VISION: 24 months
Ranibizumab 0.5 mg	Predominantly. classic CNV	41%	6%	35%	ANCHOR: 24 months
	Minimum classic + occult CNV	33%	4%	29%	MARINA: 24 months
Ranibizumab 0.5 mg (3-monthly)	All CNV types	13%	10%	3%	PIER: 12 months
Combination PDT–ranibizumab	Predominantly classic CNV	24%	5%	19%	FOCUS: 12 months

PDT, photodynamic therapy; CNV, choroidal neovascularization; TAP, treatment of age-related macular degeneration with photodynamic therapy; VIP, Verteporfin in Photodynamic Therapy study; VISION, VEGF Inhibition Study in Ocular Neovascularization; ANCHOR, Anti-VEGF antibody for the treatment of predominantly classic choroidal neovascularization in age-related macular degeneration; MARINA, Minimally classic/occult trial of the anti-VEGF antibody ranibizumab in the treatment of neovascular age-related macular degeneration; PIER, A phase IIIB multicenter, randomized, double-masked, sham injection controlled study of the efficacy and safety of ranibizumab in subjects with subfoveal CNV with or without classic CNV secondary to age-related macular degeneration; FOCUS, A phase I/II, single-masked multicenter study of the safety, tolerability, and efficacy of multiple-dose intravitreal injections of rhuFab V2 I combination with verteporfin (Visudyne) photodynamic therapy in subjects with neovascular age-related macular degeneration.

In lesions with serous detachment of the RPE, mechanical rips were observed. Expanding pigment epithelial detachments (PEDs) and those with nonhomogeneous filling may represent high-risk lesions because they may eventually exert sufficient tangential stress to result in a spontaneous tear.[38] In retinal angiomatous proliferation, RPE tears are more common when the PED exceeds 50% of the lesion. Visual recovery after RPE tear is uncommon but possible in some instances, especially when the fovea is spared and conserves the RPE.

No cases of retinal arteriole or venular nonperfusion were reported at the 50 J/cm^2 light dose used in the clinical studies or in clinical practice. However, in the phase I/II dose-finding study, retinal arteriole and venular nonperfusion were seen at a higher light dose of 150 J/cm^2. These data suggest that, to provide safe and effective treatment, the recommended light dose of 50 J/cm^2 should not be exceeded.

The most frequently reported ocular adverse events were transient visual disturbances, which were reported at an incidence of 12.4–29.8% in verteporfin-treated patients and 6.8–12.8% in placebo patients.

No clinically significant ocular adverse events occurred in either treatment group in patients with pathologic myopia or OHS.[20,21]

SYSTEMIC COMPLICATIONS AND TOXICITY

Verteporfin therapy is a particularly safe treatment in terms of systemic safety.

The most frequently reported nonocular adverse events to PDT with verteporfin are injection site reactions (including pain, edema, inflammation, extravasation, rashes, hemorrhage, and discoloration).[37]

Table 43.3 show the ocular and nonocular adverse events, listed by body system, that were reported more frequently with verteporfin therapy than with placebo therapy and occurred in 1–10% of patients.

Photosensitivity reactions were reported in 2.2% of patients. Compliance with photosensitivity protection instructions will minimize the potential for photosensitivity reactions.

Table 43.3 Adverse events, listed by body system, that were reported more frequently with verteporfin therapy than with placebo therapy and occurred in 1–10% of patients

Ocular treatment site	Blepharitis, cataracts, conjunctivitis/conjunctival injection, dry eyes, ocular itching, severe vision decrease with or without subretinal/retinal or vitreous hemorrhage
Body as a whole	Asthenia, fever, flu syndrome, infusion-related pain primarily presenting as back pain, photosensitivity reactions
Cardiovascular	Atrial fibrillation, hypertension, peripheral vascular disorder, varicose veins
Dermatologic	Eczema
Digestive	Constipation, gastrointestinal cancers, nausea
Hematic and lymphatic	Anemia, decreased white blood cell count, increased white blood cell count
Hepatic	Elevated liver function tests
Metabolic/nutritional	Albuminuria, creatinine increased
Musculoskeletal	Arthralgia, arthrosis, myasthenia
Nervous system	Hypesthesia, sleep disorder, vertigo
Respiratory	Cough, pharyngitis, pneumonia
Special senses	Cataracts, decreased hearing, diplopia, lacrimation disorder
Urogenital	Prostatic disorder

PDT with verteporfin does not appear to cause teratogenicity, mutagenicity, hepatotoxicity, or significant cardiovascular toxicity.[39]

However, PDT has been reported to result in DNA damage. No studies have been conducted to evaluate the carcinogenic potential of verteporfin. It is not known how the potential for DNA damage with PDT agents translates into human risk. No effect on male or female fertility has been observed in rats following intravenous administration of verteporfin for injection up to 10 mg/kg/day.

PDT with verteporfin has a pregnancy category of C. Studies in animals have revealed adverse effects on fetus but there are no controlled studies in women. Thus, verteporfin should be given only if the potential benefit justifies the potential risk to the fetus.

Verteporfin and its diacid metabolite have been found in the breast milk of one woman after a 6 mg/m^2 infusion. Because of the potential for serious adverse reactions in nursing infants from verteporfin, a decision should be made whether to discontinue nursing or postpone treatment, taking into account the importance of the drug to the mother.

Safety and effectiveness in pediatric patients have not been established.

Multiple-dose studies in rats and dogs given intravenous verteporfin with and without light application showed treatment-related hematopoietic effects in the bone marrow, liver, and spleen only at doses at least 66 times higher than the single 6 mg/m^2 body surface area (approximately 0.15 mg/kg) dose of Visudyne used clinically at 3-month intervals.[39]

DRUG INTERACTIONS

Drug interaction studies in humans have not been conducted with PDT with verteporfin.

Verteporfin is rapidly eliminated by the liver, mainly as unchanged drug. Metabolism is limited and occurs by liver and plasma esterases. Microsomal cytochrome P450 does not appear to play a role in verteporfin metabolism. Thus, clinically significant drug–drug interactions are unlikely, as NADPH-dependent enzymes, such as cytochrome P450 isozymes, do not play a significant role in verteporfin metabolism.[4]

Based on the mechanism of action of verteporfin, many drugs used concomitantly could influence the effect of PDT with verteporfin. Calcium channel blockers, polymyxin B, or radiation therapy could enhance the rate of verteporfin uptake by the vascular endothelium. On the contrary, compounds that quench active oxygen species or scavenge radicals (e.g., dimethyl sulfoxide, β-carotene, ethanol, formate, and mannitol), and drugs that decrease clotting, vasoconstriction or platelet aggregation (e.g., thromboxane A_2 inhibitors), may decrease PDT with verteporfin activity.

However, no obvious drug–drug interactions were seen in the pivotal placebo-controlled studies of PDT with verteporfin, in which 95% of the population received concomitant medications. including some of the above classes of agents.

It is possible that other photosensitizing agents (e.g., tetracyclines, sulfonamides, phenothiazines, sulfonylurea hypoglycemic agents, thiazide diuretics, and griseofulvin) could increase the potential for skin photosensitivity reactions.

SUMMARY AND KEY POINTS

Veteporfin is a second-generation photosensitizer, displaying rapid clearance and consequently a reduced period of skin photosensitivity compared with the first-generation photosensitizer, porfimer sodium.

PDT with verteporfin is a disease site-specific treatment modality that is particularly safe in terms of both systemic and ocular safety. It involves the local or systemic administration of a lipophilic photosensitizing drug that selectively accumulates within rapidly dividing cells, such as neovascular endothelial cells, tumor cells, as well as activated cells of the immune system, followed by irradiating the targeted disease site with nonthermal visible light of appropriate wavelength. In the presence of molecular oxygen, the activation of the photosensitizer and energy transfer can lead to a series of photochemical reactions and generation of various cytotoxic species (e.g., singlet oxygen and other reactive oxygen species), and consequently induce apoptosis and necrosis of targeted cells and tissues.

PDT with verteporfin is an established treatment for oncological disorders and nononcological disorders, such as AMD and immune-mediated conditions.

In ophthalmology, PDT with verteporfin is FDA-approved for the treatment of patients with predominantly classic subfoveal CNV due to AMD, pathologic myopia, or presumed ocular histoplasmosis.

Verteporfin therapy is a particularly safe treatment in terms of both systemic and ocular safety. In terms of general efficacy, the treatment is able to prevent further severe visual loss in patients with neovascular AMD with predominantly classic CNV.[11–14]

In patients with polypoidal choroidal vasculopathy, PDT with verteporfin seems to be the most promising treatment.[23] Further studies are needed to determine the efficacy of other treatments.

The recent development of anti-VEGF substances for use in clinical routine has markedly improved the prognosis of patients with neovascular AMD. Intravitreal treatment with substances targeting all isotypes of VEGF provide vision maintenance in over 90% and substantial improvement in 25–40% of patients.[35,36]

However, verteporfin may still play an important role in the management of these patients, as the combination with occlusive therapies like PDT with verteporfin may offer a reduction of retreatment frequency and long-term maintenance of the treatment benefit.

REFERENCES

1. Aveline B, Hasan T, Redmond RW. Photophysical and photosensitizing properties of benzoporphyrin derivative monoacid ring A (BPD-MA). Photochem Photobiol 1994;59:328–335.
2. Schmidt-Erfurth U, Hasan T. Mechanisms of action of photodynamic therapy with verteporfin for the treatment of age-related macular degeneration. Surv Ophthalmol 2000;45:195–214.
3. Li JH, Chen YP, Zhao SD, et al. Application of hematoporphyrin derivative and laser-induced photodynamical reaction in the treatment of lung cancer: a preliminary report on 21 cases. Lasers Surg Med 1984;4(1):31–37.
4. Houle JM, Strong A. Clinical pharmacokinetics of verteporfin. J Clin Pharmacol 2002 May;42(5):547–557.
5. Allison BA, Pritchard PH, Levy JG. Evidence for low-density lipoprotein receptor-mediated uptake of benzoporphyrin derivative. Br J Cancer 1994;69:833–839.
6. Chen WR, Singhal AK, Liu H, et al. Antitumor immunity induced by laser immunotherapy and its adoptive transfer. Cancer Res 2001;61:459–461.
7. Rousset N, Vonarx V, Eléouet S, et al. Effects of photodynamic therapy on adhesion molecules and metastasis. J Photochem Photobiol B 1999;52(1–3):65–73.
8. Pervaiz S, Olivo M. Art and science of photodynamic therapy. Clin Exp Pharmacol Physiol 2006;33:551–556.
9. Bissonnette R, McLean DI, Reid G, et al. Photodynamic therapy of psoriasis and psoriatic arthritis with BPD verteporfin. 7th Biennial Congress of the International Photodynamic Association; 1998 Jul 7–9; Nantes France, RC87: abstract no. 87.
10. Hendrich C, Huttmann G, Vispo-Seara JL, et al. Experimental photodynamic laser therapy for rheumatoid arthritis with a second generation photosensitizer. Knee Surg Sports Traumatol Arthrosc 2000;8(3):190–194.
11. Kaiser PK. Treatment of Age-Related Macular Degeneration with Photodynamic Therapy (TAP) Study Group. Verteporfin therapy of subfoveal choroidal neovascularization in age-related macular degeneration: 5-year results of two randomized clinical trials with an open-label extension: TAP report no. 8. Graefes Arch Clin Exp Ophthalmol 2006 Sep;244(9):1132–1142.
12. Bressler NM. Photodynamic therapy of subfoveal choroidal neovascularization in age-related macular degeneration with verteporfin: two-year results of 2 randomized clinical trials. TAP report 2. Arch Ophthalmol 2001;119:198–207.
13. Pieramici DJ, Bressler SB, Koester JM, et al. Occult with no classic subfoveal choroidal neovascular lesions in age-related macular degeneration: clinically relevant natural history information in larger lesions with good vision from the Verteporfin in Photodynamic Therapy (VIP) trial: VIP report no. 4. Arch Ophthalmol 2006;124:660–664.
14. VIP Study Group. Verteporfin therapy of subfoveal choroidal neovascularization in age-related macular degeneration: two-year results of a randomized clinical trial including lesions with occult with no classic choroidal neovascularization. Am J Ophthalmol 2001;131:541–560.
15. Kaiser PK. Visudyne In Occult CNV (VIO) study group. Verteporfin PDT for subfoveal occult CNV in AMD: two-year results of a randomized trial. Curr Med Res Opin 2009 Aug;25(8):1853–1860.
16. Schmidt-Erfurth U, Schlötzer-Schrehard U, Cursiefen C, Michels S, Beckendorf A, Naumann GO. Influence of photodynamic therapy on expression of vascular endothelial growth factor (VEGF), VEGF receptor 3, and pigment epithelium-derived factor. Invest Ophthalmol Vis Sci 2003 Oct;44(10):4473–4480.
17. Maberley D, Canadian Retinal Trials Group. Photodynamic Therapy and Intravitreal Triamcinolone for Neovascular Age-Related Macular Degeneration A Randomized Clinical Trial. Ophthalmology 2009 Sep 11. [Epub ahead of print]
18. Schmidt-Erfurth UM, Richard G, Augustin A, et al. Guidance for the treatment of neovascular age-related macular degeneration. Acta Ophthalmol Scand 2007 Aug;85(5):486–494.
19. Frank Holz. Preliminary results of the MONTBLANC study. The 2009 International AMD and Retina Congress. Athens, Greece. October 2009.
20. Verteporfin in Photodynamic Therapy Study Group. Photodynamic therapy of subfoveal choroidal neovascularization in pathologic myopia with verteporfin. 1-year results of a randomized clinical trial-VIP report no. 1. Ophthalmology 2001;108:841–852.
21. Saperstein DA, Rosenfeld PJ, Bressler NM, et al. Verteporfin therapy for CNV secondary to OHS. Ophthalmology 2006 Dec;113(12):2371.e1–2371.e3.
22. Ruiz-Moreno JM, Montero JA, Arias L, et al. Photodynamic therapy in subfoveal and juxtafoveal idiopathic and postinflammatory choroidal neovascularization. Acta Ophthalmol Scand 2006 Dec;84(6):743–748.
23. Gomi F, Tano Y. Polypoidal choroidal vasculopathy and treatments. Curr Opin Ophthalmol 2008 May;19(3):208–212.
24. Chan WM, Lai TY, Lai RY, et al. Half-dose verteporfin photodynamic therapy for acute central serous chorioretinopathy: one-year results of a randomized controlled trial. Ophthalmology 2008 Oct;115(10):1756–1765.
25. Michels S, Michels R, Simader C, et al. Verteporfin therapy for choroidal hemangioma: a long-term follow-up. Retina 2005 Sep;25(6):697–703.
26. Blasi MA, Scupola A, Tiberti AC, et al. Photodynamic therapy for vasoproliferative retinal tumors. Retina 2006 Apr;26(4):404–409.
27. Ziemssen F, Voelker M, Inhoffen W, et al. Combined treatment of a juxtapapillary retinal capillary haemangioma with intravitreal bevacizumab and photodynamic therapy. Eye 2007 Aug;21(8):1125–1126.
28. Eskelin S, Tommila P, Palosaari T, Kivelä T. Photodynamic therapy with verteporfin to induce regression of aggressive retinal astrocytomas. Acta Ophthalmol 2008 Nov;86(7):794–799.
29. Shields CL, Materin MA, Mehta S, et al. Regression of extrafoveal choroidal osteoma following photodynamic therapy. Arch Ophthalmol 2008 Jan;126(1):135–137.
30. Barbazetto IA, Lee TC, Rollins IS, et al. Treatment of choroidal melanoma using photodynamic therapy. Am J Ophthalmol 2003;135:898–899.
31. Stephan H, Boeloeni R, Eggert A, et al. Photodynamic therapy in retinoblastoma: effects of verteporfin on retinoblastoma cell lines. Invest Ophthalmol Vis Sci 2008 Jul;49(7):3158–3163.
32. Sears KS, Rundle PR, Mudhar HS, et al. The effects of photodynamic therapy on conjunctival *in situ* squamous cell carcinoma – a review of the histopathology. Br J Ophthalmol 2008 May;92(5):716–717.
33. Yoon KC, You IC, Kang IS, et al. Photodynamic therapy with verteporfin for corneal neovascularization. Am J Ophthalmol 2007 Sep;144(3):390–395.
34. Parodi MB, Iacono P, Ravalico G. Verteporfin photodynamic therapy for anterior segment neovascularization secondary to ischaemic central retinal vein occlusion. Clin Experiment Ophthalmol 2008 Apr;36(3):232–237.
35. Rosenfeld PJ, Brown DM, Heier JS, et al. Ranibizumab for neovascular age-related macular degeneration. N Engl J Med 2006;355:1419–1431.
36. Brown DM, Kaiser PK, Michels M, Soubrane G, Heier JS, Kim RY, Sy JP, Schneider S, ANCHOR Study Group. Ranibizumab versus verteporfin for neovascular age-related macular degeneration. N Engl J Med 2006 Oct 5;355(14):1432–1444.
37. Azab M, Benchaboune M, Blinder KJ, et al. Verteporfin therapy of subfoveal choroidal neovascularization in age-related macular degeneration: meta-analysis of 2-year safety results in three randomized clinical trials: treatment of age-related macular degeneration with photodynamic therapy and verteporfin in photodynamic therapy study report no. 4. Retina 2004 Feb;24(1):1–12.
38. Chang LK, Flaxel CJ, Lauer AK, Sarraf D. RPE tears after pegaptanib treatment in age-related macular degeneration. Retina 2007 Sep;27(7):857–863.
39. QLT Inc. Clinical Investigator's Brochure. BPD-MA (verteporfin). 2003 (Data on File).

CHAPTER

44

Chemotherapy for malignant intraocular tumors

Chirag P. Shah, MD, MPH, Carol L. Shields, MD, and Jerry A. Shields, MD

KEY FEATURES

Chemotherapeutic approaches, including chemoreduction (CRD), chemothermotherapy, periocular and intravitreal chemotherapy, and intra-arterial chemotherapy, are effective tools in managing different types of ocular tumors. Treatments are often individualized to patient and tumor types to yield best possible outcomes.

INTRODUCTION

Chemotherapy for intraocular malignancies has evolved since 1953, when nitrogen mustard (chlormethine) was first used to treat retinoblastoma.[1] This chapter discusses chemotherapy for retinoblastoma, uveal metastases, uveal melanoma, and intraocular lymphoma.

RETINOBLASTOMA (Tables 44.1 and 44.2)

GENERAL CONSIDERATIONS

Retinoblastoma is the most common primary intraocular malignancy in children, with an incidence of 1 in 15 000 live births.[2] Treatment of this tumor has evolved over the last several decades, increasing rates of survival, globe salvage, and visual preservation. Currently available options include laser photocoagulation, thermotherapy, cryotherapy, intravenous CRD, subconjunctival chemotherapy (carboplatin), plaque radiotherapy, external beam radiotherapy (EBRT), and enucleation.

Most experts consider enucleation to be the standard of care for advanced unilateral disease, defined as eyes with large tumors (20 mm in base, 10 mm in height), long-standing retinal detachment, neovascular glaucoma, iris neovascularization or seeding, suspicion of optic nerve or choroid invasion or extrascleral extension, or no expectation for useful vision.[3] Enucleation affords greater than a 99% cure rate in cases of unilateral retinoblastoma without extraocular disease.[4]

Retinoblastoma is a radiosensitive tumor, responding to plaque radiotherapy or EBRT. Episcleral plaque radiotherapy can help treat small solitary lesions up to 18 mm in diameter.[5] Low-energy plaques, those using iodine-125 or palladium-103, provide localized irradiation and minimize effect to the orbit and surrounding soft tissues.[2,5,6] Historically, EBRT was a common and effective treatment alternative to enucleation. Recurrence after EBRT is low, usually occurring within 2 years of treatment.[7,8]

Several reasons contributed to the emergence of CRD as an alternative to EBRT, including risk of disfiguration and secondary tumors.[9] These tumors are mostly osseous and soft-tissue sarcomas,[10] and are more common in children carrying the Rb-1 germline mutation.[9,11] Moreover, children younger than 12 months of age are more prone to the soft-tissue and bone tumors of the head associated with EBRT[12]; CRD can delay its use.

The selection of an appropriate treatment strategy for an individual patient is based on multiple factors, including risk of metastases or second cancers, laterality of disease, systemic status, size and location of tumor(s), and estimated visual prognosis.[13] One group of experts offers a general guideline. For unilateral retinoblastoma, International Classification of Retinoblastoma (ICRB) group A is usually treated with cryotherapy or laser photocoagulation; groups B and C are treated with either CRD or plaque radiotherapy; group D lesions receive CRD plus subconjunctival carboplatin or enucleation, and group E eyes are enucleated. For bilateral retinoblastoma, which is managed according to the worse eye, group A tumors are usually treated with cryotherapy or laser photocoagulation; groups B and C receive CRD; group D eyes receive CRD plus subconjunctival carboplatin or enucleation; group E eyes are enucleated unless both eyes are advanced, in which case CRD with subconjunctival carboplatin and low-dose EBRT is attempted.[13]

CHEMOREDUCTION

CRD is a strategy that combines chemotherapeutic tumor debulking with localized ophthalmic treatment (laser photocoagulation, thermotherapy, cryotherapy, or plaque radiotherapy). The strategy involves administration of intravenous chemotherapy for several cycles, coupled with focal therapy after the second or third cycle once adequate reduction in tumor size and subretinal fluid has been achieved.[14–18]

The indications for CRD have not yet been clearly established. CRD has been used for all retinoblastomas except in unilateral cases undergoing primary enucleation or in certain ICRB group A cases that can be treated with cryotherapy or laser photocoagulation alone. Some experts use CRD for all nonenucleated eyes.[19] One group[11] classifies the indications for CRD into three general categories: eyes with visual potential containing tumors too large to treat with focal treatments, children less than 1 year of age to avoid or postpone the adverse risks of EBRT, and, by some experts, any advanced unilateral or bilateral retinoblastoma.

AGENTS

CRD protocols vary in regimen and duration per center, precluding a universally accepted standard recommendation. Regimens generally use three agents: alkylating agents (carboplatin, cisplatin), DNA topoisomerase II inhibitors (etoposide, teniposide), and vinca alkaloids (vincristine). Most recent studies use vincristine, etoposide, and carboplatin (VEC) for six cycles.[20] Excluding etoposide for its potential oncogenic risk, CRD regimens using only carboplatin and vincristine do elicit tumor response. However, when compared to regimens employing etoposide as a third agent, two-agent regimens have inferior recurrence and ocular salvage rates (83% ocular salvage rate in total for Reese–Ellsworth I–III, 63% without EBRT).[21] Other experts selectively choose between two- and three-agent regimens, treating ICRB group B tumors with two agents and more advanced tumors with three agents.[13] Carboplatin has been used as a single agent, proving effectiveness against retinoblastoma but less so than multiagent regimens.[22] Almost half (47%) of eyes initially treated with carboplatin developed new tumors.[23]

Table 44.1 Reese–Ellsworth classification of retinoblastoma

Group I: very favorable for maintenance of sight

(a) Solitary tumor, smaller than 4 disc diameters, at or behind the equator
(b) Multiple tumors, none larger than 4 disc diameters, all at or behind the equator

Group II: favorable for maintenance of sight

(a) Solitary tumor, 4–10 disc diameters at or behind the equator
(b) Multiple tumors, 4–10 disc diameters behind the equator

Group III: possible for maintenance of sight

(a) Any lesion anterior to the equator
(b) Solitary tumor, larger than 10 disc diameters behind the equator

Group IV: unfavorable for maintenance of sight

(a) Multiple tumors, some larger than 10 disc diameters
(b) Any lesion extending anteriorly to the ora serrata

Group V: very unfavorable for maintenance of sight

(a) Massive tumors involving more than one-half the retina
(b) Vitreous seeding

Table 44.2 International classification system for intraocular retinoblastoma[13]

Group	Quick reference	Specific features
A	Small tumor	Retinoblastoma up to ≤ 3 mm in size
B	Larger tumor Macula Juxtapapillary Subretinal fluid	Retinoblastoma > 3 mm in size, macular location (≤ 3 mm to foveola), juxtapapillary location (≤ 1.5 mm to disc), or minor subretinal fluid (≤ 3 mm from margin)
C	Focal seeds	Retinoblastoma with localized subretinal and/or vitreal seeds (≤ 3 mm from tumor)
D	Diffuse seeds	Retinoblastoma with diffuse subretinal and/or vitreal seeds (> 3 mm from tumor)
E	Extensive	Extensive retinoblastoma occupying > 50% of the globe; or neovascular glaucoma; or opaque media from hemorrhage in anterior chamber, vitreous, or subretinal space; or invasion of postlaminar optic nerve, choroid (> 2 mm), sclera, orbit, anterior chamber

Cyclosporine is an adjuvant agent employed by some experts for CRD. *In vitro,* cyclosporine blocks the multidrug-resistant P-glycoprotein (an adenosine triphosphate membrane transport protein) found in 30% of untreated, enucleated retinoblastoma eyes, thereby blocking a cell's ability to clear antineoplastic drugs.[16,24] A study treated 40 eyes that would have otherwise undergone enucleation or EBRT with variable chemotherapeutic regimens that included cyclosporine. The authors reported an 85% rate of tumor control, better than the 37% rate reported in their prior study that did not use cyclosporine.[25] Further, 7 of 9 cases responded to the regimen with cyclosporine after failing prior CRD without cyclosporine.

Though experts agree that tumor control with CRD requires local consolidation with laser photocoagulation, thermotherapy, cryotherapy, or plaque radiotherapy, there is no consensus on its timing. Several authors have suggested that focal treatments can usually be administered after two to three cycles of CRD, given that tumors have nearly reached their maximal reduction after two cycles.[16,26] The type and timing of focal treatments require clinical judgment to tailor management for individual patients.

RESULTS

Ocular salvage rates have improved with the advent of CRD.[18] Six cycles of CRD with vincristine, etoposide, and carboplatin plus local treatment with thermotherapy or cryotherapy are highly successful in avoiding enucleation or EBRT, particularly for tumors with lower ICRB classifications. A series of 249 eyes reported success in 100% of group A, 93% of group B, 90% of group C, and 47% of group D eyes. Group E eyes were managed with primary enucleation.[6] For Reese–Ellsworth group V eyes treated with CRD, a meta-analysis of nine studies found only 37% avoided both enucleation and EBRT; 41% required EBRT but avoided enucleation; and 40% required eventual enucleation[11] (Figures 44.1 and 44.2).

Moreover, CRD may decrease the incidence of intracranial neuroblastic malignancy (trilateral retinoblastoma), a highly fatal malignancy associated with retinoblastoma.[27] It remains possible, though, that the absence of EBRT, and not the addition of CRD, deserves credit for decreased incidence of intracranial neuroblastic malignancy.[28]

CHEMOREDUCTION FAILURE

There are several possible explanations owing to CRD failure. The presence of subretinal seeds at time of CRD portends a higher risk of retinal tumor and vitreous seed recurrence.[29] Subretinal and vitreal seeds initially respond to CRD, but can recur later, requiring additional treatment.[18,20,29] Most cases can be managed with cryotherapy or plaque brachytherapy, but some require EBRT or enucleation. Some experts feel seed dispersion can be induced or exacerbated by CRD, as tumors can fragment while they regress, dispelling seeds into the vitreous.[30] Further, persistent seeds may represent inadequate chemotherapeutic penetration into the vitreous cavity or avascular subretinal areas.[4] Another explanation for failure is that CRD does not appear to have a prophylactic effect against new retinoblastoma tumors, possibly representing primary tumor resistance, selection of a resistant tumor cell line, or inadequate chemotherapeutic concentrations within small, minimally vascularized tumor foci.[31] Tumors unresponsive to CRD may be well-differentiated.[32,33]

SIDE-EFFECTS

The adverse effects of chemotherapeutic agents must be considered in counseling patients. Common side-effects include fatigue, nausea, vomiting, diarrhea, fever, leucopenia, thrombocytopenia, anemia, and vincristine neurotoxicity.[34] Ototoxicity is a potential side-effect of carboplatin, though clinically this risk appears to be minimal. A study examining 164 children who received six cycles of carboplatin (18.6 mg/kg every 4 weeks) failed to reveal any carboplatin-related hearing impairment.[35] Secondary acute myelogenous leukemia may be associated with chemotherapy.[36] Patients with hereditary, or germline, retinoblastoma are already at increased risk for secondary malignancy.[10,37] The largest study evaluating secondary acute myelogenous leukemia, a retrospective multicentered study of 15 cases, suggested that this rare secondary malignancy might be associated with topoisomerase II inhibitor and epipodophyllotoxin therapy for retinoblastoma.[36] Ophthalmic

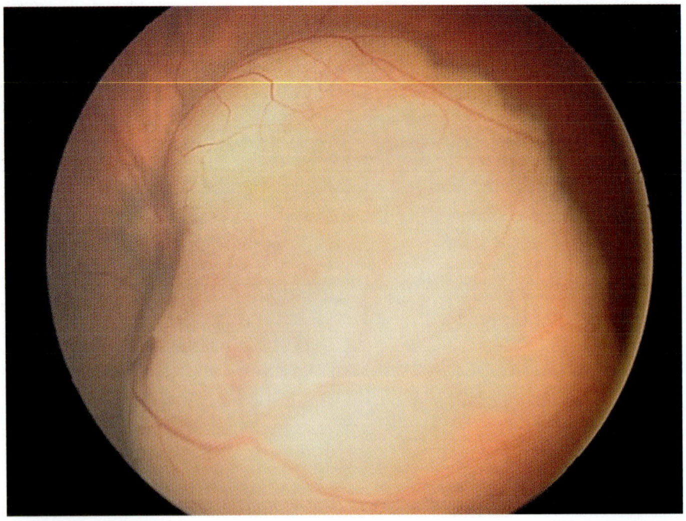

Figure 44.1 Retinoblastoma before chemoreduction.

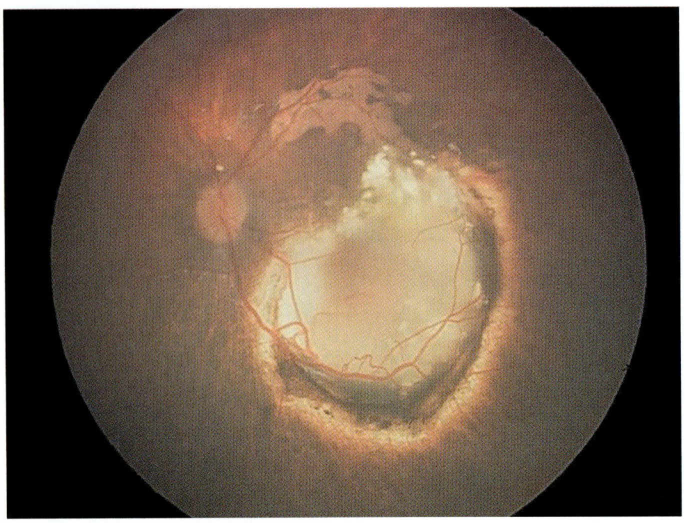

Figure 44.2 Retinoblastoma after chemoreduction.

complications include rhegmatogenous retinal detachment noted next to cryotherapy scars[38] and intraocular cholesterolosis.[39]

CHEMOTHERMOTHERAPY

Chemothermotherapy involves laser thermotherapy in conjunction with intravenous carboplatin. This technique is used for smaller retinoblastomas, those with minimal seeding or subretinal fluid, in effort to limit the amount of chemotherapy administered. In a study of 103 small to medium-sized tumors (1.5–12 mm in diameter), 92% were treated without EBRT.[40]

PERIOCULAR AND SUBCONJUNCTIVAL CHEMOTHERAPY

In primates, peribulbar and episcleral carboplatin was found to have increased intraocular concentrations compared to intravenous delivery.[41] Subconjunctival carboplatin was administered to 13 human eyes with retinoblastoma. Vitreal seeds responded well, unlike subretinal lesions.[42] There was one case of optic neuropathy. A subsequent study reported four cases of optic nerve atrophy after periocular carboplatin treatment, finding ischemic necrosis and atrophy in the retrobulbar optic nerve along with dystrophic calcification and inflammation in the surrounding fibrovascular tissue.[43] Subtenon carboplatin administered through a conjunctival incision was associated with significant fibrosis of orbital soft tissue, restricting ocular motility and complicating subsequent enucleation.[44] The authors of the initial subconjunctival carboplatin trial now suggest that peribulbar injections may have a role in salvaging advanced retinoblastoma eyes, particularly those with vitreous and subretinal seeds, but further study is needed to determine the safety and applicability of this treatment option.[4]

INTRAVITREAL CHEMOTHERAPY

Intravitreal chemotherapy has been used in an attempt to salvage an only eye with recurrent retinoblastoma unresponsive to conventional therapy. Of note, intraocular injection or surgery increases the risk of extraocular tumor seeding. Intravitreal thiotepa, an alkylating agent, had mixed success in two case series evaluating this agent. Four of six total eyes required eventual enucleation or exenteration, while two eyes appeared stable after vitrectomy and intravitreal thiotepa injections.[45,46] Another group[47] used intravitreal melphalan for recurrent vitreal seeds in 41 patients, reporting tumor control in 56% of eyes. No extraocular dissemination of tumor cells was experienced, but further study is needed to evaluate the safety and applicability of this technique.

INTRA-ARTERIAL CHEMOTHERAPY

Using selective intra-arterial cannulation, some experts have pioneered the delivery of melphalan directly into the ophthalmic artery.[47] At the present time, this technology remains experimental but may hold promise as a novel treatment modality for retinoblastoma and other intraocular tumors in the future.

ADJUVANT CHEMOTHERAPY

In the absence of overt metastatic disease, there are some definitive conclusions – and some controversial considerations – regarding the role of postenucleation adjuvant chemotherapy based on histopathologic findings. Such findings thought to be associated with increased risk of relapse include involvement of the choroid, sclera, or cut margin of the optic nerve.[48] Other debatable risk factors for metastases include anterior-chamber seeding, iris infiltration, ciliary body infiltration, and invasion of the optic nerve lamina cribrosa.[49] There is no consensus on the best chemotherapy regimen for adjuvant treatment. Though treatment protocols vary by center, many experts use cyclophosphamide and vincristine with or without EBRT.[50–52] Others have used vincristine, doxorubicin, and cyclophosphamide, or vincristine, etoposide, and carboplatin.[49]

NO CHOROIDAL, SCLERAL, OR POSTLAMINAR OPTIC NERVE INVOLVEMENT

Patients with no risk factors for extraocular relapse, those with at most prelaminar optic nerve invasion without choroidal or scleral involvement, boast excellent survival rates and no relapse after enucleation alone. Adjuvant chemotherapy is not recommended for this cohort.[48]

CHOROIDAL INVASION

Adjuvant chemotherapy for patients with isolated choroidal invasion remains controversial. The overall survival is greater than 95%, with low rates of extraocular relapse.[49,53,54] Some authors recommend adjuvant treatment only for massive choroidal involvement,[55] though the definition of "massive" is variably defined in the literature.[48] In a study of 55 patients, 94% were relapse-free at 3 years. All patients survived, including the three who relapsed and were then treated. Given the low mortality and relapse rates, the researchers did not recommend adjuvant chemotherapy for any degree of isolated choroidal invasion.[48]

POSTLAMINAR OPTIC NERVE INVASION

The greatest controversy exists for patients with postlaminar optic nerve invasion without involvement of the cut margin. Some experts report that, in the absence of choroidal or scleral invasion, patients with postlaminar optic nerve involvement and a negative margin have a very low rate of relapse (0 out of 21 patients[53]) and therefore they do not recommend adjuvant chemotherapy for this subgroup. Further, in the absence of choroidal invasion, optic nerve involvement alone is not a significant risk factor for metastatic disease.[56] On the other hand, prior studies did not stratify postlaminar optic nerve invasion based on choroidal and scleral involvement, and many experts therefore recommend adjuvant chemotherapy for all patients with postlaminar optic nerve invasion.[49,55]

TUMOR AT CUT OPTIC NERVE MARGIN

Experts agree that patients with tumor at the cut optic nerve margin are at very high risk of relapse and require adjuvant chemotherapy.[49,53–55] However, few studies effectively address adjuvant treatment for retinoblastoma extending beyond the cut margin of the optic nerve, precluding definitive recommendations.[52,54] In a study of 51 patients, doxorubicin was added to cyclophosphamide, vincristine, and EBRT if the tumor extended beyond the cut margin of the optic nerve or through the sclera into the orbit.[52] In patients with central nervous system (CNS) involvement, the authors added intrathecal chemotherapy (methotrexate, cytarabine, hydrocortisone) and cranial radiotherapy. The survival rate was 90.6% for patients with unilateral and 84.2% for patients with bilateral disease.

METASTATIC RETINOBLASTOMA

Metastatic retinoblastoma carries a dismal prognosis, though the prognosis for distant metastases is better than that for CNS metastases. Rates of metastases are higher in developing countries. Retinoblastoma can metastasize to regional lymph nodes, CNS, and distant organs, usually bone and bone marrow.[57,58] A study evaluating nine patients with CNS metastases and five with concomitant CNS and distant metastases reported 100% mortality in both groups. Four patients were treated with cyclophosphamide, doxorubicin, vincristine, carboplatin, and etoposide, along with intrathecal methotrexate, cytarabine, and hydrocortisone. Some studies have questioned the benefit of intrathecal chemotherapy.[59,60] As such, ifosfamide, carboplatin, etoposide (ICE) was used in patients with CNS metastases because of its potential to penetrate possible metastatic retinoblastoma sites. Ifosfamide and carboplatin have high CNS penetration; carboplatin also penetrates bone marrow well. All patients underwent craniospinal EBRT. Unfortunately, all 10 patients with CNS metastases died from their disease. In comparison, four patients with only distant metastases were treated with ICE chemotherapy and survived.[57]

UVEAL METASTASIS

GENERAL CONSIDERATIONS

Metastatic carcinoma to the uveal tract remains the most common intraocular malignancy.[61] Lung carcinoma is the most common primary source in men, while breast carcinoma is most common in women. Together lung and breast carcinoma account for 71–92% of cases.[62] Treatment options include systemic chemotherapy, EBRT, proton beam radiotherapy, hormonal therapy, biological therapy, brachytherapy, laser photocoagulation, transpupillary thermotherapy, photodynamic therapy, anti-vascular endothelial growth factor treatment, enucleation, or a combination of these.[62,63]

The decision to treat uveal metastases depends upon the individual case. Lesions that do not threaten vision or the status of the globe can be observed while the patient undergoes systemic treatment. Systemic treatment alone can induce tumor regression.[64]

CHEMOTHERAPY

Metastatic breast carcinoma is managed with cytotoxic chemotherapy with or without hormonal therapy. Anthracyclines, like doxorubin and epirubucin, represent a potent class of agents limited by their cardiotoxicity. Taxanes such as paclitaxel and docetaxel are often used in tandem or sequentially with other agents to improve effectiveness against breast cancer. Alkylating agents include cyclophosphamide and temozolomide, the latter boasting excellent CNS penetration. Antimetabolite fluorouracil and capecitabine (both pyrimidine analogues) and methotrexate (folic acid analogue) are also used. Hormonal therapies include aromatase inhibitors and antiestrogen agents (e.g., tamoxifen).[62] The largest case series for metastatic breast carcinoma to the uvea (85 cases) reports a 65% rate of tumor regression with chemotherapy and/or hormonal therapy.[65]

Small-cell lung carcinoma is commonly treated with a combination of platinum-based agents (cisplatin, carboplatin), etoposide, cyclophosphamide, doxorubicin, methotrexate, and vincristine. By comparison, nonsmall-cell lung cancer is less sensitive to chemotherapy; treatment is usually palliative. Chemotherapeutic agents for nonsmall-cell lung cancer include cisplatin, carboplatin, gemcitabine, vinorelbine, paclitaxel, and docetaxel.[62] Bevacizumab, an anti-vascular endothelial growth factor monoclonal antibody, and erlotinib, a tyrosine kinase inhibitor, are novel targeted agents proven to increase survival in nonsmall-cell lung cancer[66] (Figures 44.3 and 44.4).

PROGNOSIS

Unfortunately, uveal metastases tend to occur later in the course of carcinoma, portending a poor prognosis. At the time of uveal metastasis diagnosis, up to 88% of patients will have metastases elsewhere. Life expectancy for patients with uveal metastases ranges between 0.2 and 48 months (median 6–9 months).[62]

UVEAL MELANOMA

Uveal melanoma is most commonly treated with enucleation, episcleral plaque brachytherapy, proton beam radiotherapy, transpupillary thermotherapy, or local resection. To date, no convincing evidence exists for chemotherapy to treat primary uveal melanoma. One patient with bilateral primary choroidal melanoma was unsuccessfully treated with systemic interferon-α, temozolomide, paclitaxel, and carboplatin.[67] A trial of adjunctive subconjunctival interferon-α for uveal melanoma failed to find a protective effect for this experimental treatment.[68]

METASTATIC UVEAL MELANOMA

Mortality rates for uveal melanoma have remained unchanged despite improvements in diagnosis. Though only 2% of patients have evidence of metastases at the time of uveal melanoma diagnosis, 35–50% will develop metastases within 5 years of enucleation. Most experts feel this is related to subclinical micrometastases at time of diagnosis.[30] Unfortunately, median survival for metastatic uveal melanoma is only 2–15 months.[69–71]

No standard chemotherapy regimen exists for metastatic uveal melanoma. Moreover, treatment outcomes remain disappointing without compelling evidence of a survival advantage. Carboplatin- or dacarbazine-based regimens have low efficacy.[72] A multicenter study evaluating the efficacy of BOLD (bleomycin, vincristine, lomustine, dacarbazine) therapy with subcutaneous interferon-α found no response.[73] Chemoembolization of the hepatic artery with carmustine

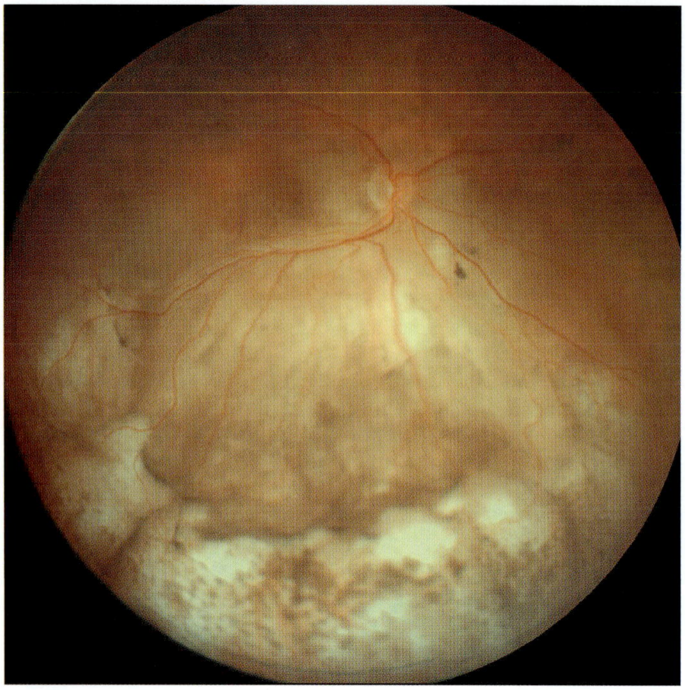

Figure 44.3 Uveal metastasis before chemotherapy.

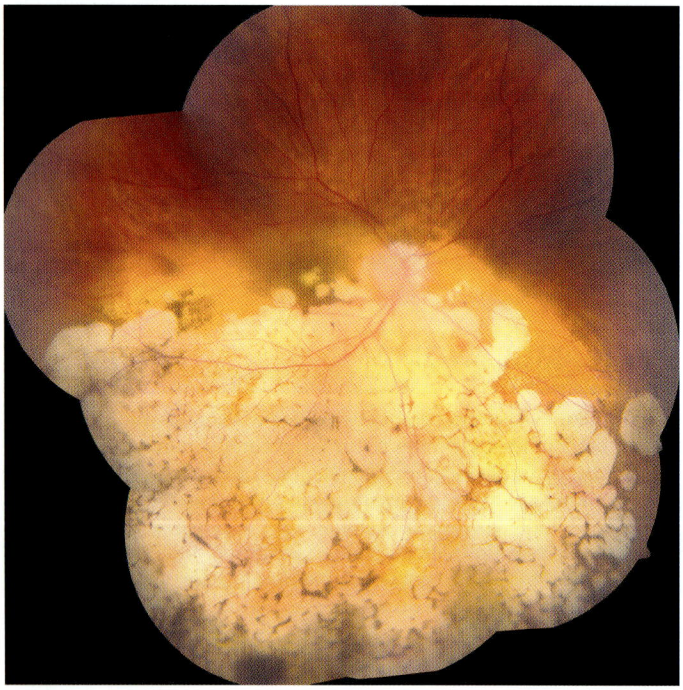

Figure 44.4 Uveal metastasis after chemotherapy.

(BCNU) using gelatine sponges for temporary arterial occlusion results in a median survival of only 5.2 months.[74] Intra-arterial intrahepatic fotemustin, a third-generation nitrosourea, delivers a 36% response and 15-month median survival for patients with hepatic metastases.[75] Including one of 24 patients showing a partial response, 33% of patients exhibited disease stabilization after gemcitabine plus treosulfan.[76] The addition of cisplatin to the gemcitabine plus treosulfan regimen does not improve efficacy, with a median survival of 7.7 months at the expense of excessive hematological toxicity.[77] A study evaluating the combination of dacarbazine and treosulfan failed to find any objective tumor response.[78]

INTRAOCULAR LYMPHOMA

GENERAL CONSIDERATIONS

Primary intraocular lymphoma is a rare entity involving the retina, vitreous, subretinal pigment epithelial space, or optic nerve head.[79] Almost always, histopathology reveals diffuse large B-cell lymphoma, though occasionally it can be of T-cell origin.[80] Many experts consider primary intraocular lymphoma a subset of primary CNS lymphoma. Though primary intraocular lymphoma presents independently of primary CNS lymphoma, 60–85% of patients eventually develop intracranial involvement. Of patients with primary CNS lymphoma, 15–25% will have concomitant ocular involvement.[80] Many patients with primary intraocular lymphoma are misdiagnosed with uveitis, resulting in a delay of diagnosis of 6–13 months.[81,82] Patients show initial response to corticosteroids and often develop brain involvement at the time of correct diagnosis.[81] Diagnosis is usually made by vitreous or direct choroidal/retinal biopsy. In a cohort of 83 variably treated patients without initial brain involvement, median overall survival was 58 months. Fifteen percent of patients had positive cerebrospinal fluid cytology at time of ocular diagnosis, and 56% ultimately progressed to develop brain lymphoma.[81] When the brain is involved, prognosis is poorer.

TREATMENT

Given the rarity of primary intraocular lymphoma, optimal treatment standards have not been established. Current options include ocular radiotherapy, intravitreal methotrexate, whole-brain radiotherapy, and intravenous or intrathecal chemotherapy. The largest study of primary intraocular lymphoma in the literature ($n = 83$) retrospectively found no difference in outcome between those treated with ocular radiotherapy and/or intraocular methotrexate versus more extensive treatments, including whole-brain radiotherapy, systemic chemotherapy, and/or intrathecal chemotherapy. Of note, all patients with positive CSF cytology were treated with more extensive measures. For patients with primary intraocular lymphoma, the researchers recommend focused ocular treatment with close follow-up for ocular, CNS, or systemic relapse.[81]

Intravitreal methotrexate has shown encouraging response rates, with almost 100% tumor eradication.[83] Adverse effects include conjunctival irriation, corneal epitheliopathy, cataract, vitreous hemorrhage, maculopathy, optic atrophy, sterile endophthalmitis,[83] and neovascular glaucoma.[84]

Case reports of patients undergoing intrathecal methotrexate and cytarabine for intraocular and CNS lymphoma are encouraging, reporting tumor regression and suggesting improved survival.[85]

Systemic chemotherapy for primary intraocular lymphoma is often methotrexate-based.[81] For primary cerebral lymphoma, regimens including high-dose methotrexate confer a better survival than radiation alone or other chemotherapy regimens (cytarabine or nitrosurea).[86] Primary intraocular lymphoma has been treated with high-dose methotrexate, high-dose cytarabine, trofosfamide, and ifosfamide.[87,88] Experts recommend high-dose methotrexate alone or in combination with other active chemotherapy agents for primary CNS lymphoma, followed by whole-brain radiotherapy unless contraindicated.[89]

Rituximab is a genetically engineered chimeric murine/human monoclonal antibody directed against the CD 20 antigen on the surface of normal and malignant B lymphocytes.[90] Animal and case reports of intravitreal rituximab fail to reveal toxicity; this may hold promise as a future treatment option for primary intraocular lymphoma.[91] Intrathecal rituximab was evaluated in a phase I study of 10 patients with recurrent CNS lymphoma, reporting meningeal responses in six, intraocular responses in two, and resolution of brain parenchymal lymphoma in one. This treatment modality warrants further investigation.[92]

SUMMARY AND KEYPOINTS

CRD, a strategy combining chemotherapeutic tumor debulking with localized ophthalmic treatment (laser photocoagulation, thermotherapy, cryotherapy, or plaque radiotherapy), successfully obviates the need for enucleation or EBRT for many patients with retinoblastoma. Chemotherapeutic regimens typically include VEC for six cycles.

Metastases to the uveal tract represent the most common intraocular malignancy, often from breast and lung carcinomas. Metastatic breast carcinoma is managed with cytotoxic chemotherapy with or without hormonal therapy. Small-cell lung carcinoma is commonly treated with a combination of platinum-based agents, etoposide, cyclophosphamide, doxorubicin, methotrexate, and vincristine.

There is no convincing evidence to support chemotherapy for uveal melanoma. Several agents have been used for metastatic uveal melanoma, though without a clear survival advantage.

Intraocular lymphoma has been treated with intravitreal methotrexate or rituximab. Intrathecal methotrexate and cytarabine may improve survival for intraocular and CNS lymphoma. Systemic chemotherapy is often methotrexate-based.

REFERENCES

1. Kupfer C. Retinoblastoma treated with intravenous nitrogen mustard. Am J Ophthalmol 1953;36:1721.
2. Finger PT, Czechonska G, Demirci H, et al. Chemotherapy for retinoblastoma: a current topic. Drugs 1999;58:983–996.
3. Shields JA, Shields CL. Management and prognosis of retinoblastoma. In: Shields JA, Shields CL, editors. Intraocular tumors: a text and atlas. Philadelphia: WB Saunders; 1992. p. 377–392.
4. Kim JW, Abramson DH, Dunkel IJ. Current management strategies for intraocular retinoblastoma. Drugs 2007;67:2173–2185.
5. Shields CL, Shields JA, Cater J, et al. Plaque radiotherapy for retinoblastoma: long-term tumor control and treatment complications in 208 tumors. Ophthalmology 2001;108:2116–2121.
6. Shields CL, Mashayekhi A, Au AK, et al. The International Classification of Retinoblastoma predicts chemoreduction success. Ophthalmology 2006;113:2276–2280.
7. Toma NM, Hungerford JL, Plowman PN, et al. External beam radiotherapy for retinoblastoma: II. Lens sparing technique. Br J Ophthalmol 1995;79: 112–117.
8. Hungerford JL, Toma NM, Plowman PN, et al. External beam radiotherapy for retinoblastoma: I. Whole eye technique. Br J Ophthalmol 1995;79: 109–111.
9. Kleinerman RA, Tucker MA, Tarone RE, et al. Risk of new cancers after radiotherapy in long-term survivors of retinoblastoma: an extended follow-up. J Clin Oncol 2005;23:2272–2279.
10. Abramson DH, Ellsworth RM, Kitchin FD, et al. Second nonocular tumors in retinoblastoma survivors. Are they radiation-induced? Ophthalmology 1984;91:1351–1355.
11. Abramson DH, Schefler AC. Update on retinoblastoma. Retina 2004;24:828–848.
12. Abramson DH, Frank CM. Second nonocular tumors in survivors of bilateral retinoblastoma; possible age effect on radiation-related risk. Ophthalmology 1998;105:573–580.
13. Shields CL, Shields JA. Basic understanding of current classification and management of retinoblastoma. Curr Opin Ophthalmol 2006;17:228–234.
14. Shields CL, De Potter P, Himelstein BP, et al. Chemoreduction in the initial management of intraocular retinoblastoma. Arch Ophthalmol 1996;114:1330–1338.
15. Kingston JE, Hungerford JL, Madreperla SA, et al. Results of combined chemotherapy and radiotherapy for advanced intraocular retinoblastoma. Arch Ophthalmol 1996;114:1339–1343.
16. Gallie BL, Budning A, DeBoer G, et al. Chemotherapy with focal therapy can cure intraocular retinoblastoma without radiotherapy. Arch Ophthalmol 1996;114:1321–1328.
17. Murphree AL, Villablanca JG, Deegan WF 3rd, et al. Chemotherapy plus local treatment in the management of intraocular retinoblastoma. Arch Ophthalmol 1996;114:1348–1356.
18. Shields CL, Meadows AT, Leahey AM, et al. Continuing challenges in the management of retinoblastoma with chemoreduction. Retina 2004;24: 849–862.
19. Zelter M, Damel A, Gonzalez G, et al. A prospective study on the treatment of retinoblastoma in 72 patients. Cancer 1991;68:1685–1690.
20. Shields CL, Mashayekhi A, Cater J, et al. Chemoreduction for retinoblastoma. Analysis of tumor control and risks for recurrence in 457 tumors. Am J Ophthalmol 2004;138:329–337.
21. Rodriguez-Galindo C, Wilson MW, Haik BG, et al. Treatment of intraocular retinoblastoma with vincristine and carboplatin. J Clin Oncol 2003;21:2019–2025.
22. Dunkel IJ, Lee TC, Shi W, et al. A phase II trial of carboplatin for intraocular retinoblastoma. Pediatr Blood Cancer 2007;49:643–648.
23. Lee TC, Hayashi NI, Dunkel IJ, et al. New retinoblastoma tumor formation in children initially treated with systemic carboplatin. Ophthalmology 2003;110:1989–1994.
24. Chan HSL, Thorner PS, Haddad G, et al. Multi-drug resistance phenotype in retinoblastoma correlates with P-glycoprotein expression. Ophthalmology 1991;98:1425–1431.
25. Chan HSL, Thorner PS, Haddad G, et al. Effect of chemotherapy on intraocular retinoblastoma. Int J Pediatr Hematol Oncol 1995;2:269–281.
26. Abramson DH, Lawrence DS, Beaverson KL, et al. Systemic carboplatin for retinoblastoma: change in tumor size over time. BJO 2005;89:1616–1619.
27. Shields CL, Meadows AT, Shields JA, et al. Chemoreduction for retinoblastoma may prevent intracranial neuroblastic malignancy (trilateral retinoblastoma). Arch Ophthalmol 2001;119:1269–1272.
28. Moll AC, Imhof SM, Schouten-van Meeteren AY, et al. Chemoreduction for retinoblastoma. Arch Ophthalmol 2003;121:1513.
29. Shields CL, Hanovar SG, Shields JA, et al. Factors predictive of recurrence of retinal tumors, vitreous seeds, and subretinal seeds following chemoreduction for retinoblastoma. Arch Oph 2002;122:1316–1323.
30. Wilson MW, Czechonska G, Finger PT, et al. Chemotherapy for eye cancer. Surv Ophthalmol Oph 2001;45:416–444.
31. Shields CL, Shelil A, Cater J, et al. Development of new retinoblastomas following six cycles of chemoreduction for retinoblastoma in 162 eyes of 106 consecutive patients. Arch Ophthalmol 2003;131:1571–1576.
32. Mashayekhi A, Shields CL, Eagle RC Jr, et al. Cavitary changes in retinoblastoma: relationship to chemoresistance. Ophthalmology 2005;112:1145–1150.
33. Singh AD, Shields CL, Shields JA. Lack of response to chemoreduction in presumed well differentiated retinoblastoma. J Pediatr Ophthalmol Strabismus 2002;39:107–109.
34. Friedman DL, Himelstein B, Shields CL, et al. Chemoreduction and local ophthalmic therapy for intraocular retinoblastoma. J Clin Oncol 2000;18:12–17.
35. Lambert MP, Shields CL, Meadows AT. A retrospective review of hearing in children with retinoblastoma treated with carboplatin-based chemotherapy. Pediatric Blood Cancer 2008;50:223–226.
36. Gombos DS, Hungerford J, Abramson DH, et al. Secondary acute myelogenous leukemia in patients with retinoblastoma: is chemotherapy a factor? Ophthalmology 2007;114:1378–1383.
37. Abramson DH, Melson MR, Dunkel IJ, et al. Third (fourth and ?fth) nonocular tumors in survivors of retinoblastoma. Ophthalmology 2001;108:1868–1876.
38. Anagnoste SR, Scott IU, Murray TG, et al. Rhegmatogenous retinal detachment in retinoblastoma patients undergoing chemoreduction and cryotherapy. AJO 2000;129:817–819.
39. Gombos DS, Howes E, O'Brien JM. Cholesterosis following chemoreduction for advanced retinoblastoma. Arch Oph 2000;118:440–441.
40. Lumbroso L, Doz F, Urbieta M, et al. Chemothermotherapy in the management of retinoblastoma. Ophthalmology 2002;109:1130–1136.
41. Mendelsohn ME, Abramson DH, Madden T, et al. Intraocular concentrations of chemotherapeutic agents after systemic or local administration. Arch Ophthalmol 1998;116:1209–1212.
42. Abramson DH, Frank CM, Dunkel IJ. A phase I/II study of subconjunctival carboplatin for intraocular retinoblastoma. Ophthalmology 1999;106: 1947–1950.
43. Schmack I, Hubbard GB, Kang SJ, et al. Ischemic necrosis and atrophy of the optic nerve after periocular carboplatin injection for intraocular retinoblastoma. AJO 2006;142:310–315.
44. Mulvihill A, Budning A, Jay V, et al. Ocular motility changes after subtenon arboplatin chemotherapy for retinoblastoma. Arch Oph 2003;121:1120–1124.
45. Seregard S, Kock E, af Trampe E: Intravitreal chemotherapy for recurrent retinoblastoma in an only eye [letter]. Br J Ophthalmol 1995;79:194–195.
46. Raina J, Logani S, Hungerford JL: Intravitreal chemotherapy for vitreous seeding in recurrent retinoblastoma. Invest Ophthalmol Vis Sci 1998;39(Suppl):S816 (abstract).
47. Suzuki S, Kaneko A. Management of intraocular retinoblastoma and ocular prognosis. Int J Clin Oncol 2004;9:1–6.
48. Chantada GL, Dunkel IJ, de Davila MTG, et al. Retinoblastoma patients with high-risk ocular pathological features: who needs adjuvant therapy? BJO 2004;88:1069–1073.
49. Honavar SG, Singh A, Shields CL, et al. Post enucleation adjuvant therapy in high risk retinoblastoma. Arch Ophthalmol 2002;120:923–931.
50. Keith CG: Chemotherapy in retinoblastoma management. Ophthalmic Paediatr Genet 1989;10:93–98.
51. Howarth C, Meyer D, Hustu HO, et al. Stage-related combined modality treatment of retinoblastoma. Results of a prospective study. Cancer 1980;45:851–858.
52. Acquaviva A, Barberi L, Bernardini C, et al: Medical therapy of retinoblastoma in children. J Neurosurg Sci 1982;26:49–52.
53. Chantada G, Fandino A, Davila MTG, et al. Results of a prospective study for the treatment of retinoblastoma. Cancer 2004;100:834–842.
54. Schvartzman E, Chantada G, Fandino A, et al. Results of a stage-based protocol for the treatment of retinoblastoma. J Clin Oncol 1996;14:1532–1536.

55. Khelfaoui F, Validire P, Auperin A, et al. Histopathologic risk factors in retinoblastoma: a retrospective study of 172 patients treated in a single institution. Cancer 1996;15:1206–1213.
56. Shields CL, Shields JA, Baez K, et al. Optic nerve invasion of retinoblastoma. Metastatic potential and clinical risk factors. Cancer 1994;73:692–698.
57. Gündüz K, Müftüoglu O, Günalp I, et al. Metastatic retinoblastoma clinical features, treatment, and prognosis. Ophthalmology 2006;113: 1558–1566.
58. Finger PT, Harbour JW, Karcioglu ZA. Risk factors for metastasis in retinoblastoma. Surv Ophthalmol 2002;47:1–16.
59. Pratt CB, Fontanesi J, Chenaille P, et al. Chemotherapy for extraocular retinoblastoma. Pediatr Hematol Oncol 1994;11:301–309.
60. Pratt CB. Use of chemotherapy for retinoblastoma. Med Pediatr Oncol 1998;31:531–533.
61. Chan RVP, Young LH. Treatment options for metastatic tumors to the choroid. Semin Ophthalmol 2005;20:207–216.
62. Kanthan GL, Jayamohan J, Yip D, et al. Management of metastatic carcinoma of the uveal tract: an evidence-based analysis. Clin Experiment Ophthalmol 2007;35:553–565.
63. Shields CL. Plaque radiotherapy for the management of uveal metastasis. Curr Opin Ophthalmol 1998;9:31–37.
64. Nicolo M, Calabria G. Choroidal metastasis from a cutaneous malignant melanoma regressed after cisplatic therapy. Retina 2004;24:622–624.
65. Demirci H, Shields CL, Chao AN, et al. Uveal metastasis from breast cancer in 264 patients. Am J Ophthalmol 2003;136:264–271.
66. Herbst RS, O'Neill VJ, Fehrenbacher L, et al. Phase II study of efficacy and safety of bevacizumab in combination with chemotherapy or erlotinib compared with chemotherapy alone for treatment of recurrent or refractory non small-cell lung cancer. J Clin Oncol 2007;25:4743–4750.
67. Kitzmann AS, Pulido JS, Mohney BG, et al. Intraocular use of rituximab. Eye 2007;21:1524–1527.
68. Richtig E, Langmann G, Schlemmer G, et al. Safety and efficacy of interferon alfa-2b in the adjuvant treatment of uveal melanoma. Ophthalmologe 2006;103:506–511.
69. Gragoudas ES, Egan KM, Seddon JM, et al. Survival of patients with metastases from uveal melanoma. Ophthalmology 1991;98:383–389.
70. Kath R, Hayungs J, Bornfeld N, et al. Prognosis and treatment of disseminated uveal melanoma. Cancer 1993;72:2219–2223.
71. Bedikian AY, Legha SS, Mavligit G, et al. Treatment of uveal melanoma metastatic to the liver: a review of the M. D. Anderson Cancer Center experience and prognostic factors. Cancer 1995;76:1665–1670.
72. Flaherty LE, Unger JM, Liu PY, et al. Metastatic melanoma from intraocular primary tumors: the Southwest Oncology Group experience in phase II advanced melanoma clinical trials. Am J Clin Oncol 1998;21: 568–572.
73. Kivelä T, Suciu S, Hansson J, et al. Bleomycin, vincristine, lomustine and dacarbazine (BOLD) in combination with recombinant interferon alpha-2b for metastatic uveal melanoma. Eur J Cancer 2003;39:1115–1120.
74. Patel K, Sullivan K, Berd D, et al. Chemoembolization of the hepatic artery with BCNU for metastatic uveal melanoma: results of a phase II study. Melanoma Res 2005;15:297–304.
75. Peters S, Voelter V, Zografos L, et al. Intra-arterial hepatic fotemustine for the treatment of liver metastases from uveal melanoma: experience in 101 patients. Annals of Oncology 2006;17:578–583.
76. Schmittel A, Schmidt-Hieber M, Martus P, et al. A randomized phase II trial of gemcitabine plus treosulfan versus treosulfan alone in patients with metastatic uveal melanoma. Ann Oncol 2006;17:1826–1829.
77. Schmittel A, Scheulen ME, Bechrakis NE, et al. Phase II trial of cisplatin, gemcitabine and treosulfan in patients with metastatic uveal melanoma. Melanoma Res 2005;15:205–207.
78. O'Neill PA, Butt M, Eswar CV, et al. A prospective single arm phase II study of dacarbazine and treosulfan as first-line therapy in metastatic uveal melanoma. Melanoma Res 2006;16:245–248.
79. Levy-Clarke GA, Chan CC, Nussenblatt RB. Diagnosis and management of primary intraocular lymphoma. Hematol Oncol Clin N Am 2005;19: 739–749.
80. Dunleavey K, Wilson WH. Primary intraocular lymphoma: Current and future perspectives. Leukemia and Lymphoma 2006;47:1726–1727.
81. Grimm SA, Pulido JS, Jahnke K, et al. Primary intraocular lymphoma: an international primary central nervous system lymphoma collaborate group report. Annals of Oncology 2007;18:1851–1855.
82. Hormigo A, Abrey L, Heinemann MH, et al. Ocular presentation of primary central nervous system lymphoma: diagnosis and treatment. Br J Haematol 2004;126:202–208.
83. Smith JR, Rosenbaum JT, Wilson DJ, et al. Role of intravitreal methotrexate in the management of primary central nervous system lymphoma with ocular involvement. Ophthalmology 2002;109:1709–1716.
84. Goldberg S, Frenkel S, Blumenthal EZ, et al. Intraocular lymphoma. Ophthal 2007;114:1236–1237.
85. Mason JO, Fischer DH. Intrathecal chemotherapy for recurrent central nervous system intraocular lymphoma. Ophthalmology 2003;110: 1241–1244.
86. Blay JY, Conroy T, Chevreau C, et al. High-dose methotrexate for the treatment of primary cerebral lymphomas: analysis of survival and late neurologic toxicity in a retrospective series. J Clin Oncol 1998;16:864–871.
87. Jahnke K, Bechrakis NE, Coupland SE, et al. Treatment of primary intraocular lymphoma with oral trofosfamide: report of two cases and review of the literature. Graefes Arch Clin Exp Ophthalmol 2004;242: 771–776.
88. Jahnke K, Korfel A, Komm J, et al. Intraocular lymphoma 2000–2005: results of a retrospective multicentre trial. Graefes Arch Clin Exp Ophthalmol 2006;244:663–669.
89. Bessell EM, Hoang-Xuan K, Ferreri AJ, et al. Primary central nervous system lymphoma: biological aspects and controversies in management. Eur J Cancer 2007;43:1141–1152.
90. Pulido JS, Bakri SJ, Valyi-Nagy T, et al. Rituximab penetrates full-thickness retina in contrast to tissue plasminogen activator control. Retina 2007;27:1071–1073.
91. Kitzmann AS, Buettner H, Pulido JS, et al. Failure of immunotherapy and chemotherapy for a patient with primary choroidal melanoma. Retinal Cases and Brief Reports 2007;1:30–32.
92. Rubenstein JL, Fridlyand J, Abrey L, et al. Phase I study of intraventricular administration of rituximab in patients with recurrent CNS and intraocular lymphoma. J Clin Oncol 2007;25:1350–1356.

CHAPTER

45 Antibiotics

Seenu M. Hariprasad, MD and William F. Mieler, MD

Key points

The Endophthalmitis Vitrectomy Study (EVS) provided ophthalmologists with evidence-based management strategies to deal with endophthalmitis for the first time. However, since the completion of the EVS, numerous unresolved issues remain. The use of oral antibiotics has important implications for the ophthalmologist, particularly in the prophylaxis and/or management of postoperative, posttraumatic, or bleb-associated bacterial endophthalmitis. One can reasonably conclude that significant intraocular penetration of an antibiotic after oral administration may be a property unique to the newer generation of fluroquinolones. Prophylactic use of mupirocin nasal ointment resulted in significant reduction of conjunctival flora with or without preoperative topical 5% povidone-iodine prep. Ocular fungal infections have traditionally been very difficult to treat due to limited therapeutic options both systemically and intravitreally. Because of its broad spectrum of coverage, low MIC_{90} levels (minimum inhibitory concentration of antibiotic required to kill 90% of isolates) for the organisms of concern, good tolerability, and excellent bioavailability, voriconazole through various routes of administration may be useful to the ophthalmologist in the primary treatment of or as an adjunct in the current management of ocular fungal infections.

INTRODUCTION

In spite of significant advances in endophthalmitis management over the past two decades, numerous unresolved issues remain. There is no doubt that approximately 20 years ago, the advent of intravitreal antibiotics paved the way for notably improved visual and anatomic outcomes. In the mid-1990s, the EVS readily addressed the role of vitrectomy versus vitreous tap in the treatment of postoperative endophthalmitis, and documented that patients with hand motion or better vision fared equally well with either a complete pars plana vitrectomy or a vitreous tap.[1] If the visual acuity was light perception, then outcomes were better with a complete vitrectomy. Both procedures employed intravitreal antibiotics consisting of vancomycin and amikicin. This study provided ophthalmologists with evidence-based management strategies to deal with this difficult condition for the first time.

The EVS also provided us with very important data regarding the pathogens which most commonly cause postoperative endophthalmitis (Figure 45.1). Additionally, the study determined that there was no apparent benefit from the use of intravenous (IV) antibiotics (cephalosporins and aminoglycosides).[1] The chosen systemic antibiotics in the EVS were the best available at the time; however, several studies following the completion of the EVS revealed that systemically administered cephalosporins and aminoglycosides do not readily achieve therapeutic intraocular concentrations in the vitreous cavity.[2,3]

Unfortunately, even within the confines of a well-conceived and thought-out multicenter, prospective clinical trial like the EVS, a number of pertinent issues remain unresolved or were not fully addressed in the original study. These include the choice of the intravitreal antibiotics (ceftazidime was not employed, and today it has virtually replaced the use of intravitreal amikacin), the management of types of endophthalmitis not specifically studied in the EVS (filtering bleb-associated, posttraumatic, indolent, and fungal endophthalmitis), the role of intravitreal corticosteroids, and inpatient versus outpatient management of infection.

Additionally, since the completion of the EVS, new antibiotics such as the fourth-generation fluoroquinolones have been developed, and these agents will most likely play a key role in the treatment of proven infection or in the prophylaxis against infection in the near future (as will be described below).

THE ENDOPHTHALMITIS VITRECTOMY STUDY

In the mid-1990s, the EVS group set out to determine the role of vitrectomy versus vitreous tap in the treatment of postoperative endophthalmitis, and to address the role of IV antibiotics versus no IV antibiotics in treating endophthalmitis. Vitrectomy was introduced in the 1970s and many surgeons began to employ it in conjunction with intravitreal antibiotics for treating endophthalmitis. There were several theoretical advantages to vitrectomy, including the removal of infecting organisms and their toxins, better distribution of antibiotics, clearing of tractional membranes that could lead to retinal detachment, clearing of opacities in the vitreous, and providing a good volume of vitreous material for microbiologic culture. Prior to the EVS, small human studies were inconclusive to the benefits of vitrectomy and in previous studies it appeared that only the most advanced cases of endophthalmitis underwent vitrectomy. Therefore, visual outcomes were poor and it was uncertain if vitrectomy would yield superior outcomes in eyes with better presenting vision. In the early 1990s, the role of vitrectomy in the management of endophthalmitis was quite controversial. During this time, the role of systemic IV antibiotics in the management of endophthalmitis was uncertain. It was the standard of care; however, it was questioned whether the theoretical benefit outweighed the systemic side-effects of antibiotics used at the time, as well as costs associated with the drug and hospitalization for administration of these antibiotics. These unresolved issues served as the impetus for the largest prospective study on endophthalmitis management to date.[4]

Clinical centers in 25 US cities enrolled 420 patients over a 3½-year period. Entry criteria were stringent and were limited to patients who had a clinical diagnosis of endophthalmitis within 6 weeks of cataract extraction or secondary intraocular lens placement and had vision worse than 20/50 but at least light perception. Additionally, included patients were required to have a hypopyon and clouding of anterior chamber or vitreous media sufficient to obscure clear visualization of second-order retinal arterioles. Patients were excluded that did not have a cornea and anterior chamber clear enough to visualize some part of iris. Furthermore, the cornea was to be clear enough to allow the possibility of pars plana vitrectomy.[4] All eyes in the EVS underwent immediate cultures of the anterior chamber and vitreous. Intravitreal amikacin and vancomycin were administered, as were subconjunctival vancomycin and ceftazadime. Topical vancomycin, amikacin, and cycloplegics were administered in all patients as well.[1]

Patients were randomized to the following groups: (1) three-port pars plana vitrectomy with IV antibiotics (ceftazadime and amikacin); (2) three-port pars plana vitrectomy without IV antibiotics; (3) vitreous tap with IV antibiotics; and (4) vitreous tap without IV antibiotics.[1]

The EVS found no difference in outcomes between immediate three-port pars plana vitrectomy versus vitreous tap/biopsy for patients with hand motion or better vision. For patients with a presenting visual acuity of only light perception, much better visual results occurred in the immediate three-port pars plana vitrectomy group versus the vitreous tap/biopsy group. These patients were three times more likely to achieve greater than 20/40 vision (33% versus 11%), twice as likely to achieve greater than 20/100 vision (56% versus 30%), and less likely to incur vision less than 5/200 (20% versus 47%). No difference in final visual acuity or media clarity was experienced whether or not systemic antibiotics were employed.[1]

Confirmed bacterial growth isolates were more likely to be positive in the vitreous compared to aqueous specimens. Figure 45.1 demonstrates that 94.2% of confirmed growth isolates were Gram-positive organisms (the vast majority due to one organism alone: *Staphylococcus epidermidis*, 70%). Gram-negative organisms only comprised 5.9% of confirmed growth isolates. At the time of the EVS, all Gram-positive organisms were sensitive to vancomycin. However, 2 of 19 Gram-negative organisms were resistant to both amikacin and ceftazadime.[5–8]

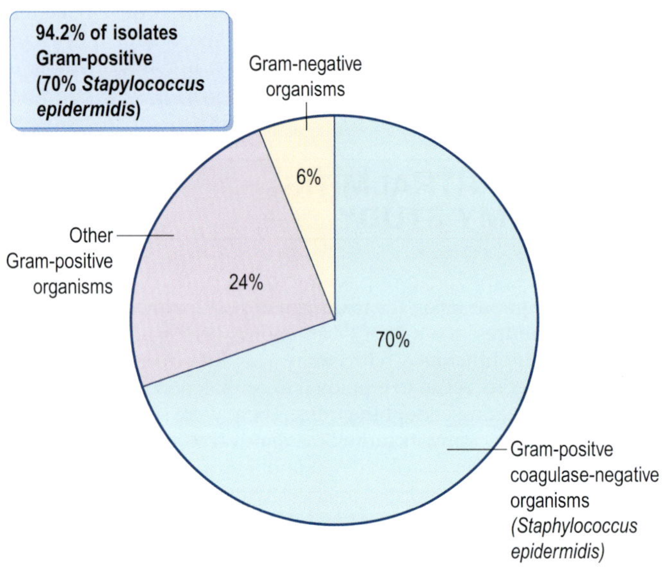

Figure 45.1 Endophthalmitis Vitrectomy Study-confirmed growth isolates. Reproduced from Endophthalmitis Vitrectomy Study Group. Results of the Endophthalmitis Vitrectomy Study: a randomized trial of immediate vitrectomy and of intravenous antibiotics for the treatment of postoperative bacterial endophthalmitis. Arch Ophthalmol 1995; 113:1479–1496, with permission.

A subset analysis of diabetic patients included in the EVS resulted in two interesting findings. First, diabetes was associated with a higher yield of *S. epidermidis*. Secondly, only 39% of diabetic patients had a final visual outcome of greater than 20/40 versus 55% of nondiabetic patients. As a group, diabetic patients fared worse and attained a less desirable visual outcome compared to nondiabetic patients.[1]

The EVS answered some of the most controversial issues surrounding endophthalmitis management at the time. It was a very well-designed study that utilized antibiotics that were the best available in the early 1990s. Additionally, the EVS has taught us valuable information regarding the spectrum of infecting organisms in postoperative endophthalmitis. The EVS clearly was a landmark study which provided ophthalmologists with evidence-based outcomes and strategies to manage postoperative endophthalmitis.

POTENTIAL NEW TREATMENT REGIMENS

TOPICAL FLUOROQUINOLONES

While topical antibiotics were not specifically studied in the EVS, they may soon play an increasingly important role in the management and prophylaxis of ocular infection. In the early 1990s, topical ciprofloxacin was released as the first ophthalmic fluoroquinolone – this agent was embraced by corneal, cataract, and refractive surgeons as a powerful weapon against ocular infection. Other topical fluoroquinolones were subsequently released; however, some of our most powerful weapons have lost a portion of their effect due to increasing levels of resistant organisms each year, especially against the Gram-positive organisms. A serious clinical problem could arise if current trends of resistance to older-generation fluoroquinolones continue. The rise in resistant organisms has challenged empiric monotherapy, creating the need for newer topical antibiotics with a broader spectrum of coverage and less risk for resistance.

During the spring of 2003, topical gatifloxacin 0.3% (Zymar, Allergan Pharmaceuticals) and topical moxifloxacin 0.5% (Vigamox, Alcon Laboratories) were released for clinical use (Figure 45.2). These fourth-generation fluoroquinolones have been engineered to be effective against a number of currently resistant organisms; thus, theoretically they should be able to delay the development of new resistant strains more effectively than their older-generation predecessors. Concerns, however, have recently been raised regarding the development of resistant strains of staphylococcal endophthalmitis isolates to topical fourth-generation fluoroquinolones, specifically in the last 5 years.[8]

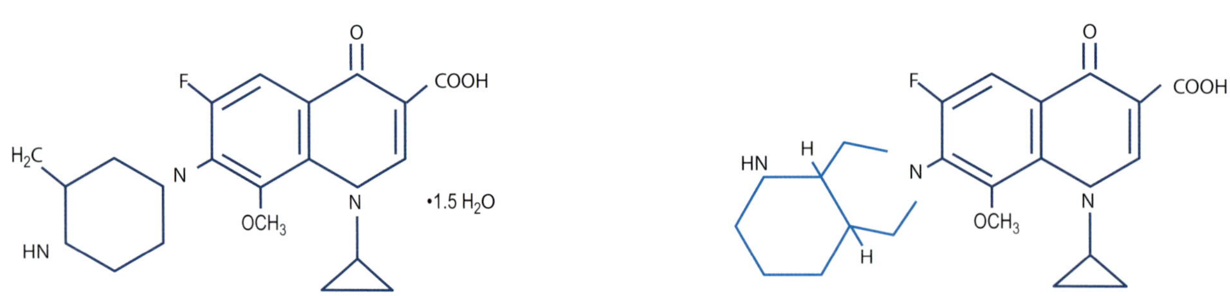

Gatifloxacin **Moxifloxacin**

Figure 45.2 Structures of gatifloxacin and moxifloxacin.

The structure of gatifloxacin and moxifloxacin gives these drugs the capacity to delay resistance through a two-pronged approach that inhibits both the prokaryotic DNA gyrase and topoisomerase IV. The structure increases hydrophobicity, which decreases resistance due to efflux pumps. Overall, the fourth-generation fluoroquinolones have enhanced Gram-positive and atypical coverage while retaining Gram-negative coverage essentially identical to the older-generation flurorquinolones.[9,10]

Topical fourth-generation fluoroquinolones are poised to be a powerful weapon for the corneal, cataract, and refractive surgeon for various anterior-segment indications. Unfortunately, there are limited data regarding the intraocular penetration of these new-generation agents in humans. Several prior studies of earlier-generation agents have demonstrated that topically administered agents do not achieve adequate intraocular concentrations to be effective against the pathogens most commonly responsible for bacterial endophthalmitis.[11]

We completed two investigations to determine the intraocular penetration of moxifloxacin 0.5% in humans to see if therapeutic concentrations of drug could be achieved in the aqueous and vitreous after topical or collagen shield route administration.[12,13] In these studies we obtained aqueous and vitreous samples in noninflamed eyes after topical or collagen shield administration of moxifloxacin 0.5%.

In the topical study, moxifloxacin was administered either every 2 hours (Q2H) or every 6 hours (Q6H), for 3 days prior to surgery. We found that mean moxifloxacin concentrations in the Q2H group for aqueous ($n = 9$) and vitreous ($n = 10$) were 2.28 ± 1.23 and 0.11 ± 0.05 µg/ml, respectively. Mean moxifloxacin concentrations in the Q6H group for aqueous ($n = 10$) and vitreous ($n = 9$) were 0.88 ± 0.88 and 0.06 ± 0.06 µg/ml, respectively (Figure 45.3). MIC_{90} levels were far exceeded in the aqueous for a wide spectrum of key pathogens. Concentration of moxifloxacin in the vitreous did exceed the MIC_{90} for several organisms; however, the MIC_{50} (minimum inhibitory concentration of antibiotic required to kill 50% of isolates) was exceeded in the Q2H group for *Staphylococcus epidermidis, S. aureus, Streptococcus pneumoniae, Haemophilus influenzae, Bacillus cereus,* and other Gram-negatives.

In the second study, delivery of moxifloxacin via a collagen shield revealed a mean aqueous concentration of 0.30 ± 0.17 µg/ml 4 hours after placement ($n = 5$). Vitreous levels at 4 hours and aqueous and vitreous levels at 24 hours were negligible using this route of administration. Peak aqueous moxifloxacin levels occurred soon after shield placement. Theoretically this is when high concentrations of moxifloxacin are most needed to clear the aqueous of bacteria. The MIC_{90} levels were exceeded for organisms commonly responsible for endophthalmitis in the 4-hour aqueous group; however, negligible concentrations of moxifloxacin were detected at 24 hours. Although aqueous moxifloxacin levels achieved through the use of a collagen shield delivery device are lower than via topical drops, there are several advantages to this route of delivery that make it appealing in the immediate postoperative period.

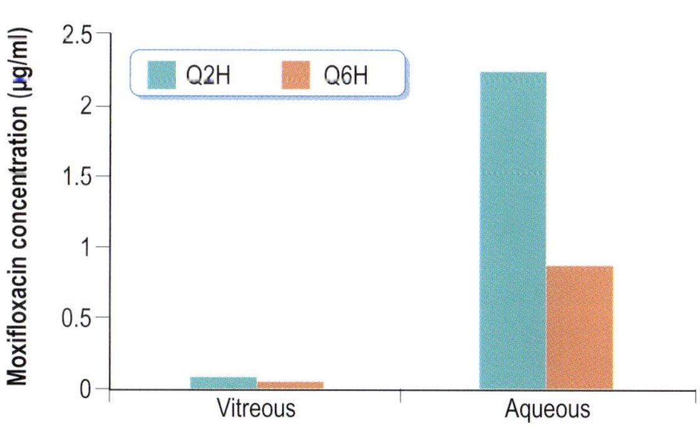

Figure 45.3 Intraocular concentrations of moxifloxacin after topical administration. Q2H, one drop every 2 hours for 3 days; Q6H, one drop every 6 hours for 3 days. Reproduced from Hariprasad SM, Blinder KJ, Shah GK, et al. Penetration pharmacokinetics of topically administered 0.5% moxifloxacin ophthalmic solution in human aqueous and vitreous. Arch Ophthalmol 2005; 123: 39–44, with permission.

Further studies will determine the precise role of topical and collagen shield administration of moxifloxacin 0.5% in the management and/or prophylaxis of intraocular infections. These data may be of significance when considering antibiotic prophylaxis against the development of infection in settings such as after ocular surgery and after intravitreal injections.

ORAL AND INTRAVENOUS ANTIBIOTICS

While intravitreal antibiotic injections are clearly the most effective way to achieve therapeutic antibiotic levels in the vitreous, using certain orally administered antibiotics can be a potential alternative/adjunct as they have been shown to achieve vitreous concentrations exceeding the MIC_{90} level for the organisms most commonly involved in bacterial endophthalmitis. Hence, use of oral antibiotics has important implications for the ophthalmologist, particularly in the prophylaxis and/or management of postoperative, posttraumatic, or bleb-associated bacterial endophthalmitis.

As previously noted, the EVS investigated the use of IV amikacin and ceftazidime in conjunction with intravitreal antibiotic injection for managing acute postoperative endophthalmitis and found no improved outcomes with the use of systemic antibiotics.[1] According to later published studies, amikacin and ceftazidime were found to have very limited intravitreal penetration.[2,3] Therefore, the only conclusion which can be inferred from the EVS data regarding systemic antibiotic use is that IV amikacin and ceftazidime specifically have no apparent role in managing postoperative endophthalmitis. Therefore, do EVS data still apply, given the recent advancements in the development of antimicrobials? The answer is: most likely not.

Over the past 10 years there has been mounting evidence in the literature that agents in the fluoroquinolone class of antibiotics are able to achieve effective concentrations in the vitreous after oral administration (Table 45.1).[14–19] Our group has reported that orally administered gatifloxacin (Tequin, Bristol-Myers Squibb) can achieve therapeutic aqueous and vitreous levels in the noninflamed human eye and the activity spectrum appears to encompass appropriately the most frequently encountered bacterial species involved in the various causes of endophthalmitis.[14,15] The fourth-generation fluoroquinolones, gatifloxacin and moxifloxacin, have high oral bioavailability of greater than 90% and reach peak plasma concentrations 1–2 hours after oral dosing. Both are well tolerated with minimal side-effects.

We designed a prospective, nonrandomized clinical study of 24 patients scheduled for elective pars plana vitrectomy surgery to investigate the aqueous and vitreous concentration of gatifloxacin achieved after oral administration of two 400 mg tablets taken 12 hours apart before surgery. The percentages of plasma gatifloxacin concentration achieved in the vitreous and aqueous were 26.17% and 21.02%, respectively. Mean inhibitory vitreous and aqueous MIC_{90} levels were achieved against a wide spectrum of bacteria (e.g., the vitreous concentration of gatifloxacin achieved with this dosing regimen exceeded the MIC_{90} for *Staphylococcus epidermidis* by over fivefold).

Garcia-Saenz and colleagues reported that orally administered moxifloxacin (Avelox, Bayer) can achieve therapeutic levels in the human aqueous; however, vitreous concentration data were not obtained in this study.[17] To address this, we designed a second prospective, nonrandomized clinical study of 15 patients scheduled for elective pars plana vitrectomy surgery to investigate the aqueous and vitreous concentration of moxifloxacin achieved after oral administration of two 400 mg tablets taken 12 hours apart before surgery. The percentages of plasma moxifloxacin concentration achieved in the vitreous and aqueous were 37.6% and 44.3%, respectively. Mean inhibitory vitreous and aqueous MIC_{90} levels were achieved against a wide spectrum of bacteria.[18]

Moxifloxacin has an inherent advantage over gatifloxacin for Gram-positive organisms. Table 45.1 reviews the mean vitreous penetration of several fluoroquinolones along with their respective MIC_{90} levels for the organisms we are most concerned about in endophthalmitis. Upon reviewing this table, it is readily apparent that moxifloxacin has roughly 50% lower MIC_{90} levels compared to gatifloxacin for Gram-positives. Although our studies have shown similar vitreous

Table 45.1 *In vitro* susceptibilities of moxifloxacin, gatifloxacin, levofloxacin, ofloxacin, and ciprofloxacin showing minimum inhibitory concentration at which 90% of isolates are inhibited (μg/ml)

	Moxifloxacin[18]	Gatifloxacin[14]	Levofloxacin[16]	Ofloxacin[17]	Ciprofloxacin[19]
Mean vitreous penetration	1.34 ± 0.66 μg/ml	1.34 ± 0.34 μg/ml	2.39 ± 0.70 μg/ml	0.43 ± 0.47 μg/ml	0.56 ± 0.16 μg/ml
Gram-positive organisms					
Staphylococcus epidermidis	0.13	0.25	0.50	0.50	1.00
Staphylococcus aureus (MSSA)	0.06	0.13	0.25	0.50	0.50
Streptococcus pneumoniae	0.25	0.50	2.00	2.00	2.00
Streptococcus pyogenes	0.25	0.50	1.00	2.00	1.00
Bacillus cereus	0.13	0.25	–	0.50	–
Enterococcus faecalis	1.00	2.00	2.00	4.00	4.00
Gram-negative organisms					
Proteus mirabilis	0.25	0.25	0.25	0.125	0.06
Pseudomonas aeruginosa	32.0	32.0	32.0	4.00	0.78
Haemophilus influenzae	0.06	0.016	0.06	4.00	0.016
Escherichia coli	0.008	0.008	0.03	0.125	0.016
Klebsiella pneumoniae	0.13	0.13	0.13	0.50	0.06
Neisseria gonorrhoeae	0.016	0.016	0.016	0.06	0.008
Anaerobic organisms					
Bacteroides fragilis	2.00	1.00	2.00	4.00	8.00
Propionibacterium acnes	0.25	0.50	0.75	1.50	–

– Data not available.
MSSA, methicillin-sensitive *Staphylococcus aureus*

penetration of the two agents after oral administration, moxifloxacin may have a theoretical advantage given its activity against Gram-positive organisms.

Based on previous studies, we can reasonably conclude that significant intraocular penetration of an antibiotic after oral administration may be a property unique to the newer-generation fluroquinolones. For example, a study demonstrated that cefipime administered orally does not achieve therapeutic levels in the noninflamed human eye.[20]

To demonstrate proof of principle that orally administered fourth-generation fluoroquinolones could be used to treat intraocular infection in humans, we assessed the use of oral gatifloxacin in the treatment of localized filtering bleb infection in six consecutive patients with blebitis. These six patients were treated with oral gatifloxacin 400 mg tablets for 1 week (BID loading dose for 1 day followed by QD thereafter) in conjunction with a topically administered antibiotic QID (ofloxacin, ciprofloxacin, fortified ceftazidime, or fortified tobramicin). Excluded were those patients with frank bleb-associated endophthalmitis. Cultures of the superior conjunctiva were obtained in two patients, revealing *Streptococcus pneumoniae* in one and *Staphylococcus aureus* in the other. All patients had prompt resolution of bleb purulence, none developed clinical features of endophthalmitis, and all patients tolerated the treatment regimen well.[21]

The ideal oral anti-infective agent has several characteristics: it offers a broad spectrum of coverage for the organisms of concern, is bactericidal, is well tolerated, has excellent bioavailability with oral administration, and has rapid kill curves. We believe that these properties are intrinsic to the fourth-generation fluoroquinolones. Experience with these agents over time and further investigations will help elucidate the precise role of oral antibiotics in the management of endophthalmitis.

NASALLY APPLIED ANTIBIOTICS

It has been demonstrated that organisms isolated from the vitreous were genetically indistinguishable from those recovered from the eyelids, conjunctiva, or nose in 14 of 17 cases of endophthalmitis.[22] Gram-positive organisms are part of the normal flora of the skin, nares, and conjunctiva and, interestingly, the EVS demonstrated that 94% of isolates recovered from eyes with postoperative endophthalmitis had Gram-positive organisms, 70% of which were due to coagulase-negative staphylococci.[1]

Mupirocin (Bactroban, GlaxoSmithKline) is a unique antibiotic that exerts bactericidal action by interfering with the action of isoleucyl-transfer RNA synthetase. Mupirocin is active against Gram-positive organisms, including *Staphylococcus* and *Streptococcus* spp. It is available as a nasal ointment, and is used for the eradication of methicillin-resistant *Staphylococcus aureus*.[23] Nasal carriage of *S. aureus* was eliminated in 91% of colonized health care workers 2–4 days following treatment with mupirocin ointment.[24]

Nasal carriage of Gram-positive organisms is a well-established risk factor for surgical site infections. In a large multicenter study of *S. aureus* bacteremia, greater than 80% of the blood isolates were identical to those from the anterior nares.[25] Perioperative elimination of nasal carriage using mupirocin ointment significantly reduced the surgical site infection rate in one study of cardiothoracic surgery patients.[26] Additionally, the use of mupirocin nasal ointment was effective in reducing the incidence of *S. aureus* infections in hemodialysis patients, as well as in those patients who undergo continuous ambulatory peritoneal dialysis.[27]

There is evidence in the literature of nonophthalmologic specialties that the rates of surgical site infections can be reduced with mupirocin nasal ointment. Therefore, we sought to determine if using mupirocin ointment to eliminate nasal bacterial carriage prior to intraocular surgery was effective in reducing conjunctival bacterial flora. If successful, we hypothesize that rates of postoperative endophthalmitis could be reduced with improved sterilization of the ocular surface.[28]

We designed a prospective, double-arm, blinded clinical trial of 37 eyes of 37 patients undergoing intraocular surgery (cataract extraction or pars plana vitrectomy) randomized to either control or mupirocin treatment groups.[29] Treated group patients received mupirocin nasal ointment twice daily for 5 days prior to surgery. Nasal cultures were obtained in all patients. All patients received a standard 5% povidone-iodine prep before the surgical procedure, and conjunctival cultures were obtained in all patients before and after the povidone-iodine prep.

All 37 patient nasal swabs were positive for bacterial growth (cultures were obtained prior to the use of mupirocin ointment in the treatment group). One of 15 eyes (6.7%) in the treatment group had positive conjunctival cultures prior to povidone-iodine prep, compared with 9 of 22 eyes (41%) in the control group ($P < 0.05$). Even after povidone-iodine prep, 8 of 22 eyes (36%) in the control group demonstrated persistent positive cultures, while only 1 (6.7%) of the treatment eyes exhibited growth ($P < 0.05$) (Figure 45.4).

The use of mupirocin nasal ointment prior to intraocular surgery or intravitreal injections is a novel method for reducing conjunctival contamination rates. Lower conjunctival contamination rates should theoretically reduce the incidence of postoperative endophthalmitis. Prophylactic use of mupirocin nasal ointment resulted in significant reduction of conjunctival flora with or without preoperative topical 5% povidone-iodine prep. Future studies will be needed to define precisely the role of mupirocin nasal ointment for prophylaxis against intraocular infections.

ORAL, TOPICAL, AND INTRAVITREAL ANTIFUNGAL AGENTS

Although fungal endophthalmitis is rare in the grand scheme of intraocular infection, it remains an important clinical problem in ophthalmology due to the potentially devastating consequences resulting from these infections. Additionally, ocular fungal infections have traditionally been very difficult to treat due to limited therapeutic options both systemically and intravitreally.

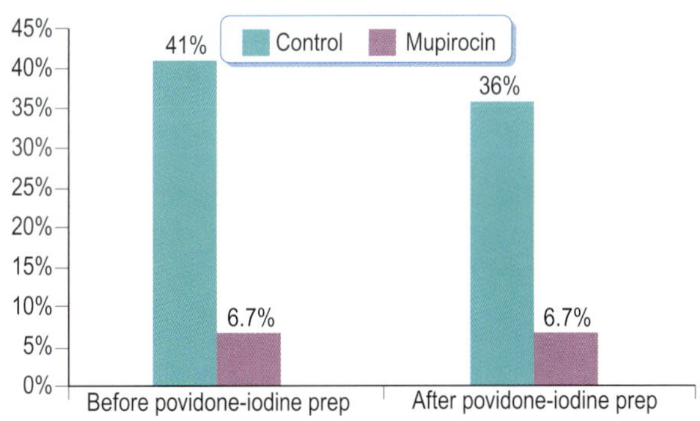

Figure 45.4 Conjunctival culture positivity in control group versus nasal mupirocin-treated group before and after povidone-iodine preparation.

In the past few years there have been major strides in the development of antifungal agents, and their potential use in the treatment of fungal endophthalmitis needs to be explored. The new-generation triazoles such as voriconazole, posaconazole, and ravuconazole represent advances in the evolution of the triazole antifungal class and have been developed to address the increasing incidence of fungal infections and the limitations of the currently available agents.[29,30]

Voriconazole (VFend, Pfizer Pharmaceuticals) is a second-generation synthetic derivative of fluconazole. It was developed by Pfizer Pharmaceuticals as part of a program designed to enhance the potency and spectrum of activity of fluconazole (i.e., *in vitro* potency of voriconazole against yeasts is 60-fold higher than for fluconazole). Voriconazole differs from fluconazole by the addition of a methyl group to the propyl backbone and by the substitution of a triazole moiety with a fluoropyrimidine group, resulting in a marked change in activity (Figure 45.5). Voriconazole has 96% oral bioavailability and reaches peak plasma concentrations 2–3 hours after oral dosing. Previous *in vitro* studies have shown voriconazole to have a broad spectrum of fungistatic action against *Aspergillus* species, *Blastomyces dermatitidis*, *Candida* species, *Paecilomyces lilacinus*, *Coccidioides immitis*, *Cryptococcus neoformans*, *Histoplasma capsulatum*, *Penicillium* species, *Scedosporium* species, *Curvularia* species, and others.[29,30]

We designed a prospective, nonrandomized clinical study of 14 patients scheduled for elective pars plana vitrectomy surgery to investigate the aqueous and vitreous concentration achieved after oral administration of two 400 mg doses of voriconazole taken 12 hours apart before surgery. The percentages of plasma voriconazole concentration achieved in the vitreous and aqueous were 38.1% and 53.0%, respectively. Mean inhibitory vitreous and aqueous MIC_{90} levels were achieved against a wide spectrum of yeasts and molds (e.g., the vitreous concentration of voriconazole achieved with this dosing regimen exceeded the MIC_{90} for *Candida albicans* by over 13-fold).[31] To determine if voriconazole could be used safely for intravitreal injection, our group also performed a histopathologic and electoretinographic study using a rodent model. Our studies demonstrated that voriconazole did not cause retinal toxicity on either electroretinogram or histology studies when intravitreal concentrations were 25 μg/ml or less. This represents a level of antibiotic that is 50-fold greater than commonly encountered MIC_{90} levels. When the concentration reached 50 μg/ml, focal retinal necrosis was occasionally noticed on histological exam (Figure 45.6).[32] While further studies are needed to delineate the appropriate level of voriconazole to use in humans, we have utilized this agent in select cases alone or with another novel IV antifungal (caspofungin), without evidence of apparent toxicity.[33] In another paper, postoperative fungal endophthalmitis was successfully treated using intravitreal and intracameral voriconazole as a single agent without combination therapy (Figure 45.7).[34]

The incidence of corneal ulceration secondary to *Fusarium* has increased dramatically in the past 3 years. One report identifies a sevenfold increase over the reported 11-month period at two tertiary eye care centers in the northeastern USA compared with the previous 30 months. There seems to be an association between the recent outbreak

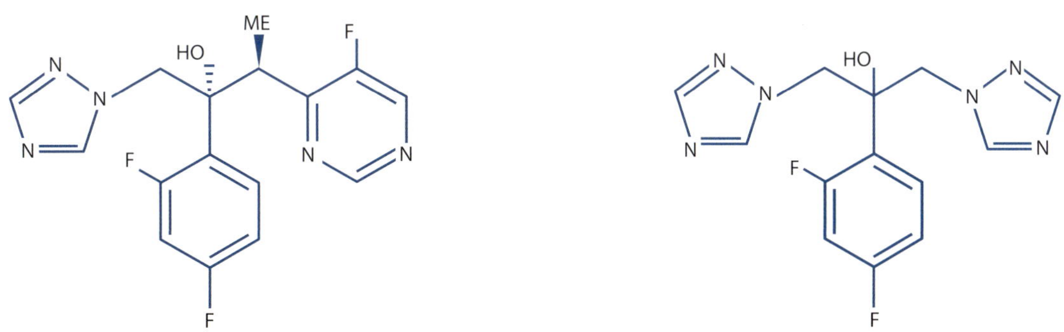

Figure 45.5 Structures of voriconazole and fluconazole.

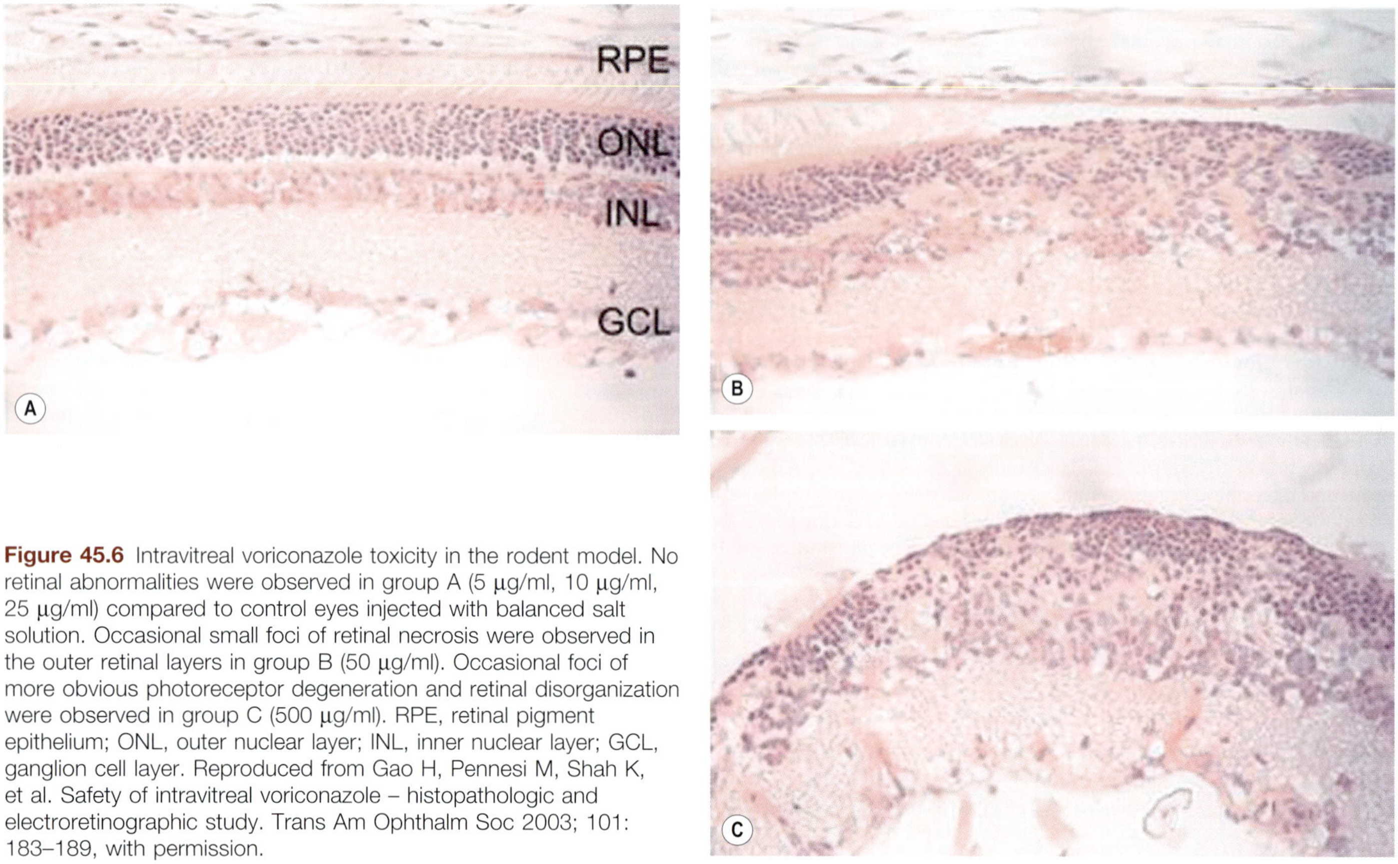

Figure 45.6 Intravitreal voriconazole toxicity in the rodent model. No retinal abnormalities were observed in group A (5 μg/ml, 10 μg/ml, 25 μg/ml) compared to control eyes injected with balanced salt solution. Occasional small foci of retinal necrosis were observed in the outer retinal layers in group B (50 μg/ml). Occasional foci of more obvious photoreceptor degeneration and retinal disorganization were observed in group C (500 μg/ml). RPE, retinal pigment epithelium; ONL, outer nuclear layer; INL, inner nuclear layer; GCL, ganglion cell layer. Reproduced from Gao H, Pennesi M, Shah K, et al. Safety of intravitreal voriconazole – histopathologic and electroretinographic study. Trans Am Ophthalm Soc 2003; 101: 183–189, with permission.

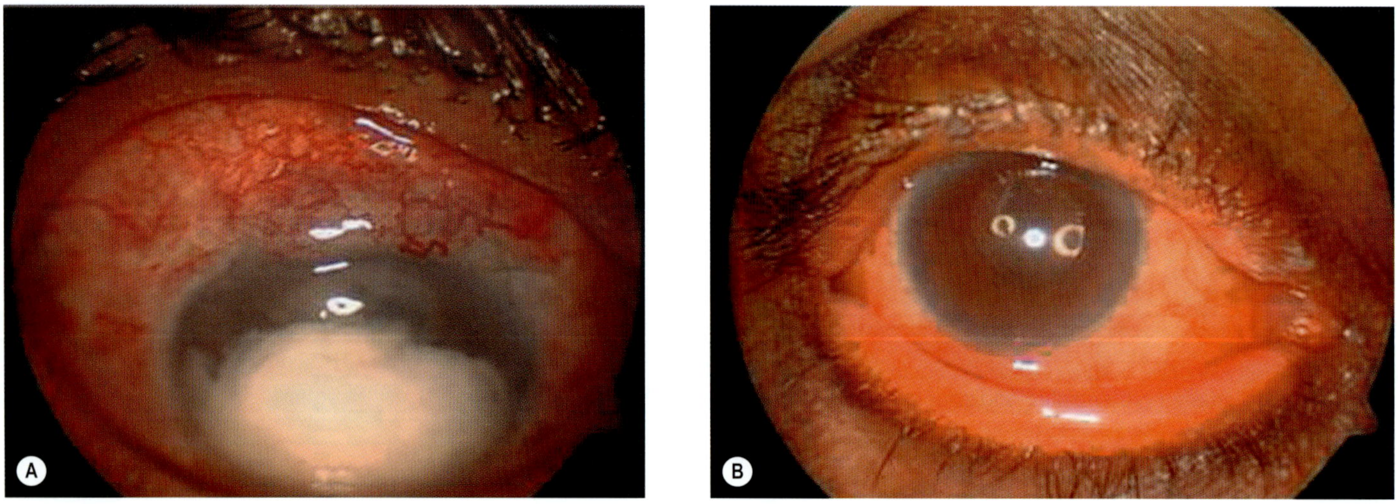

Figure 45.7 (A) Ten days after cataract surgery. Large mycotic hypopyon with ocular inflammation. (B) Five months after vitrectomy: anterior-chamber washout, intracameral and intravitreal voriconazole. Note clearing of hypopyon.

of *Fusarium* keratitis among contact lens users and the use of ReNu contact lens solution. Medical treatment of *Fusarium* keratitis may be ineffective, and emergent penetrating keratoplasty may be required in some patients.[35]

Treatment options for fungal keratitis are limited. Natamycin, a polyene compound, is the only commercially available antifungal agent approved for topical ocular use in the USA. It has limited efficacy due to poor corneal penetration, and is typically used in nonsevere superficial keratitis. While amphotericin B has reasonable activity against *Candida* and *Aspergillus*, it is not effective against *Fusarium* species, a common cause of posttraumatic fungal eye infection.

To address the unmet need in topical antifungal therapy, we conducted a study to determine the penetration of 1% voriconazole solution into the human aqueous and vitreous following topical administration. This was a prospective, nonrandomized clinical study in which aqueous and vitreous samples were obtained and analyzed after topical administration of voriconazole 1% every 2 hours for 24 hours prior to planned vitrectomy surgery.[36]

We found mean voriconazole concentrations in aqueous and vitreous were 6.492 ± 3.042 and 0.156 ± 0.082 μg/ml, respectively. Aqueous concentrations exceeded inhibitory MIC_{90} levels for a wide spectrum of fungi and mold, including *Aspergillus*, *Fusarium*, and *Candida* species. Vitreous levels of voriconazole exceeded the MIC_{90} for *Candida albicans*. Topically administered voriconazole achieves therapeutic levels in the aqueous of the noninflamed human eye for many fungi and molds, and achieves therapeutic levels in the vitreous for *Candida*. Because of its broad-spectrum coverage, high potency against organisms of concern, good tolerability, and intraocular penetration with topical administration, topical voriconazole may be a useful agent for the management of fungal keratitis and prophylaxis against the development of fungal endophthalmitis.

Orally and topically administered voriconazole achieves therapeutic aqueous and vitreous levels in the noninflamed human eye and the activity spectrum appears to encompass appropriately the most frequently encountered fungal species involved in the various causes of exogenous and endogenous fungal endophthalmitis. In addition, oral or intravitreal voriconazole may present an alternative management technique for fungal endophthalmitis by which the risk of retinal toxicity associated with intravitreal amphotericin B injection can be avoided.[37] Because of its broad spectrum of coverage, low MIC_{90} levels for the organisms of concern, good tolerability, and excellent bioavailability, voriconazole through various routes of administration may be useful to the ophthalmologist in the primary treatment of, or as an adjunct in, the current management of ocular fungal infections.[38]

CONCLUSION

In the past 20 years, numerous significant advances and the availability of new-generation anti-infectives have undoubtedly paved the way for improved outcomes in our management of ocular infections. The EVS provided us with excellent evidence-based data; however, numerous questions remain.

The fourth-generation fluoroquinolones are already playing a key role in the management of ocular infection, as well as in prophylaxis against infection. Additionally, advances in antifungal therapy, specifically the new-generation triazoles, will help improve outcomes through various routes of administration for patients with ocular fungal infection.

We need to rethink the applicability of the EVS data given the availability of these "new weapons in the arsenal of ophthalmic antibiotics."[10] So, while we do have evidence-based data from the EVS, with time the data may have lost some significance, due to the new developments noted above. Our next step is to develop new strategies for the management of ocular infection utilizing these new fluoroquinolone and triazole agents, with a goal of limiting the impact of proven infection, or ideally eliminating the development of endophthalmitis in a cost-effective manner.

Even with the advancements over the past decade, unparalleled opportunities for prevention and/or reduction of morbidity from intraocular infection continue to exist. While we truly would like to base all of our therapeutic decisions on evidence-based data, we will still be forced to rely on data from a variety of clinical sources.

REFERENCES

1. Endophthalmitis Vitrectomy Study Group. Results of the Endophthalmitis Vitrectomy Study: A randomized trial of immediate vitrectomy and of intravenous antibiotics for the treatment of postoperative bacterial endophthalmitis. Arch Ophthalmol 1995;113:1479–1496.
2. el-Massry A, Meredith TA, Aguilar HE, et al. Aminoglycoside levels in the rabbit vitreous cavity after intravenous administration. Am J Ophthalmol 1996;122:684–689.
3. Aguilar HE, Meredith TA, Shaarawy A, et al. Vitreous cavity penetration of ceftazidime after intravenous administration. Retina 1995; 15:154–159.
4. Doft BH. The Endophthalmitis Vitrectomy Study. Arch Ophthalmol 1991;109:487–489.
5. Han DP, Wisniewski SR, Wilson LA, et al. Spectrum and susceptibilities of microbiologic isolates in the EVS. Am J Ophthalmol 1996;122:1–17.
6. Endophthalmitis Vitrectomy Study Group. Microbiologic factors and visual outcomes in the Endophthalmitis Vitrectomy Study. Am J Ophthalmol 1996;122:830–846.
7. Johnson MW, Doft BH, Kelsey SF, et al. The Endophthalmitis Vitrectomy Study. Relationship between clinical presentation and microbiologic spectrum. Ophthalmology 1997;104:261–272.
8. Miller D, Flynn PM, Scott IU, et al. *In vitro* fluoroquinolone resistance in staphylococcal endophthalmitis isolates. Arch Ophthalmol 2006;124: 479–483.
9. Bannerman TL, Rhoden DL, McAllister SK, et al. The source of coagulase-negative staphylococci in the Endophthalmitis Vitrectomy Study: A comparison of eyelid and intraocular isolates using pulsed-field gel electrophoresis. Arch Ophthalmol 1997;115:357–361.
10. Mather R, Karanchak LM, Romanowski EG, et al. Fourth generation fluoroquinolones: new weapons in the arsenal of ophthalmic antibiotics. Am J Ophthalmol 2002;133:463–466.
11. Fiscella RG, Shapiro MJ, Solomon MJ, et al. Ofloxacin penetration into the eye after intravenous and topical administration. Retina 1997;17: 535–539.
12. Hariprasad SM, Blinder KJ, Shah GK, et al. Penetration pharmacokinetics of topically administered 0.5% moxifloxacin ophthalmic solution in human aqueous and vitreous. Arch Ophthalmol 2005;123:39–44.
13. Hariprasad SM, Shah GK, Chi J, et al. Determination of aqueous and vitreous concentration of moxifloxacin 0.5% in humans after delivery via a dissolvable corneal collagen shield device. J Cataract and Refractive Surg 2005;31(11):2142–2146.
14. Hariprasad SM, Mieler WF, Holz ER. Vitreous and aqueous penetration of orally administered Gatifloxacin in humans. Arch Ophthalmol 2003;121: 345–350.
15. Hariprasad SM, Mieler WF, Holz ER. Vitreous penetration of orally administered Gatifloxacin in humans. Tr Am Ophth Soc 2002;100: 153–160.
16. Fiscella RG, Nguyen TK, Cwik MJ, et al. Aqueous and vitreous penetration of levofloxacin after oral administration. Ophthalmol 1999;106:2286–2290.
17. Garcia-Saenz MC, Arias-Puente A, Fresnadillo-Martinez MJ, et al. Human aqueous humor levels of oral ciprofloxacin, levofloxacin, and moxifloxacin. J Cataract Refract Surg 2001;27:1969–1974.
18. Hariprasad SM, Shah GK, Mieler WF, et al. Vitreous and aqueous penetration of orally administered moxifloxacin in humans. Arch Ophthalmol 2006;124:178–182.
19. Keren G, Alhalel A, Bartov E, et al. The intravitreal penetration of orally administered ciprofloxacin in humans. Invest Ophthalmol Vis Sci 1991;32:2388–2392.
20. Aras C, Ozdamar A, Ozturk R, et al. Intravitreal penetration of Cefepime after systemic administration to humans. Ophthalmologica 2002;216: 261–264.
21. Hariprasad SM, Mieler WF, Orengo-Nania S, et al. The use of oral Gatifloxacin in the treatment of localized filtering bleb infections. Eye 2009 (in press).
22. Speaker MG, Milch FA, Shah MK, et al. Role of external bacterial flora in the pathogenesis of acute postoperative endophthalmitis. Ophthalmology 1991;98:639–649; discussion 650.
23. Kluytmans JA, Wertheim HF. Nasal carriage of *Staphylococcus aureus* and prevention of nosocomial infections. Infection 2005;33:3–8.
24. Doebbeling BN, Breneman DL, Neu HC, the Mupirocin Collaborative Study Group. Elimination of *Staphylococcus aureus* nasal carriage in health care workers: analysis of six clinical trials with calcium mupirocin ointment. The Mupirocin Collaborative Study Group. Clin Infect Dis 1993;17:466–474.
25. von Eiff C, Becker K, Machka K, et al. Nasal carriage as a source of *Staphylococcus aureus* bacteremia. N Engl J Med 2001;344:11–16.
26. Kluytmans JA, Mouton JW, VandenBergh MF, et al. Reduction of surgical-site infections in cardiothoracic surgery by elimination of nasal carriage of *Staphylococcus aureus*. Infect Control Hosp Epidemiol 1996;17:780–785.
27. The Mupirocin Study Group. Nasal mupirocin prevents *Staphylococcus aureus* exit-site infection during peritoneal dialysis. J Am Soc Nephrol 1996;7:2403–2408.
28. Alexandrou TJ, Hariprasad SM, Benevento J, et al. Reduction of preoperative conjunctival bacterial flora with the use of mupirocin nasal ointment. Trans Am Ophth Soc 2006;104:196–201.
29. Ghannoum MA, Kuhn DM. Voriconazole – better chances for patients with invasive mycoses. Eur J Med Res 2002;7:242–256.
30. Sabo JA, Abdel-Rahman SM. Voriconazole: A new triazole antifungal. Ann Pharmacother 2000;34:1032–1043.
31. Hariprasad SM, Mieler WF, Holz ER, et al. Determination of vitreous, aqueous, and plasma concentration of orally administered voriconazole in humans. Arch Ophthalmol 2004;122:42–47.
32. Gao H, Pennesi M, Shah K, et al. Safety of intravitreal voriconazole histopathologic and electroretinographic study. Tr Am Ophth Soc 2003;101:183–189.
33. Breit SM, Hariprasad SM, Mieler WF, et al. Management of endogenous fungal endophthalmitis with voriconazole and caspofungin. Am J Ophthalmol 2005;139:135–140.

34. Lin RC, Sanduja N, Hariprasad SM. Successful treatment of postoperative fungal endophthalmitis using intravitreal and intracameral voriconazole. J Ocul Pharmacol Ther 2008;24(2):245–248.
35. Gorscak JJ, Ayres BD, Bhagat N, et al. An outbreak of *Fusarium* keratitis associated with contact lens use in the northeastern United States. Cornea 2007;26:1187–1194.
36. Vemulakonda GA, Hariprasad SM, Mieler WF, et al. Aqueous and vitreous concentrations following topical administration of 1% voriconazole in humans. Arch Ophthalmol 2008;126(1):18–22.
37. Axelrod AJ, Peyman GA, Apple DJ. Toxicity of intravitreal injection of amphotericin B. Am J Ophthalmol 1973;76:578–583.
38. Hariprasad SM, Mieler WF, Lin TK, et al. Voriconazole in the treatment of fungal eye infections: a review of current literature. Br J Ophthalmol 2008;92:871–878.

CHAPTER 46

Rheotherapy (rheopheresis; therapeutical apheresis)

Helen Dede Ayertey, MD, Richard Brunner, MD, and Bernd Kirchhof, MD

KEY FEATURES (PHARMACOLOGY)

Rheopheresis is a form of therapeutic plasma apheresis that utilizes a novel nanopore, hollow-fiber, membrane technology configured in a differential filtration array with two single-use, in-line, membrane filters (Figure 46.1). It is designed to deplete excess concentrations of soluble high-molecular-weight plasma components by mechanically sieving circulating species larger than 25 nm (as measured across their shortest linear axis) or approximately 500 kDa by weight from the blood. As such, the therapy provides physiologic depletion of a targeted bandwidth of plasma species, including immune complexes, immunoglobulin M (IgM), α_2-macroglobulin, fibrinogen, von Willenbrand factor, low-density lipoprotein (LDL) cholesterol, and others.[1,2]

INTRODUCTION AND HISTORY

The Center of Ophthalmology of the University of Cologne has been employing various strategies to decrease fibrinogen and high-molecular plasma proteins in ocular diseases in interdisciplinary cooperation since 1988. Besides other effects, blood circulation capacity is improved and this in turn leads to a measurable upgrading of the ocular hemodynamics.[4,5]

The simultaneous elimination of a defined spectrum of high-molecular-weight rheologically relevant plasma proteins (>25 nm or 500 kDa, i.e., alpha-2-macroglobulin, fibrinogen, fibronectin, LDL cholesterol, IgM, von Willebrand factor, putatively multimeric vitronectin) immediately results in the pulsed reduction of plasma and whole-blood viscosity.[1,6–9]

Thus, rheopheresis is successfully used to improve microcirculatory impairment. Rheopheresis treatment appears to restore and activate or stabilize the functional reserve of the retina at microcirculatory levels. Results from clinical trials, evaluations of patients suffering from age-related macular degeneration (AMD) and other microcirculatory disorders (e.g., diabetic retinopathy, central retinal vein occlusion (CRVO), and uveal effusion syndrome) and basic research in the field of AMD pathogenesis describing structural and functional features of impaired microcirculation in AMD can all be referenced as proof of principle. Serial pulses of plasma protein elimination reduce plasma viscosity and thus lead to a sustained improvement in microcirculation.[1,2,4,6,9–11]

RHEOPHERESIS IN RETINAL DISEASES

AGE-RELATED MACULAR DEGENERATION

AMD is one of the leading causes of blindness in the elderly in the industrial world and is therefore of increasing socioeconomic interest. The pathogenesis of AMD is, however, not yet fully understood.[2,10–13] Pigment epithelium detachment or clumping, atrophy of the choriocapillaris, and a decrease in choroidal perfusion are common and consistent findings in AMD.[10] The diminished perfusion of the choroid seems to play a decisive role in the pathogenesis of pigment epithelium damage, leading to worsening of the visual function and the progression of morphological changes. It is thus receiving greater attention.[10,14]

Even in its early stages, AMD showing drusen and changes in the pigment epithelium can cause considerable impairment of central vision, including distortions and difficulties in reading. Risk factors for AMD besides old age are, for example, obesity, hypertension, elevated serum cholesterol, diabetes, and smoking, which further indicate a correlation between AMD and perfusion or microcirculation.[15–17]

The treatment of age-related maculopathy and the early stages of dry AMD, based on current diagnostic findings, aims at the stabilization and improvement of central vision in order to enhance patients' quality of life and level of independence. Due to a lack of generally accepted therapies, in many cases only good cardiovascular adjustment controls and ophthalmologic follow-up are recommended.

Rheopheresis has been clinically investigated over the past years and shown to have a positive influence on the natural course of AMD. Long-term evaluations have further proven that the improvements brought about by rheopheresis are stable over a period of years.[2,10,11]

MAC-1 trial

Findings of a nonblind randomized trial evaluating 40 patients treated with 10 rheopheresis treatments have been documented in the eye journal *Retina*.[10] AMD patients with soft drusen benefited most greatly from the rheopheresis treatments and demonstrated an average 2.3 lines of improvement compared to the control group (no treatment). One year posttreatment, 30% of the control group lost ≥ 3 lines of acuity, compared with only 10% of the rheopheresis group.[2]

In addition, 15% of the rheopheresis group's vision improved by ≥ 2 lines compared with only 5% of the control group. With respect to patients with vision worse than 20/40 prior to treatment, 37% of patients in the rheopheresis group gained at least 20/40 vision after treatment, compared with only 10% of the control group. (The 20/40 vision threshold is important because it defines the legal driving limit imposed by most countries.[2])

Multicenter investigation of rheopheresis for AMD (MIRA-1)

The most extensive study on rheopheresis application was performed in the USA as part of an ongoing Food and Drug Administration (FDA) trial. Over 1200 procedures were administered to 150–180 patients.[2,11]

MIRA-1 was designed to provide type 1 evidence-based information on the safety and efficacy of the rheopheresis procedure for select patients with dry AMD. The primary aim of the study was to compare the results between the rheopheresis group (which received rheopheresis) and the placebo group (which did not receive active treatment).[2,11]

In the autumn of 2001, the company in question received authorization from the FDA to conduct an interim analysis of the first 43 patients in the form of a 12-month follow-up. A total of 29 rheopheresis patients and 14 placebo patients were included in the analysis. The primary objective of the procedure is to slow down or completely stop the disease. At the 12-month postbaseline interval, rheophoresis-treated

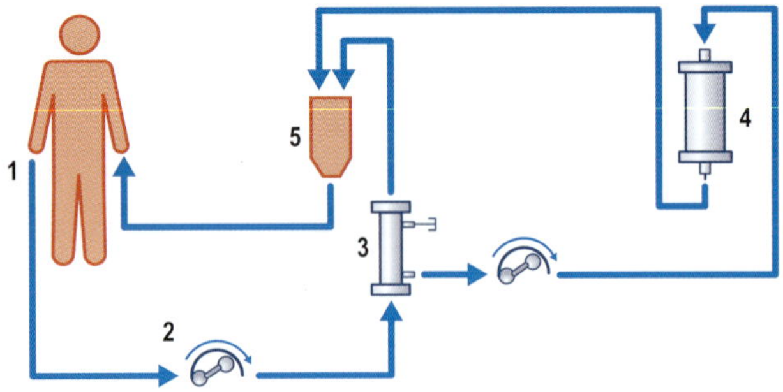

Figure 46.1 Blood circulation was established from one forearm to the other by bilateral insertion of needles into each antecubital vein (1). The whole blood is pumped (2) into a separate pressurized circuit. Here the plasma is driven through a two-stage filtration process provided by the plasma separator (3) connected in series to the plasma component separator (4). Then the sieved plasma is recombined with the cellular fraction of the blood (5) to be reinfused into the patient (1).[2,3]

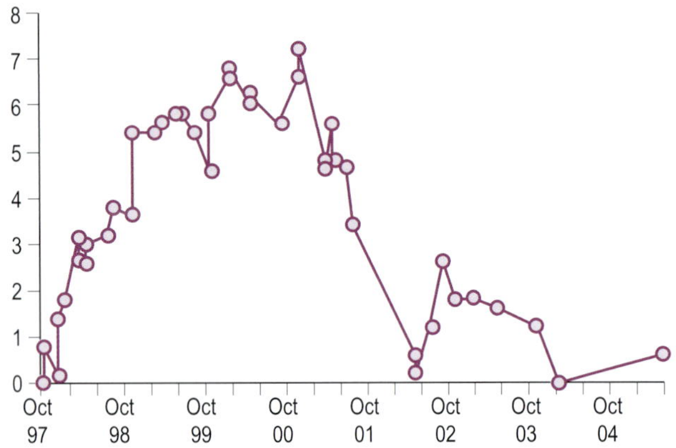

Figure 46.2 Change in visual acuity in lines (ETDRS) in patient PH, aged 66 years. Right eye initial visual acuity 20/200.

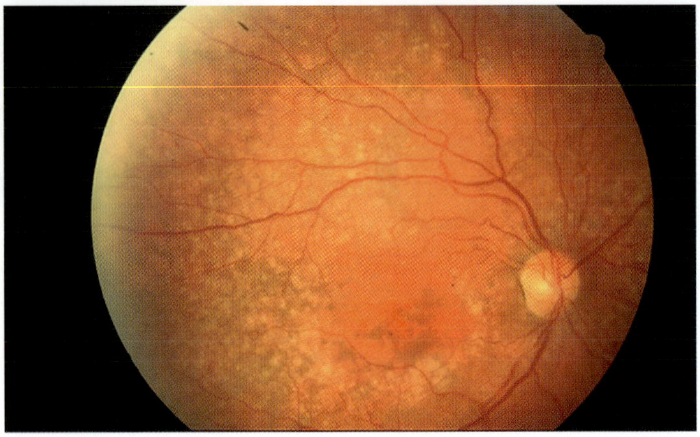

Figure 46.3 Fundus photograph of patient PH; right eye 1997.

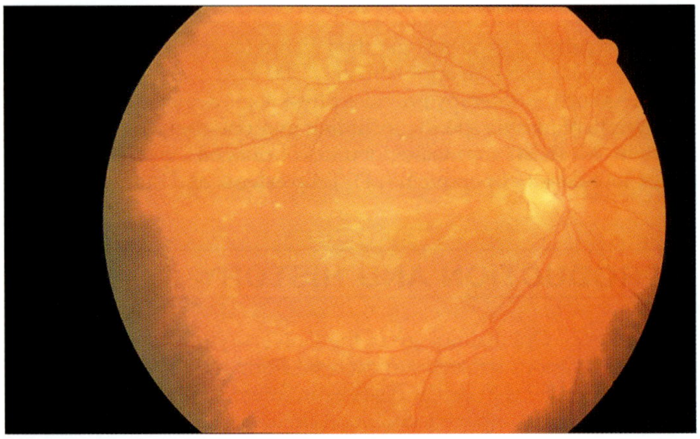

Figure 46.4 Fundus photograph of patient PH; right eye 2003.

eyes (n = 29) demonstrated an average improvement of 0.7 lines of vision compared with an average loss of 0.9 lines in the control group (n = 14) (no treatment). The mean difference of 1.6 lines between the two groups is significant (P = 0.0011, repeated-measures analysis). In the subgroup of patients with baseline vision worse than 20/40, the rheophoresis-treated eyes (n = 19) demonstrated an average improvement of 1.1 lines of vision compared with an average loss of 1.9 lines in the control group (n = 7) (no treatment). Despite the relatively small sizes of the two groups, the mean difference of 3.0 lines between the two groups is statistically significant (P = 0.0014, repeated-measures analysis).[2,11]

In our clinic we have followed several patients over a number of years and the long-term results of treatment with rheopheresis seem promising. The decrease in visual function can be prevented and an increase in visual function can be observed for a number of years. At a certain point in time, the ongoing morphological changes again lead to a reduction in visual function. Nevertheless, these patients gained between several years and a decade of better visual function and therefore improved quality of life with reading and driving capabilities (Figures 46.2–46.4).

In our opinion, patients with the following diagnostic findings and informed consent are suitable for treatment with rheopheresis.

The eye intended for treatment should show:

- dry AMD
- soft drusen (Figure 46.3), changes in the pigment epithelium
- visual acuity of between 0.1 (20/200) and 0.63 (20/32) and no exudation, bleeding, fibrosis, or advanced atrophy.

Diagnosis, indication, examination, and follow-up of the patients are the responsibility of the treating ophthalmologist.

DIABETIC MACULOPATHY

The increasing incidence of type 2 diabetes leads to an astonishing number of diabetic eye disease cases, of which diabetic maculopathy is of the greatest concern. Diabetic maculopathy is by far the most common cause of poor vision in our society and among people of working age.[18] The pathogenesis is not fully understood and satisfactory therapy is not yet available. Malfunction of the blood–retinal barrier plays a central role in the disease, leading to retinal edema and photoreceptor dysfunction. Diabetic vascular leakage and macular edema are regulated by a distinct combination of direct paracellular transport, alterations in endothelial intercellular junctions, and endothelial cell death. The distribution and relevance of these three factors for diabetic maculopathy vary over the course of the disease. Cumulative endothelial cell death becomes more relevant after prolonged diabetic conditions.[19]

Unfortunately, and unlike macrovascular diseases, the medical treatment of microvascular disease in diabetes and particularly in diabetic retinopathy is still at an early stage. Given the rapid global increase in the prevalence of diabetes and the morbidity rate caused by diabetic microvascular disease, it is important to increase the efforts in this field.

There are several indications that patients with higher baseline total cholesterol, LDL cholesterol, or triglycerides are at greater risk of developing diabetic maculopathy.

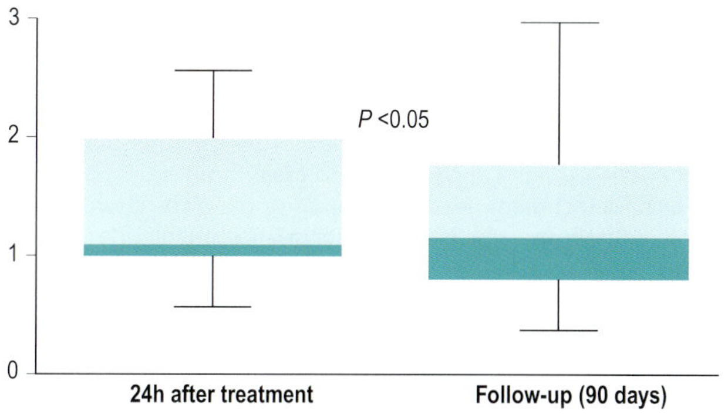

Figure 46.5 Changes in visual acuity in lines ETDRS in 10 eyes with diabetic maculopathy treated with membrane differential filtration.[3]

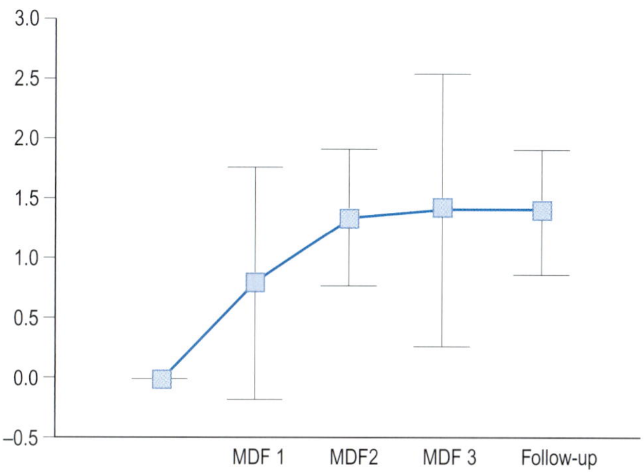

Figure 46.6 Changes in visual acuity in lines ETDRS in 11 patients with diabetic maculopathy treated with membrane differential filtration (MDF) for 18 weeks.[21]

Rheopheresis can reduce rheologically relevant plasma proteins such as LDL cholesterol and triglycerides and also improve microcirculatory impairment.[20] In combination with laser coagulation against ischemic retinopathy, rheopheresis treatment can help to restore and activate or stabilize the functional reserve of the retina at microcirculatory levels (Figures 46.5–46.7).

CENTRAL RETINAL VEIN OCCLUSION

With a prevalence of between 0.1% and 0.4%, CRVO is one of the most common causes of visual loss in adults over 40 years.[22] Risk factors for CRVO are hypertension, diabetes, and glaucoma.[23]

The Central Retinal Vein Occlusion Study (CVOS) found that the visual outcome for enrolled patients was largely dependent on initial visual acuity. Patients who had poor visual acuity (<20/200) were shown to have an 80% chance of a final acuity score of less than 20/200 on their final visit.[23,24]

Therapeutic options are still rare and most surgical and medical interventions bring with them a high risk of complications.[23]

Several random clinical trials have proposed hemodilution as a therapeutic option for CRVO. The rationale for the use of hemodilution is based on observations of increased plasma viscosity and increased hematocrit and fibrinogen levels in some patients with CRVO. The reduction of hematocrit, fibrinogen, and plasma viscosity may lead to improved retinal microcirculation.[22]

Rheopheresis has the immediate effect of simultaneously eliminating a defined spectrum of high-molecular-weight rheologically relevant plasma proteins, resulting in the pulsed reduction of plasma and whole-blood viscosity.[1,6–9] Serial pulses of plasma protein elimination, reducing plasma viscosity, can result in sustained improvement to the microcirculation.[1,2,4,6–11] Therefore, the chances of reperfusion and an improvement in visual acuity, even from low initial levels, are high (Figures 46.8–46.10).

UVEAL EFFUSION SYNDROME

Uveal effusion syndrome is a rare disease that largely affects middle-aged male subjects. The onset is spontaneous and the progression of

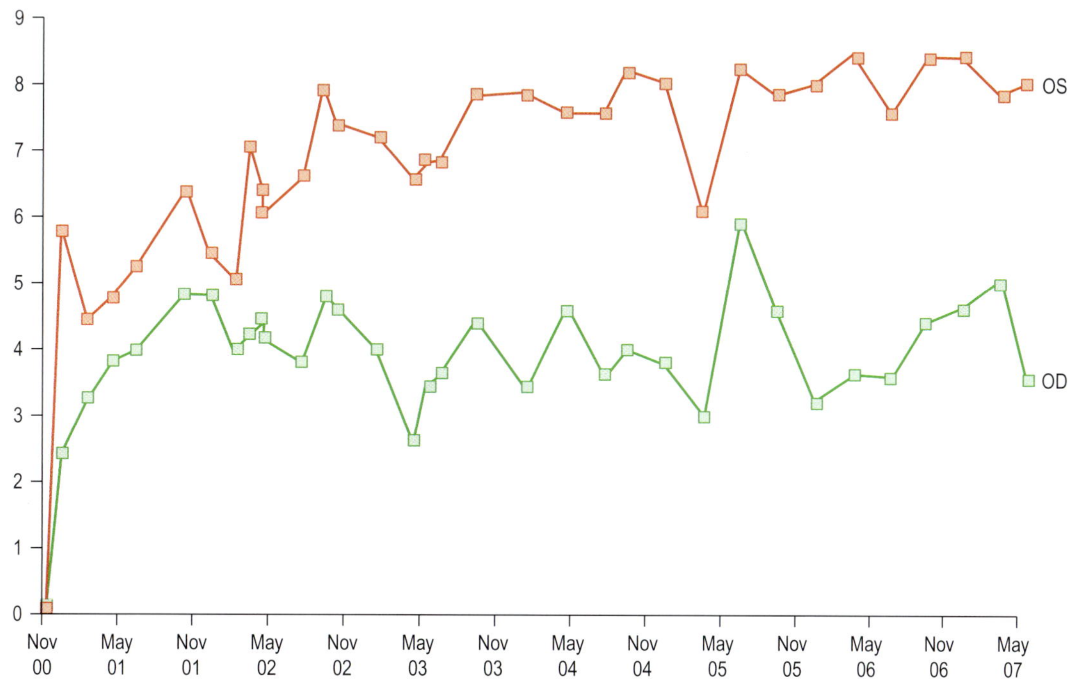

Figure 46.7 Changes in visual acuity in lines ETDRS in patients with diabetic maculopathy and treated with rheopheresis twice a year. Initial visual acuity: right eye (OD) 20/200, left eye (OS) 5/100; last visual acuity: OD 20/80, OS 20/63.

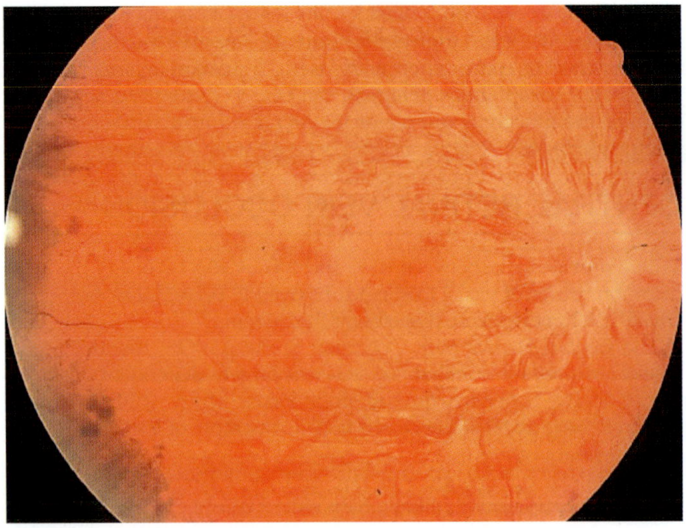

Figure 46.8 Central retinal vein occlusion in a 54-year-old man; decrease in visual acuity in right eye since 8 weeks; visual acuity 20/200.

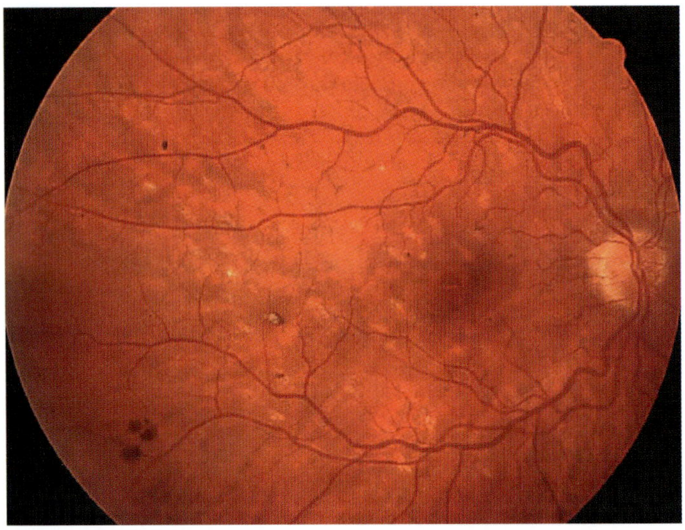

Figure 46.9 Follow-up after 27 months: Right eye after 18 rheopheresis treatments over a period of 12 months and laser coagulation 8 weeks after first visit. Visual acuity 20/25.

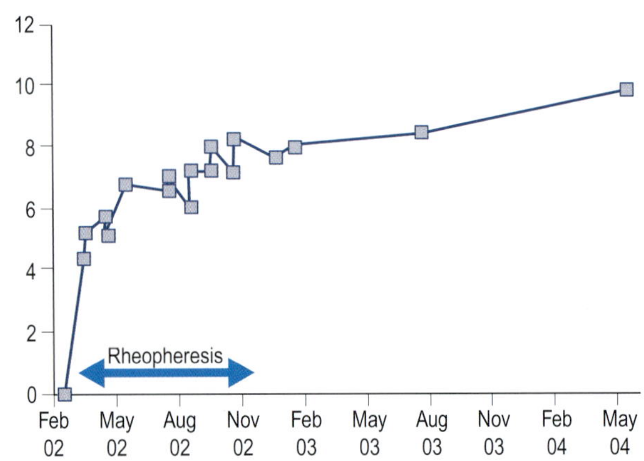

Figure 46.10 Central retinal vein occlusion in a 54-year-old man. Change of visual acuity in lines (ETDRS); initial visual acuity 0.1, current visual acuity 0.8.

the disease is slow, often leading to bilateral serous choroidal detachment and concomitant retinal detachment, shifting subretinal fluid and, in severe cases, total loss of visual acuity. Retinal holes or breaks cannot be found.[25–27]

Resistance to steroid treatment[25] and surgical intervention[28] in a number of cases is a major problem and the natural course often shows a long-term detachment, leading to an atrophy of the choroid and the pigment epithelium, which even after reattachment does not allow good functional results.[25,27]

Even in 1977 Paulmann and Heimann raised the question of the influence decreased microcirculation could have on maintenance of the detachment. They tried vascular dilatators and steroids combined with plasma expander, which led to improvement of visual acuity without recurrence.[28] Later, Brunner et al. published the successful use of therapeutic apheresis on uveal effusion syndrome resistant to steroid application.[25]

Therefore, we treated patients with idiopathic uveal effusion syndrome with repetitive therapeutical apheresis. Figures 46.11–46.13 show the case of a 43-year-old man with total serous choroidal detachment and concomitant serous amotio retinae in the left eye, which was completely resolved after treatment.

Complications

Rheopheresis is among the therapeutical apheresis procedures (double-filtration plasmapheresis) that have been performed to high technical

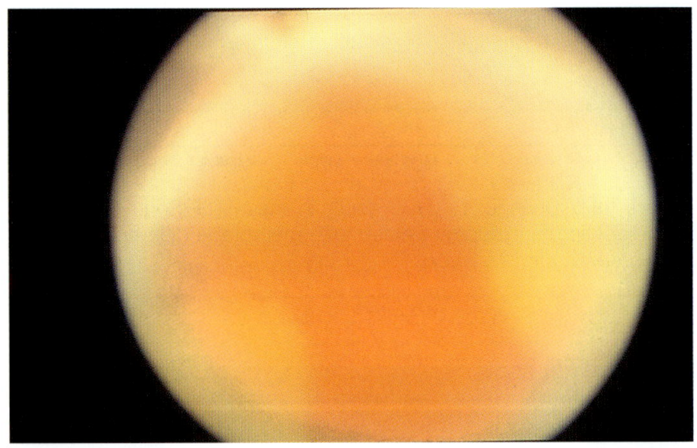

Figure 46.11 Uveal effusion syndrome in a 43-year-old man. OS before repetitive therapeutic apheresis with complete serous choroidal detachment; visual acuity: hand movement.

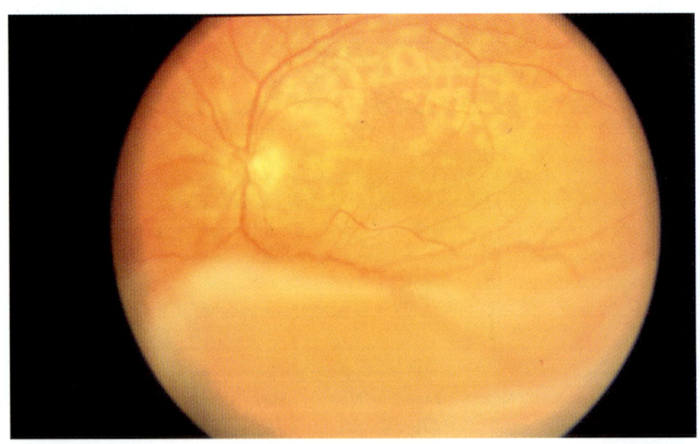

Figure 46.12 OS after start of repetitive therapeutic apheresis with partial reattachment of the choroidea; visual acuity: 20/125.

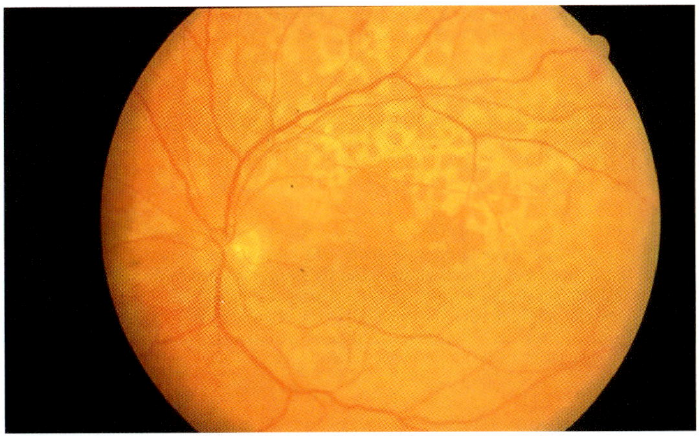

Figure 46.13 OS after 17 therapeutic apheresis with completely attached choroidea. The fundus shows the characteristic leopardiform pattern due to the long detachment of the choroidea; visual acuity: 20/50.

and safety standards in internal medicine for decades.[12] Rheopheresis's reliability has been extensively documented in the international RheoNet register, which includes data of over 7000 rheopheresis treatments, of which more than two-thirds were treatments of AMD patients. There were no severe adverse events reported. In 5.7% of treatments adverse events occurred, but only 0.5% necessitated termination of the treatment. Transient hypotension was the most frequently reported adverse event.[13,29]

SUMMARY

Rheopheresis is a safe and effective method of improving rheological parameters such as erythrocyte aggregation, plasma viscosity, and whole-blood viscosity due to the elimination of high-molecular proteins and lipoproteins. The therapy is well received by patients and, as no severe side-effects are mentioned, they appear to be rare.[10,12,13,25,30]

Rheopheresis can eliminate known vascular risk factors and suspected pathophysiologically relevant factors of AMD, CRVO, and diabetes by decreasing plasma viscosity and depleting the serum of soluble high-molecular proteins such as immune complexes, IgM, fibrinogen, LDL and very LDL cholesterol, von Willebrand factor, and α_2-macroglobulin.[1,2]

Friedman[6] has suggested a hemodynamic model of AMD pathogenesis. He hypothesized that impaired choroidal perfusion results from increases in vascular resistance in the choroid, possibly as a consequence of decreased compliance of the sclera and choroidal vessels with increased age, combined with lipidization of Bruch's membrane and accompanying drusen biosynthesis. Such effects would necessarily degrade the metabolic transport function of the pigment epithelium and other supporting posterior retinal tissues. Therapeutic apheresis may therefore be a way to improve the choroidal outflow. The reabsorbtion of subretinal fluid maintaining the serous choroidal and concomitant retinal detachment in uveal effusion syndrome leads to fast reattachment with good functional results, as shown in the aforementioned case.

Furthermore, inference of a possible systemic influence can be found in the reports of generalized risk factors that have been associated with AMD, CRVO, and diabetes in several trials. These risk factors include a history of smoking, systemic hypertension, increased body mass index, elevated fibrinogen levels, increased serum cholesterol, increased hemorheologic factors, elevated von Willebrand levels, and elevated α_2-macroglobulin levels.[15–17,25,31] Klingel and colleagues[1] state that the clinical consequences of impaired microcirculation are due to the complex interactive relationships between plasma components, blood cells, cells of the vessel wall (endothelium, vascular smooth-muscle cells, and fibroblasts), and the compartments of the surrounding tissues (cells and extracellular matrix).

Brunner and colleagues studied pulsatile ocular blood flow using a noninvasive quantitative assessment of the ciliary choroidal blood flow immediately preceding, and then subsequent to, rheopheresis treatment in 10 patients with AMD.[32] They found a statistically significant 22% increase in ocular blood flow ($P = 0.028$).

Rheopheresis as a treatment for selective patients with dry AMD, CRVO, nonproliferative diabetic maculopathy, or idiopathic uveal effusion syndrome appears to be safe and well tolerated by most patients. Long-term results show that the treatment benefits for eyes with CRVO, nonproliferative diabetic maculopathy, or idiopathic uveal effusion syndrome generally remain stable for years, or at least delay the natural course of events, as expected with dry AMD.

REFERENCES

1. Klingel R, Fassbender C, Fassbender T, et al. Rheopheresis: Rheologic, functional and structural aspects. Ther Apher 2000;4:348–357.
2. Multicenter Investigation of Rheopheresis for AMD (MIRA-1) Study Group and Pulido JS. Multicenter prospective, randomised, double-masked, placebo-controlled study of rheopheresis to treat nonexudative AMD: interim analysis. Trans Am Ophthalmol Soc 2002;100:85–108.
3. Widder RA, Brunner R, Walter P, et al. Improvement of visual acuity in patients suffering from diabetic retinopathy after membrane differential filtration: a pilot study. Transfus Sci 1999;21:201–206.
4. Brunner R, Widder RA, Fischer RA, et al. Clinical efficacy of hemorheological treatment using plasma exchange, selective adsorption and cascade filtration in maculopathy, retinal vein occlusion and uveal effusion syndrome. Transfus Sci 1997;17:493–498.
5. Soudavar F, Widder RA, Brunner R, et al. Changes of retinal haemodynamics after elimination of high molecular weight proteins and lipids in patients with age-related macular degeneration. Invest Ophth Vis Sci 1998;39:386.
6. Friedman E. A hemodynamic model of the pathogenesis of age-related macular degeneration. Am J Ophthalmol 1997;124:677–682.
7. Pulido JS, Sanders D, Klingel R. Rheopheresis for age-related macular degeneration: clinical results and putative mechanism of action. Can J Ophthalmol 2005;40:332–340.
8. Pulido J, Sanders D, Winters JL, et al. Clinical outcomes and mechanism of action for rheopheresis treatment of age-related macular degeneration (AMD). J Clin Apher 2005;20:185–194.
9. Widder RA, Brunner R, Borberg H. Changes of haemorheological parameters when using plasma exchange, selective adsorption and membrane differential separation. Transfus Sci 1996;17:505–510.
10. Brunner R, Widder RA, Walter P, et al. Influence of membrane differential filtration on the natural course of age-related macular degeneration – a randomized trial. Retina 2000;20:483–491.
11. Boyer DS. Summary of long-term interim results of MIRA-I trial: comparison of rheopheresis blood filtration vs. placebo control for the treatment of dry AMD. Retina 2001. Subspecialty Day, New Orleans, 9–10 November 2001; abstract.
12. Norda R, Stegmayr BR, Swedish Apheresis Group. Therapeutic apheresis in Sweden; update of epidemiology and adverse events. Transfus Apheresis Sci 2003;29(2):159–166.
13. Klingel R, Fassbender C, Göhlen B, et al. Rheonet – an international apheresis registry for rheopheresis: update 2004. Kidney Blood Press Res 2004;27(5-6):286.
14. Hyman L. Epidemiology of AMD. In: Hampton GR, Nelson PT, editors. Age Related Macular Degeneration. Principles and Practice. New York: Raven Press; 1993. p. 1–35.
15. Tomany SC, Wang JJ, Van Leeuwen R, et al. Risk factors for incident age-related macular degeneration: pooled findings from 3 continents. Ophthalmol 2004;111:1280–1287.
16. Klein R, Deng Y, Klein BE, et al. Cardiovascular disease, its risk factors and treatment, and age-related macular degeneration: Women's Health Initiative Sight Exam ancillary study. Am J Ophthalmol 2007;143: 473–483.
17. Tan JS, Mitchell P, Smith W, et al. Cardiovascular risk factors and the long-term incidence of age-related macular degeneration: the Blue Mountains Eye Study. Ophthalmol 2007;114:1143–1150.
18. Chowdhury TA, Hopkins D, Dodson PM, et al. The role of serum lipids in exudative maculopathy: is there a place for lipid-lowering therapy? Eye 2002;16:689–693.
19. Joussen AM, Smyth N, Niessen C. Pathophysiology of diabetic macular edema. Dev Ophthalmol 2007;39:1–12.
20. Klingel R, Mumme C, Fassbender T, et al. Rheopheresis in patients with ischemic diabetic foot syndrome: results of an open label prospective pilot trial. Ther Apher Dial 2003;7(4):444–455.
21. Lueke C, Widder RA, Soudavar F, et al. Improvement of macular function by membrane differential filtration in diabetic retinopathy. J Clin Apheresis 2001;16:23–28.

22. Mohamed Q, McIntosh RL, Saw SM, et al. Interventions for central retinal vein occlusion: an evidence-based systematic review. Ophthalmol 2007;114:507–519, 524.
23. Sharma A, D'Amico DJ. Medical and surgical management of central retinal vein occlusion. Int Ophthalmol Clin 2004;44:1–16.
24. The Central Vein Occlusion Study Group. Natural history and clinical management of central vein occlusion. Arch Ophthalmol 1997;115: 486–491.
25. Brunner R, Widder RA, Fischer RA, et al. Efficacy of haemorheological treatment using plasma exchange, selective adsorption and membrane differential filtration in maculopathy, retinal vein occlusion and uveal effusion syndrome. Transfus Sci 1996;17:493–498.
26. Schepens CL, Bockhurst RJ. Uveal effusion. Arch Ophthalmol 1963;70:189–201.
27. Gass JD. Uveal effusion syndrome: a new hypothesis concerning pathogenesis and technique of surgical treatment. Retina 1983;23S:159–163.
28. Paulmann H, Heimann K. The uveal effusion syndrome. BerZusammenkunft Dtsch Ophthalmol Ges 1977;74:545–550.
29. Heibges A, Fassbender C, Erdtracht B, et al. (2007): Assessment of safety and efficacy of rheopheresis for age-related macular degeneration (AMD) by RheoNet-Registry analysis. Nephro-News September: 30.
30. Brunner R, Heidner K, Borberg H, et al. Einfluß unterschiedlicher Plasmaspiegel von Fibrinogen und Plasmaproteinen auf hämorheologische Parameter. In: Landgraf H, Jung F, Ehrly M, editors. Klinische Mikrozirkulation und Hämorheologie. Berlin: Blackwell Wissenschaft; 1993. p. 179–186.
31. Lip PL, Blann AD, Hope-Ross M, et al. Age-related macular degeneration is associated with increased vascular endothelial growth factor, hemorheology and endothelial dysfunction. Ophthalmol 2001;108:705–710.
32. Brunner R, Widder RA, Fischer RA. Clinical efficacy of extracorporeal hemorheological treatment in age related macular degeneration. Jpn J Apheresis 1997;16:31–34.

CHAPTER

47 Enzymatic vitrectomy and pharmacologic vitreodynamics

David T. Goldenberg, MD and Michael T. Trese, MD

INTRODUCTION AND HISTORY

The field of vitreoretinal surgery has evolved substantially over the last several decades. Scientific advances have improved our understanding of disease pathophysiology and new surgical adjuncts and techniques have decreased surgical time and improved patient outcomes. Pharmacologic agents have recently been developed for intraocular use in order to enhance vitreous removal. Pharmacologic vitreodynamics is a new concept which describes the use of pharmacologic agents to manipulate the vitreous. In addition, and perhaps more importantly, it also describes the complex interactions that take place at the vitreoretinal interface.

Pharmacologic compounds that are developed for manipulation of the vitreous are designed to cleave the vitreoretinal junction and/or to increase vitreous liquefaction. This concept of lysing the vitreoretinal juncture and core vitreous has been described as pharmacologic vitreolysis.[1] Two enzymatic agents have been shown to cause both vitreous liquefaction and complete separation of the vitreoretinal interface, leading to the development of a posterior vitreous detachment (PVD).[2–5] These substances can eliminate vitreoschisis and lead to a clean internal limiting membrane (ILM), as shown in animal and human studies.[6,7] Enzymatic vitrectomy is an evolving modality that will likely be used more frequently for therapy and preventive measures.[8]

For many years, ophthalmologists have researched and utilized enzymatic agents, one of the earliest being alpha-chymotripsin and its effect on zonular proteins during intracapsular cataract extraction. Many substances have been proposed to cleave the vitreoretinal juncture and liquefy the central vitreous as an adjunct to vitreoretinal surgery. Both enzymatic and nonenzymatic agents have been developed to resolve vitreous traction and accelerate the clearance of a vitreous opacity, such as vitreous hemorrhage. The search for an appropriate agent to manipulate the vitreous has included several enzymes, most of which are autologous enzymes that activate other endogenous enzymes. Many of the earliest-studied agents were fraught with failure due to lack of efficacy, retinal toxicity, or difficult preparation. Nevertheless, several enzymes appear to be promising for pharmacologic manipulation of the vitreous. Significant progress has been made in the field of pharmacologic vitreodynamics, and this chapter will provide a summary of recent findings.

PHARMACOLOGY AND BIOCHEMISTRY

Recent advances in biochemistry have improved our understanding of the complex arrangement of the vitreoretinal interface. Until recently, the vitreous gel was long seen as unimportant and noncontributory to retinal pathology.[9] It is now commonly believed that the vitreous gel has a significant influence on retinal diseases. The vitreous is a clear, semisolid gel containing hyaluronic acid interspersed in a framework of parallel collagen fibrils.[9] The vitreous cortex contains the greatest concentrations of collagen and hyaluronic acid. These collagen fibrils form an outer layer of the vitreous cortex which is adherent to the ILM.[10] The glycoproteins laminin and fibronectin bind vitreous collagen fibers between the posterior vitreous cortex and the ILM,[11] and they are thought to play a role in areas of vitreoretinal adhesion. An age-related PVD is thought to occur as the vitreous becomes syneretic, such that the gel consistency is lost to become partially or completely fluid. Pools of fluid collect in the premacular region, and a tear in the posterior cortical vitreous facilitates this fluid then to pass through the vitreous cortex and separate the surrounding cortical vitreous from the retina. Similar to the progression of an age-related PVD, two events must occur in order to ensure successful pharmacologic vitreolysis: (1) vitreous liquefaction and (2) complete vitreoretinal interface separation (PVD).[8] Multiple pharmacologic compounds have been designed with this goal in mind, and they have been met with variable success.[9,12]

Chondroitinase, one of the earliest-studied enzymes, lyses the proteoglycan chrondroitin sulfate which is associated with the vitreoretinal interface.[13] A recent masked, placebo-controlled, *in vivo* study concluded that a dose of 1 IU chondroitinase failed to produce a PVD.[14] Dispase was initially thought to be a good candidate for pharmacologic vitreolysis due to its ability to hydrolyze type IV collagen and fibronectin. Dispase is able to create a PVD at a dose of 0.025 IU[15,16]; however, it also causes intraocular inflammation, retinal hemorrhages, electroretinogram (ERG) amplitude reductions, epiretinal membranes, cataract, and ultrastructural damage to the retina.[15–17] The retinal toxicity associated with dispase is thought to be due to the broad range of proteins that are subject to its action,[9] and this toxicity has limited its clinical use.

Hyaluronidase (Vitrase, ISTA Pharmaceuticals) is commercially available for off-label use as an adjunct to increase the absorption and dispersion of other injected drugs, such as local anesthetics. It works by primarily digesting the proteoglycan hyaluronan which makes up a large component of the vitreous body. Hyaluronidase has been shown to cause vitreous liquefaction in animal models,[9] and a recent phase III trial was conducted.[18,19] In this study, the percentage of patients achieving clearance of vitreous hemorrhage sufficient to see underlying pathology by 3 months was 33% in patients receiving hyaluronidase 55 IU and 26% for saline-treated controls ($P = 0.025$).[19] Despite the authors' conclusions that hyaluronidase is safe, approximately one-third of patients were noted to have moderate or severe iritis and approximately 10% developed a retinal detachment following injection with hyaluronidase 55 IU. Furthermore, multiple studies have concluded that an intravitreal injection of hyaluronidase cannot induce a PVD in animal models.[20–22] As mentioned earlier, successful enzymatic vitrectomy requires both vitreous gel liquefaction and complete vitreoretinal separation. Sebag[1,9] has used the term "anomalous PVD" to describe the situation when vitreous liquefaction occurs without a PVD, as is seen with hyaluronidase. Anomalous PVD may lead to traction at the vitreoretinal interface with the development of multiple pathologic conditions.[1,9] Thus, hyaluronidase has not been considered an ideal agent for enzymatic vitrectomy, and it has not been approved for intraocular use by the Food and Drug Administration.

Plasmin enzyme is a nonspecific, endogenous protease capable of creating a PVD by hydrolyzing laminin and fibronectin at the vitreoretinal interface.[23,24] Its ability to cause vitreous liquefaction is thought to be due to its activity on collegenases[25] and endogenous matrix metalloproteinase-2.[26] In animal models, a single injection of plasmin enzyme creates a PVD without causing morphological changes to the retina, and the degree of vitreoretinal separation is dose- and time-dependent, with a peak activity at approximately 30 minutes.[6,24] Autologous plasmin enzyme (APE) can be isolated from the patient's serum via

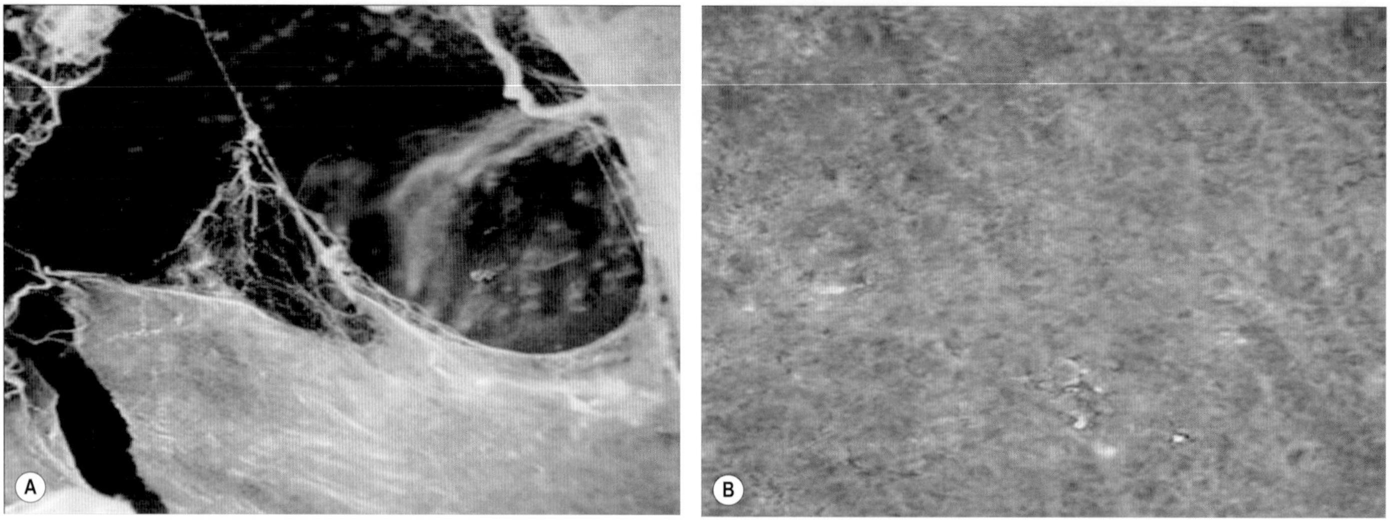

Figure 47.1 (A) Scanning electron micrograph of a porcine eye showing vitreous collagen on retinal surface. (B) Scanning electron micrograph of a porcine eye after intravitreal microplasmin injection showing no evidence of vitreous collagen fibrils on the surface of the internal limiting membrane.

trained personnel and laboratory preparation. Multiple reports have confirmed that APE 0.4–1.2 IU can successfully cause vitreous liquefaction and induce a PVD in humans.[3–5,7,27,28] No ERG abnormalities or ultrastructural changes to the ILM and retina are seen at concentrations up to 10 times the effective dose.[16]

Nattokinase (subtilisin NAT) is a serine protease that is produced by *Bacillus subtilis* (natto). It hydrolyzes collagen fibers, enhances plasminogen activators, and inactivates a plasminogen activator inhibitor.[29,30] Nattokinase has been shown to cause a PVD in rabbit eyes without histologic damage to the retina at a dose of 0.1 fibrin degradation units.[30] Despite these findings, its use in research studies is limited, and there are no reports of nattokinase use in humans.

Microplasmin (ThromboGenics, Dublin, Ireland) is a recombinant protein that is a truncated form of human plasmin.[31] It is approximately one-third the size of plasmin enzyme (29 versus 88 kDa), but it retains its active protease site.[31] This smaller size is thought to allow for increased epiretinal tissue penetration.[2] In contrast with plasmin enzyme, it can be prepared quickly without the need for venepuncture. Animal models have demonstrated microplasmin's ability to induce vitreous liquefaction[8,9] and a complete PVD[2,20,32] with a single intravitreal injection in a dose- and time-dependent fashion (Figure 47.1). A dose of 125 μg has been shown to cause a PVD in human cadaver and rabbit eyes.[2,32] In addition, this dose appears to be nontoxic as it does not alter the ultrastructure of the inner retina in postmortem human[2] and *in vivo* animal eyes,[2,32] and it does not cause significant ERG changes.[32] It is interesting to note that plasmin, microplasmin, and nattokinase appear to be the most effective enzymes for PVD induction, and all three compounds may utilize the same mechanism of action via plasmin.

INDICATIONS

SURGICAL ADJUNCT

An abnormal vitreoretinal interface plays an important role in the pathogenesis of many retinal disorders and may contribute to significant patient morbidity. Traction at this interface has been implicated in the development of vitreomacular traction (VMT), diabetic macular edema, macular pucker, proliferative diabetic retinopathy, proliferative vitreoretinopathy, macular holes, retinal detachments, and other conditions. The surgical management of such disorders often targets the abnormal vitreoretinal junction by separating the posterior hyaloid from the ILM, thereby creating a mechanical PVD. The creation of a mechanical PVD with vitrectomy may not remove all of the vitreous or completely separate the vitreoretinal junction, as cortical vitreous fibrils are left behind on the ILM.[33] Incomplete removal of the vitreous may result in surgical failure.[34,35]

Vitrectomy with removal of the ILM requires direct mechanical manipulation of the macula.[15,16] Although it is generally safe, surgical separation of the posterior hyaloid from the retina may cause retinal or optic disc trauma.[36] Therefore, creating a PVD with an intravitreal injection of a pharmacologic agent may enhance surgical separation of the posterior hyaloid, thus reducing intraoperative time and potential complications. Enzyme-assisted vitrectomy may be indicated in many retinal disorders involving abnormal vitreoretinal adhesions.

NONSURGICAL INDICATIONS

In addition to its use as a surgical adjunct, a pharmacologically induced PVD may be indicated for prophylactic treatment or as a substitute for surgical intervention. For example, a complete PVD is a strong negative risk factor for the progression of diabetic retinopathy.[37] In addition, it has been suggested that complete posterior vitreous separation allows for resolution of diabetic macular edema.[5] Thus, a pharmacologic PVD has the potential to reduce diabetic macular edema and remove the vitreous scaffold for neovascularization. This may even eliminate the need for surgery in select cases. Furthermore, persistent attachment of the posterior vitreous cortex to the macula has been suggested to be a risk factor for the development of exudative age-related macular degeneration (AMD).[38] If this theory is upheld, then the induction of a prophylactic PVD may significantly alter the natural history of AMD.

Microplasmin is currently being investigated in phase II clinical trials. The European Microplasmin for Vitrectomy IIT (MIVI-IIT) study is a phase II, randomized, double-masked clinical trial of intravitreal microplasmin injection for the nonsurgical treatment of VMT. Early results from this study have demonstrated encouraging findings (P. Stalmans, presentation at the annual meeting of the American Society of Retina Specialists, 2007). In some cases, the closure of macular holes and complete resolution of VMT were seen after microplasmin injection (Figure 47.2). The US microplasmin clinical trial (MIVI-III) is a phase IIb study that has completed patient enrollment to determine the use of microplasmin as a surgical adjunct in vitrectomy surgery. A phase III study is actively recruiting participants to determine if microplasmin can be used instead of surgical therapy for patients with pathologic vitreoretinal adhesions.

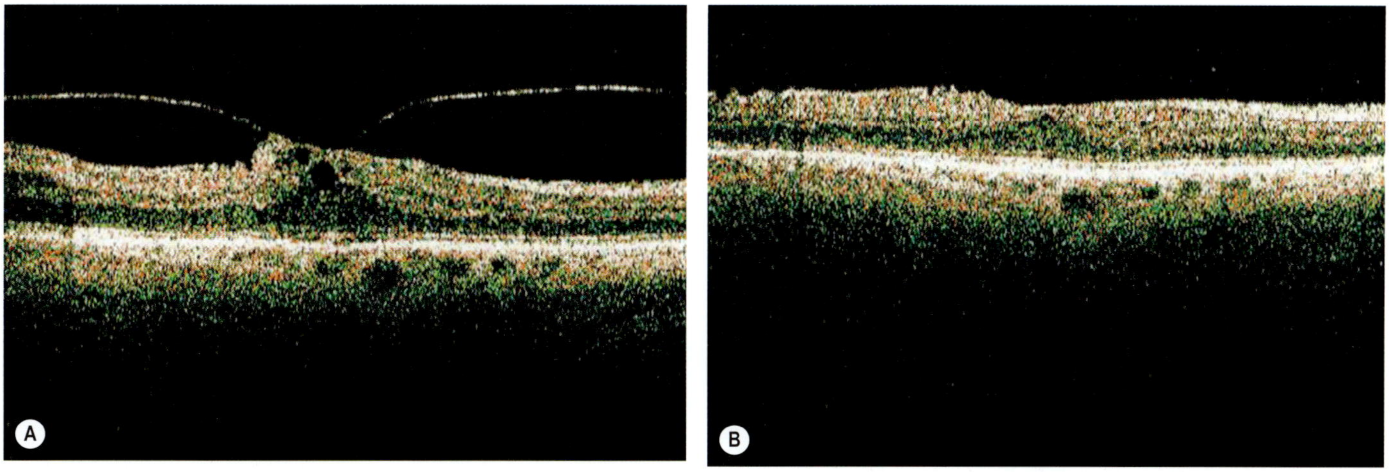

Figure 47.2 Results of Microplasmin for Vitrectomy IIT (MIVI-IIT) study. (A) Optical coherence tomography (OCT) demonstrating vitreomacular traction with visual acuity (VA) of 20/100. (B) OCT image 3 months after microplasmin intravitreal injection. There is resolution of the vitreous traction and VA has improved to 20/16.

Recent studies suggest that a pharmacologic PVD may alter the flow of molecules across the vitreoretinal interface. A microplasmin-induced PVD in animals has been shown to increase vitreal oxygen levels and increase the rate of oxygen exchange within the vitreous cavity.[20] This effect is not seen with hyaluronidase and liquefaction of the vitreous cavity alone.[20] This observation suggests that an attached posterior hyaloid may present a semipermeable barrier at the vitreoretinal junction. The change in oxygen molecular flux may be seen as a marker for the behavior of other molecules in the extracellular matrix of the vitreous cavity, particularly the vitreous cortex. In fact, preliminary data from cat models suggest a microplasmin-induced PVD leads to decreased levels of vitreal vascular endothelial growth factor,[39] which is an important factor in the pathogenesis of diabetic macular edema and neovascularization.[40,41] It is possible that an age-related PVD or a pharmacologic-induced PVD may alter the flux of molecules in the vitreous cavity and influence the concentration of other vitreal growth factors. Prospective clinical trials will be needed to address this theory.

OPERATIVE TECHNIQUES

The ability to induce a complete PVD in 30 minutes with plasmin or microplasmin is significant. This seems to be an acceptable amount of delay for pharmacologic vitreolysis to have a clinical effect. Microplasmin could feasibly be injected in the operating room or in the clinic prior to surgery. In the operating room, this injection would not cause an insurmountable delay prior to beginning a vitrectomy; in the clinic setting, it would be reasonable for a patient to wait 30 minutes or longer for a possible repeat examination in order to ensure the agent's efficacy and to identify potential complications. Both plasmin and microplasmin are clear solutions that do not alter surgical planning or techniques.

OUTCOMES

Plasmin and microplasmin are the most widely used agents for enzymatic vitrectomy. Multiple small case series have reported favorable results with APE as a surgical adjunct,[3–5,28,42–45] and clinical trials are currently under way with microplasmin.

APE and microplasmin may be most beneficial as a surgical adjunct in pediatric cases, whereby the vitreous is especially adherent to the retina and poses an increased risk of complications with mechanical separation. APE-assisted vitrectomy allows for easier peeling of the vitreous gel with a reduced risk of causing iatrogenic retinal breaks in cases of pediatric traumatic macular holes,[4] stage 5 retinopathy of prematurity,[44] congenital X-linked retinoschisis,[45] and other pediatric vitreoretinopathies.[43]

Plasmin enzyme has also shown promising results with adult vitreoretinal disorders. APE-assisted vitrectomy for stage 3 macular holes allows for easier removal of the posterior hyaloid, increased spontaneous PVD, and reduced operative time.[3] APE-assisted vitrectomy may also improve removal of the posterior hyaloid,[5,42] reduce surgical time,[42] and reduce iatrogenic retinal tears[42] in patients with diabetic tractional retinal detachments. Furthermore, patients with diabetic macular edema have shown improved visual acuity after APE-assisted vitrectomy but with mixed results regarding the resolution of edema.[5,28]

COMPLICATIONS AND HOW TO AVOID THEM

A retinal tear is an intrinsic risk during PVD creation, especially in patients with abnormal vitreoretinal adhesions, such as lattice degeneration. Thus, enzymatic vitrectomy presents the inherent risk of causing a retinal tear and subsequent retinal detachment. Although a retinal tear has not been reported as a result of pharmacologic manipulation of the vitreous, closely monitoring patients following microplasmin injection would be prudent in order to identify retinal tears early. Prophylactic laser retinopexy around suspicious lesions prior to enzyme injection may be advisable.

Intravitreal injections also present the inherent risk of infection. The incidence of endophthalmitis after enzymatic vitrectomy has not been reported; however, it is very rare (0.029%) in patients receiving intravitreal injections for other indications.[46] Prophylactic antiseptic solutions, sterile technique, and topical antibiotics are appropriate for the prevention of such infections.

SUMMARY

The emerging field of pharmacologic vitreodynamics presents a new frontier in vitreoretinal surgery. The ability to induce vitreous liquefaction and a complete PVD with a single intravitreal injection has potential implications for the management of multiple vitreoretinopathies. Enzymatic vitrectomy may help to reduce vitreous viscosity, thereby facilitating removal during vitrectomy and reducing surgical time, especially when using smaller-gauge vitrectomy instruments. The induction of a PVD also has the potential to reduce intraoperative complications. As we improve our understanding of the molecular flux in the vitreous cavity, pharmacologic vitreodynamics will likely become more important as it may allow for improved manipulation of intravitreal molecules.

Key points

- Pharmacologic agents have been developed to create vitreous liquefaction and a PVD.
- Intravitreal surgical adjuncts may facilitate vitreous removal and reduce intraoperative complications.
- APE can successfully cause vitreous liquefaction and induce a PVD.
- Microplasmin is a recombinant protein that can create a PVD in animal models. It is currently being investigated in clinical trials.
- A Food and Drug Administration phase III clinical trial is currently under way to determine if microplasmin can be used as a substitute for surgical intervention in patients with abnormal vitreoretinal adhesions.

REFERENCES

1. Sebag J. Pharmacologic vitreolysis. Retina 1998;18(1):1–3.
2. Gandorfer A, Rohleder M, Sethi C, et al. Posterior vitreous detachment induced by microplasmin. Invest Ophthalmol Vis Sci 2004;45(2): 641–647.
3. Trese MT, Williams GA, Hartzer MK. A new approach to stage 3 macular holes. Ophthalmol 2000;107(8):1607–1611.
4. Margherio AR, Margherio RR, Hartzer M, et al. Plasmin enzyme-assisted vitrectomy in traumatic pediatric macular holes. Ophthalmol 1998;105(9): 1617–1620.
5. Williams JG, Trese MT, Williams GS, et al. Autologous plasmin enzyme in the surgical management of diabetic retinopathy. Ophthalmol 2001; 108(10):1902–1905.
6. Verstraeten TC, Chapman C, Hartzer M, et al. Pharmacologic induction of posterior vitreous detachment in the rabbit. Arch Ophthalmol 1993;111(6): 849–854.
7. Asami T, Terasaki H, Kachi S, et al. Ultrastructure of internal limiting membrane removed during plasmin-assisted vitrectomy from eyes with diabetic macular edema. Ophthalmol 2004;111(2):231–237.
8. Sebag J, Ansari RR, Suh KI. Pharmacologic vitreolysis with microplasminin increases vitreous diffusion coefficients. Graefe's Arch Clin Exp Ophthalmol 2007;245(4):576–580.
9. Sebag J. Molecular biology of pharmacologic vitreolysis. Trans Am Ophthalmol Soc 2005;103:473–494.
10. Gass JD. Macular dysfunction caused by vitreous and vitreoretinal interface abnormalities. In: Gass JD, editor. Stereoscopic atlas of macular diseases: Diagnosis and treatment (Volume 2). St. Louis: Mosby, Inc.; 1997. p. 903–973.
11. Kohno T, Sorgente N, Ishibashi T, et al. Immunofluorescent studies of fibronectin and laminin in the human eye. Invest Ophthalmol Vis Sci 1987;28(3):506–514.
12. Trese MT. Enzymatic-assisted vitrectomy. Eye 2002;16(4):365–368.
13. Hageman GS, Russell SR. Chondroitinate-mediated disinsertion of the primate vitreous body. Invest Ophthalmol Vis Sci 1994;35(suppl):28.
14. Hermel M, Schrage NF. Efficacy of plasmin enzymes and chondroitinase ABC in creating posterior vitreous separation in the pig: a masked, placebo-controlled *in vivo* study. Grafes Arch Clin Exp Ophthalmol 2007;245(3):399–406.
15. Zhu D, Chen H, Xu X. Effects of intravitreal dispase on vitreoretinal interface in rabbits. Curr Eye Res 2006;31(11):935–946.
16. Wang F, Wang Z, Sun X, et al. Safety and efficacy of dispase and plasmin in pharmacologic vitreolysis. Invest Ophthalmol Vis Sci 2004;45(9): 3286–3290.
17. Jorge R, Oyamaguchi EK, Cardillo JA, et al. Intravitreal injection of dispase causes retinal hemorrhages in rabbit and human eyes. Curr Eye Res 2003;26(2):107–112.
18. Kuppermann BD, Thomas EL, De Smet MD, et al. Safety results of two phase III trials of an intravitreous injection of highly purified ovine hyaluronidase (Vitrase®) for the management of vitreous hemorrhage. Am J Ophthalmol 2005;140(4):585–597.
19. Kuppermann BD, Thomas EL, De Smet MD, et al. Pooled efficacy results from two multinational randomized controlled clinical trials of a single intravitreous injection of highly purified ovine hyaluronidase (Vitrase®) for the management of vitreous hemorrhage. Am J Ophthalmol 2005;140(4): 573–584.
20. Quiram PA, Leverenz VA, Baker RM, et al. Microplasm-induced posterior vitreous detachment affects vitreous oxygen levels. Retina 2007;27(8): 1090–1096.
21. Wang Z, Zhang X, Xu X, et al. PVD following plasmin but not hyaluronidase: Implications for combination pharmacologic vitreolysis therapy. Retina 2005;25(1):38–43.
22. Hikichi T, Kado M, Yoshida A. Intravitreal injection of hyaluronidase cannot induce posterior vitreous detachment in the rabbit. Retina 2000;20(2):195–198.
23. Liotta LA, Goldfarb RH, Brundage R, et al. Effect of plasminogen activator (urokinase), plasmin, and thrombin on glycoprotein and collagenous components of basement membrane. Cancer Res 1981;41(11 Pt 1): 4629–4636.
24. Uemura A, Nakamura M, Kachi S, et al. Effect of plasmin on laminin and fibronectin during plasmin-assisted vitrectomy. Arch Ophthalmol 2005;123(2):209–213.
25. Dano K, Andreasen PA, Grondahl-Hansen J, et al. Plasminogen activators, tissue degradation, and cancer. Adv Cancer Res 1985;44:139–266.
26. Takano A, Hirata A, Inomata Y, et al. Intravitreal plasmin injection activates endogenous matrix metalloproteinase-2 in rabbit and human vitreous. Am J Ophthalmol 2005;140(4):654–660.
27. Rizzo S, Pellegrini G, Benocci F, et al. Autologous plasmin for pharmacologic vitreolysis prepared 1 hour before surgery. Retina 2006;26(7):792–796.
28. Azzolini C, D'Angelo A, Maestranzi G, et al. Intrasurgical plasmin enzyme in diabetic macular edema. Am J Ophthalmol 2004;138(4):560–566.
29. Urano T, Ihara H, Umemura K, et al. The profibrinolytic enzyme subtilisin NAT purified from *Bacillus subtilis* cleaves and inactivates plasminogen activator inhibitor type I. J Biol Chem 2001;276(27):24690–24696.
30. Takano A, Hirata A, Ogasawara K, et al. Posterior vitreous detachment induced by nattokinase (subtilisin NAT): A novel enzyme for pharmacologic vitreolysis. Invest Ophthalmol Vis Sci 2006;47(5):2075–2079.
31. Nagai N, Demarsin E, Van Hoef B, et al. Recombinant human microplasmin: production and potential therapeutic properties. Thromb Haemost 2003;1(2):307–313.
32. Sakuma T, Tanaka M, Mitzota A, et al. Safety of *in vivo* pharmacologic vitreolysis with recombinant microplasmin in rabbit eyes. Invest Ophthalmol Vis Sci 2005;46(9):3295–3299.
33. Gandorfer A, Ulbig M, Kampik A. Plasmin-assisted vitrectomy eliminates cortical vitreous remnants. Eye 2002;16(1):95–97.
34. Sebag J. Diabetic vitreopathy. Ophthalmology 1996;103(2):205–206.
35. Schwartz SD, Alexander R, Hiscott P, et al. Recognition of vitreoschisis in proliferative diabetic retinopathy: A useful landmark in vitrectomy for diabetic traction retinal detachment. Ophthalmology 1996;103(2):323–328.
36. Russell SR, Hageman GS. Optic disc, foveal, and extrafoveal damage due to surgical separation of the vitreous. Arch Ophthalmol 2001;119(11):153–1658.
37. Ono R, Kakehashi A, Yamagami H, et al. Prospective assessment of proliferative diabetic retinopathy with observations of posterior vitreous detachment. Int Ophthalmol 2005;26(1–2):15–19.
38. Krebs I, Brannath W, Glittenberg C, et al. Posterior vitreomacular adhesion: A potential risk factor for exudative age-related macular degeneration? Am J Ophthalmol 2007;144(5):741–746.
39. Quiram PA, Leverenz V, Baker R, et al. Enzymatic induction of a posterior vitreous detachment alters molecular vitreodynamics in animal models. Invest Ophthalmol Vis Sci 2007. Abstract no. 83.
40. Patel JI, Tombran-Tink J, Hykin PG, et al. Vitreous and aqueous concentrations of proangiogenic, antiangiogenic factors and other cytokines in diabetic retinopathy patients with macular edema: implications for structural differences in macular profiles. Exp Eye Res 2006;82(5):798–806.
41. Boulton M, Gregor Z, McLeod D, et al. Intravitreal growth factors in proliferative diabetic retinopathy: correlation with neovascular activity and glycaemic management. Br J Ophthalmol 1997;81(3):228–233.
42. Hirata A, Takano A, Inomata Y, et al. Plasmin-assisted vitrectomy for management of proliferative membrane in proliferative diabetic retinopathy: A pilot study. Retina 2007;27(8):1074–1078.
43. Joshi MM, Ciaccia S, Trese MT, et al. Posterior hyaloid contracture in pediatric vitreoretinopathies. Retina 2006;26(7):S38–S41.
44. Tsukahara Y, Honda S. Autologous plasmin-assisted vitrectomy for stage 5 retinopathy of prematurity: A preliminary trial. Am J Ophthalmol 2007; 144(1):139–141.
45. Wu W, Drenser KA, Capone A, et al. Plasmin enzyme-assisted vitreoretinal surgery in congenital X-linked retinoschisis: Surgical techniques based on a new classification system. Retina 2007;27(8):1079–1085.
46. Pilli S, Kotsolis A, Spaide RF, et al. Endophthalmitis associated with anti-vascular endothelial growth factor therapy injections in an office setting. Am J Ophthalmol 2008;145:878–882.

CHAPTER

48 The use of vital dyes during vitreoretinal surgery – chromovitrectomy

Michel Eid Farah, MD, Maurício Maia, MD, PhD, Fernando M. Penha, MD, PhD, and Eduardo Büchele Rodrigues, MD

KEY FEATURES, INTRODUCTION, AND HISTORY

The term "chromovitrectomy" refers to the use of vital dyes during vitreoretinal surgery to assist in the identification of preretinal tissues and membranes.[1] The modern approach was first introduced in 2000, when the dye indocyanine green (ICG) was used to stain the thin semitransparent internal limiting membrane (ILM). Following initial experience with ICG, clinical and experimental studies demonstrated signs of the retinal toxicity of ICG, which stimulated research on alternative dyes for chromovitrectomy. Some additional alternative biostains, including trypan blue (TB), patent blue (PB), or brilliant blue (BriB), have been added to the surgical armamentarium for chromovitrectomy.[2] This chapter presents the latest data on chromovitrectomy in regard to the biochemical properties, indications, and clinical experience with various vital dyes available for chromovitrectomy.

RATIONALE

The introduction of ILM peeling to treat idiopathic macular holes enhanced closure rates to approximately 95% based on recent publications, compared with 60–90% closure rates in eyes without ILM peeling. However, surgical removal of ILM could lead to anatomic and functional retinal damage, and the two main postoperative clinical signs of complications of ILM removal are: (1) visual field defects and (2) retinal pigmented epithelium (RPE) damage.[3]

The basic rationale for the application of dyes during vitreoretinal surgery is that simple, preretinal membranes and tissues such as the ILM are very thin and semitransparent and thus difficult to detect. The application of dyes during vitreoretinal surgery indeed improved the visualization of several thin and transparent tissues in the vitreoretinal interface, such as the ILM.

PHARMACOLOGY AND BIOCHEMISTRY

Dyes are complex organic molecules containing chromophores, chemical moieties responsible for their color. By definition, vital staining refers to the coloration of living cells or tissues. In order to evaluate the various dyes currently available, the staining agents may be classified according to several criteria, where the most commonly applied include chemical classification. Some of the groups of dyes already applied in chromovitrectomy are: (1) azo dyes; (2) arylmethane dyes; (3) cyanine dyes; (4) xanthene dyes; and (5) colored corticosteroids.

Azo dyes are a class of synthetic organic dyes with nitrogen in the azo form of –N=N– in their structure. TB is an anionic hydrophilic azo dye which has the molecular formula $C_{34}H_{24}N_6Na_4O_{14}S_4$ and a molecular weight of 960 Da. TB crosses the cell membranes of dead cells only, thereby staining dead tissues/cells blue. The application of TB in ocular surgery has been widespread for vitrectomy and cataract surgery. For chromovitrectomy, TB may be commercially available at a concentration of 0.15% for vitreoretinal surgery, called Membrane Blue (DORC International, Zuidland, Netherlands).

Cyanine dyes are a class of dyes containing a –CH= group linking two heterocyclic rings containing nitrogen. ICG is a tricarbocyanine anionic vital dye with a molecular formula of $C_{43}H_{47}N_2NaO_6S_2$ and a molecular weight of 775 Da. The cyanine agent has amphiphilic properties and thereby binds to both cellular and acellular elements in living tissues. The hydrophilic dye is provided as a sterile powder and represents a very useful contrast agent in angiography, allowing imaging of choroidal and retinal tissues. For ophthalmology, ICG is commercially available under the names of ICG-Pulsion (Pulsion Medical Systems, Munich, Germany; 25- and 50-mg vials), ICV Indocianina Verde (Ophthalmos, São Paulo, Brazil; 5-, 25-, and 50-mg vials), Diagnogreen (Daiichi Pharmaceutical, Tokyo, Japan; 25-mg vial), and IC-Green (Akorn, Buffalo Grove, USA; 25-mg vial). The dye is commercially provided as a powder in the above amounts (from 5 to 50 mg) to achieve final concentrations of 0.05–0.5%. Infracyanine green (IfCG) is a green dye with the same chemical formula and similar pharmacologic properties as ICG. IfCG is commercially available under the brand name of Infracyanine (Laboratoires SERB, Paris, France; 25-mg vial), it contains no sodium iodine in the final solution and its final dilution in 5% glucose produces an iso-osmotic solution of around 310 mmol/kg.

Arylmethane dyes are a group of stains which are formed by one carbon linked to benzene or naphthalene groups; they are commonly used in modern inks. BriB is a blue anionic arylmethane compound which has the chemical formula of $C_{47}H_{48}N_3S_2O_7Na$ and a molecular weight of 854 Da. Animal and human data on the use of BriB for application in vitreoretinal surgery and anterior lens capsule staining have been described. The dye gained approval for intraocular use in Europe in 2007 under the brand name of Brilliant Peel (Geuder, Heidelberg, Germany), and it is provided in vials containing 2 mg/ml of the vital dye. Bromophenol blue (BroB) is another arylmethane color marker dye with a molecular weight of 670 Da and the chemical formula of $C_{19}H_{10}Br_4O_5S$. BroB has been applied in ocular surgery: the dark-blue stain may represent a novel useful adjunct for both cataract and vitreoretinal surgery, although there is no commercially available product in the USA. PB is a hydrophilic anionic triarylmethane dye with the chemical formula of $C_{27}H_{31}N_2NaO_6S_2$ and a molecular weight of 582 Da. PB has been certified in Europe since 2003 for capsule staining in cataract surgery in a ready-to-use solution at a concentration of 0.24% under the brand name of Blueron (Geuder, Heidelberg, Germany), whereas it has also been applied as an off-label agent in vitreoretinal surgery.

The term "xanthenes" may be applied to yellow heterocyclic organic compounds with the chemical formula $C_{13}H_{10}O$. Xanthene molecule is the basis of xanthene dyes; for instance, fluorescein is derived from its structure. Fluorescein is a xanthene fluorophore with the chemical structure $C_{20}H_{12}O_5$ and a molecular weight of 332 Da. Fluorescein may be found in nature conjugated with over 50 salt molecules or derivates, including fluorescein sodium (FS) and fluorescein diacetate (FD). Fluorescein is used extensively as a diagnostic tool in the field of ophthalmology mainly as FS, while for ocular surgery the xanthene compound has been shown to stain the vitreous gel in the form of either FS or FD.

Corticosteroids are hormones produced naturally in the cortex of the adrenal gland, whose derivates may be synthetically produced to be applied as drugs in the treatment of human diseases. Some of these potent drugs are triamcinolone, dexamethasone, and fluorometholone. Triamcinolone acetonide (TA) is a synthetic insoluble corticosteroid with the empirical formula $C_{24}H_{31}FO_6$ and a molecular weight of 434 Da, whereas fluorometholone acetate (FMA) is a synthetic fluorinated glucocorticosteroid with the chemical formula $C_{24}H_{31}FO_5$ and a molecular weight of 418 Da. In ocular surgery, both TA and FMA have demonstrated good staining of the vitreous because of the crystal composition of the drug deposits on to the transparent gel.

INDICATIONS, OUTCOMES, AND COMPLICATIONS – VITAL DYES IN CHROMOVITRECTOMY

INDOCYANINE GREEN

ICG has a great affinity for extracellular matrix components of the ILM, such as collagen and fibronectin, and facilitates its intraoperative removal in vitreoretinal surgery (Figure 48.1). Initially, chromovitrectomy with ICG-guided ILM peeling gained worldwide acceptance as a surgical technique for macular holes. However, controversial clinical reports regarding the potentially toxic effects of ICG to the retina have been reported in recent years, including RPE changes, visual field defects, and optic nerve atrophy. Our group recently published a meta-analysis regarding ICG application for ILM peeling in comparison to no staining involving 837 eyes; the meta-analysis showed similar anatomic outcomes but worse functional outcomes when ICG had been used in chromovitrectomy for macular hole treatment.[4] Nevertheless, controlled clinical studies have been performed to compare ILM removal with and without ICG staining in MH surgery in recent years, providing evidence that ICG in low doses and with careful surgical technique may not cause serious retinal toxicity.

Variations in techniques such as dye incubation time, concentration, and osmolarity should also be noted when performing ICG-guided chromovitrectomy. Incubation time may vary from immediate removal to 5 minutes after dye injection. It may be important to note that unwanted postoperative RPE changes have been found in the literature, mainly in studies reporting an ICG incubation time over 30 seconds. More frequent RPE toxicity can also be observed in those clinical and experimental studies in which the ICG solution has an osmolarity below 270 mOsm and concentration above 0.5%. Some studies have demonstrated the use of ICG at a concentration of 0.05% and osmolarity around 290 mOsm with few or no signs of RPE toxicity.[5]

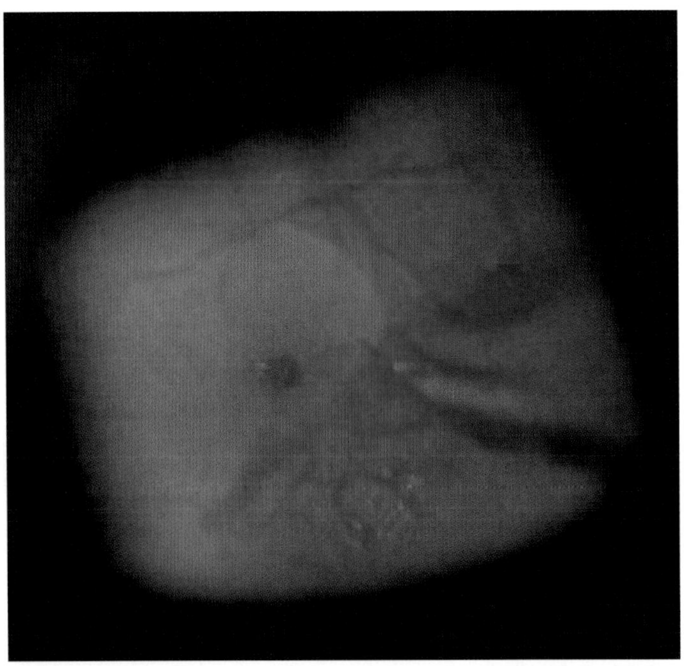

Figure 48.1 Internal limiting membrane (ILM) staining with indocyanine green enables a clear distinction between the unstained retina and the stained overlying fine ILM tissue.

ICG has also been used to facilitate ILM peeling in other diseases, such as diabetic macular edema (DME). Consecutive surgical experience determined that the use of ICG-assisted ILM peeling in DME induced no sign of retinal toxicity by visual acuity measurements when comparing vitrectomy with and without ILM peeling. A small case series examined ILM peeling with ICG for persistent macular edema from different causes, such as central retinal vein occlusion, DME, Irvine–Gass syndrome, and vitreomacular traction syndrome; besides no signs of retinal toxicity, significant improvement in visual acuity was observed just in patients with DME. A large-scale controlled investigation should determine the indications and safety of ICG-guided ILM peeling in those various macular diseases.[6]

Although the best indication for ICG use in chromovitrectomy is for ILM staining in MH surgery, ICG has been proposed for better visualization of epiretinal membranes (ERMs) in vitrectomy for proliferative diabetic vitreoretinopathy, idiopathic ERMs, and proliferative vitreoretinopathy. However, the green dye may stain the acellular ILM better; as for the task of ERM staining, other vital stains may be better.

In regard to toxicity issues, ICG may come in contact with neuroretinal cells such as photoreceptors as well as RPE cells through an MH during ICG-assisted peeling of the ILM. Several animal studies have examined the potential retinal toxicity of subretinal ICG injections, and most studies used electroretinogram (ERG) and histological findings to show a concentration-dependent retinal toxicity associated with ICG. Penha et al. evaluated the effects of subretinal injection of 0.02 ml of either iso-osmolar 0.05% ICG (279 mOsm) or hypo-osmolar ICG at 0.046% ICG (251 mOsm) with fluorescein angiography, fundus evaluation, and histologic studies. Both solutions caused severe damage to all retinal layers during the entire follow-up, but the damage induced by hypo-osmolar solutions was greater than that caused by the iso-osmolar solutions.[7]

Many authors have determined the effects of intravitreal ICG injections, and most studies have found a concentration-dependent retinal toxicity associated with ICG. In a rabbit model, Maia et al.[8] studied the effects of intravitreal injection of 0.1 ml of ICG at three different concentrations: 0.5 mg/ml (250 mOsm), 5 mg/ml (270 mOsm), and 25 mg/ml (170 mOsm). They reported impairment of retinal function and morphology proportional to the progressively increasing ICG dosages. Although differences within the species may hamper extrapolation of those results, most studies favored dose-dependent toxicity of intravitreal ICG as well as a role of osmolarity in dye-induced toxicity.

Experimental *in vitro* studies have also been reported showing that ICG causes cytotoxicity to cultured human RPE cells, retinal ganglion cells, and Müller cells in a dose- and time-dependent manner. Narayanan et al.[9] treated human ARPE-19 and R28 cells with four different concentrations of ICG in combination with light exposure. Various concentrations of ICG with light exposure were found to cause a significant decrease in cellular activity, and moreover, some evidence of RPE toxicity has also been reported with light exposure. In contrast, several additional studies in cell culture demonstrated that ICG at low concentrations (<1 mg/ml) and short incubation times (<5 min) as used in clinical practice appeared to be well tolerated. Most authors agree that ICG-related cytotoxic effects are determined by osmolarity and phototoxicity. In conclusion, although much evidence suggests that ICG may exert toxic effects on the retina, the staining agent in low doses should be safe for chromovitrectomy.

INFRACYANINE GREEN

IfCG also binds with high affinity to the acellular ILM and facilitates its visualization similar to ICG. IfCG dye possesses two pharmacologic differences compared to ICG, which may indicate its safer profile in chromovitrectomy. IfCG is produced in a synthetic manner without sodium iodine, and high-dose topical or intraocular iodine has been shown to induce severe corneal and retinal damage. As a second difference, iodine-free IfCG is dissolved in 5% glucose, giving an iso-osmotic solution of around 310 mmol/kg. In contrast, ICG is usually dissolved in water before further dilution in balanced salt solution (BSS), which produces a hypo-osmolar solution. Indeed, osmolarity changes at the vitreoretinal interface or subretinal space induced by various types of solutions, including ICG dye, have been shown to promote remarkable histological toxicity to retinal cells.[2]

Several recent clinical investigations have shown positive results with IfCG application without signs of retinal toxicity. In the clinical setting, IfCG-assisted ILM peeling for macular hole surgery demonstrated high closure rates of macular holes in over 90% of eyes and enhanced visual acuity. Conversely, one recent investigation showed the presence of remnants of footplates from Müller or glial cells and neural or ganglion cells respectively after analysis of the ILM peeled with IfCG during macular hole surgery. Therefore, despite that IfCG and ICG may facilitate ILM removal, unwanted retinal alterations may be generated, such as neurosensory RPE and visual field defects. In summary, IfCG with a presumably safer profile may represent an outstanding alternative to ICG use for ILM peeling during chromovitrectomy in humans. IfCG at a concentration of 0.5 mg/ml results in adequate ILM identification and less toxic effects.[10]

TRYPAN BLUE

TB has been proposed to stain preretinal tissues such as ILM and ERM in chromovitrectomy (Figure 48.2). Although the use of TB for ILM staining may also be feasible, in our experience ILM visualization is much more difficult than with the ICG- or BriB-guided procedure. Currently, state-of-the-art TB usage recommends blue dye application mainly for ERM staining. TB exhibits outstanding affinity for ERM because of the strong presence of dead glial cells within those membranes. TB staining of the ERM may minimize mechanical trauma to the retina during ERM removal and should allow the recognition of the whole extent of the ERM, which has led to good surgical outcomes and minimization of the recurrence of ERM in several clinical studies.[11]

The usefulness of intracameral or intravitreal injection of TB to highlight vitreous gel has been recently proposed. The blue dye in various doses may enhance the ability to detect both the prolapsed vitreous to the anterior chamber and the posterior vitreous remaining in the vitreous cavity. However, in one comparative analysis TB demonstrated an inferior ability to stain the vitreous in comparison to TA and FS.[12]

TB in vitreoretinal surgery was initially proposed for injection after an air–fluid exchange, allowing for better dye dropping on to the retinal surface. To enhance dye penetration on to retinal surface in an air–fluid exchange, TB may be mixed with glucose at higher than 5%, for instance 10% or 25%, thereby creating a "heavy" TB, denser than water. However, high glucose concentrations should be avoided; for instance, glucose 50% has a highly toxic osmolarity of 2020 mOsm/l. Experimental injection of 0.05 ml of a 1000 mOsm solution caused rapid whitening of the posterior retina followed by the development of a large detachment and permanent retinal degeneration. Indeed, osmolarity should be taken into consideration in planning the amount and location of any vitreous injection of dyes and drugs.

Consecutive clinical studies have revealed that TB exerts little or no toxic effect on the retina. For ERM surgery, TB caused no RPE defects or signs of retinal toxicity in most studies in the literature until now. Histopathological analysis of excised ERM showed no retinal cells on the retina side of the ERM or signs of apoptosis, while functional analysis by multifocal ERG also showed no signs of retinal toxicity. Comparative studies evaluated the anatomical and visual outcomes after vitrectomy and ILM peeling for treatment of patients with macular hole using ICG or TB. Their success rate for MH closure was the same; however, visual recovery has been better in the TB group.

In animal experiments, TB has demonstrated a reasonably good retinal biocompatibility in most investigations at the concentration proposed for intravitreal application from 0.06% to 0.15%. Grisanti et al. used fresh hemisected porcine eyes and applied TB 0.15% to the posterior pole after vitreous removal followed by illumination with a standard surgical light probe and source at maximum power for 10 minutes; the procedure caused no histologically detectable damage. These results imply that TB at concentrations of 0.15% or lower represents a safe adjuvant in vitreoretinal surgery.[13]

Various laboratory studies have evaluated the retina biocompatibility of TB alone or in comparison to ICG. In cultured human RPE and Müller cells, some authors have reported that exposure to TB at concentrations up to 0.3% *in vitro* induced no toxic effect.[14] In accordance with these studies, recent investigations revealed that TB is toxic to cultured RPE cells at concentrations higher than 0.5%. However, ICG may cause more toxicity to the retina, especially to human RPE cell cultures, than TB, independent of any phototoxic potentiating effect of fiberoptic light or solvent toxicity. Our research group showed that subretinal injection of 0.05% ICG results in more substantial retinal damage than that associated with subretinal injection of 0.15% TB.[15]

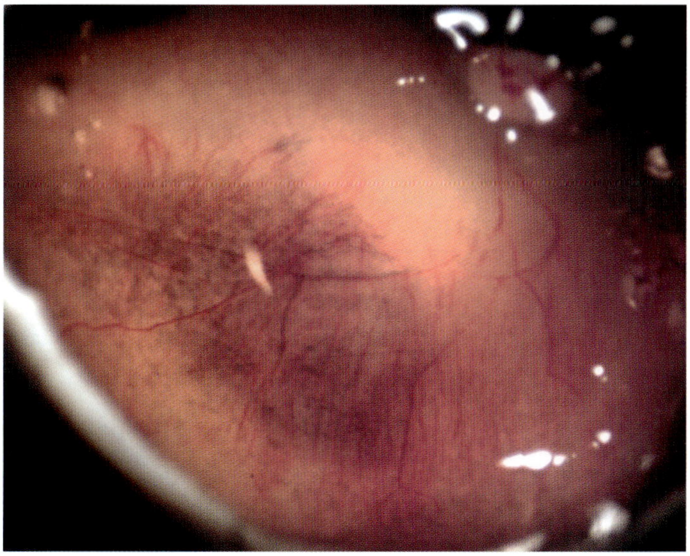

Figure 48.2 In porcine eyes, the internal limiting membrane is fine-colored with trypan blue. However, intraoperatively the blue azo agent stains rather the glial epiretinal membranes.

PATENT BLUE

PB has been certified for capsule staining during cataract surgery at a concentration of 0.24%. Animal studies and preliminary clinical data demonstrate moderate affinity of PB for ERM and vitreous, but a poor affinity for the ILM. Our recent clinical data revealed PB as an appropriate vital dye for staining the glial ERM from various causes in a similar manner to TB.[16]

Toxicology studies revealed conflicting data regarding retinal toxicity of PB. In one study PB was found to induce only mild and reversible retinal toxicity, whereas RPE cells exposed *in vitro* to PB showed no toxicity.[15] Our rabbit subretinal toxicity model demonstrated clinically on FA examination no RPE defects in positions related to the subretinal PB injection in rabbits as seen in the control BSS group. Histologically, subretinal injection of PB resulted only in mild ultrastructural retinal damage during follow-up; the histological damage induced by TB and ICG was more severe than that by PB. The exact safe dosage for intravitreal PB injection remains uncertain.[15]

BRILLIANT BLUE

In the last few years, the stain BriB has been introduced as a surgical adjuvant for chromovitrectomy and anterior lens capsule staining. In order to enable anterior capsule visualization for capsulorrhexis, BriB may be applied in an iso-osmolar solution at a concentration of 0.25 mg/ml or higher. In humans, BriB also produced adequate ILM staining when using an iso-osmolar solution of 0.25 mg/ml during macular hole surgery, while no signs of damage were noticed. Cervera et al. showed similar outcomes with good ILM staining and clinical results and no signs of toxicity in multifocal ERG. In brief, BriB represents a great alternative for ICG and IfCG in chromovitrectomy due to its suitable affinity for ILM.[17]

Experimental investigation in rat eyes revealed no damage of corneal endothelial cells in the long term after BriB exposure. In rat and primate eyes, no significant retinal pathologic changes were observed with light microscopy and electron microscopy after low-dose BriB injection; there was also no reduction in the amplitude of the ERG waves.[18] Our workgroup performed experiments with intravitreal injection of two doses of BriB and five other dyes in rabbit eyes. We found that BriB at the lower dose induced no major retinal changes, while at the higher dose some alterations of the photoreceptors were encountered. Collectively, these data imply that BriB represents an adequate and safe staining agent for clinical evaluation in humans.[2]

SODIUM FLUORESCEIN (SF)

SF has been found to be highly safe for fundus angiography at concentrations of 5–25%, even when leakage through the retina occurred. Because of its hydrophilic properties, SF is highly absorbed by the vitreous gel, as most available data indicate that intravitreal 0.20% SF dye improves the visualization of clear vitreous fibers through a green staining during chromovitrectomy. In addition, there are so far no side-effects reported in regard to the use of SF in chromovitrectomy. While so far the main indication of SF in chromovitrectomy remains the vitreous staining, further clinical experience should determine whether there is any role for SF application in the visualization of preretinal membranes.[12]

TRIAMCINOLONE ACETONIDE

Various clinical investigations have shown that TA produces the best vitreous visibility in comparison to other stains. The crystals of the crystalline steroid adhere avidly to the acellular tissue, thereby enabling a clear contrast between the empty vitreous cavity compared to areas where the vitreous fibers are still present (Figure 48.3). The currently reported surgical technique for TA application consists of a simple injection of the agent into the vitreous cavity directed toward the area of visualization. In addition to its effect on vitreous visualization, a TA injection during vitrectomy has been proposed to prevent fibrin reaction and postoperative proliferative vitreoretinopathy. Following the initial report, a list of consecutive clinical studies showed the efficacy of TA for staining the transparent vitreous, whereas anatomic or functional signs of complications have rarely been observed. A recent multicenter controlled clinical trial performed in Japan showed decreased risk of postoperative retinal detachment but increased need for postoperative antiglaucoma eye drops with intravitreal TA application.[19]

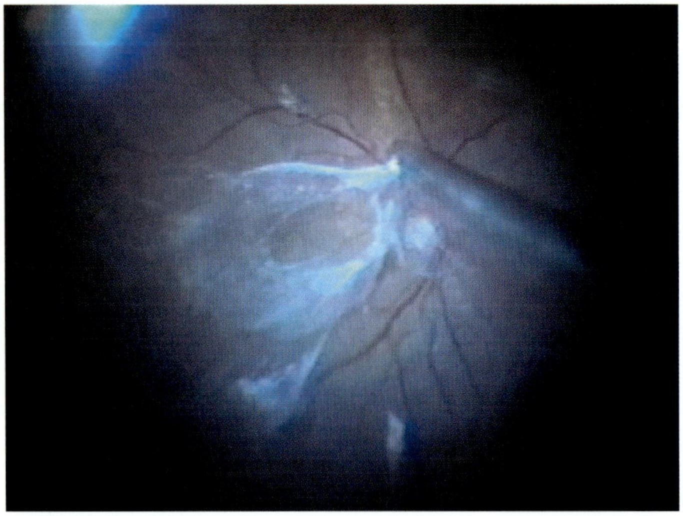

Figure 48.3 The steroid triamcinolone acetonide stains the acellular vitreous strongly and thereby ensures that the whole posterior vitreous cortex is removed during vitreoretinal surgery.

In the clinical setting, TA arose as an alternative stain for ILM peeling, since the white specks and crystals may deposit over the ILM, thereby facilitating ILM removal. Afterward, a few clinicopathologic studies disclosed the presence of ILM ultrastructures after TA-assisted peeling. Clinical studies have shown that TA-assisted ILM removal enables good clinical results, with no adverse effects noticeable in the follow-up evaluation period. However, recent data raised concern regarding the use of TA for MH surgery. Crystals of TA have been detected up to 40 days postsurgery with chromovitrectomy for MH surgery. Some authors suggest that postoperative residual TA could diminish the healing process necessary for MH closure.[20] Currently available preservative-free TA may be better for vitreous staining as a deposit to enhance visualization.

Contradicting results from a considerable number of animal experiments have recently been released regarding retinal toxicity after intravitreal TA injection. Various studies of intravitreal TA injection at concentrations varying from 4 to 30 mg TA have normal morphologic and ERG retinal findings up to 6 months' follow-up. In contrast to those reports, others examined escalating doses from 0.5 to 20 mg of suspended preservative-free TA in rabbits, and found prominent retinal damage manifested by destruction of photoreceptor outer segments and RPE/photoreceptor interdigitation at a dosage of 4 mg or higher.

There is still uncertainty as to whether TA itself or the vehicle plays the more significant role in retinal damage. In order to elucidate this question, one study compared a group of TA with vehicle to another with preservative-free TA and demonstrated severe damage to photoreceptor only in the group with vehicle.[21] In contrast to those outcomes, other investigators revealed a safer profile of the vehicle only: they described normal retinal structure after intravitreal injection of vehicle only in animals. Our investigation disclosed disturbance to photoreceptor segments after subretinal injection of preservative-free TA; however, no clinical abnormality on fundoscopy or fluorescein angiography was detected.[20] Future studies should clarify if the vehicle alone, TA alone, or both chemicals produce retinal damage in humans.

Consecutive laboratory studies examined the effects of TA on various types of retinal cells including ARPE19, human glial cells, neurosensory cells, ganglion cells, and choroidal fibroblasts.[21] A few studies have indicated that TA may cause severe toxicity to chorioretinal cells. In contrast, some investigators proposed a safe *in vitro* profile of the white steroid to RPE cells. These conflicting results may highlight the importance of many variables in chemical-induced retina toxicity in the clinical setting.

OPERATIVE TECHNIQUES AND MODIFICATIONS

DYE INJECTION

Several different surgical approaches have been used to inject vital dyes in the vitreous cavity in chromovitrectomy. One technique has been named the "dry method" or "air-filled technique." By either name, this technique consists of removing the liquid in the vitreous cavity by a fluid–air exchange before dye injection. Although the technique has the advantage of concentrating the dye in the posterior pole and avoiding contact at the posterior capsule of the lens, it may expose the retinal surface to the injected concentration of the dye. The second proposed technique to inject dyes is called the "wet method" or "fluid-filled technique." In this method, the intravitreal fluid is left inside the vitreous cavity while the surgeon infuses the dye. The amount of dye in contact with the retinal surface becomes much lower because it is diluted and washed out earlier by the fluid in the vitreous cavity. The disadvantage to this technique is the dispersion of biological stain leading to unwanted staining of the retina elsewhere. A further concern after dye administration may be the incubation time of the dye on the retinal surface. There is a recent trend toward washing out the dye no later than a few seconds after its injection.[4]

A novel painting brush to avoid unnecessary and nonselective staining of the entire retina during chromovitrectomy has recently been introduced. The commercially available applicator instrument called VINCE (Vitreoretinal INternal limiting membrane Color Enhancer, Dutch Ophthalmic, The Netherlands) consists of a modified backflush needle, containing an adjustable silicone tube surrounded by a metal cannula. The tube is connected to a reservoir in the handpiece filled with vital dye. The customized cartridge loading system contains the already prepared and diluted vital dye. This new device may provide a better visualization of fine, delicate, semitransparent preretinal tissues during chromovitrectomy.

MACULAR HOLE PROTECTION

There are some alternatives to avoid dye injection directly through the MH: slow injection of the dye, selective painting instrument (VINCE), or some substances over the MH, such as perfluorocarbon liquid (PFCL), autologous whole blood, or sodium hyaluronate. A known complication of their use, however, is liquid entering the subretinal space via a retinal break which can compress and disorganize the retina. In chromovitrectomy, PFCL has been used as a protective agent for the macular hole to avoid the direct contact of ICG with the subretinal space. Besides the apparent safety of this technique, the use of PFCL increases the costs and operative time while the meticulous use of a small-tip fluted needle is essential to prevent residual PFCL which could lead to retinal toxicity.

Some authors have described the use of autologous blood as a protective agent for the retina during ICG-assisted macular hole surgery.[22] Clinically, small noncomparative case series showed that whole blood used in ICG-assisted vitrectomy for macular hole surgery is apparently safe, with no signs of retinal damage or residual ICG detected after 1 month.[23] Whole blood could protect against physical contact of ICG with the macular hole/RPE and also could reduce the ICG retention time, thereby diminishing the risk of toxicity.

Viscoelastic in ICG-assisted vitrectomy can be used to control where the dye settles on the retinal surface to avoid staining outside the macular region. Although good visual and anatomic outcomes could be achieved with this technique, it requires more surgical time to perform fluid–air exchange and could potentially be more toxic because no additional ICG dilution occurs, as is seen with fluid-filled globe.

SUMMARY AND KEY POINTS

For vitreoretinal surgery, vital dyes enable easier identification of the semitransparent preretinal membranes. Current recommendations for the application of dyes during vitreoretinal surgery indicate that ICG, IfCG, BriB, and BroB may be the best stains for the ILM, while TB and PB may be preferred for staining the glial ERM. The highly aqueous composition of the vitreous implies that most hydrophilic vital dyes such as TB, ICG, and PB may stain the vitreous well. In addition, an excellent staining agent for vitreous visualization is the white steroid TA.

In regard to the toxicity issues in chromovitrectomy, a large number of experimental and clinical investigations in this challenging field with vital dyes have yielded many controversial results, but nonetheless, some preliminary conclusions may be drawn at this time. First, every vital dye injected intravitreally poses a rather dose-dependent toxicity to the retinal tissue. In addition, there is strong evidence that light exposure, osmolarity, and the presence of ions such as Na^+ and iodine may exert further damage to the retina. Therefore, some recommendations include very low amount of dye injection on to the preretinal membrane, avoidance of long macular exposure to endoillumination, and removal of sodium and iodine from staining solutions.

REFERENCES

1. Rodrigues EB, Meyer CH, Kroll P. Chromovitrectomy: a new field in vitreoretinal surgery. Graefes Arch Clin Exp Ophthalmol 2005;243:291–293.
2. Rodrigues EB, Maia M, Meyer CH, et al. Vital dyes for chromovitrectomy. Curr Opin Ophthalmol 2007;18:179–187.
3. Karacorlu M, Karacorlu S, Ozdemir H. Iatrogenic punctate chorioretinopathy after internal limiting membrane peeling. Am J Ophthalmol 2003;135:178–182.
4. Rodrigues EB, Meyer CH, Farah ME, et al. Intravitreal staining of the internal limiting membrane using indocyanine green in the treatment of macular holes. Ophthalmologica 2005;219:251–262.
5. Haritoglou C, Gass CA, Schaumberger M, et al. Long-term follow-up after macular hole surgery with internal limiting membrane peeling. Am J Ophthalmol 2002;134:661–666.
6. Gandorfer A, Haritoglou C, Kampik A. Staining of the ILM in macular surgery. Br J Ophthalmol 2003;87:1530.
7. Penha FM, Maia M, Farah ME, et al. Effects of subretinal injections of indocyanine green, trypan blue, and glucose in rabbit eyes. Ophthalmology 2007;114:899–908.
8. Maia M, Kellner L, de Juan Jr E, et al. Effects of indocyanine green injection on the retinal surface and into the subretinal space in rabbits. Retina 2004;24:80–91.
9. Narayanan R, Kenney MC, Kamjoo S, et al. Toxicity of indocyanine green (ICG) in combination with light on retinal pigment epithelial cells and neurosensory retinal cells. Curr Eye Res 2005;30:471–478.
10. Penha FM, Maia M, Farah ME, et al. Morphologic and clinical effects of subretinal injection of indocyanine green and infracyanine green in rabbits. J Ocul Pharmacol Ther 2008; in press.
11. Vote BJ, Russell MK, Joondeph BC. Trypan blue-assisted vitrectomy. Retina 2004;24:736–738.
12. Guo S, Tutela AC, Wagner R, et al. A comparison of the effectiveness of four biostains in enhancing visualization of the vitreous. J Pediatr Ophthalmol Strabismus 2006;43:281–284.
13. Grisanti S, Szurman P, Tatar O, et al. Histopathological analysis in experimental macular surgery with trypan blue. Br J Ophthalmol 2004;88:1206–1208.
14. Farah ME, Maia M, Furlani B, et al. Current concepts of trypan blue in chromovitrectomy. Dev Ophthalmol 2008;42:91–100.
15. Maia M, Penha F, Rodrigues EB, et al. Effects of subretinal injection of patent blue and trypan blue in rabbits. Curr Eye Res 2007;32:309–317.
16. Mennel S, Meyer CH, Tietjen A, et al. Patent blue: a novel vital dye in vitreoretinal surgery. Ophthalmologica 2006;220:190–193.
17. Cervera E, Diaz-Llopis M, Salom D, et al. Internal limiting membrane staining using intravitreal brilliant blue G: good help for vitreo-retinal surgeon in training. Arch Soc Esp Oftalmol 2007;82:71–72.
18. Enaida H, Hisatomi T, Hata Y, et al. Brilliant blue G selectively stains the internal limiting membrane/brilliant blue G-assisted membrane peeling. Retina 2006;26:631–636.
19. Yamakiri K, Sakamoto T, Noda Y, et al. Reduced incidence of intraoperative complications in a multicenter controlled clinical trial of triamcinolone in vitrectomy. Ophthalmology 2007;114:289–296.
20. Takasu I, Shiraga F, Otsuki H. Triamcinolone acetonide-assisted internal limiting membrane peeling in macular hole surgery. Retina 2004;24:620–622.
21. Maia M, Farah ME, Belfort Neto R, et al. Effects of intravitreal triamcinolone acetonide injection with and without preservatives. Br J Ophthalmol 2007;91(9):1122–1124.
22. Maia M, Penha FM, Farah ME, et al. Subretinal injection of preservative-free triamcinolone acetonide and supernatant vehicle in rabbits: an electron microscopy study. Graefes Arch Clin Exp Ophthalmol 2008;246:379–388.
23. Lai CC, Wu WC, Chuang LH, et al. Prevention of indocyanine green toxicity on retinal pigment epithelium with whole blood in stain-assisted macular hole surgery. Ophthalmology 2005;112:1409–1414.

CHAPTER

49

Epimacular and external radiotherapy

Gildo Y. Fujii, MD, PhD and Juliana V. Rossi, MD

KEY FEATURES

- Radiation is a local, targeted therapy designed to kill cancer cells or abnormal tissues such as neovascularization. Radiation therapy can be effectively used to treat several types of tumors.
- Treatment planning and strategy are paramount to obtain positive clinical results. For each case there is a specific preferred treatment plan.
- The total amount of radiation dosage is based on the type and size of tumor.
- Radiotherapy is continuously evolving and newer techniques are allowing for greater energy control, broadening its clinical use.
- Combined therapy using vascular endothelial growth factor (VEGF) inhibition and radiation is emerging as a potential new treatment modality for eyes with exudative age-related macular degeneration.
- Many radiation side-effects are long-term and have an impact on clinical results.

INTRODUCTION AND HISTORY

The use of radiation to treat eye diseases was pioneered by Verhoeff and Reese in the early 1900s.[1] In 1930, Moore described the use of radon seeds to treat choroidal sarcoma.[2] Since these early reports, several forms of radiation have been developed to treat eye tumors and, despite the significant complications from various sources of radiation, it remains a reasonable alternative to enucleation. Although ocular radiotherapy is mostly used for the treatment of melanomas, it has also been used to treat other ocular tumors.

Radiation therapy to treat subfoveal choroidal neovascularization (CNV) secondary to age-related macular degeneration was first described in 1993 by Chakravathy et al. reporting the preliminary results of a series of 19 patients treated with external beam radiation.[3] Since then, there have been numerous studies evaluating the effects of radiation for the treatment of age-related macular degeneration but its use remains controversial. Studies using an anti-VEGF drug combined with radiotherapy were published by Mauceri et al. in 1998 and 1999 for the treatment of tumors.[4–6] These studies demonstrated that the efficacy of radiation therapy may be potentiated by brief concomitant exposure of anti-VEGF drugs. Recently, this new treatment paradigm combining angiogenesis inhibitors and radiotherapy is showing promise for the treatment of eyes with exudative age-related macular degeneration. One new strategy involves the intravitreal administration of two injections of the anti-VEGF antibody (Lucentis or bevacizumab) combined with a single treatment with 24-Gy beta-radiation (strontium-90 (Sr-90)).[7]

BIOLOGICAL EFFECTS

The radiation effects on tumors include necrosis, tumor blood vessel damage, inflammation, and fibrosis. Tumor irradiation lowers the mitotic rate,[8] the proliferative activity,[9] and the microvascular density.[10] Irradiation causes blood vessel damage, necrosis, and hypoxia, resulting in tumor shrinkage.[11]

Histopathologic studies in eyes with melanoma enucleated after plaque therapy include tumor cell necrosis, vascular obstruction, fibrosis, inflammatory cells (macrophages), vacuolization, and balloon cell degeneration.[11] Radiation changes in other ocular structures have also been reported and include subretinal gliosis, chorioretinal atrophy, scleral necrosis, and iris neovascularization.[12]

In a study by Maureci et al., the authors combined radiation with angiostatin to target tumor vasculature that is genetically stable.[4] Their results showed an antitumor interaction between ionizing radiation and angiostatin for four distinct tumor types, at doses of radiation that are used in radiotherapy. Importantly, the combination produced no increase in toxicity towards normal tissue. *In vitro* studies showed that radiation and angiostatin have combined cytotoxic effects on endothelial cells, but not tumor cells. *In vivo* studies showed that these agents, in combination, target the tumor vasculature. These results provided support for combining ionizing radiation with anti-VEGF drugs to improve the cytotoxic effects of tumor endothelial cell without increasing deleterious effects.

Another study by Gorski et al. in 1999 showed in four separate tumor model experiments a more significant tumor growth delay with combined therapy compared to either anti-VEGF therapy or radiotherapy alone.[6] This group concluded that radiation up-regulates endothelial cell production of VEGF, which in turn acts as a survival factor, and that VEGF inhibition counters this survival effect.

Lee et al. were able to demonstrate a significant reduction in tumor microvessel density (36–60%) and interstitial fluid pressure (approximately 75%), and an increase in PO_2 with anti-VEGF therapy compared to controls. The increase in PO_2 may have been due to an improvement in the quality of oxygen delivery, partly owing to a decreased interstitial fluid pressure. They hypothesized that anti-VEGF therapy should decrease interstitial fluid pressure, resulting in radiosensitization.[13]

In a study by Geng et al. it was demonstrated that VEGF receptor may be a therapeutic target to improve susceptibility to radiotherapy. The authors concluded that anti-VEGF drugs, in certain conditions, act synergistically with radiotherapy.[14]

Additional work by Griffin et al.[15] and Ning et al.[16] found a greater than additive effect on tumor growth delay with combined therapy using SU6668, a broader tyrosine kinase antagonist of VEGF, and one group confirmed an increase in PO_2 after treatment with SU6668.[15,16] Furthermore, SU6668 was found to have a greater therapeutic effect than SU5416 by almost doubling the tumor growth delay from 6.5 to 11.9 days. Griffin et al. concluded that SU6668 increased the radiosensitivity of tumor blood vessels.[15] Ning et al concluded that inhibition of VEGF, fibroblast growth factor, and platelet-derived growth factor receptor function by SU5416 and SU6668 can enhance the efficacy of irradiation.[16]

By examining the anti-VEGF strategy combined with radiotherapy for tumors, several general conclusions can be drawn. The first is that combination therapy with VEGF inhibitors is probably more effective than radiotherapy alone in many types of tumors. The second is that the effect appears to be at least partly due to an elevation in PO_2, which may be mediated through a change in microvessel density and/or interstitial fluid pressure. As VEGF is a growth factor that is up-regulated by radiotherapy and acts as a survival factor for endothelial cells, it is plausible that VEGF inhibition results in blockade of this survival signal, leading to a greater radiation therapeutic effect.

Extrapolating this analysis for the treatment of eyes with exudative age-related macular degeneration, it is conceivable that the combined treatment strategy using focal brachytherapy and anti-VEGF therapy has more than an additive effect, in part due to the same mechanisms observed in the combined treatment for tumors.

INDICATIONS

CHOROIDAL MELANOMA

Radiation is the most widely used method to treat posterior uveal melanoma; brachytherapy and external beam irradiation are the two most common methods of radiotherapy employed.

The most commonly used form of radiotherapy has been the use of radioactive plaques. Treatment of a malignant tumor of the uvea by brachytherapy was first reported in 1930.[2] The preferred isotope has changed over the years and iodine-125 and ruthenium-106 plaques have largely replaced cobalt-60 at most institutions. Radioactive plaques were originally conceived to be used for the treatment of small and medium-sized melanomas that were outside the retinal vascular arcade and posterior to the ora serrata. More recently, studies have presented a rationale for using plaque radiotherapy for macular melanoma,[17] ciliary body melanoma,[18] large melanoma,[19] and melanoma with extrascleral extension.[20]

Another method of radiotherapy is external beam radiation (charged-particle irradiation).[21] This technique was originally believed to provide a collimated beam that would limit the radiotherapy selectively to the area of the tumor. However, this theory has not been substantiated by clinical experience. Radiation complications in the eye and adnexa have been described at a rate comparable to those reported using radioactive plaques.

Current data show that patients treated with radiotherapy have a survival rate similar to those treated by enucleation.[22] Mortality rates following brachytherapy have not differed from mortality rates following enucleation for up to 12 years after treatment.[22] The power of the Collaborative Ocular Melanoma Study (COMS) randomized study has allowed clinicians confidently to recommend radiation for appropriate medium size melanomas, recognizing that enucleation does not offer a greater chance of survival with follow-up to 12 years.

The optimal radiation dosage for the treatment of uveal melanoma remains controversial, but doses between 50 and 100 Gy have been accepted as appropriate. The American Brachytherapy Society has currently presented the COMS dose recommendation as the guideline for the treatment of choroidal melanoma.[23] Considerations regarding properties of half-life, shielding, tissue penetration, and physical form have made iodine-125 a preferred choice of isotope for brachytherapy in many institutions.

EXUDATIVE AGE-RELATED MACULAR DEGENERATION

Ocular radiation therapy has been explored as a treatment modality for exudative age-related macular degeneration for many years. Since proliferative tissue is more susceptible to the effects of ionizing radiation than nonproliferative tissue, choroidal neovascular membranes, which are composed of endothelial cells and proliferate more rapidly than the endothelial cells of the retina, are more sensitive to radiation treatment than the retinal vasculature and nonproliferating capillary endothelial cells and larger vessels. Early reports on the treatment of CNV with brachytherapy describe resolution of subretinal fluid, hemorrhages, and exudates after radiation therapy.

Currently, the use of radiation for the treatment of subfoveal CNV remains controversial.

The scientific rationale for using radiation therapy for a nonmalignant disease characterized by neovascular growth is based on experimental and clinical evidence. Reports in peer-reviewed publications indicate that localized radiation treatment has the ability to prevent proliferation of vascular tissue. More specifically, low-dose radiation has been shown to inhibit neovascularization. After low-dose radiation, vascular endothelium demonstrates morphologic and DNA changes, inhibition of replication, increased cell permeability, and apoptosis. Fibroblast proliferation and subsequent scar formation, a hallmark of end-stage neovascular age-related macular degeneration, are also inhibited.

Choroidal neovascular membranes, which are composed of endothelial cells and proliferate more rapidly than the endothelial cells of the retina, are more sensitive to radiation treatment than the retinal vasculature and nonproliferating capillary endothelial cells and larger vessels. Early studies examining the effect of radiation in the eye have demonstrated that low-dose radiation, while altering the biology of choroidal neovascular membranes, may affect the natural history of eyes with exudative age-related macular degeneration.

Recently, a new form of localized epimacular delivery of radiation directly to the site of the proliferative, neovascular tissue could theorectically minimize the well-established side-effects of treatment with both ionizing and nonionizing radiation. This technique has a shielded and directional applicator which will be placed just over the retina to give a dose to the CNV believed to have therapeutic benefit, while limiting the dose to the critical ocular tissues, i.e., retina outside the macular region, optic nerve, and lens.

The radiation source in the Neovista VIDION brachytherapy system is based on an Sr-90/yttrium-90 (Y-90) beta-irradiating isotope (Figure 49.1). The Sr-90/Y-90 isotope has a 28-year half-life and a relatively limited depth of effective penetration. This provides the ability to deliver the therapeutic dose to the treatment area, while limiting the exposure to nontarget tissues (Figure 49.2). With a source activity of approximately 11 mCi the treatment duration will be relatively short, approximately 2–4 minutes.

The source consists of a cylindrical aluminum insert that is doped with the Sr-90/Y-90 isotope and resides inside a stainless-steel canister. Initial studies have indicated promising results with the use of localized epimacular Sr-90 brachytherapy delivered concomitantly with intravitreal bevacizumab to treat exudative age-related macular degeneration.[7]

OTHER OCULAR TUMORS

Although radiotherapy is mostly used to treat choroidal melanomas, it has also been used to treat various ocular tumors.

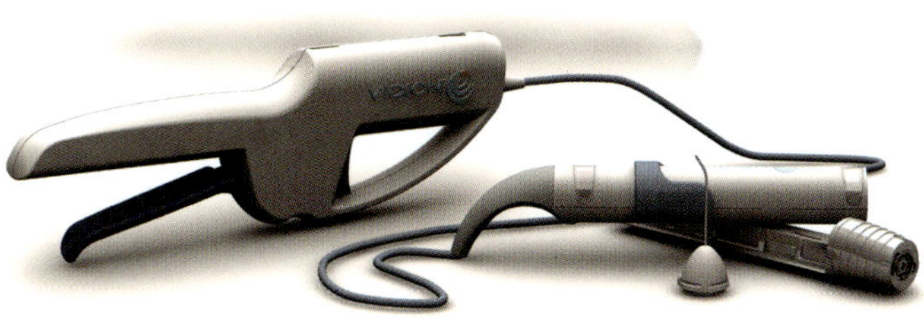

Figure 49.1 Neovista VIDION brachytherapy system based on a strontium/yttrium-90 beta-irradiating isotope for focal epimacular delivery of beta-radiation.

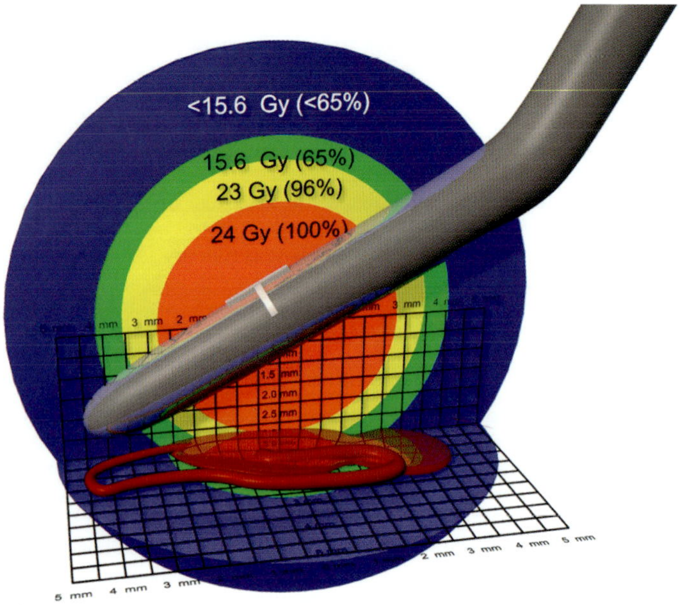

Figure 49.2 Neovista VIDION brachytherapy system dose profile. It was designed to have therapeutic radiation levels at the neovascular complex in eyes with exudative age-related macular degeneration while limiting the radiation exposure to nontarget tissues.

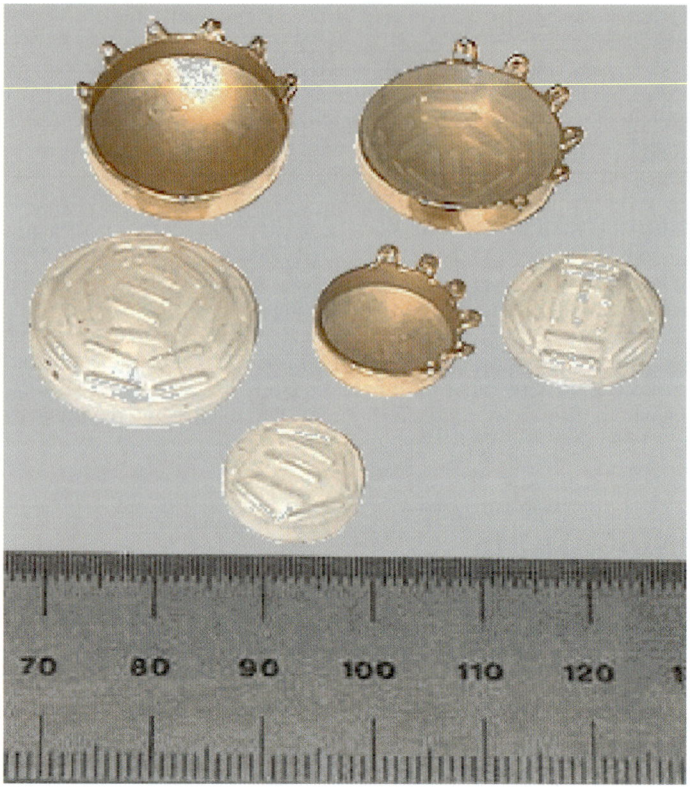

Figure 49.3 Radiation plaques used in the Collaborative Ocular Melanoma Study (COMS). These plaques consist of gold housing and seed carrier insert for iodine-125 isotopes.

Radiation has been used in several forms to treat intraocular retinoblastoma. External beam radiotherapy has been extensively used since Verhoeff and Reese pioneered the method in the early 1900s. Because retinoblastoma is a radiosensitive tumor, its control and eye preservation rates are relatively high. Intensity-modulated radiation therapy is an alternate method of delivering radiotherapy that reduces the dose to normal tissues and has been reported effective to control retinoblastoma.[24] Brachytherapy is the treatment of choice in certain types of retinoblastoma[25] and its use has increased as the danger of external beam therapy in genetically predisposed patients with heritable retinoblastoma has been recognized.

Radiation has been used to treat serous retinal detachment secondary to circumscribed choroidal hemangiomas.[26] The radiation has been delivered by external beam, proton bean, and brachytherapy. The resolution of subretinal fluid has been successfully achieved in most cases. Combined chemotherapy with radiotherapy is also recommended for patients with primary intraocular lymphoma.[27]

Radiotherapy has also been used in cases of retinal and choroidal metastasis for palliation or prevention of symptoms in patients with concomitant systemic therapy and for those untreated patients for whom effective systemic therapy is not available.[28] Most retinal and choroidal metastasis responds to treatment and regression of tumor and associated retinal detachment can be assessed in most cases, avoiding the need for enucleation.

Although not common, ocular radiotherapy has been described in the treatment of cavernous hemangioma of the retina and retinal capillary hemangioma in patients with von Hippel–Lindau disease.[29]

OPERATIVE TECHNIQUES

PLAQUE PLACEMENT TECHNIQUE

Before placing an iodine-125 plaque it is important to obtain the best estimate of the tumor size, including base and height dimensions. These dimensions will determine the size of the plaque containing iodine-125 (Figure 49.3). The most important measurement is the base diameter of the tumor.

The tumor size can be estimated by using retinal photographs or measuring grids. During photograph measurements, the horizontal diameter of the optic disc head can be used as a unit of measurement equivalent to 1.5 mm. An alternative is to use a measuring grid, as described by Hilton.[30] The measuring grid is designed so that each grid square overlies an area equivalent to approximately 1 disc diameter (DD). The image of the tumor is viewed monocularly using indirect ophthalmoscopy with a measuring grid placed over a 20-D Nikon lens, and the number of squares (DDs) overlying the tumor is counted. Then, it is converted into millimeters.

The size of the iodine-125 plaque is determined using the estimate tumor diameter plus a tumor-free perimeter of 2 mm or more. For example, a tumor with a 10-mm base diameter should be treated with a plaque that is 14 mm in diameter. Standardized A-scan ultrasonography is used to determine the thickness of the tumor.

During the surgical placement of the plaque, a peritomy should be performed and the surface of the tumor area exposed. If extraocular extension of more than 2 mm is observed, enucleation should be considered.

At surgery, the tumor base can be localized using transillumination. There are several methods to outline the scleral borders of the tumor area. Frequently it is possible to visualize the shadow of the tumor while the globe is transilluminated through the cornea. The perimeter of the tumor base should be verified with indirect ophthalmoscopy. Another technique involves the use of the MIRA diathermy transillumination unit. The intense light of the angled fiberoptic transilluminator allows the operator to visualize the tumor with indirect ophthalmoscopy while simultaneously visualizing the transsclerochoroidal illumination from the fiberoptic light tip as it is moved to localize the perimeter of the tumor. When the fiberoptic light is visualized at the perimeter of the tumor, a diathermy mark can be made on the sclera. These marks should be made more visible using a surgical marking pencil. A caliper is then used to measure the tumor diameter. In order to simulate the placement of the radiation plaque, a transparent acrylic dummy plaque with a diameter equal to the planned therapeutic plaque should be placed on the sclera, covering the scleral marks that identify the tumor perimeter as well as a tumor-free perimeter of 2 mm or more. If the therapeutic plaque is the same size as or smaller than the boundary of the tumor base as marked on the sclera, the procedure should be halted, and a larger plaque is prepared for a future procedure. If the dummy plaque is large enough to cover the tumor area plus 2 mm of tumor-free area, a surgical marking pencil should be used to mark the perimeter of the dummy plaque in the appropriate treatment position on the sclera. After the perimeter of the dummy is removed, the radioactive plaque is placed within the dummy plaque scleral mark and anchored with two or three scleral sutures.

The location of the radioactive plaque can be confirmed by transillumination examination. Examination with indirect ophthalmoscopy can be performed while transscleral transillumination is performed using a fiberoptic light source to visualize the boundary of the plaque relative to the tumor. After confirming proper plaque positioning the conjunctiva is sutured over the plaque.

After surgery, confirmation of the plaque position relative to the tumor can be performed by B-scan ultrasonography or magnetic resonance imaging.

Typically, treatment duration is about 3–6 days. After completion of the treatment period the plaque is surgically removed.

EPIMACULAR BRACHYTHERAPY FOR AGE-RELATED MACULAR DEGENERATION

SURGICAL TECHNIQUE

The subject is prepared as per standard eye surgery and the procedure is accomplished through a standard vitrectomy procedure.

Surgery begins with a standard vitrectomy procedure. An infusion cannula is inserted and secured in the sclera about 3–4 mm from the surgical limbus, usually in the inferotemporal quadrant (Figure 49.4A).

An appropriate lens for vitreoretinal surgery is placed and a limited vitrectomy performed. After vitrectomy, the treatment probe is placed in the vitreous cavity and under microscopic visualization, the surgeon places the tip of the probe directly above the macula to evaluate hand positioning better during treatment (Figure 49.4B). Once the proper probe positioning is determined by the surgeon, the probe is positioned back in the mid vitreous position and the radiation source is then advanced by pushing the sliding mechanism towards the tip of the probe (Figure 49.4C). The probe is then positioned back to the proper treatment location (Figure 49.4D) just above the neovascular membrane, with the center marker directly above the center of the choroidal neovascular complex (Figure 49.4E).

The appropriate treatment time is previously determined by the radiation source activity in order to deliver 24 Gy to the target area. Typically, treatment time varies between 2 and 5 minutes. After treatment time is reached, the surgeon pulls the sliding mechanism back to the storage position and locks it in place. After the slider mechanism is in the storage and locked position, the delivery probe will be removed from the eye and the sclerotomies closed. A radiation survey is performed to ensure that the source has been fully retracted to its storage position.

OUTCOMES

CHOROIDAL MELANOMA

Typically, choroidal melanomas treated with brachytherapy are expected to reduce in size to approximately 50% of their pretreatment thickness over a period of approximately 2 years.[22,31] Only a small percentage of medium-sized and large-sized melanomas become relatively flat scars. As the tumor contracts, increased internal ultrasonographic reflectivity and decreased vascularity are observed.

The maximum tumor size that can be effectively treated with radiation without causing severe radiation complications is still uncertain. The COMS guidelines recommend that the radioactive plaque should extend beyond the recognized tumor base by a 2-mm margin. Following these guidelines, a maximum basal dimension of a tumor treatable with brachytherapy is approximately 21 mm. The COMS reported that enucleations were more common for tumors with greater thicknesses and greater base dimensions, although percentages were not given.[31]

The COMS medium-size tumor trial enrolled 1317 patients and randomized between enucleation and iodine-125 brachytherapy.[22] The mortality rate was not statistically different 12 years after treatment. The all-cause 5-year mortality rates were reported to be approximately 20% and the estimated tumor-specific mortality was 10%.[22]

Between 5% and 10% of patients treated with radiotherapy ultimately require enucleation because of tumor recurrence or radiation complications. In the COMS, 10% of eyes were enucleated because of suspected or documented tumor recurrence. Importantly, tumor recurrences have consistently been reported to be associated with an increased rate of metastases, even when subsequently treated with enucleation. The COMS calculated a metastasis risk ratio of 1.5% when there was a local recurrence.[31] Although eyes with recurrences are often managed with enucleation, local edge recurrences may sometimes be controlled with photocoagulation or transpupillary thermotherapy.

Eyes with juxtapapillary tumors comprise a distinct group with poorer prognosis. The recurrence rate is significantly higher (15%), resulting in a greater incidence of enucleation.[32]

The visual outcome in eyes treated with iodine-125 is similar to that reported for other forms of radiation therapy (helium ion, 53% 20/200 or less; proton beam, 42% 20/200 or less) and suggests that research efforts should continue to be directed toward ways to reduce the complications of radiation.

BRACHYTHERAPY FOR AGE-RELATED MACULAR DEGENERATION

Reports in the more recent published literature describe mixed results. In a pooled analysis of eight phase I studies, results indicated that radiotherapy may only act to slow or delay the progress of the disease. A dose–response relationship was noted in at least one observational study, and better vision outcomes were reported with higher radiation doses in three recently published randomized clinical trials. External photon beam radiation was used in all of these studies.

In 1998, Bergink et al.[33] reported that, 1 year following treatment with four fractions of 6 Gy, 52% of observed eyes versus 32% of treated eyes experienced a 3-line loss of vision. In 1999, Char et al.[34], in a small clinical trial involving 27 patients with varying lengths of follow-up, reported fewer incidences of vision loss among patients treated with one fraction of 7.5-Gy photon beam irradiation than among observed patients. In 2000, Kobayashi and Kobayashi reported successful treatment of patients with smaller neovascularized regions with 20-Gy photon beam divided in 10 fractions of 2 Gy over 14 days in a randomized prospective double-blind study.[35] A total of 101 eyes were randomized to radiation treatment versus observation. Patients with classic CNV were also included. A statistically significant difference in change of logMAR visual acuity was found for follow-up of 6, 12, and 24 months ($P < 0.0001$; $P < 0.0001$; $P < 0.0001$, respectively). The increase in CNV size for 1 and 2 years in the treatment group was significantly smaller than that in the control group ($P = 0.0147$; $P = 0.0008$), showing that radiation was effective in reducing CNV leakage and size. No CNV regression was noted in the control group. No serious treatment side-effects were reported in any of the studies.

In contrast, the Radiation Therapy for Age-related Macular Degeneration study group trial used eight fractions of 2 Gy; Marcus and colleagues used seven fractions of 2 Gy; and Hart et al. used six fractions of 2 Gy but none of these studies demonstrated a clear clinical benefit.[36–38]

Although the cumulative doses (16, 14, and 12 Gy) of radiation in the trials showing no effect do not seem appreciably less than those in the

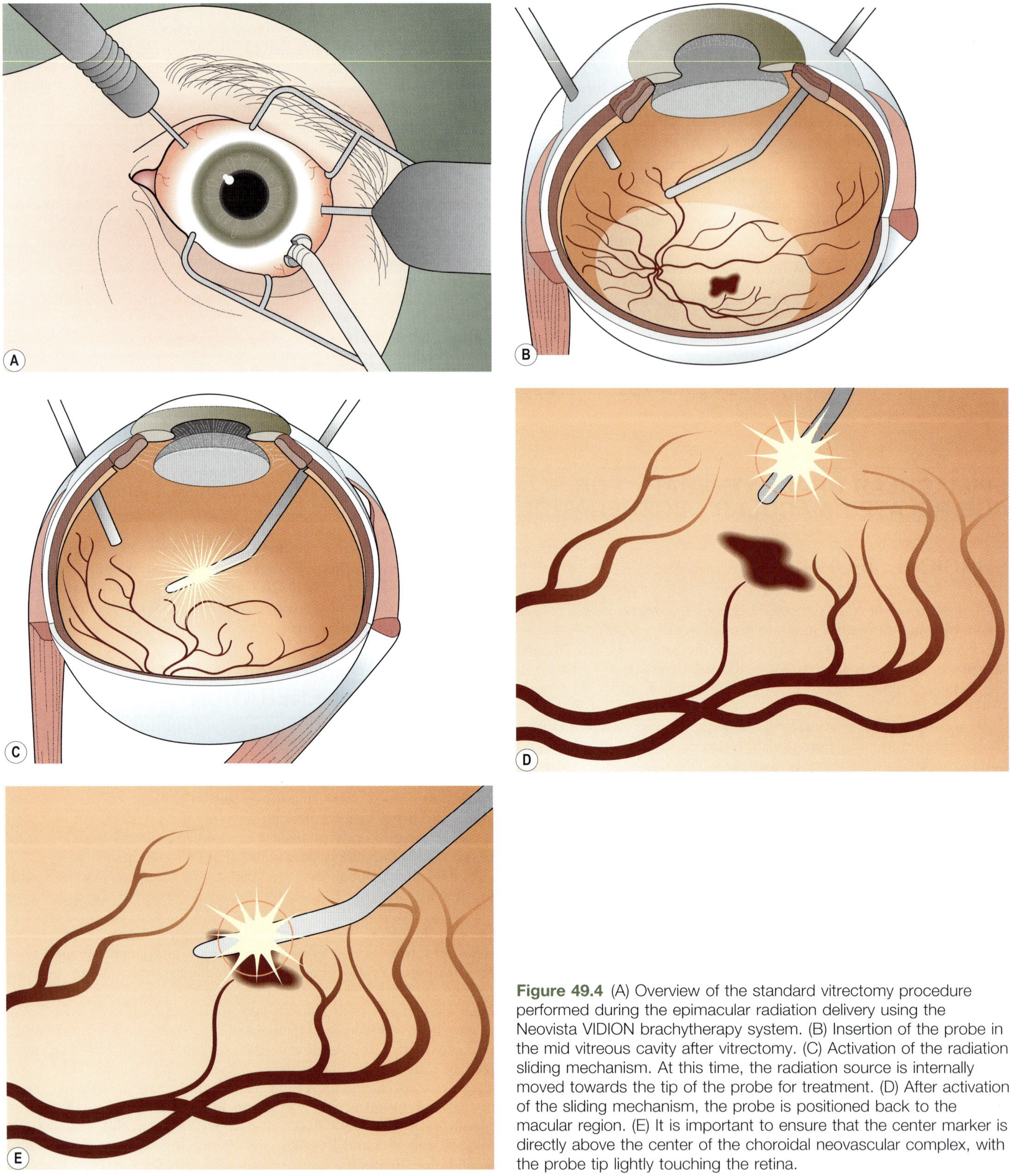

Figure 49.4 (A) Overview of the standard vitrectomy procedure performed during the epimacular radiation delivery using the Neovista VIDION brachytherapy system. (B) Insertion of the probe in the mid vitreous cavity after vitrectomy. (C) Activation of the radiation sliding mechanism. At this time, the radiation source is internally moved towards the tip of the probe for treatment. (D) After activation of the sliding mechanism, the probe is positioned back to the macular region. (E) It is important to ensure that the center marker is directly above the center of the choroidal neovascular complex, with the probe tip lightly touching the retina.

Bergink et al.[33] and Kobayashi and Kobayashi[35] studies (24 and 20 Gy, respectively), the differences in biological effect could be appreciable. With radiation therapy, the biological effect depends on the dose per fraction, the number of fractions, and the time between fractions. For example, the biological effect of the dose used in the study by Bergink et al. may be as much as three times the biological effect of the dose used in the study by the RAD research group.

A study by Flaxel et al. has shown the development of radiation retinopathy in 11 of 27 eyes receiving proton beam 14 cobalt gray equivalent within a year.[39] This study demonstrated efficacy in terms of neovascular closure in eyes with age-related macular degeneration but was limited by radiation retinopathy at 1 year.

Jaakkola et al. evaluated Sr-90 plaque brachytherapy in a prospective, nonrandomized clinical trial.[40] A single dose of 15 Gy at a depth of

1.75 mm was used, with the plaque placed using an applicator with an 8-mm diameter and 12-mm radius curvature. The disc was attached to a handle via a steel shaft. The applicator was surgically introduced in the episcleral surface, under the macula, and held in place manually for the treatment period of 54 minutes. Twenty patients with recently diagnosed CNV received plaque brachytherapy treatment and 12 patients were followed as controls. At 12-month follow-up, 3 (15%) of the 20 brachytherapy-treated eyes experienced a decrease of 6 or more lines of visual acuity, as compared to 6 (50%) of the 12 nontreated eyes (P = 0.057). The mean number of lines lost was 2.6 (SD 3.7) for treated eyes and 5.3 (SD 3.2) for nontreated eyes (P = 0.024). No radiation-related adverse effects were noted.

In the radiation treatments to date, namely photon and proton external beam and plaque brachytherapy, most of the critical ocular tissues received doses similar to that intended for the target area. Therefore, there was a small window between toxicity and effectiveness. Although there were several attempts to mitigate the side-effects by fractionating the total dosage in multiple applications over a period of time, the ideal and effective therapeutic window was not established. In several reports either the dosage was too small to provide therapeutic benefit, or the side-effects relating to neighboring structures exceeded the limited benefits.

Recently, a new form of localized epimacular delivery of radiation directly to the site of the neovascular tissue combined with anti-VEGF agents is being evaluated. This new epimacular brachytherapy strategy is being evaluated in eyes with exudative age-related macular degeneration. This technique has a shielded and directional applicator that limits the radiation dose to critical ocular tissues, i.e., retina outside the macular region, optic nerve, and lens. Initial studies have shown promising results with the use of a single treatment using the localized epimacular brachytherapy associated with anti-VEGF therapy (two injections of bevacizumab) to treat exudative age-related macular degeneration. After 12 months of follow-up the mean change in best corrected visual acuity was a gain of 8.9 letters.[7] This new regimen is being evaluated in a large multicenter phase III study.

COMPLICATIONS

Preservation of good vision following brachytherapy is inversely related to the occurrence of complications. Complications associated with brachytherapy include radiation retinopathy, optic neuropathy, and cataracts. Other long-term side-effects reported include neovascular glaucoma, vitreous hemorrhage, radiation choroidopathy, scleral necrosis, retinal detachment, keratitis, conjunctivitis, ptosis, enophthalmos, wound-healing abnormalities, bone necrosis, soft-tissue necrosis, cellulitis, and dry eye.

The incidence of radiation-induced complications is clearly dependent on the total amount of radiation delivered to the eye and the proximity of the tumor relative to macula and optic nerve. Importantly, radiation retinopathy and optic neuropathy are dose-related, fraction-related, and time-related. Importantly, the dose required is directly related to the size and location of the tumor.

RADIATION RETINOPATHY

The effect of radiation on the retina is well known and numerous reports have shown that radiation retinopathy can occur with radiation doses of 20 Gy or higher. In general, visual prognosis is less favorable when foveal or optic nerve radiation is in excess of 50 Gy.[41] Most studies also show that the higher the dosage, the higher the incidence of radiation retinopathy. In a study by Takeda et al., the retina in 21 eyes was exposed to a dose of 50 Gy or more.[42] Eight of the 21 eyes (38%) developed severe retinal complications. In contrast, none of the 22 eyes that received less than 50 Gy developed retinal complications through at least 2 years of follow-up (range, 2–11 years). More recent data indicate that 45–50 Gy delivered to half or more of the retina results in clinically apparent retinopathy.

There are isolated reports of radiation-induced radiation retinopathy at lower radiation doses. However, it is believed that some predisposing factors lower the threshold for radiation retinopathy development. These factors included chemotherapy and diabetes. It is believed that radiation should be used with caution in individuals with these conditions.

In general, radiation dose and area irradiated are the most important factors in the development of severe complications. In two reports by Finger, plaque radiation of anterior melanomas was more likely to cause reversible vision loss secondary to cataract while treatment of posterior tumors is more likely to be associated with irreversible visual loss secondary to radiation retinopathy.[43,44] Another study by Summanen et al. indicated that the risk for maculopathy and optic neuropathy was greater with increased proximity of the posterior tumor margin to the fovea and the optic disc.[45] In a multivariate analysis, the strongest risk indicator for radiation retinopathy was location of posterior tumor margin within 2 mm of the fovea (relative risk (RR) 3.4, 95% confidence interval (CI) 2.0–6.0) and for radiation optic neuropathy was location of tumor within 1 DD of the optic disc (RR 6.1, 95% CI 3.0–12.4). The area of retina receiving radiation is also a risk factor for retinopathy. In a report by Midena et al., patients with orbital tumors had a higher incidence of radiation retinopathy compared to patients with periorbital tumors treated with external beam radiotherapy (63.6% versus 36.3%).[46]

We have conducted a preclinical study with 160 pigmented rabbits (160 eyes) with the objective of evaluating and quantifying the effects of various dosages of beta-radiation in the retina and underlying tissues. All rabbits underwent pars plana vitrectomy and received focal epimacular radiation with the following dosages: 0, 13, 19, 26, 32, 38, 41, 51, 62, 77, 82, 103, 123, 164, and 246 Gy. All rabbits underwent the following pre- and postoperative exams: color fundus photography, fluorescein angiography, and electroretinography. After the pre-established follow-up all rabbits were sacrificed and underwent light and electron microscopy. The acute effects of selective focal radiation in the retinal and subretinal tissues were determined. Significant acute changes were observed in eyes that received dosages ≥ 51Gy. These results show that retinal and subretinal tissues, including retinal pigment epithelium, Bruch's membrane, choriocapillaries, and choroid, are relatively resistant to high dosages of radiation for a period of at least 6 months.

OPTIC NEUROPATHY

As for all other radiation-related complications, the incidence of radiation neuropathy also increased with increased exposure to radiation. In a prospective study by Kellner et al. to evaluate the incidence of optic neuropathy following Ru^{106}/Rh^{106} brachytherapy, no patient with peripheral tumor (peripheral melanomas with a central tumor margin of more than 60° to the optic disc) had clinical signs of optic neuropathy or pathological pattern visual evoked potential.[47] In contrast, 18% of patients with central melanoma (tumor within 15° of the optic disc) had clinical signs of optic neuropathy and 50% developed pathological pattern visual evoked potential. Most reports indicated that the threshold for radiation optic neuropathy is above 50 Gy. Jiang et al. evaluated a series of 219 patients that received radiation therapy for tumors of the nasal cavity and paranasal sinuses.[48] They found that the total radiation dose was the predominant determinant for optic toxicity. While no patient receiving a dose of less than 50 Gy developed radiation optic neuropathy or chiasm injury, the 10-year actuarial incidence of optic nerve chiasm injury was approximately 5% and 30% for patients receiving 50–60 Gy and 61–78 Gy, respectively. A study by Lommatzsch et al. has evaluated 93 patients with juxtapapillary choroidal melanomas that were treated with plaque brachytherapy.[49] In this study, the probability of developing complete radiation optic neuropathy after a median dose of 51.2 Gy was 23% and 53% at 5 and 10 years, respectively. In another study by Parsons et al., evaluating the risk of radiation-induced optic neuropathy, none of the 106 patients receiving a total dose to the optic nerve less than 59 Gy developed optic neuropathy after a minimum of 3 years of follow-up (range, 3–21 years). In contrast, the 15-year actuarial risk of optic neuropathy after doses of > 60 Gy ranged from 11% to 47%.[50]

LENS TOXICITY

The incidence of cataract development following radiation treatment for tumors has been reported to be as low as 3.4% and as high as 86%. This variance is believed to be the result of different lens exposures for the radiation and dosage regimens. Protocols using lens-sparing techniques or lower radiation dosage have lower incidence of cataract while eyes with greater exposure during radiation treatment have higher incidence of cataract development.

Several studies indicate that the radiation dosage threshold for cataract development is between 5.5 and 8 Gy.

SCLERA/CHOROID TOXICITY

The underlying sclera and choroid tolerate radiation well, as evidenced by several studies. A study by Gragoudas et al. in 15 owl monkeys (30 eyes) with a long-term follow-up (3½ years or more) showed that the choroid is not affected at doses below 4275 rad (approximately 42.75 Gy).[51] At 42 months after receiving 42.75 Gy, obliteration of the choriocapillaris and small choroidal vessels was observed, but some medium-sized and most large choroidal vessels were preserved. Gragoudas et al. also observed decreased thickness of the choroidal layer compared with the adjacent normal choroid. There were no scleral changes observed in any specimen evaluated. In addition, in a study by Brady and Hernandez using brachytherapy for choroidal melanomas, scleral complications occurred only at doses above 50 Gy.[52] In a study by Amoaku et al. ultrastructural changes were described in rats 1 hour to 1 month following X-ray radiation with single doses between 2 and 20 Gy.[53] No choroidal or scleral changes were observed at follow-up. In another study by Amoaku et al., late ultrastructural changes were described in rats 3–12 months after X-ray radiation with single dosages of 2–20 Gy.[54] At 12 months, there was no evidence of radiation damage in the choroidal vessels in any subgroup. No scleral complications were reported at the maximum dose of 20 Gy in this study.

SUMMARY AND KEY POINTS

Radiotherapy has become a quite successful treatment modality in several types of ocular diseases. There are many forms of radiation administration and, currently, external beam radiotherapy and brachytherapy are the most commonly used. Advantages and disadvantages of each should be considered for each clinical scenario.

A number of questions remain unanswered regarding the appropriate form of administration, dosage for each type of tumor, and administration strategy regarding dose fractioning and intervals. Regardless of some toxic-related controversies, there is extensive information in the literature regarding thresholds for ocular toxicity. Radiation retinopathy and optic neuropathy remain the main concerns affecting the preservation of vision in eyes treated with radiation and are clearly dose-dependent. Radiation-related complications commonly become apparent about 2 years after therapy. Efforts to develop new techniques to eliminate or to minimize radiation-related complications are warranted.

A thorough review of the literature has shown that many antiangiogenic agents administered concurrently with radiotherapy result in synergistic effect. Early warnings of a theoretical disadvantage to this combined approach due to hypoxia have been disproved. However, much still needs to be learned in both preclinical and clinical trials. For example, timing of drug administration, duration of drug exposure, and combination antiangiogenic drug therapies must be investigated. It is of concern that there are no data concerning the late effects in normal tissues of antiangiogenic agents in combination with radiotherapy. This new treatment paradigm has led to the investigation of localized epimacular brachytherapy combined with anti-VEGF therapy and a multicenter clinical trial is under way to determine its role in the treatment of exudative age-related macular degeneration.

Although radiotherapy is effective in maintaining vision and preserving eyes in many cases of ocular tumor, adjuvant forms of therapy including chemotherapy or immunotherapy may decrease complications and improve survival rates. In patients at high risk for metastasis, new systemic therapies are necessary.

REFERENCES

1. Marcus DM, Craft JL, Albert DM. Histopathologic verification of Verhoeff's 1918 irradiation cure of retinoblastoma. Ophthalmology 1990;97:221–224.
2. Moore RF. Choroidal sarcoma treated by the intraocular insertion of radon seeds. Br J Ophthalmol. 1930;14:145–152.
3. Chakravarthy U, Houston RF, Archer DB. Treatment of age-related subfoveal neovascular membranes by teletherapy: a pilot study. Br J Ophthalmol 1993;77:265–273.
4. Mauceri HJ, Hanna NN, Beckett MA, et al. Combined effects of angiostatin and ionizing radiation in antitumour therapy. Nature 1998;394:287–291.
5. Gorski DH, Mauceri HJ, Salloum RM, et al. Potentiation of the antitumor effect of ionizing radiation by brief concomitant exposures to angiostatin. Cancer Res 1998;58:5686–5689.
6. Gorski DH, Beckett MA, Jaskowiak NT, et al. Blockage of the vascular endothelial growth factor stress response increases the antitumor effects of ionizing radiation. Cancer Res 1999;59:3374–3378.
7. Avila MP, Farah ME, Santos A, et al. Twelve-month short-term safety and visual acuity results from a multicentre, prospective study of epiretinal strontium-90 brachytherapy with bevacizumab for the treatment of subfoveal choroidal neovascularisation secondary to age-related macular degeneration. Br J Ophthalmol 2009 Mar;93(3):305–309.
8. Augsburger JJ, Eagle Jr RC, Chiu M, et al. The effect of pre-enucleation radiotherapy on mitotic activity of choroidal and ciliary body melanomas. Ophthalmology 1987;94:1627–1630.
9. Chiquet C, Grange JD, Ayzac L, et al. Effects of proton beam irradiation on uveal melanomas: a comparative study of Ki-67 expression in irradiated versus nonirradiated melanomas. Br J Ophthalmol 2000;84:98–102.
10. Toivonen P, Makitie T, Kujala E, et al. Macrophages and microcirculation in regressed and partially regressed irradiated choroidal and ciliary body melanomas. Curr Eye Res 2003;27:237–245.
11. MacFaul PA, Morgan G. Histopathological changes in malignant melanomas of the choroid after cobalt plaque therapy. Br J Ophthalmol 1977;61:221–228.
12. Messmer E, Bornfeld N, Foerster M, et al. Histopathologic findings in eyes treated with a ruthenium plaque for uveal melanoma. Graefes Arch Clin Exp Ophthalmol 1992;230:391–396.
13. Lee CG, Heijn M, di Tomaso E, et al. Anti-Vascular endothelial growth factor treatment augments tumor radiation response under normoxic or hypoxic conditions. Cancer Res 2000;60:5565–5570.
14. Geng L, Donnelly E, McMahon G, et al. Inhibition of vascular endothelial growth factor receptor signaling leads to reversal of tumor resistance to radiotherapy. Cancer Res 2001;61:2413–2419.
15. Griffin RJ, Williams BW, Wild R, et al. Simultaneous inhibition of the receptor kinase activity of vascular endothelial, fibroblast, and platelet-derived growth factors suppresses tumor growth and enhances tumor radiation response. Cancer Res 2002;62:1702–1706.
16. Ning S, Laird D, Cherrington JM, et al. The antiangiogenic agents SU5416 and SU6668 increase the antitumor effects of fractionated irradiation. Radiat. Res 2002;157:45–51.
17. Gunduz K, Shields CL, Shields JA, et al. Radiation complications and tumor control after plaque radiotherapy of choroidal melanoma with macular involvement. Am J Ophthalmol 1999;127:579–589.
18. Gunduz K, Shields CL, Shields JA, et al. Plaque radiotherapy for management of ciliary body and choroidal melanoma with extraocular extension. Am J Ophthalmol 2000;130:97–102.
19. Shields CL, Naseripour M, Cater J, et al. Plaque radiotherapy for large posterior uveal melanomas (> or =8-mm thick) in 354 consecutive patients. Ophthalmology 2002;109:1838–1849.
20. Gunduz K, Shields CL, Shields JA, et al. Plaque radiotherapy for management of ciliary body and choroidal melanoma with extraocular extension. Am J Ophthalmol 2000;130:97–102.
21. Gragoudas ES, Goitein M, Verhey L, et al. Proton beam irradiation. An alternative to enucleation for intraocular melanomas. Ophthalmology 1980;87:571–581.
22. Diener-West M, Earle JD, Fine SL, et al. The COMS randomized trial of iodine 125 brachytherapy for choroidal melanoma, III: initial mortality findings. COMS Report No. 18. Arch Ophthalmol 2001;119:969–982.
23. Nag S, Quivey JM, Earle JD, et al. The American Brachytherapy Society recommendations for brachytherapy of uveal melanomas. Int J Radiat Oncol Biol Phys 2003;56:544–555.
24. Reisner ML, Viegas CM, Grazziotin RZ, et al. Retinoblastoma – comparative analysis of external radiotherapy techniques, including an IMRT technique. Int. J Radiat Oncol Biol Phys 2007;67:933–941.

25. Shields CL, Shields JA, De Potter P, et al. Plaque radiotherapy in the management of retinoblastoma. Use as a primary and secondary treatment. Ophthalmology 1993;100:216–224.
26. Levy-Gabriel C, Rouic LL, Plancher C, et al. Long-term results of low-dose proton beam therapy for circumscribed choroidal hemangiomas. Retina 2009 Feb;29(2):170–175.
27. Grimm SA, McCannel CA, Omuro AM, et al. Primary CNS lymphoma with intraocular involvement: International PCNSL Collaborative Group Report. Neurology 2008;71:1355–1360.
28. Kreusel KM, Wiegel T, Stange M, et al. [Intraocular metastases of metastatic breast carcinoma in the woman. Incidence, risk factors and therapy.] Ophthalmologe 2000;97:342–346.
29. Bornfeld N, Kreusel KM. [Capillary hemangioma of the retina in cases of von Hippel–Lindau syndrome. New therapeutic directions.] Ophthalmologe 2007;104:114–118.
30. Hilton GF. Measuring grid for indirect ophthalmoscopy. Trans Am Acad Ophthalmol Otolaryngol 1972;76:530–531.
31. Jampol LM, Moy CS, Murray TG, et al. The COMS randomized trial of iodine 125 brachytherapy for choroidal melanoma: IV. Local treatment failure and enucleation in the first 5 years after brachytherapy. COMS report no. 19. Ophthalmology 2002;109:2197–2206.
32. De Potter P, Shields CL, Shields JA, et al. Plaque radiotherapy for juxtapapillary choroidal melanoma. Visual acuity and survival outcome. Arch Ophthalmol 1996;114:1357–1365.
33. Bergink GJ, Hoyng CB, van der Maazen RW, et al. A randomized controlled clinical trial on the efficacy of radiation therapy in the control of subfoveal choroidal neovascularization in age-related macular degeneration: radiation versus observation. Graefes Arch Clin Exp Ophthalmol 1998 May;236(5): 321–325.
34. Char DH, Irvine AI, Posner MD, et al. Randomized trial of radiation for age-related macular degeneration. Am J Ophthalmol 1999 May;127(5): 574–578.
35. Kobayashi H, Kobayashi K. Age-related macular degeneration: long-term results of radiotherapy for subfoveal neovascular membranes. Am J Ophthalmol 2000 Nov;130(5):617–635.
36. A prospective, randomized, double-masked trial on radiation therapy for neovascular age-related macular degeneration (RAD Study). Radiation Therapy for Age-related Macular Degeneration. Ophthalmology 1999 Dec;106(12):2239–2247. [No authors listed]
37. Marcus DM, Sheils W, Johnson MH, et al. External beam irradiation of subfoveal choroidal neovascularization complicating age-related macular degeneration: one-year results of a prospective, double-masked, randomized clinical trial. Arch Ophthalmol 2001 Feb;119(2):171–180.
38. Hart PM, Chakravarthy U, Mackenzie G, et al. Visual outcomes in the subfoveal radiotherapy study: a randomized controlled trial of teletherapy for age-related macular degeneration. Arch Ophthalmol 2002 Aug;120(8): 1029–1038.
39. Flaxel CJ, Friedrichsen EJ, Smith JO, et al. Proton beam irradiation of subfoveal choroidal neovascularisation in age-related macular degeneration. Eye 2000 Apr;14(Pt 2):155–164.
40. Jaakkola A, Heikkonen J, Tommila P, et al. Strontium plaque irradiation of subfoveal neovascular membranes in age-related macular degeneration. Graefes Arch Clin Exp Ophthalmol 1998 Jan;236(1):24–30.
41. Cruess AF, Augsburger JJ, Shields JA, et al. Visual results following cobalt plaque radiotherapy for posterior uveal melanomas. Ophthalmology 1984;91:131–136.
42. Takeda A, Shigematsu N, Suzuki S, et al. Late retinal complications of radiation therapy for nasal and paranasal malignancies: relationship between irradiated-dose area and severity. Int J Radiat Oncol Biol Phys 1999;44:599–605.
43. Finger PT. Tumour location affects the incidence of cataract and retinopathy after ophthalmic plaque radiation therapy. Br J Ophthalmol 2000 Sep;84(9):1068–1070.
44. Finger PT, Berson A, Szechter A. Palladium-103 plaque radiotherapy for choroidal melanoma: results of a 7-year study. Ophthalmology 1999 Mar;106(3):606–613.
45. Summanen P, Immonen I, Kivela T, et al. Radiation related complications after ruthenium plaque radiotherapy of uveal melanoma. Br J Ophthalmol 1996;80:732–739.
46. Midena E, Segato T, Piermarocchi S, et al. Retinopathy following radiation therapy of paranasal sinus and nasopharyngeal carcinoma. Retina 1987;7:142–147.
47. Kellner U, Bornfeld N, Foerster MH. Radiation-induced optic neuropathy following brachytherapy of uveal melanomas. Graefes Arch Clin Exp Ophthalmol 1993;231:267–270.
48. Jiang GL, Tucker SL, Guttenberger R, et al. Radiation-induced injury to the visual pathway. Radiother Oncol 1994;30:17–25.
49. Lommatzsch PK, Alberti W, Lommatzsch R, et al. Radiation effects on the optic nerve observed after brachytherapy of choroidal melanomas with 106Ru/106Rh plaques. Graefes Arch Clin Exp Ophthalmol 1994;232: 482–487.
50. Parsons JT, Bova FJ, Fitzgerald CR, et al. Radiation optic neuropathy after megavoltage external-beam irradiation: analysis of time–dose factors. Int J Radiat Oncol Biol Phys 1994;30:755–763.
51. Gragoudas ES, Zakov NZ, Albert DM, et al. Long-term observations of proton-irradiated monkey eyes. Arch Ophthalmol 1979;97:2184–2191.
52. Brady LW, Hernandez JC. Brachytherapy of choroidal melanomas. Strahlenther Onkol 1992;168:61–65.
53. Amoaku WM, Frew L, Mahon GJ, et al. Early ultrastructural changes after low-dose X-irradiation in the retina of the rat. Eye 1989;3(Pt 5):638–646.
54. Amoaku WM, Mahon GJ, Gardiner TA, et al. Late ultrastructural changes in the retina of the rat following low-dose X-irradiation. Graefes Arch Clin Exp Ophthalmol 1992;230:569–574.

CHAPTER 50

Current status of human retinal pigment epithelial transplantation

Boris V. Stanzel, MD and Susanne Binder, MD

Human retinal transplantation has followed many years of experimental research showing that transplanted retinal pigment epithelial (RPE) cells have the potential to rescue photoreceptors. This article reviews the current status of human retinal transplantation, surgical techniques, and outcome of clinical studies. The mechanisms leading to RPE dysfunction, as well as future tissue engineering strategies for Bruch's membrane prosthetics, stem cell applications, and deconstructive reaction induced by retinal detachment are also discussed. By overviewing the current literature on retinal transplantation this should also allow us to anticipate the part it will play relative to new treatments such as photodynamic therapy (PDT), angiostatic steroids, antivascular endothelial growth factor agents, gene therapy, and the artifical retina – some available, some only proposed.

INTRODUCTION

Anatomically relatively well isolated, the RPE is a self-contained monolayer that can be readily accessed with a retinotomy through the subretinal space. As the RPE orchestrates metabolism between photoreceptors and the choriocapillaries, it was considered to be a logical experimental starting point, in any attempt to repair or reconstruct the retina through transplantation.[1]

The RPE and Bruch's membrane (BM) suffer cumulative damage over a lifetime; this is thought to induce age-related macular degeneration (AMD) in susceptible individuals. As AMD is the leading cause of blindness in the population over 50 years old and about 30 million people will suffer one form of AMD over the next 20 years, the social and economic burden of this disease will increase enormously, especially in countries with aging populations.

Two main routes of the disease occur: a slower-progressing atrophic form where most patients have limited therapeutic options and a rapidly blinding neovascular form. The intravitreal injection of antiangiogenic therapies now offers a highly effective, yet palliative, treatment for many forms of wet AMD. Still, long-term effects remain to be elucidated, and "nonresponders" do exist. Whether curative treatments can involve targeting a single component in the inflammatory cascade of neovascular AMD is not very likely.

The use of the RPE cell as a "therapeutic agent" is an attractive strategy, as healthy RPE cells would, in theory, restore all of the functions of their degenerated counterparts. The success of these cellular replacement strategies, however, clearly depends on delivery and maintenance of cells in a properly polarized state, capable to perform most, if not all, complex functions of the RPE.

This chapter describes the current state and some future prospects for RPE transplantation. Our hope is that achievements described within this chapter will foster more contributions to the growing field of RPE replacement and tissue engineering to benefit our patients.

RPE DISEASE AND INDICATIONS FOR TREATMENT BY TRANSPLANTATION

Dysfunction of RPE may alter the extracellular environment for photoreceptors and BM and thereby contribute to a variety of sight-threatening diseases. These include AMD, a multifactorial and complex genetic disorder, yet also a number of monogenetic diseases involving the RPE, such as gyrate athrophy and chorioderemia. The high blood perfusion of the choroid puts the RPE at risk for toxic side-effects from systemic medications (e.g., chloroquine).

Monogenetic diseases, such as Leber's congenital amaurosis (LCA), which is an early-onset form of retinitis pigmentosa, are in future more likely to be treated with gene therapy. Such clinical trials for a variant of LCA with a mutation in the RPE65 gene are currently underway in the UK and USA.

With long-standing disease and/or associated structural damage to the RPE and surrounding structures, a more invasive treatment with RPE transplantation, if necessary combined with gene therapy, is justified.[2] Diseases such as AMD or Best's disease would fall into this category. In these instances, a remodeling of the submacular architecture or maculoplasty would represent a curative treatment.[3,4]

BRUCH'S MEMBRANE AS A SUBSTRATE FOR TRANSPLANTED RPE

Early animal studies involving RPE transplantation into areas where normal native RPE and undisturbed BM were present do not accurately reflect the clinical situation of most patients. In an experimental study, Tezel and associates have shown that the survival of cultured RPE seeded on BM is partially dependent on the layer on which the cells are seeded. The authors found lesser apoptosis and improved proliferation on the basal lamina when compared to deeper layers or BM.[5] However, they also state that the microenvironment of RPE cells seeded on to BM in tissue culture may be different from the subretinal space in clinical situations, because the neurosensory retina, choriocapillaris, and choroid were not present in their *in vitro* experiments. Subsequent studies from this group were able to demonstrate reversal of the aforementioned observation by removal of age-related debris in different layers of BM.

In contrast to the previous work, Wang et al.[6] demonstrated with RPE wound-healing experiments on aged human BM explants closure of localized monolayer defects, albeit with a dedifferentiated cell morphology. The deeper portion of the inner collagenous layer of aged submacular human BM were more limited and variable in their ability to support RPE resurfacing when compared to superficial portions of the RPE basement membrane.

Wang's experiment may in part reflect age-related changes in the ability of the RPE to differentiate. Gullapalli et al.[7] therefore grew fetal human RPE on isolated aged submacular BM. Within a week of seeding, the RPE phenotype deteriorated compared to controls seeded on a basal laminar equivalent.

Thus the pathologic observations by all the above investigators may be deriving from BM and are commonly referred to as dynamic reprocity reactions. While the *in vivo* situation may differ from laboratory conditions, alterations of BM (e.g., advanced glycation endproducts accumulation) presumably compromise attempts to restore a physiologic subretinal environment.

HISTORICAL DEVELOPMENT OF RPE TREATMENT

Peyman and colleagues[8] were the first to transplant RPE in 2 patients suffering from terminal AMD in 1991. In 1994, Algvere et al.[9] treated 5 patients with neovascular AMD by using a patch of cultured human fetal RPE to compensate for the lesion after subretinal choroidal neovasculariztion (CNV) removal. At 3 months macular edema and rejection were observed; after 12 months mild visual loss was registered. Four dry AMD cases received very small circular patches of human fetal RPE outside the fovea, attempting to reach overgrowth of the foveal area. No visual improvement along with a milder rejection was observed, and this was explained by the more intact blood–retinal barrier in dry AMD. When different amounts of cell suspensions of fetal human RPE were used to cover larger RPE defects, rejection seemed related to higher numbers of cells.

IMMUNE REACTION AND RPE TRANSPLANTATION

Like the anterior chamber, the subretinal space was shown to possess qualities of an immune-privileged site (anterior chamber-associated immune deviation), and initial reports on RPE allografts in the Royal College of Surgeons (RCS) rat suggested that there was no rejection in eyes with up to 1-year follow-up.[10] The former seems contingent on an intact RPE monolayer and the observed tolerance is therefore unexpected, since blood–retinal barrier breakdown occurs relatively early in this animal. A subsequent study then demonstrated evidence of chronic rejection mediated through major histocompatibility complex (MHC) II expression.[11] Evidence for MHC II-mediated rejection had already been suggested in an earlier study, where interferon-γ (IFN-γ)-activated cultured RPE transplants were acutely rejected. IFN-γ stimulation of RPE induces MHC II expression in the RPE and thereby renders these as antigen-presenting cells for T cells. Alternative pathways for T-cell activation in the scenario of insufficient MHC molecule expression have also been described. It was further demonstrated that the immunologic response was related to the amount of transplanted cells and increases over time, perhaps related to the amounts of MHC. Taken together, these mechanisms may in part explain why fetal allografts transplanted into patients with dry AMD enjoyed a more prolonged survival than cases with wet AMD.[12]

Strategies have subsequently been devised to improve RPE graft survival. Cyclosporine given to rabbits receiving RPE allografts, was not able to prevent RPE allograft destruction in the subretinal space. Similarly disappointing results were obtained even using a triple immune suppression for fetal pig RPE xenografts into albino rabbits.

Conceivably, from the above discussion the foundation for the use of syngeneic (autologous) cells has been laid. Their advantages and limitations are further discussed.

AUTOLOGOUS TREATMENT

IRIS PIGMENT EPITHELIUM

Harvesting autologous RPE is challenging, so the first startegy to eliminate rejection was the use of iris pigment epithelium (IPE) cells. At that time several investigators had demonstrated the ability of IPE to phagocytose outer segments. IPE and RPE share a common embryogenesis, yet develop early distinct molecular markers. IPE cells have been mainly used by groups in Japan and Germany.[13,14]

In a clinical study of 20 eyes with exudative macular degeneration IPE transplantation showed stabilization of vision or improvement along with a low CNV recurrance rate which remained stable up to 3 years.[15]

RETINAL PIGMENT EPITHELIUM

Suspension

The delivery of a RPE cell suspension subretinally (Figure 50.1) can be improved as follows:

1. A gentle localized retinal detachment to avoid RPE damage is achieved by a Ca^{2+}-, Mg^{2+}-free solution.
2. A new instrument was developed to improve cell harvesting (Binder–Parel–Lee cannula).[3]
3. After membrane removal the subretinal area is cleaned of blood and debris, and rebleeding is avoided with a small perfluorocarbon bubble.
4. The subfoveal delivery of cells is also done under perfluorocarbon and in a soft eye to avoid reflux.
5. A small air bubble is initially aspirated in the tuberculin syringe to ensure that all harvestered RPE cells are transplanted and no residuals remain in the cannula.

In a pilot study consisting of 14 eyes where we applied the former technique, a 2-line or more improvement was achieved in 57%; 21% regained useful reading vision between Jaeger (Jg) 1 and 4. There was neither intraoperative complication nor recurrent CNV after a mean of 17 months of observation in this series.[16] However, this study was performed at a time when PDT was not available and lesions were smaller and mainly classic. A prospective trial was conducted then, in which transplantation after membrane excision was compared with a control group in which membrane excision alone was performed. Although the results after 12 months ($n = 54$) showed improvement of 2 or more lines in 52.5% in the group with RPE transplants ($n = 40$), in the statistical analysis there was a trend in favor of the transplanted group, but no significant difference between both groups. Reading acuity and multifocal electroretinogram however showed significantly better results in the transplanted group.[17] These results showed that membrane excision combined with simultaneous transplantation of an autologous suspension of RPE cells was superior to membrane excision alone. Furthermore, the CNV recurrence rate was very low – 4.4% after 12 months, 13.3% after 24 months, and 15.4% after 36 months. As a major complication retina detachments occurred in 8.6% but could be managed with a second surgery. A different suspension technique was used by van Meurs et al. in 8 eyes: they harvested the cells inferiorly and added 2 μg poly-L lysine subretinally to improve cell adhesion. Meurs et al. reported proliferative vitreopathy (PVR) in 3/8 eyes and no visual gain.[18]

RPE-BM Choroid Sheet

Transplanted intact RPE sheets come as a polarized monolayer (Figure 50.2). In human eyes the technique has improved over time and surgical trauma has decreased. The first autologous transplant series taken from ajacent areas of the CNV lesion was performed by Aylward's group.[19] The group of Jan van Meurs reported about 6 cases where the transplant was excised from the midperiphery of the retina and translocated under the fovea after subretinal membrane removal. They reported fixation on the transplant in 4 of the 6 cases. Experimental studies on pig eyes from the same group showed vascularization of such grafts. With larger numbers now treated, stabilization of vision or mean gain of 1 line has been reported by the same group.[20]

Joussen et al. also reported on 45 cases after patch transplantation: 3 of them were dry AMD, 16 had PED, and the rest had neovascular AMD.[21] Only 8.8% had a 15-letter improvement, PVR rate was 37.7%, and revision surgery was needed in 48.8%. Also MacLaren performed a similar procedure in a small series, showing very limited visual improvement and a high PVR rate of more than 40%.[22]

Bindewald et al. suggested in a small case series a modified technique,[23] whereby choroidal vessels of the RPE/choroid sheets is ablated with a 308-nm excimer laser. The rationale was to reduce diffusion distance from the choroidal wound bed, the graft, and outer retinal layers, as well as untoward cellular reactions that would limit subsequent visual recovery. *In vitro* studies have demonstrated safety of the

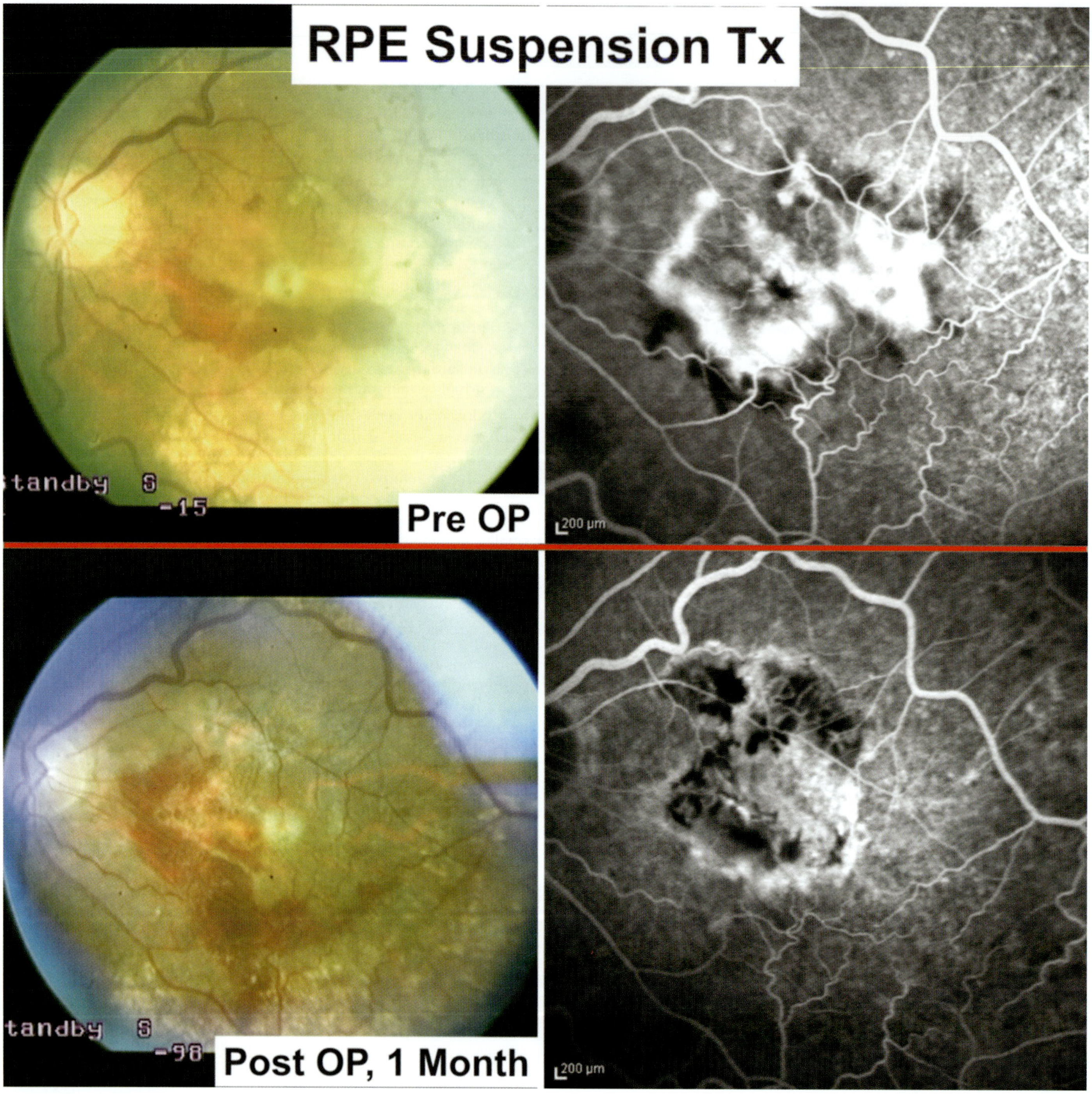

Figure 50.1 Retinal pigment epithelium (RPE) suspension transplant in exudative age-related macular degeneration (AMD). A patient with a preoperative vision of 0.05 at 2 m (ETDRS) and a large choroidal neovascularization due to AMD received a suspension of autologous RPE harvested in the nasal periphery. One month postoperatively, her vision remained stable at 0.06 at 2 m (ETDRS).

laser irradiation. Postoperative function was demonstrated with microperimetry, which showed stable fixation and maintained retinal sensitivity over the transplant.

Overall, a mean decline of visual loss is reported if postoperative complications are included. If these cases are excluded from visual analysis, the mean gain in visual acuity is 2–3 lines.[2] Van Meurs' group underscored the latter correlation in a prospective statistical analysis of 48 cases.[20] As long as the complication rates remain high, the possible gain of vision limits this surgical technique to cases otherwise not treatable with pharmacologic treatments.[24] It is therefore encouraging that mere mechanical ablation, analogous to Holz's technique, by Ma and associates was able to demonstrate low PVR rates (14.3%) at 1-year follow-up and good functional outcomes in hemorrhagic AMD patients.[25]

TISSUE ENGINEERING AND RPE REPLACEMENT STRATEGIES

PROSTHESIS OR TISSUE ENGINEERING OF BRUCH'S MEMBRANE

Cellular replacement strategies of the RPE could be beneficial to patients with AMD or related diseases, but may not be effective if BM has been damaged by disease, age, and/or surgery. Delivery and long-term survival of these transplants may require a biocompatible substrate that patches or entirely replaces diseased BM.

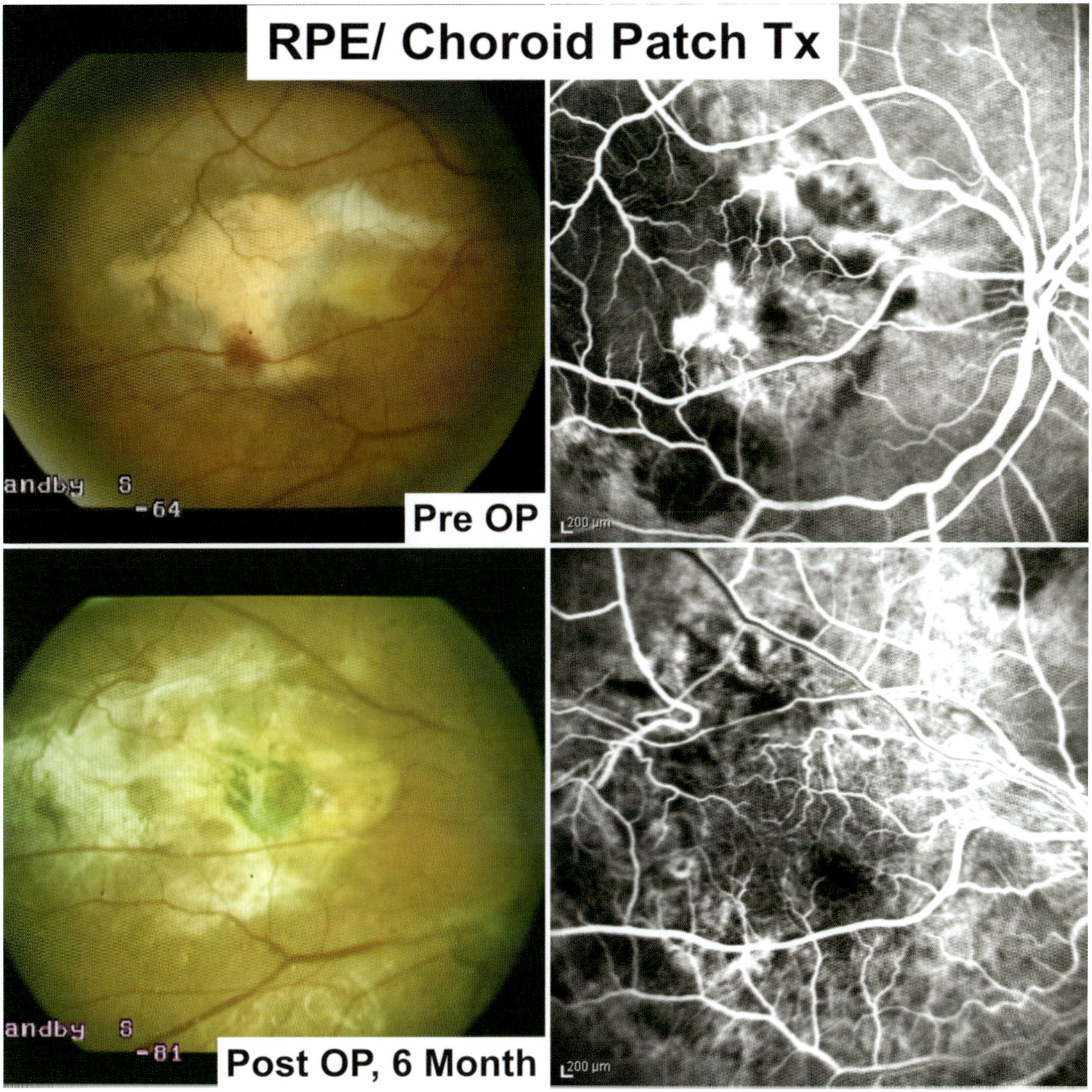

Figure 50.2 Retinal pigment epithelium (RPE)/choroid patch transplant in exudative age-related macular degeneration. A patient with extensive extrafoveal subretinal fibrosis and an active neovascular lesion with a preoperative vision of 0.28 at 2 m (ETDRS) received a subfoveal autologous patch transplant of RPE/choroid. Postoperative vision was 0.08 at 4 m (ETDRS); the fluorescent angiography leakage was no longer seen.

In contrast to animal experiments,[26] *in vitro* data suggested that freshly harvested or cultured RPE cell suspensions may fail to survive or function on a damaged BM.[27] While histopathologic studies have demonstrated integration of cultured cell suspensions in the subretinal space in animals, formation of multilayered clumps that damaged the overlying neural retina has been reported. Moreover, delivery of cell suspensions to epithelially denuded BM using the bleb technique often showed uneven distribution, with most of the cells settling in the periphery of the RPE lesion. Thus restoration of a continous monolayer using a cell suspension in the subretinal space appears challenging.

Many groups have tried to develop a RPE carrier substrate, which at the same time would serve as either a temporary or a permanent BM prosthesis. Having such an arrangement enables delivery of an intact epithelial patch that is simultaneously protected from hostile influences of aged BM.

Various biologic and artificial substrates have been proposed to date (Table 50.1 and Figure 50.3). Details of particular approaches are beyond the scope of this article and the interested reader is referred to Binder et al.[3] Nevertheless, some unifying technical considerations are given. Perhaps the foremost criterion for a carrier material is maintenance of a clinically relevant epithelial phenotype, both *in vitro* and subsequently

Table 50.1 **List of proposed retinal pigment epithelium (RPE) transplantation carrier substrates**

Literature reference	Material	RPE phenotype*	Thickness	Permeability/ pore size	Biodegradable	Surgical handling	Tissue reaction
Bhatt 1994[39]	Cross-linked collagen	Poor	NA	Poor	No	Good	Retinal atrophy
Bhatt 1994[39]	Noncross-linked collagen	Good	10 μm	NA	Yes	Good	Tolerated
Thomson 1996[40] Hadlock 1999[41]	Poly-L-lactic acid (PLLA)	Good	12 μm	No	Yes	Good	Retinal damage?
Thomson 1996[40] Hadlock 1999[41]	Poly-DL-lactic-co-glycolic acid (PLLA)	Good	3–12 μm	No	Yes	Good	Retinal damage?
Thumann 1997[42]	Descemet's membrane	Good	10–12 μm in adults	Permeable	Maybe	NA	NA
Ho 1997[43]	Gelatin	*In situ*, no culturing	NA	NA	Yes	Good	NA
Oganesian 1999[44]	Fibrinogen	Good	NA	NA	Yes	Good	Tolerated
Farrokh Siar 1999[45]	Cryoprecipitate	Good	NA	NA	Yes	NA	NA
Hartmann 1999[46]; Nicolini 2000[47]; Lee 2002[48]; Turowski 2004[49]	Lens capsule	Good	~15 μm	Not permeable (in native state)	Maybe	Good	Retinal damage
Singh 2001[50]	Hydrogel	Good	25 μm	Permeable	No	NA	NA
Tezel 2002[51]	Cadaveric Bruch's membrane	NA	2–4 μm	Permeable	Partially	Good	NA
Leng et al. 2003[52]	Bucky carbon paper	Supports cell line	NA	Permeable	No	Good	Tolerated
Tezcaner 2003[53]	Poly(hydroxybutyrate-co-hydroxyvalerate) or PHBV8 film	Supports cell line	5–10 μm	NA	Yes	NA	NA
Capeans 2003[54]; Stanzel 2005[55]; Ohno-Matsui 2005[56]; Singhal 2005[57]	De-epithelialized amniotic membrane	Good	~100 μm	Limited permeability due to long diffusion distance	Yes	Challenging	Retinal atrophy
Yeung 2004[58]	Collagen gel	Supports cell line	NA	Permeable	Yes	Feasible	NA
Yellachich 2004[59]	Cellulose acetate	Good (IPE)	25 μm	100 kDa	No	Good	Tolerance
Lombardi 2005[60]; Molnar 2005[61]	Polycarbonate	Good for fetal, poor for aged hRPE	10 μm	0.4 μm	No	Good	Unclear
Williams 2005[62]	Polyurethane	Supports cell line	10^2–10^3 μm	Not permeable	No	Good	NA
Stanzel 2006[63]	Polyester	Good for fetal, poor for aged hRPE	10 μm	0.4 μm	No	Good	Tolerance
Lu 2007[64]	Collagen films	Supports cell line	2.4 μm	Tested for 71.2 kDa	NA		NA
Stanzel 2007[65]	Polyamide electrospun nanofibers	Good support for fetal and aged hRPE	≥1 μm	Permeable	No	NA	Tolerance
Thumann 2009[66]	Collagen foil	Supports cell line	≤10 μm	Permeable	Yes	Good	Tolerance

**Note that many studies listed are confounded by the use of either cell lines or animal-derived RPE cells, which may differ in culture behavior to primary human RPE.*

IPE, iris pigment epithelium; hRPE, human retinal pigment epithelium.

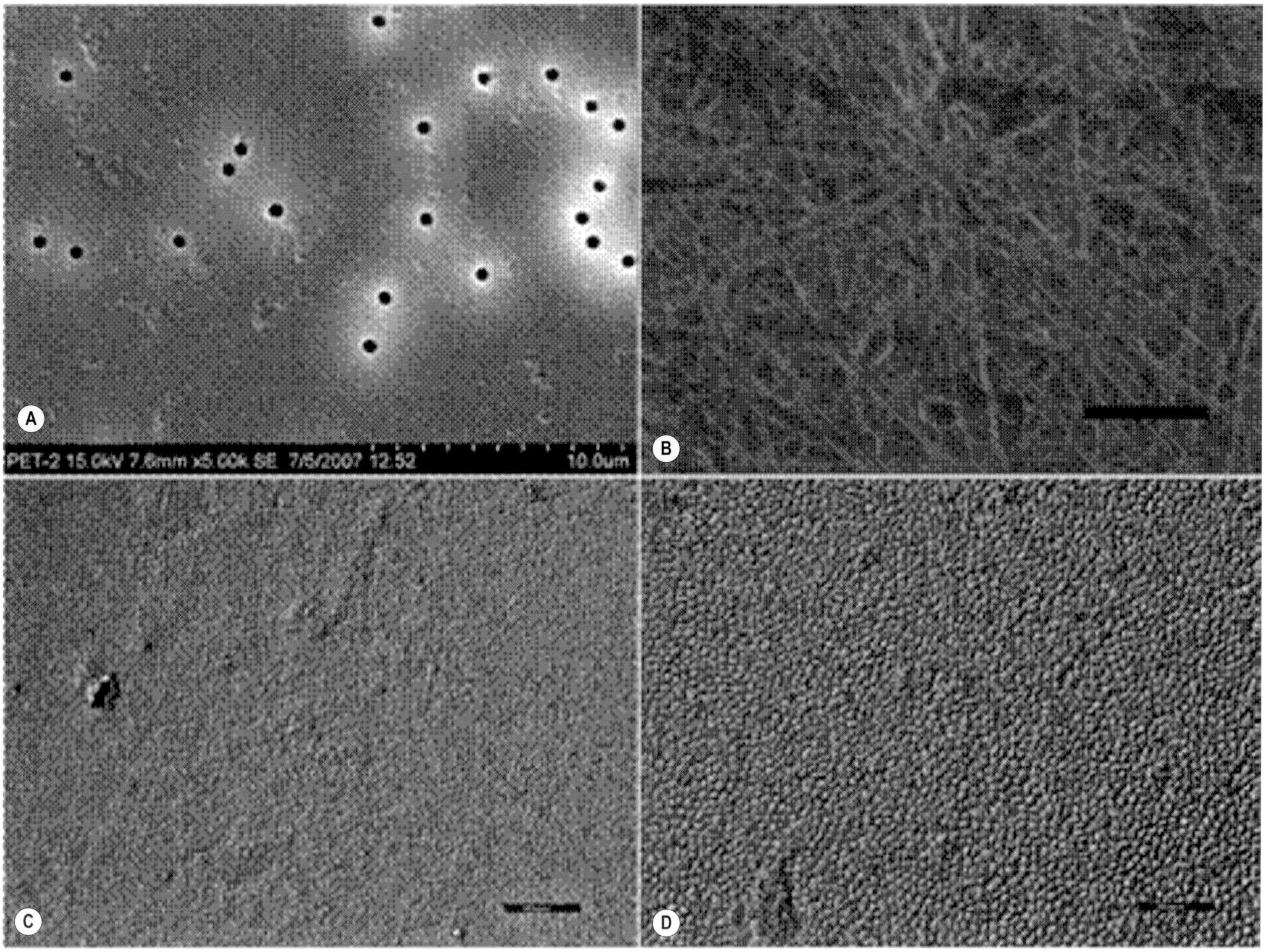

Figure 50.3 Tissue engineering for an artificial Bruch's membrane. Scanning electron micrograph images of two surface variants (smooth versus fibrillar) for potential use in an artificial Bruch's membrane prosthesis (A, B). Both substrates supported differentiation of cultured fetal human retinal pigment epithelium at 2 weeks (C, D). Micrographs in (A) and (B) were taken at the same 5000-fold magnification; the representative scale bar in B is 5 μm. Images C and D were taken at 100-fold magnification; the scale bars are 100 μm.

in vivo (Figure 50.3). Easy surgical manipulation, perhaps using specialized instrumentation, is of equal importance.[28] An elegant facilitation of surgical delivery was recently proposed using magnetite nanoparticles ingested by RPE cells prior to transplantation.[29] The RPE is a polarized epithelial cell and the prosthesis should therefore either readily facilitate nutrient flow or biodegrade rapidly, so that physiologic processes such as vitamin A, glucose, and fatty acid transport can be restored.

Taken together, while aspects of material science, culture techniques, instrumentation, and surgical delivery have been studied, a clinically applicable method of delivering cells on a prosthestic BM to restore RPE defects has not been developed thus far.[3] Given that BM is frequently affected during RPE disease, the development of prosthetic BM materials is of great significance. Besides the obvious use as a carrier for RPE transplanation, upcoming stem cell-based therapies or stimulation of RPE wound healing may equally make use of such "instrument."

STEM CELLS

Reports are accumulating about cells derived from mammalian stem cells, which acquire RPE-like phenotypes. These are very exciting new horizons for cellular replacement strategies of the RPE in the light of immunologic challenges for homologous grafts and aging changes for autologous RPE. Prosthetic replacements of BM will likely be required for their delivery or long-term function in the subretinal space. Five different sources (embryonic stem cells, ciliary margin stem cells, adipose mesenchymal stromal cells, neural stem cells, and bone marrow-derived cells) have been reported to date, of which two are briefly reviewed below.

Embryonic stem cells

Embryonic stem cells are derived from the inner cell mass of very-early-stage embryos. These cells have the potential to give rise to all cell types in the body. *In vitro*-generated RPE-like cells derived from monkey and human embryonic stem cells express RPE markers closely resembling cultured and *in situ* fetal RPE.[30,31] Transplantation of these cells into RCS rats provides long-term rescue under immunosuppression without loss of RPE phenotype or signs of tumor formation.

Application in patients may, besides ethical concerns, be complicated by their expression of MHC molecules and thus cause immune rejection. Here, homologous recombination methods may reduce immunogenicity prior to differentiation or alternatively somatic cell nuclear transfer (SCNT) can create syngeneic transplants. The challenge of the SCNT field remains the efficacy of the cloned embryos to reach the blastocyst stage (when embryonic stem cells can be harvested from the inner cell mass), yet recent developments in the field may show promise in this route.

Bone marrow-derived cells

Bone marrow-derived stromal cells have recently been shown to differentiate into a wide variety of tissues and were also demonstrated to participate in the regeneration of many acutely injured tissues in the adult. Many groups have now shown recruitment of bone marrow-derived cells into subretinal space in CNV or sodium iodate mice models, with the acquisition of RPE-like properties.[32,33]

Uncommitted hematopoietic stem cells and so-called facilitating cells have previously been more specifically implicated in the phenomenon. Coculture of green fluorescent protein-labeled, Sca+ bone marrow cells with mitomycin C-treated RPE leads to acquisition of RPE-specific proteins of the former.[34] An enriched CD133+ fraction of hematopoietic progenitor cells injected intravitreally in albino mice adopted RPE characteristics such as pigmentation or expression of RPE-specific proteins in the subretinal space.[35] Further elucidation of the mechanisms leading to these promising observations is important, since this would eventually provide a good source for autologous cells in elderly patients.

MANAGING DECONSTRUCTIVE REACTIONS INDUCED BY RETINAL DETACHMENT

RPE transplantation requires manipulation in the subretinal space and thus unavoidably creates temporary retinal detachments (RD). It is therefore important to discuss the consequences of this maneuver.

Work over the past two decades has elucidated many remodeling changes occurring with separation of both retinal layers; these changes are described in depth in a splendid review by Fisher et al.[36] Virtually all cell types of the retina, including the RPE, have been shown to participate in "deconstructive" processing upon detachment. Müller and photoreceptor reactions have been studied most widely. Alterations in both cell populations are early avenues to retinal gliosis, which in turn causes synaptic "rewiring."[37] This phenomenon may explain why anatomically reattached patients often require many months until normal vision returns.

Although candidates for RPE transplantation will already have a retinal pathology and the dimension of surgical trauma might be small or negligible, retinal detachment-related phenomena may need consideration.

Given that macular translocation surgery creates panretinal detachments and some patients are able to recover up to 20/30 vision, this suggests that clinically the retina is able to tolerate such interventions. In analogy to the latter technique, the retina can be relatively atraumatically detached with a Ca and Mg-free solution. Reattachment is expected to be relatively rapid, as was shown in the rabbit. Neuroprotective strategies during detachment and reattachment, as recently proposed by Kubay et al.,[38] will also be a future key to success for RPE replacement strategies.

CONCLUSIONS AND FUTURE DIRECTIONS

Cellular replacement strategies for the RPE have the potential of being a curative therapy for all AMD forms and related retinal degenerations, yet clinical protocols show only modest success to the present date. Research over more than two decades in this and related fields has elucidated many potential mechanisms, in addition to challenges and drawbacks. Encouraging early RPE transplantation experiments under controlled laboratory settings were soon challenged by a variety of factors in patients with AMD. The unconditional eventual rejection and/or lack functional recovery with homologous transplants had set the stage for autologous transplants. Here then, many mechanisms came into play, aging and AMD-related alterations of the RPE and BM perhaps being the foremost. Nevertheless, transplantation of uncultured autologous RPE in patients with neovascular AMD has demonstrated some success. Firstly, there is evidence that suggests improved visual rehabilitation along with a low complication rate after RPE suspension transplantation, when compared to membrane removal alone. Further, the transplantation of a full-thickness patch of RPE and choroid for the first time demonstrates long-term survival of transplanted RPE cells in the subretinal space of patients with neovascular AMD. However, the technically challenging surgery and high complication rate ethically question this treatment modality at present.

The shortcomings of freshly harvested RPE for transplantation could be overcome with tissue engineering to deliver RPE on a BM prosthesis. Stem cell-derived RPE-like cells were generated from several stem cell sources. They represent promising new sources for RPE replacement. However, in analogy, somatic RPE transplantation, cellular delivery, and aging changes in BM need to be addressed with prosthetics to ensure long-term function of stem cell-derived RPE. The need for an effective cell-based therapy is undisputable, since patients will always present at different stages of disease progression. Whether RPE transplantation ultimately represents a curative solution is unclear, but its potential application to all forms of AMD and related entities make it a worthwhile therapeutic endeavor.

ACKNOWLEDGMENTS

The authors would like to thank Jean-Marie Parel and Wiliam Lee from the Ophthalmic Biophysics Center at the Bascom Palmer Eye Institute for developing cannulas for RPE suspension transplantation. Dr. Stanzel is grateful for support received via an E. Schrödinger postdoctoral fellowship (J2463-B13) from the Austrian Science Foundation (FWF), and Adele Rabensteiner Awards in 2002, 2005, and 2006 from the Austrian Ophthalmic Society and Rüdiger Foundation, Germany in 2009.

REFERENCES

1. Gouras P. Transplantation of the retinal pigment epithelium. In: Marmor MF, Wolfensberger TJ, editors. The retinal pigment epithelium. New York: Oxford University Press; 1998. p. 492–507.
2. da Cruz L, Chen FK, Ahmado A, et al. RPE transplantation and its role in retinal disease. Prog Retin Eye Res 2007;26(6):598–635.
3. Binder S, Stanzel BV, Krebs I, et al. Transplantation of the RPE in AMD. Prog Retin Eye Res 2007;26(5):516–554.
4. Del Priore LV, Tezel TH, Kaplan HJ. Maculoplasty for age-related macular degeneration: reengineering Bruch's membrane and the human macula. Prog Retin Eye Res 2006;25(6):539–562.
5. Tezel TH, Kaplan HJ, Del Priore LV. Fate of human retinal pigment epithelial cells seeded onto layers of human Bruch's membrane. Invest Ophthalmol Vis Sci 1999;40(2):467–476.
6. Wang H, Ninomiya Y, Sugino IK, et al. Retinal pigment epithelium wound healing in human Bruch's membrane explants. Invest Ophthalmol Vis Sci 2003;44(5):2199–2210.
7. Gullapalli VK, Sugino IK, Van Patten Y, et al. Retinal pigment epithelium resurfacing of aged submacular human Bruch's membrane. Trans Am Ophthalmol Soc 2004;102:123–137; discussion 137–138.
8. Peyman GA, Blinder KJ, Paris CL, et al. A technique for retinal pigment epithelium transplantation for age-related macular degeneration secondary to extensive subfoveal scarring. Ophthalmic Surg 1991;22(2):102–108.
9. Algvere PV, Berglin L, Gouras P, et al. Transplantation of fetal retinal pigment epithelium in age-related macular degeneration with subfoveal neovascularization. Graefes Arch Clin Exp Ophthalmol 1994;232:707–716.
10. Yamamoto S, Du J, Gouras P, et al. Retinal pigment epithelial transplants and retinal function in RCS rats. Invest Ophthalmol Vis Sci 1993;34(11): 3068–3075.
11. Zhang X, Bok D. Transplantation of retinal pigment epithelial cells and immune response in the subretinal space. Invest Ophthalmol Vis Sci 1998;39(6):1021–1027.
12. Algvere PV, Berglin L, Gouras P, et al. Transplantation of RPE in age-related macular degeneration: observations in disciform lesions and dry RPE atrophy. Graefes Arch Clin Exp Ophthalmol 1997;235(3):149–158.
13. Tamai M, Abe T, Tomita H. Autologous iris pigment transplantation in age related macular degeneration. In: Das T, editor. Retina: Current practice and Future Trends. Hyderabad, India:PARAS; 1999. p. 151–161.
14. Thumann G, Aisenbrey S, Schraermeyer U, et al. Transplantation of autologous iris pigment epithelium after removal of choroidal neovascular membranes. Arch Ophthalmol 2000;118(10):1350–1355.

15. Aisenbrey S, Lafaut BA, Szurman P, et al. Iris pigment epithelial translocation in the treatment of exudative macular degeneration: a 3-year follow-up. Arch Ophthalmol 2006;124(2):183–188.
16. Binder S, Stolba U, Krebs I, et al. Transplantation of autologous retinal pigment epithelium in eyes with foveal neovascularization resulting from age-related macular degeneration: a pilot study. Am J Ophthalmol 2002;133(2):215–225.
17. Binder S, Krebs I, Hilgers RD, et al. Outcome of transplantation of autologous retinal pigment epithelium in age-related macular degeneration: a prospective trial. Invest Ophthalmol Vis Sci 2004;45(11):4151–4160.
18. van Meurs JC, ter Averst E, Hofland LJ, et al. Autologous peripheral retinal pigment epithelium translocation in patients with subfoveal neovascular membranes. Br J Ophthalmol 2004;88(1):110–113.
19. Stanga PE, Kychenthal A, Fitzke FW, et al. Retinal pigment epithelium translocation after choroidal neovascular membrane removal in age-related macular degeneration. Ophthalmology 2002;109(8):1492–1498.
20. Maaijwee K, Missotten T, Mulder P, et al. Influence of intraoperative course on visual outcome after an RPE-choroid translocation. Invest Ophthalmol Vis Sci 2008;49(2):758–761.
21. Joussen AM, Heussen FM, Joeres S, et al. Autologous translocation of the choroid and retinal pigment epithelium in age-related macular degeneration. Am J Ophthalmol 2006;142(1):17–30.
22. MacLaren RE. Autologous transplantation of the retinal pigment epithelium and choroid in the treatment of neovascular age-related macular degeneration. Ophthalmology 2007;114:561–570.
23. Bindewald A, Roth F, Van Meurs J, et al. [Transplantation of retinal pigment pithelium (RPE) following CNV removal in patients with AMD. Techniques, results, outlook.] Ophthalmologe 2004;101:886–894.
24. Stanzel BV, Bindewald-Wittich A, Holz FG, et al. Vitreoretinale Eingriffe bei fortgeschrittener altersabhängiger Makuladegeneration. Spektrum der Augenheilkunde 2008;22(6):348.
25. Ma Z, Han L, Wang C, et al. Autologous transplantation of retinal pigment epithelium–Bruch's membrane complex for hemorrhagic age-related macular degeneration. Invest Ophthalmol Vis Sci 2008;50:2975–2981.
26. Phillips SJ, Sadda SR, Tso MO, et al. Autologous transplantation of retinal pigment epithelium after mechanical debridement of Bruch's membrane. Curr Eye Res 2003;26(2):81–88.
27. Tsukahara I, Ninomiya S, Castellarin A, et al. Early attachment of uncultured retinal pigment epithelium from aged donors onto Bruch's membrane explants. Exp Eye Res 2002;74(2):255–266.
28. Thumann G, Aisenbrey S, Schaefer F, et al. Instrumentation and technique for delivery of tissue explants to the subretinal space. Ophthalmologica 2006;220(3):170–173.
29. Ito A. Construction and delivery of tissue-engineered human retinal pigment epithelial cell sheets, using magnetite nanoparticles and magnetic force. Tissue Eng 2005;11:489–496.
30. Haruta M, Sasai Y, Kawasaki H, et al. *In vitro* and *in vivo* characterization of pigment epithelial cells differentiated from primate embryonic stem cells. Invest Ophthalmol Vis Sci 2004;45(3):1020–1025.
31. Klimanskaya I, Hipp J, Rezai KA, et al. Derivation and comparative assessment of retinal pigment epithelium from human embryonic stem cells using transcriptomics. Cloning Stem Cells 2004;6(3):217–245.
32. Harris JR, Brown GA, Jorgensen M, et al. Bone marrow-derived cells home to and regenerate retinal pigment epithelium after injury. Invest Ophthalmol Vis Sci 2006;47(5):2108–2113.
33. Atmaca-Sonmez P, Li Y, Yamauchi Y, et al. Systemically transferred hematopoietic stem cells home to the subretinal space and express RPE-65 in a mouse model of retinal pigment epithelium damage. Exp Eye Res 2006;83(5):1295–1302.
34. Li Y, Atmaca-Sonmez P, Schanie CL, et al. Endogenous bone marrow derived cells express retinal pigment epithelium cell markers and migrate to focal areas of RPE damage. Invest Ophthalmol Vis Sci 2007;48(9): 4321–4327.
35. Harris JR, Fisher R, Jorgenssen M, et al. CD133 Progenitor cells from the bone marrow contribute to retinal pigment epithelium repair. Stem Cells 2008;27:457–466.
36. Fisher SK, Lewis GP, Linberg KA, et al. Cellular remodeling in mammalian retina: results from studies of experimental retinal detachment. Prog Retin Eye Res 2005;24(3):395–431.
37. Marc RE, Jones BW, Watt CB, et al. Neural remodeling in retinal degeneration. Progress in Retinal & Eye Research 2003;22:607–655.
38. Kubay OV, Charteris DG, Newland HS, et al. Retinal detachment neuropathology and potential strategies for neuroprotection. Surv Ophthalmol 2005;50(5):463–475.
39. Bhatt NS. Experimental transplantation of human retinal pigment epithelial cells on collagen substrates. Am J Ophthalmol 1994;117:214–221.
40. Thomson RC. Manufacture and characterization of poly(alpha-hydroxy ester) thin films as temporary substrates for retinal pigment epithelium cells. Biomaterials 1996;17:321–327.
41. Hadlock T. Ocular cell monolayers cultured on biodegradable substrates. Tissue Eng 1999;5:187–196.
42. Thumann G. Descemet's membrane as membranous support in RPE/IPE transplantation. Curr Eye Res 1997;16:1236–1238.
43. Ho TC. Tissue culture of retinal pigment epithelium following isolation with a gelatin matrix technique. Exp Eye Res 1997;64:133–139.
44. Oganesian A. A new model of retinal pigment epithelium transplantation with microspheres. Arch Ophthalmol 1999;117:1192–1200.
45. Farrokh Siar L. Cryoprecipitate: An autologous substrate for human fetal retinal pigment epithelium. Curr Eye Res 1999;19:89–94.
46. Hartmann U. Human and porcine anterior lens capsule as support for growing and grafting retinal pigment epithelium and iris pigment epithelium. Graefes Arch Clin Exp Ophthalmol 1999;237:940–945.
47. Nicolini J. The anterior lens capsule used as support material in RPE cell-transplantation. Acta Ophthalmol Scand 2000;78:527–531.
48. Lee CJ. Microcontact printing on human tissue for retinal cell transplantation. Arch Ophthalmol 2002;120:1714–1718.
49. Turowski P. Basement membrane-dependent modification of phenotype and gene expression in human retinal pigment epithelial ARPE-19 cells. Invest Ophthalmol Vis Sci 2004;45:2786–2794.
50. Singh S. Natural and artificial substrates for retinal pigment epithelial monolayer transplantation. Biomaterials 2001;22:3337–3343.
51. Tezel et al. Bruch's membrane as a support for RPE transplantation. 5. annual vision research conference; Ft. Lauderdale, 2002;5.
52. Leng T, Huie P, Bilbao KV, Blumenkranz MS, Loftus DJ, Fishman HA. Carbon Nanotube Bucky Paper as an Artificial Support Membrane and Bruch's Membrane Patch in Subretinal RPE and IPE Transplantation. Invest Ophthalmol Vis Sci 2003;44(5):481.
53. Tezcaner A. Retinal pigment epithelium cell culture on surface modified poly(hydroxybutyrate-co-hydroxyvalerate) thin films. Biomaterials 2003;24:4573–4583.
54. Capeans C. Amniotic membrane as support for human retinal pigment epithelium (RPE) cell growth. Acta Ophthalmol Scand 2003;81: 271–277.
55. Stanzel BV. Amniotic membrane maintains the phenotype of rabbit retinal pigment epithelial cells in culture. Exp Eye Res 2005;80:103–112.
56. Ohno-Matsui K. The effects of amniotic membrane on retinal pigment epithelial cell differentiation. Mol Vis 2005;11:1–10.
57. Singhal S. Primary adult human retinal pigment epithelial cell cultures on human amniotic membranes. Indian J Ophthalmol 2005;53: 109–113.
58. Yeung CK. The transfer of ocular cells using collagen. Cell Transplant 2004;13:585–594.
59. Yellachich D. Autologous iris pigment epithelium cultured on cellulose acetate membrane transplanted into the subretinal space of rabbits. ARVO Meeting Abstracts 2004;45:5168.
60. Lombardi L. Full Thickness Retinal Pigment Epithelium Explants Proliferate Into Epithelial Monolayers on Synthetic Bruch's Membrane Substitutes. Invest Ophthalmol Vis Sci 2005;46:4152 [abstract].
61. Molnar FE. Synthetic Bruch's Membrane Substitutes: Comparisons After Subretinal Transplantation With Cultured Iris Pigment Epithelium. Invest Ophthalmol Vis Sci 2005;46:4154 [abstract].
62. Williams RL. Polyurethanes as potential substrates for sub-retinal retinal pigment epithelial cell transplantation. J Mater Sci Mater Med. 2005;16: 1087–1092.
63. Stanzel BV. Culture of Human RPE From Aged Donors on a Potential Bruch's Membrane Prosthesis. Invest Ophthalmol Vis Sci 2006;47:1407 [abstract].
64. Lu JT. Thin collagen film scaffolds for retinal epithelial cell culture. Biomaterials 2007;28:1486–1494.
65. Stanzel BV. Perspektive: Tissue engineering bei RPE-Transplantation in AMD. Spektrum der Augenheilkunde. 2007;21:212.
66. Thumann G. The *in vitro* and *in vivo* behaviour of retinal pigment epithelial cells cultured on ultrathin collagen membranes. Biomaterials 2009;30:287–294.

CHAPTER 51

Off-label drugs and the impact of the Food and Drug Administration in the treatment of retinal disease

George A. Williams, M.D

INTRODUCTION

The pharmacotherapy of blinding retinal disease is replete with examples of off-label drug use (Table 51.1). The history of this off-label drug use is testimony to the innovation, persistence, and even courage of ophthalmologists in their continuing efforts to improve vision for those afflicted with retinal disease. Sometimes, off-label drug use is employed to treat relatively rare conditions such as endophthalmitis or uveitis, for which a Food and Drug Administration (FDA) label is unlikely. Other times, off-label drugs are used to treat common disorders such as diabetic retinopathy or age-related macular degeneration when approved therapies are suboptimal. Off-label drug use is also employed in combination therapy with approved treatments. Regardless of the indication, the use of off-label drugs may prove to be the best available treatment for an individual patient. However, off-label retinal pharmacotherapy places additional regulatory, legal, and economic burdens upon the ophthalmologist. This chapter will discuss the regulatory, legal, and coverage implications of off-label retinal pharmacotherapy.

OFF-LABEL DRUG USAGE AND THE FOOD AND DRUG ADMINISTRATION

HISTORICAL PERSPECTIVES

The advent of ocular photodynamic therapy with verteporfin in 2000 initiated a new era in the management of age-related macular degeneration. Although this novel therapy provided a safe and effective treatment for many patients with previously untreatable subfoveal choroidal neovascularization, the FDA label restricted its use to predominantly classic neovascular lesions. This limited label was used as the basis for the Centers for Medicare and Medicaid Services (CMS), coverage as outlined in a National Coverage Determination (NCD).[1,2] Although this NCD was the first exposure for many ophthalmologists to the confusing and arcane regulations that govern off-label drug use, most ophthalmologists had been using approved drugs off-label for years for the treatment of endophthalmitis, uveitis, proliferative vitreoretinopathy, and cystoid macular edema. Even the use of preoperative and postoperative antibiotics for endophthalmitis prophylaxis is off-label.

FDA APPROVAL PROCESS

An understanding of the issues involving off-label drug use requires a review of the FDA approval process.[3] The FDA is a public health agency whose mission is to oversee the use and marketing of regulated medical products. The FDA reviews the toxicology and clinical research from phase I, phase II, and phase III studies which is presented in an investigational new drug (IND) application and, when appropriate, approves a drug for use and marketing. When a drug is approved, the FDA issues a label that describes and defines the drug's specific medical indication(s), dose, dosage form, side-effects, and chemical structure. For some drugs, the FDA may include a "black box" warning in the label to emphasize potential complications associated with severe morbidity or mortality. The format of the FDA label has received widespread criticism for its confusing and almost impenetrable structure and syntax. Recently, FDA announced a more "user-friendly" format designed to facilitate use by both patients and physicians.[4] Although this new format is an improvement, it remains difficult.

THE CONCEPT OF "OFF-LABEL"

Any use of a drug not listed in the label is considered off-label. Off-label uses include giving an approved drug for a disease or indication other than that for which it is approved; at a different dose, frequency, or route of administration than specified in the label; or to treat a child when the product is approved to treat only adults. However, the use of an approved product by physicians is not restricted by the FDA to the limitations of the label. Physicians are allowed to use FDA-approved drugs in the treatment of an individual patient as medical practice. The FDA recognizes that off-label use of drugs by physicians is often appropriate and may represent the standard of care. The most obvious example of off-label drug use constituting the standard of care in ophthalmology is the use of intravitreal antibiotics for endophthalmitis despite the fact that no antibiotics are approved for intravitreal injection or for the treatment of endophthalmitis. The FDA has issued specific guidance on off-label drug use:

Good medical practice and the best interests of the patient require that physicians use legally available drugs, biologics and devices according to their best knowledge and medical judgment. If physicians use a product for an indication not in the approved labeling, they have the responsibility to be well informed about the product, to base its use on firm scientific rationale and on sound medical evidence and to maintain records on the product's use and effects. Use of a marketed product in this manner when the intent is in the practice of medicine does not require the submission of an Investigational New Drug Application … or review by an Institutional Review Board (IRB). However, the institution at which the product will be used may, under its own authority, require IRB review or other institutional oversight.[4]

In addition to the FDA, medical organizations such as the American Medical Association (AMA) and the American Academy of Ophthalmology are on record supporting off-label drug use when there is appropriate evidence-based medicine, expert consensus opinion, or unmet medical need.[5,6] The AMA policy on off-label drug use is "The AMA confirms its strong support for the autonomous clinical decision-making authority of a physician and that a physician may lawfully use an FDA-approved drug product or medical device for an unlabeled indication when such use is based on sound scientific evidence and sound medical opinion."[5]

If the FDA recognizes off-label drug use as appropriate and if the FDA does not regulate medical practice in the treatment of an individual patient, what role does the FDA play in off-label drug use? One important role is that the FDA precludes drug sponsors from marketing drugs to physicians or patients for off-label use. "Pharmaceutical manufacturers cannot proactively discuss off-label uses, nor may they distribute written materials (promotional pieces, reprints of articles,

Table 51.1 Common off-label retinal pharmacotherapies

Drug class/name	Indication
Antibiotics	Endophthalmitis treatment or prophylaxis by topical, subconjunctival, intravitreal, or oral administration
Corticosteroids	Macular edema, retinal vasculitis, uveitis
Nonsteroidal anti-inflammatory agents	Cystoid macular edema
Antimetabolites	Proliferative vitreoretinopathy treatment and prophylaxis, uveitis
Hyaluronidase	Vitreous hemorrhage
Pegaptanib sodium	Diabetic retinopathy
Bevacizumab	Neovascular age-related macular degeneration (AMD), diabetic retinopathy, retinal vascular occlusions, neovascular glaucoma
Ranibizumab	Diabetic retinopathy, retinal vascular occlusions, choroidal neovascularization not related to AMD, retinal tumors

etc.) that mention off-label use."[6] Therefore, the FDA label has important marketing implications because pharmaceutical companies are not allowed to market drugs for off-label use. Currently, this limitation applies to any formal marketing such as media advertising or drug detail information. Recently, the FDA has proposed a controversial relaxation on the restrictions for the marketing of off-label indications.[7] Regardless of the status of off-label marketing, the FDA does not restrict other parties such as physicians or specialty societies from discussing off-label uses or distributing written materials concerning them.[8,9]

"INVESTIGATIONAL USAGE OF DRUGS"

The FDA also becomes involved in off-label drug use when the drug is in "investigational use." The term "investigational use" suggests the use of an approved drug in the context of a clinical study protocol. When the primary intent of the investigational use is to develop information about a drug's safety or efficacy, or if the off-label use involves a route of administration or dosage level or use in a subject population or other factor that significantly increases the risks associated with the use of the drug, submission of an IND is required. Physicians can obtain the IND application (form 1571) from the internet.[3] The application process is self-explanatory, though rather tedious. Most investigational review boards will require an IND for a clinical trial involving off-label drug use.

COMPOUNDING PHARMACIES

Another regulatory issue involving off-label drugs is the formulation of ophthalmic preparations by compounding pharmacies. Any drug product prepared by a compounding pharmacy is considered by the FDA to be either off-label or a new drug. Compounding pharmacies are licensed by individual states to provide drugs to individual patients at the prescription request of a physician. In ophthalmology, compounding pharmacies provide multiple drugs for retinal pharmacotherapy, such as antibiotics, corticosteroids, and bevacizumab. Compounding pharmacies prepare approved drugs at dosages which are relevant for ocular administration and prepare preservative-free drugs. Although the FDA states: "Traditional compounding typically is used to prepare medications that are not available commercially", the FDA has recently expressed concerns about the legality of some compounding pharmacy practices related to retinal pharmacotherapy.[10] These issues are related primarily to the marketing of compounded retinal drugs and the need for a patient-specific prescription for each dose. The role of the FDA in regulating the state-controlled compounding pharmacies is also a concern. At the time of this writing, these issues are under litigation. As a result, legislation has been introduced in Congress to clarify the role of the FDA in the regulation of compounding pharmacies. The implications of this legislation to retinal pharmacotherapy are unknown.

RISK MANAGEMENT ISSUES

The legal implications of off-label drug use primarily involve risk management issues. The keys to addressing these risk management issues are patient selection and informed consent. As discussed above, FDA approval status does not necessarily define appropriate medical practice, nor does the FDA regulate medical practice. Medical practice is the therapeutic relationship between a physician and an individual patient. The physician must decide what the appropriate medical care is for each patient and this decision must fall within the standard of care. The question then becomes: "When does off-label drug use become the standard of care?" The answer depends on who is defining the standard of care. Payers may use specific definitions of the standard of care to establish coverage determinations, which will be discussed later. From a risk management perspective involving malpractice, a jury, judge, or arbitrator determines whether treatment is within the standard of care. This determination is based upon factors such as supporting authoritative literature, expert consensus, scientific rationale, and local or national medical practice patterns.

INFORMED CONSENT

An important factor in establishing the standard of care is informed consent. This is particularly critical with off-label drug use. The Ophthalmic Mutual Insurance Company (OMIC) recommends that physicians inform patients about the off-label status of a proposed treatment.[11] This discussion should include the known and potential unknown risks as well as the rationale for the off-label drug use. The physician should also discuss why any available FDA-approved or CMS-covered therapies are not appropriate. This discussion should be well documented in the chart. OMIC also recommends that a specific off-label informed consent be used. OMIC provides a specific consent for bevacizumab and triamcinolone acetonide with useful suggestions concerning patient selection, preparation of the medication, and informed consent and documentation.[11]

MEDICAL PAYMENT/COVERAGE

Perhaps the most difficult issue concerning off-label drug use concerns coverage for the drug and associated services. In ophthalmology, this often means coverage by Medicare. Coverage by Medicare can be established either by the local Medicare carrier via a local carrier decision (LCD) or by the CMS as an NCD. The Medicare Benefit Policy Manual provides that individual carriers may establish on a case-by-case basis coverage for off-label drug use based upon their assessment of the medical indication as reasonable and necessary.

FDA-approved drugs for indications other than what is indicated on the official label may be covered under Medicare if the carrier determines the use to be medically accepted, taking into consideration the major drug compendia, authoritative medical literature and for accepted standards of medical practice[12]

Some carriers have outlined criteria they consider when determining coverage of off-label drug use on a case-by-case basis. These criteria consider the following factors:

1. Whether alternative treatments were tried before considering off-label use
2. Whether there are published recommendations from specialty societies or in other authoritative-based guidelines
3. Whether authoritative medical literature supports the off-label use. Such literature must include peer-reviewed publications that demonstrate efficacy. Such studies may not include case reports, opinions, book chapters, or abstracts
4. Whether there is other evidence of broad scientific support
5. Whether the use is an accepted standard of medical practice.[13]

For some off-label drug use such as the use of intravitreal antibiotics for endophthalmitis, the above criteria are easily satisfied. For others, such as intravitreal injection of triamcinolone acetonide as either monotherapy or in combination therapy, the evidence is less compelling. As a result, there are variable coverage policies between Medicare carriers concerning off-label retinal pharmacotherapy. Currently, there is considerable controversy involving the off-label use of anti-VEGF agents such as pegaptanib sodium, ranibizumab, and bevacizumab. All Medicare carriers cover pegaptanib sodium and ranibizumab for the labeled treatment of neovascular age-related macular degeneration. All but one of the Medicare carriers covers bevacizumab for the off-label treatment of neovascular age-related macular degeneration as well. However, the coverage for other off-label uses, such as proliferative diabetic retinopathy, diabetic macular edema, retinal vascular occlusions, and neovascular glaucoma, is variable. This irregular coverage is frustrating to both ophthalmologists and patients since many of these conditions have no approved or consistently effective therapy. Medicare carriers often look to professional organizations such as the American Academy of Ophthalmology for guidance on these coverage issues. The American Academy of Ophthalmology in turn looks to the scientific literature for appropriate evidence to support recommendations for coverage, particularly in situations of unmet medical need. The strong support of the American Academy of Ophthalmology for the use of off-label bevacizumab was instrumental in obtaining Medicare coverage.[5]

NATIONAL COVERAGE DETERMINATION

CMS can establish a national coverage mandate to all Medicare carriers through an NCD. CMS uses a NCD to determine whether an item or service is "reasonable and necessary." While there is no statutory or regulatory definition of "reasonable and necessary," CMS has generally interpreted the term to mean that the item or service should improve health outcomes for Medicare beneficiaries.[12] CMS may consider an NCD when:

1. There are questions about the safety, effectiveness or appropriateness of a therapy, including off-label use of drugs
2. Local coverage policies are inconsistent
3. There is wide variation in billing practices not related to variation in clinical need
4. The health technology represents a substantial clinical advance and is likely to result in significant health benefits if it diffuses more rapidly to all patients for whom it is indicated.

To address the above issues, CMS relies on generally accepted principles of evidence-based medicine.[12] For drug coverage, an NCD typically requires strong evidence from clinical trials on safety and efficacy for the indication. Interestingly, FDA approval of the indication is not required for CMS coverage. This is the case for the coverage of photodynamic therapy with verteporfin for the treatment of occult with no classic and minimally classic subfoveal choroidal neovascularization and evidence of recent disease progression.[2] This indication is not listed in the verteporfin FDA label. However, this NCD is based on multiple clinical trials, an independent review by CMS of the clinical trial data, and the recommendation of a Medicare Carrier Advisory Committee. Such a process typically takes a year or longer. At the present time, CMS believes there are insufficient data to warrant an NCD for either off-label triamcinolone or bevacizumab (personal communication, CMS coverage team). CMS therefore has deferred these coverage decisions to the local carriers.

CLINICAL TRIALS

A relatively new mechanism by which CMS may cover off-label drug use is through a clinical trial. To be eligible for coverage, the clinical trial must meet a variety of requirements, including:

1. The principal purpose of the trial should be to test whether the intervention improves the participant's health outcome.
2. The trial should either be well supported by available scientific and medical information, or be intended to clarify or establish the health outcomes of interventions already in common clinical use.
3. The trial must not duplicate existing studies.
4. The trial must be appropriately designed and sponsored by a credible organization.

One obvious way to conduct such a trial is through the National Eye Institute and such trials on off-label drug use are in progress and include the Comparison of Age-related macular degeneration Treatment Trials (CATT) and the Diabetic Retinopathy Clinical Research Network.[14]

Currently, nearly all off-label drug use in ophthalmology is at the discretion of the local Medicare carriers. Usually, coverage will hinge on whether the carrier considers the off-label drug use reasonable and necessary. The Medicare Carrier Manual states that if a medication is determined not to be reasonable and necessary, the carrier excludes the entire charge, including any charges for services that were primarily for the purpose of administering a noncovered medication. This means that for intravitreal injection of a therapeutic agent (CPT code 67028), if the drug is not covered then neither is the injection.

Considering the above aspects of off-label drug coverage, how should ophthalmologists proceed when they believe off-label drug is in a patient's best interest? For Medicare beneficiaries, ophthalmologists should seek specific guidance from their local Medicare carrier. If the carrier declines coverage, the ophthalmologist may bill the patient for noncovered services associated with the off-label drug use by using an advance beneficiary notice (ABN). The necessary ABN form is available on the CMS website (www.cms.medicare.gov). The use of an ABN requires that the patient be informed about why the proposed treatment is not covered by Medicare and that the ABN form be signed prior to the performance of the service. The ABN form is then submitted to the local Medicare carrier with the bill on form 1500, using either the GA or GY modifier. Physicians should contact their local carrier to determine which modifier is preferred and to confirm how the carrier handles the ABN process. With an appropriate ABN, physicians can bill the patient for the noncovered services. For payers other than Medicare, ophthalmologists must contact the individual payer to determine payment policy for off-label retinal pharmacotherapy. Many payers have established payment policy based on the criteria discussed above.

SUMMARY AND KEY POINTS

With the continued development of new and more effective drugs for retinal disease, off-label drug use will escalate as ophthalmologists attempt to optimize treatment outcomes. This is particularly true for combination therapies in which drugs with different mechanisms of action are combined to improve visual outcomes and minimize complications. This increase in off-label drug use carries the responsibility to establish both safety and efficacy in order to allow off-label drugs to become the standard of care. Our patients deserve nothing less.

REFERENCES

1. Off-label use of non-oncology drugs and biologicals LCD No. L18709 AdminiStar Federal, Inc (February 10, 2005).
2. CMS Manual System. Pub 100-103. Medicare National Coverage Determinations. April 1, 2004. Change request 3191.

3. Feinsod M, Chambers WA. A primer on successfully navigating the waters of the Food and Drug Administration. Ophthalmology 2004;111: 1801–1806.
4. US Food and Drug Administration. Available online at: www.fda.gov.
5. American Academy of Ophthalmology. Available online at: www.aao.org.
6. Patient access to treatments prescribed by their physician. H-120.988. Available online at: www.ama-assn.org.
7. US Food and Drug Administration. Off-label and investigational use of marketed drugs. Biologics and medical devices. Available online at: www.fda.gov/oc/ohrt/irbs/offlabel.html.
8. US Food and Drug Administration. Good reprint practices for the distribution of medical journal articles and medical or scientific reference publications on un-approved new uses of approved drugs and approved or cleared medical devices: draft guidance, Feb 2008. Fed Regist 2008;74(34):9342. Available online at: http://www.fda.gov/oc/op/goodreprint.html.
9. Psaty BM, Ray W. FDA guidance on off-label promotion and the state of literature from sponsors. JAMA 2008;299:1949–1951.
10. Food and Drug Association. Available online at:www.fda.gov/foi/warning_letters/g6147d.htm.
11. Ophthalmic Mutual Insurance Company. Available online at: www.omic.com.
12. CMS Draft Guidance for NCDSs. Available online at: www.cms.gov; accessed March 9, 2005.
13. Off-label use of non-oncology drugs and biologicals LCD No. L18709 AdminiStar Federal, Inc (February 10, 2005).
14. Diabetic Retinopathy Clinical Research Network. Available online at: www.clinicaltrials.gov.

CHAPTER 52

Value-based medicine and pharmacoeconomics

Gary C. Brown, MD, MBA and Melissa M. Brown, MD, MN, MBA

INTRODUCTION

HISTORY

In 1972, Archie Cochrane advocated the randomized clinical trial to promote higher-quality medical evidence.[1] But it was not until the last decade of the 20th century that the term "evidence-based medicine" came into vogue.[2,3] Evidence-based medicine is essentially what the name implies – the practice of medicine based upon the highest-quality and most reproducible evidence available.

More recently, the term "value-based medicine" has been introduced into health care by our group of researchers at the Center for Value-Based Medicine.[5–8] Value-based medicine incorporates the highest level of evidence-based medicine and takes it to a higher level by incorporating patient-based quality-of-life preferences to measure the value conferred by an intervention. This value is then amalgamated with the resources expended upon an intervention to produce a cost–utility ratio. Value and cost–utility ratio are the most important measures in value-based medicine. As the reader will see, value-based medicine allows a quality of health care heretofore not possible.

This article will briefly discuss evidence-based medicine and then elaborate on the various forms of pharmacoeconomic analyses. The last of the pharmacoeconomic analyses is cost–utility analysis, the most sophisticated variant and the foundation for value-based medicine. Value-based medicine pharmacoeconomic analyses standardize the input variables used in cost–utility analysis to allow a comparison of comparative effectiveness (value) and cost-effectiveness of a drug across all specialties in medicine.

KEY CONCEPTS

EVIDENCE-BASED MEDICINE

There are essentially five levels of medical interventional evidence.[4] The higher the level, the greater the confidence the clinician can have that the information is reproducible (reliable).

The highest level of evidence, level 1, is that supplied by the randomized clinical trial with low type 1 and type 2 errors. This means a *P*-value of <0.05, and a β of <0.20, or a power $(1 - \beta)$ of 80% or more to detect a predetermined difference among groups. Level 2 evidence is supplied by the randomized clinical trial with a type 1 error >0.05 and/or a type 2 error >0.20. Level 3 evidence occurs with a nonrandomized clinical trial, while the case series provides level 4 evidence and the case report provides level 5, or anecdotal evidence. A summary of the levels of interventional evidence is shown in Table 52.1.[4]

In addition to the level of evidence, the clinician should also be cognizant of whether a study is properly masked and has an acceptable dropout rate.[2] Masking can occur in the form of a single-blind study in which a patient typically does not know which treatment is being given, and the double-blind study, in which neither the researcher nor the patient knows which treatment is being given. A double-blinded study is preferable, but may not always be possible.

A dropout rate of <5% is considered excellent, while a rate of 5–15% is acceptable and a rate greater than 20% casts suspicion upon the validity of a study.[2] For example, a 10% event rate can be misleading if there is a 30% dropout rate and half of those who dropped out (15% of all participants) also had an event. Thus, the true event rate might have been 25%, or 250% higher than found in the study with a 30% dropout rate. An intent-to-treat study keeps in all patients who are randomized,[2] thereby allowing the reader to know the dropout rate. Importantly, the quality of evidence incorporated into a pharmacoeconomic analysis is only as strong as its weakest link.

Lastly, the reader should be aware of the terms "criterion validity" and "construct validity." Criterion validity measures how well an intervention measures up to a criterion, or "gold standard." For example, how does a new drug for the treatment for neovascular macular degeneration measure up to the gold standard of vascular endothelial growth factor (VEGF) inhibitors? Construct validity assesses how effectively something measures what it is supposed to measure. For example, how well does the quality-of-life instrument National Eye Institute Visual Functioning Questionnaire 25 (NEI-VFQ-25)[9] for ocular diseases actually measure the quality of life associated with neovascular macular degeneration?[5,10]

TYPES OF PHARMACOECONOMIC ANALYSIS

There are essentially four types of pharmacoeconomic analyses. In order of increasing complexity, these are: (1) cost minimization analysis; (2) cost–benefit analysis; (3) cost-effectiveness analysis; and (4) cost–utility analysis.[5,10]

COST MINIMIZATION ANALYSIS

Cost minimization analysis compares the cost of two similar interventions to ascertain which is less expensive. Cost minimization analysis, however, suffers from the problem that it often compares two different interventions that may initially seem similar but are not. For example, two VEGF inhibitors for the treatment of neovascular age-related macular degeneration (AMD) may have similar visual results. Nonetheless, the types of adverse events associated with each may differ very significantly, as may the incidence of each of the adverse events. Thus, even though they may superficially seem very similar, the drugs are often not exactly comparable. Thus, this form of analysis is used infrequently today.

An example of a reasonable cost minimization analysis would be one that compares the administration of the same VEGF inhibitor, with the same administration technique, in the hospital outpatient setting versus that in a private office. Here the exact same intervention is performed in a different setting and the cost is compared to ascertain which is less expensive.

Table 52.1 Levels of interventional evidence	
Level	**Description**
1	Randomized clinical trial with type 1 error ≤ 0.05 and type 2 error ≤ 0.20
2	Randomized clinical trial with higher type 1 and/or type 2 error
3	Nonrandomized clinical trial
4	Case series
5	Case report

COST–BENEFIT ANALYSIS

Cost–benefit analysis compares the dollars expended for an intervention with the dollars gained from the intervention. For example, let us assume that a VEGF inhibitor treatment for neovascular AMD has direct medical costs of $10 000/year. The treatment may greatly decrease the human burden of suffering, but the key factor here is the costs expended and the costs saved. On the gain side, the treatment may allow 40% of treated individuals to reach a vision of 20/40, thereby allowing many who might be on disability to obviate a disability scenario. Thus, the weighted disability gain per patient might be $600 per month, or $7200/year. Furthermore, let us assume that the treatment allows 20% of treated individuals to work and contribute to the gross domestic product (GDP: the sum of all final products and services produced annually in the USA), resulting in a weighted gain per patient of $700/month, or $8400/year. With this societal cost perspective, these disability and unemployment costs saved ($15 600/year) exceed the cost of treatment ($10 000/year) by $5600 a year, indicating a positive cost–benefit for the intervention.

Most often, cost–benefit analysis fails to take into account the quality of life associated with a health state, although a methodology of utility analysis, known as willingness to pay, does allow quantification of quality-of-life changes by assessing how much of a person's salary, savings, retirement plan, and so forth, a person would be willing to pay in return for perfect health. Nonetheless, this form of utility analysis to measure quality of life is not often used since those who have greater assets are often willing to pay proportionately more for the same therapeutic intervention than those with minimal assets.[5]

COST-EFFECTIVENESS ANALYSIS

Cost-effectiveness analysis measures the resources expended for a given endpoint. The endpoint may be years of life gained, years of good vision gained, disability-free years, level of vision gained (such as 20/25), or any other endpoint.

Confusion has arisen with this term since certain authors use cost-effectiveness analysis synonymously with cost–utility analysis.[11–13] Others reserve cost–utility analysis for those studies which measure the improvement in length of life and/or quality of life for the resources expended using dollars expended per quality-adjusted life-year ($/QALY). The present authors agree that the term cost–utility analysis should be used to describe the latter, rather than cost-effectiveness analysis.

Cost-effectiveness analysis

Tengs et al.[14] have produced an excellent treatise on 500 life-saving treatments published in the form of cost-effectiveness analysis. In each of these instances the analysis was performed using cost per year of life saved. Adjusting the 1993 US dollars from the study of Tengs et al.[14] to year-2007 dollars reveals that the median cost to save a year of life with a medical intervention is approximately $28,350, while that for injury reduction is $72,500, and that for toxin control is $4.2 million. Injury reduction includes entities such as seat belt use and setting speed limit, while toxin control includes setting maximum levels of arsenic in water and benzene emissions in tire plants. Needless to say, medical interventions appear to be far more cost-effective than injury reduction interventions and efforts at toxin control.

COST–UTILITY ANALYSIS

Cost–utility analysis is the most sophisticated form of pharmacoeconomic analysis in that it takes into account the improvement in quality of life and/or length of life conferred by an intervention for the resources expended. The increase in longevity conferred by an intervention can generally be ascertained from evidence-based data in the literature. Measurement of the quality of life conferred by an intervention is more difficult.

Quality of life: Function-based instruments

Numerous instruments have been used to assess the quality of life associated with a health state. Among the general medical instruments are the Medical Outcomes Short-Form-36 (SF-36),[15] the Sickness Impact Profile (SIP),[16] and the Quality of Well-Being Scale.[17] Included among the ophthalmic instruments are the VF-14[18] and the NEI-25.[19] The general medical instruments are generally not applicable to ophthalmic disease health states and the ophthalmic tests are not applicable to medical disease health states.[5] All of these tests primarily measure the function associated with a given health state.[5]

Quality of life: Preference-based instruments

Utility analysis provides a measure of the quality of life associated with a health state and is believed to be more all-encompassing than function-based quality-of-life measures in that it incorporates function, psychological overlay, caregiver availability, socioeconomic conditions, occupational aspects, and virtually every other aspect that comprises quality of life.[20–22] The time tradeoff methodology appears to have the best construct validity and correlates most closely with visual acuity, particularly that of the better-seeing eye.[5,8,23–27]

A time tradeoff utility value is calculated by asking two questions:

1. How many additional years do you expect to live?
2. How many of those remaining years, if any, would you be willing to trade for an intervention that would immediately return your health state to a normal health state on a permanent basis?

The utility is then calculated by subtracting the proportion of years traded from 1.0. For example, if a person with diabetes and 20 theoretical remaining years of life is willing to trade 3 of the 20 years in return for a normal health state, the utility is $1.0 - 3/20 = 0.85$. Because patients can have a preference to trade time for better health or trade no time and remain in the same health state, utility analysis is referred to as a preference based quality-of-life instrument.

Utilities associated with visual acuity in the better-seeing eye are shown in Table 52.2, while utilities associated with general medical conditions are shown in Table 52.3. The ocular utilities are directly comparable with the general medical utilities. Of note is the fact that ocular utilities appear to correlate more with the visual acuity in the better-seeing eye, rather than the underlying cause of visual loss.[24]

Utility gain

The improvement from one health state to another after an intervention can also be measured using utility analysis. For example, if the vision in the better-seeing eye improves from 20/200 (utility of 0.66) to 20/25 (utility of 0.87), the utility improvement is 0.21 (0.87 – 0.66). Decision analysis is often helpful in amalgamating the benefits of a drug with its adverse events, as well as the incidences of adverse events, to demonstrate more effectively the utility associated with use of a drug (Figure 52.1).

Table 52.2 Time tradeoff utilities associated with visual acuity in the better-seeing eye[8,23,27]

Acuity	Utility
20/20 OU permanently	1.00
20/20–20/25 OU	0.97
20/20	0.92
20/25	0.87
20/30	0.84
20/40	0.80
20/50	0.77
20/70	0.74
20/100	0.67
20/200	0.66
20/400	0.54
20/800	0.52
HM-LP	0.35
NLP	0.26

OU = both eyes
HM = hand motions
LP = light perception
NLP = no light perception

Table 52.3 Time tradeoff utilities for general medical health states[8]

Health state	Utility
Mild angina	0.88
Moderate angina	0.83
Severe angina	0.53
Diabetes mellitus	0.88
Myocardial infarction, mild	0.91
Myocardial infarction, moderate	0.80
Myocardial infarction, severe	0.30
Hemodialysis	0.49
Renal transplant	0.79
Stroke, minor	0.89
Stroke, major	0.30
Ulcerative colitis, severe	0.58
Ulcerative colitis (1 year after surgery)	0.98
Impotence and incontinence after TURP	0.60

TURP, transurethral resection of the prostate.

Value gain

The improvement in utility can be multiplied by the years of duration of treatment benefit to arrive at the total value conferred by an intervention.[5,10] This value is measured in QALYs gained. A utility improvement of 0.21 for 10 years (0.21 × 10) equals 2.1 QALYs gained. Value, however, can also be measured in percentage gain. For most ophthalmologic interventions value is conferred by improvement in quality of life rather than gain in length of life. Thus, the percentage gain for ophthalmic interventions is equivalent to quality-of-life gain.

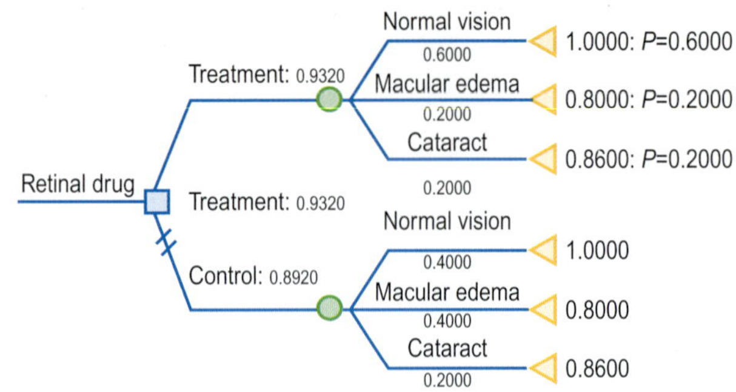

Figure 52.1 Example of decision analysis showing the resultant utilities associated with the use of a drug (utility = 0.932) and the control group not treated with the drug (utility = 0.893). Utilities for each of the adverse event outcomes are located to the right of the triangular terminal nodes and the incidence of each outcome is listed, below its respective branch. Treatment reduces the incidence of macular edema from 40% to 20%, resulting in a utility gain of (0.9320 – 0.8920) = 0.04.

The tree is read from left to right. The square is a decision node when one must decide whether to treat or not treat. The O is a chance node, for which the incidences are listed under the arms of the subtrees. The triangle indicates a terminal node, to the right of which are located the utilities associated with each of the possible outcomes.

Value trumps cost

All patients should want and deserve the intervention which confers the greatest value. Only when the value conferred by interventions is the same should cost be a consideration; in this instance the intervention which is least expensive is the preferred intervention. At the current time, the VEGF inhibitors appear to deliver the greatest value among interventions for neovascular AMD (Table 52.4).

A good example of the clinical benefit of value-based medicine, pharmacoeconomic analyses is demonstrated by the head-to-head comparison of intravitreal pegaptanib and photodynamic therapy (PDT) with verteporfin for the treatment of classic, subfoveal, neovascular AMD. The final vision in the Treatment of AMD with PDT (TAP) trial was 20/160 + 1 in the treatment cohort versus 20/320 + 1 in the control group, while in the pegaptanib VEGF inhibition study (IS) trial the final vision was 20/126 – 1 in the treatment cohort versus 20/200 + 1 in the control group.[28] Comparing these results, much less the associated adverse events and incidences of the adverse events, is virtually impossible without a value-based medicine analysis. Value-based data clearly demonstrate that PDT confers the greatest value with an 8.1% improvement in quality of life, while pegaptanib confers inferior value with a 5.9% improvement in quality of life (Table 52.4).

Cost–utility ratio

The total number of QALYs gained from an intervention is then amalgamated with the costs associated with the intervention to arrive at a cost–utility ratio, which is measured using dollars expended per QALY gained. The cost–utility of an intervention can be compared with that of any other intervention in health care. Thus, the value of all health care interventions given for the resources expended can be compared on an equal playing field.

Cost-effectiveness standards

An intervention is typically thought to be cost-effective if its cost–utility ratio is < $100 000/QALY and very cost-effective if it costs <$50 000/QALY.[5] World Health Organization standards suggest <$40 000/QALY as very cost-effective and < $120 000/QALY as cost-effective.[29] In general, despite the fact that we use the cost–utility ratio to assess cost-effectiveness, we speak of an intervention as being cost-effective, rather

Table 52.4 Value gain conferred by health care interventions

Intervention	Value gain ($/QALY gained)
Laser, subfoveal choroidal neovascularization[28]	4.4%
Pegaptanib therapy for subfoveal choroidal neovascularization[28]	5.9%
Photodynamic therapy for classic subfoveal choroidal neovascularization[28]	8.1%
β-blockers for systemic arterial hypertension*	6.3–9.1%
Cataract surgery, second eye[33]	12.7%
Ranbizumab, intravitreal, subfoveal neovascular AMD, minimally classic and occult choroidal neovascularization[30]	15.8%
Ranbizumab, intravitreal, subfoveal neovascular AMD, minimally classic and occult choroidal neovascularization*	17.0%
Cataract surgery, first eye[32]	20.8%
Antidepressants (SSRIs)*	20–24%
Proton pump inhibitors, acute erosive esophagitis*	13.3–26.2%

**Data from the Center for Value-Based Medicine Pharmaceutical Value Index internal files.*

QALY, AMD, age-related macular degeneration; SSRI, selective serotonin reuptake inhibitor.

than being cost-utilitarian. The cost utilities of various nonophthalmic, health care interventions and interventions for neovascular ARMD are shown in Table 52.5.[28,30]

Table 52.5 Cost–utility of various health care interventions[8]

Intervention	Cost–utility ($/QALY gained)
Laser, threshold ROP	$879
SSRIs, depression*	$1060–10 700
PPV, diabetic vitreous hemorrhage	$2347
β-blockers for systemic arterial hypertension*	$2400–25 400
Cataract extraction, first eye	$2444
Cataract surgery, second eye	$3245
Laser, DME	$3810
Laser, subfoveal CNVM[28]	$8179
Cochlear implant, children	$11 621
Photodynamic therapy with verteporfin for subfoveal neovascular AMD[28]	$31 544
Rx, occupational HIV exposure	$48 660
Ranbizumab, intravitreal, subfoveal neovascular AMD, minimally classic and occult choroidal neovascularization[30]	$50 691
Surgery for PVR, C_3F_8 gas, no previous vitrectomy[34]	$56 780
Pegaptanib therapy, classic, minimally classic and occult subfoveal choroidal neovascularization[28]	$66 798
Simultaneous kidney and pancreas transplant	$143 655
Acute CRAO Rx with AC paracentesis and $CO_2:O_2$ inhalation	$4.65 million

QALY, quality-adjusted life year; ROP, retinopathy of prematurity; SSRI, selective serotonin reuptake inhibitor; PPV, pars plana vitrectomy, DME, diabetic macular edema; CNVM, choroidal neo-vascular membrane; AMD, age-related macular degeneration; Rx, treatment; HIV, human immunodeficiency virus; PVR, proliferative vitreoretinopathy; C_3F_8, perfluoropropane; CRAO, central retinal artery obstruction; AC, anterior-chamber; CO_2, carbon dioxide; O_2, oxygen.

Discounting[5]

Both costs and value outcomes (QALYs) are discounted in a net present value (NPV) analysis to account for the time value of money and of good health. In essence a dollar is now worth more than a dollar in 10 years' time, since that dollar can now be invested to yield more dollars. Good health can now also be used to create dollars that can be invested to yield more dollars.

Value-based medicine

Value-based medicine is the practice of medicine based upon the value conferred by health care interventions, especially drugs.[5] Theoretically, it enables the practice of higher-quality care since it integrates patient utilities, thus incorporating patient preferences for health states and quality-of-life parameters often ignored in the outcomes of evidence-based medicine clinical trials.[5] In addition, it incorporates all benefits associated with an intervention, as well as all adverse events using decision analysis (Figure 52.1).

A critical aspect of value-based medicine is the fact that it standardizes the input criteria and outcomes used in pharmacoeconomic analysis.

Standardization

Unfortunately, most of the cost–utility studies in the current literature are not comparable since they use different utility methodologies, different utility respondents, as well as different cost perspectives and cost bases.[5] Value-based medicine cost–utility analyses use the standards listed in Table 52.6 to allow a comparison of studies across all specialties.

Patient respondents

Value-based medicine specifically uses patient utilities since community and expert (physician) surrogate values often differ considerably. For AMD, physicians who treated the disease underestimated its burden upon the quality of life of patients with the condition by anywhere from 96% to 750%.[31]

COST PERSPECTIVE

The third-party insurer perspective includes only those costs the insurer has to pay, or the direct medical costs. The societal perspective includes the third-party insurer costs, but also includes direct nonmedical costs such as caregiver costs and travel costs, as well as indirect costs such as loss of wages and disability payments obviated.

Thus, the third-party perspective and the societal perspective are quite different and difficult to compare without a thorough breakdown. A thorough cost–utility analysis is more complete if it offers ratios utilizing both the third-party insurer cost perspective and the societal cost perspective. Typically the societal cost perspective yields a more favorable cost–utility ratio versus the third-party insurer cost perspective. One note of caution, however, is that societal costs are not as standardized and readily available as the direct medical costs.

Table 52.6 Cost–utility analyses to allow comparability across studies: summary of recommended cost–utility variable standards

Perspective – third-party insurer (using direct health care costs) + societal (direct medical, direct non-medical and indirect costs)

Population analysis – reference case

Utilities

Methodology: time tradeoff

Source: patients

Comorbidities: should not be used to discriminate against those who are disabled

Costs: direct health care costs

Direct health care cost	Standardized reference source
Provider reimbursement	Average national Medicare payment
Hospital, acute reimbursement	Average national Medicare payment
Ambulatory surgical center	Average national Medicare payment
Skilled nursing facility	Average national Medicare payment
Rehabilitation	Average national Medicare payment
Home health care	Average national Medicare payment
Clinical tests	Average national Medicare payment
Durable goods	Average national Medicare payment
Nursing home care	Average national Medicaid payment
Pharmaceuticals	Average Sales Price (ASP)

Annual discount rate – 3% for quality-adjusted life-years (QALYs) and costs

Sensitivity analysis – should be performed at least one way, and often two way. Those input variables in which there is the least confidence should be analyzed.

Adapted from Brown MM, Brown GC, Sharma S. Evidence-Based to Value-Based Medicine. Chicago: AMA Press, 2005: pp. 1 324.

IMPLICATIONS FOR RETINAL PHARMACOTHERAPY

Pharmacoeconomics has already had a huge impact on the use of retinal pharmacologic agents,[35,36] a phenomenon that will only become more pronounced in the near future as the USA adopts cost–utility principles.[37] Pharmacoeconomic principles are currently used in public policy in the UK, Canada, Australia, Estonia, Latvia, and Lithuania, and will be adopted in other countries as well.

The National Institute for Health and Clinical Excellence (NICE), the agency which recommends whether new therapies should be adopted by the National Health Service in the UK, originally recommended the use of ranibizumab for only second eyes with classic subfoveal neovascular AMD, or approximately 10% of eyes which might benefit.[35] When the conferred value and cost–utility of ranibizumab for the treatment of all forms of subfoveal choroidal neovascularization became apparent in NICE analyses and through cost–utility analyses in the peer-reviewed literature,[30] the policy was changed to allow 14 injections of ranibizumab per eye for cases of subfoveal choroidal neovascularization.[36]

It is very likely that combination therapies for neovascular AMD will be undertaken in the near future.[38] When this is the case, value-based medicine will objectively assess the value and cost-effectiveness of these interventions so the clinician will be able to provide the highest-quality care to patients for the most reasonable cost.

SUMMARY AND KEY POINTS

Value-based medicine pharmacoeconomics, as applied to vitreoretinal interventions and across all of medicine, signals a new era of quality in the health care arena.

The advantages of value-based pharmacoeconomic analyses include the facts that they:

1. integrate all benefits and adverse events associated with a drug to demonstrate its overall value
2. incorporate patient quality-of-life preferences often ignored in clinical trials
3. allow physicians to appreciate better what patients consider most relevant so they can provide higher-quality care
4. identify drugs with superior value, an aspect especially important for drug companies that often have done poorly in demonstrating the value of their drugs
5. demonstrate the often underappreciated benefits of drugs, such as the facts that they prevent disability and allow patients to continue to work
6. allow a head-to-head comparison of the value conferred by drugs and other interventions
7. assess the cost of comparator drugs of similar value so the least expensive can be identified.

In essence, value-based medicine pharmacoeconomics provides an information system which allows all stakeholders the ability to appreciate the value conferred by drugs, as well as the costs expended for that value. It will bring a new era of quality care to medicine as it takes evidence-based medicine outcomes to a higher level, and is a methodology to facilitate the most efficient use of scarce health care resources.

REFERENCES

1. Cochrane AL. Effectiveness and Efficiency. Random Reflections on Health Services. London: Nuffield Provincial Hospitals Trust; 1972. (Reprinted in 1999 for Nuffield Trust by the Royal Society of Medicine Press, London.)
2. Sackett DL, Straus SE, Richardson WS, et al. Evidence-Based Medicine. How to Practice and Teach EBM. 2nd ed. Philadelphia: Churchill Livingstone; 2000.
3. Evidence-Based Medicine Working Group. A new approach to teaching the practice of medicine. JAMA 1992;268:2420–2425.
4. Sharma S. Levels of evidence. Evidence-Based Eye Care 2002;3:175–176.
5. Brown MM, Brown GC, Sharma S. Evidence-Based to Value-Based Medicine. Chicago: AMA Press; 2005. p. 1–324.
6. Brown MM, Brown GC, Sharma S. Value-based medicine. Evidence-Based Eye Care 2002;3:8–9.
7. Brown MM, Brown GC. Outcome of corneal transplantation. Value-based health care. Br J Ophthalmol 2002;86:2–3.
8. Brown MM, Brown GC, Sharma S, et al. Health care economic analyses and value-based medicine. Surv Ophthalmol 2003;48:204–223.
9. National Eye Institute Visual Functioning Questionnaire – 25 (VFQ-25). Available online at: www.nei.nih.gov; accessed April 2, 2008.
10. Drummond ME, O'Brien B, Stoddart GL, et al. Methods for the Economic Evaluation of Health Care Programmes. 2nd ed. New York: Oxford University Press; 1999.
11. Gold MR, Patrick DL, Torrance GW, et al. Identifying and valuing outcomes. In: Gold MR, Siegel JE, Russell LB, et al. editors. Cost-Effectiveness in Health and Medicine. New York: Oxford University Press; 1996. p. 82–134.
12. Weinstein MC, Siegel JE, Gold MR, et al. Recommendations of the Panel on Cost-Effectiveness in Health and Medicine. JAMA 1996;276:1253–1258.
13. Siegel JE, Weinstein MC, Russell LB, et al. Recommendations for reporting cost-effectiveness analyses. Panel on Cost-Effectiveness in Health and Medicine. JAMA 1996;276:1339–1341.
14. Tengs TO, Adams ME, Pliskin JP, et al. Five-hundred life-saving interventions and their cost-effectiveness. Risk Analysis 1995;15:369–390.
15. Edelman D, Williams GR, Rothman M, et al. A comparison of three health status measures in primary care patients. J Gen Intern Med 1999;14:759–762.
16. Bergner M, Bobbitt RA, Carter WB, et al. The Sickness Impact Profile: Development and final revision of a health status measure. Med Care 1981;119:787–805.

17. Kaplan RM, Ganiats TG, Sieber WJ, et al. The Quality of Well-Being Scale: Critical similarities and differences with the SF-36. Int J Qual Health Care 1998;10:509–520.
18. Steinberg EP, Tielsch JM, Schein OD, et al. The VF-14. An index of functional impairment in patients with cataract. Arch Ophthalmol 1994;112:630–638.
19. National Eye Institute Visual Functioning Questionnaire – 25 (VFQ-25). Available online at: http://www.nei.nih.gov/resources/visionfunction/vfq_ia.pdf; accessed 4-16-08.
20. Torrance GW, Thomas W, Sackett D. A utility maximization model for evaluation of health care programs. Health Services Research 1972;7:118–133.
21. Klarman H, Francis J, Rosenthal G. Cost-effectiveness applied to the treatment of chronic renal disease. Medical Care 1968;6:48–55.
22. Redelmeier DA, Detsky A. A clinician's guide to utility measurement. Med Decis Making 1995;22:271–281.
23. Brown MM, Brown GC, Sharma S, et al. Utility values associated with blindness in an adult population. Br J Ophthalmol 2001;85:327–331.
24. Brown MM, Brown GC, Sharma S, et al. Quality of life with visual acuity loss from diabetic retinopathy and age-related macular degeneration. Arch Ophthalmol 2002;120:481–484.
25. Brown GC, Brown MM, Sharma S, Kistler J: Utility values associated with age-related macular degeneration. Arch Ophthalmol 2000;118:47–51.
26. Brown MM, Brown GC, Sharma S, et al. Utility values and diabetic retinopathy. Am J Ophthalmol 1999;128:324–330.
27. Brown GC. Vision and quality of life. Trans Am Ophthalmol Soc 1999;97:473–512.
28. Brown GC, Brown MM, Brown HC, et al. A value-based medicine comparison of interventions for subfoveal neovascular macular degeneration. Ophthalmology 2007;114:1170–1178.
29. World Health Organization. The World Health Report 2002. Reducing Risks, Promoting Healthy Life. Geneva: WHO; 2002. p. 101–144.
30. Brown GC, Brown MM, Brown H, et al. A value-based medicine analysis of ranibizumab (MARINA Study) for the treatment of subfoveal neovascular macular degeneration. Ophthalmology 2007 Oct 31; [Epub ahead of print].
31. Brown GC, Brown MM, Sharma S. Difference between ophthalmologist and patient perceptions of quality-of-life associated with age-related macular degeneration. Can J Ophthalmol 2000;35:27–32.
32. Busbee B, Brown MM, Brown GC, et al. Incremental cost-effectiveness of initial cataract surgery. Ophthalmology 2002;109:606–612.
33. Busbee B, Brown MM, Brown GC, et al. A cost–utility analysis of cataract surgery in the second eye. Ophthalmology 2003;110:2310–2317.
34. Brown GC, Brown MM, Sharma S, et al. A cost–utility analysis of interventions for proliferative vitreoretinopathy. Am J Ophthalmol 2002;133:365–372.
35. Reuters UK. NICE backs Lucentis for blindness treatment. Available online at: http://uk.reuters.com/article/domesticNews/idUKL1388321720070614; accessed 4-19-08.
36. National Institute for Health and Clinical Excellence. Press release. NICE consults for proposal on dose-capping scheme to make Lucentis available on the NHS. http://www.nice.org.uk/media/D46/26/2007068ConsultationonproposalLucentis.pdf; accessed 4-18-08.
37. CBO Testimony. Statement of Peter Orszag, Director. Research on the comparative effectiveness of medical treatments: Options for an expanded federal role. Before the Subcommittee on Health, Committee on Ways and Means, U.S. House of Representatives, June 12, 2007. From the Internet @ http://www.cbo.gov/ftpdocs/82xx/doc8209/Comparative_Testimony.pdf, accessed April 19, 2008.
38. Brown MM, Brown GC, Brown HC, et al. Comparative effectiveness and cost-effectiveness analyses of VEGF-A inhibitor and ^{90}Sr brachytherapy for neovascular macular degeneration, Submitted for publication.

CHAPTER 53

Future perspectives: agents on the horizon

R. C. Andrew Symons, MB, BS, PhD, FRANZCO, Peter K. Kaiser, MD, Glenn L. Stoller, MD, and Quan Dong Nguyen, MD, MSc

INTRODUCTION

As demonstrated in the previous chapters of this textbook, retinal pharmacotherapeutics is a rapidly developing area. The enormous burden of disease in an aging population will hopefully be met by significant improvements in our understanding and treatment of disease processes such as age-related macular degeneration (AMD) and diabetic retinopathy.

KEY FEATURES

This chapter will provide some perspectives on select antiangiogenic drugs currently in development, as well as therapies directed against the complement cascade for the treatment of AMD, and an anti-inflammatory monoclonal antibody for the treatment of diabetic macular edema (DME). One of the exciting possibilities is that the use of a combination of these modalities will enable earlier and more complete control of disease processes. For instance, the use of complement cascade inhibitors in addition to the use of vascular endothelial growth factor (VEGF) inhibition may lead to a reduction in ongoing accumulated damage to the Bruch's membrane and retinal pigment epithelium (RPE), as well as allowing more complete control over neovascular AMD. The mechanism of action of a number of the discussed drugs differs enough to give the potential to control neovascularization in several different ways, potentially allowing more effective management of this process with fewer treatments.

Multidrug combination therapy is employed throughout medicine, often exploiting synergistic therapeutic effects to allow reduction of dosages, thus minimizing side-effects. Examples are the use of multidrug cocktails of antineoplastic agents in oncology, the use of multiple immunosuppressants in the management of autoimmune disease and transplants, and the use of multidrug therapy to control infectious disease. Fortunately, today's most commonly used pharmacotherapeutic modality for the treatment of ocular neovascularization and for some causes of macular edema, VEGF inhibition, has had minimal clinically manifested side-effects. However, VEGF inhibition is usually accomplished by intravitreal injection, and this procedure is not without risk. Combination therapy may lead to a reduction in the number of treatments required.

VEGF inhibition has a number of theoretical possible adverse effects on the retina. VEGF is a neurotrophic agent, and there is a possibility that inhibition may lead to loss of retinal tissue. In some conditions where VEGF inhibition is used, such as diabetic retinopathy, obliterative retinal vasculitides, and vein occlusions, VEGF inhibition may potentially place macular capillaries at risk if they are VEGF-dependent.

In the following section, select drugs and categories of drugs (listed in Table 53.1), which are currently under development and which may play an important role in the therapeutic armamentarium for retinal vascular diseases in the future, will be discussed according to the disease processes that they may modulate.

ANGIOGENESIS AND NEOVASCULAR AGE-RELATED MACULAR DEGENERATION

TYROSINE KINASE INHIBITORS

All three VEGF receptors are tyrosine kinases and cause downstream activation of additional tyrosine kinases in a cascade that leads to gene transcription and downstream effects, including leakage, proliferation, migration, and angiogenesis. Thus, blocking this downstream activation is an appealing target. In addition, the receptors for fibroblast growth factor and platelet-derived growth factor (PDGF) are also tyrosine kinases. Thus, tyrosine kinase inhibitors may offer the potential to inhibit angiogenesis via the VEGF pathway and other angiogenic pathways. Inhibition of all three of these receptor tyrosine kinases also raises the possibility of inhibition of the development of subretinal fibrosis associated with choroidal neovascularization (CNV). As an example of this concept, it has been demonstrated that in rats, an inhibitor of these three tyrosine kinases attenuates the development of bleomycin-induced pulmonary fibrosis.[1] A number of tyrosine kinase inhbitors are under investigation and are discussed below.

Intravitreal injections of AG013764 and AG013711, which inhibit the kinase domains of VEGF receptor 1 (VEGFR-1), receptor 2 (VEGFR-2), and PDGF receptor (PDGFR), have been demonstrated to reduce the area of CNV induced by subretinal injections of a viral vector carrying the gene for the 165-kDa isoform of VEGF (AAV-VEGF(165)).[2] Vatalanib (PTK787) inhibits the kinase domain of VEGFR-1, -2, and -3. It is being extensively studied as a chemotherapeutic agent for solid tumors. Oral vatalanib administered daily has undergone a phase I/II study for the treatment of subfoveal CNV secondary to AMD: this study was sponsored by Novartis and was concluded in 2007. The study estimated that it would enroll 47 patients. It was to assess safety over 12 months as well as comparing the effects of vatalanib on visual acuity and retinal anatomic measures with the effects of standard therapy. Initially, patients were randomized to vatalanib or photodynamic therapy with verteporfin. As the standard of care has changed since the study was commenced, the second cohort of patients has been randomized between vatalanib and ranibizumab.

Vatalanib has a high oral bioavailability, which makes the elimination of intravitreal injections with their associated adverse effects a possibility. However, systemic administration would make systemic adverse effects of VEGF inhibition more likely. Vatalanib must be evaluated for the side-effects that have been experienced with systemic bevacizumab and VEGF-Trap, including hypertension, proteinuria, intestinal perforation, reversible posterior leukoencephalopathy syndrome (RPLS), and a trend towards delayed surgical wound healing.[3] The CONFIRM-2 trial evaluating vatalanib in the treatment of metastatic colorectal cancer reported adverse effects likely related to VEGF antagonism, including hypertension, thrombotic and embolic events, and RPLS. Other adverse effects that occurred in a higher proportion of vatalanib-treated patients than of those treated with placebo included diarrhea, fatigue, nausea, vomiting, and dizziness.[4]

Table 53.1 Categories of pharmacologic agents

Neovascular age-related macular degeneration
Tyrosine kinase inhibitors
PDGF inhibitors
Integrin inhibitors
Insulin-like growth factor receptor inhibitors
Nicotinic acetylcholine receptor antagonists
Mammalian target of rapamycin inhibitor
Small interfering RNA (siRNA)
Bioactive lipids
Nonneovascular age-related macular degeneration
Complement inhibitors
Diabetic macular edema
Inhibitors of inflammation

Imatinib, which inhibits both the alpha and beta receptors of PDGF, has been proposed as an adjunctive treatment to VEGF inhibition with ranibizumab. A trial of this combination approach is under way. There is now considerable experience with the use of imatinib in oncology. It is generally well tolerated, although less so in blast crises in chronic myeloid leukemia, and is of importance for retinal disease in the elderly. Most of the significant side-effects derive from fluid retention, and pleural effusion, pulmonary edema, renal failure, and congestive cardiac failure may all occur. Rash and muscle cramps also occur. TG100801 is an ocular formulation of the prodrug 4-chloro-3-(5-methyl-3+1,2,4-benzotriazin-7-yl) phenyl benzoate, an inhibitor of the VEGFR-2, Rous sarcoma oncogene (SRC) and Yamaguchi sarcoma oncogene (YES) kinases. Studies from knockout mice suggest that SRC and YES play an important role in vascular permeability. This prodrug has been formulated so as to maximize the drug concentration in the posterior pole resulting from topical administration.[5] The formulation has already undergone toxicity studies in healthy volunteers, and is currently under investigation for the treatment of subfoveal CNV secondary to AMD. The study participants are randomized between two doses of the prodrug administered twice daily for 30 days. The effect on central retinal thickness and on visual acuity will be compared.

PDGF INHIBITORS

In addition to the use of tyrosine kinase inhibitors to target the PDGF receptor, E10030 (Ophthotech), a pegylated aptamer which is antagonistic to PDGF function, is in phase I clinical trials in eyes with subfoveal CNV secondary to AMD. PDGF is an appealing target in neovascular AMD since PDGF is required for recruitment of pericytes to developing endothelial cells. Without pericyte recruitment and attachment, neovascular vessels do not mature. Thus, by blocking PDGF a crucial step in the angiogenesis cascade is blocked. The phase I study is an ascending-dose study of intravitreal injections of E10030 used either as monotherapy or in combination with ranibizumab. The endpoints are dose-limiting ocular toxicities and adverse events.[6] Although PDGF inhibitors may hold potential in the treatment of CNV, their potential in treating proliferative diabetic retinopathy, where PDGF likely has a pathogenic role,[7] is limited by the requirement for PDGF for pericyte retention and recruitment.[8]

INTEGRIN INHIBITORS

Integrins are adhesion molecules by which cells attach themselves to the extracellular matrix (ECM). They also have a signal transduction role in that they mediate the effect of the ECM on cellular function. Inhibitors of $\alpha_5\beta_1$,[9] $\alpha_v\beta_3$,[10] and $\alpha_v\beta_5$ [11] integrins have all been demonstrated in some systems to have antiangiogenic properties. Only an antagonist of $\alpha_5\beta_1$ integrin (JSM6427) has been demonstrated to have antiangiogenic properties in mouse laser-induced CNV.[12] This molecule is now undergoing an ascending-dose phase I trial sponsored by Jerini Pharmaceuticals for the treatment of subfoveal neovascular AMD.

Volociximab is a chimeric monoclonal IgG_4 antibody that binds $\alpha_5\beta_1$ integrin. It was developed for the treatment of solid tumors and is being tested for the treatment of CNV by Ophthotech. This molecule has been demonstrated to inhibit endothelial cell proliferation and angiogenesis in *in vitro* assays. When administered by intravitreal injection concurrently with laser-induced Bruch's membrane rupture and then weekly, it inhibits the development of laser-induced CNV in cynomolgus monkeys.[13]

INSULIN-LIKE GROWTH FACTOR RECEPTOR INHIBITORS

Insulin-like growth factor 1 (IGF-1) has been implicated in the pathogenesis of both diabetic retinopathy and CNV. In rats made diabetic with the use of streptozotocin, intravitreous injections of IGF-1 increased retinal activity of Akt, JNK, HIF-1α, NF-κB, and AP-1, and also increased retinal VEGF levels, while systemic inhibition of the IGF-1R caused reduction of Akt, JNK, HIF-1α, NF-κB, and AP-1 activity, decreased VEGF levels, decreased retinal vascular leukostasis, and reduced breakdown of the blood–retinal barrier.[14] IGF-1 and its receptor (IGF-1R) are expressed throughout the retina and RPE in normal eyes. IGF-1 mRNA and both IGF-1R mRNA and protein have been detected in endothelial cells of CNVs and in associated RPE in a majority of lesions.[15] IGF-1 increases VEGF expression by cultured RPE cells from surgically excised CNV lesions.[16] The cyclolignan picropodophyllin, an inhibitor of the IGF-1R, reduces the size of laser-induced CNV lesions in mice, and reduces the expression of VEGF in the choroid.[17]

NICOTINIC ACETYLCHOLINE RECEPTOR ANTAGONISTS

Nicotinic acetylcholine receptors (nAChr) occur on vascular endothelial cells. Nicotine acts on these receptors to enhance angiogenesis in response to limb ischemia. Nicotine also causes angiogenesis in tumors and atherosclerotic plaques at the concentrations found in the serum of smokers.[18] nAChr have been demonstrated on human retinal and choroidal vascular endothelial cells.[19] Mecamylamine completely inhibits VEGF-induced angiogenic activity of human retinal and choroidal endothelial cells in an *in vivo* assay by blocking nAChr. Nicotine increases the size of CNV in mice secondary to laser-induced Bruch's membrane rupture. This effect is abrogated by inhibition of nAChr by subconjunctival mecamylamine. At least in the cerebral microcirculation, nicotine acts on endothelial cells to alter the distribution of tight junctions, and thus to increase the permeability of the blood–brain barrier.[20] Blockade of nAChr inhibits endothelial cell migration induced by both basic fibroblast growth factor and VEGF.[21] This raises the possibility that nAChr inhibition may block angiogenesis mediated by other factors in addition to VEGF.

Mecamylamine (Comentis) is a specific inhibitor of nAChr. Studies of the pharmacological distribution of topically administered mecamylamine in the rabbit eye have demonstrated significant retinal and choroidal concentrations and much lower plasma concentrations. A topical mecamylamine formulation (ATG-003) has undergone phase I toxicity studies in healthy volunteers. ATG-003 is currently being evaluated in a phase II clinical trial involving 330 patients with CNV (Optima). Published results are expected in 2010. A more limited phase II safety and efficacy trial in the treatment of DME with endpoints of visual acuity and retinal thickness as measured by optical coherence tomography (OCT) is also under way.

MAMMALIAN TARGET OF RAPAMYCIN INHIBITOR

Rapamycin (sirolimus) is a macrolide antibiotic that is produced naturally by *Streptomyces hygroscopicus*. Rapamycin binds to FKBP12. The resulting complex binds to the mammalian target of rapamycin (mTOR), inhibiting the function of mTOR in the mTORC1 complex.[22] The mammalian target of rapamycin is a key component in a cell's response to insulin, insulin-like growth factors, nutrient levels, hypoxia, and redox status. mTOR forms the complexes mTORC1 and mTORC2, where only mTORC1 is susceptible to regulation by rapamycin. mTORC1 promotes mRNA translation by phosphorylating and activating the p70-S6 kinase 1 (S6K1) and phosphorylating and inactivating eukaryotic initiation factor 4E (eIF4E) binding protein 1(4E-BP1), which is a repressor of mRNA translation.[23] By a separate mechanism, in the presence of activated mTOR, the regulatory-associated protein of mTOR (Raptor), which is part of the mTORC1 complex, interacts with HIF-1α to activate it.[24] Thus sirolimus has an inhibitory effect on HIF-1α. Rapamycin inhibits mTORC1 activity and has antiproliferative, antiangiogenic, and immunosuppressive functions.[25] Rapamycin (Macusight) underwent phase I testing in neovascular AMD as a sustained-release intravitreal or subconjunctival injection in a dose escalation study. Currently, Macusight is sponsoring a phase II trial that is randomizing 120 patients between three different doses of subconjunctival sirolimus and placebo. The main outcomes will be visual acuity and central macular thickness. The National Eye Institute is also conducting a study assessing the role of immunomodulatory agents in combination with routine care using antiangiogenic therapies for the treatment of subfoveal CNV secondary to AMD. Twenty patients will be randomly assigned to one of four study arms. Patients will receive intravenous daclizumab, intravenous infliximab, oral sirolimus, or no study medication. The study will assess recurrence of neovascularization, as well as changes in visual acuity and retinal thickening as measured by OCT over a 24-week interval.

A phase I/II study of ocular sirolimus is being conducted. Patients will be randomized between three subconjunctival injections of 1320 μg or three intravitreal injections of 352 μg of sirolimus. Visual acuity will be assessed over 180 days, and safety endpoints over 1 year.[26]

The role of sirolimus in the treatment of DME is also being investigated in two trials. Sirolimus is an excellent candidate for treating DME due to its anti-inflammatory action, effect on HIF-1α levels, and reduction of vascular permeability. The National Eye Institute is evaluating the efficacy of subconjunctival injections of 440 μg of sirolimus at baseline and at 2 months on visual acuity and macular edema, as measured by OCT in 5 patients.[27]

SMALL INTERFERING RNA

PF-04523655 (Quark/Pfizer) is a small interfering RNA inhibitor of RTP801. RTP801 is a hypoxia-inducible gene which acts via the TSC1/TSC2 tumor suppressor complex to inhibit mTOR.[28,29] PF-04523655 has been demonstrated to be efficacious in inhibiting the development of CNV in a murine laser-induced CNV model. Moreover, the drug appeared to have an additive effect when used in combination with pegaptanib or an antibody against mouse VEGF. The drug has been studied in mouse, rat, rabbit, and monkey systems, and a human phase I study has been performed. A phase II prospective, randomized, dose-ranging study of PF-04523655 in comparison with ranibizumab for the treatment of subfoveal CNV secondary to AMD is currently recruiting patients. The study has two stages, where the first will determine whether an initial injection of ranibizumab is required before starting PF-04523655. The structure of the second stage will depend on the results of the first stage. If a "first-line" design is used, 160 patients will be randomized 1:1:1:1 between three different doses of PF-04523655 or ranibizumab, and will receive the study drug on a monthly basis until week 44 of the trial. If an "induction" design is implemented, all patients will receive an initial treatment with ranibizumab, and will then receive monthly injections of the study drug to which they have been randomized. The primary endpoint of the study will be best corrected visual acuity at 48 weeks. Secondary endpoints will be changes in fluorescein angiography and OCT parameters, and requirement for rescue therapies. Other pharmacologic agents that employ small interfering technology, such as siRNA-027 and bevasiranib, have been described elsewhere in this book.

BIOACTIVE LIPIDS

There is increasing recognition that many classes of lipids, especially metabolites of cell membrane components, have a role in signal transduction and in the regulation of multiple cellular processes. Lipids with these roles are known as "bioactive lipids." The sphingolipids, formed from the condensation of serine and palmitate, are of particular interest in the regulation of the vascular endothelium. The sphingolipid sphingomyelin is an important component of cellular membranes. It is synthesized from and broken down to ceramide, which in turn is broken down by ceramidase to yield sphingosine, and then phosphorylated by the sphingosine kinases (SK1 and SK2) to yield sphingosine 1-phosphate (S1P). S1P is the ligand for five different cell surface S1P receptors. S1P, S1P receptors, and sphingosine kinases have all been demonstrated to be present in the eye.[30]

S1P is intimately involved in regulation of endothelial function. $S1P_1$ receptors are required for recruitment of vascular smooth-muscle cells and pericytes during mouse embryonic vessel formation.[31] S1P induces proliferation and migration of human endothelial cells,[32] and regulates basal and angiopoietin-1-mediated endothelial permeability.[33] There is extensive cross-talk between S1P and VEGF receptors: S1P can activate VEGFR-2 in the absence of VEGF; VEGF sensitizes endothelium to the action of S1P by up-regulating its receptors; activated PDGF receptor activates sphingosine kinase 1 to the cell membrane, activating S1PR1.

S1P has a role in animal models of retinal disease. In mice, an anti-S1P monoclonal antibody inhibits the development of laser-induced CNV.[30] $S1P_2$ receptor knockout mice demonstrate reduced angiogenesis in the oxygen-induced retinopathy model.[34] Systemic treatment with a small-molecule inhibitor of sphingosine kinase significantly reduced retinal fluorescein leakage in diabetic rats.[35] A monoclonal antibody against S1P has been humanized and is in phase I trials as an antiangiogenic agent in cancer treatment. A phase I trial for neovascular AMD is planned. If the antibody is well tolerated, its function in human diabetic retinopathy will also be of interest.

NONNEOVASCULAR AGE-RELATED MACULAR DEGENERATION

COMPLEMENT INHIBITORS

The complement cascade is part of the innate immune system.[36] The complement system consists of a cascade of cleavage enzymes, regulatory molecules, and the components of the membrane attack complex. The membrane attack complex forms a pore through the cellular surface membranes, and if sufficient numbers of pores are present, cell death will ensue. Many of the cleavage products of the complement cascade have biological functions in addition to their enzymatic role in the cascade. Complement component C3b (where the complement components are designated by "C" followed by a number and then, where appropriate, "a" or "b" to indicate the cleavage products) enhances opsonization. C5a is chemotactic for inflammatory cells, and activates macrophages. C3a and C5a trigger mast cell degranulation. C5b initiates the formation of the membrane attack complex.

Activation of the complement cascade may occur via one of three pathways. The classical pathway is initiated when complement component C1q binds to IgM– or IgG–antigen complexes, or when it binds directly to the surface of a pathogen. The lectin pathway is similar: it is activated by the binding of either ficolins or mannose-binding lectin to the surface of a pathogen. The alternative pathway is triggered by the

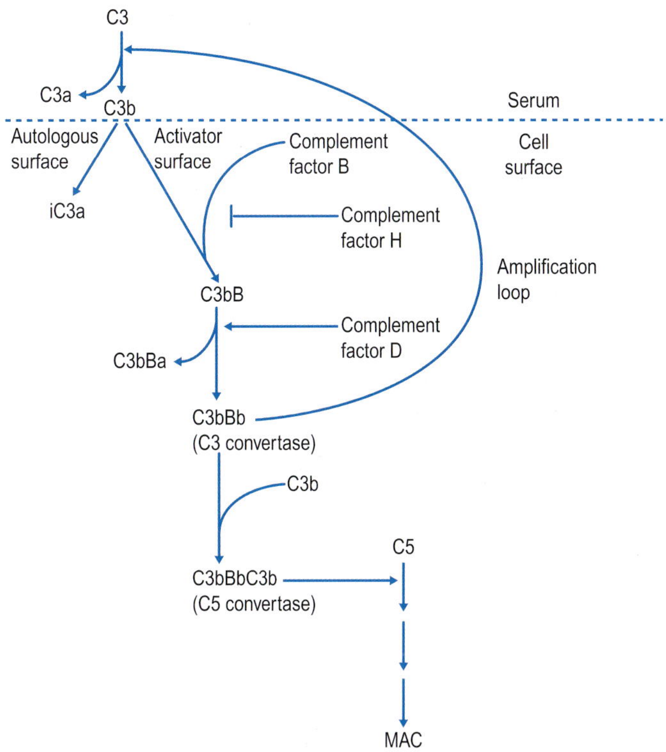

Figure 53.1 The alternative complement pathway (simplified to aid in conceptualization).

The principal components of the alternative complement pathway to the stage of C5 convertase production are shown in detail. Initially, C3 is converted spontaneously to C3a and C3b, making C3b available for binding to cell surfaces. On binding to an activator (pathogen) surface, C3b is converted to C3 convertase (C3bBb) through the several steps shown here, of which C3bBa is a byproduct, which in turn upregulates the conversion of C3 to C3b. On binding to an autologous cell surface, C3b is inactivated (iC3b) and the amplification loop is not entered. Complement factor H acts as one of the primary regulators of this pathway by inhibiting the binding of complement factor B to C3b and also by degrading C3b. Reprinted from DeWan A, Bracken MB, Hoh J. Two genetic pathways for age-related macular degeneration. Curr Opin Genet Dev 2007;17,228–233, with permission.

hydrolysis of complement component C3 on the surface of a cell membrane. Once the cleavage product C3b has covalently bonded to a cell it binds factor B, which is then cleaved by factor D. This results in formation of the alternative pathway C3 convertase, C3bBb, which in turn leads to signal amplification by further C3 cleavage, and formation of C5 convertase, and consequently C5 cleavage and formation of the membrane attack complex. Host cells are protected from alternative pathway activation by the presence of complement receptor 1, factor H, the decay-accelerating factor, and the plasma protease, factor I (Figure 53.1).

Genetic polymorphism associations and analysis of the composition of drusen suggest that dysregulation of the complement cascade plays a key role in the development of AMD. In particular, the presence of the complement factor H 402H risk allele appears to be one of the most significant risk factors for the development of soft drusen in some populations.[37] Because there is evidence that polymorphisms in many components of the complement cascade are associated with AMD, proposed therapeutic strategies attempt either to block activation of the alternative pathway by inactivating C3, or to inhibit the cascade downstream by binding C5.

POT-4 (Potentia Pharmaceuticals) is a cyclic peptide that binds and inactivates complement component 3. A dose-escalating phase I safety and tolerability trial of intravitreal POT-4 injections in patients with subfoveal CNV is being conducted.

ARC1905 (Ophthotech) is a pegylated RNA aptamer that inhibits complement component 5. This molecule is also undergoing a dose-escalating phase I trial of multiple intravitreal injections in eyes with subfoveal CNV. All patients will be treated with ARC1905. Patients will also be treated with either a single induction dose of ranibizumab or multiple doses of ranibizumab.

Although safety studies are being performed in eyes with neovascular AMD, it is hoped that complement cascade inhibitors may slow the progression of nonneovascular AMD.

DIABETIC MACULAR EDEMA

INHIBITION OF INFLAMMATION

It is hypothesized that inflammatory processes are involved in the pathogenesis of DME, and intravitreal triamcinolone has been demonstrated to be efficacious in improving visual acuity and reducing macular thickness of eyes affected by DME.[38] The role of intraocular steroids in DME needs further investigation, as a recent 3-year study has indicated that laser photocoagulation may have better safety and efficacy for DME compared to intravitreal triamcinolone.[39] Lymphocyte function-associated antigen-1 is composed of CD11a and CD18. It mediates leukocyte adhesion by binding intercellular adhesion molecules 1–3 and also functions in lymphocyte co-stimulatory signaling.[40]

The hypothesis that blockade of CD11a by the monoclonal antibody efalizumab may be beneficial in the treatment of DME is being examined in the Combined Approach to Treatment Using Ranibizumab and Efalizumab for Diabetic Macular Edema (CAPTURE DME) study. In this phase I study, the primary endpoint is the evaluation of adverse events. The secondary endpoints are visual acuity and anatomical measures by OCT and fluorescein angiography at 6 and 12 months. In the study, a three-way comparison of efficacy between efalizumab, ranibizumab, and combination therapy of ranibizumab and efalizumab will be performed.

SUMMARY AND KEY POINTS

As the field of pharmacotherapeutics continues to expand for retinal and ocular inflammatory diseases, *Retinal Pharmacotherapy* has been prepared to provide comprehensive ophthalmologists and retina specialists the basic understanding of relevant ophthalmic drugs and their characteristics. This chapter has given the reader a glimpse of selected future agents in clinical testing, and is not meant to be all-inclusive. It is expected that by the time the first edition of *Retinal Pharmacotherapy* is printed, preparation of the second edition will have begun in order to accommodate the additional therapeutic agents. In addition, there are several significant areas of therapeutic need that are not met by the therapies described in this book. Such areas include repair of areas of RPE loss, repair of atrophied choriocapillaris, elimination of the fibrotic component of CNV, protection against loss of retinal tissue in diabetic maculopathy and both neovascular and nonneovascular AMD, and protection against macular capillary loss in diabetic retinopathy. Hopefully, with the continuing advancements of basic and clinical research, pharmacotherapy for these and other areas will be covered in future editions of *Retinal Pharmacotherapy*.

ACKNOWLEDGMENT

The Cole Eye Institute receives research grant support on behalf of Dr. Kaiser from Allergan, Alcon, Genentech, Quark, Pfizer, Novartis, and QLT. Dr. Kaiser has received honoraria that have been disclosed to the conflict of interest committee of the Cleveland Clinic from Alcon, Genentech, Novartis, Allergan, and QLT.

REFERENCES

1. Chaudhary NI, Roth GJ, Hilberg F, et al. Inhibition of PDGF, VEGF and FGF signalling attenuates fibrosis. Eur Respir J 2007;29:976–985.
2. Wang FE, Shi G, Niesman MR, et al. Receptor tyrosine kinase inhibitors AG013764 and AG013711 reduce choroidal neovascularization in rat eye. Exp Eye Res 2007;84:922–933.
3. Nguyen QD, Shah QD, Hafiz G, et al. A phase I trial of an IV-administered vascular endothelial growth factor trap for treatment in patients with choroidal neovascularization due to age-related macular degeneration. Ophthalmology 2006;113:1522.e1–1522.e14.
4. Los M, Roodhart JM, Voest EE. Target practice: lessons from phase III trials with bevacizumab and vatalanib in the treatment of advanced colorectal cancer. Oncologist 2007;12:443–450.
5. Palanki MS, Akiyama H, Campochiaro P, et al. Development of prodrug 4-chloro-3-(5-methyl-3-{[4-(2-pyrrolidin-1-ylethoxy)phenyl]amino}-1,2,4-benzotriazin-7-yl)phenyl benzoate (TG100801): a topically administered therapeutic candidate in clinical trials for the treatment of age-related macular degeneration. J Med Chem 2008;51:1546–1559.
6. Ophthotech Corporation. A phase I, safety, tolerability and pharmacokinetic profile of intravitreous injections of e10030 (anti-PDGF pegylated aptamer) in subjects with neovascular age-related macular degeneration. www.ClinicalTrials.gov NCT00569140.
7. Simo R, Carrasco E, Garcia-Ramirez M, Hernandez C. Angiogenic and antiangiogenic factors in proliferative diabetic retinopathy. Curr Diabetes Rev 2006;2:71–98.
8. Betsholtz C. Insight into the physiological functions of PDGF through genetic studies in mice. Cytokine Growth Factor Rev 2004;15:215–228.
9. Kim S, Bell K, Mousa SA, Varner JA. Regulation of angiogenesis *in vivo* by ligation of integrin alpha5beta1 with the central cell-binding domain of fibronectin. Am J Pathol 2000;156:1345–1362.
10. Brooks PC, Clark RA, Cheresh DA. Requirement of vascular integrin alpha v beta 3 for angiogenesis. Science 1994;264:569–571.
11. Friedlander M, Brooks PC, Shaffer RW, et al. Definition of two angiogenic pathways by distinct alpha v integrins. Science 1995;270:1500–1502.
12. Umeda N, Kachi S, Akiyama H, et al. Suppression and regression of choroidal neovascularization by systemic administration of an alpha5beta1 integrin antagonist. Mol Pharmacol 2006;69:1820–1828.
13. Ramakrishnan V, Bhaskar V, Law DA, et al. Preclinical evaluation of an anti-alpha5beta1 integrin antibody as a novel anti-angiogenic agent. J Exp Ther Oncol 2006;5:273–286.
14. Poulaki V, Joussen AM, Mitsiades N, et al. Insulin-like growth factor-I plays a pathogenetic role in diabetic retinopathy. Am J Pathol 2004; 165:457–469.
15. Lambooij AC, van Wely KH, Lindenbergh-Kortleve DJ, et al. Insulin-like growth factor-I and its receptor in neovascular age-related macular degeneration. Invest Ophthalmol Vis Sci 2003;44:2192–2198.
16. Rosenthal R, Wohlleben H, Malek G, et al. Insulin-like growth factor-1 contributes to neovascularization in age-related macular degeneration. Biochem Biophys Res Commun 2004;323:1203–1208.
17. Economou MA, Wu J, Vasilcanu D, et al. Inhibition of VEGF secretion and experimental choroidal neovascularization by picropodophyllin (PPP), an inhibitor of the insulin-like growth factor-1 receptor. Invest Ophthalmol Vis Sci 2008;49:2620–2626.
18. Heeschen C, Jang JJ, Weis M, et al. Nicotine stimulates angiogenesis and promotes tumor growth and atherosclerosis. Nat Med 2001;7: 833–839.
19. Kiuchi K, Matsuoka M, Wu JC, et al. Mecamylamine suppresses basal and nicotine-stimulated choroidal neovascularization. Invest Ophthalmol Vis Sci 2008;49:1705–1711.
20. Hawkins BT, Egleton RD, Davis TP. Modulation of cerebral microvascular permeability by endothelial nicotinic acetylcholine receptors. Am J Physiol Heart Circ Physiol 2005;289:H212–H219.
21. Ng MK, Wu J, Chang E, et al. A central role for nicotinic cholinergic regulation of growth factor-induced endothelial cell migration. Arterioscler Thromb Vasc Biol 2007;27:106–112.
22. Wan X, Helman LJ. The biology behind mTOR inhibition in sarcoma. Oncologist 2007;12:1007–1018.
23. Hay N, Sonenberg N. Upstream and downstream of mTOR. Genes Dev 2004;18:1926–1945.
24. Land SC, Tee AR. Hypoxia-inducible factor 1alpha is regulated by the mammalian target of rapamycin (mTOR) via an mTOR signaling motif. J Biol Chem 2007;282:20534–20543.
25. Tee AR, Blenis J. mTOR, translational control and human disease. Semin Cell Dev Biol 2005;16:29–37.
26. MacuSight Inc. Phase 1/2 study of an ocular sirolimus (Rapamycin) formulation in patients with age-related macular degeneration. www.ClinicalTrials.gov NCT00712491.
27. National Eye Institute. Sirolimus to treat diabetic macular edema. www.ClinicalTrials.gov NCT00711490.
28. Brugarolas J, Lei K, Hurley RL, et al. Regulation of mTOR function in response to hypoxia by REDD1 and the TSC1/TSC2 tumor suppressor complex. Genes Dev 2004;18:2893–2904.
29. Corradetti MN, Inoki K, Guan KL. The stress-inducted proteins RTP801 and RTP801L are negative regulators of the mammalian target of rapamycin pathway. J Biol Chem 2005;280:9769–9772.
30. Caballero S, Swaney J, Moreno K, et al. Anti-sphingosine-1-phosphate monoclonal antibodies inhibit angiogenesis and sub-retinal fibrosis in a murine model of laser-induced choroidal neovascularization. Exp Eye Res Mar 2009;88(3):367–377.
31. Liu Y, Wada R, Yamashita T, et al. Edg-1, the G protein-coupled receptor for sphingosine-1-phosphate, is essential for vascular maturation. J Clin Invest 2000;106:951–961.
32. Kimura T, Watanabe T, Sato K, et al. Sphingosine 1-phosphate stimulates proliferation and migration of human endothelial cells possibly through the lipid receptors, Edg-1 and Edg-3. Biochem J 2000;348(Pt 1):71–76.
33. Li X, Stankovic M, Bonder CS, et al. Basal and angiopoietin-1-mediated endothelial permeability is regulated by sphingosine kinase-1. Blood 2008;111:3489–3497.
34. Skoura A, Sanchez T, Claffey K, et al. Essential role of sphingosine 1-phosphate receptor 2 in pathological angiogenesis of the mouse retina. J Clin Invest 2007;117:2506–2516.
35. Maines LW, French KJ, Wolpert EB, et al. Pharmacologic manipulation of sphingosine kinase in retinal endothelial cells: implications for angiogenic ocular diseases. Invest Ophthalmol Vis Sci 2006;47:5022–5031.
36. Janeway CA, Travers P, Walport M, et al. Immunobiology: the immune system in health and disease. New York: Garland Publishing; 2001.
37. DeWan A, Bracken MB, Hoh J. Two genetic pathways for age-related macular degeneration. Curr Opin Genet Dev 2007;17:228–233.
38. Shimura M, Nakazawa T, Yasuda K, et al. Comparative therapy evaluation of intravitreal bevacizumab and triamcinolone acetonide on persistent diffuse diabetic macular edema. Am J Ophthalmol 2008;145:854–861.
39. Beck RW, Edwards AR, Aiello LP, et al. Three-year follow-up of a randomized trial comparing focal/grid photocoagulation and Intravitreal Triamcinolone for diabetic macular edema. Arch Ophthalmol Mar 2009;127(3):245–251.
40. de Fougerolles AR, Qin X, Springer TA. Characterization of the function of intercellular adhesion molecule (ICAM)-3 and comparison with ICAM-1 and ICAM-2 in immune responses. J Exp Med 1994;179:619–629.

INDEX